Diseases of the
Nose, Throat
and Ear

Diseases of the Nose, Throat and Ear

JOHN JACOB BALLENGER, M.S., M.D.

Associate Professor of Otolaryngology and Maxillofacial Surgery, Northwestern University School of Medicine; Head, Division of Otolaryngology, Evanston Hospital, Evanston, Illinois

AND CONTRIBUTORS

TWELFTH EDITION

LEA & FEBIGER · *Philadelphia*

To Constance

The illustration on the cover is one of five tapestries entitled collectively "The Lady and the Unicorn." This example of the Lady and the Unicorn is traditionally thought to symbolize the sense of hearing. Other tapestries in the series represent taste, odor, touch and sight. They were woven between 1480 and 1500, but by whom and where is unknown. They now reside at the Musée de Cluny, Paris.

This tapestry depicts a Lady playing an organ while a young maidservant works at the bellows. Both the lion and the unicorn listen intently and function also as heraldic supporters. It may be that the tapestry was offered to Claude Le Viste, by Jean de Chabanne, as an engagement present.

Library of Congress Cataloging in Publication Data

Ballenger, John Jacob, 1914–
    Diseases of the nose, throat, and ear.

    Bibliography: p.
    Includes index.
    1. Otolaryngology. I. Title. [DNLM: 1. Otorhinolaryngologic diseases.   WV100 D612]
RF46.B2 1977   616.2′1   77–2674
ISBN 0–8121–0549–4

Published in Great Britain by Henry Kimpton Publishers, London

PRINTED IN THE UNITED STATES OF AMERICA

Print No.   3   2

Preface

Continuing demand has afforded me the opportunity, which is a privilege and pleasure, to contribute, both as author and editor, to a new edition of Diseases of the Nose, Throat and Ear.

My desires for the 12th edition of this textbook are symbolized in the tapestry appearing on the cover. Though entitled *Hearing* it suggests the entire field of study of otorhinolaryngology. The text, it is hoped, is well woven and constructively and beautifully presented.

Personal investment in the 69-year history of this textbook has made it inevitable that I would make whatever sacrifices necessary to continue this tradition and to produce a work that was comprehensive, current, and accurate. I believe the present volume accomplishes this goal, and be it noted the weeks and months devoted to this end are untold and unregretted.

Having served in the dual capacity of contributing author myself, as well as the editor, I realize how indebted I am to the other twenty contributing authors who have assisted me and thank them profusely for their excellent efforts. Of these contributors, twelve also wrote for the previous volume and eight are new to this one. Topics new to the 12th edition include cryosurgery, immunology and chemotherapy of head and neck neoplasms, and polytomography of the facial bones and paranasal sinuses. The subject matter of bronchoesophagology and reconstructive surgery of the head and neck has been completely rewritten. The entire book has been thoroughly revised.

I have been particularly pleased to note the wide distribution achieved by the 11th edition, produced in 1969, to Spanish speaking peoples through Editorial Jims of Barcelona; to India and England and other English speaking countries through Henry Kimpton of London; as well as to the United States and Canada through the admirable efforts of Lea & Febiger to whom I once again extend my gratitude. I have every hope that the present volume will be as well received and widely distributed.

Chicago, Illinois   John J. Ballenger

Contributors

Thomas B. Abbott, Ph.D.
Professor of Speech Pathology
Director of Speech Pathology and Audiology
University of Florida
Gainesville, Florida 32611

Bobby R. Alford, M.D.
Professor and Chairman,
  Department of Otorhinolaryngology
  and Communicative Sciences
Baylor College of Medicine
Houston, Texas 77025

David F. Austin, M.D.
Professor of Otolaryngology
Abraham Lincoln School of Medicine
University of Illinois
Chicago, Illinois 60602

John J. Ballenger, M.D.
Associate Professor of Otolaryngology and
  Maxillofacial Surgery
Northwestern University School of Medicine
Head, Division of Otolaryngology
Evanston Hospital
Evanston, Illinois 60201

Oscar J. Becker, M.D.†
Clinical Professor of Otolaryngology
University of Illinois
Chicago, Illinois 60612

Alfred C. Coats, M.D.
Professor of Physiology and Otorhinolaryngology
  and Communicative Sciences
Baylor College of Medicine
Houston, Texas 77025

Meyer S. Fox, M.D.
Clinical Professor, Department of Otolaryngology
University of Wisconsin Medical School
Madison, Wisconsin 53706

†Deceased

Robert Frisina, Ph.D.
Senior Vice President
Rochester Institute of Technology
One Lomb Memorial Drive
Rochester, New York 14623

Harry B. Harding, M.D.†
Emeritus Head of Division of Microbiology
Evanston Hospital
Evanston, Illinois 60201

James Jerger, Ph.D.
Professor and Head, Division of Audiology
  and Speech Pathology
Baylor College of Medicine
Houston, Texas 77025

Janardan D. Khandekar, M.D.
Head, Medical Oncology
Assistant Attending Physician
Evanston Hospital
Evanston, Illinois 60201

Imre Laszlo, M.D.
Associate Professor of Radiology
Head of Radiology
Pulmonary Institute of MAV
Budapest, Hungary

Richard Mallen, M.D.
Professor and Chairman
Division of Otolaryngology
University of Alberta
Edmonton, Alberta, Canada

Daniel Miller, M.D.
Associate Clinical Professor of Otolaryngology
Harvard Medical School
Consulting Surgeon, Massachusetts Eye
  and Ear Infirmary
Boston, Massachusetts 02114

William W. Montgomery, M.D.
Professor of Otolaryngology, Harvard
    Medical School
Senior Surgeon, Massachusetts Eye and
    Ear Infirmary
Boston, Massachusetts 02114

G. Paul Moore, Ph.D.
Emeritus Professor, Department of Speech
University of Florida
Gainesville, Florida 32601

H. Bryan Neel III, M.D., Ph.D.
Mayo Clinic, Division of Otolaryngology
Rochester, Minnesota 55901

Joseph Ogura, M.D.
Lindberg Professor and Head
Department of Otolaryngology
Washington University School of Medicine
St. Louis, Missouri 63110

James B. Snow, M.D.
Professor and Chairman, Department of
    Otorhinolaryngology and Human
    Communication
University of Pennsylvania School of Medicine
Philadelphia, Pennsylvania 19104

Gershon J. Spector, M.D.
Professor, Department of Otolaryngology
Washington University School of Medicine
St. Louis, Missouri 63110

M. Eugene Tardy, Jr., M.D.
Associate Professor of Otolaryngology
Abraham Lincoln School of Medicine
University of Illinois
Chicago, Illinois 60602

Galdino Valvassori, M.D.
Professor of Radiology
Abraham Lincoln School of Medicine
University of Illinois
Chicago, Illinois 60602

Contents

PART III.   DISEASES OF THE LARYNX

PART IV.   THE EAR

PART V. BRONCHOESOPHAGOLOGY

PART 1
THE NOSE AND ACCESSORY SINUSES

Chapter 1
The Clinical Anatomy and Physiology of the Nose and Accessory Sinuses

John J. Ballenger

The External Nose

The more or less pointed tip of the nose is known as the apex. Extending superiorly and somewhat posteriorly from the apex is the dorsum, leading to the root of the nose where the dorsum merges with the forehead. The *membranous columella* extends from the apex posteriorly to the center of the lip and is located just distal to the cartilages of the nasal septum. The point where the columella strikes the lip is known as the base of the nose. The upper lip at this point bares a shallow, rounded trench, known as the *philtrum,* that stretches from above downward. On either side of the columella are the right and left anterior *nares* bounded laterosuperiorly by the *alae* of the nose and inferiorly by the floor.

The supporting framework of the external nose consists of the two nasal bones, the frontal process of the maxillary bones (*processus frontalis maxillae*), the upper lateral cartilage, the paired lower lateral (greater alar) cartilages, and the anterior (ventral) edge of the cartilaginous nasal septum (Fig. 1–1). The support of the nose is probably afforded primarily by the first four named structures. The upper lateral cartilages at their medial ends blend with the cartilaginous septum and at their cranial ends are firmly attached to the undersurface of the nasal bones and frontal processes.

The lower or caudal margins of the upper lateral cartilages lie under the upper or craniad margin of the lower lateral cartilages. On elevation of the lower lateral cartilage with a retractor, this margin, the limen nasl, of the upper lateral cartilage is visible. At times the opposing margins of the upper and lower lateral cartilages may not be adjacent at their medial extremities. In such a case, the support of the external nose is potentially less secure at this point. Between the upper and lower lateral cartilages laterally are found one or more sesamoid cartilages. The lower lateral cartilage has a horseshoe shape. The lateral crus of this is broad and strong and provides the framework of the ala of the nose. The medial portion is weak and extends partly along the free caudal edge of the cartilaginous septum and partly within the membranous columella.

In the bony skull the pear-shaped nasal opening is called the piriform aperture. The superior lateral margins are formed by the nasal bones and frontal processes of the maxilla. The base is formed by the alveolar process of the maxilla. In the midline of this last structure is a prominence called the anterior nasal spine.

The alar muscles consist of two sets, the dilators comprising the *dilator naris* (anterior and posterior), the *m. procerus,* and the *caput angulare* of the *quadratus labii*

1

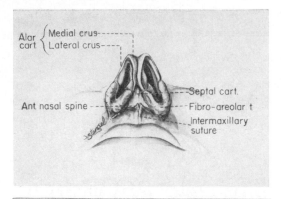

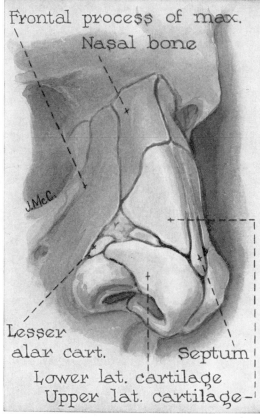

FIG. 1–1. The external framework of the nose.

superioris; and the constrictors comprising the *m. nasalis* and the *depressor septi.*

The Nasal Septum

The septum divides the nose into two cavities or chambers, the right and the left. The septum (Fig. 1–2) is formed superiorly by the perpendicular plate of the ethmoid bone; anteriorly by the septal (quadralateral) cartilage, premaxilla, and membranous columella; and inferiorly and posteriorly by the vomer, the maxillary crest, the palatine crest, and the sphenoidal crest.

The Nasal Chambers

The Floor. The floor of the nose is formed by the palatal process of the maxilla and the horizontal process of the palate bones.

The Roof. The roof from before backward is composed of the upper and lower lateral cartilages, the nasal bone, the nasal process of the frontal, the body of the ethmoid, and the body of the sphenoid bones. The lamina cribrosa or the cribriform plate of the ethmoid, which forms the major portion of the roof of the nose, transmits the filaments of the olfactory nerve as they descend from the undersurface of the olfactory bulb to their distribution in the mucous membrane covering the uppermost portion of the nasal septum down to and including the cranial surface of the superior turbinate.

The Lateral Wall. The lateral wall is formed by the inner surface of the frontal process of the maxilla, the lacrimal, the superior and middle nasal turbinates of the ethmoid bone, the inferior nasal turbinate, the perpendicular plate of the palate bone, and the medial pterygoid plate.

The Turbinates (Conchae). The nasal fossa is divided into three meatuses by the three turbinates (Fig. 1–3); the space situated between the inferior turbinate and the floor is called the inferior meatus, the space between the middle turbinate and the inferior turbinate is known as the middle meatus, and above the middle turbinate is the superior meatus. Occasionally a fourth turbinate (supreme turbinate) is observed. The supreme, superior, and middle turbinates originate from the lateral mass of the ethmoid bone. The inferior turbinate, a separate bone, is attached to the superior maxilla and to the palate.

The inferior turbinates are two elongated, shell-like laminae of bone, attached by their superior borders to the lateral wall of the nasal cavity on either side. They have curved borders separating a medial and a lateral

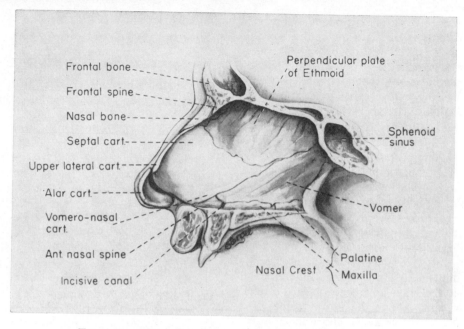

FIG. 1–2.   The nasal septum denuded of its membrane.

surface. The inferior or free portion is curved from before backward and from above downward, with the convex surface facing the septum. The bone that forms the turbinate is deeply pitted and of somewhat cellular character, which gives a slightly rough and pitted appearance. The anterior and posterior extremities are somewhat pointed. The surface of the turbinate is per-

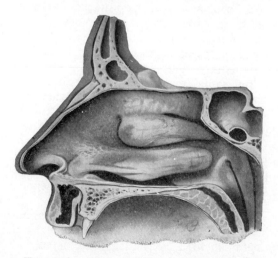

FIG. 1–3.   The middle and inferior turbinates. The superior turbinate, which may be absent or rudimentary, is not shown.

forated in numerous places by apertures through which the blood supply is transmitted. Longitudinal grooves or partial canals also help to distribute the large blood supply. The mucous membrane is thick, vascular, and adherent to the underlying perichondrium or periosteum.

Both the middle and inferior turbinates are covered with pseudostratified ciliated columnar epithelium, and the anterior tip of either the middle or the inferior turbinate in the adult may be replaced by low cuboidal or squamous cell epithelium. The stroma of the middle turbinate is characterized by the presence of many glands, whereas that of the inferior turbinate is characterized by many blood lakes. Glands, too, are found in the inferior concha but not to the extent they are in the middle. These blood lakes or venous plexuses constitute the erectile tissue of the nose and are distributed chiefly along the inferior border of the inferior turbinate and the posterior ends of both the middle and inferior turbinates.

The Superior Meatus. The superior meatus or ethmoid fissure is a narrow, slit-like space situated between the septum and the lateral mass of the ethmoid above the middle turbinate. The posterior group of ethmoidal cells drains by one or more orifices of variable size into the central portion of the meatus. Above and behind the superior turbinate and in front of the body of the sphenoid is the **sphenoethmoidal recess,** into which opens the sphenoidal sinus.

The Middle Meatus. The middle meatus, a much more roomy space than the superior meatus, contains the orifices of the frontal and maxillary sinuses and of the anterior group of ethmoidal cells. Hidden by the anterior half of the overhanging middle turbinate and situated on the external wall is a deep crescentic groove, the **infundibulum.** The crescentic opening or fissure leading from the middle meatus into the infundibulum is called the **hiatus semilunaris.** The inferior and median wall of the infundibulum forms a shelflike ledge known as the **uncinate process.** Above the infundibulum is a hemispherical prominence, the **ethmoid bulla,** formed by one of the ethmoidal cells.

The orifices of the frontal sinus, maxillary antrum, and anterior ethmoidal cells usually drain into the infundibulum. The frontal sinus and anterior ethmoidal cells usually drain into the anterior upper portion, and the maxillary sinus drains posteriorly to the frontal sinus. However, certain ethmoidal cells may have openings located above the ethmoid bulla, and the frontonasal duct sometimes has an independent orifice anterior to the infundibulum.

The Inferior Meatus. The inferior meatus, the largest of the three, contains the orifice of the nasolacrimal duct located on the lateral wall from 3 to 3.5 cm behind the posterior margin of the nostril.

The Nares. The posterior nares or choanae through which the nasal fossae and the nasopharynx communicate are oval-shaped apertures located one on each side of the nasal septum. Each opening is formed inferiorly by the horizontal plate of the palate bone, internally by the vomer, superiorly by the vaginal process of the sphenoid and the ala of the vomer, and externally by the medial pterygoid plate of the sphenoid.

The anterior nares provide communication of the nasal cavity with the outside. They are considerably smaller than the posterior nares or choanae, the latter being about 2.5 cm in height and 1.25 cm in width.

THE NASAL ACCESSORY SINUSES

The nasal sinuses are eight in number, four on each side of the nose: the right and left frontal sinuses, the right and left ethmoidal sinuses (anterior and posterior), the right and left maxillary sinuses (antra of Highmore), and the right and left sphenoidal sinuses. The sinuses are lined with mucous membrane continuous with that of the nasal cavity; all are filled with air, and all communicate with the nasal fossa through their various ostia.

The sinuses are divided for clinical purposes into two groups, anterior and posterior. The anterior group consists of the frontal and maxillary sinuses and the anterior ethmoidal cells of the ethmoidal sinus. The posterior group is made up of the posterior ethmoidal cells and the sphenoidal sinus. The line of attachment of the middle turbinate to the lateral wall of the nose marks the division between the two. The anterior group drains below the middle turbinate into or near the infundibulum and the posterior group at several locations above the middle turbinate.

The Frontal Sinus

The frontal sinus varies greatly in size and form, and in many instances the sinus differs in extent and shape from its fellow, one sinus appearing to develop at the expense of the other. Occasionally the sinus is rudimentary but never entirely wanting. Bony septa may partially subdivide the sinus into one or more compartments. The sinus communicates with the middle meatus of the nose by means of the frontonasal duct (Fig. 1–4), which passes downward and backward and opens into or near the upper portion of the infundibulum. The frontonasal canal opens directly into the middle meatus in some instances.

The average measurements of the frontal sinus are: height 3 cm, width 2 to 2.5 cm, depth 1.5 to 2 cm, and average capacity 6 to 7 ml.

The anterior plate of the frontal sinus is almost always diploetic, especially in the re-

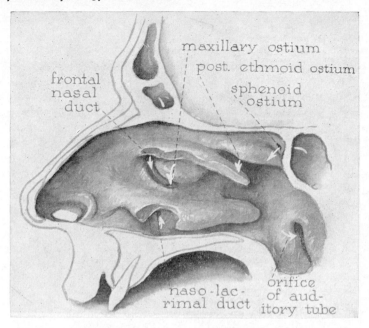

FIG. 1–4.   Sagittal section through the nose. Portions of the middle and inferior turbinates have
been removed to show various structures.

gions of the external or inferolateral angle and the superior sulcus where the anterior and posterior plates fuse.

The Ethmoidal Cells

The ethmoidal cells or labyrinth lies on either side just lateral to the superior one half or one third of the nasal cavity and medial to the bony orbit (Figs. 1–5 to 1–7). The ethmoid bone has a horizontal plate and a vertical plate that are at right angles to each other. The vertical plate has a superior portion called the *crista galli* and an inferior portion called the *perpendicular plate of the ethmoid,* a part of the nasal septum. The horizontal plate is comprised of a medial portion, the thin perforated *cribriform plate,* and a more lateral, thicker portion that forms the roof of the ethmoidal cells.

The cribriform plate is not covered by the ethmoidal cells but is freely exposed in the attic of the nose. While the bone is dense and not easily fractured by ordinary force exerted during an operation, its numerous openings render it a possible atrium for the conveyance of infection to the meninges, especially if the ethmoid is operated upon in

the presence of an acute upper respiratory infection. The outer wall of the ethmoidal sinus is the *os planum,* or *lamina papyracea,* of the ethmoid and the lacrimal bones. These plates of bone are extremely thin and form the inner wall of the orbital cavity. Should this plate of bone be perforated, orbital cellulitis, with protrusion of the eyeball, might result.

The ethmoidal cells, first seen in the fourth month of fetal life, are present in the newborn, developing in size with advancing years until puberty. In the adult the sinus is a series of pneumatic cells of variable size and number. Anterior ethmoidal cells not uncommonly encroach upon and narrow the nasofrontal duct. The volume of the two sinuses together is about 14 ml but may vary considerably from this figure. Two groups of cells may be differentiated: an anterior group, which drains into the middle meatus, and a posterior group, which drains into the superior meatus.

The anterior cells are separated from the posterior cells by a thin, transverse, bony partition. The attachment of the middle turbinate to the lateral wall of the nose also marks the line of division between the ante-

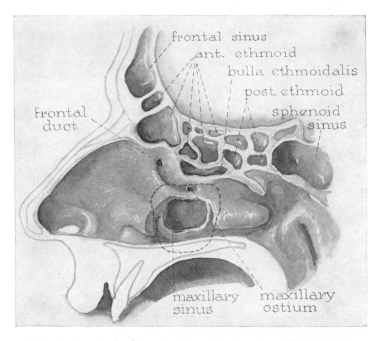

FIG. 1–5.   Sagittal section through the ethmoidal labyrinth.

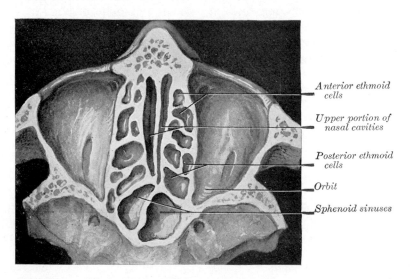

FIG. 1–6.   Horizontal section through the ethmoidal labyrinth.

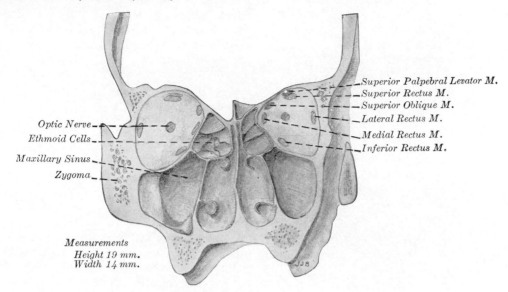

Superior Palpebral Levator M.
Superior Rectus M.
Superior Oblique M.
Lateral Rectus M.
Medial Rectus M.
Inferior Rectus M.

Optic Nerve
Ethmoid Cells
Maxillary Sinus
Zygoma

Measurements
Height 19 mm.
Width 14 mm.

Fig. 1–7.   Coronal section through the ethmoidal labyrinth.

rior and posterior groups of cells. The anterior cells lie in front of and below it, while the posterior cells lie above and behind it.

The two groups may be found to differ greatly in size when specimens are examined, but usually the posterior ethmoidal cells are fewer in number and larger in size than the anterior cells.

It is not uncommon to find cells beyond the confines of the ethmoidal sinus proper. The middle turbinate frequently is the site of a posterior ethmoidal cell, *concha bullosa,* whereas the anterior group frequently extends into the agger nasi and the uncinate process. Frontoethmoidal cells may encroach on the lumen of the frontal sinus, in which case they are termed the frontal bulla, or they may extend above the sinus to form supraorbital cells. Occasionally the body of the maxilla is the site of ethmoidal cells. Ethmoidal cells may also be found on the body of the sphenoid bone, with encroachment on the sphenoidal sinus.

The Maxillary Sinus

At birth the maxillary antrum occupies a small space to the inner side of the orbit. At first its floor is above the nasal floor, descending continually, until at 8 years it is on the same level. The subsequent development is downward, its full shape being assumed after eruption of the permanent teeth. Maximum development is attained between the fifteenth and eighteenth years. The maxillary sinus, or the *antrum* of *Highmore,* the largest of the nasal accessory sinuses, is an irregularly shaped pyramid with its base presenting to the nasal fossa and its apex corresponding to the zygomatic process of the maxilla. Morris's Human Anatomy gives the following average dimensions for the newborn—7–8 × 4–6 mm—and for the individual of 15 years—31–32 × 18–20 × 19–20 mm. In the adult the capacity of the sinus is approximately 15 ml.

The median wall or base of the antrum is formed by the vertical plate of the palate bone, the uncinate process of the ethmoid, the maxillary process of the inferior turbinate, and a small portion of the lacrimal bone (Fig. 1–8). The upper wall separates the cavity from the orbit. The posterior-inferior wall or floor is normally the thickest and is formed by the alveolar portion of the superior maxilla and by the outer part of the hard palate. The anterior wall corresponds with the canine fossa.

The antrum communicates with the infundibulum in the middle meatus by means of a small opening, the maxillary ostium, located in the upper and anterior part of the

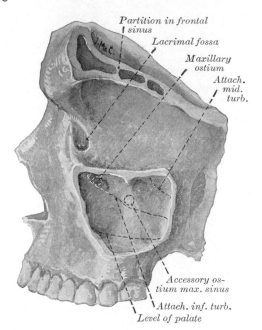

Partition in frontal sinus
Lacrimal fossa
Maxillary ostium
Attach. mid. turb.
Accessory ostium max. sinus
Attach. inf. turb.
Level of palate

FIG. 1–8. Medial antral wall showing the relationship of the intranasal structures.

median sinus wall. The ostium is usually membranous. Thus the bony ostium is larger than the actual orifice, a fact that provides the rhinologist with an area of easy access for purposes of irrigation of the sinus. In a small percentage (10%) of cases, an additional opening (accessory ostium) is present, lying posterior to the major opening. In the majority of cases, the ostium is a canal of 3 mm or more in length. The accessory ostium is in almost all instances an orifice or true ostium. Most nerves and blood vessels enter the sinus by way of the ostium or the membranous portion of the nasoantral wall.

The second bicuspid and the first and second molar teeth are in close relation to the floor of the sinus. Indeed, they sometimes project into the bony cavity, being covered at times by mucous membrane only. A suppurative process around the root of either of these teeth might affect the mucous membrane of the sinus through the lymphatics and blood vessels, and removal of these teeth may create an opening into the sinus with resultant sinusitis.

The superior wall or roof of the sinus is crossed in its central portion by the infra-

orbital nerve, which lies in a groove on the broad inferior side of the plate of bone. The nerve may be covered by mucous membrane or by thin bone and may be injured during the curettage of the sinus.

The Sphenoidal Sinus

The sphenoidal sinuses are small before the third year but are fully developed by the twelfth to fifteenth year. They are situated within the body of the sphenoid bone and are variable in size and often in shape. They are separated from each other by a thin, bony partition or septum that frequently deviates to one side or the other, producing one large and one small cavity.

Each sphenoidal sinus communicates with the superior meatus of the nose by means of a small aperture that empties into the sphenoethmoidal recess. The size of the ostium of the sphenoid varies from 0.5 to 4 mm and is located usually 10 to 20 mm above the sinus floor, thus being disadvantageously placed for gravity drainage. The dimensions of the sinus are approximately as follows: at 1 year 2.5 × 2.5 ×1.5, and at 9 years 15 × 12 × 10.5 mm. The average capacity is about 7.5 ml (0.05 to 30 ml).

The ostium is practically always membranous, its bony circumference being considerably larger than its actual orifice. It is near the septum of the nose and is hidden from view by the approximation of the middle turbinate to the septum. If there is marked atrophy of the turbinate, or if the septum deviates to the opposite side, it may be seen by anterior rhinoscopy. The purulent secretion flowing from the ostium drains either directly through the posterior choana into the nasopharynx or onto the posterior end of the middle turbinate.

The optic nerves and the hypophysis lie above the sinus, and the pons lies posteriorly. External and lateral to the sinus are found the cavernous sinus, the internal carotid artery, the superior orbital fissure, and related cranial nerves. The sphenoidal sinus may present a bony dehiscence so that the mucous membrane lies in direct contact with the subjacent structures. Thus curetting of the sinus must be done with great care. The nerve of the pterygoid canal (vidian) may encroach upon the lumen of the sinus.

Development of the Sinuses

The primordia (anlagen) of the sinuses originate rather late during the prenatal period, especially that of the frontal sinus. During the first and second months of embryonic life, the main features of the nasal cavities are differentiated. The sinuses arise as localized epithelial sprouts or recesses of the nasal mucosa after the second month. The recesses later become the ostia of the various sinuses.

The maxillary and sphenoidal sinuses arise as mucosal recesses during the third prenatal month. At this time glandular sprouts develop from the mucosal recess in the hiatus semilunaris of the middle meatus to form the future maxillary sinus. At birth the maxillary sinus is a fairly well developed tubular sac with its floor slightly below the superior border of the inferior meatus. After the seventh year the expansion of the maxillary sinus to its adult size and shape is relatively fast.

The sphenoidal sinuses originate during the third fetal month as paired evaginations of the mucosa in the superior posterior portion of the nasal cavity. The development of the mucosal evaginations is slow. Even at birth the mucosal cavities are not in relation to the posterior nasal cartilage or bony sphenoid. Pneumatization of the sphenoid bone occurs during middle childhood, proceeding rapidly after 7 years to its final form and extent, which is usually attained between 12 and 15 years or even earlier.

The ethmoidal cells originate during the fifth and sixth fetal months from the superior and supreme meatus to form the anterior and posterior groups of cells. The anterior group of cells derived from the middle meatus lies anterior, as a rule, to those cells originating from the superior meatus. These cell groups expand unequally with great individual and group variations. The various groups of cells are fairly well formed at birth. The rounded epithelial recesses forming the cells are separated from each other by interspaces and bony septa. Growth of the cells is relatively rapid, especially dur-

ing the second year of life. At 7 years most or all of the available space is pneumatized. Between 12 and 14 years the cells have attained their final form.

Pneumatization of the frontal bone begins at the end of the first year of life in one of three ways: (1) by expansion of the frontal recess in the upper anterior portion of the infundibulum; (2) by development of one of the frontal cells; or (3) by growth and expansion of a bullar cell. The location of the adult frontal ostium would vary somewhat, depending upon the origin of the frontal sinus. The growth of the frontal sinus is slow (size of a pea) up to the seventh year of life; the sinus does not attain its adult size and form until 15 to 20 years.

The Pterygopalatine Fossa

This fossa, or space, is an elongated triangular area that lies between the rounded posterior border of the maxillary sinus and the pterygoid process. Its boundary is formed medially by the perpendicular plate of the palatal bone and superiorly by the undersurface of the sphenoid bone.

The sphenopalatine foramen is situated on the junction of the roof and medial walls, close to the posterior tip of the middle turbinate. Through this foramen pass most of the vessels and nerves to the nasal cavity. The sphenopalatine ganglion is just lateral to the foramen.

Also communicating with the sphenopalatine space are the foramen rotundum, the pharyngomaxillary fissure, and the infraorbital fissure. A wire passed up the greater or lesser palatine canal enters the fossa from below. Within the fossa, in addition to the sphenopalatine ganglion, are found the second division of the fifth cranial nerve, the third division of the internal maxillary artery, and the vidian nerve.

The Nasal Mucous Membrane

The nasal fossa, nasopharynx, and sinuses are lined by a continuous mucous membrane of varying thickness and character. Above the level of the superior turbinate (approximately), it is olfactory in type; below, it is respiratory.

The Respiratory Region. The mucosa, as well as its covering epithelium, in the respiratory region varies according to whether it is in an exposed or protected location. "Typical" respiratory mucous membrane is found in the latter portion of the nose. It consists of four types of cells. First are the tall, columnar, pseudostratified cells bearing approximately 275 cilia per cell. The action of the cilia is described under Physiology of the Nose. Irregularly spaced in the epithelium and between the ciliated cells are the goblet cells. Between the ciliated and goblet cells are found cells bearing microvilli—so-called brush cells. The function of these cells is unknown, but it has been suggested that they perform three functions: offer some support to the ciliated cells, provide nutritional elements to the ciliated and goblet cells, and perhaps provide the low-viscosity medium in which the cilia beat. Lastly, the basal (replacement) cells are noted above the basement membrane.

The Olfactory Region. The brownish olfactory epithelium consists of three types of cells: supporting, basal, and olfactory. In the tunica propria, numerous branched, tubuloalveolar glands of Bowman are found. A discussion of the olfactory region is contained under Physiology of the Nose.

The Mucous Membrane Lining the Sinuses. The mucosa of the paranasal sinuses (see Fig. 10–8) is continuous with that of the nasal fossa, although it is thinner and contains fewer glands. It is composed of pseudostratified, ciliated, columnar epithelium resting on a thin basement membrane and tunica propria somewhat adherent to the underlying periosteum. The beating of the cilia, which are more abundant near the ostia, moves the overlying blanket of mucus to the nose via the respective ostia.

Nerve Supply of the Nose

Sensory Nerves. The sensory nerves of the nose (in addition to the olfactory nerves) consist mainly of the ophthalmic and maxillary divisions of the trigeminal or fifth cranial nerve. The first branch of the trigeminal nerve, the ophthalmic, gives rise to the nasociliary nerve, of which the chief branches are the anterior and posterior ethmoid (Fig.

1–9) and infratrochlear nerves. The anterior ethmoidal nerve passes over the anterior portion of the cribriform plate (Fig. 1–10) and enters the nose along with the anterior ethmoidal artery by way of the anterior ethmoidal foramen, where it divides into the medial and lateral internal nasal branches. The medial branch passes forward and downward on the septum to supply the anterior margin of the septum, while the lateral branch supplies a similar part of the lateral wall and also sends a branch, the external nasal nerve, to the external surface of the nose.

Branches from the maxillary division of the trigeminal nerve give rise to the posterior superior nasal nerves and enter the nose by way of the sphenopalatine foramen, passing in close proximity to the lateral and medial (septal) walls into the sphenopalatine ganglion. They divide into branches. The most prominent of the medial branches is the *nasopalatine nerve* (nerve of Cotunnius); it ends in the region of the incisive foramen where it communicates with the anterior palatine nerves (see Figs. 1–9 and 1–10).

The maxillary division of the trigeminal nerve also gives rise to the posterior inferior nasal nerves, which, after entering the nose via the sphenopalatine foramen, pass downward and distribute on the inferior turbinate.

The description of the sphenopalatine (Meckel's) ganglion suffers from lack of

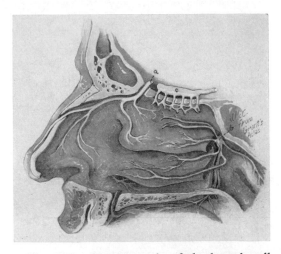

FIG. 1–9. Nerve supply of the lateral wall of the nose: *a,* anterior ethmoidal nerve; *b,* sphenopalatine ganglion; *c,* olfactory nerves.

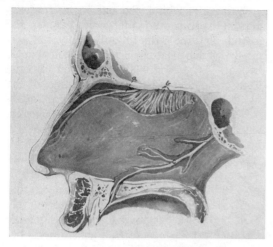

FIG. 1–10. Nerve supply of the nasal septum: *a,* anterior ethmoidal nerve; *b,* olfactory nerve; *c,* nasopalatine nerve.

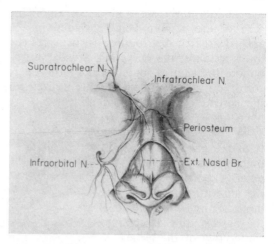

FIG. 1–11. Nerve supply to the external surface of the nose (Oscar Becker).

accurate knowledge. It lies deeply within the pterygopalatine fossa just lateral to the sphenopalatine foramen and is usually described as suspended from the maxillary nerve above. Entering into the ganglion are the great deep petrosal nerve (sympathetic) and the great superficial petrosal nerve (parasympathetic). Larsell states that the fibers of the fifth nerve and sympathetic system pass through the ganglion without interruption. The great superficial petrosal nerve, on the other hand, extends from the superior salivatory nucleus and terminates in the ganglion. The postganglionic fibers of the greater superficial petrosal nerve are distributed to the lacrimal gland and the mucosa of the upper respiratory tract; their function is vasodilation and stimulation of the lacrimal and nasal secretions.

From anatomical studies it would appear that the sphenopalatine ganglion plays little or no part in mediating vague face pains. Securing anesthesia of the ganglion itself by local applications to the sphenopalatine foramen or by injection into the ganglion probably accomplishes little as far as control of pain is concerned. The fibers of the second division of the fifth nerve are in proximity, and relief of pain may accompany anesthesia of these fibers.

Other branches from the second division of the trigeminal nerve descend in the ptery-gopalatine canal to emerge at the greater palatine foramen on the undersurface of the hard palate; they are distributed to the hard and soft palates, the uvula, and the tonsil and reach forward to the incisive canal.

The infratrochlear nerve arises from the first division of the trigeminal nerve, and its branches are distributed to the eyelids and the skin of the upper part of the side of the nose (Fig. 1–11).

The external nasal nerve, after its origin from the anterior ethmoid, runs downward in a groove on the inner surface of the nasal bone, a groove that must be distinguished on the x-ray film from a fracture line. It pierces the wall of the nose between the nasal bone and the upper lateral cartilage and supplies the skin of the lower part of the dorsum as far as the tip of the nose.

The infraorbital nerve emerges on the cheek below the eye at the infraorbital foramen to supply a portion of the lateral wall of the nose and other structures of the face.

Olfactory Nerve. The olfactory nerve descends through the cribriform plate *(lamina cribrosa)* from the undersurface of the olfactory bulb and is distributed in the mucous membrane covering the upper portion of the superior turbinate and a corresponding portion of the septum. Formerly it was thought that the distribution of the olfactory nerve in man covered a much more extensive area, the upper and median surfaces of

(2) a rigid airway to the lower respiratory tract, (3) an organ for the preparation of inspired air for the pulmonary surfaces, and (4) a self-cleaning structure. Thus the nose offers the body a protective barrier to inhaled noxious agents. The part that the nose plays as a resonator during phonation is obvious to all who have suffered from the common cold.

Olfaction

The brownish pseudostratified olfactory epithelium consists of three types of nerve cells: supporting, basal, and olfactory. At the free surface of the slender supporting cells, small "cuticular plates" or terminal webs are found that form firm attachments of one cell to another. The free surface of the cell bears numerous microvilli that project into the overlying blanket of mucous. There is a small Golgi complex in the apical cytoplasm, and brownish pigment granules impart the typical color to the epithelium. The lamina propria of the olfactory area also contains the branched, tubuloalveolar, olfactory glands of Bowman. Both supporting cells and Bowman's glands (Graziadei) produce a thin mucus covering the olfactory region that is relatively different from that covering the respiratory region of the nose; the histochemical composition is not known, however. Between the bases of the supporting cells are the basal cells, which probably function as replacement cells for the supporting elements and perhaps the olfactory cells.

Distributed evenly between the supporting cells are bipolar olfactory nerve cells. At the apical portion of each cell is a modified dendrite. It extends to the epithelial surface, just above which a bulbous enlargement, the olfactory rod or vesicle, is formed. Radiating from this rod are six to eight olfactory cilia that are essentially nonmotile and 50 to 200μ in length. On cross section the proximal one fifth of the ciliary shaft is about 250 mμ in diameter and contains the usual nine doublet peripheral fibrils and two singlet central fibrils. Distal to this the cilium is about 150 mμ in diameter and contains 11 singlet fibrils. The number of fibrils is progressively reduced as the tip of the cilium is approached, and near the tip only two fibrils are present. The significance of this arrangement is unknown. The cilia lie *parallel* to the mucosal surface and are covered by the mucous blanket. They arise from basal bodies located distally in the cell and often are not provided with rootlets; when present, these are randomly arranged rather than regularly oriented (see description of respiratory cilia).

According to the stereochemical theory of olfaction, each of the seven primary odors or modalities of the sense of smell possesses a molecule of unique size and shape and of an electrophilic or nucleophilic nature. The olfactory epithelium is then presumed to possess receptor sites that have definite shapes and dimensions, so that a specific odor-molecule is required for a particular receptor. The primary odors are: ethereal, camphoraceous, musky, floral, pepperminty, pungent, and putrid. Additional odors, including the almond odor, are supposed to be complex combinations caused by the molecules fitting two or more different primary receptor sites.

An alternative theory of olfaction involves the basic assumption that the molecular quality perceived as odor lies in certain vibrational movements of the odorous molecules. Some sort of interaction occurs between this vibration and the receptor organ. Each primary odor (perhaps as many as 25 according to Wright) would correspond to a small range of frequencies.

It is likely that the first event in the initiation of an impulse in the olfactory nerve is excitation of the olfactory rods or cilia, perhaps with a solution of the odorous particle in the mucous. Pinocytotic vacuoles often are found in association with the rods. Upon stimulation of the receptor cells, a change in electric potential is produced that causes an impulse to travel to the olfactory bulb where the mitral cells are stimulated. The change in membrane potential, the electro-olfactogram, can be measured. The amplitude varies in different regions of the olfactory epithelium, and the shape, duration, and latency periods are related to the intensity of the stimulus. The olfactory bulb has a continuous-background electric activity and is interrupted by brief or long bursts of increased activity during olfactory stimulation. Quality may depend upon the pattern of excitation of the receptor or mitral cells.

The proximal end of the olfactory cell tapers into a filament 1 μ thick, the axon. It joins with other axons to form about 20 grossly visible filaments, the fila olfactoria, that pass through openings in the cribriform plate and enter the olfactory bulb of the brain. The fila are unmyelinated. The olfactory epithelium is also provided with myelinated fibers from the trigeminal nerve. The distal fibers of the trigeminal arborize between the supporting cells under the epithelial surface, and here they are unmyelinated. They respond to sensory (but not odorous) stimuli.

Within the olfactory bulb the axons from the olfactory nerves make contact with the mitral cells, and these axons leave the bulb to form the olfactory tract, which passes along the base of the frontal lobe to enter in a complex pattern the piriform cortex, the anterior commissure, the caudate nucleus, the olfactory tubercle, and the anterior limbus of the internal capsule, with secondary connections.

Animals can be divided into microsomatic and macrosomatic, depending on the acuteness of the sense of smell. In the former, to which man belongs, the olfactory sense is poorly developed and is not of importance to the safety of the animal or its ability to procure food. In the latter group the sense of smell is well developed and is of great importance to the animal.

Airway

The nose provides a rigid passageway through which the incoming and outgoing air may pass. If the passageway were not rigid, the walls would collapse on deep inspiration when the pressure falls. The pathway that incoming air and outgoing air traverse is determined largely by three factors: the directing effect exerted by the anterior nares on the air current, the shape of the nasal vault, and the fact that the anterior nares, particularly at the limen nasi, are almost invariably smaller than the posterior choanae. Thus a relative obstruction exists at the anterior nares, and alterations in

intranasal pressure (resistance) will occur during nasal respiration.

During inspiration the air is directed upward toward the nasal vault by the anterior nares. It then passes posteriorly in a wide arc, reaching as high as the olfactory area (Fig. 1–14). As the air passes posteriorly, it is in the form of a thin sheet, but there are eddy currents as well, so that the air is in intimate contact with the wet mucosal surfaces. The expiratory route is, in general, the reverse of the inspiratory, but because of the relative obstruction at the anterior nares, there is more eddying.

During quiet respiration the intranasal resistance varies from about +5 to −7 mm of water, but these figures mean little since the resistance varies from moment to moment, depending largely on the turgescence of the

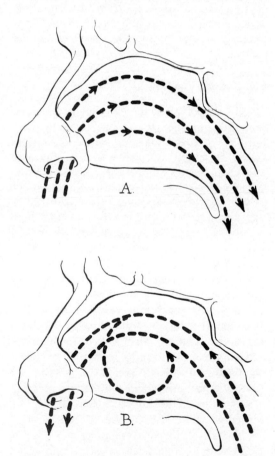

FIG. 1–14. Physiologic airway. *A*, Inspiratory current. *B*, Expiratory current with partial eddying (after Proetz).

nasal mucosa and turbinates. There is no correlation between nasal resistance and age, sex, or race. It is increased by both hot and cold air, more by the latter. Evidence has accumulated that there is a cyclical change in the nasal resistance from side to side. Excursion of intranasal pressure is reflected in the membrana tympani via an overly patent eustachian tube.

It has been shown that the resistance offered by the nose to the inflow and outflow of air comprises 50 to 60% of the total airway resistance, including tissue viscous resistance. Thus it is clear that the condition of the nose must be carefully considered in relation to the respiratory tract. A recent report demonstrated increased bronchial airway resistance when the nasal and nasopharyngeal mucosa was irritated by silica dust. Luke et al. reported abnormal increased nasal obstruction as a cause of cardiomegaly, cor pulmonale, and pulmonary edema.

Protection of the Lung

The principal ways in which the nose modifies the respired air are by tempering, humidifying, and cleaning. Heat is radiated from the blood vessels located in the subepithelial tissues of the turbinates and mucosa. The vessels lie in parallel rows much like a radiator, the veins more superficially and the arteries more deeply situated. This is an efficient arrangement for dispersing heat.

Measurements made at the glottis of an individual inspiring air via the nose at room temperature (20°C) showed a temperature of 32°C at a relative humidity of 98%. This had occurred in the fraction of a second it takes the inspired air to pass through the nose. With oral respiration, the corresponding figures are 30°C and 80% relative humidity. Not much more heat or moisture needs to be added to warm the air to body temperature at 100% relative humidity.

The nasal mucous membrane is varying degrees cooler than the warm, humid, expiratory air that passes upward into the nose. The expiratory air is cooled by contact with the mucosa, moisture condenses, and the nasal mucosa is warmed. This is called the regenerative heat and moisture exchange.

The inferior turbinate, which contains the majority of the blood spaces, acts primarily not as a radiator of heat but as a valve that controls the capacity of the nose. Its numerous blood spaces are adapted to this purpose. Inspired air also can be heated by mouth breathing, but not so well as by nasal breathing. Undesirable mouth dryness is incurred by mouth breathing.

Cleansing of the inspired air is inextricably bound up with the self-cleansing mechanism discussed below. That this is done efficiently is indicated by the fact that, in health, cultures from the nasopharynx are sterile despite the wide variety of challenges in the inhaled air.

Particulate matter of a diameter of 5 to 10 μ is about 85% filtered out by the vibrissae or is trapped on the wet mucosal surfaces above the glottis. Material smaller than this reaches the tracheal and bronchial airways. It may be that the phenomenon of adsorption plays a part in this cleansing process. Once entrapped by the blanket of mucus, the foreign material is removed by a process to be described below.

Of great interest is how efficiently the nose cleanses the air of gases. Brain, using dogs, has provided some pertinent answers. When SO_2 at a level of 1.0 ppm was administered nasally (inspiration only) at the rate of 3.5 L per minute, 99.9% was removed by the nose, oropharynx, and larynx. Others have reported that the upper respiratory tract of dogs inhaling gases at "smog" concentrations removes 73% of nitric oxide, 100% of ozone, and 0% of CO and hydrocarbons. It is little wonder that in polluted areas exposed individuals complain of rhinitis and pharyngitis. None of the gases mentioned above contained particles. If the gas did contain them, the particles, usually less than 5 to 6 μ, might enable the adsorbed gas to be carried beyond the glottis in a greater proportion. NO_2 is insoluble and thus is poorly removed by the nose. It has been shown that the nose absorbs a significant amount (approximately 32%) of the organic matter in tobacco smoke. Ballenger demonstrated experimentally that contamination of an otherwise innocuous balanced salt solution (e.g., Earle's or Gey's) with small amounts of cigarette smoke resulted in ciliostasis.

Self-Cleansing

While performing its other primary functions—i.e., in olfaction, as an airway, and in preparation of the air for use by the lungs —the nose also must keep itself clean. The most important factor in this is the mucociliary transport system. The successful functioning of this system not only protects the luminal surfaces from drying out but also protects the underlying cells from the deleterious effects of inhaled noxious material.

The *mucous blanket* is a thin, sticky, tenacious, adhesive sheet. In health, the pH is about 7 or slightly acid, and its approximate composition is mucin 2.5 to 3%, salts 1 to 2%, and water 95%. Mucus also contains IgA.

The mucous blanket is found throughout the nose (except the vestibule), sinuses, eustachian tube, and bronchial tree, perhaps extending to the alveoli in a related form of surfactant. The beating of the underlying cilia propels the blanket of mucus, along with trapped foreign material, in continuous movement toward the pharyngeal end of the esophagus, where it is swallowed or expectorated. Mucus is produced by both the mucous and serous glands and also by the goblet cells of the mucosa. Two layers of mucus have been described: an adhesive, stiff, transport layer (gel) into which only the tips of the cilia project on their forward, effective stroke, and a more fluid layer (sol) in which the shaft of the cilium resides during its entire cycle.

The mucous blanket in the respiratory portion of the nose moves posteriorly in a thin sheet that covers the ciliated area. The nature of movement, if any, in the olfactory area is uncertain. In the nonciliated anterior one third of the nose, the mucus either drops out of the nose or is pulled posteriorly by traction exerted by mucus in the ciliated area. In the posterior two thirds of the nose, the streaming from the middle meatus passes chiefly along the depths of the meatus, emerging under the posterior tip of the turbinate and passing down ante-

rior to the eustachian tube. From the superior meatus the mucous stream divides anteriorly and posteriorly to the torus tubarius and joins again below it. Material from the sphenoid sinus either passes over the lateral wall of the pharynx or down the posterior margin of the septum.

In the sinuses the blanket of mucus moves toward the various ostia, sometimes by a circuitous rather than a direct route. In operations on the sinuses it is important to avoid injury to the continuity of the ciliary system. Principally this means avoidance of injury in and about the ostium and sinus duct, for injury would invite ciliary stasis and stagnation of the sinus contents.

The speed of motion of the blanket of mucus varies with the position in the nose. The rate is relatively rapid in the ciliated posterior two thirds of the nose, where it may reach 10 mm per minute. In general, it can be said that the mucous blanket in the posterior two thirds of the nose renews itself every 10 minutes, whereas renewal occurs once every hour in the sparsely ciliated anterior one third.

Cilia

Phylogenetically, cilia are old structures, being first encountered in primitive unicellular organisms, where the ciliary motion propels the organism from place to place. In man respiratory cilia are found throughout the respiratory tract except for the anterior one third of the nose, the posterior oropharyngeal wall, portions of the larynx, and the terminal ramifications (alveoli) of the bronchial tree. They are located in the eustachian tube, most of the middle ear, and in the paranasal sinuses, being more concentrated near the sinus ostia.

In recent years much has been learned concerning the ultrastructure of the respiratory cilium, and this is illustrated in Figures 1–15 and 1–16. Human respiratory cilia extend about 6 μ on the average above the luminal surface of the cell and are about 0.3 μ in width. Perhaps 250 cilia are found per cell. Each cilium appears to be anchored by a basal body that is located just below the luminal cell surface. The structure of the centriole of the dividing cell and the

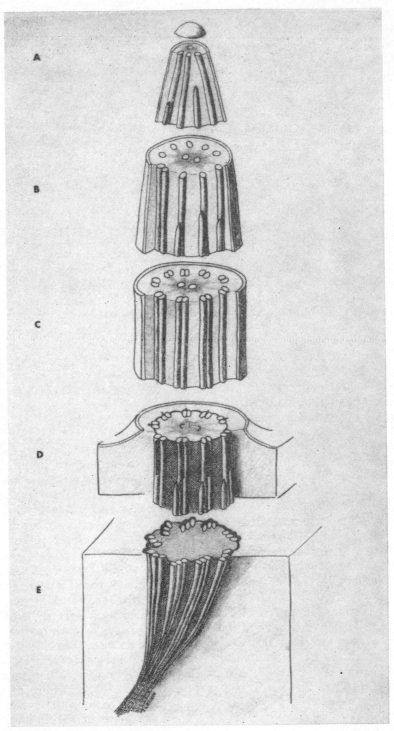

FIG. 1–15.   This drawing summarizes the fine structure of a human tracheal cilium and its basal body. It represents this author's interpretation of the three-dimensional orientation of mainly the peripheral filaments in the tip of the cilium (*A* and *B*), in the main stalk (*C*), in the transitional zone between the cilium and the basal body (*D*), and in the basal body, including the rootlets (*E*).

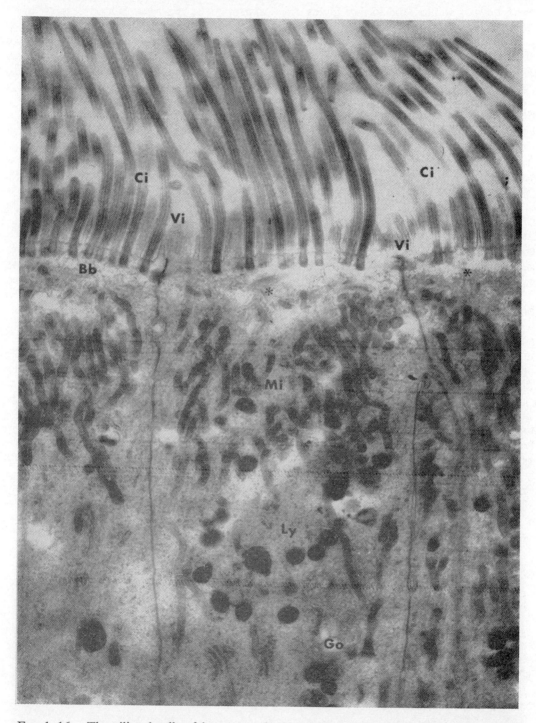

FIG. 1–16. The ciliated cells of human trachea have numerous mitochondria (Mi) clustered beneath the basal bodies (Bb) of the cilia (Ci). Several lysosomes (Ly) are usually seen between the mitochondria and the Golgi complex (Go). Fine bundles of banded fibrils (*) arise from the basal bodies and extend downward in the cell among the mitochondria. Between the cilia (Ci) are seen fine microvilli (Vi) projecting from the cell surface. × 9500.

basal body is similar, the former giving rise to the latter.

Each cilium is characterized by a system of longitudinally arranged filaments or fibrils. In the shaft of the cilium there are nine pairs of filaments arranged peripherally on a cartwheel pattern and a single central pair. Below the basal bodies the filaments are triple. The peripheral filaments do not seem to enter the basal bodies, however. Toward the tip of the cilium the peripheral fibrils become single and may fuse. Within the body of the stalk (at least in mussels and unicellular organisms), the peripheral filaments present "arms" to adjacent pairs. This and the fusing of the central pair at the tip of the cilium may be of importance in understanding conduction and contraction of the cilium.

The triple fibrils below the basal bodies are termed rootlets and extend into the interior of the cell where they may become part of a complex network of fibers that perhaps functions to pass the impulse from one cilium to adjacent cilia in such a way that metachronous rhythm is possible.

Ciliated cells are continuously being sloughed and replaced. It is most likely that the basal cells have the potentiality to differentiate into goblet cells or ciliated cells as the environment requires.

Control of ciliary action is poorly understood. In man there is no neural control, although in the frog pharynx this does not appear to be the case. Neural control, however, may influence the composition of the mucus. Acetylcholine increases the frequency of ciliary beating in the frog; 5-hydroxytryptamine (serotonin) increases ciliary beating in mollusks but appears to have little effect on mammals. Adenosine triphosphate is one energy source for mammalian ciliary activity.

The to-and-fro movement of the cilium is called its beat (Fig. 1–17). There is a more forceful forward effective stroke and a less forceful and slower backward recovery stroke. Stroboscopic measurements of excised specimens indicate that guinea pig cilia beat about 1400 to 1600 times per minute.

The cilia are closely coordinated. They act in such a fashion as to move the mucous blanket that covers them, the ones ahead carrying on the load where those behind leave off, that is, they beat metachronously, not synchronously. The nature of this nervous coordination is not known, nor is the source within each cell of the movement of the cilia of that cell understood. The cilia of a cell will continue their activity despite profound changes in their proximal cytoplasm and nucleus. Active cilia can be seen on individual epithelial cells found in the thin nasal discharge of a patient suffering from coryza. After removal of ciliated epithelium, regrowth may occur with unimpaired efficiency.

Cilia, indeed, are hardy structures. They continue their activity, with apparently un-

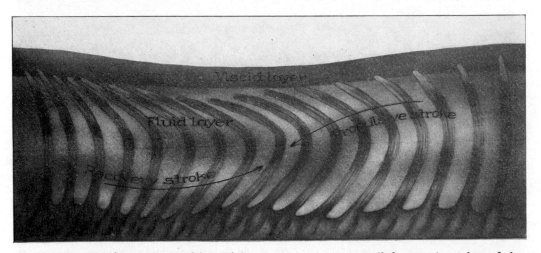

FIG. 1–17. The forward propulsive (right arrow) and recovery (left arrow) strokes of the ciliary cycle, pictured diagrammatically.

diminished vigor, though bathed in purulent secretions for months. Most bacteria seem to impede the frequency of ciliary beating very little or not at all. For more than 72 hours after death of the body itself, actively beating cilia may be found. Many parallels can be drawn between the cilia of respiratory cells and heart muscle cells. Both can continue their activity when entirely extirpated from the body if kept in a suitable environment; both are relatively indefatigable; and both exhibit a type of local neuroid control. The separate effects of temperature, hydrogen ion concentration, and the absence of calcium are the same in the two. Both heart muscle and ciliated cells continue to be active in the absence of oxygen, though less efficiently than in the presence of the gas. Cilia, like muscle, have been shown to possess the ability to split adenosine triphosphate.

Dryness exerts a permanent and rapidly deleterious effect on the cilia. It is essential that the cilia constantly be covered by a moist blanket of mucus for prolonged vigorous activity. Abnormal eddy currents created in the nose (e.g., by septal deflections) by various means may lead to dryness at various points and stasis of the cilia. This may be one mechanism whereby bacteria or other noxious agents trapped in the mucous blanket are allowed sufficient time to "settle out" and penetrate the underlying mucosa.

Some respiratory viruses, particularly the influenza virus, have the ability to interfere with ciliary activity. Electron photomicrographs of ciliated membranes exposed to these viruses show the virus particles adhered to the cilia and the cilia themselves clumped together. It is obvious that such cilia would be inefficient in performing their cleansing function. Likewise, some drugs applied topically to the ciliated nasal mucous membrane decrease the efficiency of the cleansing function by slowing the frequency of ciliary beating. This is particularly so if the drug is alkaline. It is likely that prolonged exposure to SO_2, ozone, CO, and other environmental pollutants may lead to the same reduction in efficiency. SO_2 in the gaseous state is almost completely absorbed by the nasal and nasopharyngeal mucosa. If the gas is adsorbed onto particles, it is carried to the lower respiratory tract. It is still not known what the level of the various pollutants and the length of exposure must be before ciliary injury occurs.

REFERENCES

Amoore, J. E.: Current Status of the Steric Theory of Odor. Ann. N.Y. Acad. Sci., *116*:457, 1964.

Amoore, J. E.: *Molecular Basis of Odor.* Springfield, Ill., Charles C Thomas, Publisher, 1970.

Anderson, I., *et al.*: Human Nasal Mucosal Function in a Controlled Climate. Arch. Environ. Health, *23*:408, 1971.

Ballenger, J. J.: Experimental Effect of Cigarette Smoke on Human Respiratory Cilia. New Engl. J. Med., *263*:832, 1960.

Ballenger, J. J., and Orr, M. F.: Quantitative Measurement of Human Ciliary Activity. Ann. Otol. Rhinol. Laryngol., *72*:31, 1963.

Ballenger, J. J., *et al.*: Effects of Nicotine on Ciliary Activity in Vitro. Ann. Otol. Rhinol. Laryngol., *74*:303, 1965.

Bang, F. B., *et al.*: Response of Upper Respiratory Mucosa to Drugs and Viral Infections. Am. Rev. Resp. Dis., *93*(#3, pt. 2—Symposium):142, 1966.

Brain, J. D.: The Uptake of Inhaled Gases by the Nose. Ann. Otol., *79*:529, 1970.

Cauna, N.: Electron Microscopy of the Nasal Vascular Bed and Its Nerve Supply. Ann. Otol., *79*:443, 1970.

Dalhamn, T.: Mucous Flow and Ciliary Activity in the Trachea of Healthy Rats and Rats Exposed to Respiratory Irritant Gases (SO_2, H_3N, HCHO). Acta Physiol. Scand., *36*(Suppl. 123):1, 1956.

Dalhamn, T., *et al.*: Nasal Absorption of Organic Matter in Animal Experiments. Arch. Environ. Health, *22*:554, 1971.

Dourmashkin, R. R., and Tyrrell, D. A. J.: Attachment of Two Myxoviruses to Ciliated Epithelial Cells. J. Gen. Virol., *9*:77, 1970.

Graziadei, P. P. C.: The Mucous Membranes of the Nose. Ann. Otol., *79*:433, 1970.

Hilding, D. A., and Hilding, A. C.: Electron Microscopic Observations of Nasal Epithelium After Experimental Alteration of Airflow. Ann. Otol. Rhinol. Laryngol., *79*:451, 1970.

Kilburn, K. H., and Salzano, J. V. (Eds.): Symposium on the Structure, Function and Measurement of Respiratory Cilia. Am. Rev. Resp. Dis., *93*(#3, pt. 2—Symposium):1, 1966.

22

Krahl, V. E., and Bulmash, M. H.: Studies on Living Ciliated Epithelium. Am. Rev. Resp. Dis., *99*:711, 1969.

Luke, M. J., *et al.*: Chronic Nasopharyngeal Obstruction as a Cause of Cardiomegaly, Cor Pulmonale, and Pulmonary Edema. Pediatrics, *37*:762, 1966.

Morris Human Anatomy, 12th ed. Ed. by Barry Anson, New York, McGraw-Hill, 1966.

Ohloff, G., and Thomas, A. F. (Eds.): *Gustation and Olfaction*. New York, Academic Press, 1971.

Rhodin, J. A. G.: Ultrastructure and Function of the Human Tracheal Mucosa. Am. Rev. Resp. Dis., *93*(#3, pt. 2—Symposium):1, 1966.

Ritter, F. N.: The Paranasal Sinuses, 2nd ed. St. Louis, C. V. Mosby Co., 1978.

Sleigh, M. A.: *The Biology of Cilia and Flagella*. Oxford, Pergamon Press, 1962.

Takagi, Y., *et al.*: Effects of Cold Air and Carbon Dioxide on Nasal Air Flow Resistance. Ann. Otol. Rhinol. Laryngol., *78*:40, 1969.

Westerberg, S. C., Smith, C. B., Wiley, B. B., and Jensen, C. G.: Pathogenesis of Influenza Virus Infection in Mouse Tracheal Organ Cultures. Proc. Soc. Exp. Biol. Med., *140*:856, 1972.

Wright, R. H.: Odor and Molecular Vibration: The Infrared Spectra of Some Perfume Chemicals. Ann N.Y. Acad. Sci., *116*:552, 1964.

Chapter 2

Surgical Correction of Facial Deformities

M. Eugene Tardy and Oscar J. Becker

FACIAL FRACTURES

High-speed vehicular trauma and an increasingly violent society have created a rising incidence of facial fractures, many involving one or more sinus cavities. Well-equipped trauma units and paramedical emergency assistance teams now salvage many lives previously lost because of lack of immediate medical care; the complex facial fractures resulting after the patient's vital functions have been stabilized present a considerable reconstructive challenge.

Trauma and secondary deformities of the bones of the face and skull may involve single sites but more commonly involve multiple fractures of adjacent bony structures when the trauma is severe. Multiple fractures should therefore always be suspected.

Examination and Findings. Although the patient may complain of few symptoms, certain common findings should be sought. When emergency measures to establish life support have been accomplished, a *systematic* examination of the face and skull is in order. The *facial traumagram* provides a basic pattern for examination.

Ecchymosis, crepitus, and pain or tenderness upon palpation should be detected and recorded. Deformity, malocclusion, abnormal motion, and trismus are diagnostic findings. Important concomitant findings may include epistaxis, diplopia, anesthesia (or hypoesthesia), and subconjunctival hemorrhage. Any midface injury may be responsible for

---

FACIAL TRAUMAGRAM

1. ECCHYMOSIS
2. DEFORMITY
3. PAIN (TENDERNESS)
4. MALOCCLUSION
5. EPISTAXIS

6. CREPITUS
7. DIPLOPIA
8. ANESTHESIA
9. CONJUNCTIVAL HEMORRHAGE
10. CSF RHINORRHEA

2

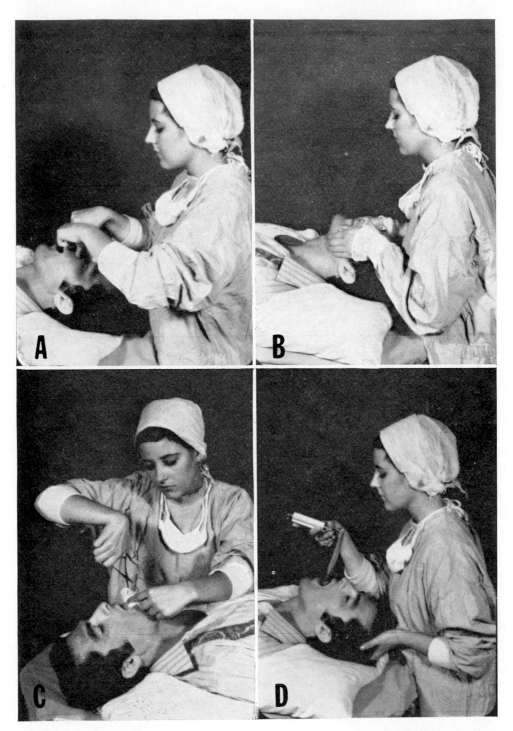

FIG. 2–1.   *A*, Manual control of maxilla (anterior traction). *B*, Manual control of mandible (anterior traction at angle of jaw).   *C*, Emergency manual control of tongue with finger or towel clip (anterior traction).   *D*, Upper airway inspection with laryngoscope, providing visualization and temporary support of upper airway.

cerebrospinal fluid rhinorrhea, signaling a loss of integrity in the cribriform plate or frontal area.

In fractures of the maxilla, mandible, or larynx, the airway may be actually or potentially embarrassed by retropositioning of the unstable jaw fragments, edema or hemorrhage in the tongue and floor of the mouth, or laryngotracheal hematoma. In all types of head injuries, neurogenic shock may be present. Airway stabilization *must* precede any x-ray corroborative studies.

Emergency Treatment. Initial considerations in the treatment of major injury to the face and neck include immediate provision for an adequate airway, control of hemorrhage, and reversal of neurogenic shock. The latter two measures are futile without airway development and maintenance.

Maxillary fractures with an unstable upper jaw may be temporarily maintained by any medical or paramedical person aware of the mechanism of airway blockade. Forward (anterior) finger traction on the upper jaw fragment(s) (Fig. 2-1, *a*) provides tempo-

rary and often life-saving control. Similar anterior manual traction applied to the unstable mandible (Fig. 2-1, *b*) serves to clear the upper airway of tongue and soft tissues, retrodisplaced by loss of mandibular integrity. Additional control of flaccid tongue airway blockade may require temporary anterior stabilization with a safety pin or towel clips (Fig. 2-1, *c*). Immediate inspection for actual or potential airway foreign bodies (dentures, fractured teeth, bony fragments) requires adequate suctioning and lighting (Fig. 2-1, *d*).

Equally important in the immediate assessment of the airway is early identification and palpation of the hyoid, laryngeal, and cricoid cartilage landmarks (Fig. 2-2). Palpable deformity, crepitus, subcutaneous emphysema, pain, and dysphonia are all clues to actual or impending laryngeal airway obstruction.

Finally, tracheotomy may be immediately required in severe injury involving multiple severe facial fractures and/or severe neurologic damage.

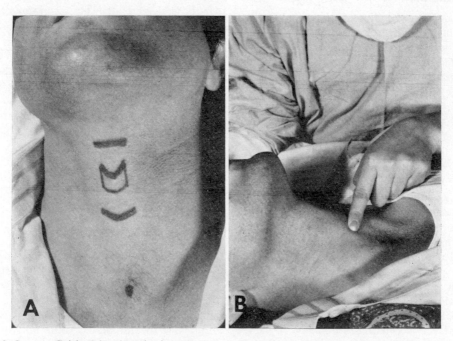

FIG. 2–2. *A,* Critical landmarks in anterior neck: hyoid, laryngeal, and cricoid cartilages. *B,* Palpation of anterior neck landmarks in assessment of trauma. Suspicious findings include tenderness, deformity, crepitus, and subcutaneous emphysema.

Nasal Fractures

Exposed, unprotected, and occupying the central portion of the face, the nose sustains fractures more frequently than any other bone in the body. Often unrecognized and undiagnosed are variable fractures of the cartilaginous framework of the septum, creating septal hematoma and deflection. Palpation and intranasal inspection allow diagnosis without the need for nasal bone radiographs. Concomitant injuries involving the ethmoidal or orbital region demand radiologic evaluation.

Topical and infiltration local anesthesia allows closed reduction of many nasal fractures, provided ecchymosis, swelling, and deformity are minimal. Increasingly, we rely on a modified rhinoplastic open reduction procedure to realign malpositioned bony and cartilaginous fragments. Stabilization of the fragments is accomplished by using fine intranasal sutures and external plaster cast immobilization. Intranasal packing and splints are generally avoided.

Ethmoidal and Frontal Sinus Fractures

The delicate, fragile ethmoidal sinuses are particularly susceptible to fracture, often in association with nasal and frontal sinus injury. Telescoping of nasal and ethmoidal fragments posteriorly is not uncommon and requires forward replacement of comminuted fragments.

All patients with injury to the ethmoidal, frontal, or orbital regions should be initially admonished to avoid blowing the nose; marked subcutaneous orbital emphysema may develop rapidly when intranasal pressure is increased. Avulsion of the ethmoidal vessels can lead to severe orbital hematoma. The severity of fractures of both the frontal and ethmoidal sinuses is considerably increased if the cribriform plate or dura is involved, precipitating cerebrospinal fluid rhinorrhea. Fracture repair in such instances is usually deferred until the cerebrospinal fluid (CSF) leak closes spontaneously or the dural defect is repaired surgically.

Fractures through the frontal sinuses occur in approximately 5% of facial fractures. No symptoms at all may be present unless bony displacement and deformity occur.

Every effort should be made to reconstitute the anatomy of the bony margins of the sinus by careful fragment wiring. Severely crushed or infected frontal sinuses may require obliteration procedures, preferably with microscopic removal of all sinus lining epithelium and obliteration with abdominal fat.

Malar Fractures

The classic malar fracture is of a tripartite nature, usually involving fractures of the orbital rim, zygomatic arch, and zygomaticofrontal suture line. Variable deformity in facial contour results, occasionally with trismus due to impingement of the arch fracture upon the temporalis muscle. Associated fractures of the orbital floor, nose, and maxilla are not uncommon.

Reduction of the existing fractures and stabilization, often by direct wiring, are usually required. Frontozygomatic suture line displacements are approached through a brow incision for optimal camouflage; arch fractures are usually amenable to reduction and elevation by a urethral sound or elevator passed beneath the temporalis muscle fascia through a temple incision camouflaged in the hairline.

Direct approaches to the orbital rim and malar bone may require lower eyelid incisions combined with a sublabial Caldwell-Luc approach for elevation and reduction of the depressed, rotated malar segment. A heavy towel clip or hook may be used to seize the bone and move it into its normal position. The hook is passed through a small nick in the skin below the fragment. The fragment is then elevated until proper approximation is accomplished.

Maxillary Fractures

Fractures of the upper jaw may be single or multiple and not uncommonly result in a posterior or lateral displacement of the upper jaw and teeth, with consequent potential airway obstruction. Malocclusion is common, and the maxillary sinus and orbit are invariably involved. Maxillary mobility is detectable with normal manipulation.

Simple alveolar fractures respond well to reduction and interdental fixation with interdental wiring and arch bars, although damaged teeth may not survive.

Major maxillary fractures require forcible reduction to a satisfactory occlusal relationship, interdental fixation, and stabilization by bilateral suspension wiring to a more cephalic stable structure (orbital rim, zygomatic arch, or temporal scalp). Forward traction over a period of several weeks may be required; this is accomplished by wiring the retrodisplaced maxillary segment to a skull cap or headgear.

Associated fractures are treated accordingly.

Mandibular Fractures

Unlike other facial bone fractures, mandibular fractures come under the distracting influence of strong attached muscles; fragment displacement therefore depends on the number of fractures and their position relative to muscle pull. Mandibular fractures are commonly multiple; second fracture sites should always be suspected. Pain, dental malocclusion, lateral crossbite, tenderness, abnormal motion, swelling, and intraoral bleeding are common findings. Mandibular fractures generally occur at areas of relative bony weakness (foramina, condyles, etc.).

X-rays will confirm the physical findings and clearly delineate the site and extent of fractures. Airway establishment precedes any attempts at radiologic survey; tracheotomy may be required in severe comminuted mandibular fractures.

Mandibular immobilization and provision for acceptable dental occlusion during the healing period are the aims of treatment. Intermaxillary fixation with application of arch bars and intermaxillary elastic bands suffices to achieve healing in uncomplicated

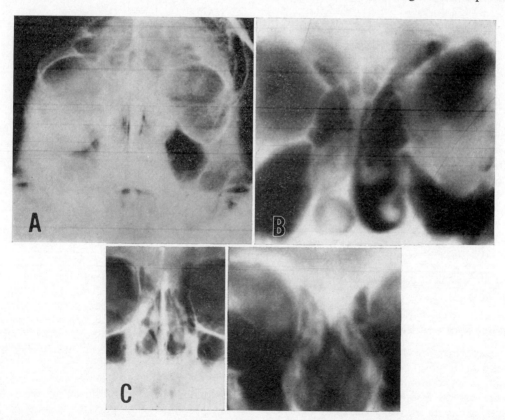

FIG. 2–3.   *A,* Orbital blowout fracture with orbital contents dehiscent into maxillary sinus (patient's right). Water's view. *B,* Polytomographic demonstration of orbital floor fracture with soft tissues prolapsed into maxillary sinus (patient's left). *C,* Fracture through lamina papyracea (patient's right). Medial blowout fracture.

mandibular fractures in patients with a reasonable dentition. Healing, generally complete at 5 to 6 weeks, is judged by lack of mobility and pain at the fracture site, since radiologic evidence of healing may not appear for many months. Edentulous patients require intermaxillary fixation of dentures or specially prepared prostheses wired circumferentially to the mandible. Open reduction and direct interosseous wiring are not uncommonly used. Similarly, fractures of the angle or multiple mandibular fractures may prove unstable with intermaxillary fixation alone; consequently, open interosseous wiring is the rule in these fracture sites. Certain unstable subcondylar fractures require similar management. Minimally displaced subcondylar or condylar fractures respond favorably to a semiliquid diet and minimal jaw motion. Indeed, immobilization of the subcondylar fracture for several weeks may

tures are persistent diplopia due to trapping of the inferior rectus muscle (or inferior oblique) in the fracture site, and early or late enophthalmos as a consequence of the relative increase in orbital volume.

A Water's view facial x-ray (Fig. 2-3, a) will often confirm the clinical diagnosis by showing depression of the orbital floor, fluid (blood) in the maxillary sinus, and possible orbital rim disruption; laminography, or polytomography (Fig. 2-3, b), delineates the precise site of questionable fractures and is commonly employed for exact diagnosis. Medial blowout fractures through the parchmentlike lamina papyracea of the ethmoid (Fig. 2-3, c) may be asymptomatic unless the patient inadvertently blows his nose, creating abrupt, frightening orbital emphysema and crepitus.

Classic but variable findings in blowout fractures are listed below.

CLASSIC FINDINGS IN BLOWOUT FRACTURES

(VARIABLE FREQUENCY)

1. VERTICAL DIPLOPIA
2. ENOPHTHALMOS
3. INFRAORBITAL NERVE HYPOESTHESIA
4. EPISTAXIS
5. PERIORBITAL ECCHYMOSIS
6. SUBCUTANEOUS EMPHYSEMA
7. OCULAR INJURY
8. ANTRAL CLOUDING ON X-RAY

---

lead to distressing ankylosis and functional disability.

Orbital Rim and Floor Fractures

Nonpenetrating hydraulic forces applied to the orbit (fist, baseball, etc.) commonly result in a comminuted "blowout" fracture of the orbital floor, with dehiscence of the orbital contents into the maxillary sinus below. Associated fractures of the orbital rim and roof may be present, particularly when trauma is sufficient to create malar fractures.

Two major concerns in orbital floor frac-

Failure to properly elevate the injured eye on upward gaze (Fig. 2-4, a,b) suggests muscle trapping, which may be confirmed by a "forced duction" test (forward traction on the inferior rectus muscle with toothed forceps). Diplopia suggests muscle dysfunction, although edema, neurapraxia, and orbital hematoma may all create temporary vertical diplopia. Hypoesthesia of the cheek signifies contusion or partial avulsion of the infraorbital nerve.

The treatment of blowout fractures is primarily surgical, although recent evidence suggests that asymptomatic fractures with no

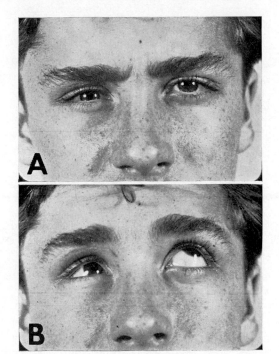

FIG. 2–4. *A*, Enophthalmos and orbital asymmetry following blowout fracture. *B*, Restriction of upward gaze due to trapping of inferior rectus muscle by blowout fracture.

bony fragments are retrieved into the orbit and stabilized with an autogenous or alloplastic implant. Bone grafts are preferred, but Supramid mesh has proved reliable and safe for bridging more extensive defects.

Certain definite contraindications to early surgical repair exist. In every patient, initial and continuing ophthalmologic assessment is mandatory.

In severe depression of orbital contents, a sublabial approach to the involved maxillary sinus is occasionally required to provide elevation and support of the dehiscent orbital contents. The majority of blowout fractures may be treated quite adequately by the orbital approach.

NASAL RECONSTRUCTION AND RHINOPLASTY

Incisions and Excisions

External nasal and paranasal incision and excision sites should be planned and positioned in areas where scar camouflage is optimum. The varying thickness and mobility of the skin in the upper three fifths of the nose contrasted with that in the lower two fifths dictates different approaches to similar problems of excision. Defects resulting from excision or trauma in the more cephalic nasal regions may be diminished considerably by circumferential epithelial undermining and advancement of the thinner mo-

muscle trapping may be treated expectantly with good results. Through a lower lid blepharoplasty incision, the floor of the orbit is gained subperiosteally and inspected carefully and gently; herniated fat, muscle, and

---

RELATIVE CONTRAINDICATIONS TO BLOWOUT FRACTURE REPAIR

1. MARKED, PERMANENT VISUAL LOSS
2. CENTRAL RETINAL ARTERY OR VEIN OCCLUSION
3. TRAUMATIC RETINAL DETACHMENT NEAR MACULA
4. BILATERAL SEVERE OCULAR TRAUMA SUFFICIENT TO PRECLUDE RECOVERY OF BINOCULAR VISION OR STEREOPSIS
5. PENETRATING INJURY TO GLOBE
6. LENS DISLOCATION
7. VITREOUS HEMORRHAGE
8. MACULAR EDEMA
9. ASSOCIATED CNS OR BRAIN INJURY

bile skin. Similar defects in the lower nasal regions near the tip are less easily decreased in extent because the thick skin is heavily laden with sebaceous glands and variably dense subcutaneous tissue.

All external nasal incisions should be planned to ultimately fall in inconspicuous areas, leading to minimal distortion of nasal features and symmetry. *Junctions of facial landmarks* hide surgical scars well; therefore, incisions situated along the *nasomaxillary groove,* the *alar-facial junction,* and the *columellar-labial* (or nasolabial) *junction* heal inconspicuously. Lesion excision in these areas should be preplanned so that the ultimate suture line(s) will symmetrically recreate these natural landmark borders. Strict attention to maintaining or recreating symmetry will lead to superior esthetic results. Local pedicle flaps transposed into these areas should be similarly designed.

Natural folds created by the synergistic interaction of muscle groups at the root of the nose provide ideal sites for incision and excision camouflage. Horizontal, oblique, and vertical wrinkles apparent in this area, blending into the glabellar region, provide wide latitude in scar camouflage in the aging patient. Redundant nasal and glabellar skin allows considerable excisional license without sacrifice of normal landmarks. It is usually possible and always preferable to reconstitute these natural folds during the course of repair.

Alternate but less ideal incision sites exist. *Anterior midcolumellar incisions* generally heal with minimal scar evidence, although the *lateral columellar incision* lends similar surgical access and creates less potential scar. *Staggered or W-shaped incisions* in the anterior midcolumellar area are acceptable for tumor excision and as an approach to infrequent external rhinoplasty procedures.

Congenital nasal tumors (dermoid cysts, lymphangiomas) in children require incisional approaches through the nasal dorsum, wide exposure being required for total excision. A precise *midline dorsal incision* or *semilunar transverse incision* creates a visible but symmetrical scar which, if meticulously repaired, fades acceptably with time.

Mature nasal scars on exposed nasal epithelium (i.e., not camouflaged in landmark junctions or natural folds) may be rendered less conspicuous by superficial mechanical dermabrasion. Minimal scars resulting from laceration repair or pedicle flap reconstruction of the lower half of the nose respond particularly well to dermabrasion techniques (widened, depressed scars due to inexact dermal healing require re-excision and meticulous repair; dermabrasion here is ineffective).

A useful technique for diminishing the extent of a large nasal excisional defect is to remove a portion of an existing nasal hump (bone and cartilage), thus creating a relative excess of skin for repair, proportionally diminishing the defect, and favorably improving the patient's profile and nasal length.

Several areas of nasal anatomy should be considered inviolate, as scars here almost always heal with unacceptable results. Incisions or lacerations cutting across the delicate alar rim remain conspicuous (notching is a common sequela), as do incisions cutting across the columella in transverse fashion. Since most incisions bridging a concavity will contract and heal as a tight, tethered bridle contracture, transverse incisions crossing the concave upper lateral nasal skin toward the inner canthus should be avoided.

Finally, the nasal defect created by traumatic laceration or lesion excision provides the surgeon with an unparalleled opportunity to study the exposed nasal anatomy and framework, aiding considerably in an understanding of the delicate, precise structural rearrangements necessarily less apparent during septorhinoplasty.

Epithelial Reconstruction

Epithelial nasal defects commonly result from minor to major excision of nasal lesions, benign or malignant. On occasion, epithelial reconstitution is necessary for replacement of irradiated nasal skin of poor quality. Traumatic avulsion defects demand immediate repair if esthetics are to be properly served and unacceptable scarring and contracture avoided. Occupying the conspicuous central portion of the face, the nose draws immediate attention to itself; nasal defects, however minor, accentuate that attention. Therefore, the camouflage repair of nasal defects deserves high esthetic and functional priority.

Until recent decades, the split-thickness or full-thickness skin graft served the surgeon well as an effective tissue for immediate epithelial replacement. Skin is readily available about the head and neck, its rate of successful "take" is high, and one-stage repairs conserve the patient's and the surgeon's time and skills. Gradually, however, the multiple advantages of adjacent or regional pedicle flaps became apparent to head and neck surgeons interested and skilled in a higher degree of esthetic camouflage, effective one-stage (or, on occasion, two-stage) repair, and superior defect effacement and color-match. Properly designed and executed, flaps should provide a near-100% take, replacing like tissue with like tissue, a fundamental concept in plastic surgery. Furthermore, flaps possess the following distinct advantages over skin grafts:

1. They provide their own blood supply.
2. They contract less than grafts.
3. Cosmetically and chromatically they are superior to grafts.
4. They provide bulk and lining.
5. They create superior protection for bone and cartilage.
6. They resist infection.
7. They undergo minimal pigment change.
8. They may incorporate cartilage, bone, or skin in composite fashion.

In their simplest form, adjacent flaps may be classified as *advancement, rotation, transposition,* and *interpolation* flaps, all designed and derived from tissue adjacent to the nasal defect. *Regional flaps* are best employed when more abundant tissue is required for repair or when adjacent skin is inadequate or unsatisfactory. Unipedicled flaps of similar texture, thickness, and color from adjacent *regions* (glabella, forehead, scalp, cheek, neck) are used. A second stage of repair is required to transect the bridge of the flap and then to make the final repair of both the defect and the donor site to render both inconspicuous. Regional flaps are invariably designed and transposed from areas of relative epithelial excess.

Adjacent Flaps. *Advancement Flaps.* Advancement flaps are created when tissue is undermined and advanced in a straight line in the same axis as the defect.

Mobile cheek skin (Fig. 2-5) may be undermined and advanced to repair heminasal defects of varying proportions. Design

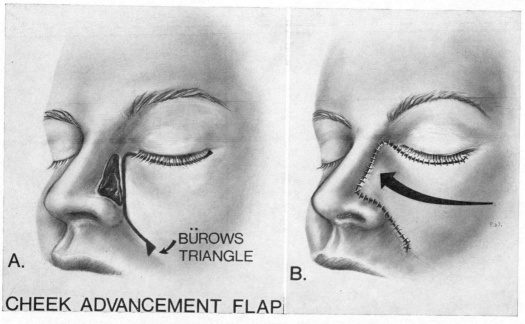

BÜROWS TRIANGLE

A.

B.

CHEEK ADVANCEMENT FLAP

FIG. 2–5.   Cheek advancement flap to nose.

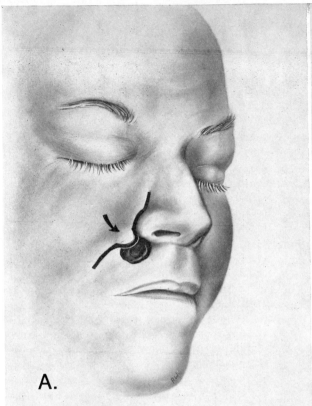

A.

CHEEK ADVANCEMENT FLAP

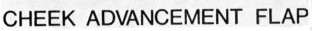

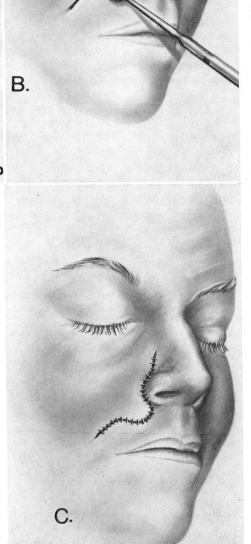

B.

C.

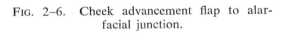

Fig. 2–6. Cheek advancement flap to alar-facial junction.

is such that ultimate closure falls in the nasolabial fold, the infraciliary area, and at the junction of the nose with the face (Fig. 2-6). Where possible, the nasolabial fold should be preserved or reconstituted to achieve bilateral facial symmetry. The inherent elasticity and redundancy of skin allow for a variety of geometric designs in creating advancement flaps whose ultimate suture lines lie in favorable areas for camouflage.

Advancement flaps along the dorsum of the nose may be created after transverse fusiform excision of lesions, the defect being diminished by shortening the nose and accomplishing hump removal.

Rotation Flaps. A local flap whose axis is created in a plane different from that of the defect is termed a "rotation flap." Rotation flaps are extremely useful in nasal repair, particularly when designed so that the donor site may be closed in an inconspicuous straight line, natural fold, or landmark junction. Typical ideal donor sites are the nasolabial fold (Fig. 2-7) and glabellar regions (Fig. 2-8).

The surgeon should approach any potential nasal defect with several alternative repair techniques in mind, choosing finally the flap or technique that possesses the most advantages and least risks for defect closure. Almost all excisional defects may be diminished in extent by circumferential undermining. The important *concept of reverse planning* is utilized, the final defect size being measured and the flap being planned accordingly before final incisions are created. Small local flaps undergo minimal shrinkage during healing (less than 10%); therefore, almost exact flaps may be tailored to reconstitute precisely the nasal defect. Flap thickness should approximate the depth of the defect for full and complete effacement. Suture technique should include key interrupted, buried, absorbable sutures in the dermis and subcutaneous tissue to match precisely the flap to the defect, with nonabsorbable fine sutures being utilized for 3 to 5 days to approximate epithelium. Tension-reducing taping (Steri-Strips) enhances wound approximation and allows earlier removal of sutures. Light compression bandages are employed for 24 to 48 hours, after

which time they are removed and replaced by an antibiotic-steroid ointment to keep the suture lines free of debris and clot.

Properly designed and executed, rotation flaps of adjacent nasal tissue may be expected to provide superior three-dimensional reconstruction of surgical and traumatic nasal defects within several weeks following repair. Defatting and "touch-up" procedures are rarely necessary. Light dermabrasion of the resulting fine nasal scars 3 to 4 months later can favorably enhance the blending effect.

Transposition Flaps. These are by far the most versatile of adjacent flaps. The transposition flap designs available for nasal repair are varied and reliable. The variety of designs possible with the use of transposed flaps provides the surgeon with many possibilities for nasal defect repair. Transposition flaps ordinarily allow primary closure of defects larger than those repaired with the simpler advancement and rotation flaps. If the flaps are properly designed, little tension is created on suture lines and "dog-ears" or "standing cones" are minimized.

In addition to the classic transposition flap design, bilobed transposition flaps, rhomboid transposition flaps, and the standard ubiquitous Z-plasty comprise superior methods of epithelial nasal reconstruction with adjacent tissue.

The classic transposition flap design is useful in the glabellar area, with redundant, lax tissue being transposed to upper lateral nasal defects. Proper design will allow the ultimate incision lines to fall in or near natural folds, creating effective camouflage. Similar designs can take advantage of redundant nasolabial fold cheek tissue by sliding tissue medially to provide ample cover for lateral nasal tissue deficits. An undesirable side effect of this maneuver is the partial obliteration of the nasolabial groove, a highly desirable landmark.

A tissue-abundant and versatile example of the transposition flap is the *bilobed flap* (Fig. 2-9), described by Zimany as "consisting of two lobes separated by more or less of an angle and based upon a common pedicle." This variety of flap design has several general applications in facial repair and two specific applications in nasal repair.

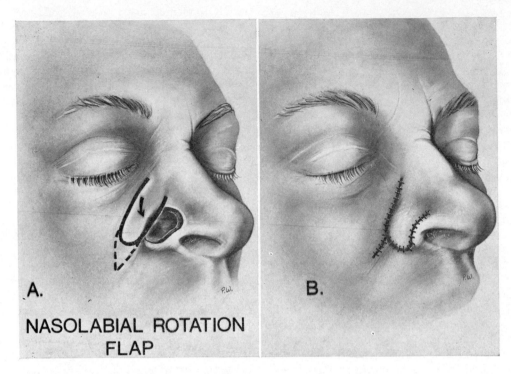

FIG. 2–7.   Nasolabial rotation flap to nose.

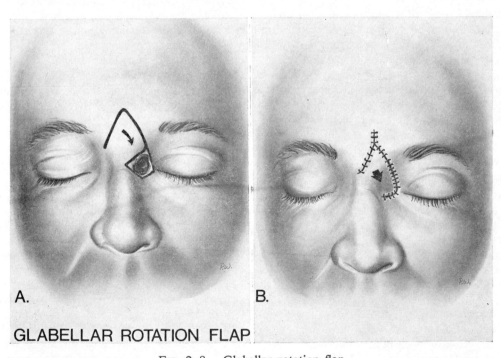

FIG. 2–8.   Glabellar rotation flap.

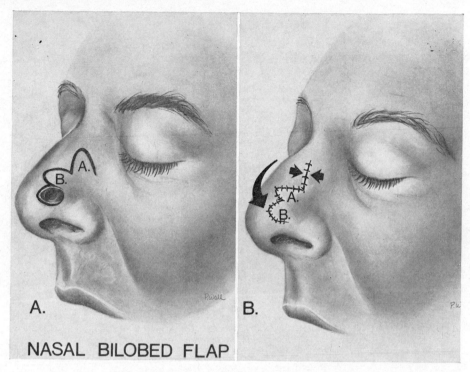

NASAL BILOBED FLAP

FIG. 2–9.   Nasal bilobed transposition flap.

Ideally, the dual flaps employed should be similar (although not necessarily exact) in size and designed to rotate approximately 90° for repair. In practice this angle can vary from 45° to almost 180°, depending on the location of the defect. Opportunities for its use exist in the upper half of the nose, where the primary donor site of the bilobed flap may be reduced in size by undermining and advancement of its edges, thus reducing the required size of the secondary donor flap. The major advantage of the bilobed flap is that it makes use of the laxity (elasticity) and redundancy of tissue along two axes at approximately right angles to each other, combining these tissues into one flap.

Abundant glabellar skin with vertical wrinkles, common in the aging face, combines favorably with the lax skin of the inner canthus area to supply tissue for the glabellar bilobed flap (Fig. 2-10). The primary lobe of the flap is of ideal thickness and color-match for dorsal nasal repair. The glabellar skin, constituting the secondary flap, is often thicker than inner canthal skin and must be carefully thinned following un-

dermining to match evenly at the suture line. Heavy, thick eyebrows extending into the glabellar midline may impair the cosmetic effectiveness of this transposition flap.

An extension of this flap design (Fig. 2-11) lends itself favorably to the repair of large lesions near the inner canthus and lateral nasal borders. A relaxing incision buried and camouflaged in the nasolabial fold frees an advancement flap of cheek skin to diminish the size of the primary recipient site, thereby reducing the effective size of the bilobed donor flap.

Similar principles are involved in deriving donor skin for nasal resurfacing from redundant nasolabial fold skin (Fig. 2-12). The secondary donor site is closed primarily in the fold, effectively camouflaging its presence. For large nasal defects especially, the cosmetic appearance of the healed flap is preferable in most situations to that of free skin or composite grafts.

The principles involved in bilobed flap design can be employed in a variety of reconstructive situations in the head and neck.

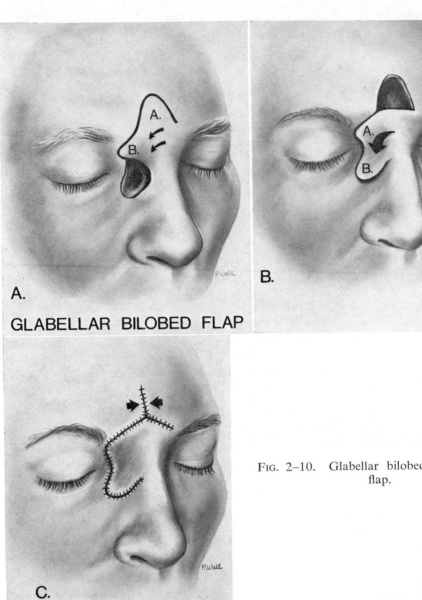

GLABELLAR BILOBED FLAP

Fig. 2–10.   Glabellar bilobed transposition flap.

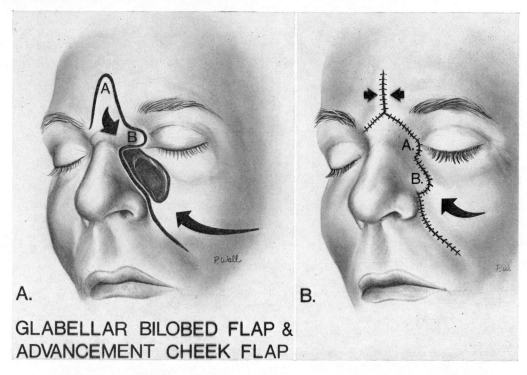

FIG. 2–11. Glabellar bilobed flap combined with advancement cheek flap.

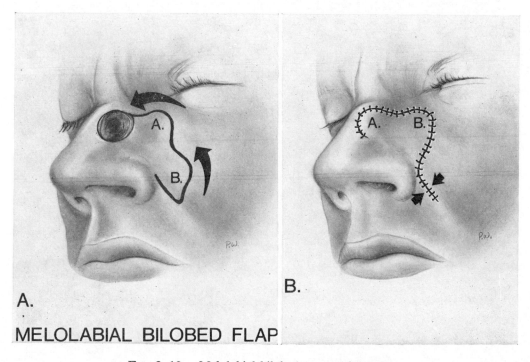

FIG. 2–12. Melolabial bilobed transposition flap.

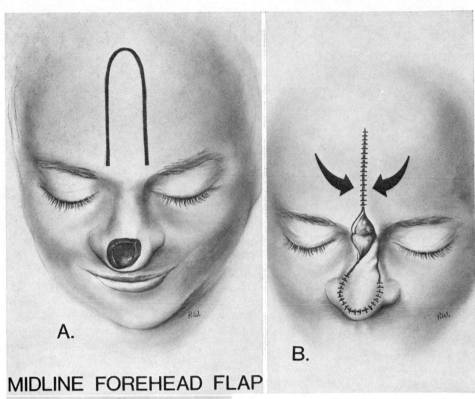

MIDLINE FOREHEAD FLAP

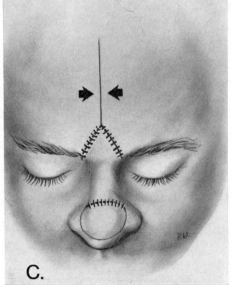

FIG. 2–13. Midline forehead flap.

Regional Flaps. Tubed pedicle skin flaps designed and transposed from head and neck *regions* other than those immediately adjacent to the nose are termed *regional flaps.* They are judiciously employed when tissue in more abundance than that provided by adjacent flaps is required, or when flap transport of buried skin, bone, or cartilage is required for framework reconstitution (in the latter incidence, the flap becomes a *composite* or *compound flap* and always requires delay and staging of 14 to 21 days before total elevation and transposition of the pedicle to the recipient site). Regional flaps are mainly designed around vigorous named vessels in the head and neck in order to allow nondelayed primary elevation and transposition. As circulatory efficiency in the flaps approaches its optimum level (14 to 21 days), the bridge of the flap is transected, final repair of the recipient site is effected, and all or a portion of the unused pedicle is either replaced in its previous anatomic bed or discarded if donor site repair is unnecessary. Regional flaps from the forehead, scalp, and temple provide excellent tissue of appropriate bulk and near-ideal color-match for nasal reconstruction. Furthermore, the ultimate donor sites in these areas are easily and effectively camouflaged, thereby making them the sites of choice for regional flap nasal repair. Tissue derived from cervical and more distant unexposed regions (shoulder, arm) lacks this ideal color-match potential.

Midline Forehead Flap. Of all the subtotal forehead flaps described for nasal reconstitution, the precise midline vertical forehead flap (Fig. 2-13) is preferred for immediate transposition. The color-match is near perfect, the midline donor site defect may be closed immediately by advancing the lateral edge of the defect, and the resultant forehead scar is negligible if closure is meticulous and free of tension. (Indeed, a midline vertical wrinkle already exists in many older patients, inviting scar camouflage.) A flap width of 2.5 to 4 cm is available, and length is limited only by the extent of the hairline widow's peak. Abundantly nourished by the supratrochlear and dorsal nasal vessels, the midline forehead flap is suitable for primary restoration of defects of nasal epithelium (Fig. 2-14), alar margin, and columella. A dressing of Adaptic gauze and antibiotic ointment substitutes for lining on the undersurface of the flap.

If desirable and appropriate, forehead tissue may be carried as a subcutaneous island pedicle flap beneath the tunnel of skin at

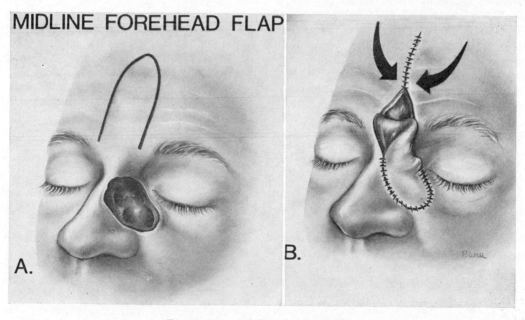

MIDLINE FOREHEAD FLAP

A.

B.

P. Wee

FIG. 2-14.   Midline forehead flap.

the root of the nose; although this design provides one-stage repair, it adds unnecessary vascular hazard to the repair and often unsightly fullness in the tunnel region.

Approximately 14 to 18 days following primary flap elevation and transfer, the vascular viability of the transposed tissue is challenged by circumferential tourniquet compression; generally, division of the flap bridge is safely accomplished at this time. The majority of the flap is discarded, and only enough tissue to reconstitute the oblique wrinkle lines at the root of the nose is restored. Camouflage is excellent.

The esthetic advantage of the midline flap is apparent to all surgeons who regularly use it. Oblique, transverse, and "off-center" forehead flaps leave more of a scar and are therefore poor esthetic choices. Midline flaps preserve forehead symmetry and expression.

In near-total nasal reconstruction, midline forehead flaps can serve as the internal epithelial lining for the new nose, underlying a scalp flap designed to reconstitute nasal form.

Scalp Sickle Flap. A variety of facial and nasal reconstructive problems can be effectively and esthetically solved by using a pedicle flap derived from the scalp-forehead junction and designed in sickle or "horseshoe" fashion (Fig. 2-15). A vigorous and tissue-abundant flap based on the superficial temporal vessels with contributions from the postauricular vessels, the sickle flap may be elevated and transposed without delay. The distal tip of the flap is composed of the non–hair-bearing bay of forehead-scalp skin, major forehead scarring and disfigurement thereby being avoided. Ambitious length to width ratios (often 6 or 8 to 1) are commonly feasible. Replacement of the unused bridge of the flap to its previous scalp position effectively camouflages donor site deformity.

The bilateral non–hair-bearing bays of forehead-scalp skin, abundant in normal scalps and more generous in patients with receding hairlines, are a choice site for donor tissue. The requirements of ideal color-match and skin texture are admirably fulfilled by the sickle flap tissue. By sparing the frontal forehead, donor site camouflage is effected by ultimate replacement of the bridge of the flap within the scalp defect, combing adjacent hair over the forehead bay, and, on occasion, lowering the frontal hairline by rotating a small adjacent rhomboid or bilobed hair-bearing flap into the bay defect. Judicious design of the flap thereby creates minimal donor site deformity, all of which may be effectively camouflaged. Normal anatomy is thus preserved.

Vigorous and reliable nourishment of the flap is derived from the superficial temporal vessels with contributions from postauricular branches, which allows nondelayed flap elevation and transposition to the recipient site. This generous blood supply permits ambitious length to width ratios of up to 8 to 1, allowing reconstruction of facial defects at great distances from the scalp. Nasal defects of major proportion are ideally suited for sickle flap reconstruction. Compound sickle flaps, transporting buried skin, bone, or cartilage to a recipient site, routinely require delay to ensure viability. Although based on the same blood supply as the classic forehead flaps, the sickle flap creates less scarring and disfigurement by sparing the central regions of the forehead.

Scalping Flaps. A great deal of scalp and forehead tissue may be primarily elevated and transposed for near-total nasal reconstitution without fear of vascular embarrassment (Fig. 2-16). In older males with balding tendencies, the donor site portion of the flap is best designed to lie upon the scalp, ideally at the vertex of the skull. In younger patients and in females, the laterally placed skin superficial to the frontalis muscle comprises the donor tissue; a postauricular full-thickness skin graft covers the forehead defect over the intact frontalis muscle. Careful flap design with a reverse planning pattern technique provides ample tissue for alar simulation by enfolding skin edges for both inner and outer nasal lining. Sufficient length must be incorporated in the design for adequate columellar length; failure to provide for ample length disallows adequate tip projection. Small local turnover flaps should be developed when possible at the lateral edges of the nasal defect to provide an enhanced vascular bed for side-to-side rather than edge-to-edge suture repair.

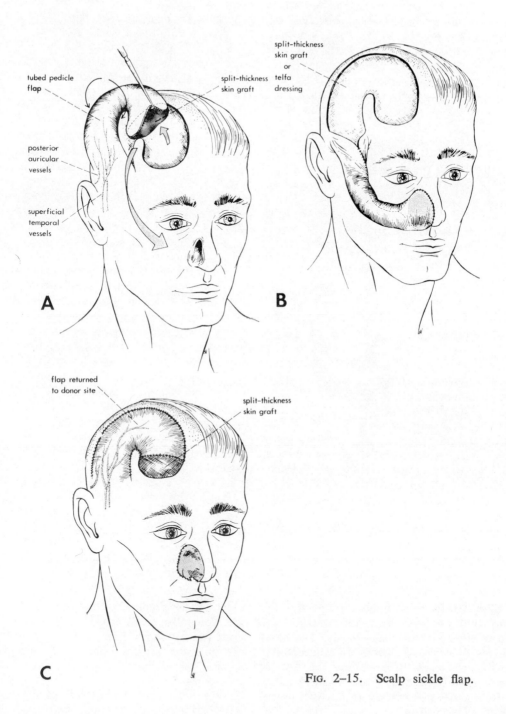

FIG. 2–15. Scalp sickle flap.

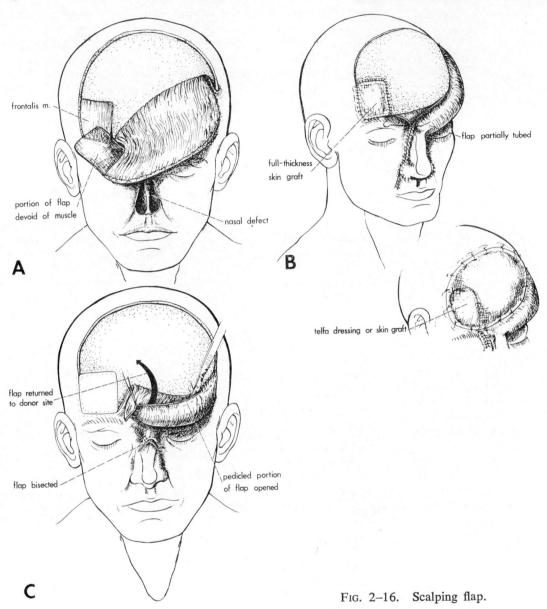

FIG. 2–16. Scalping flap.

Skin Grafts. Although infrequently utilized, split-thickness and full-thickness skin grafts are useful in nasal repair. The alternatives of primary closure or adjacent flap repair are generally preferable because of the inherent advantages previously detailed.

Skin grafts possess several distinct assets. Their use involves a one-stage repair with no sacrifice of surrounding tissue. No further incisions are required adjacent to the defect, and planning certainly is less complex and sophisticated. Normal landmarks are generally undisturbed, and should the graft fail for any reason, secondary grafting can proceed almost immediately following wound debridement, freshening, and infection control.

Superficial epithelial defects of the lower half of the nose (trauma, burns, surgical excisions) are readily repaired with skin grafts derived from postauricular, upper eyelid, or cervical skin. Skin from the latter site has proved to be a less ideal color-match than skin derived from the former two sites. An ideal but neglected donor site in older patients is the redundant skin of the nasolabial fold. Full-thickness skin donated therefrom is abundant, is of excellent color-match, and allows camouflage of the donor defect in the nasolabial crease. Similarly, the glabellar area may harbor redundant skin with similar advantages. Seldom does the need arise to graft with skin derived from the more classic distant skin graft sites (inner arm, abdomen, thigh, buttocks).

Deep shave excision repair of the nose afflicted with rhinophyma may dictate the need for near-total skin graft repair of the nose. Shave excision and dermabrasion with preservation of epithelial islands, however, uniformly lead to re-epithelialization of remarkable esthetic appearance, thereby obviating the need for grafting.

Grafts applied to the nose require delicate handling and special attention to detail in the operative and postoperative periods. Human noses are by no means inanimate; consequently, immobilization of skin grafts by means of stents, bolus dressings, and, on occasion, splints is necessary for the critical early period of 4 to 5 days. Tie-over bolus dressings of Adaptic or Telfa gauze provide light but reliable immobilization and protection of the graft. In contrast, adjacent flaps require little, if any, dressing, which is convenient for the patient and allows an early return to normal activities.

Worthy of repeated emphasis is the fact that grafts seldom satisfy the need for three-dimensional augmentation or effacement of nasal defects; they may become depressed and thinner with time, will seldom provide appropriate covering for implants of bone and cartilage, and carry with them none of their own blood supply. For these reasons and those previously outlined, adjacent flaps are preferred for immediate nasal repair. Grafts are generally inappropriate in areas of dense scarring and/or irradiation with poor blood supply.

ESTHETIC SEPTORHINOPLASTY

There is perhaps no other surgical procedure that blends artistic and technical skills to the degree required in esthetic rhinoplasty. Although it is one of the more common operations performed, only a few surgeons ever master its subtleties and nuances. Successful rhinoplasty is initially preceded by careful analytical assessment of the nasal configuration, the deformity, and its relationship to the surrounding facial features, i.e., deformity diagnosis. A realistic estimate of surgical correction, based on the possibilities and limitations imposed by the characteristics of the nasal tissues, is formulated —the preoperative "game plan." The goal of the surgery is to fashion a natural nose which is in harmony with its surrounding facial features and does not draw attention to itself. Finally, the master surgeon is separated from the novice by the ability to *predict* the favorable and *compensate for* the unfavorable healing factors which influence ultimate nasal appearance 18 to 24 months later. Only with continued experience and study, coupled with a continued impartial analysis of one's own long-term results, can the latter capability be developed and refined.

Rhinoplastic surgery, then, is more than a technique; it involves an artistic concept and the ability to envision the final result of the operation. Strict adherence to basic principles will not necessarily produce the ideal result. It is essential that an understanding of dynamic nasal structure transcend the components of static bone and cartilage. The relationship of shape and form to muscle tension and skin texture, the relationship of bone and cartilage to surrounding structures, the degree of postoperative thickening and/or relaxation of tissues, and the role of interrelated structures in the production of the deformity must be realized and evaluated.

Variations in rhinoplasty are manifold, ranging from minor corrections to complete reconstruction of the nose. Esthetic rhinoplasty aims at the creation of a nose that can be considered ideally proportioned; proper physiologic function is essential. In post-traumatic deformities and in many developmental and congenital deformities, the correction of respiratory derangements is paramount, and esthetics, though significant, are secondary. Some congenital deformities, such as the cleft lip or bifid nose, encompass both functional and cosmetic requirements of a special nature.

Esthetic Rhinoplasty. The objective of esthetic nasal plastic surgery is the creation of a nose that will be in harmony with the other features of the face. This simple statement represents a complex problem. What is "beautiful" or "ideal" is an age-old question, and the answer involves a multiplicity of emotional reactions and prejudices. In addition, values and assessments of beauty vary within different age groups and social structures. To evaluate what is beautiful entails a study of physical and cultural anthropology, ethnology, psychology, and esthetics, the ramifications of which may be endless.

Perhaps Anatole France was right when he declared, "I believe that we shall never know exactly why a thing is beautiful." However, we may allow ourselves certain elusive generalities by which to gauge the terms "beauty" or "ideal" and to emphasize some known facts, one of which was aptly stated by Francis Bacon when he said, "There is no excellent beauty which hath not some strangeness of proportion." It is the slight disproportion which may be entrancing; however, gross disharmony of features is displeasing. The task of plastic surgery is to reduce the disproportionate to "normal" or harmonious proportions.

There are multiple factors involved in studying the face from an artistic viewpoint. As Sir Thomas Browne stated, "It is the common wonder of all men, how among so many millions of faces, there should be none alike." Ability to distinguish people by their facial characteristics is a matter of self-training and the high development of man's innate artistic sense. In all probability, we distinguish faces by variations in facial expression as well as by skeletal differences.

The variations in facial expression are a direct outgrowth of the highly complex development of speech, whereby small muscle fibers were needed superficially to allow multiple variations of facial movement. The muscles involved in facial expression are known as the mimetic muscles and have no real fascial covering as do the skeletal muscles of the body. Instead they are found below and in the panniculus adiposus or super-ficial fascia, and the fibers are inserted directly into the dermis and cutis of the skin. A thick fascial covering, such as is encountered in the nonmimetic muscles, would leave the face blank and expressionless.

Anthropometric Factors. The anthropometrist utilizes basic measurements to divide and subdivide the face; these may be noted in Figure 2-17. Designated points in the midline of the face include the *trichion,* located in the center of the forehead at the hairline; the *nasion,* located at the fronto-nasal suture line; the *subnasale,* a point at the root of the nasal spine; and the *gnathion,* the most anterior point of the symphysis of the mandible. If horizontal lines are drawn through these points, the face is normally divided into three equal parts. If, in profile view, another line is projected from the upper rim of the external auditory canal (the auricular point) to the lower rim of the orbit or infraorbital point, a line known as the Frankfort horizontal, or Reid's base line, is formed. This line divides the face into two equal parts from trichion to gnathion (see Fig. 2-17).

Many of the basic observations on the divisions of the face were originally made in the fifteenth century by Leonardo da Vinci in the section of his notebooks entitled "Of the Parts of the Face." We use the accepted statement of Leonardo da Vinci—"The space from the chin to the beginning of the bottom of the nose is the third part of the face, and equal to the nose and to the forehead"—and have set up our blocks accordingly. After dividing these three groups into equal spaces, we are immediately led to certain observations. Although this spacing is equal, it is not monotonous, for the forms lying next to each other occupy different numbers of spaces. Nevertheless, the proportions are equal, indicating a certain regularity in size, shape, and position of forms. For example, the forehead occupies one entire group, or one third of the height of the face. The eye from the brow to lower lid fills one third of the height of the nose, which is the height of the forehead, or one third of the height of the face. Thus, one could say that the forehead is to the face as the eye is to the nose, or, again, one could observe that the upper lip is to the lower

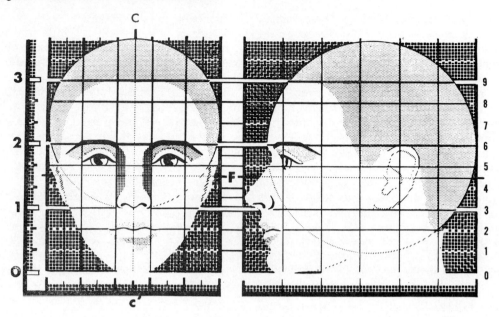

FIG. 2–17.   Anthropometric measurements of the "normal" or "ideal" face. Points in the mid-line of the face (c to c′) are the trichion (3), nasion (2), subnasale (1), and gnathion (0), divid-ing the face into three equal parts. Frankfort horizontal line (F) divides face in half. Further subdivisions of each space into thirds both horizontally and vertically reveal the eye to be a single square, the face to be five squares in width, and the space between the eyes to be one square wide. (Becker, O. J.: Trans. Am. Acad. Ophthal. Otolaryng., *60*:522, 1956.)

lip and the chin as the height of the nostril is to the remainder of the nose. In this manner one can divide and subdivide and compare indefinitely. It is rather interesting to notice that the eye tends to group a large area with a small one and to compare this grouping with other similar groupings of large and small areas.

The midline is the most obvious division of the front view. In the midline of the face, the measurement used is the width of one eye, for "the space between the eyes is equal to the size of one eye" (da Vinci). Further-more, by the size of the eye, the face is divided into five equal vertical sections. These may again be equally divided and mathematical comparisons made as before to prove pleasing points of interest. An ex-ample would be that the alae nasi occupy the space between the two inner canthi, or one eye's breadth.

Esthetic Values. Can we reduce beauty to a logical or mathematical formula by producing a so-called "norm," or is it sub-ject to an intuitive, imaginative, or concep-tual image? My opinion is that it involves both the conceptual and perceptual ap-proaches. In the logical or intellectual ap-proach, certain standards are considered ideal; however, these are modified by an overlay of subjective, intuitive, and condi-tioned thinking. There is a great deal of projection and association on the part of the viewer, and this projection is largely determined by his ethnic and cultural en-vironment. The classical beauty of ancient Greece or Egypt may not fulfill the modern ideal of Western culture, nor is it the stan-dard among the Oriental or African groups of today.

Our tastes are to a large extent of a hor-tative nature, being fostered by our culture and influenced by multiple factors, such as Madison Avenue, the cinema, and television. These have a profound influence on our esthetic judgments and preferences, almost to the point of setting unconscious standards of beauty. They deal with psychological images and make us feel or sense beauty rather than understand how we arrive at these standards or conclusions.

Since the beginning of civilization, beauty has been pursued through sculpture, painting, architecture, poetry, and music. The fine arts over the ages represent a monumental effort by man, equal, no doubt, to the energy expended on war and industry. In modern manufacturing there is a distinct effort (e.g., motivational research) to make the product appealing to our sense of beauty or to cultivate our senses into believing it is beautiful. As George Santayana stated:

There must be in our nature a very radical and widespread tendency to observe beauty, and to value it. No account of the principles of the mind can be at all adequate that passes over so conspicuous a faculty. That esthetic theory has received so little attention from the world is not due to the unimportance of the subject of which it treats, but rather to lack of an adequate motive for speculating upon it, and to the small success of the occasional efforts to deal with it.

Psychological Factors. Beauty and the concept of body image, i.e., one's attitude toward his physiognomy and body structure, are potent factors in the emotional and intellectual development of the individual. Paul Schilder in *The Image and Appearance of the Human Body* states that we should not underrate the importance of beauty and ugliness in human life.

Beauty can be a promise of complete satisfaction and can lead up to this complete satisfaction. Our own beauty or ugliness will not only figure in the image we get about ourselves, but will also figure in the image others build up about us and which will be taken back again into ourselves. The body-image is the result of social life. Beauty and ugliness are certainly not phenomena in the single individual, but are social phenomena of the utmost importance. They regulate . . . and thus become the basis for our sexual and social activities.

Beauty is interrelated and identified with the secondary sexual characteristics. Freud in *Civilization and Its Discontents* states: "The science of esthetics examines the conditions under which we experience beauty.

It cannot give an explanation of the nature and genesis of beauty. . . . It is bad that psychoanalysis also can say the least about beauty. Only its origin out of the field of sexual feelings seems assured."

Santayana similarly states: "The attraction of sex could not become efficient unless the senses were first attracted. The eye must be fascinated and the ear charmed by the object which nature intends should be pursued. Both sexes for this reason develop secondary sexual characteristics. . . ."

The nose, being a conspicuous organ, has definite secondary sexual characteristics and is frequently referred to as masculine or feminine. The patient with a poor body image, especially when there is an unconscious sexual or libidinous misidentification, may suffer a severe conflict because of a masculine or feminine appearance, or because of the erroneous belief of such an appearance. Some of the most remarkable psychological changes, often out of proportion to the surgical result, are in these individuals. Regardless of the physical change from a masculine to a feminine nose, if the patient believes that the change has wrought a new sex identification, the psychic change is spectacular. This psychic change is usually based on unconscious factors, the patient never being aware of the reasons for the dramatic change in attitude.

The psychological factors basic to an evaluation of one's appearance are instinctive and conditioned; therefore, much of the individual's reaction depends on his concept of *body image*. To a great extent this is influenced or conditioned in early life, usually by the attitude of the parents. The individual with a distorted and unrealistic self-image is usually an emotionally disturbed person. A realistic appraisal of one's own image, within reasonable limits, is usually indicative of a mature individual.

Patients seeking rhinoplastic surgery for a gross deformity usually have a realistic view of themselves and valid reason for correction of the deformity. The individual with a minor defect usually has a poor self-image, thereby exaggerating the deformity. The latter group of patients are usually, but not always, poor candidates for rhinoplastic surgery. Linn and Goldman have stated:

Psychiatrists are often troubled by the fact that the disruption in the patient's life frequently seems disproportionate to the extent of the actual nasal deformity. It is important to keep in mind that a small but real nasal deformity can immobilize a considerable quantity of psychic energy. The relief which the patient will get from the correction of the defect will be measured not by the size of the deformity but by the quantity of psychic energy bound up by it.

Shulman has contributed to the surgeon's ability to understand the motives and needs of patients seeking esthetic surgery by summarizing certain exhibited clues and characteristics. Certain diagnostic clues tending to identify the patient with a *good prognosis* include:

1. The patient with obvious disfigurement.
2. Occupational reasons for seeking surgery to improve appearance.
3. The patient who realistically wishes to appear younger.
4. The patient who has "wanted to do this for a long time."

A less ideal (or guarded) prognosis might be expected, according to Shulman, in those patients who:

1. State an unrealistic motive ("so I can look more masculine").
2. Request surgery upon sudden whim.
3. Expect surgery to be the solution to all their problems ("to save my marriage").
4. Exhibit a history of hospitalization or treatment for recurrent psychiatric illness.
5. Relentlessly surgeon-shop.
6. Have undergone repeated surgery with consistent dissatisfaction.

In summary, we can state that the motivations for and the psychological effects of rhinoplastic surgery are a complex subject. A few factors are reviewed, and an evaluation and definition of beauty from a perceptual and conceptual view are attempted. The attempt, because of its ramifications, is inconclusive. However, some of the basic precepts are discussed.

Beauty of the human face is neither abstract nor absolute; it varies between different ethnic groups and is subject to the projection of the individual. This attitude is based on a multiplicity of factors, including body image and individually conditioned cultural values, particularly during the formative years when they often become part of the unconscious mind.

In an ethnic group, beauty is the approximation of the so-called norm; for Western man this norm is depicted by mathematical proportions. It is, therefore, a form of esthetic ethnocentrism influenced by extraneous cultural factors. A great latitude in the variety and balance of features exists, so there are no absolute rules by which beauty may be determined.

Single exaggerated disproportions and the way they alter the appearance of the otherwise normal features of the face are shown in the illustrations presented here, which depict them as overlays on the drawing of the ideal norm.

Anatomic Description. The nose is the shape of a pyramid, of which approximately the upper two fifths comprise the bony vault, and the lower three fifths the cartilaginous vault (see Fig. 2-21). The upper narrow end joins the forehead at the glabella and is called the *radix nasi,* or root of the nose, and its free angle at the lower point is termed the tip or *apex nasi.* The two elliptical orifices, the *nares,* are separated from each other by a skin-cartilage septum known as the *columella.* The lateral surfaces of the nose form the dorsum by their union in the midline. The lateral surface ends below in a rounded eminence, the *ala nasi.*

The bony vault is composed of the two nasal bones, which are set on the nasal process of the frontal bone above, the frontal process of the maxilla laterally, and the perpendicular plate of the ethmoid and the septal cartilage below.

The upper portion of the cartilaginous vault consists of the two *upper lateral cartilages,* which are somewhat triangular in shape and fuse with the septum in the midline. The upper margins underride the nasal bones and the frontal process of the maxilla and are attached to them by connective tissue. The lower cartilaginous vault is composed of two *lower lateral cartilages* (alar cartilages), which are of variable shape and more or less frame the nares and help in forming the ala. The two medial crura are attached to each other by fibrous tissue and to the lower end of the septum by skin, thereby constituting the columella and the membranous septum. Fairly near the midline, the lateral crura may slightly overlap the upper lateral cartilage and are attached to its lower rim and to the septum by connective tissue. They are also intimately attached to the overlying skin. The medial crura are loosely attached to the nasal septum and to each other by connective tissue. A few small loose cartilages (minor alar cartilages) are occasionally found laterally or just above the lateral crura (Fig. 2-18).

The septum consists of both cartilage and bone. The septal cartilage is a single quadrilateral plate of cartilage which forms the anterior inferior portion of the septum. It unites with the bony portion of the septum and behind with the perpendicular plate of the ethmoid, and rests below on the groove of the vomer, the maxillary crest, and the

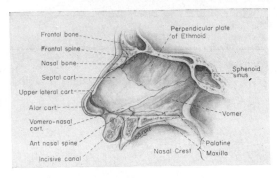

FIG. 2–19.   The nasal septum.

maxillary spine. A tail-like posterior projection of the cartilage between the perpendicular plate and vomer is known as the sphenoidal process. A small strip of cartilage, which is often absent, lies over the nasal spine and maxillary crests and is known as the vomeronasal cartilage of Jacobson (Fig. 2-19).

The skin covering the external nose is thin and contains an areolar type of subcutaneous tissue. It is loosely attached in its upper half, but in its lower portions it is intimately bound to the lower lateral cartilages and may sometimes be thick and fatty and contain many sebaceous glands. The skin continues into the naris to supply lining to the nasal vestibule.

The muscles of the nose lie directly subjacent to the skin, and occasionally muscle bundles are attached to the cutis itself. The muscles comprise the procerus, nasalis, depressor septi, dilator naris posterior, dilator naris anterior, and the angular head of the quadratus labii superioris.

The blood supply of the external nose is principally through the angular and lateral nasal branches of the external maxillary artery and the infraorbital branch of the internal maxillary artery. The internal nose is supplied by the sphenopalatine branches of the internal maxillary artery, and the ethmoidals from the ophthalmic artery. The veins terminate in the anterior facial and ophthalmic veins.

The motor nerve supply to the nose is by the facial nerve. The sensory supply includes the infratrochlear and nasal branches from the ophthalmic division of the trigeminal nerve and the infraorbital nerves from

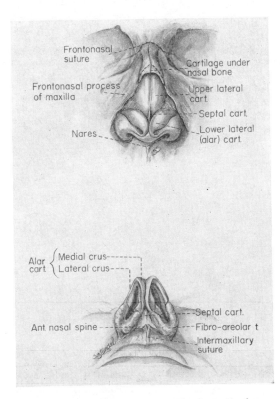

FIG. 2–18.   The nasal vault, frontal view (above) and from below.

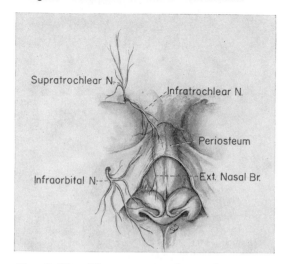

Supratrochlear N.

Infratrochlear N.

Periosteum

Infraorbital N.

Ext. Nasal Br.

FIG. 2–20.   The nerve supply to the external
nose.

the maxillary division of the trigeminal nerve. The nasal septum is innervated by the ethmoidal and nasopalatine nerves from the first and second divisions of the trigeminal nerve, respectively. The lateral wall of the internal nose receives fibers from the nasal branches of the palatine nerve, the ethmoidal nerves, and a small nasal branch from the anterior superior alveolar nerve (Fig. 2-20).

Artistic Anatomy. An artistic anatomic concept must be developed by the plastic surgeon when he approaches the study of nasal anatomy. He must take into account not only the static bone and cartilage of the nasal structure but also muscle tension, skin texture, relationship to surrounding structures, and the effect of the related and the interrelated structures on the shape of the nose. Furthermore, this concept divides the nose into an upper or immobile portion and a lower or mobile portion.

The immobile or upper portion of the nose is composed of the nasal bones and the upper lateral cartilages. The upper lateral cartilages are firmly attached to the undersurface of the nasal bones and maxillas by dense connective tissue and are fused with the septum in the midline except for a small area at its lowermost end. The nasal bones are supported by the adjacent maxillas, by the nasal process and spine of the

frontal bone, and by the septum below. Covering these structures are periosteum, perichondrium, and the procerus and transverse nasalis muscles. The overlying superficial fascia or panniculus adiposus is thin with scanty fat and fibrous tissue, thereby allowing great mobility of the skin over this area.

The lower or mobile portion of the nose is composed of the two alar (lower lateral) cartilages and occasionally by a few sesamoid cartilages superiorly and laterally. These cartilages are curved, thereby shaping the nares. The alar cartilages are more or less free-floating, being suspended and maintained in position by fibrous and muscular attachments to the two upper lateral cartilages, to the septum, to each other, and to the overlying and surrounding skin (Fig. 2-21, *A,B*).

The shape of the nasal tip is basically formed by the alar cartilages. However, depending upon the thickness of the skin, the amount of subcutaneous fat and areolar tissue, and the activity of the sebaceous glands, the configuration of the tip may vary considerably from the basic structure of the alar cartilage. Furthermore, the form of the nasal tip is dependent on its relative position in respect to the immobile or fixed structures, which suspend and hold the tip in position by firm fibrous attachments. Determining factors in the position and shape of the nasal tip include a long, short, elevated, or depressed septum; long or short upper lateral cartilages; the shape of the nasal bone and maxillary processes; the spine of the maxilla; and the direction and tension of the surrounding muscles and fibrous connective tissue.

We are frequently surprised to note what remarkable changes in shape and position are accomplished by simply dissecting the tip from the surrounding tissues. A further change is also noted when the last remaining suspensory attachment of the tip is freed by dissection of the alar cartilage from the enveloping skin. The skin at the nasal tip is immobile because of its firm adherence to the cartilage by dense, fibrous connective tissue. This firm union aids in suspending and positioning the tip; thus, to properly mobilize it, the alar cartilage is detached

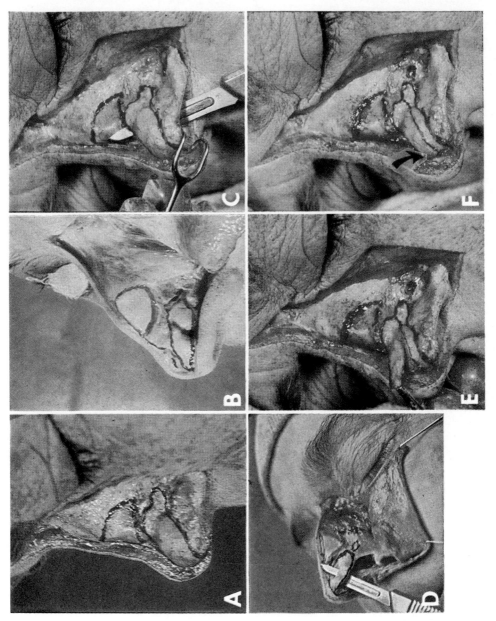

FIG. 2–21. The classic steps of rhinoplasty. *A,* Surgical anatomy of nose. *B.* Variability of upper and lower lateral cartilages. *C,* Intercartilaginous incision. *D,* Alternative approach—intracartilaginous incision. *E,* Lower lateral cartilage sculpting. *F,* Resection of cephalic portion of lower lateral cartilage; intact caudal segment preserved (arrow marks high point of dome).

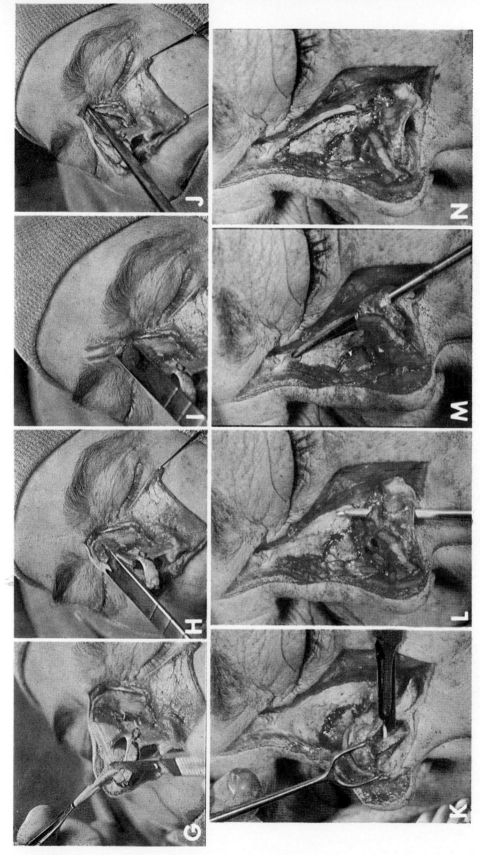

FIG. 2–21. *G*, Cartilaginous hump removal. *H*, Bony hump removal initiated. *I*, Bony hump removal completed. *J*, Medial osteotomies. *K*, Caudal septal resection. *L*, Lateral osteotomy initiated. *M*, Lateral osteotomy completed. *N*, Infracture with nasal narrowing completed.

from the overlying and surrounding skin. Frequently this may be all that is required to change the shape and direction of the tip. This is usually accomplished at the onset of the rhinoplastic operation. In thus mobilizing the alar cartilages, the muscle fibers are also detached. The muscles involved are the nasalis (transverse and alar), the dilator naris, the depressor septi, and occasionally a few slips of the caput angulare of the quadratus labii superioris. To completely mobilize the tip in a very dependent or long nose it may be necessary to do a wide blunt dissection of the skin down to the orbicularis oris and laterally to the nasolabial fold, thereby freeing portions of the quadratus muscle.

The muscles which surround and envelop the nose are part of the mimetic muscles of the face, which have no real fascial covering as do the skeletal muscles of the body. Instead, they are found below and in the panniculus adiposus or superficial fascia, and the fibers are inserted directly into the dermis and cutis of the skin. This arrangement of muscle fibers is a direct outgrowth of the highly complex development of speech, whereby small muscle fibers were needed superficially to allow multiple variations of facial movements.

Planning the Correction. In planning the correction of a nasal deformity, the component features of the face and the general body build of the patient must be considered. Frequently, failure to consider the relationship of the nose to the chin, maxilla, and forehead will mar an otherwise successful rhinoplasty and result in a nose which appears unnatural for the particular individual.

A variety of procedures for analysis of the deformity have been advocated and consist of marking angles on photographs, the employment of mechanical measuring instruments directly on the face, and the use of plaster casts. These techniques may be of value. It is difficult, however, to measure in angles and degrees so subjective an abstraction as beauty, since there are so many variables in facial physiognomy. Rather, one should strive to attain a harmonious relationship of all the features. A simple but valuable method of studying the relationship of facial features includes the use of sketches made on the reverse side of a photograph. The photograph is held up to a light or placed on a roentgen film shadow box, and by pencil sketching and shading the ultimate desired result may be visualized.

Whether or not sketches are made on the photographs, they constitute an integral part of the preoperative routine. In all plastic surgical undertakings, a photograph is absolutely essential and should form a part of the case record. A series of standardized and uniform photographs, serving as a planning and self-instructional device as well as a necessary medicolegal record, is more informative than the most carefully detailed notes.

Black and white prints combined with 2 × 2 inch color slides make ideal records in rhinoplasty photography. Preoperative photographs are followed by postoperative slides taken at 1 week and at 1, 3, 6, 12, 18, and 24 months. This carefully standardized photographic composite provides a clear, uniform panorama of the dynamics of healing, as well as a superior teaching record. The Frankfort horizontal line is utilized to position the patient properly, providing for uniformity and standardization from sitting to sitting. The following views are preferred: (1) frontal; (2) basal; (3) left lateral; (4) right lateral; (5) right lateral, smiling.

If single lens reflex cameras are used, photography, aided by properly positioned electronic flash units and a pastel background complimentary to skin tones (blue or green), is rapid and relatively simple. Use of a fast, sharp lens of approximately 105 mm focal length will avoid parallactic distortion and provide precise uniformity. Commercial photographers are frequently employed, but it is to the surgeon's advantage to master personally the details of precise photography.

THE CLASSIC STEPS OF RHINOPLASTY

Rhinoplasty remains the most challenging of all esthetic operations, since no two procedures are ever quite identical. Each patient's nasal configuration and structure requires individual and unique operative planning and surgical reconstruction. Therefore, no single technique, even though mastered, will prepare the surgeon for the varied anatomic patterns encountered. It is essential to regard rhinoplasty as an operation planned to *reconstitute and shape* the anatomic features of the nose into a new, more pleasing relationship to one another and the surrounding facial features without altering the physiologic function of the nose. Rhinoplasty should be approached as an anatomic dissection of the nasal structures requiring alteration, these elements being conservatively shaped and repositioned. Far more problems and complications arise from overcorrection of nasal abnormalities than from conservative correction. Inappropriate technique applied persistently without regard for existing anatomy creates frequent complications. One truism remains valid: "it is not what is removed in rhinoplasty that is important, but what is left behind." Furthermore, it is mandatory that the dynamic aspects of operative rhinoplasty be fully comprehended since all surgical steps in the correction of the nose are interrelated and interdependent, most maneuvers leading to a temporary deformity to be repaired by the steps that follow.

Most corrections of the long nose associated with a hump or a dorsal projection follow the basic principles formulated by Jacques Joseph in the early part of the century. His monumental treatise, *Nasenplastik und Sonstige Gesichtplastik,* published in 1931, has proved fundamentally sound for over a quarter of a century.

The procedure varies in each patient according to the amount of tissue which is excised and the relative repositioning of variable structures.

Classically, then, rhinoplasty consists of the following interrelated steps:

1. Tip remodeling, projection, and cephalic rotation (Fig. 2-21, *E,F*).
2. Hump removal (establishing the profile line) (Fig. 2-21, *G* to *I*).
3. Narrowing of the nose with osteotomies (Fig. 2-21, *L* to *N*).
4. Septoplasty.

Preoperative Preparations

Thorough, comprehensive preparation by the surgeon prior to surgery ensures a streamlined operative procedure, designed to achieve esthetic satisfaction and avoid complications. The optimum time for operation with regard to the physiologic and psychological condition of the patient (and the surgeon) should be chosen. Patients are counseled that the procedure will be a meaningful and exciting event with long-range implications rather than a necessarily unpleasant experience.

A complete physical examination is indicated, including routine laboratory tests such as blood count, urinalysis, and chemical and coagulation profiles. Untoward bleeding problems should be completely resolved before proceeding. Recent upper respiratory infections, skin pustules, or allergic exacerbations may be sufficient reasons to postpone surgery. Conditions such as anemia, metabolic disorders, or nutritional deficiency states contraindicate any elective procedure. A patient who is a poor surgical risk usually heals poorly and unpredictably.

A well-devised "game plan" should be constructed prior to surgery. Intraoperative improvisation is not recommended. Photographs of the patient's deformity can be helpful in preoperative planning. The patient should clearly comprehend the details, ramifications, limitations, and potential complications of the procedure. This informed consent discussion is purely a physician-patient encounter; no other individual, no written list of "helpful hints" supplants this critical part of the preoperative conditioning.

Preoperative Medication

The cardinal rule in preoperative medication is to use as few different categories of drugs as possible and preferably to employ drugs whose actions may be reversed or antagonized. (Too often patients scheduled for rhinoplasty are given a wide array of different drugs, confusing the pharmacologic picture considerably—certainly a therapeutic error.) Use of predictable narcotic and phenothiazine drugs only has been found safe and effective, particularly since rhinoplasty is performed using a combination of local infiltration and intravenous analgesia and anesthesia, carefully titrated, controlled, and monitored by a medical anesthesiologist. Individual drug titration in each patient, involving slow infusion of minimal intravenous increments, provides a safe and comfortable combination of euphoria, analgesia, and obtundency. Narcotic antagonists (NARCAN) provide a measure of safety but are rarely required during the operation. They are routinely administered at the conclusion of the procedure, however.

One or two small gauze pads (neurosurgical cottonoids) moistened with 5% cocaine solution are placed in each nasal passage. Surface anesthesia with intense vasoconstriction and turbinate shrinkage results.

Minimal intranasal subcutaneous infiltration of standard 1% Xylocaine with 1:100,000 epinephrine is conservatively accomplished. Infiltration occurs only as the 25-gauge needle is being withdrawn, so that the possibility of direct vessel injection is avoided. The intent is to diffuse a thin layer of anesthesia and vasoconstrictive influence in the plane just above the nasal cartilage, where most dissection will be carried out. Small amounts of infiltration anesthesia are added at the piriform aperture and columella and intraseptally. No attempt is made to create a specific block anesthesia of specific sensory nerves. This method effectively anesthetizes the operative field, creates excellent vasoconstriction, and avoids distortion of the nasal structures (a common error). Seldom is more than 4 to 5 ml of anesthetic solution required. Overaggressive injection leads to tissue ballooning, feature distortion, and consequent impaired surgical judgment.

It is essential that 10 to 15 minutes pass between the completion of injection and the initiation of surgical steps to assure intense vasoconstriction, minimal bleeding, unrestricted vision, and improved surgical technique. The surgeon who fails to make use of the improved visualization afforded by a strong headlight limits his potential surgical skills.

The face and nose are gently cleansed with hexachlorophene and thoroughly rinsed. Vibrissae are trimmed only if excessively long.

Operative Procedure

Tip Remodeling, Projection, and Rotation. The left nostril is retracted with a wide double skin hook, and counterpressure is applied over the cartilage with the middle finger. An intercartilaginous incision is created with a No. 15 blade just above and along the projecting rim of the upper lateral cartilage; the knife, preferred for atraumatic dissection, thus elevates the skin and soft tissue from the dorsal cartilaginous septum and the septal angle (Figs. 2-21, C and 2-22, A to C). A similar maneuver in the right nostril is accomplished; the two planes of dissection are connected by the knife in the same motion, and the incision is carried anterior to and around the septal angle to terminate in a partial transfixion incision (Fig. 2-22, D, E). Complete transfixion incisions, involving the entire length of the columella, are reserved for those anatomic deformities in which the caudal septum is severely deviated from the midline (Fig. 2-22, F). Complete transfixion incisions are disadvantageous in that they interrupt a particularly vital support to the tip of the nose, the intimate wraparound relationship of the feet of the medial crura and the caudal quadrangular cartilage. Elevation of the soft tissue and periosteum over the nasal bones can occur at this time (Fig. 2-22, C) but is ordinarily delayed until tip modeling is complete.

Each nostril is again retracted in turn, and a curved incision is created in the vestibular skin precisely at the caudal margin of the lower lateral cartilage. The incision extends medially past the dome area and courses variably downward along the caudal edge of the medial crus, depending upon the anatomy involved. The knife then dissects the soft tissue plane immediately superficial to the lower lateral cartilage (lateral crus), and the cartilage is subluxed from the nostril as a bipedicle flap with a thin, curved elevator.

It should be emphasized that every attempt is made to reduce surgical maneuvers within the nasal tissue to a minimum, accomplishing as much as possible with the fewest possible strokes of the knife.

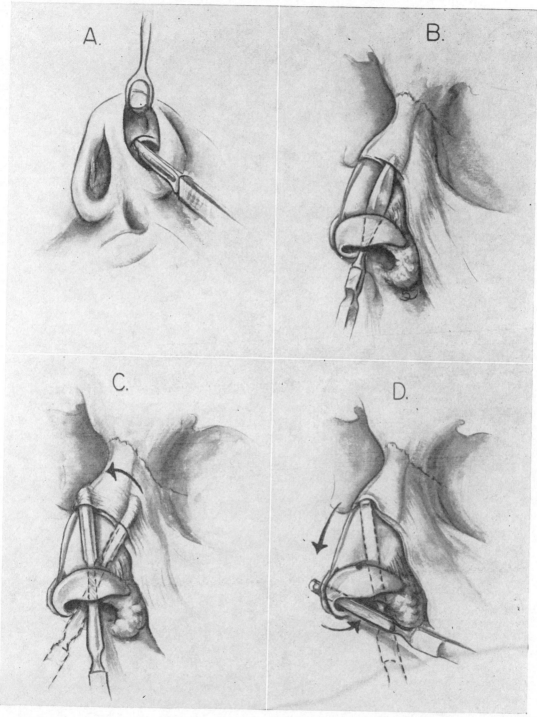

Fig. 2–22.   See legend on page 59.

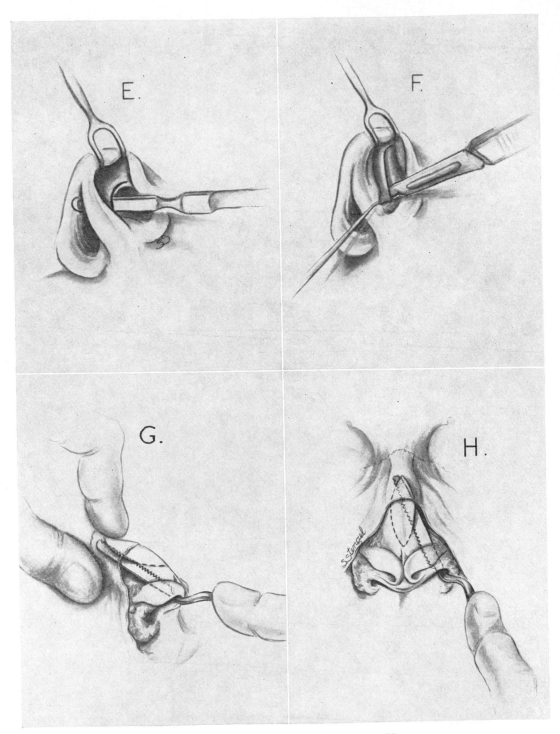

FIG. 2–22.   See legend on page 59.

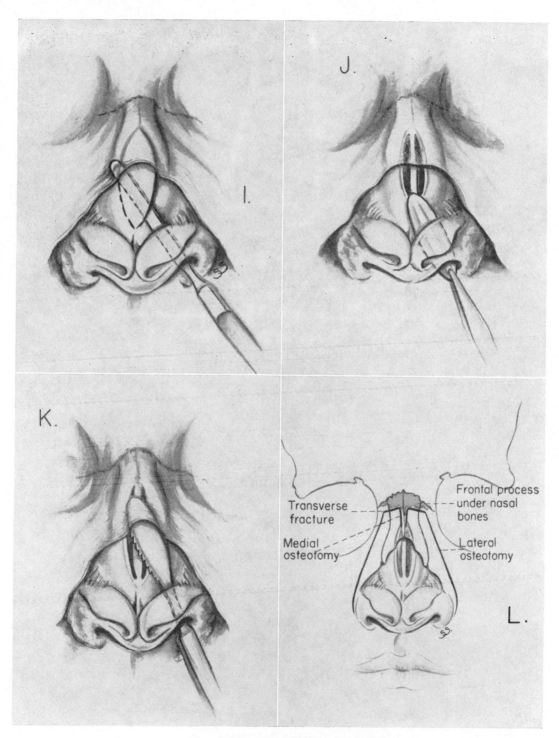

Fig. 2–22. See legend on page 59.

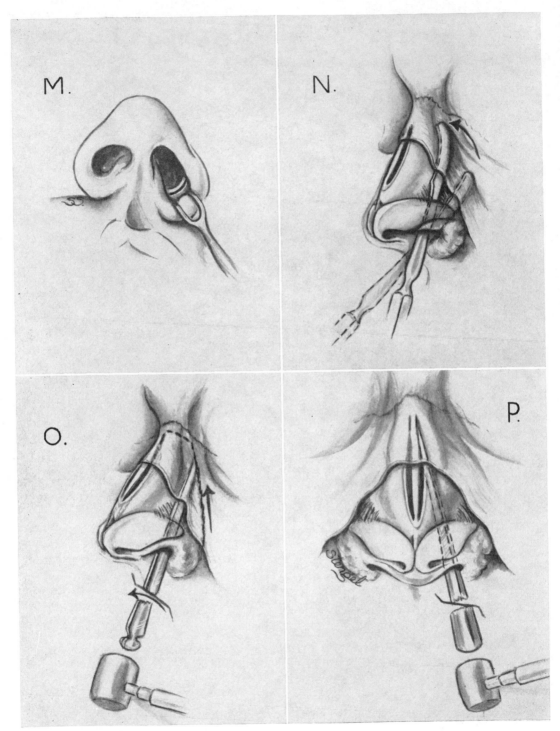

FIG. 2–22. See legend on page 59.

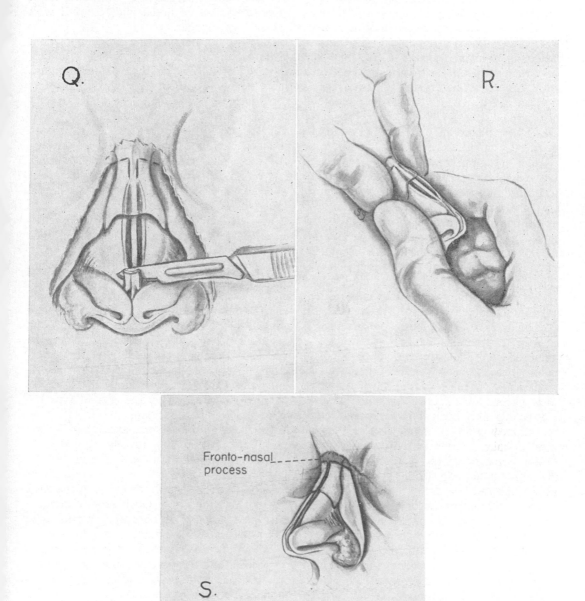

FIG. 2-22.   *A*, The intercartilaginous incision of the nasal septum. *B, C*, Elevation of the skin over the dorsum. *D* to *F*, Transfixion of the nasal columella. *G, H*, Hump removal with either saw or chisel. *I, J*, Cartilaginous hump removal. *K*, Final profile alignment with rasp. *L*, Sites of the osteotomy incisions. *M*, Mucosal incisions at the piriform margin. *N, O*, Lateral osteotomy. *P*, Medial osteotomy. *Q*, Final trimming of septal angle. *R*, Complete fractures of nasal bones insured by gentle manual manipulations.

Exposing the cartilages in this manner (intercartilaginous and marginal incisions) provides a clear comprehension of their anatomy and allows symmetrical, precise remodeling. Various geometric excisions are now removed from the dome area, combined with generally conservative excisions of a portion of the cephalic margin of the lateral crus (see Fig. 2-21, *E, F*). The cartilages are now replaced in their normal anatomic beds.

Every attempt is made to preserve an intact caudal marginal segment of the cartilage to ensure sufficient tip support and symmetry (see Fig. 2-21, *F*). This is of considerable importance; failure to observe its surgical significance will lead to a larger number of tip cartilage asymmetries and irregularities. Only in cases involving wide, box-type tips is this rule violated by cutting totally across and resecting a portion of the otherwise intact caudal segment. Throughout, the vestibular skin is religiously preserved.

Several dynamic changes will now have been effected that are critical to the surgeon's comprehension of the refinements of rhinoplasty. Freeing of the cartilages from their fibrous attachments, combined with selective cephalic segment (and partial dome) resection, creates a narrowing refinement and cephalic rotation of the nasal tip in relation to the remaining features of the nose. A new tip-supratip profile relationship is now established.

If the nasal tip is to be elevated, it is placed in the proper upward position. If the nasal tip is held in this position, the excessive length of the septum occasionally may be seen protruding beyond the columella and nasal tip. This is removed by *gradual excision* of small sections of septal cartilage from the lower portion of the septum until the septum conforms to the desired new position (Fig. 2-22, *F*). A No. 15 blade is used for this maneuver because it is more accurate than a scissors and because it also preserves mucosa and skin at the lower septal border, which may be trimmed later for accurate approximation of the columella. Varying geometric designs (triangular, rectangular, parallelogram) may be resected to create a pleasing columellar-labial angle. In any instance, conservatism is the hallmark

of expert nasal surgery. A protruding nasal spine may also be noted and removed with a chisel or rongeur.

The tip will now assume its new position. If the appearance is good, no further surgery is necessary. However, one of three things may become apparent: (1) the tip projects too much; (2) the tip is too wide; or (3) the tip does not project enough.

If the tip projects too much, an incision is made medial to the angle, but not through the skin. The cartilage is undermined for a few millimeters from the underlying skin. An overlapping of the medial crus by the lateral crus will be noted, and the excess cartilage is removed. This allows the remaining cartilage to meet and form a new angle with no defect between the crura.

Another way to lower the tip is to free the medial crus by dissection down the columella through the original rim incision. Separation of the fibrous connections and dissection down to the spine will allow the medial crus to settle downward. It may be necessary to remove a section of the lowermost portion of the medial crus as it inserts into the base of the columella. However, cutting the cartilage on the medial crus below the angle, dissecting the lateral crus from the underlying skin, and removing the resultant overlap are usually sufficient to drop the tip. Sometimes just cutting through the angle or at two or three areas on either side of the angle will drop the projection adequately. This maneuver may widen the alar base, and appropriate wedges must then be removed from the base.

If a wide tip is present, it is necessary to expose the area between the two medial crura near the angle and remove any excess connective, fibrous, or fatty tissue. An incision is then made at the angle of both alar cartilages, the underlying skin being left intact. The two medial crura are then brought together with one or more fine catgut sutures. In some patients it may be necessary to remove a narrow strip of cartilage at each angle before bringing the crura together.

If the nasal tip does not project enough, an incision is made just lateral to the angle, and the cartilage is undermined from the vestibular skin for a few millimeters under both the medial and lateral crura. The two medial crura are then united with fine catgut sutures. Often this is not sufficient to project the tip, and a section of tapered septal or alar cartilage is then sutured over the medial crura. This should be done under direct vision to make sure that the section of cartilage is placed in the midline and that it extends laterally to cover any defect which may result from rotation of a portion of lateral crus into the medial crus. It should be emphasized that this latter technique is very infrequently utilized and is not recommended for the inexperienced surgeon.

All the foregoing maneuvers, which are performed at the inferior rim border of the lower laterals, are accomplished without cutting through the vestibular skin. It is only in exceptionally thickened tip deformities that skin lining and cartilage are removed together in the lower half of the alar cartilage region.

Hump Removal (Establishing a Profile Line). Once satisfactory tip remodeling and projection, usually the most difficult and unpredictable portion of rhinoplasty, have been established, attention is focused on the establishment of the new profile line. My own preference is for a high, strong profile line, referred to at times as a "patrician" appearance. The wishes and anatomic limitations of the patient are also factors in profile planning.

The question "how do I determine how much nasal hump to remove?" is perhaps the most common query made by the student in rhinoplasty. No precise answer is possible, since degree and angulation of hump removal depend upon a variety of factors, some of which are under the control of the surgeon and some of which are not. These include skin thickness, amount of bony hump relative to cartilaginous hump, the width of the nose, the angulation of the nasal tip, the degree of inclination of the nasofrontal angle, and, most importantly, the patient's wishes regarding nasal profile. In the final analysis, it is the surgeon's ability to conceptualize and visualize the appearance of the nose after approximately 12 to 18 months of healing that allows exact and precise hump removal, with avoidance of extremes in either direction. Remember that few surgeons are capable of accom-

plishing complete hump removal in one grand flourish with the chisel or saw and that most accomplish hump removal in *controlled increments* to avoid overreduction of the hump. As much of the hump as possible should be removed under *direct vision*.

With this in mind, a safe, reliable controlled increment method of hump removal under direct vision has been developed in the course of performing and teaching rhinoplasty procedures. The soft tissues of the nose are undermined by sharp *knife dissection only* through whatever incision has been utilized to expose the bony cartilaginous nasal framework. The plane is created directly over the cartilaginous skeleton in the *lower half* of the nose to avoid the blood vessel–bearing strata of the nose.

The periosteum and the skin are elevated as one unit to allow a thick covering for the cut surface of the bone after a dorsal projection is removed (see also p. 59). As a rule, only sufficient lateral elevation is necessary to completely remove the existent hump. If periosteum and muscle are sacrificed with the hump, there is always the possibility of skin retraction and dimpling, because the skin in this area has little fibrous and fatty tissue. Should this happen and the correction is difficult, careful elevation of the skin and the insertion of a cartilage graft over the dorsum prevent a recurrence of the dimpling. Furthermore, a thick covering tends to camouflage any minor bony irregularities which may exist (or come to exist 18 to 24 months later).

Under direct vision with use of a good light and an Aufricht retractor, the cartilaginous dorsum is exposed. A knife is positioned in the midline at the junction of the caudal edge of the nasal bones and the dorsal cartilaginous septum. The blade is drawn downward to the caudal margin of the septum, thus allowing any remaining soft tissue to fall laterally and thereby expose the cartilaginous dorsum and its attached upper lateral cartilages. Under direct vision, with the knife blade at precise right angles to the cartilaginous dorsum, segmental strips of dorsal cartilage are shaved away in smooth fashion (Fig. 2-21, *G* and 2-22, *I*). This maneuver accurately establishes the supratip nasal profile in relation to the nasal tip and *precisely defines* the amount of *bony* hump requiring removal.

It is helpful to check this profile angle in relation to the tip by frequently depressing the tip using finger pressure on the upper lip. Failure to remove an adequate amount of dorsal cartilaginous hump is one of the common causes of one form of the post-rhinoplasty "polly-beak."

After sufficient removal of the cartilaginous dorsum, the upper lateral cartilages are now visually checked for their relative height in relation to the dorsal septum. Ordinarily they will require lowering by knife or scissors to a height just below that of the dorsal septum. At this point, the bony component of the hump (often less than the cartilage component) will be precisely defined and delineated for removal. We prefer a wide, sharp chisel for bony hump removal, believing it to be much less traumatic and more precise than a saw or forceps. A 12-mm chisel is seated intranasally at the caudal end of the bony hump; progressive gentle taps from a sound-deadened mallet accomplish accurate bony hump removal (Fig. 2-21, *H, I*). If any error is to be made, it should be on the conservative side, since overaggressive hump removal is extremely difficult to correct precisely. Final adjustments are made in creating the new nasal dorsal profile by smoothing with a sharp rasp (Fig. 2-22, *J*) (a dull rasp is traumatic and accomplishes nothing) and by trimming excess soft tissue under direct vision with scissors.

Whether a saw (Fig. 2-22, *G, H*) or chisel is used for bony hump removal makes little difference if the result is a smooth and nicely leveled dorsum, with excess mucous membrane trimmed to the level of the nasal bones, upper lateral cartilage, and septum.

Narrowing the Nose: Osteotomies. The hump removal will result in an excessive width of the dorsum, thereby requiring an infracture of the lateral nasal walls to narrow the bony and cartilaginous dorsum. This is accomplished by a partial medial osteotomy and a complete lateral osteotomy (Fig. 2-22, *L* to *P*). To accomplish the latter, an incision is made at the piriform margin (Fig. 2-22, *M*); the periosteum is generally not elevated along the ascending process of the superior maxilla. A saw or an osteotome is used to transect the bone along this line.

Before the lateral osteotomy is performed, the partial medial osteotomy is completed. An osteotome is inserted between the septum and lateral nasal wall and carried up the midline for a short distance until a resistance is encountered at the frontal process (Figs. 2-21, *J* and 2-22, *P*). Both medial osteotomies are directed upward and laterally at an angle of approximately 15 degrees from the midline, to more closely approach the lateral osteotomy that follows (Figs. 2-21, *L* to *N* and 2-22, *L, O*). A high medial osteotomy will allow the thick frontal process and nasal bones to interfere with the lateral infracture. The large frontal bone section will become incorporated in the lateral osteotomy, resulting in the "rocker formation" described by Wright. If this happens, it then becomes necessary to use excessive pressure to fracture the bone transversely below the heavy frontal process; in some instances this may leave a loose fragment of bone above the transverse fracture line. Instead of excessive pressure, an osteotome inserted through the original limen vestibuli incision or through an external incision to produce a fracture at the region of the junction of the heavy frontal and nasal bones may be used. Another alternative involves the use of an outfracture that will break the bone at the nasofrontal suture, thereby incorporating the thick frontal area. To eliminate this thick area, wedges of bone are removed from the frontal process to provide space for the infracture. This will in many instances produce a good and a high infracture, but there is always the grave possibility of a depression of the lateral nasal wall resulting because of excessive mobility of the bony structures. The removal of wedges may leave the area weak and somewhat mobile, so that postoperative intranasal edema, subsequent rhinitis with edema, or a slight injury may be sufficient to splay the bones outward. It is simpler to do a partial medial osteotomy, or no medial osteotomy if a large hump is removed, to eliminate the high fracture.

Firm pressure applied for several minutes over the lateral osteotomy site will minimize postoperative edema and ecchymosis (Fig. 2-22, *R*).

There are some patients with an excessively high nasion and dorsum or especially wide and thickened nasal bones, e.g., the post-traumatic nose. In these cases it is necessary to remove wedges or sections of bone, but these are special situations and are not included under the ordinary "routine" rhinoplasty.

In some patients a thick or high deviation of the septum will prevent a clean or complete infracture. It may be necessary to cut the septal cartilage vertically or to fracture the cartilage and perpendicular plate of the ethmoid with a heavy scissors or septal forceps. This should be done with circumspection. Undue removal of septal cartilage or vigorous fracturing of the septum and ethmoid plate may result in a weakening of the nasal dorsum with subsequent depression.

After the nasal bones are properly infractured, the dorsum is palpated and inspected for any irregularities. A rasp for bony irregularity and a scissors for excess upper lateral cartilage are used to equalize the dorsum.

The fracture line of the lateral osteotomy should be as low as possible to allow a large lateral wall for infracture and to prevent a steplike deformity. The bones must be mobile from side to side and must be approximated in the midline. The fractures must be complete, obviating the need for clamps and splints to hold the bones together. The external splint is applied only for protection and to aid in preventing hematoma.

Although the root of the nose may not appear high before the infracture, it may become slightly elevated after the lateral walls are moved together and should be lowered by rasping or by shaving with an osteotome. Occasionally a slight depression of the bone at the fracture line occurs just below the radix, thereby placing the radix on a slightly higher level than the newly positioned lateral walls.

At this point it is mandatory to palpate the dorsum or to inspect it was a nasal speculum, because a small portion of septum may project above the nasal bones. A scissors, a Joseph right-angle knife, or a rasp may be used to lower the septum to the level of the infractured lateral walls.

The upper lateral cartilages are left attached to the septum if they were not cut when the hump was removed. They help to stabilize the septum and, to some degree, to prevent the nasal bones from slipping down after infracture. If they are intact, the intranasal packing may be placed against them, for they help in stabilizing the dorsum. If the hump is large, the upper laterals are almost always separated from the septum after the hump removal. If the nose is excessively long, it is necessary to free them to remove the excess. However, in many cases it is possible to leave some attachment to the septum, even if it is only mucoperichondrial.

The septum is again inspected for any deviation which may interfere with nasal respiration or with complete infracture of the bones. If the septum was previously exposed and partially removed or cut, it is again inspected for any interference with proper narrowing of the dorsum and for inadequate breathing space. Further removal or cutting of the septum may be executed at this time, and ridges or spurs may be shaved with a chisel or biting forceps or fractured into position.

Another feature of importance is the projection of the lower third of the cartilaginous border. Palpation of the dorsum may reveal an excess of septal and upper lateral cartilage at the lower third of the profile line. If present, further conservative incremental cartilaginous hump removal is accomplished by shave excision (see Fig. 2-21, *G*).

The septum is again inspected to see whether any further shortening is needed to help in elevating the tip. By waiting until this stage of the operation, the danger of overshortening the septum is avoided. The upper laterals are also inspected at this time; if any excess is present, it is also removed. It is surprising how little excess upper lateral cartilage is present. The author finds that if enough of the upper portion of the alar cartilage is removed, little of the upper lateral need be sacrificed. This results in a better appearance, aids in preventing scar formation, and protects the function of the internal nasal aperture.

If the nostril is wide at its alar base, it is necessary to excise a wedge of skin and fibrous tissue from this region. A variety of excisions may be used, depending on the type of ala, but the method most commonly employed is to remove a triangular wedge with the apex into the nostril and the base toward the cheek.

Suturing the septum to the columella is accomplished with 4–0 catgut. Two sutures are used on each side to unite the septal mucosa to the skin of the columella. The mucosa of the septum must be cut almost flush with the cartilage, so that the redundant mucosa will not thicken and scar and may later relax to allow a drop in the height of the tip. The sutures have no real effect on elevation of the nose; the nose should be in the desired position without tension on the suture. The alar incisions for reducing the width of the nostril base are sutured with 6–0 nylon on an atraumatic needle. The marginal (rim) incisions of the lower lateral cartilages are sutured with fine catgut.

Intranasal packing with petrolatum gauze, antibiotic-impregnated gauze, Gelfoam, or Telfa may be employed, depending on the amount of support needed internally. An external splint is applied after the nasal tip is strapped into position with one layer of paper tape. The type of external splint is immaterial. Dental compound, copper, brass, tin, aluminum, or plaster of Paris may be used. Fast-drying plaster of Paris immersed in hot saline will dry quickly and adhere quite satisfactorily with no external taping.

The packing and splint are removed on the fifth to seventh postoperative day, at which time further strapping with adhesive can be done to hold the nose in position for another 5 or 6 days (although this is seldom necessary).

Postoperative Care

The patient is placed in a semireclining (Fowler) position, and a soft diet is prescribed for the first day. A broad-spectrum antibiotic is used for about 5 days. The use of enzymes and cortisone preparations has been of little value in my experience. Depending on the individual, the ecchymosis usually subsides in about a week or less. Subconjunctival hemorrhage, if present, may persist for almost 3 weeks but is uncommon.

The patient is discharged from the hospital on the morning following surgery with specific instruction regarding sensible home activities.

Associated Deformities

If the columella is thick, the removal of dense connective tissue between the medial crura and the base of the columella and closure with a mattress suture will result in a narrowing.

A hanging columella is due to the excessive curvature and width of the medial crus. An incision is made along the anterior rim border of the medial crus on each side, the excess skin and cartilage of the medial crura are excised, and the defect is sutured.

A retracted columella is usually the result of a short or dislocated septum and may, in the case of a dislocation, be repaired by correction of the septum. However, it is usually necessary to insert a small section of septal cartilage into a pocket between and in front of the medial crura. An incision is made at the anterior rim border of the medial crus, a pocket is dissected, and an implant is inserted. The skin is then closed with fine nylon sutures.

The flat tip with a short columella is usually associated with a wide base and occasionally with a long nose. One method or a combination of methods may be used. The nose is elevated; the medial crura are elongated by cutting the lateral crura beyond the angle and rotating them upward; the fibroadipose tissue is removed at the columellar base, and the medial crura are entirely freed to allow their elevation; the alae are cut at their base to allow mobilization of the tip; and a columellar implant of sufficient height to project beyond the tip of the nose is inserted. The apex of the implant should be covered with a tapered section of cartilage so that it does not form a sharp point. In rare instances, it may be necessary to cut the columella in a V-shaped manner at its base and advance it as a V–Y flap.

The webbed lip or hanging septum is the result of a projecting spine of the maxilla, a long septum, and/or an excess of fibrous connective tissue in the columella. After the pathologic condition is corrected, a submerged suture will bring the tissues into position and obliterate the webbing.

Prominent Nasal Frontal Angle. If the radix nasi, or root of the nose, is high, a section of bone is rasped down or removed by wedging it out with an osteotome. In this latter maneuver one must be extremely careful not to engage the bone too deeply, or a much larger section will be dislodged than anticipated; instead, the osteotome is used in a shaving fashion. If this area is unusually high, obliterating the nasofrontal indentation, the hump and radix may be removed together. The cartilaginous portion of the hump is cut with a knife. A wide osteotome is then placed along the cut borders of the bone, and with a few taps of the mallet, the hump and high radix may be removed in one section.

THE SEPTUM IN RHINOPLASTY

The role of the septum in rhinoplasty has always been subject to debate. The difficulty arises because of a lack of definition; that is, the septal operation may be performed as an entity in itself, or it may be performed as a combined operation with a rhinoplasty. Septal resection without a rhinoplasty for radical removal of the septum found many advocates at the turn of the century. These views were propounded by such authorities as Killian, St. Clair Thomson, and Freer. In 1937, Peer expressed the opinion that radical removal may be necessary for certain types of deflection but emphasized the need for a section of cartilage in the anterior position to replace the septum for nasal support. Foman et al. in 1946, 1948, and 1951 described a similar method but incorporated the rhinoplastic approach of Joseph. The adherents of this method did not clearly define the limitations of this procedure vis-à-vis rhinoplasty, although they were adumbrated. These techniques apply primarily to the correction of the deviated-dislocated sep-

tum alone and are rarely indicated when septal repair is combined with a rhinoplasty except in the badly traumatized nose.

A more complex problem arises when external repair and septal deformity correction are combined. The radical removal of the septum performed with an extensive rhinoplasty will on occasion result in a depressed nose because of lack of septal support. The exception is the severely traumatized nose. In these cases the dorsum is depressed, and it is impossible to shift the septum without sacrifice of large sections of cartilage. It is then that a radical removal of the septum may be required, but dorsal implantation of a bone or cartilage graft is necessary to correct the depression.

To correct safely a deviated-dislocated septum in conjunction with a rhinoplastic correction in the developmental type of deformity, techniques advocating the shifting and reconstruction of the septal cartilage with minimal removal of septum are currently considered preferable to radical septal resection.

Deviated or Scoliotic Nose

Deviation of the entire nose involves both the bony and cartilaginous vaults; deviations of the lower half of the nose are mainly due to septal derangements accompanied by secondary effects on the cartilaginous vault.

Associated asymmetries and deformities of the upper lateral cartilage commonly accompany severe septal scoliosis. The septal and external deformities are corrected together, whenever feasible. Since the procedures are interdependent, a better evaluation of the problem is possible when they are done together, and the patient is saved considerable time and discomfort.

Correction of the cartilaginous component precedes management of the bony deformity to allow adequate space for readjustment and infracturing of the bony vault. Furthermore, seldom can an externally twisted nose be adequately rendered straight without concomitant septal realignment. The admonition "as goes the septum, so goes the nose" holds much truth.

For a better understanding of the pathologic changes and mechanics involved in correcting this type of nasal deformity, a review of the etiologic and anatomic factors is presented.

Etiologic and Anatomic Factors. At birth, the septum is almost completely cartilaginous with the exception of the vomer and the two premaxillas and their processes. The vomer develops bilaterally on each side of the cartilaginous nasal septum from a pair of ossification centers, which are present at the beginning of the third month of fetal life. The bilateral plates of the vomer unite from behind and grow forward at the expense of the imprisoned cartilage. Their development is completed at the age of 15. The bilateral origin of the vomer is evidenced in the infant by a deep groove between the two plates. The groove is somewhat flattened in adults.

Development of the premaxilla parallels that of the vomer until the child is 6 years old, when the premaxilla develops rapidly. The ethmoid bone begins to ossify during the first year of life, and this process is not complete until the end of the seventeenth year.

At birth, neither the palatine bones nor the superior maxillas rise into a crest for the support of the lower edge of the septum, but in the adult these bones have marked crests. The upward growth of the crests, along with the development of the premaxilla and vomer, combined with the downward growth of the septum from the ethmoid ossification centers and the downward expansion of the cranial cavity, may account for many deviations and dislocations of the septum. This disproportion of growth with pressure on the cartilaginous septum was emphasized by Mosher as a causative factor in septal deformities.

The vomer and premaxilla are enveloped by a periosteal covering that separates the bony portion of the septum from the cartilaginous septum, which in turn is enveloped in perichondrium. Microscopic studies of sections removed from the junction of bone and cartilage in the vomeroseptal–maxillary crest region reveal the perichondrial envelopment of the septal cartilage and its fusion with the periosteum of the bone below. The two opposing membranes form a smooth surface between bone and cartilage, especially at the junction of vomer, maxillary crest, and maxillary spine, where the groove of the vomer is usually shallow or flat. This region is therefore a weak point and a frequent site of dislocations on a traumatic basis. Furthermore, the bones themselves form a smooth surface. The lower end of the vomer is smooth and rests on the smooth concave surface of the maxillary crest, which in turn rests on the smooth concave surface of the nasal spine.

From observations at the operating table, in the majority of patients a dislocation was accompanied by a deviation of the vomer and maxillary crest and spine along with the septal cartilage. These findings were either developmental in origin, or the patient had a history of trauma before the age of 6 or 7. Trauma in early childhood is an important factor, as the maxillary crests and vomer are not completely ossified, and a slight shifting of these tissues may cause the crest and vomer, as they develop, to grow to the side. This will result in a flattening of the vomerine groove and the loss of its lip on the side of deviation. Some of these cases may possibly have their origin in birth trauma. The cases in which the septal cartilage was displaced from the vomer and maxillary crest were usually traumatic in origin, the injury occurring, in most instances, sometime after the child reached the age of 6 or 7. The complicated septal dislocation, accompanied by a buckling, twisting, and reduplication of cartilage and marked depression and deviation, invariably had a traumatic basis.

Some developmental factors in the etiology of the dislocated septum may be gathered from the embryonal description of nasopalatal relationship and the influence of palatal development on the floor of the septum. The formation of the premaxilla, the eruption of the permanent incisor teeth, the asymmetric development of the maxillary sinuses, thumb-sucking and tongue pressure habits with resultant shifting of the alveolar ridge, mouth breathing, and congenital deformities such as cleft lip and palate are some causative factors which may account for developmental disturbances. The eruption of the permanent incisor teeth and the effect this has on the septum were well described by Mosher, who felt that deformities of the septum were rather infrequent and rarely very marked in children before eruption of the second dentition. However, the disproportion in growth between the premaxilla, vomer, and ethmoid, with downward encroachment of the cranial cavity, is probably the dominant factor.

The Developmental Type. In the developmental type of septal deformity, the cartilaginous septum is dislocated and deflected, and there is similar deviation of the underlying bony septum (Fig. 2-23). The cartilage is separated from the bone by a smooth layer of perichondrium and periosteum. Because of this smooth, sliding surface between them, the freeing of the cartilage at its junction with underlying bone may be insufficient to prevent the septum from slipping back into the original position of dislocation. Moreover, the pull of the shortened mucosa on the side of the dislocation may gradually shift the cartilage on its smooth bed back to its dislocated position.

To prevent such recurrence, the cartilage should not be cut at its junction with the vomer and maxillary bone but should be shifted as one unit with the bony septum (Fig. 2-24). This is accomplished by completely fracturing the maxillary spine and crest and lower end of the vomer from the floor of the nose and shifting the entire lower end of the septum to the midline. Complete fracture through the bone prevents recurrence of the deformity, because the bone, unlike resilient cartilage, has no tendency to move after it has been fractured and set in position. Equally important is the fact that the fracture along the floor leaves the smooth, sliding perichondrial-periosteal surface undisturbed.

To ensure further the replacement of the septum in the midline and to prevent possible scar contracture or pull due to shortening of the mucosa, which results from shifting of the bone and cartilage to the midline, an incision is made in the mucous membrane along the floor of the nose and lateral to

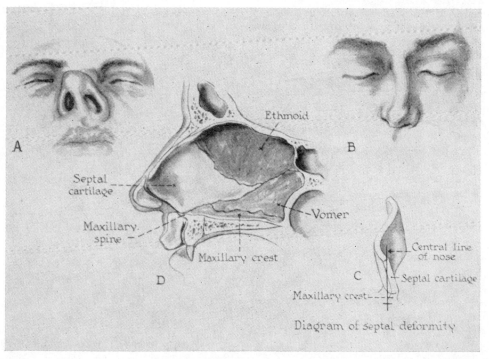

Fig. 2–23. Developmental type of septal deformity. *A,* Dislocation of septum into left nostril. *B,* Deviation of nasal tip to the right. *C,* Diagrammatic sketch of septal deformity revealing the underlying bony portion deflected along with the cartilaginous portion. Midline of nose externally indicated by solid vertical line. *D,* Lateral view of septum. (Becker, O. J.: Trans. Am. Acad. Ophthal. Otolaryng., 55:244, 1951.)

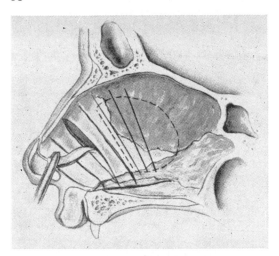

FIG. 2–24. Correction of developmental type of septal deformity. After unilateral elevation of mucoperichondrium, vertical incisions are made through the cartilage extending into the maxillary crest and vomer, which is then completely fractured through the base. A section of cartilage is removed vertically at the angle of deflection to break the spring. Posterior resection of cartilage, when indicated, is outlined by dotted line. Upper lateral cartilages are left intact at midline when the extent of the rhinoplasty permits this. (Becker, O. J.: Trans. Am. Acad. Ophthal. Otolaryng., 55:244, 1951.)

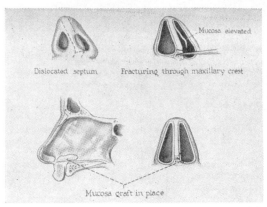

FIG. 2–25. Mucoperiosteum cut at the base of the nose to prevent recurrence of deformity by the pull of the shorter mucosa. Maxillary spine and crest and lower end of the vomer are completely fractured at the base. Scar contracture is prevented by a mucous membrane graft to cover the created defect. Smooth perichondrial-periosteal junction between bone and cartilage retains its original relationship. (Becker, O. J.: Trans. Am. Acad. Ophthal. Otolaryng., 55:244, 1951.)

the region of the fracture line. A free graft of mucous membrane or, better, a composite graft of mucosa and cartilage is placed over the raw area (Fig. 2-25). The graft takes rapidly, and by the sixth or seventh postoperative day the nasal floor is completely healed. Tissue for grafting may be obtained from the upper lateral cartilages where they are shortened (using the tissue as two grafts), or if the septum is shortened, the removed section of cartilage with attached cutaneous-mucosal surface on one side may be utilized as an alternative composite graft along the floor of the nose. If tissue is not available from either of these sources, a mucosal graft from the undersurface of the inferior turbinate of the untreated nostril or a graft of buccal mucosa may be used.

After the bony septum is fractured through completely, the septal cartilage should be cut vertically through its height, and when necessary narrow sections should be re-

moved at the bends in the cartilage. The vertical incisions are carried down into the bone to join the fracture at the base. This should be done without disturbing the perichondrium and mucosa on the opposite side. The perichondrial attachments of the opposite side are left intact, not so much to ensure the viability of the cartilage as to help prevent the anterior segment of cartilage from slipping back or down after it is cut. The perichondrial and mucosal attachment thus acts as an adherent plate to the cartilage. The mucosal attachment on the opposite side of the anterior dislocation is disturbed only when it is desirable to thin down thickened cartilage or a ridge, usually along the floor in the region of bone and cartilage approximation. The deflected posterior portion of the septum may be removed according to the indications.

The upper lateral cartilages, which often are an integral part of the septal deformity, should be freed from the septum. When the cartilages are twisted along with the septum, a readjustment may be necessary to avoid pulling by the shortened upper lateral cartilage, which may cause recurrence of the

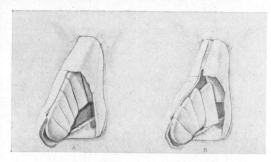

FIG. 2–26.   In the combined rhinoplasty and septal operation, when removal and cutting of the septal cartilage is indicated, extensive procedures on the dorsum may result in a depressed nose. If the upper lateral cartilages are detached from the septum in the midline or the bony arch of the nasal bones is broken, the septum will slip downward and backward resulting in a partial saddling. A lateral freeing of the upper laterals (rather than detachment in the midline) and mobilization of the nasal bones without breaking the arch will avoid this danger. If a large hump has been removed, it is safer to cut the septum and fracture it into position without the removal of any cartilage. More extensive septal correction may be done if the hump is small, thereby leaving most of the upper lateral cartilages and nasal bones intact in the midline. (Becker, O. J.: Trans. Am. Acad. Ophthal. Otolaryng., *60*:522, 1956.)

deformity and prevent complete straightening of the twisted dorsum. This may be accomplished by detaching the cartilages from the septum, but this is not advisable because the upper lateral cartilages are intimately bound to the septum and function as lateral stabilizing extensions of the septum (Fig. 2-26). These cartilages, together with the septal cartilage, maintain the stability and form of the cartilaginous dorsum. In many cases, depending on the pathologic condition of the septum and the extent of the rhinoplasty, it is not necessary to free the upper lateral cartilages, since shifting of the septum will readjust their position. In other cases, infracture of the nasal and maxillary bones plus shifting of the septum will readjust the position of the upper lateral cartilages. In still others, partial division of the upper lateral cartilages from the septum will take care of the matter. If complete division

of one or both cartilages from their dorsal attachment to the septum is necessary, the underlying mucosa and perichondrium should be left *intact* and attached to the septum to maintain some fixation or continuity between upper lateral and septal cartilages. This is referred to as central freeing of the upper lateral cartilages. After the nose has been packed and splinted, fibrous adhesions will form a fixation between the cartilages.

Since it is highly advisable not to detach the upper lateral cartilages from the septum, a lateral freeing procedure can be used to mobilize them. This consists of freeing the lateral borders of the upper lateral cartilages from the soft tissue and the maxillary bone but not from the undersurface of the nasal bone, so that the central septal attachment remains. This will prevent the septal cartilage from slipping backward after it is cut vertically, even if the septum is resected behind the thoroughly freed and cross-cut anterior segment of septal cartilage.

Absorbable sutures approximating the septum to the columella are inserted without tension. The cartilage of the septum should not be sewn into a pocket between the two medial crura, for the natural contour of the membranous septum and columella may be destroyed, resulting in an unnatural firmness of the nasal tip. Horizontal mattress transseptal sutures are placed at intervals throughout the repositioned cartilaginous septum to stabilize the residual cartilage segments and to adapt firmly the mucoperichondrial flap(s) to the septum. Dead space is thereby diminished, hematoma is avoided, and nasal packing and/or splints may be kept to a minimum. Telfa gauze strips are placed in each nasal cavity and removed in 24 to 48 hours. Seldom are paraseptal splints required.

The Traumatic Type. The septal deformities encountered after trauma may be divided into three groups: (1) the lateral type, which usually results from a lateral fracture of the nose with displacement of the septum from the vomerine groove and maxillary crest; (2) the depressed type, following a crushing frontal fracture and resulting in a bizarre septal configuration of buckling, twisting, reduplication, and fibrosis; and (3) the laterofrontal type, which

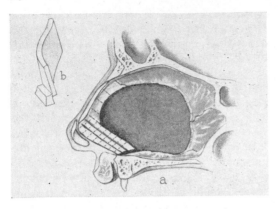

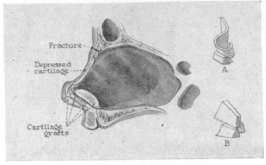

FIG. 2–27. Lateral traumatic deformity with dislocation of cartilaginous septum from bony septum (*b*). Correction by vertical cuts through anteriorly dislocated septum, and removal of a portion of bone and cartilage from base of septum to allow placement of septum in the midline (*a*). In some cases, the septum can be replaced on the vomer and maxillary crest after cutting of its attachments to the bone, removal of posterior deflected portion, and vertical cuts through remaining subdorsal septum. (Becker, O. J.: Trans. Am. Acad. Ophthal. Otolaryng., *55*:244, 1951.)

FIG. 2–28. Depressed traumatic deformity of septum with buckling, twisting, and reduplication of septum (*A* and *B*). Septum completely removed, followed by columellar grafts and a section of cartilage replaced behind the columella. These are inserted to prevent retraction of columella. A graft of bone or cartilage is placed over the dorsum to correct the depression. (Becker, O. J.: Trans. Am. Acad. Ophthal. Otolaryng., *55*:244, 1951.)

combines the first two types but more often is an accentuation of the lateral type.

The lateral type of traumatic septal deformity is corrected by methods similar to those used in treating the developmental type of deformity (Fig. 2-27). However, in this type the cartilage is shifted from the vomer and maxillary crest, in contradistinction to the complete shift of bony and cartilaginous septum found in the developmental deformity. It is therefore necessary not only to use the methods outlined for the developmental type of deformities but also to replace the septal cartilage on the vomerine groove. After the maxillary crest and vomer are fractured, the cartilage is cut at its base; the vomerine groove is cleansed of scar and periosteal tissue, and the cartilage is replaced. This may necessitate freeing or cutting the mucosa on the opposite side of the septum. In other cases, the added resection of an angulated strip of cartilage and bone at the juncture of vomer and septal cartilage may be necessary to allow placement of the septum in the midline.

The depressed type of traumatic septal deformity poses a problem different from that of developmental and lateral traumatic deformities. In most cases, it is impossible to shift the septum back into position by the foregoing procedures, and wide resection of the crushed septum is necessary (Fig. 2-28).

Whenever a wide or thorough resection is required, the stability of the nasal dorsum is endangered. However, when complete resection is necessary, the stability of the dorsum usually is not a problem, since the nose is already depressed. The procedure resolves itself into refracture of the nasal bones; thorough resection of the septum, including the dislocated lower portion; and implantation of a graft to the nasal dorsum and to the (usually) retracted columella. When the nose is both twisted and depressed, the upper lateral cartilages should not be freed from their attachment to the septum, since refracture of the nasal bones and complete resection of the septum will usually shift their position to the midline. When complete straightening does not result from refracture, either central freeing with mucoperichondrial attachments to the septum or lateral freeing of the upper lateral cartilages will adjust their position.

The laterofrontal type of traumatic deformity results in a marked twist of the lower end of the septum and nasal dorsum, but the dorsum is not especially depressed (Fig. 2-29). In this type of repair, it may be necessary to remove completely the lower end of the septum. The stability of the dorsum becomes important in such cases. Since the nasal dorsum is in a relatively good position, it is almost always necessary to leave the upper lateral cartilages attached to the septum in order to protect the projection of the nose. Resection of the dislocated anterior septum, bilateral osteotomy of the frontal processes of the

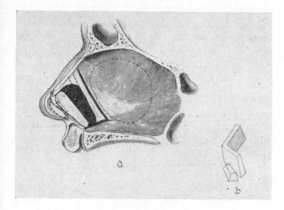

FIG. 2–29. Laterofrontal traumatic deformity with marked angulation of cartilage and displacement from underlying bony septum (*b*). This deformity may often be corrected by the procedure outlined under lateral traumatic type. In many cases, the anterior portion of septum is removed, followed by replacement of a section of cartilage (*a*). The posterior portion is cut, a vertical strip is removed at angle of deflection, and the base is fractured into position. A beam of cartilage is left under the dorsum to prevent sagging of the tip. This may be vertically cut (indicated by dotted line) to break the spring. A columellar graft is inserted to prevent retraction of the columella (indicated by dotted area in columella). In occasional cases, it may be necessary to remove the entire anterior segment, but this may necessitate correction of the dorsum for a saddle; however, this depends on the extent of the rhinoplasty, the structure of the upper and lower lateral cartilages, and whether it is necessary to free the upper lateral cartilages from the septum. (Becker, O. J.: Trans. Am. Acad. Ophthal. Otolaryng., *55*:244, 1951.)

maxilla, and lateral freeing of the upper lateral cartilages will in most cases correct the deviation and dislocation of the septum and straighten the dorsum.

During correction of the septum, it is highly advisable to maintain the support of the dorsum by leaving a narrow strip of subdorsal cartilage attached to the undersurface of the upper lateral cartilages. This strip or beam should extend to the extreme lower border of the septum to prevent sagging of the dorsum, particularly in the area which is dependent on the septum for maintenance of the dorsal projection. This beam should be cut vertically if indicated, a section of cartilage removed at the posterior angle of deflection, and the base fractured in order to shift the septum to the midline. It is possible in some cases to remove the lower portion of this cartilaginous beam and still maintain the profile, but only when the upper lateral cartilages are long, extending to the tip of the septum, and when the lower lateral cartilages are well developed and either firmly bound to the upper lateral cartilages or large enough to override the central portion of the upper lateral cartilages. Usually these conditions are lacking; instead, an area of septum about 0.75 cm long is devoid of upper lateral cartilages, and the fibrous union of lower to upper lateral cartilage in this region is often too weak to prevent a depression just superior to the tip of the nose. Furthermore, if unusually firm fibrous attachments and overlapping upper and lower cartilages hold the nose in position without any septal support, there is always the risk that some slight trauma to the nose may cause a depression at a later date. The upper lateral cartilages alone cannot withstand much trauma without the additional reserve support of the septum. However, a narrow beam of septal cartilage, extending beyond and under the upper lateral cartilages and continuous posteriorly with the ethmoid plate and vomer, will furnish adequate reserve support to resist trauma. A large section or smaller segments of cartilage used to replace the completely resected septum will not furnish the stability and support that this beam of cartilage provides. However, even when this beam is preserved, it is necessary to replace a section of cartilage just behind and into the columella, not to serve as a support but to prevent retraction of the columella.

Obviously, only a limited rhinoplasty can be combined with this type of septal correction. Many cases of this type, however, can be adequately corrected by the methods outlined under the lateral type of deformity, thereby allowing a more extensive rhinoplastic correction. This is especially true in a long nose deformity which requires shortening of the lower end of the septum.

General Considerations. The methods outlined may also be used to good advantage in cases repaired without a rhinoplastic correction but should be accomplished through the use of the rhinoplastic approach. This implies using incisions in both limina vestibuli, freeing the skin from the overlying lower half of the nasal dorsum, and in some cases transfixing the septum from the columella. With this maneuver, better exposure of the septum is obtained, and if necessary, sections of the upper lateral cartilages may be freed and trimmed. Complete transfixion incisions are generally necessary when caudal septal deflection is present.

All septal corrections are accomplished through the original transfixion incision, thus eliminating any secondary incisions inside the nose which may possibly cause scar formation. However, if it is unnecessary to elevate the nasal tip, a complete transfixion incision may not be needed. Instead, an incision on one side of the free septal border is made, i.e., on the side of the dislocation, thereby allowing a complete and continuous attachment of the mucosa of the opposite side down to the columella. In many cases a one-half or three-fourths transfixion may be all that is necessary. The latter is advantageous in some cases, as it allows a firmer attachment of the membranous and cartilaginous septum of the columella.

After administration of 5% cocaine surface anesthesia, a 1% solution of Xylocaine hydrochloride containing 1:100,000 epinephrine hydrochloride is infiltrated under the septal mucosa and perichondrium for better anesthesia, to provide hemostasis, and to facilitate dissection.

When the septum is deviated without an anterior displacement and without causing an external deviation of the nasal dorsum, a submucous resection is accomplished prior to beginning the rhinoplasty. The mucoperichondrial flap is elevated on the side of the deviation through the rhinoplastic transfixion incision. The septal resection may be necessary to aid in the narrowing of the nasal bridge and/or to correct any nasal obstruction. A complete submucous resection or excessive removal of the septum is rarely indicated.

Only the part which is deflected should be removed. This removal may be accomplished after the perichondrium of the posterior portion of the septum on the opposite side is elevated. Repositioning and reconstruction are always preferable to resection. Often the septum is straightened sufficiently merely by vertical incisions and cross cuts through the cartilage without elevation of the perichondrium on the opposite side or removal of any cartilage. Occasionally, a few vertical strips of cartilage are removed to break the spring. Transseptal sutures, irregularly positioned, maintain the new relationship and midline orientation of the remaining cartilage.

It may be necessary to remove a thick septal cartilage at its junction with the ethmoid plate to aid infracture of the nasal bones and to narrow the bridge. This is a dangerous area because it helps to maintain the nasal bones at the juncture of the upper lateral cartilages. A depression of the nasal bones will not follow this maneuver provided the nasal bones are not outfractured or separated from each other by chiseling through the junction of the two nasal bones. The bones may be shifted to the midline as one unit by infracturing them without disturbing the attachments of the septum to the frontal spine and the undersurface of the nasal bone. To mobilize the bony bridge completely without separation of the nasal bones at the midline and without outfracture, it may be necessary to fracture the bones completely by chiseling through the nasal frontal region, either through the original osteotomy incision or by the use of a small external incision at the lateral side of the nasion. If it is necessary to separate the nasal bones or to remove a wedge from the bony radix, the removal of a large section of septum in this region should not be attempted; instead, a fracture of the septum should be accomplished with an Ashe septal forceps.

Some instances of anterior dislocation of a long nose may be corrected simply by shortening the septum and lower ends of the upper lateral cartilages. Since removal of an anterior segment of septal cartilage is necessary for the correction of nasal length, it may also be sufficient to correct the dislocation. However, it is usually necessary to fracture the maxillary crest behind the area which has been removed in the shortening procedure. Any further posterior deviation of the septum is corrected by removing or cross-cutting the deviated cartilage and bone.

Bony Vault. Bilateral freeing or infracture of the bony arch is usually sufficient to realign the nasal bones after the cartilaginous vault has been corrected. A hump, if present, is removed in an unequal manner, i.e., at an angle, to equalize the length of the lateral nasal walls; a larger section of the bony hump is removed from the long or wide side of the deviation. After infracture, they will meet in the midline. In cases with or without a hump, after infracture (and sometimes after the separation of the nasal bones in the midline) a section of the longer side of bone may project above the dorsum. This is a result of the unequal length of the lateral wall and necessitates removal of the excess with a heavy bone-biting scissors or rongeur. In other instances, a double fracture line ("double osteotomy") at the base of the long side will allow a section of the lateral nasal wall to underride itself. Only rarely is removal of a triangular section of bone from the long side indicated. In rare instances, it may be necessary to comminute the bones for proper alignment. Comminution is preferable, however, to incomplete or greenstick osteotomy fractures, which commonly result in postoperative nasal deviation.

In summary, the correction of the twisted or deviated nose is a complex procedure, consisting of interrelated, interdependent surgical maneuvers. One-stage reconstruction of the septum and external nose is recommended for those who study and understand the pathophysiology and dynamics involved.

Depressed or Saddle Nose

As a result of trauma, septal infection (such as abscess, syphilis, Hansen's disease, or tuberculosis), extensive resection of the septum, or congenital deformities, the entire length or limited areas of the dorsum of the nose may become depressed.

To restore the level of the depressed profile line and the normal nasal contour requires the use of a filling substance. Bone and cartilage are the transplants most commonly employed for this purpose; many foreign body substitutes have been advocated from time to time, only to be eventually discarded. However, the results with new synthetic polymers have been favorable and encouraging but have yet to be shown superior to autogenous tissue for use in reconstruction.

Use of homogenous ("bank") bone and cartilage is advantageous in that an operation to obtain them is unnecessary, but the possibility of absorption, shrinkage, and extrusion and the lack of resistance to infection far outweigh the risk or discomfort entailed in the procurement of fresh autogenous material.

Saddle or depressed nasal deformities (without the loss of skin covering) may be classified into three types:

1. Relative saddle nose, which is not truly a saddle nose, appears as such because of an unusually high projecting tip. A high bony hump may also give the appearance of a relatively depressed lower vault deformity.
2. Partial saddle nose refers to a deformity which may be corrected by shifting and manipulating surrounding nasal tissues or by using a partial or small implant over the dorsum.
3. True saddle nose refers to a deformity requiring a complete dorsal implant for its correction.

The relative saddle nose presents a normal profile line, but the dorsum appears depressed because of the prominence of the nasal tip and/or a high bony hump. The correction is accomplished by reducing the height and the bulk of the lower lateral cartilages or by removal of the hump.

Partial saddle nose may be the result of trauma to the lower portion of the nose with depression and dislocation of the cartilaginous structure, leaving the bony portion intact. This results in a supratip depression. Quite frequently, replacement of the septum in the midline will spontaneously correct the defect. However, if the supratip depression results from overzealous removal of the septum or septal abscess, this method is not feasible. Occasionally the nasal bone projection may be removed to the level of the depression and thereby result in a straight dorsum. The excess bony hump may be positioned in the supratip area, thereby restoring satisfactory profile without the need for distant tissue grafts. If the nose is long, elevation of the tip will raise the alar cartilages into a position overriding the depression, thereby obliterating it. A combined approach utilizing these two factors is usually employed to further reinforce the depression. If elevation of the tip is not indicated, the upper half of the alar cartilage may be cut parallel to the upper lateral cartilages and rotated upward after being dissected from the vestibular skin. This is executed in a hinged fashion with the pivot at the medial attachment. A catgut suture unites the two sections of alar cartilage (Kazanjian). Another method is to free the upper lateral cartilages from their septal attachments and either spontaneously superimpose them or suture them together over the dorsum to aid in building out the depression. The latter two methods give somewhat unpredictable results and are not recommended as primary methods of reconstruction.

The use of small grafts of septal, alar, or ear cartilage is usually not advisable, since they do not maintain a stable position and often cause irregularities of the dorsum. If the defect cannot be corrected by superimposing and rotating the patient's own tissues over the defect, it is advisable to use a complete dorsal transplant; this will entail the sacrifice of a part of the bony dorsum for the preparation of a proper bed.

True saddle-nose deformity requires an implant of proper shape and dimension to restore the profile line. The implant is modeled either from a mold prepared on a plaster cast of the patient's face or directly on or in the nose at the operating table with a rotating burr. The latter method is more accurate, for the nose is already prepared to receive the implant and definite measurements can be made directly. Sterile pink base plate wax and paraffin compound which is softened in warm water may be shaped and inserted into the nose to obtain accurate dimensions, which may then be applied to modeling the graft.

Local anesthesia or general endotracheal anesthesia is used. The bone graft is procured from the patient's iliac crest with small chisels and rotating saws. Careful atraumatic technique will diminish postoperative discomfort. An incision is made along the lower rim of the alar cartilage, followed by separation of the two medial crura from each other and from the overlying skin. The midline of the dorsum is then undermined with a slightly curved blunt scissors, and the periosteum of the nasal bones is elevated to the glabella, fashioning a pocket to receive the implant. The pocket should be small enough to maintain stabilization of the implant but large enough to avoid undue pressure from the graft on the overlying thin skin. The thickest possible skin-subcutaneous tissue flap should be elevated. The advantage of the unilateral complete alar incision is that one continuous enclosed pocket is formed from the glabella down to the nasal spine of the max-

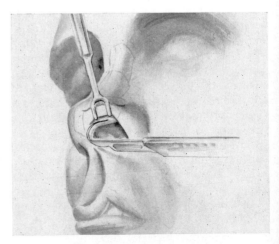

FIG. 2–30. An incision is made along the lower rim of the alar cartilage.

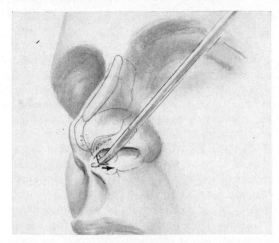

FIG. 2–31. The medial crura are separated from each other.

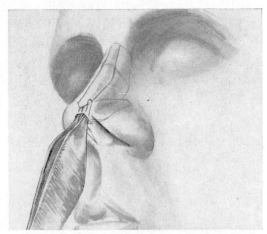

FIG. 2–34. The graft is inserted.

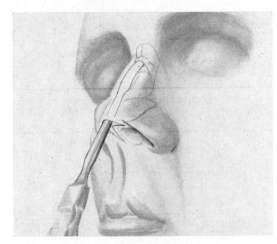

FIG. 2–32. The periosteum is elevated.

illa without an opening into the nasal fossae. Moreover, there will be no external scar. Access to the lower lateral cartilages, which frequently require modeling, may be accomplished through this approach by utilizing a similar incision on the opposite side. The lower lateral cartilages may then be modeled in conjunction with the placement of the dorsal implant (Figs. 2-30 to 2-34).

If a columellar graft is necessary, it may be inserted into position under direct vision (Figs. 2-35 to 2-37).

The graft is shaped to fit the concavity of the nose and is placed on bone, denuded of periosteum, that has been roughened and stimulated by rasping. If the dorsum of the

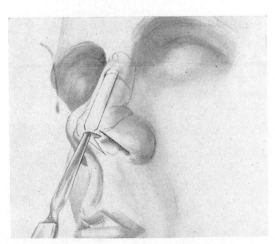

FIG. 2–33. A rasp is inserted.

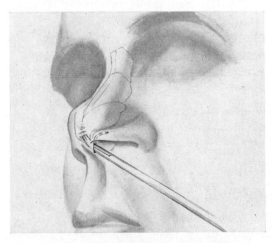

FIG. 2–35. A pocket is created down to the nasal spine.

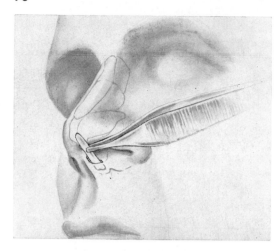

FIG. 2–36.   The graft is inserted.

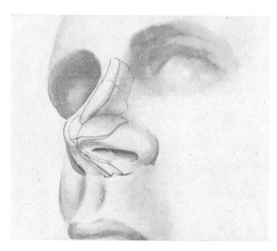

FIG. 2–37.   Both dorsal and columellar grafts
are in place.

nose presents irregularities or excessive height in any segment, it is smoothed and equalized by the use of rasps, bone-biting forceps, scissors, or saws to create a smooth bed for the reception and placement of the implant. It is advantageous to chisel a small niche in the glabella to act as a firm contact and recess for the graft.

The foregoing procedures may be difficult to perform through the alar cartilage incision. It is then advisable to use the usual intercartilaginous incisions with a partial transfixion of the septum. After the dorsal bed is prepared by rasping, a lateral osteotomy in the usual manner may be accom-

plished if the nasal bridge requires narrowing. The bone graft is then inserted and placed in the midline. The incisions between upper and lower lateral cartilages are sealed with fine catgut sutures on each side.

An alternative method is illustrated in Figures 2-38 to 2-40. In this method a midline incision is made in the columellar skin, and through this access is gained to the nasal dorsum, where a pocket is created as illustrated. A properly shaped implant is then inserted and the skin incision closed by fine sutures.

A single dorsal implant is usually all that is needed if it firmly adheres to the nasal bones. It will maintain adequate tip support

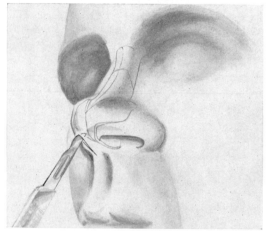

FIG. 2–38.   The midline columellar incision.

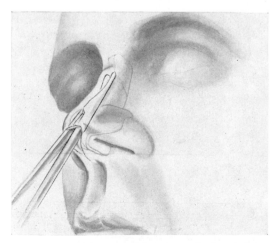

FIG. 2–39.   The overlying tissue is freed from
the cartilage and bone.

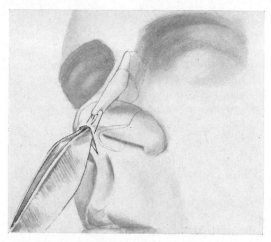

FIG. 2–40. The graft is inserted.

by acting on the cantilever principle. If this gives inadequate tip support, however, a septal cartilage or bone implant is inserted as a prop under the dorsal implant. The use of a prop or post under the dorsal implant is rarely indicated. If there is insufficient nasal tip projection, modeling of the lower lateral cartilages will usually correct this. The lower lateral cartilages are exposed and then sectioned just lateral to the junction of the medial and the lateral crura. The area between the two medial crura is cleansed of connective tissue, and the cartilages are brought together with fine catgut sutures. An alternative method employs an L-shaped graft as one solid block; it has the disadvantage of resulting in an unusually firm tip, however, and its use is therefore not advised. Furthermore, bone inserted into the columella has a tendency to absorb.

Composite Skin-Cartilage Grafts. In saddle noses in which airway collapse as well as profile depression is present, auricular skin-cartilage composite autografts present an alternative method of repair. Particularly useful in children, the auricular composite graft restores both internal epithelial lining and external reconstruction to the collapsed and foreshortened nose. Total nasal lengthening is possible; furthermore, composite grafts have been shown to grow along with the rest of the nasal structure (Dingman and Walters).

The nose and ear donor sites are prepared with sterile solutions. An intranasal intercar-

tilaginous incision is accomplished, and the soft tissue is elevated over the depressed area. The incision and elevated area are kept to a minimum to allow for later complete closure. Transfixion incisions are avoided.

An outline is created on the postauricular skin similar to the size of graft needed. A composite graft of skin and cavum conchae cartilage is then removed, leaving the anterior cavum conchae skin undisturbed. The postauricular incision may now be closed primarily or sewn onto a small defect created in the postauricular mastoid area. Neither closure, properly performed, should distort the appearance of the auricle.

The cartilage is now trimmed to the exact size required, two islands of skin being left attached to cartilage, sitting side by side. This fashions a composite skin-cartilage graft in "butterfly" design. An incomplete incision into the cartilage between the two islands of skin weakens the cartilaginous spring, creating a hinge effect. The nasal defect now receives the graft through the intercartilaginous incisions, with the islands of skin (epithelial surface down) sewn to the upper and lower edges of the mucous membrane at the intercartilaginous incision site. Properly executed, this "butterfly" composite graft lends excellent new support to the lower half of the nose, restores lost or scarred epithelial lining internally, and effaces the saddle nose. Its use in children, in whom growth potential must be considered, has been particularly gratifying.

If desired and necessary, a bony or cartilaginous columellar strut may be utilized to aid in distal tip support, when cartilaginous tip collapse is near-complete.

REFERENCES

Anderson, J. R.: New Approach to Rhinoplasty. Arch. Otolaryng., 93:284, 1971.
Becker, O. J.: Problems of the Septum in Rhinoplasty Surgery. Arch. Otolaryng., 53:622, 1951.
Becker, O. J.: The Routine Corrective Rhinoplasty Operation. Trans Am. Acad. Ophthal. Otolaryng., 68:830, 1964.
Bloom, S. M.: The Problem of Implants in Rhinoplasty, Including Technique of Obtaining Iliac Crest Grafts. Arch. Otolaryng., 71:778, 1960.

Bloom, S. M.: Rhinoplasty in Adolescence, Arch. Otolaryng., *92*:66, 1970.

Bloom, S. M.: Implants and Grafts in Nasal Reconstruction. *In* Conley, J., and Dickinson, J. (Eds.): *Plastic and Reconstructive Surgery of the Face and Neck: Proceedings of the First International Symposium, New York.* Stuttgart, Georg Thieme Verlag, 1971, pp. 156-59.

Book, H. E.: Psychiatric Assessment for Rhinoplasty. Arch. Otolaryng., *94*:851, 1971.

Cinelli, J. A.: Surgical Formulae for Common Nasal Tip Problems. Eye, Ear, Nose and Throat Monthly, *44*:99–102 (May), 1965; *44*:96–103 (June), 1965.

Converse, J. M.: Deviated Nose—Panel Discussion. Trans. Am. Acad. Ophthal. Otolaryng., *58*:741, 1954.

Converse, J. M. (Ed.): *Reconstructive Plastic Surgery.* Vols. 1–3. Philadelphia, W. B. Saunders Co., 1964.

Denecke, H. J., and Meyer, R.: *Plastic Surgery of the Head and Neck: Corrective and Reconstructive Rhinoplasty.* New York, Springer-Verlag, 1967.

Dingman, R., and Walters, C.: Use of Composite Ear Grafts in Correction of the Short Nose. Plast. Reconstr. Surg., *43*:117, 1969.

Farrior, R. T.: The Problems of the Unilateral Cleft Lip Nose. Laryngoscope, *72*:289, 1962.

Farrior, R. T.: Synthetics in Head and Neck Surgery. Arch. Ophthalmol., *84*:82, 1966a.

Farrior, R. T.: Implant Material and Restoration of Facial Contour. Laryngoscope, *76*:934, 1966b.

Farrior, R. T.: Corrective Surgery of the Nasal Framework. J. Florida Med. Assoc., *45*:276, 1968.

Farrior, R. T.: Septorhinoplasty in Children. Otolaryngologic Clinics of N.H. Pediatr. Otolaryng., *3*:345, 1970.

Fomon, S., Gilbert, J. G., Silver, A. G., and Syracuse, U. R.: Plastic Repair of the Obstructing Nasal Septum. Arch. Otolaryng., *47*:7, 1948.

Fomon, S., Goldman, I. B., Neivert, H., and Schattner, A.: Management of Deformities of the Lower Cartilaginous Vault. Arch. Otolaryng., *54*:467, 1951.

Fomon, S., Syracuse, U. R., Bolotow, N., and Pullen, M.: Plastic Repair of the Defective Nasal Septum. Arch. Otolaryng., *44*: 141, 1946.

Frye, H.: Interlocked Stresses of Cartilage. Br. J. Plast. Surg., *19*:276, 1966.

Frye, H.: Cartilage and Cartilage Grafts—Basic Properties of Tissue and Its Components Responsible for Them. Plast. Reconstr. Surg., *40*:426, 1967a.

Frye, H.: Importance of Septal Cartilage in Nasal Trauma. Br. J. Plast. Surg., *20*:392, 1967b.

Frye, H.: Nasal Skeletal Trauma and the Interlocked Stress of the Septal Cartilage. Br. J. Plast. Surg., *20*:146, 1967c.

Gilbert, J. C., and Segal, S.: Growth of the Nose and the Septorhinoplastic Problems in Youth. Arch. Otolaryng., *68*:673, 1958.

Goldman, I. B.: Analysis of Osseous Complications in Rhinoplasty. Eye, Ear, Nose and Throat Monthly, *42*:78, 1963a.

Goldman, I. B.: Nasal Plastic Surgery—Late Results. Eye, Ear, Nose and Throat Monthly, *42*:88, 1963b.

Goldman, I. B.: Nasal Tip Correction with Special Reference to the Medial Crura. Trans. Am. Acad. Ophthal. Otolaryng., *68*:854, 1964.

Goldman, I. B.: Rhinoplastic Sequelae Causing Nasal Obstruction. Arch. Otolaryng., *83*:151, 1966.

Hilger, J.: Internal Lateral Osteotomy in Rhinoplasty. Arch. Otolaryng., *88*:211, 1968.

Holmes, E. M.: Restoration of Nasal Contour Lost Through Deficient Septal Cartilage. Trans. Am. Acad. Ophthal. Otolaryng., *68*:874, 1964.

Huffman, W. C., and Lierle, D.: The Deviated Nose. Ann. Otol. Rhinol. Laryngol., *63*:62, 1954.

Huffman, W. C., and Lierle, D.: Reduction of the Prominent Nasofrontal Angle. Trans. Am. Acad. Ophthal. Otolaryng., *68*:838, 1964.

Janeke, J. B.: Studies on the Support of the Nasal Tip. Arch. Otolaryng., *93*:458, 1971.

Marquit, B.: Radiated Homogenous Cartilage in Rhinoplasty. Arch. Otolaryng., *85*:100, 1967.

Millard, D. R.: Adjuncts in Augmentation Mentoplasty and Corrective Rhinoplasty. Plast. Reconstr. Surg., *36*:48, 1965.

Parkes, M. L., and Brennan, H. G.: High Septal Transfixion to Shorten the Nose. Plast. Reconstr. Surg., *45*:487, 1970.

Peer, L. A.: An Operation to Repair Lateral Displacement of the Lower Border of the Septal Cartilage. Arch. Otolaryng., *25*:475, 1937.

Rees, T. D., *et al.*: Secondary Rhinoplasty. Plast. Reconstr. Surg., *46*:332, 1970.

Roe, J.: The Deformity Termed "Plug Nose" and Its Correction by a Simple Operation. Plast. Reconstr. Surg., *45*:78, 1970.

Rubin, F. F.: Permanent Change in Shape of Cartilage by Morselization. Arch. Otolaryng., *89*:602, 1969.

Safian, J.: Deceptive Concepts in Rhinoplasty. Plast. Reconstr. Surg., *18*:127, 1956.

Schutz, R. D.: *Facial Injuries*. Chicago, Year Book Medical Publishers, 1971.

Smith, H. W.: Septal Bone Grafts—Correction of Saddle Nose. Arch. Otolaryng., *92*:230, 1970.

Smith, T. W.: The Selection of Patients for Rhinoplasty. Arch. Otolaryng. *94*:56, 1971.

Stewart, M.: Psychological Problems of Patients Requesting Rhinoplasty. Trans. Am. Acad. Ophthal. Otolaryng., *68*:881, 1964.

Tardy, M. E.: Nasal Septal Reconstruction: Contemporary Techniques. Laryngoscope (in press).

Tardy, M. E.: Rhinoplasty Tip Ptosis: Etiology and Prevention. Laryngoscope, *83*:923, 1973.

Unger, M.: Architectural Design of the Nasal Septum. Laryngoscope, *75*:322, 1965.

Walter, C.: Composite Grafts in Nasal Surgery. Arch. Otolaryng., *90*:622, 1969.

Wright, W. K.: Lateral Osteotomy in Rhinoplasty. Arch. Otolaryng., *78*:680, 1963.

Wright, W. K.: Study on Hump Removal in Rhinoplasty. Laryngoscope, *77*:508, 1967.

Wright, W. K.: General Principles of Nasal Septum Reconstruction. Trans. Am. Acad. Ophthal. Otolaryng., *73*:252, 1969.

Chapter 3
Surgical Correction of Obstructive Lesions of the Septum

Irregularities of the nasal septum may be related to a nasal cosmetic problem (see Rhinoplasty) or cause obstruction to the nasal airway. In either case an indication for surgical correction may be present. The cause, other than obvious trauma to the nose, is unknown. Deviations are common in Caucasians but uncommon in the more primitive races. Men are more frequently affected than women, and the deviations become clinically manifest during adult life rather than in childhood. They are frequently associated with the high or "Gothic" arch of the bony palate, although the reverse may be true. It seems likely that the descent of the bony palate might push the cartilaginous palate into buckles or deviations. Some of the deviations are of no clinical importance, as illustrated in Figure 3–1.

It is important to remember that the airway proceeds from the anterior naris posteriorly in a high parabola just under the nasal bones (see Physiology of the Nose). Obstructions in this area are of more importance to a free airway than those located more inferiorly. Deviations that force the anterior end of the middle turbinate against the lateral nasal wall may prevent easy drainage from the anterior group of sinuses. At times a deviation just posterior to the naris presents a prominence that is kept constantly dry and crusted by the inspired air, the crusts in turn leading to a raw, bleeding surface.

The technique given below is that of the "classic" submucous resection of the nasal septum.

SUBMUCOUS RESECTION OF THE NASAL SEPTUM

Position of the Patient

The patient may be placed in either the sitting or reclining position, depending on the operator's preference.

Anesthesia

Either local or general anesthesia may be used. The former is attended by less bleeding and is preferred.

After the face, nose, and nasal vestibules are cleansed, cotton pledgets wound on thin metal applicators and saturated with the anesthetic solution are placed in each of three positions: (a) high in the superior meatus so as to anesthetize the anterior ethmoidal nerves (see Fig. 1-10); (b) at the posterior end of the middle turbinates opposite the sphenopalatine ganglion; and (c) just within and on the floor of the anterior nares to anesthetize the nerves issuing from the incisive canal. In addition, the posterior end of the columella and the line of incision along the caudal septal margin should be infiltrated with 1% procaine or other injectable anesthetic.

Some surgeons prefer to cover the entire septal mucous membrane with cotton strips

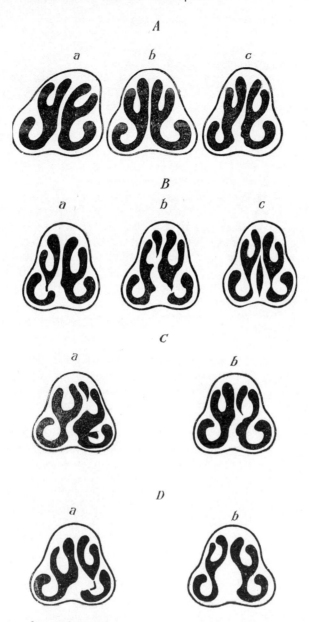

Fig. 3–1. *A*, Types of nonobstructive septa: *a*, deviated from the median line; *b*, normal straight septum in the median line; *c*, deviation of the lower portion of the septum with a concavity in the left nasal chamber but with compensatory hypertrophy of the left inferior turbinate.

B, Types of obstructive septa: *a*, ridge pressing against the inferior turbinate; *b*, ridge pressing against the left inferior turbinate and a convexity higher up on the right side obstructing the olfactory fissure on that side; *c*, a split septum causing double obstructive convexity of the septum.

C, *a*, An S-shaped septum causing obstruction in the inferior portion of the nasal chamber on the right side and the superior portion of the chamber on the left side; *b*, a high, angular deviation of the septum causing obstruction of the olfactory fissure of the left side.

D, *a*, Marked deviation of the septum along the crest, the vomer wedged firmly against the left inferior turbinate; *b*, abscess or hematoma of the septum obstructing both nasal chambers.

saturated with the topical anesthetic solution (e.g., 4% cocaine or 2% tetracaine). This method is satisfactory but entails the use of larger amounts of anesthetic solution.

The Incision

The choice of the location of the incisions should depend upon the character and location of the septal deviation. If it extends into the vestibule of the nose, Hajek's incision should be made at the extreme anterior margin of the cartilage of the septum, as shown in Figure 3-2 *a*. As the membrane of the vestibular portion of the septum is firmly attached to the fibrocartilage beneath it, this incision should be made only when the deflection is far enough forward to render it necessary to remove the anterior portion of the deflected cartilage.

When the deviation does not extend forward into the vestibule, Killian's incision (Fig. 3-2, *b*) should be made at the junction of the vestibular membrane with the mucous membrane of the septum, as the mucoperichondrium elevates with comparative ease posterior to this point.

The Killian incision is usually preferable and should be made with a sharp-pointed knife upon the left side of the septum. Many writers have recommended that it be made

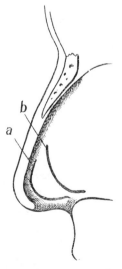

FIG. 3–2. Incisions for submucous resection of the septum: *a,* the Hajek incision; *b,* the Killian incision.

upon the side of the convexity of the septum, since they believe this allows greater freedom of access in elevating the membrane over the region of convexity. This is ill advised, as most operators are more dextrous with their right hands. Furthermore, it is unnecessary, as the tip of the nose is flexible and may be turned to one side out of the way. Hence it is recommended that the incision be made upon the left side of the septum except for left-handed or ambidextrous surgeons.

The tip of the index finger of the left hand should be introduced into the right nasal chamber to exert counterpressure while the incision is being made. The incision should extend only through the mucous membrane and perichondrium. If it is carried deeper, it interferes with the elevation of these tissues.

Elevation of the Mucoperichondrium and Periosteum

This step of the operation is often the beginning of either success or failure in the operation. If the elevation is properly done over the entire area of the deviation on both sides of the septum, the subsequent steps are comparatively easy to carry out. If, however, the elevation is not properly executed and extended over the entire field of the deviation, it may interfere with the remaining steps of the operation to such an extent as to defeat its purpose. In the average case in which the cartilage, the perpendicular plate of the ethmoid, and the vomer are involved in the deviation, the membrane should be elevated over almost the entire area of both sides of the septum. If, however, only the cartilage of the septum is affected, the elevation should be extended about 1 cm beyond the junction of the cartilage and the perpendicular plate, and down to the floor of the nose. The membrane should always be elevated at least 1 cm beyond the area of the tissue to be removed, as otherwise the membrane may be injured in the process of removing the deviated portion of the framework of the septum.

The technique in elevation of the mucoperichondrium may be accomplished in various ways. Some operators prefer small, thin, sharp elevators with which the mucoperichondrium and periosteum are dissected from the framework of the septum. Curved elevators are also used to work around curved portions of the septum. A study of the following descriptive technique will show how the heavy, blunt elevators may be used successfully to encompass curved and angular deviations of the cartilage and the perpendicular plate of the ethmoid. The chief reasons for using the blunt, heavy elevators are the greater speed and the lessened liability of tearing the membrane in the process of elevation.

To start the elevation, a sharp or semisharp elevator should be used, care being exercised to get beneath the perichondrium. If the elevator penetrates between the mucous membrane and perichondrium, the surface of the cartilage will present a velvety red appearance, as the perichondrium is still covering it. If, however, the elevator penetrates beneath the perichondrium, the exposed cartilage presents a glistening white surface. Great patience is often required to start the elevation properly; this being done, the remaining elevation is comparatively

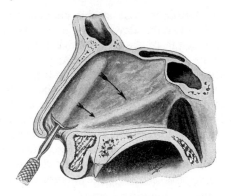

Fig. 3–4. The Hajek elevator introduced beneath the mucoperichondrium along the line of least resistance. When it is thus introduced, the elevation should be made with the whole shank of the instrument in a downward and backward direction to the crest of the vomer. The periosteum along the crest of the vomer should then by excised, as shown in Figures 3-7 to 3-9.

easy. The point of least resistance is usually at the upper portion of the Killian incision, whereas at the lower portions, the perichondrium is often so adherent as to require a knife to separate it from the cartilage.

When the elevation is begun, the sharp elevator is abandoned and the blunt one inserted (see Fig. 3-19, Ballenger's elevator) into the small pocket already made. The elevator is directed parallel with the ridge of the nose, as this is the direction of least resistance (Fig. 3-4). When the elevator is introduced almost to the cribriform plate, the elevation should be continued backward and downward with the whole length of the shank of the elevator within the pocket of the membrane. The mistake is usually made of attempting to elevate with the tip of the elevator, whereas it should be done with the shank. With the former it is easy to tear the mucoperichondrium, while with the latter the elevation may be rapidly accomplished with little danger of tearing it. As a matter of fact, the mucoperichondrium and periosteum elevate readily under moderate tension with a broad, dull instrument, whereas if a small, sharp elevator is used, extreme care must be constantly exerted to avoid making a perforation.

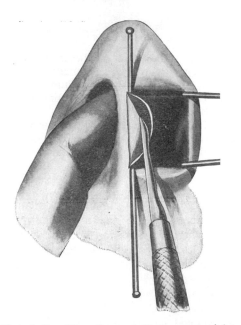

Fig. 3–3. Elevation of the mucoperichondrium upon the side of the primary incision in the mucous membrane. The elevation is begun with a sharp or semisharp elevator and is completed with the blunt elevator.

duced and passed upward parallel to the dorsum of the nose (direction of least resistance) until its tip is near the level of the cribriform plate of the ethmoid bone. The elevation should then be continued downward and backward with the shank of the instrument, as previously described, extending over an area considerably larger than the area of cartilage and bone to be removed.

Removal of the Cartilaginous Portion of the Septum

In nearly all cases this is most easily accomplished with the swivel knife (Figs. 3-10 to 3-13; see also Fig. 3-18). The advantages of the swivel knife are the ease, precision, and rapidity with which it encircles the cartilage, and the further fact that it removes it in one piece, thus allowing the operator to study the specimen as a whole.

Before the swivel knife is utilized, the mucoperichondria should be distended with a septum speculum to lift them from the cartilage and to provide room for the knife. This fully exposes the cartilage. The swivel knife may be applied to the cartilage at either the upper or lower portion of the incision. If to the upper portion, the incision will be made upward, backward, downward, and finally forward along the floor of the nose, thus completely encircling the portion

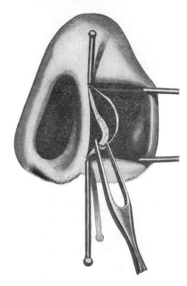

Fig. 3–11. The swivel knife in position at the lower portion of the incision of the cartilage.

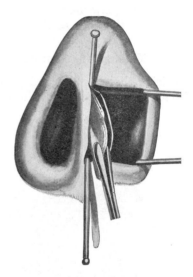

Fig. 3–12. The cartilage, having been excised submucously with the swivel knife, is removed from the mucoperichondrial pouch with dressing forceps.

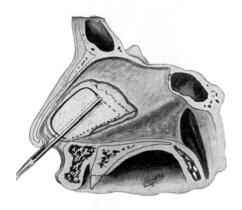

Fig. 3–10. Removal of the quadrilateral cartilage of the septum with Ballenger's swivel knife. The membrane is shown removed to expose the knife to view. In the actual operation the membrane is not removed.

of the cartilage to be removed (Fig. 3-10). If the knife is applied at the lower portion of the incision, the cut will extend backward, along the crest of the vomer, to the junction of the vomer and perpendicular plate of the ethmoid, thence upward and forward, along the anteroinferior margin of

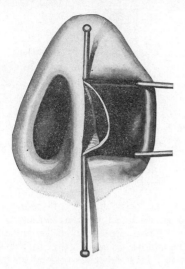

FIG. 3–13. The mucoperichondrial pouch after removal of the cartilage. The bony crest of the vomer is shown in the bottom of the pouch, while deep in the pouch is shown the perpendicular plate of the ethmoid extending upward from the crest of the vomer. This should be removed with forceps, as shown in Figure 3-11.

the perpendicular plate, and then downward, parallel with the ridge of the nose to the upper limit of the primary incision of the cartilage, thus encircling the portion of the cartilage to be removed. If the incision is begun at the lower limit of the primary incision, it may be necessary first to make a slight cut with a knife or scissors, since the cartilage is often fibrous at this point.

Determination of the amount of septum to be removed is sometimes a difficult problem. In the first place, enough of the deviated portion must be removed or replaced in the midline to create adequate airways, but on the other hand, removal of large amounts may lead to postoperative contractural deformities of the nose. These considerations do not apply to removal of the septum lying under the posterior one third of the nose, where the nasal bones furnish more than enough support even though large amounts of the septum are removed.

In the anterior two thirds of the nose, however, much greater care must be exercised. Here the support afforded by the upper and lower lateral cartilages may not

be sufficiently strong, without the septum, to maintain the shape of the nose. A cicatrix forms after removal of the cartilage from between the mucous membrane flaps. It is the contraction of this cicatrix or scar in the septum that can pull the nose out of shape in 1 or 2 months following surgery. These postoperative nasal deformities are more likely to occur either at the junction of the upper and lower lateral cartilages or in the columella, because the support is less strong in these areas. These mishaps will be less likely to occur if the following precautions are observed:

1. Unobstructing portions of the septum, particularly along the columella and under the dorsum of the nose, should not be removed.

2. If removal of a large piece of septal cartilage is necessary, the force of the cicatricial pull can be lessened by the replacement of straight pieces of cartilage between the mucous membrane flaps. The larger the area of the two flaps separated by the replaced cartilage, the less the cicatricial pull will be. The pieces of cartilage are placed between the flaps after nasal packing has been inserted snugly in the nose between the septum and turbinates and thus are held in place without sutures.

3. Lastly, the septum may be relocated as described under Rhinoplasty.

Removal of the Perpendicular Plate of the Ethmoid

This is accomplished with the Foster-Ballenger bone forceps (Figs. 3-14 and 3-20). It removes a comparatively large piece at each bite and in two or three bites removes all that is necessary. The bites may be made without removing the forceps from the mucoperichondrial pouch, a point of considerable importance, as each introduction of an instrument into the perichondrial pouch increases the chance of injury to the membranes. The perpendicular plate may also be removed by seizing it with heavy dressing forceps and twisting it from its attachments, though this is a crude and dangerous method since there is no control of the extent of the fracture.

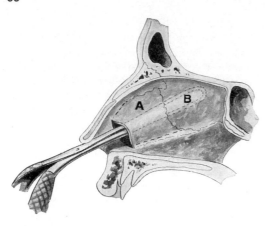

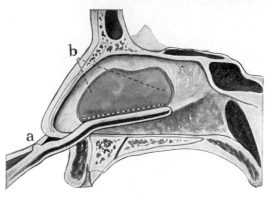

FIG. 3–14. Removal of the perpendicular plate of the ethmoid bone with the Foster-Ballenger forceps: *A,* the area of cartilage previously removed with the swivel knife; *B,* the area of perpendicular plate removed with the forceps.

FIG. 3–16. A method of removing the ridge of bone in submucous resection of the septum. *a,* The septum forceps grasping the ridge, the blades being external to the mucous membranes. The forceps is rotated on its longitudinal axis, thus fracturing the vomer from its lower attachment. *b,* The area of cartilage and perpendicular plate of the ethmoid previously removed. The mucous membrane is shown removed, although this is not actually done in the operation.

Removal of the Vomer

Various methods are used for removal of the deviated vomer, which often forms the so-called ridge of the septum. It is obviously almost impossible to elevate the mucoperiosteum beneath the crest of the ridge (vomer), as its anterior portion is near the floor of

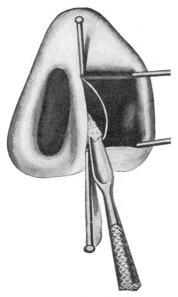

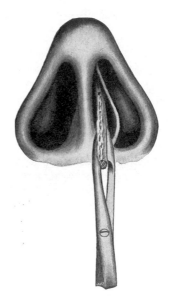

FIG. 3–17. Removal of the vomer after it is fractured as shown in Figure 3-16.

the nose, and to attempt to pass the elevator over the margin of the crest would almost certainly tear the tense mucous membrane along this line. Fortunately, the deviated or thickened bone can be removed without previous elevation of the membrane beneath the crest.

FIG. 3–15. Removal of the thickened crest of the vomer with a V-shaped gouge.

An old and approved method of removing the vomer is a gouge or some modification of it (Figs. 3-15 and 3-21). The V-shaped end of the gouge is engaged at the anterior end of the ridge of bone and driven with a mallet into its substance for a short distance; the handle of the gouge is then depressed, thus partially splintering the bone from its attachment (Fig. 3-16). The gouge is then driven farther into the ridge until the ridge is finally removed in its entirety. As the vomer is loosened, it separates from the mucoperiosteum without tearing, provided, of course, the gouge is always directed parallel to the anteroposterior direction of the crest of the vomer.

The vomer should be fractured first from the premaxillary bone at the floor of the nose and then removed with heavy dressing forceps introduced into the mucoperiosteal pouch. During the fracturing process, the mucoperiosteum separates from beneath the crest of the vomer, allowing the long ridge of bone to be removed from the pouch (Fig. 3-17). In young adults and children this method is not applicable as the vomer is not yet fully ossified. In adults it is a speedy and an almost painless procedure. The technique of the procedure is as follows:

The blades of the Asch septum forceps are introduced into the nasal chambers outside of the mucoperichondria, and the deviated vomer is firmly grasped. The forceps is twisted in its longitudinal axis, fracturing the vomer from its attachment at the floor of the nose. The blades of the forceps should be placed a little above the floor of the nose, as they may otherwise tear the mucous mem-

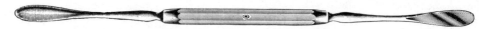

FIG. 3–18.   Ballenger's swivel cartilage knife.

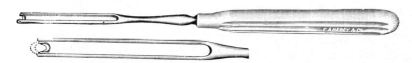

FIG. 3–19.   Hajek-Ballenger mucoperichondrium elevators.

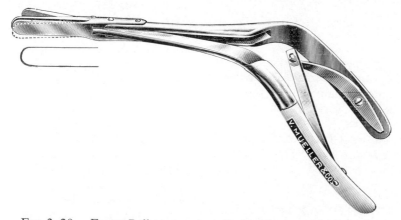

FIG. 3–20.   Foster-Ballenger perpendicular plate septum forceps.

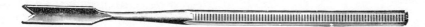

FIG. 3–21.   Ballenger's septum gouge.

brane at the junction of the vomer with the floor of the nose. The fracture should be thorough in order to permit detachment of the fragments from the floor of the nose. The Asch forceps is removed, and the tips of heavy dressing forceps are introduced into the mucoperichondrial pouch. The vomer is grasped, and with a tugging, teasing motion it is lifted from its fractured base. The mucoperiosteum remaining attached below the crest will separate readily and allow the bone to be removed.

Inspection of the Field Operated Upon

After completion of the various steps of the operation, the field operated upon should be subjected to the closest scrutiny, because if a portion of the deviated cartilage or bone is left in place, it may still cause obstruction of the nasal chambers when healing is complete. Every vestige of the deviated framework of the septum should be removed. Some type of bone-cutting forceps is usually used for this purpose in the cartilaginous and perpendicular plate portions of the septum, although the gouge may be more useful for cutting along the floor of the nose. A helpful practice is to insert a finger an inch or two into the nasal chambers, as it enables one to detect the presence of bony prominences which might otherwise have escaped notice.

The Dressing

A dressing should be placed in the nasal chambers for two purposes: (a) coaptation of the membranes, and (b) prevention of the formation of a blood clot in the mucoperichondrial pouch.

The dressing most frequently used is ½-inch selvedged-edge gauze tape soaked in petrolatum and removed in 4 to 6 days.

CORRECTION OF OBSTRUCTIVE LESIONS OF THE SEPTUM

Complications

Incision Through Both Mucous Membranes. This mistake is avoided by utilization of extreme care in incising the cartilage.

Should both mucous membranes be incised, it will be necessary to close one of them with sutures.

Tears Through Both Mucous Membranes. Sometimes during the elevation of the mucous membrane tears do occur at points exactly opposite one another. Again suturing should be done.

Postoperative Nasal Deformities. These unfortunate sequelae can be averted by avoiding too generous removal of the septal cartilage. It must be remembered that a cicatrix forms between the two mucous membrane flaps, and it is the contraction of this cicatrix that pulls the nose out of shape—usually at the junction of the upper and lower lateral cartilages, along the dorsum, or by retraction of the columella. The pull of the contracting cicatrix can be lessened by replacing flat pieces of cartilage between the two mucous membrane flaps.

Septal Abscess. Acute abscess of the nasal septum is not common. It may result from trauma, postoperatively, or as a complication of infectious disease. Pyogenic bacteria may invade a hematoma and thus convert it into an abscess.

PERFORATION OF THE SEPTUM

Etiology. The great majority of septal perforations follow trauma of some sort, usually operative. Acute infectious diseases such as diphtheria or scarlet or typhoid fever may be the cause. Occasionally a chronic granulomatous disease such as midline lethal granuloma involves a septal perforation. In the young, multiple digital ("nose picking") traumata may eventually lead to perforation. In recent years syphilitic ulceration and perforation of the nasal septum have been rare.

Symptoms. The symptoms of perforation of the septum vary with the size, cause, and location of the perforation. A small anterior perforation sometimes gives rise to a whistling sound, whereas a large one does not. Crusts, if of large size, may give rise to the feeling of a foreign body in the nose and, if forcibly blown or picked off, may cause nasal hemorrhage. Repeated epistaxis should arouse suspicion of a perforating ulcer. Syphilitic ulceration is usually accompanied by an offensive necrotic odor. Many cases will progress to complete perforation without the patient's knowledge.

Treatment. Large perforations are not amenable to surgical closure. Small ones may often be closed by proper plastic surgical procedures.

Plastic Flap Operation. A plastic flap may be used to close the perforation in two ways. First, a flap of septal mucosa may be turned to cover the perforation.

Technique

1. Topical anesthesia.
2. The rim or edge of the perforation is freshened by pairing off the epithelium and mucous membrane.
3. The mucoperichondrium is then elevated for a distance of ½ inch around the edge of the perforation.
4. A ring of cartilage is resected for ⅛ to ¼ inch from the edge of the perforation.
5. A mucous membrane flap, the area of which is considerably larger than the perforation, is dissected from the most convenient surface of the septum, turned into the perforation, and tucked between the elevated membranes around the perforation.

6. When the pedicled flap is placed, three or four stitches hold it in position. One surface is covered by epithelium, while the other is left to heal by granulation from the edges of the closed perforation (Fig. 3-22).

A second and more simple method is applicable to small perforations.

1. Topical anesthesia.
2. The edges of the perforation are freshened and the mucoperichondrium elevated, as in the submucous resection operation.
3. A long curved incision (Fig. 3-23, *b* to *b*) is made through the mucoperichondrium, ¼ to ½ inch anterior to the perforation. The ribbon-flap thus made is elevated.
4. A long curved incision (*e* to *e*) is made through the mucoperichondrium of the opposite side of the septum, ¼ to ½ inch posterior to the perforation and the flap elevated.
5. The anterior flap is sutured to the freshened posterior edge of the mucous membrane of the perforation (Fig. 3-24), and the posterior flap on the opposite side of the septum is sutured to the freshened anterior edge of the membrane of the perforation, as shown in Figure 3-25. The areas *a* and *a*, in Figures 3-24 and 3-25 respectively, heal by granulation.

When both mucoperichondria are torn during a submucous operation, making it

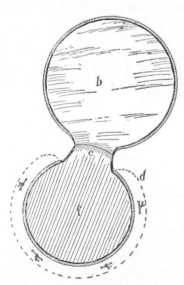

FIG. 3–22. *f*, The plastic flap sutured in the perforation; *c*, the pedicle of the plastic flap; *b*, the denuded area from which the plastic flap is removed heals by granulation; *d*, the edge of the plastic flap between the mucoperichondria of the septum.

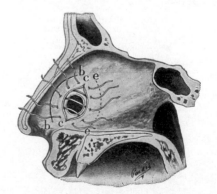

FIG. 3–23. Schema of Hazletine's plastic operation for closure of perforations of the septum: *b* to *b*, incision in front of the perforation; *e* to *e*, incision posterior to the perforation on the opposite side of the septum; *c* to *c*, the freshened edges of the perforation.

4

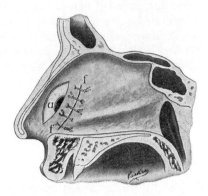

Fig. 3–24.   Detail of Figure 3-23 showing the opposite side of the septum. The flap formerly covering area *a* is sutured to the posterior margin of the perforation.

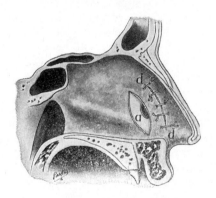

Fig. 3–25.   Detail of Figure 3-24: *a,* the denuded cartilage after the plastic flap (*d* to *d*) is sutured.

probable that a permanent perforation will follow, the cartilage removed may be reintroduced between the membranes, thus affording a bridge over which the granulating edges of the mucous membranes may extend and close the perforation. As an alternative, a 1-mm acrylic plate may be placed between the flaps to fill in the perforation. The posterior part of the plate is perforated so that the mucous membrane flaps may adhere together by fibrous tissue and thus hold the plate in position.

Nasal Synechia

Adhesions between the nasal septum and turbinates are usually the result of surgical trauma but at times may follow infections of the nasal mucosa in which ulcerative lesions occur. Most nasal synechiae are found between the septum and inferior turbinate.

Symptoms, if present, are partial obstruction to breathing on the affected side and a sensation of a foreign body in the nose.

Treatment by separation of the adhesion and application of cauterizing agents or ointments to the base of the adhesion is unsatisfactory as the adhesion usually returns. A thin segment of a sheet of dental wax inserted between the turbinate and septum after the synechia is removed will prevent its return in some cases. The sheet of wax should be removed and replaced every 2 or 3 days, but insertion should be continued for 2 or 3 weeks.

Chapter 4

Epistaxis, Rhinophyma, Furunculosis, Foreign Bodies in the Nose, Rhinoliths, Choanal Atresia

EPISTAXIS

Etiology. Epistaxis or bleeding from the interior of the nose may be primary or secondary, spontaneous or induced, and located posteriorly or anteriorly.

The exposed and unprotected state of the blood vessels of the nasal mucosa renders them particularly liable to rupture and thus hemorrhage. The septal vessels in particular are not well supported and protected from external insults but rather lie closely adjacent to bone and cartilage, protected only by a thin mucous membrane. Once injured, the blood vessel retracts poorly into the scant submucosa. Thus apparently minor injuries and erosions may cause vigorous nasal hemorrhages.

In children and younger adults the overwhelming majority of epistaxes occur from the anterior part of the nasal septum—the so-called *Little's area* or *Kiesselbach's plexus*. This area is exposed to the drying effect of inspiration as well as to multiple small traumata. An ulceration, rupture, or some other local pathologic condition occurs and bleeding commences.

In older adults the site of bleeding may be located anteriorly but more often is found to originate in the posterior part of the nose. Here the cause is usually not trauma but rather spontaneous rupture of a sclerotic vessel. The bleeding is made worse if the patient is hypertensive.

Since epistaxis may be a manifestation of a more serious local or constitutional disease, careful observation should be practiced. The historical background indicates, of course, if a recent injury or surgical procedure is to be considered etiologically. An ancient persistent septal perforation not infrequently leads to epistaxis from its margins.

Nasal angiomas, foreign bodies, and neoplasms may occasionally be present. Nasal parasites (nasal myiasis), nasal diphtheria, and rhinoliths are more rare causes.

Epistaxis due to general or constitutional factors is much less common etiologically than that due to local factors but nevertheless must always be kept in mind. The anemias and blood dyscrasias, namely, pernicious anemia, acute aplastic anemia, polycythemia vera, and acute and chronic leukemia, may number epistaxis among their early symptoms. It occurs likewise in vascular purpura, thrombocytopenic purpura, and various coagulation defects. A special statement might be made about the vascular purpura, hereditary hemorrhagic telangiectasia (Rendu-Osler-Weber disease). It is characterized by dilatation of the arterioles, capillaries, and venules into small angiomas that appear in all parts of the body, though the oral and nasal mucosa are the most common sites of predilection. Slight trauma to the nasal mucosa leads to multiple bleeding points.

Among the coagulation defects in which epistaxis occurs are those involving prothrombin and prothrombin acceleration factors and also fibrinogen and antihemophilic factor, of which hemophilia is an example. Anticoagulants are now widely used therapeutically and may promote a tendency to nasal bleeding. Epistaxis may accompany some acute infectious diseases such as influenza, measles, whooping cough, scarlet fever and rheumatic fever principally but also typhoid fever, pneumonia, erysipelas, dengue, and malaria.

Sudden decompression from a high atmospheric pressure (caisson disease) and violent exertion also occasionally cause nasal bleeding.

Site of Bleeding. Location of the exact site of bleeding is important not only for accurate placement of cautery or other form of local therapy but also for identifying the trunk blood vessel supplying this point (see Treatment). Anatomically it should be recalled that the anterior ethmoidal artery supplies the anterior and anterosuperior portion of the nose, and the sphenopalatine artery supplies the balance. Thus bleeding from above the anterior half of the middle turbinate comes from the former, and bleeding from below the middle turbinate and more posteriorly in the nose comes from the latter. *Kiesselbach's plexus* on the septum is an area of anastomosing vessels from both these sources as well as from branches of vessels in the upper lip.

Treatment. A clear appreciation of the amount and speed of blood loss is the first consideration in the treatment of epistaxis. Hematocrit, hemoglobin, and blood pressure determinations should quickly be made. If the patient is in shock, the condition must be promptly attended to. If there is suspicion of a coagulation defect, a platelet count, a prothrombin time, and a partial thromboplastin consumption time should also be obtained, and further diagnostic procedures should be carried out as the situation demands. In the event of a significant and rapid blood loss, transfusion of red blood cells, preferably packed, as well as fluid replacement should also be considered.

Most important in the local treatment of epistaxis are rigid-tube spot suction and bright, shadowless illumination. These enable the surgeon to clean the nose and to determine the exact site of bleeding. If the exact site is seen and is accessible, the hemorrhage should quickly be controlled and the emergency thus terminated.

Anterior Epistaxis. When the bleeding point has been located, the vessel may be controlled by pressure or by destruction using either chemical cautery or electrodesiccation. Pressure is easily applied by inserting a clean, dry cotton pack within the nose against the bleeding vessel. If, as is almost always the case with children, the vessel is located in Kiesselbach's plexus, enough cotton (or similar material) is inserted to make the ala of the nose bulge on that side. The material is left in place for 3 to 4 hours. Applying finger pressure to the outside of the nose provides additional pressure.

Packing of the anterior half of the nose is frequently necessary to apply pressure. The bleeding point must be determined so that the packing can be properly applied, the amount of instrumentation and discomfort to the patient thus being minimized. If the bleeding is very vigorous, widespread packing of the nose, preceded by local anesthesia if time permits, is necessary. Dry or petrolatum gauze ½-inch wide is introduced above the posterior end of the middle turbinate, and by working forward and downward, the entire nasal space is filled. The posterior end of the pack should extend almost into the nasopharynx. The packing may be impregnated with 1:1000 epinephrine and may be used to hold oxidized cellulose or similar hemostatic materials in place. Anterior nasal packing may be left in place 3 to 4 days if necessary. However, there is danger of obstructing the paranasal sinus drainage, so antibiotic coverage is prudent.

If the bleeding is small in amount and issues from one or several small points in Kiesselbach's plexus, the use of chemical cautery can be tried. This is more readily tolerated by the young patient but also is less effective than electrodesiccation, to be described subsequently. On a small cotton-mounted wooden applicator (or a bead made from silver nitrate or chromic acid crystals) 50% trichloroacetic acid is applied to the bleeding points and surrounding mucosa. The bead is made by touching the red-hot tip of a metal applicator to a crystal and then holding it vertically so that the liquid silver nitrate hardens at the tip of the applicator. Application of topical anesthesia with 2% tetracaine, 5% cocaine, or a similar drug is desirable beforehand.

In the event of more vigorous bleeding, either electrocautery (galvanocautery) or electrocoagulation (electrodesiccation) of the bleeding vessel should be instituted at once. In the former case, the cautery is heated to cherry redness, and the bleeding vessel is lightly singed until the outlines of the vessel have disappeared. Deep cautery may result in a septal perforation.

Electrocoagulation (electrodesiccation) is preferred because it affords better control. Desiccation of the bleeding vessel and immediate surrounding area takes place as soon as the mucosa is touched. It is necessary to have a reasonably dry field, and for this purpose a combination of a suction tip and a diathermy electrode is convenient. Care should be taken to avoid contact of the electrode with the metal nasal speculum. Prior local anesthesia is desirable in both electrocautery and electrocoagulation.

Simple elevation of the septal mucoperichondrium may be necessary for some persistent or recurrent septal bleeding. Presumably the cicatrix which forms between the elevated membrane and the subjacent cartilage obliterates the abnormal vessel. A more firm cicatrix is formed if the cartilage is also removed, so that the elevated membrane is in contact with its fellow on the opposite side.

Posterior Epistaxis. Control of the bleeding is greatly complicated in this area by the inaccessibility of the bleeding site. Frequently all that can be known is the side on which the bleeding is located and the fact that the exact site is near the posterior choana or perhaps in the nasopharynx itself. In either event, after any possible local anesthesia is obtained, a postnasal pack should be inserted into the posterior end of the nose on the appropriate side either by a sponge as described below or by a postnasal balloon inserted through the anterior naris and inflated to fill the posterior choana. Ideally the balloon will exert pressure against the sphenopalatine artery as it passes through the sphenopalatine foramen or as it crosses the anterior wall of the sphenoid sinus.

To insert postnasal packing, a strong silk suture or tape is attached near the pointed end of a cone or cigar-shaped sea sponge, roll of gauze, or similar material. A second suture is left attached to the packing as well and is permitted to dangle in the pharynx. It will be useful when the pack is removed. A small rubber catheter is then passed through the nose into the pharynx, where it is grasped by a forceps and pulled out of the mouth far enough so that it can be attached to one end of prepared tape or suture. Traction is then applied on the nose end of the tube, thus pulling the tampon into the posterior choana via the nasopharynx. Use of a finger to guide the pack into the nasopharynx facilitates the maneuver. The catheter is then freed and the suture holding the tampon secured firmly to the cheek by adhesive tape. Removal of the tampon, usually in 2 to 4 days, is accomplished by first using a forceps to recover the tape in the mouth and then using the tape to exert pressure posteriorly and downward on the tampon. Once the postnasal pack is in place, it usually is well to use an anterior pack in addition (Fig. 4-1).

Bluestone and Smith have recently introduced intranasal freezing for the control of severe epistaxis. Their method consists of circulating a coolant solution through a Fraser intranasal balloon, but a Fox or similar one can also be used. The outlet temperature of the coolant is maintained at −17 to −20° C, and it is left in the nose for approximately 1 hour.

A warning concerning the use of anterior and posterior nasal packing, particularly in patients with marginal cardiovascular and pulmonary disease, has been raised by Cassisi and coworkers. In a small series they have noted that pronounced nasopharyngeal obstruction (e.g., an edematous uvula) or nasal obstruction caused by anterior and posterior nasal packing was associated with a decreased arterial oxygen tension but with

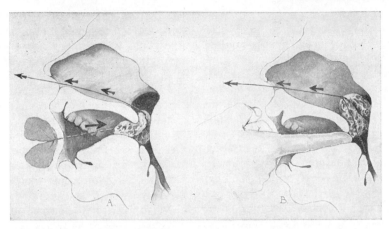

Fig. 4–1. The postnasal pack. *A*, Traction is being applied to the thread or tape extruding from the nostril, thus pulling the gauze pack into the pharynx behind the soft palate. *B*, The index finger exerts pressure on the pack to ensure a snug fit into the nasopharynx.

little change in the carbon dioxide tension. In this same connection Ogura and Harvey have reported that the pulmonary airway resistance is increased when nasal obstruction is present.

Ligation. Ligation of the vascular supply may be required if lesser measures fail, again indicating the necessity of accurately determining the precise source of the hemorrhage by adequate illumination and suction. *Ligation of the ethmoidal arteries* is begun by making a curved incision medial to the inner canthus of the eye and locating the periosteum posterior to the lacrimal bone. The periosteum is then elevated along the inner wall of the bony orbit just below the roof for a depth of 3 to 4 cm or until the ethmoidal vessels are found lying in the frontoethmoidal suture. It usually is easier to ligate with a metal clip rather than with a suture.

The approach to the *internal maxillary artery* is via the maxillary sinus. After an incision is made in the canine fossa, a 2-cm opening into the sinus is created so that the posterior sinus wall is readily accessible. Chisels and rongeurs remove a 1-cm to 2-cm segment of bone from the medial and superior portion of the posterior wall. Then by means of blunt dissection with long Metzenbaum scissors or a similar instrument, a search is made for the internal maxillary artery, which passes more or less horizontally across the posterior wall of the sinus. The artery is usually located at the level of the posterior end of the middle turbinate. The procedure is facilitated by using a microscope fitted with either a 300-mm or 400-mm lens.

Occasionally it is necessary to *ligate the external carotid artery,* though this is less efficient in controlling nasal bleeding than interrupting the flow proximal to the nose itself. Ligation of the internal carotid should be done rarely and only in extreme conditions because of the danger of hemiparesis. The approach to the carotid artery, usually with the patient under local anesthesia, is through an incision made along the anterior edge of the sternocleidomastoid muscle from the angle of the mandible to the upper margin of the thyroid cartilage. The anterior border of the muscle is freed and displaced posteriorly. By gentle upward retraction of the inferior pole of the parotid gland, the digastric tendon and the arching loop of the hypoglossal nerve (which crosses the artery at this level) are exposed. Deeper dissection discloses the pulsating artery, which should be carefully freed until a branch is found, thus distinguishing the external from the internal carotid, which has no cervical branches. Ligation of the external carotid should be as high as conveniently possible. Care must be taken to avoid the superior laryngeal nerve, which lies behind the artery.

The wound is then closed in the usual fashion without a drain.

RHINOPHYMA

Rhinophyma, also known as elephantiasis and cystadenofibroma of the nose, is a benign nodular enlargement of the skin of the lower half of the nose. The blood vessels are dilated, and fissures containing sebaceous masses are found between the nodules.

Pathologically rhinophyma is considered to be the last stage of acne rosacea. It develops slowly over a period of 10 to 15 years. Microscopic sections show greatly increased number and size of the sebaceous glands (Fig. 4-2).

Many forms of treatment have been tried without benefit. If the disease is well developed, the most success follows either subepithelial enucleation of the abnormal tissue or so-called decortication. With reasonably good skin the former is used. First, two U-shaped incisions are made through the skin on either side of the nose. The concavity of the U lies above the apex of the nose in one case and below in the second, and the arms join to form a V on the lateral aspect of the nose on either side. Then through these two incisions, the pathologic tissue is dissected free, and the two skin flaps are joined by sutures. Hemorrhage, which is likely to be extensive, is controlled by pressure. Healing is complete in 10 days.

Decortication is preferable if the skin of the nose is badly degenerated. A knife or razor is used to shave or pare the nodular enlargement down until the proper size and shape have been approximated. It is necessary to leave a rim of untouched skin around the nares; otherwise disfigurement will result from cicatricial contracture. Care must be taken to avoid injury to the cartilages. Leaving epithelial islands for regrowth of the skin is not difficult because of the deeply indented nature of the epithelium in this disease. The raw area is covered with several layers of petrolatum gauze, and a pressure dressing is used to control bleeding.

Roentgen rays and radium are of no avail once the disease has developed. They may be of some use as preventive measures. Postoperatively suberythema doses of roentgen rays are used. Two doses are given 1 week apart.

FURUNCULOSIS OF THE NOSE

Definition. Furunculosis of the nose is a superficial abscess formation that may occur

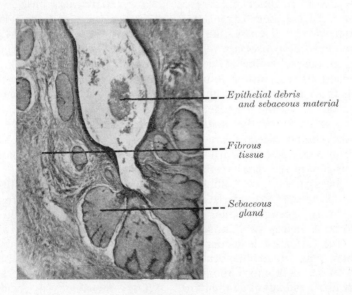

FIG. 4–2.   Rhinophyma of the nose showing a fissure with numerous large sebaceous glands at its base. × 15.

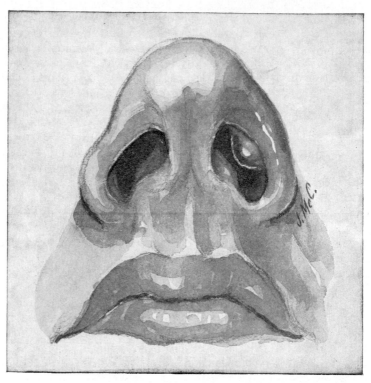

Fig. 4–3. Furunculosis of the lateral margin of the left naris.

in any part of the nose; it does not differ materially from the same process in other parts of the body. Most commonly, *Staphylococcus aureus* is the infecting organism.

Etiology. Some portal of entry must be provided before the *Staphylococcus aureus* gains entrance to the subepithelial tissues where the infection occurs. Minor injuries, such as picking the nose and thus injuring the hair follicle of the nasal vibrissae, are sufficient to permit entry of the bacteria. Diabetes and debilitating diseases are frequently accompanied by recurrent furuncles. The abscess is usually in the nasal vestibule.

Symptoms. The skin of the vestibule as well as that over the apex is characteristically tightly bound to the subjacent cartilage. Thus what appears to be a slightly swollen, somewhat red area (the furuncle) is tender and exhibits throbbing pain to an unexpectedly marked degree. Were there more room for edema (i.e., less tightly adherent epithelium), the pain and tenderness would be less

marked. When the condition is well advanced, the center of the furuncle becomes yellow and releases pus.

Furuncles around the nasal vestibule and apex as well as the upper lip are potentially dangerous because of the possibility of rupture into venous channels leading directly to the cavernous sinus. Swelling of the lids, chemosis, pupillary changes, deep-seated headache, beginning ptosis, and exophthalmos, as well as chills, fever, and symptoms of systemic spread, are all possible signs and symptoms of this dread complication.

Treatment. Most importantly, furuncles of the nose and upper lip should not be taken lightly but rather treated as a serious disease. The abscess should not be squeezed or otherwise manipulated for fear of enhancing the possibility of intracranial spread. Main reliance should be placed on heat to the area and antibiotic therapy (see p. 142).

Once the abscess is localized to a clearly defined fluctuant "head," this head can be gently incised. If spread to the cavernous sinus occurs, in addition to vigorous antibiotic therapy, anticoagulant medication should be used to produce a prothrombin time twice or more that of the control.

FOREIGN BODIES IN THE NOSE

Foreign bodies in the nose may be animate or inanimate.

Myiasis of the nose is caused by flies, such as the common blow fly (screw-worm) and the green bottle fly, depositing their eggs within the nasal cavity. The flies predominate in warm, dry climates with low elevations. The screw-worm fly (*Cochliomyia americana*) is the important infesting agent in America. The eggs usually hatch within 24 hours after being deposited within the nose.

The mucous membrane lining the nose and sinuses may be partly destroyed, with denuding of the bone and cartilage. The cranial cavity may be invaded with fatal meningitis in rare instances.

The symptoms are those of an acute sinusitis, that is: a profuse unilateral mucopurulent discharge, usually with an offensive odor; nasal stenosis, usually complete, on the affected side; pain or headache in some form; and bleeding or a bloody mucopurulent discharge in most instances. The worms cling with great tenacity to the tissues. Much destruction of tissue with bulging of the walls may occur in the more severe cases.

The diagnosis is made from the finding of eggs or worms within the secretions or cavities of the nose or sinuses.

Inanimate foreign bodies include almost every kind of inert substance small enough to be introduced into the nose and some that are too large to be introduced through the nasal opening, such as those from injuries and gunshot wounds.

In most instances the foreign body is voluntarily introduced by the patient. Young children have an inordinate desire to introduce such substances as beans, peas, and beads into their noses. Seeds, if in the nose long enough, may sprout or become greatly softened.

Removal of the foreign body may be accomplished through the anterior nasal opening without the use of a general anesthetic, though in some cases this may be necessary. Forceps with good grasping tips may be used to seize a rough or easily grasped object, but a curved probe is better for removing such objects as beads and marbles. The curved portion of the probe should be passed behind the object and pulled forward, and thus the object readily comes out. Some bleeding may result.

RHINOLITHS

Synonyms include nasal concretions and nasal calculi.

These formations are rare in the nasal spaces. They usually have a foreign body nucleus of bacteria, blood, pus cells, mucus, crusts, or some foreign material from outside the body. They are usually unilateral and are located, in the majority of instances, in the lower portion of the nasal cavity. They vary in size from small granules to those an ounce or more in weight. The condition is found more commonly in adults than in children and more often in the female than in the male. The lesions may have a gray, brown, or greenish black color. They may be soft and crumbly or hard and brittle. They are largely composed of calcium and magnesium salts, principally carbonate and phosphate, with traces of sodium chloride. The stones vary in shape but usually conform to the shape of the nasal cavities.

The presence of some nasal disease or deformity that provides varying degrees of nasal obstruction, resulting in poor drainage of the nasal cavity which favors stasis of the secretions, is an important factor in the formation of the true type of rhinolith. The inorganic salts adhere to the nucleus, and as it enlarges, it has a tendency to fill the nasal space, impacting itself in the surrounding tissues.

The symptoms of rhinolithiasis vary from a slight one-sided nasal discharge or obstruction to marked structural changes. A unilateral fetid discharge, hemorrhages, and obstruction to breathing are symptoms usually observed.

The treatment is removal, under general anesthesia if necessary.

ATRESIA OF THE POSTERIOR CHOANAE

Choanal atresia consists of abnormal membranous or bony closure of one or both posterior choanae (Fig. 4-4). The closure may be partial or complete, congenital or acquired.

Etiology. Congenital atresia is located in the posterior choanae, whereas acquired atresia is more apt to be found further toward the oropharynx. Various theories have been mentioned to explain the congenital form: persistence of the nasobuccal membrane; persistence of the buccopharyngeal membrane; a median overgrowth of the vertical and horizontal processes of the palatine bone; and an intrauterine inflammatory condition. The first is probably the most likely explanation.

The acquired type of atresia is the result either of severe uncontrolled infection (syphilis, diphtheria, etc.) with a resultant stenosing cicatrix or of inexpert surgery in the region, which is more likely nowadays.

Symptoms. The most striking result of choanal stenosis is the absence of a nasal airway; this possibility must never be overlooked in the newborn experiencing respiratory difficulties. The quick provision of a nasal airway may be lifesaving in such a case.

Such an infant can only breathe with the mouth open, and the nose is filled with an inspissated glairy mucus. Nursing is difficult or impossible for the infant because in so doing he loses his oral airway too.

The occluding obstruction, which prevents passage of a tube from the nose into the pharynx, is also revealed by digital palpation of the nasopharynx. A radiopaque liquid instilled into the nose with the patient supine can be seen on the x-ray film to be against the occluding membrane itself. In an older individual a mirror may visualize the atretic choanae.

Treatment. Treatment of atresia of the posterior choanae involves surgical removal of the obstruction. The technique employed would depend upon the type of obstruction (whether membranous or bony), the age of the patient, and the presence or absence of any associated pathologic condition.

A membranous occlusion may be removed surgically, or it may be perforated with a probe or other instrument and the opening enlarged by a series of dilatations, with good results in many instances. Destruction of the membranous type by means of electrocoagulation has been successfully accomplished.

In bony occlusions, which constitute about 90% of the congenital cases, it is necessary to perforate and break down the partition by means of chisels, drills, curettes, trephines, etc. The entire bony obstruction must be removed, as well as the posterior portion of the nasal septum. This latter procedure

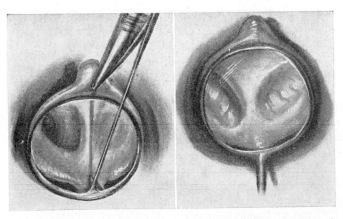

FIG. 4-4. *A*, Nasopharyngeal "mirror exposure" of a unilateral choanal atresia. *B*, Nasopharyngeal "mirror exposure" of a bilateral choanal atresia. (Kazanjian, V. H.: Ann Otol. Rhinol. Laryngol., *51*:704, 1942.)

is necessary to avoid a later cicatricial closure. In removing the occlusion, care should be taken to avoid injuring the pterygopalatine canal, which is situated above and just anterior to the choanal orifice, and the posterior palatine canal, situated just behind the choanal opening on the outer wall.

Various approaches to the obstructing wall have been tried. Von Eicken in 1911 and White in 1918 removed the posterior end of the vomer and bony occlusion by way of a submucous resection of the septum. This method would be feasible for adults only. Ruddy suggests a transpalatine approach for infants and small children and reports a successful result. Kazanjian in his adult patients incises the base of the columella and extends a through-and-through incision along the base of the septum backward to the anterior tip of the vomer. The incision is then carried upward along the junction of the quadrilateral cartilage and perpendicular plate of the ethmoid, thereby creating a movable flap of the cartilaginous septum. The vomer is then removed back to the atresia, creating a large opening through which the occluding bone is accessible for removal. The cartilaginous septum is then sutured into place. A large posterior nasopharyngeal space is thus created.

Prevention of cicatrization with subsequent closure has received much attention. Various methods have been mentioned and tried, such as nasal tampons, metal and rubber tubes or catheters, postoperative electrocoagulation, and skin grafting of the exposed areas. All have been successful in selected cases. If complete removal of the obstructing tissue, including a portion of the posterior edge of the nasal septum, is done, subsequent closure will probably not occur if excessive granulations are prevented.

Beinfield has described an operation to be used in the first 24 hours of life for bony or membranous choanal atresia. The first step is to keep the infant's mouth open by inserting an anesthetist's airway until the operation is completed. With the infant mummified, the operative procedure is carried out under local anesthesia. To destroy the bony or membranous obstruction, a No. 2 Lempert or similar curette is used (Fig. 4-5). It is inserted along the floor of the nose

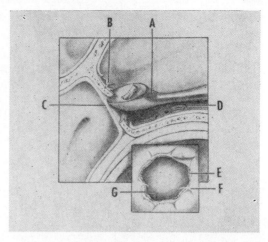

FIG. 4–5. Pharyngeal mucous membrane: *A*, Curette; *B*, shreds of nasal mucous membrane; *C*, pharyngeal mucous membrane; *D*, removed spicules of bone on floor of nose. Inset: *E*, bony atresia almost completely removed; *F*, shreds of nasal mucous membrane in front of the atresia; *G*, intact pharyngeal mucous membrane. (Beinfield, H.H.: Arch. Otolaryng., *70*:1, 1959.)

until the occluding membrane is encountered, usually 1¼ inches beyond the rim of the nostril. Beinfield emphasizes that along the floor of the nose the curette should not be inserted to a depth greater than 1¾ inches beyond the rim of the nostril because of the danger of injury to the posterior-lying vertebrae. As the curette is moved upward, the safe depth is even less.

The curette having been inserted along the floor of the nose, firm pressure is exerted against the obstruction until the bone is perforated. The nasal mucous membrane in front of the obstruction must be sacrificed with the bone. The bone perforation is then enlarged to a point at which a normal-sized opening has been created. The pharyngeal mucous membrane that covered the posterior surface of the bone atresia still remains and is now incised near the floor of the nose with a No. 11 Bard-Parker blade on a long No. 7 handle (Fig. 4-6). The incision is then enlarged in a stellate fashion so as to admit a No. 12 or larger rubber catheter. Incision of the membranous pharyngeal portion of the occlusion should be done with utmost care. A finger or metal shield in the

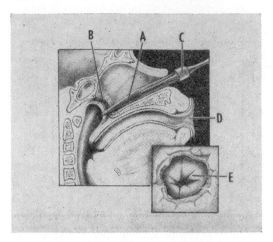

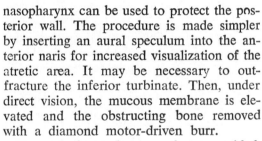

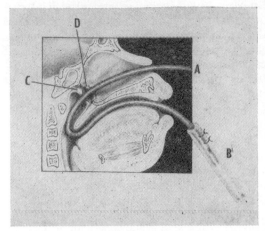

FIG. 4–6. *A*, No. 11 Bard-Parker blade cutting through pharyngeal mucous membrane near floor of nose; *B*, bony atresia completely removed; *C*, adhesive tape wrapped around handle of Bard-Parker blade 1¼ inches from tip of blade; *D*, airway still in mouth. Inset: *E*, Stellate incisions through pharyngeal mucous membrane. (Beinfield, H. H.: Arch. Otolaryng., *70*:1, 1959.)

FIG. 4–7. *A, B,* Insertion into lumen of a piece of No. 18 French polyvinyl tubing about 1 inch long, with two silk sutures passed through catheter and tubing and tied firmly near end of tubing. Note airway in mouth has been removed before catheter is passed. *C,* Incised pharyngeal mucous membrane, with No. 12 catheter passed through opening in it. *D,* Bony atresia completely removed. (Beinfield, H. H.: Arch. Otolaryng., *70*:1, 1959.)

nasopharynx can be used to protect the posterior wall. The procedure is made simpler by inserting an aural speculum into the anterior naris for increased visualization of the atretic area. It may be necessary to outfracture the inferior turbinate. Then, under direct vision, the mucous membrane is elevated and the obstructing bone removed with a diamond motor-driven burr.

A nasal airway has now been provided, and the last step is to make it permanent (Fig. 4-7). First, a No. 12 rubber catheter is passed via the nose into the pharynx, recovered, brought out through the mouth, and attached to a piece of polyvinyl tubing of slightly less than 1¾ inches in length. The diameter of this tube is the same as that of the posterior choanae, which is slightly larger than the anterior nares. The polyvinyl tube is now pulled by the rubber tube into the nasopharynx, through the perforated choanae, and into the nose, where the anterior end is wedged just within the nasal vestibule and the posterior end will, of course, lie within the nasopharynx and thus maintain the patency of the atretic area during healing. When the plastic tube is pulled

through the atretic area, the mucous membrane is also pulled anteriorly and thus tends to cover the raw bony surfaces. If the occlusion is bilateral, the same procedure is done on the second side.

Postoperatively the nasal airway tube is left in place for 1 month. It may be suctioned as necessary. If, after removal, signs of closure of the nasal airway appear, it may have to be reinserted for another month.

In the adult, congenital choanal atresia is almost invariably partly bony. For the correction to be successful an adequate amount of bone must be removed, and to prevent a stenosing cicatrix all raw surfaces of bone must be covered with either an adjacent mucous membrane flap or a split-thickness skin graft. Prevention of the postoperative stenosis is also furthered by removal of the posterior end of the bony nasal septum.

Most authors in recent years have advocated a transpalatal approach to surgical correction of choanal atresia in the older child or adult. The various methods involved in the transpalatal approach to the nasopharynx have been well reviewed by Wilson. In this approach great care must be exercised to avoid injury to the pterygopalatine and posterior palatine canals. In unilateral choanal stenosis, Wilson advises use of an inverted Y-shaped incision in the palate with the vertical stem running upward to the incisor teeth and the lateral oblique arm extending from the midportion of the palate downward to a point medial to the pterygopalatine canal. The palatal mucosa is now elevated, and, beginning posteriorly, the hard palate is removed, the mucosa on the superior surface being preserved if possible for use in covering raw bone. Sufficient bone is removed to expose the mucosa of the nose anterior to the atretic area, and a smaller area of hard palate is removed on the unaffected side to allow ease of removal of the posterior part of the bony nasal septum.

The bone of the posterior part of the septum is removed in a submucous fashion to preserve the mucosa for covering raw bone; similarly, the mucosa covering the posterior and anterior surfaces of the atresia itself is preserved. These mucosal flaps are used as seems most appropriate to the operating surgeon to cover the most important raw surfaces of the newly created choana, namely, the roof, floor, and lateral wall. Sponge rubber or a similar device may be used for 24 hours to hold the flaps in place. To complete the operation, the original incision in the palate is closed.

In the case of bilateral atresia, there is less mucosa available for flaps, and recourse must be made to free split-thickness skin grafts.

ATRESIA OR STENOSIS OF THE NASOPHARYNX

Etiology. Stenosis of the nasopharynx is usually acquired postoperatively or following acute disease processes, such as diphtheria and tuberculosis. The various chronic granulomas may at times play a role.

Pathology. The palate and posterior pillars are adherent in varying degrees to the posterior pharyngeal wall, leaving only a small connection between the pharynx and nasopharynx. The finding of normal tympanic membranes usually excludes stenosis of the nasopharynx.

Symptoms. The symptoms are dependent on the degree of obstruction, the most severe cases involving total dependence on mouth breathing at the expense of the nasal airway.

Treatment. Surgical treatment of the condition requires attention to the same principles used above for choanal stenosis, namely, removal of obstructing tissues (fibrous scar in this case) and the covering of all raw surfaces with split-thickness skin grafts since mucous membrane flaps are not available.

MacKenty some years ago devised an ingenious procedure. He developed flaps in the soft palate and, by means of sutures, doubled the flaps upward and backward, thus applying the two raw surfaces against each other. Dilatation was practiced afterward. In the event of failure or inability to secure satisfactory flaps from the posterior pharyngeal wall, he produced a cleft in the soft palate.

Technique. A horizontal incision is made along the normal palatal curve from one pillar to the other. From the center of this, a perpendicular incision is carried through the soft palate upward well beyond the upper line of the atresia. The adhesions are freed lateral to this on both sides. The soft palate is now divided into two triangular portions. The anterior and posterior mucous membranes of these flaps are united by a continuous or interrupted stitch across their raw edges. To make this more effective and to do away with tension as far as possible, a V-shaped trough is made in the edges of the flaps, a strip of tissue being removed from the two sides of each triangle. This requires a sharp knife and an assistant to keep the tissues taut.

Figi describes a method for relining a newly created nasopharyngeal opening with a skin graft and for maintaining the lumen by a self-retained obturator. A transverse incision about 4 cm long is made across the posterior pharyngeal wall just beneath the scarred attachment of the soft palate. The incision, carried upward and separating the palate from the posterior wall, is made large enough to admit the index finger into both posterior choanae.

A split-thickness skin graft from the abdominal wall is placed over a sponge-rubber mold containing two rubber breathing tubes. This is retained in the nasopharyngeal lumen by two heavy silk sutures extending from the upper surface of the mold through the nostrils and then tied together below the columella. The edge of the palate and the pharyngeal incision are then sutured to the mold. The mold, removed for inspection on the tenth day, is replaced by the self-retaining acrylic obturator after 2 weeks and is worn for 2 additional weeks.

NASAL TEETH

Etiology. The cause of nasal teeth is unknown. An obstruction to the downward growth of the teeth is thought to be a factor. Supernumerary teeth are present in the majority of cases. A single tooth, usually the maxillary first incisor or canine, is generally involved, but multiple nasal teeth may be seen at times.

Symptoms. Symptoms, if present, are possible obstruction to breathing on the affected side, crusting and ulceration, nasal discharge frequently with odor, bleeding from the region of the tooth, and neuralgic pain simulating trifacial neuralgia.

The diagnosis is made from the physical and roentgenographic examinations.

Treatment. Treatment, if indicated, is surgical removal.

ATRESIA OF THE ANTERIOR NARES

Atresia of the anterior nares is rare. It is much less common than atresia of the posterior nares. It may be congenital or acquired, unilateral or bilateral, complete or partial.

Etiology. Acquired atresia may be due to trauma, infections, caustics, or faulty surgical procedures.

The congenital form has been attributed to inflammatory processes during intrauterine life, a developmental anomaly of the pouch of Jacobson's organ, marked proliferation of the epithelium (Schaeffer), and persistence or plugging of the anterior nares during early embryonic life; according to Thomson, the condition may be caused by a "web of skin" at the junction of the vestibule and the nasal chamber. The condition may be the result of faulty dissolution of the tissues before birth, somewhat similar to the web found at times in the lower end of the nasolacrimal duct in the newborn.

Symptoms. The symptoms of complete bilateral occlusion in the infant include difficulty in nursing, mouth breathing, and possibly asphyxia.

Treatment. The treatment consists of surgical removal of the atretic membrane and at times the use of skin grafts to line the raw area to prevent granulations and contraction. Before the skin graft is applied, the field must be dry and the graft must adhere snugly to the exposed area. The graft is held in place for 10 days or more by means of a rubber tube or light packing.

REFERENCES

Beinfield, H. H.: Surgery for Bilateral Atresia of the Posterior Nares in the Newborn. Arch. Otolaryng., 70:1, 1959.

Bluestone, C. C., and Smith, H. C.: Intranasal Freezing for Severe Epistaxis. Arch. Otolaryng., 85:445, 1967.

Cassisi, N. J., et al.: Changes in Arterial Oxygen Tension and Pulmonary Mechanics with the Use of Posterior Packing in Epistaxis: A Preliminary Report. Laryngoscope, 81:1261, 1971.

Ogura, J. H., and Harvey, J. E.: Nasopulmonary Mechanics; Experimental Evidence of the Influence of the Upper Airway Upon the Lower. Acta Otolaryng. (Stockh.), 71:123, 1971.

Singleton, G. T., and Hardcastle, B.: Congenital Choanal Atresia. Arch. Otolaryng., 87:620, 1968.

Wilson, C. P.: Observations on the Surgery of the Nasopharynx. Ann. Otol. Rhinol. Laryngol., 66:5, 1957.

Chapter 5

Allergy, Hay Fever, Hyperesthetic Rhinitis, Asthma, Nasal Hydrorrhea

Allergy may be considered to be a pathologic hypersensitivity on the part of the allergic individual to substances or situations to which a nonallergic individual does not react or reacts minimally. The allergic reaction is mediated by the presence of an antibody which has been formed by the allergic individual in response to exposure to an antigen. Antibodies may be found circulating freely in the serum (humoral antibodies) or attached to the body cells (somatic antibodies) of the affected individual. Allergic reactions associated with humoral antibody are spoken of as *immediate allergic reactions* and are characterized by the familiar skin wheal and erythema reaction. Hay fever, asthma, and urticaria are all immediate reaction allergies, and positive skin tests are elicited by intradermal injections of the appropriate antigen. On the other hand, reactions involving somatic antibodies alone are termed *delayed allergic reactions* and do not give wheal and erythema formations. Delayed reactions include the tuberculin reaction, drug reactions, contact dermatitis, and perhaps certain allergic responses to focal infection. The particular antibody which is responsible for wheal formation in the immediate reaction (e.g., hay fever) is termed *reaginic antibody* and possesses the characteristic of attaching itself to the skin cells.

Allergy itself is not considered to be hereditary; rather, the existence of a family predisposition to allergic disease may be present. Reaginic antibodies may, on the other hand, be genetically related. Familial allergic disease is commonly spoken of as *atopic allergy.*

Most antigens are considered to be protein in nature, although polysaccharides attached to a protein may be allergenic. Some drugs and chemicals are thought to be capable of inducing antibody response. Sensitization can occur via parenteral, respiratory, oral, or other routes. Cooke has described the "blocking antibody" as an explanation of desensitization in patients suffering from immediate reaction allergies. This antibody appears in the serum following repeated parenteral injections of pollen antigens and is capable of reducing the wheal reaction. Blocking antibodies are more heat-stable than other antibodies and do not attach themselves to the skin, thus distinguishing them from reaginic antibody.

A great deal more needs to be learned about the chemical mechanisms involved in the allergic response. The wheal formation and anaphylactic shock are related to *histamine,* or at least injection of histamine alone can closely reproduce these conditions.

Recently, 5-hydroxytryptamine (serotonin) has been implicated in the allergic state, but again additional evidence is needed. In addition, heparin and other substances are probably involved. Roentgen irradiation, if administered before the injection of the antigen, reduces the antibody response. The tissue injury of an allergic reaction results from the union of the antigen and antibody which is still attached to the cell.

AUTONOMIC DYSFUNCTION

In 1951 Henry L. Williams introduced the concept of autonomic dysfunction in relation to allergic disease. He believed that there is an inherited abnormal activity or "dysfunction" of the autonomic nervous system (more specifically the cholinergic fibers) which predisposes the affected individual to allergic disease. The abnormal activity of the cholinergic nerves can be initiated by physical stress (including fatigue), emotional perturbation, endocrine imbalance, and perhaps such physical factors as barometric pressure change. This entity can be loosely spoken of as *physical allergy*. The term autonomic imbalance should probably not be employed in speaking of the nose, because the nasal blood vessels are under the control of the sympathetic side of the autonomic system, and the parasympathetic side plays little or no part.

In the anatomic area of autonomic dysfunction, a stereotyped reaction of the peripheral vascular bed occurs. This consists of "arteriolar spasm with atonic dilation" of the distal capillaries and venules. Because of the block produced by the arteriolar spasm, an anoxic state of the capillary loop results, with greater or lesser cellular damage, the release of histamine, increase of capillary permeability, and allergic edema or necrosis. He terms this the basic allergic unit. It may occur through the activity of the cholinergic nerves of the autonomic nervous system in the absence of conventional antibodies or antigens of any kind. In seasonal allergies in which pollens usually are the antigen, there is an antigen-antibody reaction associated with the same vascular reaction described above and characterized by a positive skin test. In delayed allergic sensitivity reactions, the same vascular reaction is presumably present, but skin tests are negative. The allergic reaction does not occur in an area devoid of blood vessels, such as the cornea of the eye.

Diagnosis of Allergy. The diagnosis of allergy rests primarily on a complete and careful history and physical examination which fit the case at hand into one of the syndromes (e.g., hay fever) to be described subsequently. The presence of the following in the history also supports a diagnosis of allergy: a positive family history, previous instances of allergy in the patient under consideration, recurrent or seasonal attacks of disability not otherwise explained, and eosinophilia of the blood or secretions. Skin tests are of great use in wheal and erythema allergies, as explained previously. They are most useful in pollen and inhalant allergies and are least useful in food allergies. Rinkel believes that skin tests are clinically accurate 40 per cent of the time.

Skin Tests. For the diagnosis of wheal and erythema allergies, scratch and intracutaneous skin tests are useful. Extracts are usually standardized on the basis of content by weight and their dilution or by content of protein nitrogen. In the latter case, one unit represents 0.01 microgram of protein nitrogen. Of the two methods, the scratch test is safer and easier to employ and thus is preferred for children. Both methods are most reliable when used for pollen type allergies and of least use when testing for food allergies.

The technique of the *scratch test* is as follows. After the skin is cleansed with alcohol and ether, a sterile needle or other scarifier is used to abrade or scratch the outer layer of the epidermis, but not deep enough to draw blood. The abrasions are 2 to 4 mm long. Into the abraded area pollen extract (1:20 dilution in 50% glycerin) or other allergen is gently rubbed. Within 10 to 20 minutes a positive reaction occurs and is characterized by a pale raised wheal measuring 0.5 to 2.5 cm in diameter, surrounded by a zone of erythema measuring 2 to 10 cm in diameter. The reaction begins to fade within 30 to 40 minutes, but some evidence remains for 6 to 24 hours or longer. False reactions occur because of the trauma itself or because of the vehicle solution.

In making the intracutaneous test, minute quantities (usually 0.05 ml) of fluid extracts of the suspected allergen are injected by small needles (usually No. 25 or 26) between the outer layers of the skin. The injection must be sufficiently superficial, so that a slightly blanched 3-mm to 4-mm elevation of the skin is created at the point of emission from the needle. If hypersensitivity to the injected substances exists, the positive reaction appears in 5 to 30 minutes and consists of a distinct urticarial wheal, having a sharply defined but irregular border, surrounded by a zone of erythema, and frequently characterized by itching. The wheal varies from 0.5 to 2.5 cm in diameter, and the erythema is several times that size. Again, false reactions may occur because of the trauma itself or the vehicle solution.

For the intracutaneous test, extracts of 1:10 million to 1:100 million are used, depending on the suspected clinical sensitivity of the patient. If after 0.05 ml of one of the more dilute extracts is tried a positive wheal is not obtained, a less dilute extract is tried. In a general way the greater the clinical hypersensitivity of the patient, the more dilute will be the extract producing a positive wheal.

Commonly, the flexor surface of the forearm or the lateral aspect of the upper arm is selected for the scratch or intradermal tests, though the posterior thorax may be used. The test sites should be 2 to 3 cm apart, and it is safer to do only eight to ten tests at a time so as to avoid severe reactions. In the event of a severe or constitutional reaction, a tourniquet is immediately applied above the site of the test and 8 to 10 minims epinephrine injected above the tourniquet. As the reaction of the patient subsides, the tourniquet is experimentally loosened for short periods, and finally its use is entirely discontinued.

It is the experience of all who have administered skin tests that clinically unimportant positive reactions occur commonly. They may indicate only that a great allergic potential is present in the particular patient involved.

Treatment of Allergy. The simplest and most effective form of treatment of allergic disease is avoidance of the offending agent when possible. When this is impossible, recourse must be had to palliative drug therapy or to attempts to desensitize the patient to the specific allergens bothering him.

Of the many palliative drugs used in the treatment of allergy, the antihistamines are the most useful. They produce satisfactory relief of symptoms in the majority of cases of pollen and inhalant sensitivity but little or no relief in the delayed reaction and food allergies. Almost all the various antihistaminic drugs now on the market produce the undesirable side effect of drowsiness. Combining the antihistamines with a vasoconstrictor drug, such as ephedrine, causes a desirable decongestant effect and combats the drowsiness.

More potent than the antihistamines in relieving severe symptoms are the adrenal cortical steroids. These drugs suppress allergic reactions, including those characterized by humoral antibodies (hay fever, urticaria, asthma, etc.) as well as those displaying cellular hypersensitivity, in many locations. The presence of diabetes mellitus, peptic ulcer, tuberculosis, hypertension, and certain mental disturbances usually contraindicates the use of the cortical steroids. The concomitant presence of infection usually requires simultaneous use of antibiotic therapy.

Techniques and methods involved in specific desensitization by multiple injections are included below in the discussion of the disease itself.

HAY FEVER

Definition. Hay fever is a recurrent seasonal ailment due to an abnormal hypersensitivity to pollens, principally, and characterized chiefly by watery rhinitis with sneezing, nasal obstruction, and itching of the nose, eyes, and throat. *Allergic rhinitis* is a more general term and is not characterized by seasonal periodicity, though it is of allergic etiology and in other respects may resemble hay fever. *Vasomotor rhinitis* is a more inclusive term denoting an abnormality of the vasomotor control of the nose; it may or may not be of allergic origin. Recurrent pollinosis is a synonym for hay fever.

Etiology. Ragweed pollen is the principal offending plant causing hay fever in the United States, but any pollinating plant that depends on the wind for cross pollination may be the offending agent, including the grasses, many weeds, and trees. Plants pollinated by insects, including most flowering plants, such as roses, goldenrod, and dandelion, are not important causes of hay fever unless the patient is in intimate contact with them. Other airborne antigenic particles have also been incriminated in the etiology of hay fever. These include feathers, dust, animal danders, facial powder, fungus, weeds, and clothing. The particular season during which symptoms appear depends on the pollinating calendar of the plant in question. Reference to books on allergy can be made for such tables. In northern and eastern parts of the United States the pollination is as follows:

1. Early spring, usually occurring in April and early May, due to pollens from trees.

2. Late spring or early summer, usually occurring in May to August, due largely to pollens from the following grasses: timothy *(Phleum pratense),* sweet vernal *(Abthoxanthum odoratum),* June or Kentucky bluegrass *(Poa pratensis),* orchard grass *(Dactylis glomerata),* redtop *(Agrostis alba* or *palustris),* and rye *(Secale cereale).*

3. Fall, occurring about the middle of August until frost, due to a large extent to the giant and dwarf ragweed pollens *(Ambrosia).*

The grasses causing the late spring or early summer hay fever, named in their order of pollination, are: sweet vernal beginning the first or second week in May; June grass the second or third week in May; orchard grass the third or fourth week in May; timothy, redtop, and rye the first or second week in June. Pollination continues in all these grasses until about the middle of July.

Timothy is the most important of the grass pollens producing mid and late summer hay fever in the northern and eastern states. Bermuda grass and Johnson grass are the most important in the southeastern states. In the Middle West, broom grass and bluegrass predominate.

The ragweed *(Ambrosia)* type of hay fever, which makes its appearance in the early fall, is the most severe and longest in duration of any of the seasonal attacks. On account of its buoyancy, this type of pollen is very widely distributed. The pollen granules are carried even by light winds several miles from their source. In the eastern part of the United States, the ragweeds (giant and common) are the most abundant members of this family. The Western ragweed, sandbur, and marsh elder are the most important causes of fall hay fever in the western States; the wormwoods (mugwort, sagebrush) and franseria predominate on the Pacific Coast. In the Southwest, the amaranths (careless weed and pigweed), saltbush, and the chenopods (lamb's quarters) are important during late summer and fall.

There are many localities to which these generalizations do not apply. In some districts other plants, less common than those named above, predominate.

Hay fever from grasses is more prevalent in England and on the Continent than in this country.

It has been estimated that the late spring and summer cases occur about eight times as frequently as the early spring type, and the fall type about twice as frequently as the summer cases. About 5% of the cases are attributed to the airborne tree pollens (particularly willow, hickory, ash, oak, elm, and black walnut). These cases are limited for the most part to a period of 1 or 2 weeks in the early spring. About 26% of hay fever sufferers have the combined summer and fall types.

The various plants that are pollinated by insects, such as clover, dandelion, daisies, honeysuckle, roses, and goldenrod, are not of great importance, as patients susceptible to these pollens are affected by intimate contact only. As a result, attacks from these pollens are few in number and more or less mild in type.

Symptoms and Pathology. The symptoms of hay fever resemble in many ways those of acute coryza, but there is no fever. The hay fever patient during a period of exacerbation of his symptoms is seized by varying degrees of malaise. His paroxysmal sneezing is bothersome, especially since it is accompanied by profuse lacrimation and a serous nasal discharge, which may excoriate the upper lip. Adding to his discomfort is the engorged, edematous nasal mucosa which causes nasal obstruction. Characteristically the upper lip of the hay fever sufferer is raised habitually in an attempt to overcome the nasal blockage. Moreover, he repeatedly wipes the anterior nares, perhaps with the palm of his hand *(allergic salute)* or a handkerchief.

Symptoms are worse on dry, sunny, windy days when the pollen can be disseminated widely. On rainy days the amount of pollen in the air is less, and symptoms are decreased. Areas relatively free of pollen are to the same degree relatively free of hay fever sufferers.

Examination of the patient reveals the nasal mucosa to be pale, wet, and edematous, so that nasal obstruction is apparent. Superimposed infection leads to the formation of purulent matter rather than a simple serous discharge containing an abundance of eosinophils, which characterizes the uncomplicated case. Nasal polyps further obstruct the nasal airway and exaggerate the infection. Many patients with hay fever eventually develop asthma.

Treatment. The successful care of a hay fever patient revolves around three factors: avoidance of the offending pollen, palliative drug therapy, and specific hyposensitization by injection of the offending allergen.

Complete avoidance of the causative pollen, for example, by temporary removal of the patient to a pollen-free area, is the simplest and most efficient way to provide symptomatic relief of hay fever. When this is not possible, partial avoidance can be obtained by use of suitable pollen filters or by air conditioning.

The most useful drugs for palliative relief of symptoms of hay fever are the so-called "antihistamines." There are a large number of these on the market, and frequently several must be tried before one is found that provides adequate relief from symptoms as well as freedom from the side effect of drowsiness, which all antihistamines possess to some degree. Combining the antihistamine with a drug such as ephedrine provides some decongestant vasoconstrictor action as well as a counterforce to the tendency to drowsiness. The antihistamines as a group are most effective in drying the nasal mucosa as well as in decreasing the tendency to sneeze.

In those situations in which the symptoms are more distressing and more acute, recourse may have to be made to adrenal cortical steroids. These drugs, given orally, frequently are extraordinarily effective in relieving the symptoms of allergic rhinitis, including hay fever, and were it not for their side effects, they would be more widely used. Hydrocortisone in doses of 25 to 100 mg each day is usually quite effective. Also prednisone, 5 to 20 mg, or methylprednisone, 4 to 12 mg orally, will usually be effective.

A variety of agents are available for "shrinking" or decongesting the nasal mucosa to provide relief from nasal obstruction. These agents can be used locally as nose drops but preferably are taken orally. Ephedrine in amounts of 15 mg (often combined with an antihistamine) taken orally four times a day will be helpful.

The use of specific desensitization should be reserved for the more severe cases of hay fever which do not respond to the above and probably all cases in which asthma plays a significant role. Desensitization is accomplished by multiple subcutaneous injections of the specific antigen in increasing dosage. Treatment is preferably begun 4 to 6 weeks before the onset of hay fever season. A controversy exists as to the size of the dose to be administered. After obtaining some idea of the degree of sensitivity of the patient from the history as well as the skin tests, safety demands that the initial dose be well below the tolerance level of the patient. Then at intervals of 4 to 7 days, increasing amounts of the specific antigen are injected. The end point is usually the point at which the patient experiences satisfactory relief of his symptoms. As the patient improves, the length of time between injections is increased to 10 to 30 days and then discontinued. Thus let us assume an intracutaneous skin test with giant ragweed (see above) in a dilution of 1:100,000 produces a wheal of 7 to 8 mm and an erythema of 3 to 4 cm in diameter. This is considered a moderately positive skin test. Treatment should begin with the same amount injected to produce the skin reaction but ten times more dilute. The second injection 4 to 7 days later is more concentrated, depending on clinical judgment. Injections are usually given subcutaneously, though in the more sensitive individual the intracutaneous method provides a greater margin of safety. In an uncomplicated case suitable injection treatment successfully alleviates symptoms in 75% of cases.

All patients should be observed for 20 to 30 minutes following an injection because of the danger of an untoward reaction. If this does occur, a tourniquet is applied above the site of the injection, and 0.3 to 0.5 ml of epinephrine 1:1000 is injected subcutaneously above the tourniquet.

PERENNIAL ALLERGIC RHINITIS

Definition. Perennial allergic rhinitis is essentially the same as hay fever except that symptoms persist unabated throughout all or most of the year. Seasonal exacerbations may be present, however. *Hyperesthetic rhinitis* is a synonym. Vasomotor rhinitis, on the other hand, designates an abnormality of the vasomotor control of the nose, which may be allergy-related or may be related to nonallergenic causes (e.g., endocrine malfunction).

Etiology. Most cases of perennial allergic rhinitis find their etiology in airborne allergens, particularly dusts, though infective agents, foods, and drugs may play a part. Dust as collected in various locations in the home and office contains a multitude of allergic factors: animal danders, feathers, down, cottonseed, orris, food, molds, etc. Commercial products are available containing a wide spectrum of these substances.

Chronic allergic rhinitis due to bacterial allergy is more likely to be accompanied by nasal polyps and hyperplastic mucosa.

Symptoms and Signs. The chief complaint is nasal blockage, perhaps alternating from side to side, throughout the year and with only minimal seasonal variation. The patient complains of a "wetness" of his nose, so that he must sniff or clear his throat repeatedly; the patient may call his condition "postnasal drip." Some of the wetness is probably due to the irritative effect of various air pollutants (see p. 21). The nasal discharge, in the absence of infection, is colorless and mucoid. In acute attacks the symptoms of perennial allergic rhinitis are virtually identical to those of hay fever.

The appearance of the nasal mucosa in perennial allergic rhinitis is that of a wet, edematous membrane which is grayish blue in color. It can be deeply indented by probe palpation. The secretions contain a high proportion of eosinophils. If infection has been superimposed, redness, pus, and other evidence of acute inflammation may be present. Quite commonly nasal polyposis accompanies any infected allergic rhinitis.

Skin tests to inhalant antigens should be done as described in the section on hay fever in an attempt to make a specific diagnosis. Positive tests must be interpreted in the light of the history and the patient's environment. Tests with food antigens are indicated only if the history suggests that a relationship is possible. Skin tests are not satisfactory for determining the existence of a bacterial allergy. Bacterial and food allergy are more easily evaluated by a careful history.

Treatment. As in the case of hay fever, the greatest success is found in those cases in which the sensitivities are few and the allergens can be completely avoided. Since this, unfortunately, is usually not the case, recourse must be made to the symptomatic palliative measures, to specific therapy, and to elimination of infections which might give rise to bacterial sensitivity.

Avoidance of Allergens. When the substance to which the patient is hypersensitive is known, it should be eliminated from the environment, if possible, whether it be a household pet or something else. If the allergen is wool, for example, this substance must be eliminated from the body clothing, bed blankets, etc. The various allergens which can be eliminated are legion.

Frequently the environment can be reasonably well controlled except for house dust, which is ubiquitous and present the year round. Bed pillows and mattresses are a potent source of dust, so nonallergenic foam rubber products may be substituted, or the pillow and mattress may be encased in a tight-fitting plastic cover. Simple wooden furniture, light washable draperies and rugs, and frequent housecleaning all help to some extent. Likewise air conditioning aids in dust control.

Palliative Measures. The use of locally administered nose drops or sprays affords temporary relief to the nasal blockage but is a measure which is easily abused and thus generally is to be discouraged. Prolonged use of nose drops may be accompanied by a *"rebound" phenomenon* in which the initial vasoconstriction is followed by a secondary congestion. This demands more nose drops, and thus their use ever increases. It is preferable to administer decongestant (vasoconstrictor) drugs by mouth (see Treatment, under Hay Fever).

Antihistamine drugs are useful in the treatment of perennial allergic rhinitis and particularly should be tried during an acute exacerbation. Between exacerbations, however, they are of limited value. Combining them with a decongestant helps to relieve the nasal blockage.

During more severe attacks of allergic rhinitis, particularly if polyps obstruct the nasal airway and the free drainage of the paranasal sinuses into the nose, the adrenal cortical steroid drugs may be used. Prednisone, 20 to 30 mg per day in four divided daily doses, frequently reduces the obstruction rapidly, so that free drainage ensues. These steroids are not suitable for prolonged use, however, because of their side effects. If secondary infection is also present, antibiotic medication should simultaneously be used.

Most frequently in the treatment of perennial rhinitis recourse must be made to specific injection treatment to lessen sensitivities to allergens that cannot be avoided. If the sensitivities are few, this is not difficult, and some measure of success follows. Many times it is necessary to assume house dust is the principal uncontrolled etiologic agent and attempts made to desensitize to this substance. By using the technique described under Hay Fever, some idea of the degree of the sensitivity to house dust can be obtained by skin tests. The first injection is then well below this degree of sensitivity, and the injections are continued at intervals of 4 to 7 days until satisfactory relief is obtained, at which point no further increase in size of dose occurs. The same dosage is then repeated every 2 to 4 weeks throughout the year, depending on the response of the patient.

Elimination of Infection. A great deal of additional accurate information is necessary before true evaluation is possible of the part played by infection of the nose and sinuses. If bacterial sensitization occurs, it is of the delayed allergic reaction type (see introductory statement on allergy). Infection of the nose and sinuses should be eliminated. During acute infections antibiotics offer the best form of treatment. Surgical measures to provide adequate drainage of the sinuses, removal of nasal polyps, adenoidectomy, and tonsillectomy may be necessary in chronic infection. Autogenous vaccines may warrant a trial, though their use is difficult to evaluate.

PERENNIAL VASOMOTOR RHINITIS

Definition. Perennial vasomotor rhinitis is a somewhat obscure disease entity indicating an abnormality of the vasomotor control of the nose and characterized mainly by nasal obstruction. The specific etiologic agent usually cannot be determined, although it seems most often to be of an allergic nature, particularly if the allergic reaction is of the delayed sensitivity type. Without doubt there is some etiologic significance to endocrine malfunction and physical allergy (see Autonomic Dysfunction), but the extent to which these agents are influential is not clear. Air pollution is likely a factor as well. In this regard it should be remembered that gaseous SO_2 is about 99% absorbed by the nasal mucosa. Nasal congestion and other evidences of irritation would not be unexpected. The presence of SO_2 adsorbed onto small particles (less than 0.3 to 0.4 $m\mu$) facilitates passage of the gas to the lower respiratory tract.

Symptoms and Signs. A history is usually obtained of frequent nasal infections and nasal blockage, frequently associated with itching of the nose and palate. The persistent nasal blockage which alternates from side to side and continues month after month despite orthodox allergic management is a commonplace complaint of the patient. The nose is "wet," so that sniffling is constantly necessary; perhaps the patient is aware of "postnasal dripping" and notes only minor relationship to the seasons, though the summer is likely an improvement over the winter. Geographic location is of little importance, though an urban environment may enhance his symptoms.

Examination of the nasal mucosa reveals moderate edema, but without superimposed infection. Skin tests fail to reveal the presence of humoral antibodies, though, as mentioned, the presence of delayed allergic sensitivity cannot be ruled out.

Treatment. If some etiologic clue has been discovered, treatment should be directed to the eradication of the same, as described under Perennial Allergic Rhinitis. When necessary, treatment must include supportive therapy for the endocrine glands (particularly the thyroid) and correction of the various factors discussed under Autonomic Dysfunction.

ASTHMA

Definition. Asthma (or bronchial asthma) is a type of pulmonary incompetence, characterized chiefly by expiratory dyspnea, cough, overinflation of the lungs, expiratory wheezing, and rhonchi. The symptoms usually occur in attacks with complete freedom between. Frequently they are seasonal in incidence.

Etiology. The majority of cases of asthma are due to extrinsic factors such as inhaled or ingested allergens. Etiologically inhalant allergens, such as pollens, animal danders, dusts, weeds, and fungi, are the most important factors. Ingested foods are of less importance. Intrinsic asthma constitutes a smaller proportion of the total number of cases and is caused by the bronchiolar response to indwelling body factors, primarily respiratory infections. Extrinsic asthma is clearly of allergic origin; there is disagreement about the origin of intrinsic asthma.

Once the allergic asthmatic pattern to intrinsic allergens has developed, other factors unrelated to the original situation may be present. These include emotional stress, atmospheric change, irritating air pollutants, and physical fatigue (see p. 21).

Pathology. Obstruction of the bronchial airway is generalized and is produced by viscid secretions containing abundant eosinophils in the lumina, mucosal and submucosal edema, hypertrophy of the bronchial walls, and contraction of bronchial smooth muscles. Varying degrees of emphysema accompany asthma, depending on the degree and chronicity of the expiratory obstruction. The bronchial epithelium shows many goblet cells and mucous glands. The number of ciliated cells available for removing the excess mucus is reduced.

The mechanism of allergic reaction for the extrinsic forms of asthma is that of the immediate erythema-wheal type. For the intrinsic form the mechanism is likely that of a delayed reaction type of allergy. Humoral antibodies usually cannot be demonstrated in intrinsic asthma.

Symptoms and Signs. In its typical form asthma occurs in an attack. The onset is marked by a sense of suffocation and cough. Soon expiratory dyspnea and wheezes are experienced and are frequently audible to the patient and bystanders alike. Often the patient prefers to sit upright or lean forward to gain maximum use of his accessory respiratory muscles. Termination of the wheezing and dyspnea usually occurs within 1 to 2 hours but is followed by a cough productive of tenacious mucus. Attacks may last for many hours (status asthmaticus).

Physical signs of asthma are obvious. The wheezing may be audible to the unaided ear and is readily apparent when a stethoscope is used, being heard throughout the chest and best during the expiratory phase. A localized area of wheezing is more suggestive of a foreign body or a patch of infection. Signs of emphysema may also be present.

Microscopic examination of the tenacious sputum usually shows large numbers of eosinophils and occasionally crystals (Curschmann's spirals). Purulent sputum is indicative of superimposed infection. Only rarely is there gross blood found in the sputum.

Hay fever sometimes precedes the development of asthma, or they may occur simultaneously. This type of asthma is observed most commonly below the age of 30 and is usually seasonal and of extrinsic origin. Individuals suffering their first attack of asthma after the age of about 30 are more likely to manifest a nonseasonal incidence and show a positive relation between attacks and infections (intrinsic).

Diagnosis. A family or personal history of allergic disease is helpful in recognizing allergic asthma. The presence of localized wheezing in the lungs of a suspected asthmatic is to be interpreted with caution, as mentioned above. Allergic asthmatic wheezing is typically an expiratory phenomenon. Between two asthmatic attacks the lungs are remarkably clear. In allergic asthma there is an increase in airway resistance, and a blood eosinophilia of 8 to 10% or more may be present.

Skin tests for humoral antibodies as described under Hay Fever are present in allergic asthma, particularly when the antigen is extrinsic. In intrinsic cases when the allergen is related to infection, the skin tests are generally negative, and the diagnosis must be made largely on the basis of history.

Treatment. Greatest success follows the removal of the offending allergens from the patient's environment. Since this is frequently impossible or the specific allergens cannot be determined, additional measures are necessary. Infections, particularly upper respiratory infections, should be eliminated and the environmental air rendered as clean and inoffensive as possible. In those cases in which the allergen is known with some certainty, specific desensitization should be tried.

Prophylactic treatment of asthma primarily involves the use of bronchodilators. Ephedrine, 15 to 25 mg, in combination with a similar amount of pentobarbital taken four times a day by mouth is frequently used. Aminophylline may be added to the above. Antihistamines are less protective in asthma than in hay fever.

Prompt relief of an acute attack usually follows 0.2 to 0.5 ml of a 1:1000 solution of epinephrine cautiously injected subcutaneously and repeated in one-half hour if necessary. The epinephrine may be used in oil, 0.5 to 1.0 ml of a 1:500 solution injected intramuscularly every 6 hours or so. In refractory situations aminophylline (0.25 to 0.5 g) in 1 liter of glucose may slowly be given intravenously. Also for the intractable case the adrenal cortical steroids are advisable and, if necessary, may be continued for long periods. Morphine is contraindicated in asthmatics because of its tendency to contract the bronchioles. In persistent severe asthma with retention of thick sputum, bronchoscopic aspiration is sometimes effective.

For home use during less severe attacks, nebulized epinephrine and its analogues can be used. The epinephrine is usually in a 1:100 solution and is deeply inhaled by the patient.

URTICARIA

Definition. Urticaria or hives is a skin eruption characterized by sharply defined and transitory elevated wheals, usually accompanied by erythema and itching.

Etiology. The allergic mechanism principally involved is the immediate hypersensitivity reaction, though such nonspecific agents as emotional tension, physical exercise, and heat occasionally seem to be the cause. Urticaria may follow allergens which are ingested, inhaled, or merely externally contacted.

Symptoms. Typically the urticarial lesion is well demarcated, 1 to 4 cm in diameter, and raised so as to be easily palpable. Individual lesions fade, usually within 6 to 24 hours. They may be localized or generalized over the body.

Treatment. When the allergen is known, it should be eliminated. Acute symptoms can usually be relieved with antihistamine drugs, but occasionally adrenal cortical steroids are required. Symptomatic relief can also be secured with epinephrine 1:1000 injected hypodermically in doses of 0.4 to 0.6 ml.

Angioedema

Angioedema (angioneurotic edema or giant hives) is an allergic phenomenon which is similar to urticaria. The edematous swellings may be localized or diffuse and are most commonly located on the face, hands, feet, and genitalia. The much more dangerous situation of possible airway obstruction occurs if the lips, tongue, pharynx, or larynx is involved, and in such cases tracheostomy may be lifesaving.

ACUTE CIRCUMSCRIBED EDEMA OF THE NOSE; CORYZA OEDEMATOSA

This affection may involve both the pharynx and larynx in the same case. It is not an inflammatory affection but is probably an edema of allergic origin. It is quite like urticaria, though it involves the mucous membrane. It is usually associated with other symptoms or diseases, such as hay fever, urticaria of the skin, headache, gastrointestinal disturbances, and itching.

The treatment should be directed to the allergic factor producing the circumscribed edema.

NASAL HYDRORRHEA; RHINAL HYDRORRHEA

Nasal hydrorrhea, usually allergic, is characterized by a thin, watery, slightly opalescent secretion more or less serous in type. The amount of discharge varies from a few drams to several ounces in 24 hours. The secretion when tested with alcohol or acetic acid throws down a stringy precipitate like mucin. When the precipitate is boiled with dilute sulfuric acid, a sugarlike material is formed, probably because of the presence of mucin. The protein is coagulated by heat; it does not reduce Fehling's solution. Peptones and proteoses are absent. The alcohol extract of the secretions contains no reducing substance. The secretion may be distinguished from normal cerebrospinal fluid by the presence of mucin and the absence of a reducing substance.

Symptoms. The clinical picture of nasal hydrorrhea may resemble that of allergic rhinitis, with symptoms of intense local irritation, or it may consist of a passive and almost painless watery discharge from the nose. It is apparently a disease of adult life, which affects males and females equally. Although it may be more marked on one side of the nose than on the other, the flow usually comes from both nostrils. When handkerchiefs are soaked with it, they generally become stiff when dry. In cerebrospinal rhinorrhea, on the other hand, the discharge is so watery that handkerchiefs dry quite soft; in this affection the discharge is limited entirely to one nostril, unless there happens to be some obstruction on the affected side, when it may make its way to the opposite nasal fossa. When the fluid is of arachnoid origin, headache or other mental symptoms are frequent but are relieved by the discharge. The latter disease is not accompanied by lacrimation or suffusion of the conjunctiva and photophobia. It may occasionally give rise to sneezing, especially in the morning.

In nasal hydrorrhea the feeling of malaise begins with the discharge and only stops with its cessation. It is frequently ushered in with sneezing, photophobia, and lacrimation. It rarely continues during sleep, while cerebrospinal rhinorrhea continues day and night. It is erratic in its onset and in its intermissions and is dependent on external influences and on conditions of health.

Treatment. The treatment should be addressed to the various etiologic factors found in hay fever or forms of hyperesthetic rhinitis or to any other pathologic condition present in the nose and accessory sinuses.

CEREBROSPINAL RHINORRHEA

King in 1834 made a notable contribution to rhinologic literature when he described for the first time the escape of cerebrospinal fluid from the nose. Such cases had been previously regarded as nasal hydrorrhea.

Etiology. The possible etiologic factors are: some pathologic change in the contents of the skull leading to increased intracranial pressure; fracture of the anterior fossa of the skull involving the cribriform plate; dehiscence in the walls of the sphenoid sinus; pressure necrosis or ulceration from tumors of the brain or infection of the sinuses; hydrocephalus internus; a defect in the craniopharyngeal canal (forced open by an increase in cerebrospinal fluid); herniation of the cerebellum and brain stem through the foramen magnum into the vertebral canal by way of the perineural sheath of the olfactory nerve and by way of the lymph passages from the arachnoid spaces.

Symptoms. The fluid is clear and watery in contrast to the slightly opalescent and more viscid fluid of nasal hydrorrhea. The dripping is usually intermittent but may be constant. It is free from sediment, odor, albumin, and mucin. It usually escapes from the same nostril day and night for many days. It may disappear and reappear suddenly.

Glucose is present in the fluid, and no precipitate (mucin) is found when acetic acid is added. It is faintly alkaline in reaction and is either tasteless or slightly salty. The specific gravity is between 1.005 and 1.010.

Chapter 6
Headache and Neuralgia of the Face and Head

HEADACHE

Headache is a prominent symptom of many disorders of the body, both organic and functional. It may be associated with some generalized disease; it may be a prominent symptom of a disordered organ or localized region; or it may be the result of frustration, resentment, and dissatisfaction on the part of the patient and thus be independent of any recognizable organic disease. In the following discussion an attempt will be made to systematize headaches, but many gaps in our knowledge exist.

Origin of Head Pain

Data collected by Wolff and others indicate that all the extracranial structures covering the head are pain-sensitive, but only portions of the intracranial structures are pain-sensitive. Of the extracranial structures particularly important as the site of origin of headache are the arteries of the scalp, the pericranium, the muscles of the scalp and upper neck, the orbital contents, the external and middle ear, and, of course, the paranasal sinuses. While pain in these structures is frequently confined to the site of origin, it may extend more widely to other parts of the head.

Intracranial structures sensitive to painful stimuli include: (1) the meningeal arteries; (2) the arteries at the base of the brain leading to and emerging from the circle of Willis; (3) the major venous sinuses; and (4) the dural floor of the anterior and posterior fossae. Insensitive to pain are the brain parenchyma, most of the pia-arachnoid and dura, the ependymal lining of the ventricles, the choroid plexus, and the cranium.

Generally speaking, a head pain located anterior to a vertical line through the external auditory meatus, if from an intracranial source, is usually transmitted by one or more of the three branches of the fifth cranial nerve and has its origin in lesions above or on the tentorium cerebelli. Head pain located posterior to this line is carried chiefly by the tenth cranial nerve, but it is also carried by the ninth, eleventh, and twelfth cranial nerves and the upper three cervical nerves and has its origin in lesions found below the tentorium. When the headache is clearly localized behind one ear, homolateral acoustic neuromas and cerebellopontile angle tumors should be considered.

Mechanisms of Headache

Extracranial mechanisms which may lead to headache include the following: (1) painful distention of cranial arteries; (2) sustained skeletal muscle contraction about the face, scalp, and particularly the neck near the occiput; (3) various disease processes of the eyes, ears, teeth, nose, and paranasal sinuses; (4) the cranial nerve neuralgias; (5) nonspecific inflammations of the cranial

115

arteries; and (6) pain incident to injury, infection, or tumors, frequently by direct pressure or indirectly by traction. The great majority of *extracranial pain* arises from either the first (the "vascular headache") or the second (the muscle "tension" or muscle contraction headache) category.

"Vascular headaches" are caused by a painful dilation of certain pain-sensitive arteries of the head. The pathology is more completely described under Migraine Headache. If the vascular headache is recurrent, it is classified as a migraine type of headache. If it is nonrecurrent, the disorder is associated with a number of conditions, chief among which is the combination of fever and systemic infection. Also associated with nonrecurrent vasodilating head pain are hypoxic states, CO poisoning, vasodilating chemical agents, caffeine withdrawal, postconcussion and postconvulsive states, "hangover" reactions, hypoglycemia, hypercapnia, and acute pressor reactions. This list could be extended.

Vascular headaches of the recurrent or migraine type are characterized by recurrent episodes of throbbing, pulsating head pain (at least at the onset). The ache is caused principally by the painful dilation of one or more extracranial branches and, probably, of the dural (intracranial) branches of the external carotid artery. Occipital neuralgia is most likely due to the painful distension of the postauricular and occipital arteries. Distension of the extracranial portion of the middle meningeal artery and of the internal maxillary artery may lead to "atypical facial neuralgias," including the "lower half headache" of Sluder and vidian neuralgia of Vail. Also included in this recurrent vasodilating group are "cluster headaches," which are probably identical to the "ciliary neuralgia" described in earlier editions of this textbook.

A steady, constant, nonpulsating ache on one or both sides of the head or neck is characteristic of muscle tension headache. It is due to long-sustained contraction of the skeletal muscles about the face, scalp, and neck and may be secondary to a vascular headache. Muscle tension and vasodilating mechanisms combined explain the great majority of all headaches.

The principal intracranial mechanisms which lead to a headache include: (1) direct pressure on a pain-sensitive nerve or structure; (2) inflammation or irritation of the pain-sensitive structure of the head or portions of the dura and pia at the base of the skull; (3) distension of the intracranial arteries; (4) traction on and displacement of the pain-sensitive arteries, including the middle meningeal; and (5) traction on or displacement of the veins that are tributary to the venous sinuses from the surface of the brain. Intracranial headaches are increased in intensity by a jolt of the head.

Traction Headache. Headache may result from traction on pain-sensitive intracranial structures by masses of various types: tumors, hematomas, abscesses, etc. The traction may result directly from local displacement or indirectly from displacement of continuous intracranial structures until a pain-sensitive structure is displaced and pain generated. In general, the site of the pain, particularly if continuous, aids in the localization of a brain tumor. In the absence of papilledema, a one-sided headache indicates a lesion on the same side. With a tumor of the posterior fossa, the ache is usually in the back of the head, and with a tumor above the tentorium, in the absence of papilledema, the lesion is usually located in the anterior part of the head.

Headache that follows lumbar puncture is included in this group of traction headaches. It is thought that the loss of spinal fluid leads to traction of the brain on various pain-sensitive structures which anchor it to the cranium. Such postpuncture headaches can be relieved by elevation of the intracranial pressure to normal.

MIGRAINE HEADACHE

Migraine headache is characterized by a periodic, unilateral (at least at the outset) headache of some hours' duration with complete freedom between attacks. Not infrequently the attack is introduced by scotomata, hemianopia, paresthesia, or speech disorders. The presence of a preheadache differentiates migraine from "cluster" headaches discussed in a later section. The length of an attack varies from a few minutes to 8 to 12 hours, but the headache may occasionally last for a few days.

Etiology. Although the true etiology of migraine headache is not known, there are certain common historical features that can be elicited. Frequently there is a family history of migraine and one in which the females are more frequently afflicted than the males. Many of these women note that the attacks are more severe during the menses but may cease during pregnancy or after the menopause. Characteristically the onset of migraine is during adolescence.

Life situations which engender stress, frustration, and dissatisfaction are quite likely to precipitate an attack. It is common to note that these patients are rigid and perfectionist in demeanor. They do not bend or adjust easily to new conditions but instead become resentful and dissatisfied. Many observers believe allergy, especially to foods, plays a part in the etiology, but the evidence to support this view is meager. Physical allergy as described by Henry Williams may contain an etiologic clue.

Symptoms. Preceding the headache an aura usually occurs and may last a few minutes to over an hour, even overlapping the headache itself. The aura most frequently consists of scintillating scotomata or other visual hallucinations but may also involve paresthesias and speech defects.

As the aura recedes, the severe unilateral (at least at the outset) throbbing headache begins. The most common time of onset is in the early morning hours, perhaps awakening the patient from sleep, and it usually dissipates in the early evening (i.e., sunup to sundown). Photophobia and phonophobia almost always accompany intense headaches.

The throbbing quality is most often noted early and may be replaced by a deep-seated ache which spreads to the other side of the head. Characteristically the pain is located in the temporal, retro-orbital, or frontal region, though it may be in the posterior part of the head. The pain is frequently accompanied by pallor, dizziness, tinnitus, tingling or numbness of the face, arms, or tongue, and disturbances of taste and smell. Nausea and vomiting are likely with all but mild migraine headaches. The attacks of migraine vary greatly in frequency and intensity,

the same individual having several attacks a month and then displaying remission for years. They may occur regularly at the same time of each month or year (see Cluster Headache).

Disturbance of water metabolism is frequently a concomitant symptom of migraine headaches. Before and during the early hours of the morning, the face and especially the lids become edematous; a watery nasal discharge and lacrimation may occur. A weight gain may be noted preceding an attack, with a corresponding weight loss several days following the head pain.

In a few patients time mitigates the frequency and intensity of the headaches. Sometimes other body disturbances, such as chest or abdominal pains, attacks of vomiting and diarrhea, fever, or disorders of the mind, replace the headache. These are termed migraine equivalents, and their true significance is not known.

During the attack striking changes in mood may occur. The patient becomes irritable and irascible, unsocial and dejected, even depressed. His judgment is poor, and he is not dependable. Following the attack there may well be a swing to the other extreme, so that abnormal good spirits and energy may prevail.

Often but not invariably, migraine attacks cease during pregnancy, and many women lose the headache at the time of the menopause. It has been reported that the taking of oral contraceptives by some women is accompanied by an increased frequency of migraine attacks.

Pathology. The symptoms of the aura preceding the head pain are most likely due to intracranial vasoconstriction. Consistent with this concept is the observation that the aura can be abolished or greatly modified by inhalation of the cerebrovasodilator, 10% CO_2, and if this is combined with O_2, the combination is even more effective.

The pulsating headache of the migraine attack is due to dilation and distension of extracranial blood vessels, particularly the extracranial portion of the external carotid artery. It is likely that in some cases the pain also arises from a distended meningeal (intracranial) vessel. Compression of the scalp vessels and the carotid artery on the affected side frequently affords temporary relief.

Treatment. Migraine headache may require no treatment other than an explanation of its causes to the patient and reassurance that it will do him no harm. Treatment is rarely required during the aura.

The patient is usually most concerned about getting relief from the severe throbbing headache. The milder attacks may respond to acetylsalicylic acid (0.6 to 0.9 g) or similar analgesia. For more severe attacks, caffeine citrate (25 mg) and codeine (60 mg) may be added to the analgesia.

The majority of the attacks are more severe and respond only to ergot preparations, chiefly ergotamine tartrate. It should be administered intramuscularly in doses of 0.25 to 0.5 mg, and relief will be obtained within 1 hour in about 90% of cases. More prompt relief occurs with intravenous administration. Ergot drugs raise the arterial pressure and should be used with care in the presence of left ventricular failure and angina pectoris. With rare exceptions, no more than 0.5 mg of ergotamine tartrate should be administered parenterally in 1 week.

Two tablets of ergotamine, 1 mg in combination with 100 mg of caffeine, may be taken by mouth every half hour until a total of six tablets are taken or until the headache is relieved. Rectal suppositories can also be used and may avoid the nausea that accompanies, to a greater or lesser degree, the use of all ergot preparations. The administration of ergot preparations should be combined with bedrest in a quiet environment. The presence of nausea justifies the injection of an antihistamine or chlorpromazine, 25 mg.

Prophylactic therapy of migraine has always principally revolved around an improvement in the response of the patient to his life situation. To accomplish this may be a time-consuming occupation for the physician (and patient), but its importance cannot be overemphasized.

Pharmacologically the use of methysergide may be of considerable value in preventing or reducing the frequency and intensity of vascular headaches which fail to respond to other means of treatment. For adults, 4 to 8 mg are given daily, with medi-cation-free intervals of 3 to 4 weeks every 6 months. Cyproheptadine is a serotonin and histamine antagonist which, though less effective, may be used for prophylaxis alone or in combination with methysergide. Generally it is employed in amounts of 8 to 12 mg daily.

TEMPORAL ARTERITIS

Temporal arteritis, also known as cranial arteritis, is a self-limited severe pain or headache following the course of one or both temporal arteries.

Etiology. The cause is unknown. It is a disease of late life, usually of 50 or more years of age. It has been reported following some acute infections or associated with a hypersensitivity state, and possibly it is related to migraine. It has also been suggested that it is a variation of periarteritis nodosa and thromboangiitis obliterans.

Pathology. The pathology consists of a panarteritis with thickening of the intima and fragmentation of the internal elastic lamina. The media is replaced by collagen and granulation tissue. The panarteritis is associated with a foreign body giant cell reaction which seems to be pathognomonic. A thrombus may form in the narrowed vessel.

Symptoms. The severe throbbing or lancinating pain is located in the region supplied by the temporal artery and is due to edema of its walls. The palpating finger easily follows its tortuous course. Systemically there is slight fever, sweating, and malaise. Ocular complications such as impaired vision or muscle paralysis may result from diminished blood flow to the orbital contents, perhaps because of arteritis of associated vessels.

Prognosis. The disease is usually self-limited, lasting a few weeks to a year. An occasional death has been reported in cases in which the arteritis is more widespread.

Treatment. The medical treatment has been largely ineffective, but adrenocorticotropic hormones and adrenal corticosteroids should be tried, although their worth is yet to be determined. Surgical resection of the affected artery yields much benefit.

CLUSTER HEADACHE

Also known as histamine cephalgia (Horton) and erythrocephalgia, cluster headache is a variety of vasodilating head pain. It may also be identical to nasociliary or ciliary neuralgia. Cluster headaches are clearly differentiated from migraine headaches by the absence of a preceding aura.

Symptoms. The disorder is characterized by a severe unilateral headache, often lasting less than an hour and often suddenly (without an aura) awakening the patient from sleep. It frequently appears in young adult males. During an attack there is scleral injection, lacrimation, rhinorrhea, and nasal obstruction on the same side, accompanied by a deep boring pain, mainly periorbital in location, which may spread to the temple, neck, and face. Nausea and vomiting are absent. There is a strange tendency for the symptoms to occur in clusters of one to five attacks in 24 hours. Thus the symptoms appear daily at the same time for some days or weeks and then inexplicably do not appear for a year or more. The typical attack may be precipitated by the subcutaneous injection of 0.35 mg of histamine base (Horton), by 1 mg of nitroglycerine taken sublingually, and at times merely by the ingestion of alcohol.

Pathology. Cluster headaches are considered to be the result of a painful vasodilation of branches of the external carotid artery.

Treatment. Most cluster headaches respond to vasoconstrictor agents given intravenously or intramuscularly, the most effective being ergotamine tartrate. Methysergide and the serotonin antagonist cyproheptadine can also be used. In past years Horton has recommended histamine desensitization, but little use is made of this treatment at the present time.

MUSCLE CONTRACTION HEADACHE

The prolonged, sustained contraction of muscles of the head, scalp, jaws, and particularly the neck is a common source of head pain. The ache is a constant, frequently bilateral, *nonpulsating* pain or tightness usually located in the occipital region, though it often extends forward and upward toward the vertex. This type of headache may last for days or weeks at a time. There is no characteristic time of onset, though most often it is present on arising in the morning or even when awakening at night. It may be aggravated by exposure to drafts and cold. Careful palpation of the nuchal muscles may reveal tender nodular areas. Active movements of the head may be limited.

Etiology. Although several factors contribute to the genesis of muscle contraction headache, the most common factor is undoubtedly *emotional tension*. These patients are frequently rigid, aggressive, hostile, and perfectionist by long habit; in short, they do not react well to the stresses and strains of life. Because of this, there frequently is an element of fatigue in the background.

The presence of a concomitant vascular headache may contribute to painful muscle contractions. Likewise, inflammation of the eye, nose and paranasal sinuses, or teeth, other disease processes involving such areas, or trauma may contribute to the contractions. A secondary element may be the habits of posture of the patient in question. For example, the flexed neck of the typist or draftsman may put undue stress on the nuchal musculature.

A special word needs to be said about *myalgias* of the head and neck, though it is questionable if they should be distinguished from muscle tension headaches. Williams believes the muscles most commonly involved are: (1) the upper border of the trapezius and its insertion; (2) the insertion of the splenius capitis into the mastoid process and that portion of the muscle just distal to the insertion; (3) the upper third of the sternocleidomastoid muscle; (4) the styloid process and the stylohyoid and anterior belly of the digastric muscle; (5) the styloglossus muscle and its insertion into the tongue, with entire freedom from tenderness of the remainder of the tongue; (6) the superior constrictor of the pharynx (when the superior constrictor of the pharynx is involved, swallowing occasionally will produce a pain in the ear so severe that it is confused with glossopharyngeal neuralgia); (7) the cricoarytenoideus posterior muscle (involvement of this muscle frequently produces pain on talking); (8) the temporalis muscle; and (9) the occipitofrontalis muscle.

Ocular Headaches

Acute Glaucoma. The headache from acute glaucoma is characterized by sudden onset of a severe pain in the eye and head in the supraorbital region. The pain is worse at night and is accompanied by blurred vision, dilated pupil, steamy cornea, shallow anterior chamber, and increased ocular tension.

Acute Iritis. Acute iritis gives rise to pain radiating to the forehead and temple on the affected side. The pain is worse at night. The eye is active and red, and the pupil is small. The iris is discolored and the tension normal. Vision is somewhat blurred.

Acute Retrobulbar Neuritis. The pain from retrobulbar neuritis is usually a unilateral discomfort or pain deep in the orbit, which is increased by rotation of the eye. The pain usually precedes the advent of blurred vision. A larger central scotoma is usually present.

Herpes Zoster Ophthalmicus. A severe neuralgic pain on one side of the face and head usually precedes the typical herpetic eruption along the ophthalmic division of the fifth nerve.

Errors of Refraction. The headache from myopia, hyperopia, astigmatism, and presbyopia may be a morning headache following an eyestrain from the preceding night or an afternoon or evening headache from strain during the day. Rest of the eyes relieves the headache.

Heterophoria. Heterophoria, or imperfect muscle balance, if marked, may produce a headache or pain in the eyes or other parts of the head. This may be accompanied by blurring of print, diplopia, nausea, and vertigo.

HEADACHES FROM SINUSITIS

By and large the pain emanating from an acute infection of the frontal or maxillary sinuses is located immediately over these structures. Pain associated with acute ethmoidal and sphenoidal sinus disease is ex-

perienced more posterior to and between the eyes and tends to be referred to the vertex of the head. Sinus pain is a moderately severe deep, steady, or pulsatile pain which only rarely is in itself associated with nausea. Commonly it is relieved by aspirin or codeine and made worse by activities that increase the engorgement of the nasal mucosa, e.g., ingestion of alcohol, bending the head forward, menstruation.

Mechanism of Sinus Pain

Wolff noted that the mucosa covering the approaches to the paranasal sinuses was the most pain-sensitive of the nasal and paranasal structures and cavities, much more so than the mucosal lining of the sinuses themselves. Thus inflammation and engorgement of the turbinates, sinus ostia, nasofrontal ducts, and superior nasal spaces leads to sinus pain. Pressure within the sinus cavity itself, long considered to be the cause of pain, does not, under clinical conditions, lead to discomfort. Negative pressure within a sinus, usually the frontal sinus, is capable of causing considerable discomfort (see Vacuum Sinusitis).

NEURALGIA OF THE FACE AND HEAD

Sphenopalatine Neuralgia

The sphenopalatine (Meckel's, pterygopalatine) ganglion (see Fig. 1–9, b) is irregular in shape and is about 1 cm in length and one half that in breadth and width. Situated in the upper part of the pterygopalatine fossa, it lies as if suspended from the maxillary nerve by two or three branches. It is in close relation to the posterior ethmoidal cells, the lateral wall of the nose, and, posteriorly, the sphenoid sinus, if that sinus extends forward far enough. The sphenopalatine ganglion is a parasympathetic ganglion and is essentially a relay station on the secretory pathway of the greater superficial petrosal nerve from the geniculate ganglion (Cr VII). The postganglionic fibers supply the lacrimal, nasal and palatine glands. Sensory and sympathetic fibers pass through the ganglion without interruption. (See sphenopalatine ganglion, Chap. 1.) The branches of the internal maxillary artery are near the ganglion. It is likely that "Sluder's" sphenopalatine neuralgia is a variant of a vascular headache and involves this artery.

Etiology. The exact cause(s) of sphenopalatine ganglion neuralgia has not been determined. It occurs in women about twice as frequently as in men and usually occurs between the ages of 20 and 50. It seems to have no seasonal incidence but is frequently seen when an acute nasopharyngitis is present. At times the condition is associated with the menopause. Williams ascribes the cause to a vasomotor imbalance or physical allergy (see Autonomic Dysfunction).

Symptoms. The clinical picture of sphenopalatine (nasal) neuralgia or "lower half headache" consists of pain about the eye, the upper jaw, and the teeth, extending to the zygoma and temple, with earache and pain in the mastoid, emphasized at a point about 5 cm behind it. According to Sluder this point is always tender on pressure, although the pain is often temporarily absent. It may extend to the occiput, neck, shoulder, scapula, arm, forearm, hand, and fingers.

There may also be a sympathetic syndrome of sneezing, rhinorrhea, lacrimation, and photophobia. The sense of taste is usually slightly diminished on the anterior half of the tongue, and occasionally there may be vertigo.

Many neurologists doubt this syndrome and believe the explanation lies in the spilling over of pain impulses from the fifth nerve.

Diagnosis. Cocainization of the sphenopalatine ganglion on the affected side with a 10% solution of cocaine gives relief from pain within 3 or 4 minutes (Fig. 6–1).

The differential diagnosis should be made from other unilateral neuralgic facial pains, such as migraine, trigeminal neuralgia, temporomandibular joint syndrome, and lesions or disturbances of the teeth, sinuses, and orbit, and from the various referred pains in general.

Treatment. These cases are extremely resistant to all forms of ordinary treatment but respond readily to cocainization of the sphenopalatine ganglion (Fig. 6–1). Frequently one or more applications will give relief, possibly because of action of the cocaine on the fifth cranial nerve.

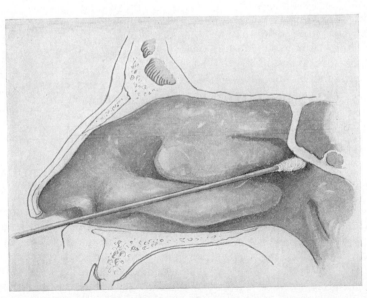

FIG. 6–1.   Cocainizing the sphenopalatine ganglion. The cotton-mounted applicator is moistened with a 10% cocaine-epinephrine solution and is applied to the posterior wall of the nasopharynx immediately behind the posterior tip of the middle turbinate.

Vidian Neuralgia

Vidian neuralgia is similar to sphenopalatine ganglion neuralgia. It is thought to be due to an irritation of the vidian nerve as it passes behind the posterior ethmoidal cells and along the sphenoidal sinus and is usually associated with infection of these areas.

Nasociliary Neuralgia

Greenfield Sluder many years ago described a syndrome of vague pain in the eyes and brow and at the root of the nose which he ascribed to neuralgia of the nasociliary nerve. He stated that the pain was usually referred to the small district bounded by the supraciliary ridge above, the supraorbital notch laterally, and the nasal bone below. "Neuritic" pains in the eyeball or orbital cavity and a unilateral rhinitis with pain at the apex of the nose have been associated with the syndrome.

TRIGEMINAL NEURALGIA

Trigeminal neuralgia (tic douloureux) is characterized by severe, darting, lancinating pain of 10 to 30 seconds' duration along the course of one or more branches of the fifth cranial nerve, although the first division is much less frequently involved than the other two. The pain rarely, if ever, crosses the midline, thus distinguishing it from many other face pains. The attacks may increase in frequency until they are almost continuous, or remissions of months or years may occur.

So-called "trigger zones" usually are present, and these, when touched, incite the sharp pains. Commonly these are located about the ala of the nose, along the gums, over the hard palate, and along the lower lip. The average age of onset is about 50 years, and females predominate.

The etiology and pathology are undetermined, though transient ischemia of trigeminal structures is said by some to be the cause.

Medical treatment has been disappointing. Vasodilating drugs (e.g., nicotinic acid in the amount of 200 mg four to five times a day) may be tried. Inhalation of trichloro-ethylene has been successful in lessening the pain during an attack.

Alcohol injection into the gasserian ganglion or one or more of its branches is in itself painful, is not always successful, and only rarely relieves the pain for more than one year. Permanent results follow the surgical division of the posterior sensory roots of the gasserian ganglion. Such a procedure, of course, also involves the permanent loss of touch sensation.

Glossopharyngeal Neuralgia

This is almost identical to trigeminal neuralgia, because the ninth and fifth nerves supply contiguous sensory areas. The "trigger" zone in glossopharyngeal neuralgia is usually located in the tonsillar fossa with pains radiating to the ear rather than along the branches of the fifth nerve, as in trigeminal neuralgia. The pain is instigated by swallowing, eating, or irritation of the tonsillar region. Cocainization of the throat causes a cessation of the glossopharyngeal pain but has no effect on the pain from trigeminal neuralgia.

Treatment. The injection of alcohol for glossopharyngeal neuralgia is not recommended because of the close proximity of the ninth cranial nerve to the great vessels of the neck and to the tenth and eleventh cranial nerves.

Peripheral avulsion of the nerve will afford relief, but the treatment of choice for severe cases is the intracranial section of the sensory root before it enters the jugular foramen. The nerve is exposed by a suboccipital craniotomy.

TEMPOROMANDIBULAR JOINT
NEURALGIA (COSTEN'S SYNDROME)

Costen believes this syndrome, first described by him in 1934, is a clinical entity related to the malocclusion, improper action, and abnormal position of the condyle of the mandible within the glenoid fossa. Symptomatically it consists of pain of moderate severity in the frontal, parietal, and occipital regions with involvement of the ear, tongue, and jaws on prolonged chewing. At times the symptoms include deafness, tinnitus, and vertigo. These symptoms arise from excessive contraction or spasm of the masseter muscles and from irritation of the nearby auriculotemporal and chorda tympani nerves. The joint itself is frequently found to be eroded, narrowed, or otherwise deformed, as well as tender to palpation.

Treatment. If deformity of the temporomandibular joint is clearly demonstrable, measures to place the joint at rest for 3 to 6 weeks are of prime importance. This is done by use of a soft diet or by elastic fixation with a suitable headgear. Attention must be paid to dental abnormalities which may interfere with joint action.

In more severe cases, 25 mg of hydrocortisone injected directly into the joint space, with the jaw open, may provide weeks to months of relief.

NEUROSES OF OLFACTION

The neuroses of olfaction are characterized by either (1) a perverted sense of smell (parosmia), (2) oversensitivity to olfactory stimuli (hyperosmia), (3) a partial loss of the sense of smell (hyposmia), or (4) a total loss of the sense of smell (anosmia).

Parosmia

Parosmia is characterized by a perception of imaginary odors and may be due to pathologic changes in the olfactory brain center. Inflammatory disease of the mucous membrane in the attic of the nose may also produce parosmia by overstimulating the nerve endings. It usually accompanies lesions of the central brain, although it occasionally occurs in hysteria, hypochondria, epilepsy, insanity, and syphilis.

Hyperosmia

Hyperosmia is characterized by an oversensitivity to olfactory stimuli—that is, the perception of odors is exaggerated. The most delicate perfumes or odors not ordinarily perceived are recognized even to the point of unpleasantness. In some cases the perception of odors persists after the source of

the odor is removed, and in this respect the condition approaches parosmia.

It may be due to an irritation of the olfactory lobes, hysteria, neurasthenia, hypochondria, sexual disorders in women (especially at the menstrual period), and wasting diseases.

Hyposmia

Hyposmia is characterized by a partial loss of smell due to an impairment of the mucous membrane of the superior meatus of the nose, the nerve endings, the bulb, or the brain center. The impairment is only great enough to obtund the perception of odors without totally destroying it.

Anosmia

Anosmia is a total loss of the sense of smell, though careful evaluation is required to establish this as a total loss.

Etiology. The causes of true anosmia can be extremely varied. Most commonly there is an interference with the intranasal diffusion of the odorous particles, so that the odors do not impinge on the approximately 500 mm² of olfactory mucosa. This commonly occurs because of obstructive nasal turgescence (e.g., the common cold) and nasal polyposis. Other organic and inorganic causes are indicated in Table 6–1.

Diagnosis. Schneider has suggested a useful clinical procedure when testing for anosmia. It is based on the fact that the olfactory epithelium contains fibers of the trigeminal nerve, and these, when properly stimulated, lead to a sensation described by the patient as hot or cold, superficial touch or superficial pain (tingling, prickling, irritation). Two odors are used: one is a strong trigeminal stimulant (ammonia), and the other is one which approximates a pure olfactory stimulus (freshly ground coffee). Normally a patient can detect both coffee and ammonia. The patient with organic anosmia cannot detect coffee but does note a tingling or slight burning with ammonia. The hysteric malingerer can detect neither, or his responses are inconsistent on successive tests. In a patient with severe and wide-

Table 6–1.   Causes of Anosmia

   I.   Intranasal airway obstruction

    A. Trauma.
    B. Allergic edema, including nasal polyps
    C. Inflammatory edema and exudate
    D. Neoplastic

  II.   Intranasal mucosal destruction

    A. Atrophic rhinitis
    B. Senile atrophy
    C. Toxic chemical poisons
       1. Zinc sulfate
       2. Lead

 III.   Intranasal surgery producing injury to the olfactory nerves

 IV.   Intracranial lesions

    A. Tumors, both neoplastic and vascular, usually bilateral and involving the undersurface of the frontal lobes and cribriform plate
    B. Vascular causing an ischemia of the olfactory apparatus
    C. Head trauma
       1. Fracture of the cribriform plate
       2. Shearing laceration of the olfactory nerves
       3. Hemorrhage causing interference with the frontal lobes, olfactory bulbs, and tracts
    D. Infection
    E. Congenital; Kallmann's syndrome (hypoplasia of the olfactory apparatus and hypogonadism)

  V.   Hysteria and/or malingering

---

spread atrophy or crusting of the nasal mucosa, both trigeminal and olfactory nerve endings may also be destroyed.

REFERENCES

Dalessio, D. J.: *Wolff's Headache and Other Head Pain.* New York, Oxford University Press, 1972.

Friedman, A. P.: *In* Baker, A. B. & Baker, C. H. Clinical Neurology, Vol. 2, 1973 New York, Harper & Row, 1973.

Schneider, R. A.: Anosmia: Verification and Etiologies. Ann. Otol., *81*:272, 1972.

Wolstenholme, G. E. W., and Knight, J. (Eds.): *Ciba Symposium on Taste and Smell in Vertebrates.* London, J. & A. Churchill, 1970.

Chapter 7
Chronic Infections of the Nasal Fossae

CHRONIC RHINITIS

It is questionable whether chronic rhinitis should be classified as a separate entity. If possible, it is preferable to uncover the etiologic agent (sinus, anatomic defect, etc.) and apply the descriptive diagnostic term.

Etiology. Frequently so-called chronic rhinitis has its basis in a low-grade chronic sinusitis or allergy. Frequent and prolonged sinusitis over the years may lead to a change in the nasal mucosa (see ozena). In recent years the presence of increasingly high levels of air pollution is suspected of leading to destructive changes in the nasal epithelium.

Pathology. In the early stages there is distension of the venous or cavernous tissue of the turbinates. If the inflammatory process continues, true hyperplasia of the tissues takes place. There is a hypertrophy of the mucous glands.

Symptoms. The symptoms are caused chiefly by transient stenosis of the airway of the nose. In addition, the mucoid element of the secretions is increased, perhaps at the expense of the serous element. Crusts may be bothersome to the patient.

Treatment. The treatment should be directed toward removal of possible allergens, appropriate care of nasal or sinus infections, and correction of any significant nasal septal deviations.

HYPERPLASTIC RHINITIS

Etiology. In the etiology of hyperplastic rhinitis, allergens are important factors. Infection is usually considered a secondary development; however, some writers maintain that the hyperplastic changes are due to a primary bacterial infection. The opinion that the inhalant and food allergens are the principal etiologic factors is based on the fact that eosinophilic cells are usually found in the membranes, nasal secretions, and blood, and a positive allergic history is obtained in the majority of patients.

Nasal abnormalities such as marked septal deflections may be a predisposing cause in some instances. The sinuses, especially the ethmoids, may be diseased independent of the septal deviation and may thus be the primary cause of the hyperplasia. In either event the irritation from dust, smoke, and so forth, or the irritation resulting from the secretions constantly flowing over the mucous membrane of the middle and inferior turbinates causes the pathologic changes in these structures.

Pathology. Hyperplastic rhinitis is characterized by thickened and edematous changes in the mucous membrane and periosteum. It is usually associated with polypoid masses of the soft tissues and rarefaction and osteoporosis of the bone.

The allergic reaction in the tissues of the nose, especially the inferior turbinate, consists of dilatation of the blood vessels, increased capillary permeability, edema of and cellular infiltration, particularly of eosinophils.

Symptoms. The symptoms of hyperplastic rhinitis are often complex, as the disease is frequently associated with an allergy or with a suppurative inflammation of one or more of the sinuses. They are chiefly obstructive in nature.

Anterior rhinoscopy shows the middle or inferior turbinate to be enlarged and paler than normal, or it may be red and boggy and somewhat nodular in outline. Polypi may be seen growing from the middle turbinate, ethmoid, or maxillary ostium. Many of the ethmoidal cells removed at operation may show a beginning polypoid degeneration. In view of these findings, it is obvious that the removal of the visible polypi may fail to relieve the patient completely, as the small budding polypi within the cells might later extend through the ostia into the nasal chambers. If the septum is deviated, a ridge corresponding to the crista nasalis and the crest of the vomer may be present on one side, while there is a bowing of the septum toward the opposite side in the region of the middle turbinate. The mucous membrane covering the septum is often thickened just below the inferior border of both the middle turbinates, thereby obstructing both olfactory fissures.

If empyema of the posterior ethmoidal cells is present, pus may be seen in the olfactory fissure as well as in the lower portion of the nose. If there is hyperplastic ethmoiditis, the anterior end of the middle turbinate may be red and boggy in texture. Patients with this type of ethmoidal inflammation at times complain of fissures at the margins of the vestibules.

Treatment. Complete sensitivity tests for allergy should be done and appropriate treatment instituted. Obstructive polyps, septal deviations, or other obstructive nasal lesions should be treated, as well as any sinusitis or latent infection present. If nasal obstruction persists, especially from hyperplasia of the inferior turbinate, a submucosal or linear cauterization of the inferior turbinate should be tried. This will give relief in most instances. If much hyperplastic tissue remains along the inferior borders of the inferior or middle turbinates after adequate cauterization, and if obstructive symptoms persist, the excessive redundant tissue may be removed by means of a straight or curved nasal scissors or snare. Care should be taken

to leave the turbinates themselves and the nasal mucous membrane in as nearly intact a condition as possible; otherwise, marked disturbances of the nasal physiology might occur.

Cauterization of the Inferior Turbinate

Various methods for cauterizing or scarring the intumescent or hyperplastic inferior turbinate have been used. One of the earliest methods was linear cauterization using silver nitrate, chromic acid beads, or trichloroacetic acid. These agents, when successful, frequently resulted in marked destruction of the nasal mucosa. Linear cauterization by means of the actual cautery is much more effective and does not have this disadvantage to as great a degree. Diathermy or high-frequency current has been used for coagulation of the venous spaces with some good results, but severe reactions and sloughing have occurred in some instances.

Electrocauterization. The technique of electrocauterization is as follows:

Local anesthesia is induced by the application of a 4% solution of cocaine on a thin pledget of cotton to the swollen free border of the inferior turbinate for a period of 10 minutes.

The electric current is turned on until the point of the cautery electrode is of a bright cherry-red color.

The cold electrode is introduced into the nasal chamber and placed on the free border of the inferior turbinate (Fig. 7–1). It is

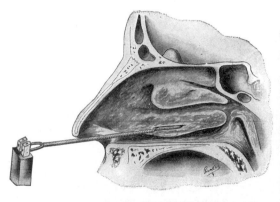

FIG. 7–1. Lateral view showing the cautery electrode in position for cauterizing the inferior turbinate.

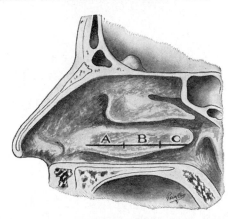

FIG. 7–2. Lines for linear cauterization in chronic rhinitis, *A, B,* and *C* representing the first, second, and third cauterizations, respectively, which should be made 1 week apart.

then moved backward and forward while still cold, until its correct position is determined. The to-and-fro motion is maintained, and the contact spring of the cautery handle is pressed for 1 or 2 seconds, after which the contact should be broken. The to-and-fro motion should be continued until the electrode is cold, that is, for 2 or 3 seconds after the spring contact is broken, and then it should be removed from the nose.

If these instructions are followed, the procedure is painless and does not tear the eschar from the turbinate. If the to-and-fro motion is not maintained before, during, and after the electrode is heated, the eschar will be torn off and the cautery effect lost.

The cauterization should be linear and

should be about 1 inch in length. The whole length of the inferior turbinate should be cauterized in two or three sittings (Fig. 7–2), never in one, as too great a reaction and sloughing may follow.

The sittings should be from 5 to 10 days apart. A week after the first cauterization, the opposite side may be treated in like manner. At the end of another week, the middle portion of the inferior turbinate first cauterized may be thus treated. In many instances one cauterization over the most swollen portion may be sufficient.

Hyperplasia of the Inferior Turbinate

If the hyperplastic tissue of the inferior turbinate blocks the nasal passage and other methods of treatment have failed to reduce the hyperplasia, the excess portion on the lower or free border may be removed by means of the serrated nasal scissors.

Technique. Local anesthesia is induced by the application of a 5% solution of cocaine by means of a thin pledget of cotton, which is placed over the hyperplastic area for 10 minutes.

With nasal scissors the necessary portion of the hyperplastic membrane is cut off (Fig. 7–3).

If bleeding occurs, the nose should be packed with tampons of petrolatum gauze. If severe hemorrhage occurs from the posterior portion, it may become necessary to introduce a postnasal tampon. A long strip of gauze should then be packed against it

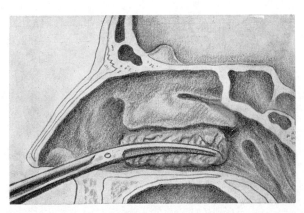

FIG. 7-3.   Removal of the excess hyperplastic tissue from the lower border of the inferior turbinate by means of curved scissors. The turbinate bone is not removed.

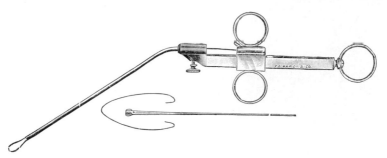

FIG. 7-4.   Krause's nasal snare.

through the anterior nares. The tampon should be removed in from 2 to 4 days. It may be renewed if necessary.

Submucous Turbinectomy

Under local anesthesia an elliptical incision is made over the most prominent portion of the inferior turbinate. This portion of the mucous membrane is resected. The excess mucous membrane and as much bone as necessary are removed. The flaps are sutured and a tampon inserted if desired.

Partial Turbinectomy with Scissors and Snare

Removal by the scissors and snare is probably the most universally used method. It is safe and rapid when part or all of the middle turbinate is being removed.

Technique. Cocaine-epinephrine anesthesia is sufficient.

The attachments of the anterior two thirds of the middle turbinate are severed, with Knight's or other nasal scissors, as close to the outer nasal wall as possible.

The loop of a Krause (Fig. 7-4) or other snare is engaged in the severed portion of the middle turbinate, the unengaged portion of the loop being carried backward so as to include all or any desired portion of the middle turbinate. By tightening of the snare, the turbinate is severed from its attachment. It is removed by grasping with a suitable nasal forceps.

Packing may be used if bleeding is profuse.

With curved scissors of the Holmes or similar type the snare is not necessary, as the blades are so curved that the cut made with them extends backward and downward until it emerges from the tissue (Figs. 7-5 to 7-7).

Fracture of the Middle Turbinate

In most instances removal of all or part of the middle turbinate is not necessary. Fracture of the middle turbinate away from

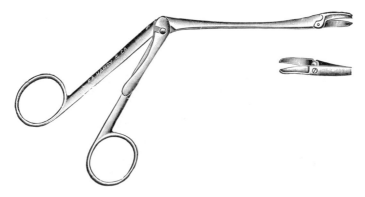

FIG. 7-5.   Holmes' middle turbinate scissors.

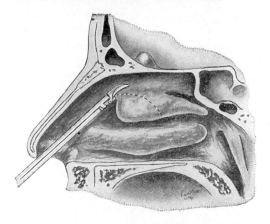

FIG. 7–6.   Removal of the anterior half of the middle turbinate with Holmes' scissors.

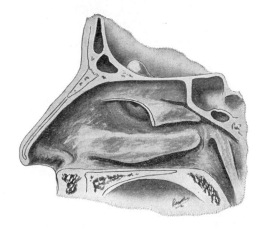

FIG. 7–7.   Anterior half of the middle turbinate removed with Holmes' scissors, exposing the bulla ethmoidalis.

the sinus ostia may give the necessary drainage and aeration.

Technique. After local anesthesia, the middle turbinate is grasped by a broad, smooth-bladed nasal forceps (Fig. 7–8) and is rotated in an inward and upward direction so that the inferior border and body of the turbinate are turned away from the outer nasal wall and toward the septum. A small strip of gauze may be placed between the inner portion of the fractured turbinate and the outer wall to keep the turbinate in the new position. The gauze should be renewed daily. Many times the turbinate will maintain its position without the use of the support.

CHRONIC ATROPHIC RHINITIS; OZENA

Definition. Atrophic rhinitis is characterized by a sclerotic change in the mucous membrane and occasionally in the underlying bone and by the presence of crusts and an offensive nasal breath.

Etiology. Many theories and hypotheses have been advanced in the explanation of chronic atrophic rhinitis. No one of the theories explains a sufficiently large number of the cases to be generally accepted. Any one of the theories will explain in a satisfactory manner some of the cases.

Probably one of the most extensively discussed theories is that of Grunwald; he claims the disease is the result of a long-continued suppurative sinusitis in childhood. A proliferation of the connective tissue cells

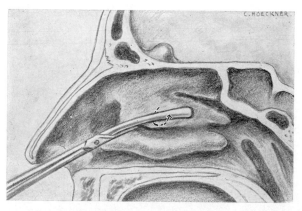

FIG. 7–8.   Forceps grasping middle turbinate, preparatory to fracturing away from the outer nasal wall. The forceps is rotated in an inward and upward direction.

occurs; these later contract, thereby reducing the nourishment to the mucous membrane, with atrophy and shrinkage as a later manifestation.

Pathology. The histologic changes of atrophic rhinitis are, in the early stages, a chronic inflammatory process, and in the late stages, a thickening and fibrosis of the arterial walls, especially an obliterating endarteritis. There is an early loss of the columnar epithelial cells and cilia. The epithelium may undergo early stratification and a characteristic squamous cell type of metaplasia (Fig. 7–9). In the late stage, a considerable portion of the epithelium is of the squamous cell type. Subepithelially, a dense fibrous tissue is present.

"The bone undergoes fibrosis and resorption; the nerve structures undergo fibrous and degenerative changes, and the glands are degenerated and replaced by undifferentiated fibrous tissue" (Fabricant).

Symptoms. The symptom complained of most frequently is the odor or "stench" emanating from the patient's breath. The odor is usually not noticed by the patient, as a partial or complete anosmia is present; however, it is most evident to others in the near vicinity. The odor seems to be present in varying degrees, depending upon the amount of crusting present. If daily nasal cleanliness is practiced, the odor is lessened greatly or is absent.

Nasal obstruction due to crust formation is present in nearly all patients. The crusts or dried secretions may fill the nasal chamber completely, forming a cast which may obstruct nasal respiration. If the crusts are removed, a fluid mucopurulent secretion is found beneath and over the nasal mucosa. Frequently the crusts are so hard it is necessary to soften them before they can be removed. If they are attached to the mucosa, as frequently occurs in the anterior or other portions of the nares, slight bleeding may occur. The crusting and odor may disappear after many years, usually during or after middle age.

Examination. Examination of the nasal cavity reveals greenish gray or grayish black dried crusts covering the turbinates and septum. The crusts may fill the nasal fossae, especially the inferior meatus, or may cover all or a portion of the mucosa without blocking the airway to any extent. If the crusts are removed, a marked atrophy of the inferior turbinate becomes evident. A clear view of the posterior nasopharynx and the upper portions of the soft palate is obtained. The nasal mucosa has a pale, shiny appearance.

Treatment. The treatment is essentially that of intranasal cleanliness. This is obtained by nasal douching at necessary intervals, usually once or twice a day to two or three times a week. The douche may be administered by means of a douche bag, a fountain syringe, some form of a siphon douche, or the Birmingham glass douche in which the flow is determined by a vent in the top of the glass container. The solutions used are usually a normal salt or sodium bicarbonate. The patient should be told how to inject fluids in the nose without strangling and without forcing the fluids or secretions into the sinuses or eustachian tubes.

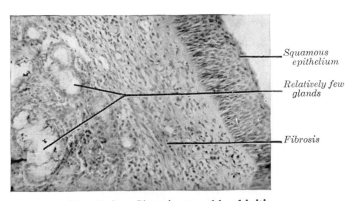

FIG. 7–9. Chronic atrophic rhinitis

Spraying the nose two or three times daily with an oily estrogenic solution for a period of several months has been tried by a number of investigators with some good results. The exact value of this substance has not yet been determined. It is possible that the improvement is due to the increased attention, such as the preliminary douching, rather than to the estrogenic substance which follows the douching.

Mild astringent, stimulating solutions may be of value in reducing the local infection. Any associated sinus disease should be treated as indicated. In recent years acetylcholine used locally, with or without pilocarpine hypodermically, has been advocated on the assumption that acetylcholine produces a vasodilatation and reactivity of the mucous glands.

RHINITIS CASEOSA

Synonyms. Synonyms include coryza caseosa, ozena caseosa, rhinitis cholesteatoma, and caseous purulent rhinorrhea.

Rhinitis caseosa is a rare type of unilateral nasal disease characterized by the accumulation in the nose and sinuses of an extremely offensive, cheeselike mass, by the presence of a seropurulent discharge and other manifestations of chronic suppurative sinusitis and last by intranasal and frequently by extranasal deformity.

Etiology. The usually accepted explanation is that the disease is secondary to a nasal stenosis which blocks the nasal discharge. Owing to mechanical and chemical changes and continued exfoliation of the mucosa, the bottled up secretion is transformed into the caseous material. The condition is invariably unilateral. It is about equally divided between the sexes. It may occur at any age, but the greatest number of patients are seen in the third and fourth decades of life.

Symptoms. The early symptoms are those of a chronic nasal or sinus infection. Examination may reveal polypi or occasionally the presence of a foreign body. Cheeselike particles may be observed in the early stage. As the disease advances, the discharge is more profuse and offensive. Rhinoscopic examination reveals the characteristic cheesy mass with intranasal pressure deformity and erosions.

The late stage is characterized by facial disfigurement and discharging bony fistulas. The disfigurement consists of swelling of the cheek, widening of the bridge of the nose, and at times displacement of the eyeball forward and laterally. A fistulous tract in the canine fossa or frontal process of the superior maxilla may be present.

Prognosis. The prognosis is excellent if the cheesy debris is completely removed and the nose is kept properly cleansed.

RHINITIS SICCA ANTERIOR

Dry anterior rhinitis, a relatively common disease, is atrophic in character and confined to the anterior part of the nasal septum. It is characterized by a dry whitish mucous membrane, usually covered by a crust or a thin, dry pseudomembrane more or less firmly adherent to the underlying mucosa. The removal of the crusts or membrane may cause an occasional slight bleeding. Constant irritation of the mucous membrane from forceful removal of the crusts or dry secretions perpetuates the trouble and leads to permanent changes in the mucous membrane and perichondrium. The ciliated columnar epithelium is replaced by a flat squamous type with a decrease or absence of glandular function. Superficial ulceration frequently occurs. If extensive or long-continued, these ulcers may lead to perforation of the cartilaginous septum.

Treatment. Forceful removal of the crusts and dry exudate should be avoided. A bland ointment should be prescribed. If excessive bleeding occurs, the bleeding points should be cauterized, preferably with the platinum tip electric cautery. Slight bleeding may be controlled by small cotton plugs or by cotton pledgets soaked in epinephrine placed over the bleeding area for a few minutes.

Chapter 8

Etiology of the Inflammatory Diseases of the Upper Respiratory Tract

Harry B. Harding and John J. Ballenger

ACUTE VIRAL INFECTIONS OF THE UPPER RESPIRATORY TRACT

The term "upper respiratory infection" (URI) has come into common use in recent years in an attempt to characterize certain usually mild diseases of the pharynx, nasopharynx, sinuses, eustachian–middle ear apparatus, larynx, and trachea. The causative agents for these number at least 180, with more viruses being discovered each year. The clinical entities they cause are almost as numerous (see Table 8–1). On occasion, certain of these agents may invade the lung, giving rise to a pneumonitis or lower respiratory infection, which also varies in severity.

One should appreciate the impact of these diseases on the national and worldwide economy. In the United States alone, in a survey conducted in 1971, 255 million respiratory infections occurred, of which over 56 per cent were the "common cold" (coryza). However, since so many viruses can cause or be found in association with certain clinical entities, the proof of etiology lies with the laboratory. One can no longer classify viral disease on the basis of clinical observations alone. Viruses can now be observed morphologically with the electron microscope in specially prepared mounts employing phosphotungstic acid.

Tissue culture methods available today, with bacterial contamination controlled by antibiotics and the availability of a multiplicity of host cell types, make the isolation of viruses routine. Likewise, refinements of antibody detection, including fluorescent antibody techniques, make the virus laboratory as practical as the bacteriology laboratory. Studies with two drugs—amantadine (influenza) and the deoxyuridine variants (herpes simplex)—indicate that we will soon have antiviral drugs of clinical significance. Then it will become necessary to test viruses against drugs, just as we now test bacteria for their antibiotic susceptibilities.

Adenoviruses

Adenoviruses were first isolated in 1953 from tonsillar tissue taken from those carrying the latent agents. They are 60 to 85 nanometers (nm)* in size and have a naked cubic icosahedral structure with rodlike structures emanating from the apices. Since 1953, 30 distinct serotypes pathogenic for man have been recognized. Still other types have been recovered from animals, but definite proof of their infectiousness for man is lacking.

* Nanometer (nm) = 1/1000 of 1/1000 of a millimeter; a more acceptable term for millimicron.

All adenoviruses possess a common complement-fixing antigen in addition to type-specific antigens. Use is made of this fact in the indirect detection of these agents when disease occurs sporadically in civilian populations. These viruses multiply well in tissue cultures derived from epithelial tissue but have not been adapted to the common laboratory animals.

Types 1, 2, and 5 adenovirus may be isolated from approximately 50% of the tonsils and adenoids that are surgically removed, but the significance of this is not clear. It is possible that these viruses remain latent in the lymphoid tissue and with the proper stimulus initiate an infection in the person harboring them.

Serologic surveys have shown that a high percentage of adults have antibodies to one or more types of adenovirus, indicating previous infections. The proportion of persons exhibiting antibodies increases with age. The epidemiology of adenovirus infections varies with the type of population studied. Adenoviruses, particularly types 3, 4, and 7, are the most important causal agents of acute respiratory illnesses in military recruits. In the civilian population, adenoviruses are responsible for only 3 to 4% of all respiratory illnesses. Why there is such a marked difference between civilian and military populations is not clear.

Adenoviruses have been recovered from patients suffering from many diseases. These include acute respiratory disease, pneumonitis, nonbacterial pharyngitis, pharyngoconjunctival fever, follicular conjunctivitis, and the common cold.

The relationship of adenoviruses to the acute respiratory disease (ARD) syndrome of military recruits was established by Hilleman and Werner in 1954. These investigators isolated type 4 adenovirus from ARD cases occurring during an epidemic in a military establishment. Other studies have shown that outbreaks were caused by types 4 and 7 adenovirus. The mode of epidemic propagation is considered respiratory in nature and to some extent dependent upon close contact and stress.

Clinical, laboratory, and epidemiologic data accumulated to date indicate that type 3 adenovirus is the causal agent of nonbac-terial pharyngitis and pharyngoconjunctival fever.

Influenza Viruses

Influenza is of viral etiology, the causal agents being among the classified myxoviruses. In fact, it is now classified as an orthomyxovirus in contrast to the paramyxoviruses, which will be discussed subsequently. As is typical of these viruses, the influenza agent consists of spherical to pleomorphic rodlike structures having an external diameter of approximately 110 nm. There is an envelope composed of three layers. There is a double lipid layer at a radius of 35 nm, attached to the outside of which are projecting spikes. One type of spike is the hemagglutinating antigen so important in the routine diagnosis of influenza. There are about half as many drumstick-shaped spikes, which give rise to neuraminidase, an enzyme which destroys the mucoid layer riding over the surface of susceptible cells, thus allowing the virus to enter the cell. Deep to the second lipid layer is a layer of protein subunits, inside of which exists a ropelike structure (the nucleocapsid). The nucleocapsid reminds one of the structure of the tobacco mosaic virus. This latter structure contains the ribose nucleic acid of the virus, which is reproduced within the nucleus of the host cell and then is pushed outside, very much like a reverse pinocytosis. The protein, lipid, and "spike" coats are then added, the first two within the host cell cytoplasm and the spikes from the host cell membrane. Influenza virus, therefore, is quite complex.

At present, there are three immunologically distinct types of influenza viruses—A, B, and C—and within these types are several immunologically distinct strains. A fourth serologic type of virus, formerly known as influenza D, has now been classified as a parainfluenza virus.

With the exception of the 1945, 1952, and 1954–55 outbreaks, influenza A virus strains have been responsible for the major outbreaks of influenza during the past 5 to 6 decades. Strains of type A virus tend to mutate rather frequently, thus initiating new serotypes and concomitantly new epidemic waves of the disease. This phenomenon was

Table 8–1. Viruses Concerned with Upper Respiratory Infection

Name and Group	Size	Type of Nucleic Acid	Shape and Structure	Immunologic Types	Diseases and Syndromes
Adenoviruses Some human types can cause malignant disease in mice, and others act as helper viruses to produce malignancies in animals.	70–90 nm	DNA (double-stranded)	Icosahedral, triangular faces, 12 pentons at the triangle apices naked; 252 capsomeres.	Types 1–30.	Adenopharyngeal conjunctival fever; conjunctivitis; keratoconjunctivitis caused by type 8 becomes epidemic; can cause permanent damage; common cold; viral pneumonitis; acute respiratory disease (ARD).
Picornaviruses; Enteroviruses 1. Polioviruses	25–28 nm	RNA	Form is really a rhombic tricontahedron; 32 capsomeres.	Types 1, 2, and 3.	Common cold; meningism and abortive disease; true poliomyelitis, spinal and/or bulbar.
2. Coxsackie A viruses	28 nm	RNA	Same as above.	More than 30 types.	Herpangina; pleurodynia; aseptic meningitis; mild paresis; neonatal disease; common cold; hand, foot, and mouth disease; some strains produce polio-type disease; myositis (widespread) condition.
3. Coxsackie B viruses	28 nm	RNA	Same as polioviruses.	Types 1–6.	Common cold; aseptic meningitis; meningoencephalitis; myocardiopathy, which may be severe; focal myositis; necrotizing steatitis.
4. ECHO viruses (enteric cytopathic human orphan viruses)	24–30 nm	RNA	Same as polioviruses.	More than 32 types.	Gastroenteritis; pharyngitis; aseptic meningitis; meningoencephalitis; paresis; mild paralysis; skin rashes; febrile illness; conjunctivitis; Boston exanthem disease.

5. Rhinoviruses (not enterovirus); "common cold" agents	20–30 nm	RNA	Naked viruses with picornavirus structure.	Over 90 serotypes recognized.	Common cold; acute respiratory disease; pharyngitis.
Myxoviruses 1. Influenza (ortho-myxovirus)	100–110 nm	RNA	A spherical complex virus, three-layered outer envelope, internal nucleocapsid rod-shaped, wound into a regular sphere.	Types A, B, and C; A, most epidemic; type **B** often endemic.	Common cold; mild **ARD**; acute laryngotracheobronchitis; influenza, pharyngitis; fatal viremia with encephalitis.
2. Paramyxoviruses a. Mumps virus	175–200 nm	RNA (single-stranded)	They possess a helical capsid about 18 nm by 1 nm and an ether-sensitive envelope between 150–300 nm in diameter. Contain RNA-dependent polymerase.	Only one serotype known at present.	Parotid mumps; orchitis; oophoritis; pancreatitis; encephalomyelitis; common cold-like syndrome in abortive cases.
b. Measles virus	140 nm	RNA	The nucleocapsid is about 65 nm.	Only one type known at present, although it shares an antigen in common with distemper (dog) and rinderpest (bovine).	Measles (red measles); common cold-like onset; giant cell pneumonia; subacute sclerosing panencephalitis.
c. Parainfluenza viruses (also known as the hemadsorption viruses)	90–200 nm	RNA	They appear similar to influenza except that the nucleocapsid **is** very irregularly wound. They both lyse and agglutinate erythrocytes.	There are 4 types: hemadsorption 2; croup-associated virus; hemadsorption 1; M–25 virus.	Febrile colds, particularly in children; acute laryngotracheobronchitis; bronchiolitis; bronchopneumonia in children.

135

Table 8–1. Viruses Concerned with Upper Respiratory Infection (cont.)

Name and Group	Size	Type of Nucleic Acid	Shape and Structure	Immunologic Types	Diseases and Syndromes
d. Respiratory syncytial virus	90–140 nm	RNA	Same as above, though smaller.	Slight variability in seasonal-type strains.	Bronchiolitis and pneumonia, characterized by formation of large syncytia in the affected parts; mild illness in older children.
e. Rubella virus (German measles)	60 nm	RNA	Round and smaller than others. The internal nucleocapsid is 33 nm in diameter.	One type as far as is known. (May be transferred to the togavirus group.)	Common cold onset; rubella is a systemic disease accompanied by rash and occipital lymphadenopathy. It has a high propensity for producing monster malformed fetuses. This danger is greatest during the first trimester of pregnancy.
Diplornaviruses 1. Reoviruses (double-layered capsid)	75–80 nm	RNA	The nucleocapsid has a double layer of capsomeres with 92 subunits in the outer visible layer. They are icosahedral in shape with an envelope.	These viruses were formerly classified among the ECHO viruses but have been separated for reasons of size and immunity. Types 1, 2, and 3 are found.	Type 1: minor winter febrile illness in children. Type 2: diarrhea or steatorrhea in children. Type 3: febrile upper respiratory disease in children.
2. Coronaviruses (double-layered capsid)	70–250 nm	RNA	Round to elliptical particles with petal-shaped projections resembling a solar corona. Very fastidious growth requirements.	Infectious bronchitis virus (IBV) of adults in man. IBV of avians. IBV of swine. Mouse hepatitis virus.	Infectious bronchitis of adults; common cold in abortive cases.

	Nucleic acid	Size	Morphology	Viruses / types	Disease / clinical notes
3. Papovaviruses (included because they are the third grouping of double-layered capsid viruses; lesion viruses do occur in the ear, nose, and throat)	DNA (double-stranded)	40–50 nm	Viruses have double-stranded DNA. Exhibit icosahedral symmetry, naked capsid with 72 capsomeres.	Papilloma virus of man, rabbit, cow, and dog. Polyoma virus of mice. Vacuolating virus of monkeys.	Papilloma viruses cause warts (benign tumors) in all species marked. The polyoma virus of mice causes many different types of malignant tumors in this species. The last virus causes vacuolating lesions in cells.
Herpesviruses (at least 25 viruses in this group) 1. Herpes simplex virus	DNA (double-stranded)	Naked virus, 100 nm; enveloped, 150–180 nm	Contain 16 capsomeres in the capsid, which is icosahedral. A rather prominent envelope is present.	Herpes simplex virus of man. Occurs in two types —(1) oral, and (2) genital.	Type 1: can cause abortive unrecognized disease in infants between ages of 1 and 3. Often causes acute gingivostomatitis, generalized eczema, herpeticum (Kaposi's varicelliform eruption). Keratoconjunctivitis; meningoencephalitis; chronic herpes febrilis. Type 2: has been associated with carcinoma of the cervix. It may be transmitted to and cause serious to fatal infection in infants. Both types can cause mild meningitis or fatal encephalitis.
2. Varicella-zoster	DNA (double-stranded)	150–180 nm	Identical in morphology with the simplex type.	One type, as far as is known at this time, regardless of the clinical entity.	Varicella or chickenpox varies widely in the severity of the clinical disease. Ranges from unrealized infection to fatal disseminated type. Repeat infection likely. May cause encephalitis zoster. Herpesvirus zoster causes disease in a partially immune host. Pain is sometimes severe, followed by outbreak of macules, papules, and very thin-walled vesicles along the skin over distribution of a sensory nerve.

137

Table 8-1. Viruses Concerned with Upper Respiratory Infection (cont.)

Name and Group	Size	Type of Nucleic Acid	Shape and Structure	Immunologic Types	Diseases and Syndromes
3. Cytomegalovirus	150–180 nm	DNA	Identical in morphology with the simplex virus. Inclusion bodies most prominent in certain cells.	One type for man. Cannot infect lower animals with this agent and vice versa.	Congenitally acquired disease as a rule. Sometimes without symptoms. Can be severe; as encephalitis; can give rise to kernicterus. Can be acquired later in childhood or young adulthood. Can cause cytomegaloid mononucleosis. *No heterophile antibodies found.* May be seen in children and adults, either spontaneous or after blood transfusion.
4. EB virus (Epstein-Barr) confirmed by Henle	150–180 nm	DNA	Under the electron microscope it is indistinguishable from herpes forms. Very few enveloped forms have been observed.	Only one type known thus far.	This Epstein-Barr virus is now thought to be the cause of Burkitt's lymphoma, most often seen in young boys in Central Africa. Also incriminated as the cause of nasopharyngeal carcinoma. Recently evidence is gathering that this agent causes typical infectious mononucleosis.
5. Herpesvirus "B" of old world monkeys; herpesvirus simiae	110 nm	DNA	Morphologically identical with other agents of this group.	Only one type known.	This disease is mild to inapparent in monkeys. In man, particularly after a monkey bite, it often produces a highly fatal disease.

responsible for the A_2 or Asian mutant, which resulted in the 1957 pandemic and is probably related to the A/New Jersey and A/Victoria outbreaks.

Influenza B infections have been found to occur sporadically and to be present in a somewhat endemic fashion. Extensive outbreaks due to influenza B occur less frequently than those caused by type A strains. In some instances influenza B has been more prevalent in military populations, suggesting that crowding and fatigue are factors in the epidemiology of these infections.

Although antibody surveys have shown influenza C to have a worldwide distribution, only widely scattered and localized outbreaks have been attributed to this type. Generally, the only clinical manifestations of an influenza C infection are those of a mild upper respiratory infection.

Immunity to influenza can be established with a vaccine. In well-controlled studies in the military, this has been proved several times. The criteria for success in this effort include the following:

1. The most recent mutants of any strains of type A and type B must be present in the vaccine.

2. Sufficient concentration of each of the viral antigens, calculated in chick red cell–agglutinating units, must be present.

3. Adsorption of the vaccine on calcium phosphate particles used as adjuvant improves the effectiveness of the preparation.

4. The dose of vaccine should be large enough to give a sufficient stimulus for above-threshold levels of antibody to be formed.

5. The recommendation at present is to give 0.5 ml of vaccine annually in the early fall by the subcutaneous route. (Persons with overt sensitivity to egg protein should not be given the vaccine, or at least not given it in this manner.)

6. Some authors recommend giving 0.2 ml intradermally, followed by two more such doses at 2-week intervals. This takes advantage of the possibility of producing a booster effect while giving more time to combat hypersensitivity in a patient whose history is unknown.

Parainfluenza Viruses

The parainfluenza viruses are now considered to be a separate subgroup of viruses classified as the paramyxoviruses. Included in this group are four viruses, some of which are associated with upper respiratory illnesses. They are similar to the influenza viruses in their ability to agglutinate mammalian and avian erythrocytes. They differ from the true influenza viruses, however, in their slightly larger size and their tendency to lyse as well as agglutinate erythrocytes. These viruses are also known as hemadsorption viruses because of their ability to cause the adsorption of erythrocytes in infected tissue cultures. Since a complete discussion of the biologic properties of these agents is beyond the scope of this book, only the salient features of these viruses which would be of interest to clinicians are presented below.

Parainfluenza Virus Type 1 (Hemadsorption Type 2, Influenza D, Sendai Virus). This virus has been reported to be the causal agent of pneumonitis in newborn children and one of the chief etiologic agents of acute laryngotracheobronchitis in children. In adults it has been reported to cause symptoms similar to those of the common cold.

Parainfluenza Virus Type 2 (Croup-associated Virus). This agent has been associated with acute laryngotracheobronchitis in children. It also causes croup in children.

Parainfluenza Virus Type 3 (Hemadsorption Virus Type 1). This virus has been isolated from children suffering from mild respiratory illness and acute laryngotracheobronchitis. Infections with parainfluenza type 3 virus are more prevalent and occur earlier in life than infections with parainfluenza types 1 and 2. This agent exhibits a predilection for the lower respiratory tract, and first infections frequently result in bronchitis, bronchiolitis, or bronchial pneumonia.

Parainfluenza Virus Type 4. The sum total of the clinical knowledge about this virus is very scant. Clinically, all that can be said about this virus at present is that it is associated with malaise in young children. It is also known as the M–25 virus.

Respiratory Syncytial Virus (RS Virus)

This agent has been so named because it causes the formation of syncytial masses in serially propagated tissue cultures which have been derived from human sources. It is the chief cause of bronchiolitis and viral pneumonia in infants less than 6 months of age. Infections occurring after the first 6 months of life are much less severe than those occurring earlier. The severity of the infections in the younger children appears to be correlated with the inability of the patients to develop antibodies against this virus. It has been reported that only 20% of the infants infected with this virus develop complement-fixing antibodies during convalescence. Preexisting antibodies in young children and adult volunteers do not appear to afford complete resistance to subsequent lower respiratory infections with this agent.

The epidemiology of RS virus infections is different from that observed in the influenza viruses and the parainfluenza 1 and 3 viruses. Infections with the RS virus occur extensively in children during the winter months of every year, while outbreaks of influenza A and B viruses recur at intervals of 2 to 3 years. Illnesses caused by parainfluenza virus types 1 and 3 appear to be endemic in a community throughout the year.

Rhinoviruses

The rhinoviruses now number 55 distinct serologic types, and it is likely many more will be added in the future. Association of these viruses with respiratory illnesses, particularly the so-called common cold, is well-documented; in adults and older children the rhinoviruses are the most common cause of the cold. Because of the multiplicity of serotypes, developing a vaccine is difficult.

Rhinoviruses are small, ether-resistant viruses containing ribonucleic acid. They belong to the picornavirus group, from whose other members they are distinguished by their acid lability and possibly by their higher density. One rhinovirus, ECHO 28, was previously thought to be an enterovirus but is now properly classified as a rhinovirus.

Etiology of the Common Cold

The possibility that a filterable virus caused the common cold was suggested by Kruse in 1914. In 1923 Olitsky and McCartney, using bacteria-free filtrates from nasal secretions of patients, transmitted the common cold to chimpanzees. Dochez and coworkers confirmed this work in 1930.

The extensive use of tissue culture techniques during the past decades has resulted in the isolation of many viruses from persons with colds. Viruses capable of causing the common cold or coldlike symptoms in man are legion and are summarized in Table 8–1. A recent addition is the herpesvirus, which is more commonly associated with vesicular diseases of the upper respiratory tract.

Little doubt remains concerning the viral etiology of the common cold, but the possibility still exists that allergenic substances, fungi, or bacteria may operate in concert with a virus in producing this syndrome. Of the many viruses causing the common cold, rhinoviruses are most frequently encountered, especially in older children and adults.

The significance of excessive dryness in the pathogenesis of the common cold is not clear. An intact, actively moving blanket of mucus usually provides an efficient first line of defense for the mucosal surface. In addition to its flushing action, nasal mucus contains IgA, which is probably responsible for the specific antiviral activity of the healthy nose. Nasal secretions also contain the bactericidal enzyme lysozyme. Areas of dryness may lead to stasis of the blanket of mucus, which in turn provides an opportunity for penetration by noxious organisms into the deeper tissues. Banks has experimental evidence, produced in chickens, suggesting that alteration of the mucus blanket in the nose leads to an increased susceptibility to infection with a myxovirus called Newcastle disease virus. It does not seem unlikely that such areas of dryness are encouraged by abnormal convection currents, low humidity, or autonomic imbalance. Ideal environmental humidity in health is considered to be in the range of 45 to 50%. Humidities in the range of 80 to 90% are desirable in some acute upper respiratory diseases (e.g., laryngotracheobronchitis).

Vesicular Viral Diseases of the Upper Respiratory Tract

Two groups of viruses, Coxsackie A and herpesvirus, are the chief causal agents of the viral vesicular diseases of the upper respiratory tract. The etiologic agents and the syndromes they produce are presented in Table 8–1. Detailed accounts of the etiology and pathogenesis of these diseases follow. The clinical picture and treatment of these diseases are discussed in Chapter 9 under Diseases of the Pharynx and Fauces.

Herpesvirus. The two clinical stages of herpetic infections, primary and recurrent herpes simplex, are caused by the same virus. The primary stage usually occurs as an asymptomatic infection but may occur as a localized or systemic infection in young children. The recurrent stage is a localized vesicular eruption caused by the activation of latent virus in the tissues of a person with circulating antibody. In the majority of cases, the reactivated virus produces herpes labialis (fever blisters, cold sores).

There are only two antigenic types of herpes virus, and this virus replicates primarily in the cell nucleus. Man is the only natural host, although the virus is easily adaptable to laboratory animals and tissue cultures derived from other vertebrates.

The binomial Latin nomenclature of *Herpesvirus hominis* has been proposed for this virus. Also included in this group are *Herpesvirus simiae,* the etiologic agent of monkey B disease, and the viruses causing varicella-zoster and cytomegalic inclusion disease. Also included in the herpesvirus group are viruses associated etiologically with Burkitt's lymphoma, nasopharyngeal carcinoma, and infectious mononucleosis.

The primary infection with herpes simplex virus generally occurs during the first 5 years of life, but maternal antibodies offer a high degree of protection during the first 6 months of age. An increased incidence of childhood primary herpetic infections has been noted in lower socioeconomic groups. Epidemics are rare, but institutional outbreaks are known. The virus has been found to be intermittently present in the oropharynx of healthy carriers. Serologic surveys have shown that 90% of adults possess circulating antibodies against herpesvirus. While these antibodies prevent spread of the virus to other tissues, they do not preclude viral multiplication or localized lesion development.

In the primary stage of the disease, the virus multiplies at the portal of entry, resulting in either a localized lesion or an asymptomatic infection. Viremias have been detected in nonimmune individuals. Recurrent herpetic infections tend to occur at the site of the original lesion. This occurs as a result of the activation of the latent virus by a stress, such as exposure to sunlight, minor febrile illness, gastrointestinal disturbance, trauma, menstruation, pregnancy, physical exertion, or even strong emotion.

Histologically the lesions of varicella-zoster (shingles), primary herpes, and recurrent herpes are indistinguishable from one another. Histologic sections or tissue scrapings from all of these lesions exhibit degenerating epithelial cells with ballooned cytoplasm, eosinophilic intranuclear inclusion bodies, and multinucleated giant cells of the Tzanck variety.

Coxsackie Viruses. The Coxsackie viruses are causal agents of myocarditis, herpangina, vesicular stomatitis, epidemic pleurodynia, aseptic (nonbacterial) meningitis, acute respiratory illnesses, and epidemic exanthemata (meningoencephalitis with rash). These viruses are members of the enterovirus group and, like the other members of this group, are most prevalent during the late summer. Epidemics in institutions or summer camp populations are frequently seen during this time of the year.

The term "Coxsackie virus" was proposed in 1949 to provide a name for the new group of agents isolated in Coxsackie, New York, during a poliomyelitis outbreak. This term had no anatomic or clinical significance, since little was known of the pathogenesis of Coxsackie infections. The Coxsackie viruses are now included in the picornavirus group because of their similarity to its other members. The other viruses in this group are the poliovirus, ECHO (enteric cytopathic human orphan) virus, and rhinovirus.

Twenty-nine distinct serotypes of this virus have been recognized since Dalldorf and Sickles isolated the first agent in 1948. The Coxsackie agents are classified into two groups, A and B, on the basis of the lesions produced in newborn mice. The 23 group A viruses produce a severe and generalized myopathy in the striated muscles of newborn mice. The six group B viruses produce localized and less severe muscle lesions, in addition to pancreatitis, hepatitis, myocarditis, and encephalitis. The Coxsackie viruses may also be grouped on the basis of their ability to replicate in primary (first invitro passage) monkey kidney (PMK) tissue cultures. The six group B types, as well as types A7 and A9, replicate in PMK, whereas the remainder of the A types will not replicate in tissue culture.

The similarity in the epidemiology of Coxsackie virus and poliomyelitis is striking. Both viruses may be present in healthy carriers. They may be carried for varying periods of time and cause an inapparent or clinically recognized disease. Both agents may be recovered from man, sewage, and flies. Both agents may be recovered from the same specimen. When this occurs in a patient with a clinically recognizable infection, it is impossible to determine which agent is contributing to the observed symptoms. Both viruses are disseminated by oropharyngeal secretions and feces.

BACTERIAL DISEASES OF THE UPPER RESPIRATORY TRACT

Streptococcal Infections

The streptococci are frequent causal agents of diseases in man, particularly those of the upper respiratory tract. These organisms were divided into three varieties on the basis of their hemolytic activity by Schöttmuller in 1903. This classification is convenient, since blood-agar is the medium of choice for the propagation of these organisms. The three varieties are:

1. Alpha-hemolytic streptococci, which produce a zone of green discoloration (incomplete hemolysis) in the medium immediately surrounding the colony. In addition to the discoloration, the colony size of organisms in this group is larger than that seen in the beta-hemolytic variety.

2. Beta-hemolytic streptococci, which completely hemolyze the blood cells in the area surrounding the colony, resulting in a clear zone within the red opaque medium.

3. Anhemolytic or gamma variety of streptococci, which produce no hemolytic change in the surrounding medium.

The beta-hemolytic streptococci have been divided into a number of immunologically distinct groups by Lancefield on the basis of a heat-stable, acid-extractable polysaccharide termed C substance. This polysaccharide is group-specific and is found in all streptococci except those of the viridans group. Lancefield's groups are termed A, B, C, D, E, F, G, H, J, K, L, M, and N. Of these groups, members of group A are the most frequently isolated organisms in human streptococcal diseases. The streptococci were further classified by Griffith into immunologically distinct types on the basis of a type-specific M substance, which is a protein in group A but is probably a polysaccharide in the other groups.

The hemolytic classification and the Lancefield classification have been utilized in a further method of considering streptococci, namely, a clinicophysiologic grouping as follows:

1. **The Pyogenic group of streptococci.** This grouping includes all members of Lancefield groups A, B, C, F, G, H, and K which give rise to acute fulminating pyogenic infections in man. Of these, the group A infections give rise to the most important diseases, such as scarlet fever, septic sore throat, mastoiditis, erysipelas, acute rheumatic fever, and acute glomerulonephritis.

2. **The Group D or Enterococci.** Though these organisms are classifiable as members of the Lancefield grouping and many are hemolytic, some are definitely of the alpha-hemolytic type. Some are even of the gamma type in 24 hours, only to become slightly alpha in 48 to 72 hours. These organisms include streptococci known as *Streptococcus faecalis* and the enterococci. They are involved in genital infections and peritonitis.

3. **The Viridans Group of Streptococci.** This group includes microorganisms such as *Streptococcus salivarius, streptococcus MG,*

Streptococcus sanguis, streptococcus of subacute bacterial endocarditis *(S.B.E.)* and *Streptococcus mitis,* which can be alpha-hemolytic or nonhemolytic. They are associated with subacute bacterial endocarditis and many types of focal infection. Though much slower than group A streptococci in their invasive character, they result just as often in fatal diseases.

4. **The Lactis Group of Streptococci.** These organisms belong to Lancefield groups L, M, and N and are usually utilized to make cottage cheese, cheese, yogurt, and other partially fermented foods. Two species, *Streptococcus lactis* and *Streptococcus cremoris,* can hemolyze human blood and have been pathogenic to man in a very few instances in the host with compromised or greatly lowered resistance.

5. **The Microaerophilic Streptococci.** These organisms are usually resident within the skin of man. Though not highly invasive, they can cause postpartum or generalized infection. They are capable of causing abscesses, Meleny's gangrene, peritonitis, focalized infection, and pulmonary suppuration. They are strictly anaerobic on primary isolation but later become microaerophilic. Many belong to the genus *Peptostreptococcus* and cause brown hemopeptic zones around their colonies on blood-agar. These streptococci are usually quite small in size.

6. **The Anaerobic Streptococci.** The members of this group are also members of the *Peptostreptococcus* genus but are obligate anaerobes. About seven species have been recognized. They are found normally in the feces and in the vagina of females. They have been associated with puerperal fever, peritonitis, empyema, and Meleny's gangrene. They usually produce foul odors. They may be associated with *Clostridium* sp. and/or spirochetes in peritonitis or pulmonary abscess formation.

In addition to immunologic antigens and hemolysins, the streptococci also possess a number of exotoxins. These include leucocidin, hyaluronidase, erythrogenic toxin, fibrinolysins, and streptolysins.

Leucocidin. An enzymelike substance, leucocidin is toxic for leukocytes and therefore may prevent or inhibit phagocytosis. There is some evidence that the leucocidin produced by the group A streptococcus is identical to another of its toxins, streptolysin O.

Hyaluronidase. This factor was at one time thought to have a correlation with the invasive action of the streptococci. At present it occupies a somewhat paradoxical position in that it has been shown to digest the capsule of streptococcal organisms, thus making them less virulent and more susceptible to phagocytosis.

Erythrogenic Toxin. This toxin is responsible for the rash of scarlet fever and is also known as the Dick or scarlatinal toxin. It differs from the classic exotoxins in that it is partially resistant to boiling.

Fibrinolysin. Fibrinolysin (streptokinase) is an activator of a serum protease and may be associated with the invasive characteristic of the microorganism.

Streptolysins. In addition to the alpha and beta hemolysins previously described, Todd in 1938 described two additional hemolysins. These are different in that the type designated S is heat-labile and acid-labile, while streptolysin O is inactivated only by oxygen. This oxygen inactivation is reversible by the addition of a mild reducing agent. The immune response to streptolysin O, *anti–streptolysin O titer (ASO),* is a useful criterion in the laboratory diagnosis of streptococcal infections. The presence of a rising titer during a febrile illness is confirmatory evidence of a streptococcal etiology. Low titers reflect a past streptococcal infection. A direct correlation exists between the severity of a streptococcal infection and the height and duration of the ASO titer.

The production of the aforementioned toxins is a characteristic of beta-hemolytic streptococci as a group. Not all strains of group A streptococci will produce all the above toxins, but those that do are generally more virulent. Likewise, there is no specific streptococcus of scarlet fever, septic sore throat, cellulitis, erysipelas, or puerperal sepsis, although in any given season one particular type of streptococcal organism may be the etiologic agent of the many and varied infections observed.

The most commonly observed group A streptococcal infections of the upper respiratory tract are scarlet fever, pharyngitis, and tonsillitis. These are most commonly observed in children of 5 to 15 years of age. Transmission of group A streptococci is usually by direct contact, and significant extrahuman reservoirs do not exist, although many outbreaks due to food contamination (often milk) have been reported. The epidemiologic chain in cases of milk-borne streptococcal infections is mainly one of man to cow to milk to man.

Members of group A hemolytic streptococci are the chief etiologic agents of erysipelas. Some cases due to group C organisms have also been reported. Although persons suffering from erysipelas harbor large numbers of group A streptococci in their nasopharynx, the pathogenesis of the disease is unknown. In the spontaneous type of erysipelas, the infecting organism is apparently transferred from the patient's own nose or pharynx. In the postsurgical type of this disease, group A streptococci are apparently spread to the patient from hospital personnel who are healthy carriers of this organism.

Suppurative complications of group A streptococcal diseases can usually be readily prevented by appropriate therapy. Present interest is centered on the poststreptococcal, nonsuppurative complications. Most important among these are rheumatic fever, glomerulonephritis, and mesenteric adenitis, which are believed by some investigators to be the result of inappropriate immunologic reactions.

Treatment. Most important in the management of streptococcal disease is the immediate institution of antimicrobial therapy. The drug of choice is penicillin, although erythromycin and tetracyclines may be used. Sulfonamides are not effective against group A beta-hemolytic streptococci. When tetracyclines are prescribed it should be remembered that 20 to 40% of streptococci isolated from hospitalized patients are resistant to tetracyclines.

Satisfactory therapy is accomplished by:

1. Benzathine penicillin G, 900,000 to 1,200,000 units, as a single injection.

2. Oral penicillin V or G, 250 mg (adult), four times daily for 10 days.

3. Procaine penicillin, 600,000 units, by injection every second day for four to five doses.

4. When penicillin is contraindicated, oral erythromycin, 250 mg, four times a day for 10 days may be used.

5. Recently a new synthetic penicillin, ampicillin, has been introduced for oral use. It has the same general spectrum of antibacterial activity as the other penicillins but seems more effective against certain gram-negative bacteria than the others. It is not to be considered a broad-spectrum antibiotic. Ampicillin is useful in controlling infections caused by *Hemophilus influenzae* and *Diplococcus pneumoniae*. If the alpha-hemolytic streptococci are the causative agents, the Group III penicillins, such as oxacillin and cloxacillin, or the Group IV drugs, such as cephloradine, should be used.

Abscess formation, though diminished in antibiotic-treated infections, still requires drainage.

Staphylococcal Infections

The classification of the staphylococci, like that of many other organisms, is unsatisfactory. These organisms are classified on the basis of their pathogenicity and pigment production. The pigments produced by the more important members of this group are as follows: *Staphylococcus aureus,* golden yellow; *S. albus,* white; and *S. citreus,* lemon yellow. Most human staphylococcal diseases are caused by *Staphylococcus aureus.*

The staphylococci, like the streptococci, form a number of toxins. These toxins include hemolysins, leucocidins, coagulase, hyaluronidase, staphylokinase, and an enterotoxin. Brief descriptions of these toxins are presented below.

The pyogenic staphylococci, on primary isolation on blood-agar, are generally beta-hemolytic. The colonies are surrounded by a clear zone of hemolysis (see Streptococcal Infections). This hemolytic activity has been shown to be due to an exotoxin and consists of several distinct hemolysins. The first hemolysins differentiated were the alpha and beta lysins, which differ in their spectra of hemolytic activity. The alpha lysin lyses sheep and rabbit erythrocytes but not those of humans or guinea pigs. The beta lysin is active against sheep but not rabbit red blood cells and is a hot-cold lysin, i.e., the cells do not lyse when incubated at 37°C but do when chilled following this incubation. The delta lysin differs from the first two in that it lyses the erythrocytes of man, monkeys, horses, rats, and guinea pigs, as well as those of sheep and rabbits.

Three toxins, active against leukocytes and termed leucocidins, have been reported. The effects of these toxins include inhibition of respiration, swelling, and lysis of the affected leukocytes.

Many staphylococci possess an enzyme, *coagulase*, which is capable of clotting the plasma of man and other animals. Strains possessing this enzyme are said to be coagulase-positive. The high correlation between virulence and coagulase production has made these terms virtually synonymous.

Some strains of staphylococci produce an enzyme, hyaluronidase, which depolymerizes hyaluronic acid. This depolymerization of the ground substance of tissue permits the spread of infecting organisms.

Staphylokinase, like streptokinase, activates a protease which causes fibrinolysis. It is distinguishable from coagulase in that it is heat-labile. Staphylokinase differs from streptokinase in its fibrinolytic spectrum; it acts on the plasma of other animal species as well as on the plasma of man.

There have been reports of the formation of a scarlatinal or similar toxin which produces a scarlet fever of staphylococcal etiology.

Staphylococci are present in relatively large numbers on the skin and in the upper respiratory tract. These organisms, except in cases of staphylococcal pneumonias, invade the body of man via the hair follicles and sebaceous glands. Virtually all adults possess staphylococcal antibodies in the skin, but the role of humoral immunity, if it exists at all, is not clear. There is no satisfactory evidence to indicate that vaccine prophylaxis or desensitization is effective in preventing staphylococcal infections. However, treatment of chronic antibiotic-resistant staphylococcal infections with autogenous vaccines may be of value.

Pathogenic strains of staphylococci, i.e., *Staphylococcus aureus,* can be isolated from the anterior nares ("picking area") and skin of 50 to 60% of humans. Hospital personnel have an even higher incidence of colonization. The indiscriminate use of antibiotics has led to the development of antibiotic-resistant strains of staphylococci. These resistant strains are seen more frequently in hospital personnel and patients than in individuals in other walks of life. Resistance to penicillin, streptomycin, tetracycline, chloramphenicol, erythromycin, oleandomycin, and novobiocin have been reported. Resistance to bacitracin, neomycin, kanamycin, ristocetin, and vancomycin is frequent. Recently sodium methicillin (Staphcillin) has been reported to be the drug of choice in the treatment of antibiotic-resistant staphylococci. The recommended dosage is 1 g given intramuscularly or intravenously every 4 to 6 hours for adults, and 100 mg per kg body weight per day for children. The oral drug Prostaphylin (sodium oxacillin) may be administered in 500-mg doses every 4 to 6 hours for adults; 50 to 100 mg per kg body weight per day in four divided doses is given for children.

PLEUROPNEUMONIA-LIKE ORGANISMS

Primary Atypical Pneumonia

Although primary atypical pneumonia is a disease of the lower respiratory tract, it is included in this text because of the highly significant studies carried out with this organism during the past several years.

Primary atypical pneumonia (PAP) is an acute respiratory disease characterized by cough, pulmonary infiltration, and self-limiting constitutional symptoms. These symptoms are nonspecific and are often found in such viral and rickettsial infections as psittacosis, Q fever, and influenza, as well as some of the pneumonias caused by the adenoviruses. Because of the possibility that more than one agent might produce an infection classified as atypical pneumonia, the accepted practice has been to refer to this entity as a syndrome rather than as a specific disease. Although formerly there were no specific agents associated with this syndrome, it was noted that cold agglutinins and streptococcus MG agglutinins developed in some cases during convalescence. Eaton in 1944 recovered a filterable agent from the sputum of PAP patients which produced pneumonia in experimental laboratory animals and which was neutralized by the serum of patients recovering from the disease. This agent, thought to be a virus, was known as Eaton's agent.

The status of the Eaton agent was unresolved until 1962, when Chanock, Hayflick, and Barile successfully grew the organism on artificial media. This organism produced colonies of typical pleuropneumonia-like organisms (PPLO) on agar supplemented with high concentrations of horse serum. The relationship of these organisms to the PAP syndrome was documented by human volunteer infection experiments and by specific fluorescence in the fluorescent antibody test. This organism is now accepted as the etiologic agent of PAP. *Mycoplasma pneumoniae* has been suggested as the name for the PPLO of primary atypical pneumonia by Sommerson and coworkers.

Mycoplasma pneumoniae produces small homogeneously granular colonies easily differentiated from the "nippled" or "fried egg" colonies of other oral PPLO's. This organism may also be differentiated from other human PPLO's by the production of beta hemolysis in a guinea pig erythrocyte-agar overlay or by specific neutralization with antiserum.

BACTERIAL VARIANTS

The term "bacterial variant" refers to cell wall–defective, morphologically altered bacteria. They are variously called spheroplasts, protoplasts, and L-forms.

They arise from normal bacteria, either spontaneously or in the presence of converter substances (e.g., penicillin) that have the capacity of altering the cell wall. Thus by virtue of the deficient cell wall, they are resistant to antimicrobials that act by interruption of cell wall synthesis (e.g., penicillin, cephalosporin, cycloserine, and bacitracin). Though morphologically similar to organisms of the genus *Mycoplasma,* the bacterial variants are separate and distinct from them.

It is thought that L-forms are able to revert to the original bacterial form.

The pathogenicity of L-forms is apparently low, though they may be responsible for recrudescence of infection by reversion to the intact bacterial form. L-forms may be the etiologic agents of aphthous ulcers.

REFERENCES

Burrows, W.: *Textbook of Microbiology.* 20th ed. Philadelphia, W. B. Saunders Co., 1973.

Chanock, R. M., *et al.*: Growth of an Agent Associated with Atypical Pneumonia and its Identification as a PPLO. Proc. Natl. Acad. Sci. USA, *48*:41, 1962.

Dalldorf, G., and Sickles, G. M.: An Unidentified, Filterable Agent Isolated from the Feces of Children with Paralysis. Science, *108*:61, 1948.

Dalldorf, G., *et al.*: The Coxsackie Virus Group. In Rivers, T. M., and Horsfall, F. L. (Eds.): *Viral and Rickettsial Diseases of Man.* 4th ed. Philadelphia, J. B. Lippincott Co., 1965.

Dingle, J. H., and Ginsberg, H. S.: The Adenovirus Group. In Rivers, T. M., and Horsfall, F. L. (Eds.): *Viral and Rickettsial Infections of Man.* 4th ed. Philadelphia, J. B. Lippincott Co., 1965.

Dunnet, W. N., and Schallibaum, E. M.: Scarlet Fever-like Illness due to Staphylococcus Infection. Lancet, *2*:1227, 1960.

Eaton, M. D., *et al.*: Studies on the Etiology of Primary Atypical Pneumonia. A Filterable Agent Transmissible to Cotton Rats, Hamsters and Chick Embryos. J. Exp. Med., *79*:649, 1944.

Francis, T.: Influenza. In Rivers, T. M., and Horsfall, F. L. (Eds.): *Viral and Rickettsial Infections of Man.* 4th ed. Philadelphia, J. B. Lippincott Co., 1965.

Hilleman, M. R., and Werner, J. H.: Recovery of New Agent from Patients with Acute Respiratory Illness. Proc. Soc. Exp. Biol. Med., *85*:183, 1963.

Jackson, G. G., *et al.*: Respiratory Diseases of Viral Etiology. VII. Present Concepts of The Common Cold. Am. J. Public Health, *52*:940, 1962.

Jawetz, E., *et al.*: Viral Diseases of the Respiratory Tract and Parotid Glands. In *Review of Medical Microbiology.* 5th ed. Los Altos, Lange Medical Publishing Co., 1962.

Kapian, A. Z.: Rhinoviruses: A Numbering System. Nature (Lond.), *213*:761, 1967.

Liu, C., *et al.*: Studies on Primary Atypical Pneumonia. II. Observations Concerning the Development and Immunological Characteristics of Antibody in Patients. J. Exp. Med., *109*:545, 1959.

Mufson, M. A., *et al.*: Acute Respiratory Diseases of Viral Etiology. V. Eaton, Agent; A Review. Am. J. Public Health, *52*:925, 1962.

Negro, R. C., *et al.*: Escarlatina par *Staphylococcus aureus*. An. Fac. de Med. Montevideo, *41*:263, 1956.

New Drugs. Chicago, American Medical Association, 1966.

Pelon, W., and Mogabgob, W. J.: A Cytopathogenic Agent Isolated from Naval Recruits with Mild Upper Respiratory Illness. Proc. Soc. Exp. Biol. Med., *94*: 262, 1957.

Price, W. H.: The Isolation of a New Virus Associated with Respiratory Clinical Disease in Humans. Proc. Natl. Acad. Sci. USA, *42*:892, 1956.

Rowe, W. P., *et al.*: Isolation of a Cytopathogenic Agent from Human Adenoids Undergoing Spontaneous Degeneration in Tissue Culture. Proc. Soc. Exp. Biol. Med., *84*:570, 1953.

Sommerson, N. L., *et al.*: Hemolysin Production as an Aid in the Identification and Quantitation of Eaton Agent *(Mycoplasma pneumoniae)*. Am. J. Hygiene, *77*:122, 1963.

Chapter 9

Acute Inflammatory Diseases of the Nose and Sinuses

John J. Ballenger and Harry B. Harding

THE COMMON COLD

The common cold is an acute, recurrent, relatively mild infection of the upper respiratory tract. The etiology was discussed in Chapter 8.

Signs and Symptoms. The onset of a cold is usually abrupt and may be heralded by a sense of dryness, tickling, or burning in the nose or nasopharynx. Chills and malaise are soon noted and are accompanied by sneezing and a watery nasal discharge. Fever is usually not present at this time. A mild headache or feeling of fullness between the eyes is frequently present.

The full-blown cold usually develops within 48 hours and is marked by a husky voice, suffusion of the eyes, watery nasal discharge, and diminished or absent sense of smell and taste. The greatly reduced nasal airway in a patient with a cold is the most disturbing symptom. The low-grade ache about the forehead, eyes, and sometimes the cheeks is related to the turgescence of the nasal mucosa.

The course of a well-developed cold is variable. The illness may subside in 3 to 4 days, but more commonly secondary bacterial invaders appear which prolong illness another 6 to 8 days. When this occurs, the nasal discharge becomes yellow-purulent or mucopurulent. This is accompanied by a productive cough caused by the nasal drainage entering the larynx.

The mucosa of the nasal sinuses participates in the inflammatory reaction of the common cold. Purulent nasal discharge is noted when secondary (bacterial) infection supervenes. Vertigo, transitory deafness, and otitis media may occur if the eustachian tubes become obstructed.

Physical examination of the patient during the first days of a cold reveals a hyperemic but not a fully turgescent nasal mucosa. Within the first hours, the mucosa is abnormally dry and sometimes glazed in appearance. Later the mucosa becomes edematous, and a thin watery or mucoid discharge is obvious. In this latter state, the mucosa may be pale and boggy and resembles that seen in the allergic state. An allergic etiology is suggested when stained smears of the nasal secretions show many eosinophils. Redness and excoriation of the anterior nares are frequently noted. Coryzal symptoms may herald the onset of measles, and a search for Koplik's spots may be in order.

Laboratory Findings. In the uncomplicated cold the leukocyte and erythrocyte counts are normal. Urinalysis is normal, and cultures from the upper respiratory tract yield no pathogenic bacteria.

Pathology. Microscopic sections of nasal and nasopharyngeal tissue exhibit edema and hypersecretion with comparatively little cellular infiltration. As in influenzal infections, an appreciable amount of desquamation, particularly of ciliated epithelium, occurs.

Treatment and Prophylaxis. The treatment of the common cold is largely symptomatic. Antibiotics and sulfonamides are of no benefit to the patient in the absence of bacterial complications. Aqueous ephedrine nose drops, 1%, are helpful in relieving nasal congestion. Since lysozyme is inactivated in an alkaline environment, any intranasal medication should have a slightly acid pH to prevent interference with ciliary and lysozyme activity. Highly effective symptomatically is the oral administration, every 4 hours, of a capsule containing:

Ephedrine sulfate	0.015g
Pentobarbital	0.015g
Acetylsalicylic acid*	0.300g

Several years ago the use of antihistaminic drugs in treating common colds was widespread, but in the absence of the allergic state their use has been disappointing.

Attempts to increase the resistance of individuals by a "hardening" process, bacterial vaccines, vitamins, heat lamps, and so forth have proved disappointing. There are no specific vaccines commercially available for immunization against colds. However, the efficacy of a polyvalent cold vaccine is currently being evaluated in several clinical trials in this country.

The immunity conferred by a common cold is of a low order, of short duration, and type-specific for the infecting virus. Considering the low-grade immunity and the large number of viruses causing the common cold, one can understand why many people suffer repeated colds.

INFLUENZA

Influenza is an acute infectious respiratory disease of man commonly encountered in epidemic form. Epidemics are characterized by a rapid onset, irregular spread, high

---

* Acetaminophen, 300 mg, may be substituted for acetylsalicylic acid.

morbidity, and low mortality except in infants and the aged. In addition to the clinical disease, a relatively high incidence of subclinical infection can be detected by serologic testing.

Signs and Symptoms. Clinically, influenza is characterized by a sudden onset of fever, myalgia, headache, pharyngitis, and a dry cough. The constitutional symptoms of this disease far overshadow the respiratory features. Patients, particularly children, complain of accompanying gastrointestinal symptoms. Retrobulbar pain and pain in the lower back and legs occur. The disease is usually self-limiting and runs its course in 3 to 5 days. The chief complication of influenza is secondary bacterial infection of the paranasal sinuses, middle ear, bronchi, and lungs. Encephalitis due to influenza viruses has also been reported, as well as an overwhelming viremia.

Physical examination usually reveals a temperature elevated to 101° to 104° F, nonexudative pharyngitis, and suffusion of the eyes. The fever usually lasts about 5 days. A watery nasal discharge may be present. Scattered rales are sometimes encountered upon examination of the chest. A leukopenia is usually present, while a leukocytosis is indicative of a secondary bacterial invasion.

Treatment. Except in the case of the A_2 strains (amantadine), the treatment of uncomplicated influenza is symptomatic. Penicillin and broad-spectrum antibiotics are not indicated in the absence of secondary complications.

PARAINFLUENZA

In parainfluenza virus infections, as in other viral diseases, antibiotic therapy is of no benefit to the patient. However, appropriate antibiotic therapy is indicated in the presence of secondary bacterial invasion. No vaccines are commercially available for immunization against the parainfluenza organisms.

ERYSIPELAS

Erysipelas is an acute group A streptococcal infection of the skin. The face and head are usually involved, but other areas of the body may also be affected. Two types of erysipelas, spontaneous and surgical, are recognized.

Signs and Symptoms. The onset of erysipelas is characterized by an abrupt fever accompanied by a shaking chill. A history of recent febrile illness may be obtained from one third of adult cases and more frequently in children. During the first 24 hours of the disease, the lesion is minimal. Shortly thereafter the affected areas become erythematous and edematous and exhibit the characteristically elevated and progressing border. The bridge of the nose or the cheeks are most commonly involved in facial erysipelas, whereas the areas around surgical incisions are affected in the postsurgical type of disease.

Laboratory findings show a leukocytosis with an accompanying shift to the left. Bacterial cultures from the lesion *border* and nasopharynx reveal large numbers of group A beta-hemolytic streptococci.

Treatment. The treatment of erysipelas is the same as that recommended for other streptococcal diseases (see Chapter 8, Streptococcal Infection). The application of cold saline compresses to the affected areas decreases the discomfort somewhat. The spread of the lesion stops abruptly, and the temperature usually returns to normal within 48 hours after starting treatment.

Complications associated with untreated erysipelas are abscess formation, rheumatic fever, and glomerulonephritis. While it is thought that these complications may be prevented by adequate antibiotic therapy, detailed studies of erysipelas cases managed with modern antibiotics are not available. Erysipelas is not seen as often as it formerly was.

DISEASES OF THE PHARYNX AND FAUCES

Acute Respiratory Disease (ARD)

This is an infection of the respiratory tract in which constitutional symptoms and fever are prominent. It is common in recently recruited military groups but uncommon in "seasoned" military and civilian populations.

Signs and Symptoms. The onset may be gradual or sudden. Chief complaints include sore throat, headache, general malaise, cough, and chest discomfort. Physical examination reveals a moderately hyperemic pharynx with prominent lymph follicles. Mild cervical adenopathy and mucous membrane edema may be seen. The temperature generally is in the range of 100°F but may rise to 103 to 104°F. The leukocyte and differential counts are usually normal. Bacteriologic studies of the throat and sputum reveal a normal flora. Respiratory symptoms persist for 1 to 2 weeks, but the constitutional symptoms subside with defervescence. Recovery is uneventful and complete.

Treatment and Prophylaxis. The treatment of ARD is symptomatic. Antibiotics are of no value in uncomplicated cases. A vaccine containing adenovirus types 3, 4, and 7 has been used successfully in the armed forces, but the smaller number of adenovirus infections in civilians does not warrant its general use.

Nonbacterial Pharyngitis and Pharyngoconjunctival Fever

Nonbacterial pharyngitis is an acute respiratory disease in which an exudate is present on the tonsils or pharynx. In some instances a conjunctivitis is also present. When this occurs some authors name the syndrome pharyngoconjunctival fever.

Signs and Symptoms. With the exception of localized symptoms of pharyngitis and conjunctivitis, the clinical picture of this syndrome is similar to that seen in ARD. The onset is gradual after an incubation period of 5 to 7 days. The chief symptoms include fever, chills, headache, sore throat, hoarseness, cough, and malaise. Conjunctivitis, if present, is follicular in nature and may be either unilateral or bilateral. Physical examination reveals an acutely but not severely ill person. The pharynx may be normal or slightly red. A slight exudate may be present on the tonsils or posterior pharyngeal wall. If an exudate is present, it is grayish white and pinpoint in appearance. Throat and sputum cultures reveal only normal bacterial flora. When conjunctivitis is present, the examiner may notice preauricular lymphadenopathy. Otitis media and moderate cervical lymphadenopathy may also be present.

Treatment. As in ARD, the treatment is symptomatic and supportive. Recovery is complete and usually occurs in 4 to 5 days.

Acute Tonsillitis and Pharyngitis

Symptoms and Signs. The onset of streptococcal pharyngitis is usually abrupt in older children and more gradual in younger patients. Prior to the onset there may be a sense of malaise or chilliness, followed by soreness of the throat, particularly on swallowing. The symptoms frequently are largely unilateral at first, and palpation of the lymph nodes near the angles of the jaw may reveal tenderness and enlargement. Coryza does not occur early, and its presence suggests a viral etiology.

Examination of the patient reveals a prostrate and febrile individual whose pharynx is red, uvula edematous, and pharyngeal lymphoid tissue greatly swollen. The tonsils are greatly enlarged and covered with a scattered exudate. The leukocyte count is in the range of 12,000 to 13,00 per cu mm with a left shift. A culture of the pharynx usually reveals group A beta-hemolytic streptococci.

Differential Diagnosis. Differentiation must be made from diphtheria, nonbacterial exudative pharyngitis, infectious mononucleosis, and rarely staphylococcal pharyngitis.

Treatment. If group A streptococci are suspected or demonstrated by culture, antimicrobial therapy should be begun at once and continued for 10 days. Penicillin is the drug of choice (see Chapter 8, Streptococcal Infections). Various general measures should be employed. Bedrest and an adequate intake of fluids to promote diuresis, thus eliminating bacterial toxins, are encouraged. Hot saline solution (110 to 115°F) or 5% glucose throat irrigations every 2 hours will help the sore throat. Acetylsalicylic acid, 0.3 to 0.9 g every 3 to 4 hours, is of symptomatic benefit.

Primary Atypical Pneumonia

Primary atypical pneumonia (PAP) is an acute respiratory disease characterized by cough, pulmonary infiltration of both alveoli and interstitial tissue, and self-limiting constitutional symptoms.

Signs and Symptoms. Primary atypical pneumonia has an insidious onset with an incubation period of 1 to 3 weeks. The early complaints are referable to either the upper or lower respiratory tract or may be constitutional in nature. Respiratory symptoms include sore throat and a dry paroxysmal cough. After 3 to 5 days the cough becomes productive and mucoid or mucopurulent in character. Patients may complain of substernal chest pain which appears to be related to the severity of the cough. Constitutional symptoms include headache, fever, anorexia, chills, and fatigue.

Physical examination reveals few abnormal findings. The temperature range is usually between 102 and 104°F, and the pulse rate is slowed. Examination of the chest reveals decreased breath sounds and minimal dullness to percussion. These appear minimal in relation to roentgenographic evidence of pulmonary infiltration. The characteristic finding of fine subcrepitant rales appears later in the disease. The disparity between minimal physical findings and roentgenographic involvement is a constant feature in almost every case of PAP.

A significant finding in recent human volunteer infection experiments was the production of myringitis, characterized by bullae and hemorrhage formation, in 48% of the test volunteers who had no demonstrable antibody to *Mycoplasma pneumoniae*. This high incidence of myringitis, compared to a 4% incidence in a similar number of volunteers with preexisting antibody, suggests that the organism was responsible for the observed pathology. This finding has not been reported in naturally occurring PAP, although Mufson and coworkers observed myringitis in 6% of a military recruit population ill with PAP.

Treatment. Many investigators have advocated the use of tetracyclines in the treatment of PAP. This recommendation could not be adequately evaluated, in the absence of a specific diagnostic test, by studying a heterogeneous group of respiratory illnesses. The development of a specific immunologic test, the fluorescent antibody test, paved the way for specific diagnosis and drug trials. A recent study by Mufson and coworkers in a military recruit population demonstrated the efficacy of demethylchlortetracycline (Declomycin) in the treatment of PAP. These authors reported that treatment with Declomycin significantly reduced the duration of the febrile period, positive x-ray findings, cough, anorexia, fatigue, malaise, and bedrest. A 5-day course of 125 mg of Declomycin every 6 hours is recommended for the treatment of PAP.

Primary Herpes Simplex

Under Herpesvirus (Chapter 8), the pathology of oral disease caused by this virus was discussed and should be considered in conjunction with this description. In 90% of herpes simplex infections, the primary infection is inapparent. Occasionally, however, varied lesions do develop at multiple mucosal and cutaneous sites. Herpetic gingivostomatitis is characterized by swollen gingivae, salivation, pain, and fetid breath. Vesicles 2 to 4 mm in diameter develop on the gingivae, tongue, lips, and buccal mucosa. Posteriorly, the pharyngeal mucous membrane may be affected as well. With rupture of the vesicles, a shallow painful erosion covered by a yellow pseudomembrane develops and is surrounded by an erythematous margin.

Rarely, in the newborn, a complicating meningoencephalitis or generalized herpes simplex (Kaposi type of eruption) may develop which is usually fatal. Herpetic conjunctivitis or keratitis also is occasionally found but is self-limited and heals without scarring. One exception to this, which is much more troublesome, is herpes simplex following the use of contact lenses.

Recurrent Herpes Simplex

This disease is thought to occur at the same site as the primary infection. Generally the reactivation of the latent virus assumes the form of herpes labialis (cold sore, fever blister). The lesions are clear vesicles with an erythematous base and are usually found at the mucocutaneous junction but may spread to surrounding cutaneous areas in

severe cases. Constitutional symptoms are rare in recurrent herpes. Pain, a burning sensation, and itching at the lesion site are frequently encountered and may be severe. The vesicles may rupture and release a serous or serosanguineous fluid. The lesions most often heal within a week in the absence of secondary bacterial infection.

Rarely recurrent herpesvirus infection takes the form of keratoconjunctivitis and more rarely still of herpes meningoencephalitis. It has been mistakenly assumed that aphthous ulcers located posteriorly in the mouth and in the pharynx were due to the herpesvirus. It is more likely that cell wall–deficient (L-form) bacteria are the cause (see Chapter 8, Bacterial Variants).

Treatment. Antimicrobial drugs have no effect on the course of herpes simplex infections uncomplicated by secondary bacterial infection. Soothing dressings and topical anesthesia are usually sufficient to control the pain. Corticosteroids are contraindicated in keratoconjunctivitis because of the possibility of causing spread of virus to the brain.

Herpetic Stomatitis

Herpetic stomatitis is a more extensive form of herpes simplex viral stomatitis. It is characterized by fever, pharyngitis, and malaise accompanied by severe pain and tenderness of the oral cavity. Opiates may be required for adequate relief. The pain is often so severe that it limits the oral intake of solid foods or liquids. White plaques and vesicles erupt on the buccal mucosa, tongue, and palate. These may sometimes extend to the posterior pharynx. The vesicles soon rupture, leaving areas of desquamated epithelium. Subsequent bacterial infection causes bleeding gums, fetid breath, pain, and cervical adenopathy. About one fourth of these cases exhibit a maculovesicular rash that involves the buttocks, genitals, feet, hands, and legs. Differential diagnosis includes herpangina, aphthous ulcer, apthous fever (hand, foot, and mouth disease), Vincent's angina, and thrush. Herpes simplex around the oral cavity is usually of immunologic type 1, unless oral sex is practiced. Urogenital lesions are due to type 2.

Laboratory Diagnosis of Herpetic Infections. Serologic studies, virus isolation, and cytologic studies are of value in the diagnosis of primary infections. The serologic diagnosis of recurrent herpes simplex is of questionable value because the complement-fixing and neutralizing antibodies do not exhibit consistent rises in titer. In these instances, virus isolation and cytologic studies are the diagnostic procedures of choice. Herpetic lesions may be diagnosed histologically by examining Giemsa-stained preparations of the lesion scrapings for the presence of Tzanck cells or typical intranuclear inclusion bodies.

Treatment of Herpetic Infections. Antibiotics are of no value in the treatment of herpetic lesions not secondarily infected with bacteria. However, chlortetracycline or erythromycin, 250 mg four times a day for three days, is effective in treating herpetic lesions severely infected with secondary invaders. Although 5-iodo-2-deoxyuridine, a metabolic antagonist, is effective in acute ocular herpes, its efficacy in extraocular herpes is not considered adequate. Some hope is derived from the fact that many modifications of the original molecule are now undergoing clinical tests. Topical anesthetic ointments are effective in reducing the severe pain and itching at localized herpetic lesion sites.

Lactinex, a viable suspension of *Lactobacillus acidophilus* and *Lactobacillus bulgaricus,* has been reported to be effective in treating herpetic gingivostomatitis. This treatment is empirical, and its mode of action is not known.

Herpangina

Definition. Herpangina is a specific infectious disease caused by group A Coxsackie viruses and characterized by small papulovesicular lesions, usually six or seven in number, on the soft palate and anterior tonsillar pillars. There is some question whether group B viruses might not also be involved.

Signs and Symptoms. Herpangina is a common infection occurring predominantly in the summer and early fall and usually in infants and young children. It is characterized by a sudden onset of fever of 101 to 105°F. In the posterior pharynx, discrete papulovesicular lesions, 1 to 2 mm in size, on an erythematous base are seen, and these may progress to larger ulcers. The disease is self-limiting, and complete recovery commonly occurs in 5 to 7 days. Herpangina must be differentiated primarily from acute infectious gingivostomatitis resulting from recurrent herpes simplex infection. In the latter case, the lesions are located on the gums, lips, buccal mucosa, and tongue.

Hand, Foot, and Mouth Disease (Vesicular Stomatitis)

In 1950 Robinson and coworkers observed a clinical syndrome caused by Coxsackie A viruses affecting chiefly infants and children and occasionally young adults. It is characterized by vesicular and ulcerative lesions of the mouth and oropharynx or fauces and a vesicular eruption of the hands, feet, and legs. Healing occurs within 5 to 10 days. Some authorities consider this disease identical to aphthous fever, and others reserve the latter for the foot-and-mouth disease of cattle, which rarely also involves man. In such a case, vesicular lesions are also present on the palms, soles, and oropharyngeal mucosa.

Laboratory Findings. Routine laboratory findings are usually within normal limits. Laboratory diagnosis is made by isolating Coxsackie group A viruses from the stool or throat washings obtained during the acute stage of the disease. Serologic diagnosis is established by demonstrating a rise in complement-fixing or neutralizing antibodies in paired sera specimens, obtained in the acute and the convalescent stages of the disease, to the virus isolated.

Treatment. There is no specific treatment for the disease or its complications. Symptomatic treatment consists of administration of antipyretics and analgesics. Antibiotics are of no value in Coxsackie infections. Bedrest is essential during the symptomatic stages of the illness. Complications of herpangina are encephalitis and orchitis. The incidence of both these complications is increased in patients who are ambulatory during the acute stage of herpangina.

REFERENCES

Abbott, P. L.: Viable Mixture of *Lactobacillus acidophilus* and *bulgaricus* in Treatment of Herpetic and Aphthous Stomatitis. J. Oral Surg. Anesth. Hosp. D. Service, *19*:310, 1961.

Dingle, J. H., and Ginsberg, H. S.: The Adenovirus Group. In Rivers, T. M., and Horsfall, F.L. (Eds.): *Viral and Rickettsial*

Infections of Man. 4th ed. Philadelphia, J. B. Lippincott Co., 1965.

Huebner, R. J.: Herpangina. In Beeson, P. B., and McDermott, W. (Eds.): *Cecil-Loeb Textbook of Medicine.* 13th ed. Philadelphia, W. B. Saunders Co., 1971, pp. 77, 78.

Mufson, M. A., *et al.*: Acute Respiratory Diseases of Viral Etiology. V. Eaton, Agent: A Review. Am. J. Public Health, *52*:925, 1962.

Wagner, R. R.: Herpes Simplex. In Beeson, P. B., and McDermott, W. (Eds.): *Cecil-Loeb Textbook of Medicine.* 13th ed. Philadelphia, W. B. Saunders Co., 1971.

Chapter 10
Paranasal Sinus Infections

ETIOLOGY

The paranasal sinus may be nothing more than residual olfactory surfaces dating from that period eons ago when man was dependent on keen olfaction for food and safety. Whatever the original function of the sinuses may have been (and no dogmatic statement can be made), the paranasal sinuses are directly continuous portions of the upper respiratory tract and thus often participate in infections of the latter. A description of the etiology of upper respiratory tract infections will not be repeated here, but it applies equally well to the sinuses. There are no microorganisms which have a special affinity for sinus infections, although the sinuses often are the site of a prolonged residue of what earlier was a more generalized respiratory infection. Why this is so is not clear, but local factors listed below may be of etiologic significance.

Any anatomic or physiologic feature which one way or another obstructs free drainage from the sinuses permits stasis of secretions and thus infections. Figures 10–1 to 10–7 indicate several such possibilities.

Another local cause which predisposes to sinusitis is the presence of unfavorably located allergic polyps. Perhaps most typically is a polyp located in or near the semilunar hiatus which thus causes relative obstruction to drainage from the anterior group of sinuses.

Quite obviously apical infection of a tooth root which projects into the floor of the

maxillary sinus can lead to infection. This is particularly likely if such an infected tooth is removed and a fistula created into the maxillary sinus, or if a portion of the root of the tooth is inadvertently lost within the sinus lumen.

Impaired ciliary activity may so interfere with the cleansing of the sinus that infections occur. In addition to smoking and air pollution (see Chapter 1, p. 17), septal devia-

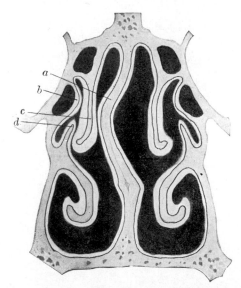

FIG. 10–1. A high deviation of the septum, causing closure of the infundibulum: *a,* high deviation of the septum; *b,* inner wall of the bulla ethmoidalis; *c,* middle turbinate crowded against the outer wall of the nose and blocking the drainage of the infundibulum; *d,* uncinate process.

6

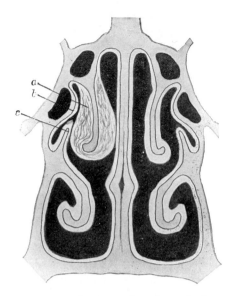

Fig. 10–2.   Cross section through the nose: *a*, hyperplasia of the middle turbinate, which crowds upon the uncinate process and closes the infundibulum (*c*); *b*, bulla ethmoidalis.

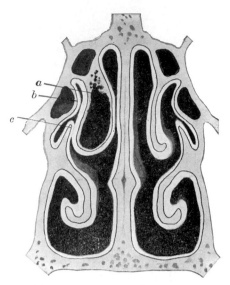

Fig. 10–4.   A large cell in the middle turbinate occluding the infundibulum: *a*, cell in the middle turbinate; *b*, the inner wall of the bulla ethmoidalis; *c*, the uncinate process or inner wall of the infundibulum or gutter.

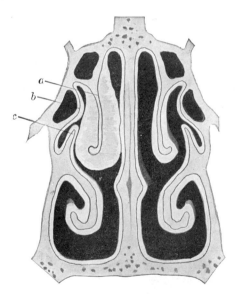

Fig. 10–3.   Edema of the mucous membrane of the middle turbinate blocking the infundibulum: *a*, edematous middle turbinate; *b*, bulla ethmoidalis; *c*, uncinate process or inner wall of the infundibulum.

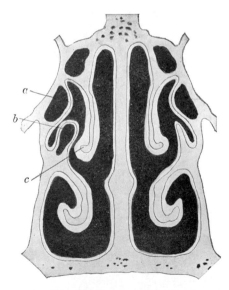

Fig. 10–5.   Cell in the uncinate process (*b*) blocking the infundibulum: *a*, bulla ethmoidalis; *c*, middle turbinate.

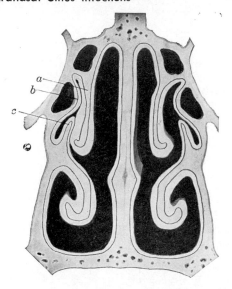

FIG. 10–6. The middle turbinate (a) cling-
ing to the outer wall of the nose and blocking
the infundibulum; b, inner wall of the bulla
ethmoidalis; c, uncinate process or inner wall
of the infundibulum.

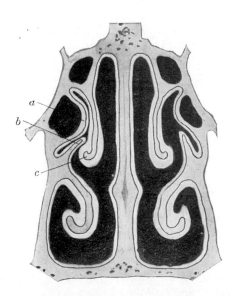

FIG. 10–7. Enlargement of the bulla ethmoidalis blocking the infundibulum: a, the inner and distended wall of the bulla ethmoidalis, crowding inward and downward against
the uncinate process and blocking the infundibulum; b, the uncinate process; c, the middle
turbinate, which, on account of the bulging
bulla, appears to be the cause of the blockage.

tions may change convection currents of inspired air in such a way that spots of dryness destroy ciliary activity. Thus a chain of
events, beginning with stasis of secretions
and ending with infection, is initiated.

It is probable that most persons succumb-
ing to sinusitis after swimming are infected
by their own pathogenic organisms, perhaps
mechanically driven into these cavities by
the force of water pressure. Avoidance of
swimming when suffering from an active or
latent respiratory disease would avoid such
sequelae.

PATHOLOGY

The pathologic changes which occur in
the mucous membrane and bony walls of
the sinuses in the course of suppurative inflammation are what might be expected in a
mucus-lined cavity (Figs. 10–8 to 10–13).

There are four different types of nasal
sinus infection: acute congestive, acute purulent, chronic purulent, and chronic hyperplastic.

Chronic suppurative sinus disease may be
classified microscopically as (1) edematous;
(2) granular or infiltrating; (3) fibrous; or
(4) a mixture of any or all of these forms.
Connective tissue changes are common, with
much thickening in the subepithelial layer.
This thickening in the cellular structure is
composed of spiral, round, star-formed, plasma, eosinophil, and pigment cells.

For didactic purposes, the changes which
occur in the tissues may be studied in the
following order, which represents the usual
sequence of pathologic events:

1. The submucous tissue is infiltrated
with serum, while the surface is dry. Leukocytes also fill the meshes of the submucous
tissue.

2. The capillaries are dilated, and the
mucous membrane is greatly thickened and
red as a result of the edema and engorgement of the subepithelial structures. At this
stage there is usually no defect in the epithelium.

3. After a few hours or a day or two,
the serum and leukocytes escape through
the epithelial covering of the mucosa, where
they become admixed with bacteria, epithelial debris, and mucus. In some instances

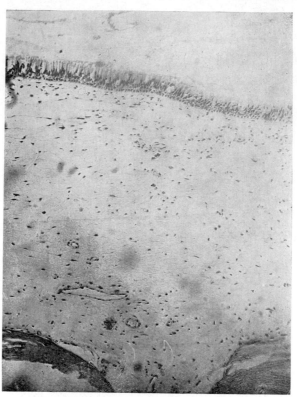

FIG. 10–8. Normal mucous membrane taken from the floor of the maxillary antrum shows a ciliated columnar epithelium resting on a delicate basement membrane. The tunica propria consists of fibrous connective tissue which superficially is arranged somewhat loosely, while deeper it is more compact and blends with the periosteum. The glands are found in the tunica propria and are most numerous near the ostium of the antrum. × 63. (Courtesy of Dr. Leroy A. Schall.)

capillary hemorrhage occurs, and blood becomes mixed with the secretions. The secretions, at first thin and watery, later become thicker and tenacious, on account of the coagulation of the fibrin of the serum.

4. In many cases resolution by the absorption of the exudate and the cessation of the discharge of the leukocytes take place in 10 to 14 days.

5. In other cases, however, the inflammation passes from the congestive to the purulent type, the leuokocytes being thrown out in immense numbers. Resolution is still possible, although not probable, as the tissue changes are not yet of a fixed type. Unless the process is speedily arrested, the tissue changes become permanent, and chronicity is established. The underlying bone may show an osteitis and in places a definite bony necrosis.

Extension of the infection from the sinuses to other parts may occur: (1) by a thrombophlebitis of the perforating veins; (2) by a direct extension through an ulcerating or necrotic portion of the sinus wall; (3) by way of dehiscence; and (4) through the vascular channels in the form of a bacteremia. It is questionable whether an infection may be transmitted from the sinuses by way of the lymphatics.

In chronic sinusitis the surface changes are similar to those in acute suppurative inflammation affecting other mucous membranes and bone tissue. The mucous membrane may present a granular surface, villous and fungoid excrescences, granular, cushionlike thickenings, etc. In cases of long standing there are hyperplastic thickenings. The membrane may be destroyed in spots by ulceration, exposing smooth, bare bone,

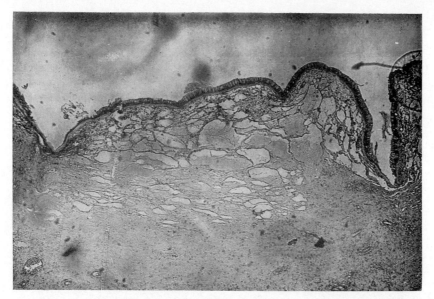

FIG. 10–9. Chronic inflammation of the maxillary antrum. The characteristic feature is the immense amount of edema in the superficial portion of the stroma. The epithelium does not show much change. In places it is lacking, which is due to an artifact in the preparation of the specimen. In the deeper portion of the tunica propria there is profuse round cell infiltration with thickening of the blood vessels. ×27. (Courtesy of Dr. Leroy A. Schall.)

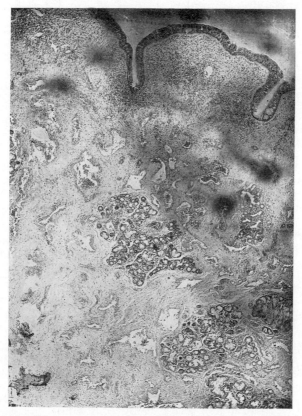

FIG. 10–10. Chronic inflammation of the maxillary antrum. The epithelium is intact but with profuse round cell infiltration of the stroma and proliferation of fibrous tissue. There is marked activity of the glands. ×27. (Courtesy of Dr. Leroy A. Schall.)

159

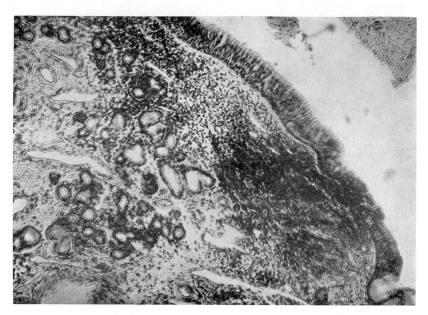

Fig. 10–11. Chronic proliferative inflammation of the maxillary antrum. Marked round cell infiltration with superficial abscess formation. Marked activity of the glands and slight fibrosis. ×63. (Courtesy of Dr. Leroy A. Schall.)

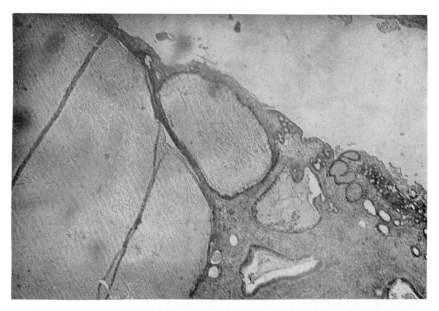

Fig. 10–12. Cystic degeneration of the maxillary antrum. ×63.
(Courtesy of Dr. Leroy A. Schall.)

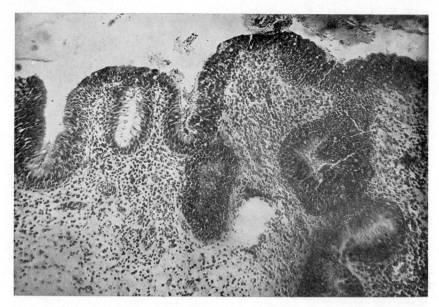

FIG. 10–13.   Chronic inflammation of the maxillary antrum. There is much round cell infiltration throughout the entire stroma with marked activity around the glands. × 63. (Courtesy of Dr. Leroy A. Schall.)

or it may be soft or rough from caries. In some cases necrosis and bone sequestra are present, or they may be absorbed.

A microscopic examination of the sections of the mucous membrane sometimes shows a loss of the epithelium and glands, which are replaced by connective tissue. Ulcerations of the membrane are often surrounded by granulation tissue, especially if there is necrosis of the bone. Granulation buds may encroach upon the periosteum and thus unite the bone and mucous membrane. When this happens the bone is superficially absorbed and somewhat roughened in consequence. Osteophytes, or bony scales or plaques, resulting from plastic exudation sometimes form on the surface of the bone.

Polypi in the Sinuses

Polypi have been found in all the sinuses, although they are more common in the antrum and ethmoidal cells. They are much more common in the ethmoidal cells than is generally supposed. Their hidden location within the small ethmoidal spaces renders their diagnosis rather difficult. In the antrum, however, they are more easily diag-

nosed, as they may be exposed through the canine fossa. A polypoid degeneration of the mucosa of the maxillary antrum may occur without any change in the normal appearance of the nasal mucosa even in the ethmoidal region. The local symptoms depend upon the amount of hyperplastic changes which have occurred within the sinus cavity. As the hyperplastic area spreads, the symptoms, such as serous discharge, occlusion of the nostril, and sometimes sneezing, become more pronounced, often simulating mild attacks of hay fever. When this hyperplasia becomes well advanced, polypi begin to show themselves in the nasal cavities. As in hyperplastic ethmoiditis, they may give rise to a recurrent polyposis of the middle meatus. Hirsch believes this form of disease is the most frequent cause of recurrent nasal polypi. Iodized oil will be of great help in diagnosing this type of antrum pathology. Polypi have been found in the frontal and sphenoidal sinuses, although not so frequently as in the antrum and ethmoidal cells. The polypi in the ethmoidal cells are usually quite small, on account of the limited space within the cells, whereas in the antrum they are much larger.

The microscopic changes in the epithelium of chronic hyperplastic sinusitis are thickening, polypoid degeneration, metaplasia, and areas of ulceration. The basement membrane shows thickening. The tunica propria reveals edema, round cell infiltration, fibrosis, dilatation or compression of the glands, and thickening of the blood vessel walls. The periosteum is thickened. The underlying bone may show osteoblastic or osteoclastic activity, with fibrosis, hyperostosis, osteomalacia, and necrosis.

SYMPTOMS AND DIAGNOSIS

Subjective Symptoms

Pain. Pain referable to the region of the sinus involved may or may not be present. In active inflammation of the maxillary or frontal sinus, pain is usually referred to the region involved. In the deeper sinuses, such as the posterior ethmoidal and sphenoidal sinuses, the pain is vaguely deep-seated in the head, or it is referred to the periphery of the head without reference to the location of the sinus. For example, sphenoidal inflammation may give rise to pain in the occipital or frontal region. As a matter of fact, inflammation in any or all of the sinuses usually causes pain in the frontal region. These pains are almost universally called headaches by the patient.

Anatomically the apices of the upper anterior teeth (excepting the incisor teeth) may be separated from the sinus lumen by a thin layer of bone or by no bone and only mucous membrane. For this reason maxillary sinusitis frequently causes painful aching of these teeth.

Headache. Headache is one of the most common and significant signs of sinusitis. Wolff states that head pain arising in the nose has its origin in congestion and edema in and around the sinus ostia. The local use of vasoconstrictor medication (e.g., 1 to 2% ephedrine) to reduce this edema should abolish the pain. Headache has multitudinous causes and is not, therefore, pathognomonic of inflammatory or other diseased conditions of the sinuses.

Headache, if due to eye strain, is usually bilateral and worse at the end of the day, whereas in sinus disease it is more often unilateral or, if not unilateral, more pronounced on one side, or it begins as a unilateral headache and extends to the other side. The headache which originates in a sinus is increased upon stooping forward and upon sudden jarring of the body. It may persist upon closing the eyes upon retiring or in a darkened room, whereas if it is of ocular origin, it disappears under such conditions.

The pains and headache due to disease of the frontal sinus may assume the form of sharp, shooting pains through the eyes, or they may be dull and heavy and nearly constant. They may consist of a dull feeling in the forehead, which is aggravated by leaning forward. In the acute form of frontal sinusitis, daily pain beginning at 10 or 11 A.M. and ending by 3 or 4 P.M. is quite characteristic. These attacks of periodic pain may last for a week or more. The patient generally complains of frontal headache which is limited to or originates on the side affected. Pressure under the floor of the sinus at the inner angle of the orbit usually elicits pain in these cases.

In the chronic form of sinusitis, pain and headache may be absent unless drainage and ventilation are impaired.

Vacuum Frontal Sinusitis. A number of years ago Sluder called attention to the existence of what he called "the vacuum frontal headache." This type of headache is usually frontal, low-grade, and made worse by the use of the eyes for close work. The nose contains no pus and no pathologic condition other than a possible redness or swelling of the nasal mucosa in the region of the middle turbinate. His explanation is that obstruction in the inlet of the frontal sinus causes its contained air to be absorbed and a partial vacuum to be produced. Hilding has demonstrated that in a dog, approximately -35 mm of water can be produced by ciliary activity. He excluded the possibility of blood absorption by obtaining the same results using an exsanguinated dog or a decapitated head. The author (J.J.B.) demonstrated that by closing the frontonasal ducts in dogs, the oxygen of the contained air in the frontal sinus seems to be absorbed under special circumstances, and a partial vacuum results. The vacuum frontal headache is probably a clinical entity. There is as logical a reason for its existence in the frontal sinus as for a similar condition in the middle ear.

Tenderness Upon Pressure. Tenderness and pain upon finger pressure may be present in disease of those sinuses contiguous to the surface of the face, namely, the frontal, anterior ethmoidal, and maxillary sinuses.

Tenderness over the frontal bone is rarely present in frontal sinusitis except in acute cases with obstructed drainage. Tenderness is often present, however, when pressure is exerted against the floor of the affected sinus near the inner angle of the orbital cavity (Fig. 10–14). The fingertip or thumb should be placed well under the roof of the orbit and the pressure directed upward. Pain is thus often elicited even in chronic congestive cases. Tenderness in this region does not, however, always indicate disease of the frontal sinus, as the anterior ethmoidal cells sometimes project beneath the floor of the sinus.

When such an anatomic deviation is present, the surgeon may be led to a wrong conclusion. This difficulty may be obviated by having a roentgen-ray film made, as it will aid in determining the position and condition of the frontal and anterior ethmoidal cells.

In the examination of the anterior ethmoidal cells, pressure should be made at the inner angle of the orbit against the orbital plate of the ethmoid. In the examination of the maxillary sinus, pressure should be made over the canine fossa of the superior maxilla.

In sphenoiditis the anterior surface of the sphenoidal sinus is sensitive to palpation, and frequently as the examining probe causes pressure over the sphenoidal sinus, the patient will state that pain in the occiput or temporal region is elicited.

Disturbances of Smell. The olfactory sense may be perverted (parosmia), the patient apparently perceiving odors that are not evident to normal noses. A more common symptom is the loss of olfaction (anosmia). This is accounted for by the blocking of the olfactory fissure by the tissues in the region of the middle turbinate. Ventilation of the superior meatus of the nose is thereby prevented, hence the loss of the sense of smell. In some chronic cases this may be due to the degeneration of the terminal filaments of the olfactory nerve, although in most cases the sense of smell is regained after the infectious process has subsided.

Objective Symptoms

Swelling and Edema. If the sinuses contiguous to the skin (frontal, maxillary, and anterior ethmoidal) are acutely involved, some slight swelling of the skin due to a periostitis with edema may occur. Palpation with the finger gives the sensation of a slight

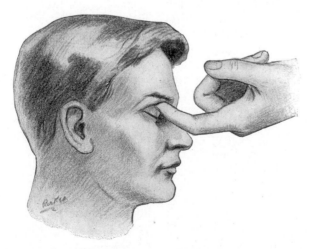

FIG. 10–14. Pressure should be made under the floor of the frontal sinus. Pressure is often made under the supraorbital ridge, whereas it should be made much deeper.

thickness or velvety feeling. This swelling is more commonly found over the frontal sinus.

Nasal Discharge. Pus within the nasal chambers usually indicates empyema of the sinuses. The nasal mucosa is rarely the focal center of suppurative inflammation, whereas the sinuses are commonly the focal center of such an inflammation. The presence of pus in the nasal chambers should therefore excite suspicion of the existence of an inflammation of the sinuses. Pus in the middle meatus usually signifies an involvement of the frontal, anterior ethmoidal, or maxillary sinus, as these cells drain into the middle meatus. If pus is seen in the olfactory fissure (between the septum and middle turbinate), the posterior ethmoidal or the sphenoidal cells are presumed to be involved, as these cells drain into the superior meatus above the middle turbinate. Pus is usually absent from the nose in hyperplastic sinusitis.

Transillumination. Transillumination of the sinuses affords objective information as to the condition of the maxillary and the frontal sinuses, but none in reference to the other sinuses.

In transillumination of the maxillary sinuses, a hooded light is placed in the mouth in a dark room with the patient's eyes open. If a sinus is normal, three points should be noted: (1) the red pupillary reflex, (2) the crescent of light corresponding to the position of the lower eyelid, and (3) the sense of light in the eye when closed. If the red pupillary reflex and the crescent of light are absent, the antrum is probably affected. Note both sides at once and thus determine which one, if either, is affected. A comparison of the lower portion of the field of illumination may be very misleading, as the anterior wall of the antrum varies greatly in density, irrespective of the disease present. The orbital or upper wall of the antrum is, however, more nearly uniform in its density in all cases and affords a fair opportunity for a comparison of the transilluminated light through the two orbital plates; that is, when both orbital plates of the antrum are normal, the amount of light transmitted through them is about equal. When one is thickened by an inflammatory exudate, however, the transmission of light is interfered with; hence, the crescent of light is dimmed or altogether absent. Likewise, when both orbital plates are normal (antral disease absent), the light transmitted into the interior of the eyeball is shown in the red pupillary reflex in each eye, whereas if one antrum is involved, the pupillary reflex is absent upon that side and present on the other. The sense of light (eyes closed) is present on the healthy side and absent upon the diseased side in maxillary diseases.

The antrums may be transilluminated from above by placing a small light above the infraorbital ridge and slightly within the orbit. The beam of light is directed downward through the orbitoantral plate. The reflected light is viewed over the palate by looking through the mouth if the sinus is healthy. If a thickened mucosa or secretions are present in the sinus, the transmitted light is absent or diminished.

Transillumination of the frontal sinuses is a satisfactory means of diagnosis in adults with well-developed sinuses. In children with small sinuses or in adults with bilateral involvement, transillumination is not so reliable. The hooded lamp should be placed under the floor of the frontal sinus at the upper and inner angle of the orbit and the two sides compared. If the lamp is not placed well under the supraorbital ridge, the skin transmits the light and may thus lead to a false deduction.

Radiopaque Solutions. Radiopaque solutions injected into the sinuses are of distinct value in the diagnosis of many cases. They are of special value in the sphenoidal and maxillary sinuses. By their use the cavity of the sinus may be sharply outlined, so that the thickness of the mucous membrane and the presence of polypi may be determined (Fig. 10–15), and irregularities of size and shape can be accurately outlined. Diseased mucous membrane is shown by an unfilled zone between the oil mass and the bony outlines. It is also of value as an aid in the detection of extensions of the sphenoidal sinuses into the greater wings of the sphenoid bone. The radiopaque material may be injected directly by cannulation of the sinus or by displacement irrigation described elsewhere.

Displacement Method. At about the same time, Proetz and Frazer, independent of each

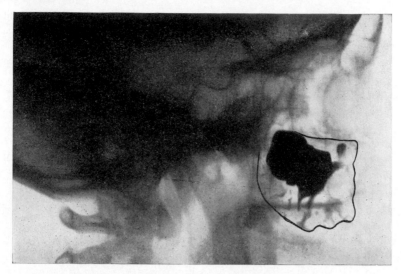

Fig. 10–15.   Defective filling with iodized oil of the left maxillary sinus. The left side of the face is next to the film, and the oil has collected toward the zygoma. The irregular rivulets in the anterior and inferior portions outline the polypi in these areas. Numerous polypi were found at operation.

other, introduced the displacement method of diagnosis and treatment of sinus disease. It is the only method by which medication may enter the ethmoidal cells. The frontal sinus is more difficult to fill by displacement, the maxillary, ethmoidal, and sphenoidal sinuses less so.

For the method to be effective, (1) the ostia must be covered by the displacement fluid, (2) the ostia must be patent and in normal relation to the sinuses, and (3) there must be a negative pressure produced at the ostia.

The technique is as follows: the patient's head is lowered posteriorly until the chin and the external auditory canal occupy the same vertical line (see Fig. 12–1). While the head is in this position and while the patient refrains from swallowing, the nasal cavity on one side is filled with 2 to 3 ml of the radiopaque displacement fluid. Inclining the head to the homolateral side increases the certainty of covering the sinus ostia. While the patient elevates the soft palate by repeating the letter "K," intermittent negative pressure of 180 mm Hg is applied to the naris on the filled side, and the other side is occluded by digital pressure. Following the procedure the patient is returned to the erect position, and roentgen-ray pictures are taken at 24 and 72 hours to determine the emptying time. Normally the sinuses should be empty by 96 hours.

Diagnostic Irrigations.   In many instances a definite opinion concerning the presence or absence of pus cannot be formed without a diagnostic irrigation. This is done in the same manner as for therapeutic purposes, either through the natural ostium or by puncture. Cultures and smears of the fluid may be taken from the washings.

SINUSITIS IN CHILDREN

Etiology.   Sinusitis in children usually is seen between the fourth and tenth years of age. Climatic conditions play a great part.

The ethmoidal sinus is well developed at birth and probably is involved more frequently than the other sinuses. The maxillary sinus is not fully developed until puberty, however, and rarely gives trouble before the tenth year. The sphenoidal sinus has clinical significance from the third year on but does not reach full development until the twelfth year. Involvement of the frontal sinus is rare prior to the sixth year.

Many local conditions may be the offending factors causing the apparent "sinusitis" and must be kept uppermost in mind. These factors include adenoidal obstruction of the nasal airway, foreign bodies and tumors located in the nasal cavities, septal deflections, etc. An allergic respiratory mucosa must also be considered.

Pathology. The histopathology of chronic sinusitis in children is similar to that in the adult. Two general forms may be recognized: hyperplastic (polypoid, edematous, etc.) and atrophic (fibrotic). The hyperplastic form of sinusitis is suggestive of an allergic background.

Rarefaction, resorption, or atrophy of the bone is frequently seen. It begins as an erosion of the ethmoidal septa or the nasoantral wall. It is frequently associated with fibrosis and proliferative fibrous connective tissue changes. The bony atrophy is usually due to an endarteritis and vascular thrombosis, causing a shutting off of the blood supply. Necrosis and hypertrophy of the bone are not so commonly seen. Necrosis may be found in chronic antrum suppuration involving the nasoantral wall. Bone hypertrophy is usually observed involving the inferior turbinate.

In atrophic sinusitis the epithelial layer of the nasal mucosa and turbinates usually shows dissolution, exfoliation, or absence of the surface epithelium. The subepithelial layer is thickened as a rule. A round cell infiltration is usually present.

The tunica propria in atrophic sinusitis shows a low-grade chronic inflammatory process with glandular atrophy. The periosteum may be thickened and infiltrated. The bone usually shows a retarded growth or underdevelopment with sclerosis of the bony framework.

Symptoms. Sinusitis in children is characterized by a chronic nasal discharge from one or both sides of the nose. Frequent colds and earaches occur as a rule. Examination frequently will disclose a malnourished and underweight child. The child may be inattentive and not do well in school.

A discharge in the middle meatus in a child under 6 years of age usually means involvement of the ethmoidal or maxillary sinuses, as the frontal sinuses are not fully developed before this time and seldom become involved earlier. Discharge coming from above the middle turbinate before 3 years of age is indicative of a posterior ethmoiditis, as the sphenoid sinus is not fully developed or does not often become infected before this age. Nasal discharge is most profuse on the side affected. It may be mucoid, mucopurulent, or purulent.

Nasal obstruction on the involved side is usually present. It is more or less constant but may be intermittent.

Headache is a symptom of much diagnostic value in the acute cases in children over 5 years of age. Frontal headache most often indicates disease of the anterior group of cells. Occipital headache most often indicates disease of the posterior group of cells. Morning frontal headache diminishing in intensity toward afternoon usually indicates a frontal involvement in an older child. Pain in the upper jaw or teeth increasing in intensity toward the afternoon usually indicates maxillary sinuses. Tenderness to pressure over the thin areas of the sinus walls is of great assistance in the diagnosis in older children. These areas are the same as in the adult.

Diagnosis. Sinus infections in children are frequently overlooked. This may be due to the fact that the roentgen ray and transillumination as a means of diagnosing sinus disease in early childhood are not so reliable as in adults. The diagnosis is also more difficult than in adults because subjective symptoms cannot be expressed. In older children, indefinite pains around the head and face with headache may be complained of, although these symptoms are not always present. Any chronic cold with a nasal discharge should arouse suspicion of infection in these structures. Sneezing, headache, irritability, and depression are important symptoms. The maxillary and especially the ethmoidal sinuses chiefly concern us in children.

Treatment. Acute sinusitis requires the same general measures as any acute respiratory illness. The patient should be at bedrest in a humidified room (45 to 55%) and at a temperature of 21 to 22°C (70 to 72°F). Pain can usually be controlled with acetylsalicylic acid or a similar preparation.

In more severe cases of sinusitis in which the temperature is elevated 1 to 2°F above normal and there are signs of systemic toxicity, recourse should be made to one of the sulfonamides or the antibiotics.

Some help in the early stages is obtained by the oral administration of ephedrine in small doses three to four times per day. The vasoconstricting action of this drug may alleviate some of the generalized head fullness and tightness.

Local Measures. After the initial edema and inflammation have subsided, local measures may be useful. Marked nasal obstruction is relieved by vasoconstricting nose drops, such as ephedrine, 1%. More thorough vasoconstriction ("shrinkage") is obtained by placing an ephedrine-saturated pledget about the anterior end of the middle turbinate. Ephedrine, 0.25% in 0.85% saline solution, or some other gentle, bland vasoconstricting drug may be introduced into the sinuses by displacement irrigation. Profuse nasal secretions may be removed by direct suction through a cannula or by gentle nasal irrigation with warm saline solution.

In older children the maxillary sinus can be irrigated through the natural ostium in many instances. Local anesthesia is sufficient. Occasionally the sinus must be irrigated by forcing a trochar through the naso-antral wall. In this case the trochar is inserted high near the attachment of the inferior turbinate and directed upward because the floor of the antrum in children is frequently above this point.

Surgical Procedures. If used at all, surgical procedures should be conservative. The establishment of ventilation and drainage with the least possible trauma is of the greatest importance.

Operative procedures on the sinuses themselves in children are not often indicated, the acute infections of these cavities usually disappearing of themselves. Those cases which are classified as chronic empyemas yield much more readily than in the adult to nonoperative procedures as a result of two factors: (1) the age of the patient excludes long chronicity; (2) nasal obstructive lesions at this age are not common.

If the maxillary infection does not clear up after a thorough trial by conservative treatment, additional ventilation and drainage may be obtained by making an opening beneath the lower turbinate. Such openings usually close rapidly in children.

A suitable antrum trocar is inserted under the inferior turbinate, and the nasal wall of the antrum is pierced in an upward and outward direction. The opening is enlarged with a rasp or small biting forceps to permit the introduction of a rubber catheter. The catheter should extend from the interior of the antrum into the vestibule of the nose.

Irrigations or instillations are made through the tube. The tube is removed on the fifth or sixth day. Subsequent irrigations are made with a straight needle or a curved trocar.

AVIATION SINUSITIS; AERO-SINUSITIS

Acute inflammation of the lining mucous membrane of the sinuses, hemorrhaging into the sinuses, or even sinusitis may result from rapid barometric changes in altitudinal flights. These pathologic changes may occur if the ostia of the sinuses are closed by redundant tissue or are covered by a purulent secretion. During ascent the air within the sinuses is reduced in conformity with the changed barometric pressure, but during descent redundant tissue may be sucked within the sinus ostium and act as a ball-and-flutter valve. The temporarily reduced air pressure within the sinus may result in an acute swelling, inflammation, or bleeding of the mucosa. Acute pain in the region of the affected sinus is usually experienced until the air equilibrium is restored.

Chapter 11
Radiology of the Paranasal Sinuses

Imre Laszlo

Roentgenographic examination of the patient with possible paranasal sinus disease or other pathologic processes of the facial bones usually requires a series of different views. From the anatomic topography of the facial bones, it is evident that each paranasal sinus is better visualized on one projection than on another. Different projections are necessary, however, for obtaining more exact details of each of the sinuses. In addition, the various projections offer different superimpositions of the other bony structures of the skull. Radioanatomic orientation is needed to recognize the pathologic processes and to differentiate pathologic processes from normal anatomic variations.

Four basic views (Caldwell, Waters, lateral and submentovertical) are generally used for visualization of the paranasal sinuses. Additional views of the facial bones and the base of the skull are available, however. Whenever available a radiographic head unit should be used. The upright position, using this unit, is more comfortable for the patient and films taken in this position provide more exact details for the radiologist (fluid level, mucosal changes, etc.).

TECHNIQUE AND PROJECTIONS

Six basic conventional x-ray views of the paranasal sinuses are used.

Caldwell View (Fig. 11–1). This projection is accomplished by placing the nose and the forehead on the table top so that the orbital meatal line (joining the outer canthus of the eye to the superior margin of the external auditory canal) is perpendicular to the film. The angulation of the x-ray beam is at 15 degrees craniocaudally, and the exit point is at the nasion. This projection offers the best view of the frontal sinus and a fairly good visualization of the ethmoidal cells, with a partial superimposition of the sphenoidal sinuses. It is to be realized that the contour of the medial orbital wall is formed by the posterior aspect of the lamina papyracea, which means that the posterior ethmoidal cells are better visualized on this projection than are the anterior cells.

Modification of the angulation of the x-ray tube may offer several advantages. A 30-degree craniocaudal tilting of the x-ray beam allows better visualization of the bony contour of the orbit as well as of the infraorbital rim and floor (Fig. 11–2). In addition, this view allows a better visualization of the anterior (and superior) ethmoidal cells, since the sphenoidal sinuses are not superimposed on them.

Waters View (Fig. 11–3). This view is the most frequently used. Its purpose is to project the petrous bone below the maxillary antrums. It is obtained by extending the patient's head so that the chin touches the

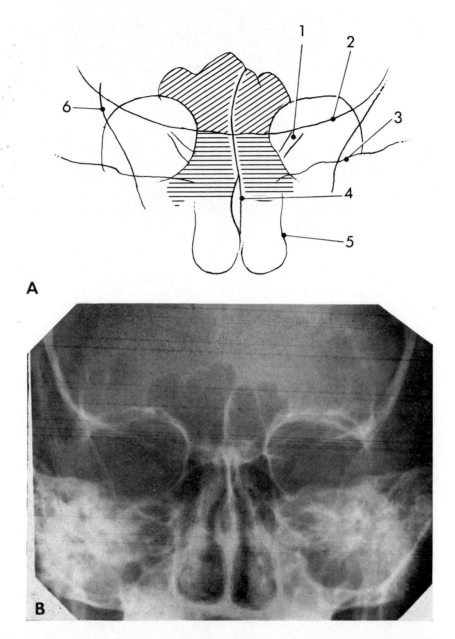

FIG. 11–1. Caldwell view: (*1*) superior orbital fissure; (*2*) lesser wing of the sphenoid; (*3*) petrous ridge; (*4*) nasal septum; (*5*) nasal aperture; (*6*) temporal line. (The right oblique lined area outlines the frontal sinus, the horizontal lined area the ethmoidal cells.)

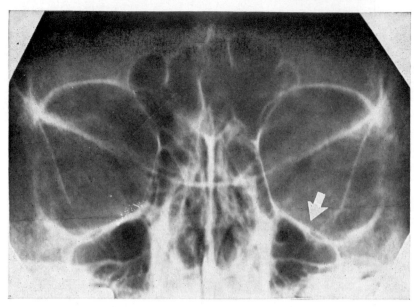

FIG. 11–2.   Modified Caldwell view.   Arrow points to the superimposed contour of the
infraorbital rim and floor.

table top. The plane extending from the outer canthus of the eye to the tragus forms an angle of approximately 35 degrees with the film. For better visualization of both the zygomatic body and the arch, the patient's head could be further extended.

The Waters view obtained with mouth open allows visualization of all the paranasal sinuses including the sphenoidal sinuses. It provides the best view of the maxillary antrums, permitting exact evaluation of even mild changes in the sinus cavities. The x-ray beam in this projection is usually perpendicular to the posterior (cerebral) wall of the frontal sinus. This means that the size of the frontal sinus depends not only on its height—as is the case in the Caldwell projection—but also upon the depth of the sinus.

The medial bony wall of the orbit is formed by the anterior aspect of the lamina papyracea, so that the ethmoidal cells projected between the two orbits represent the anterior cells. The posterior cells are projected into the maxillary antrums, together with the superior orbital fissure and the sphenoidal sinuses.

Lateral View (Fig. 11–4). The cassette and therefore the film are placed parallel to the main sagittal plane of the skull. The lateral view is of less value because of the superimposition of the right and left paranasal sinuses, either when located relatively far apart, such as the maxillary sinuses, or when separated only by bony septa, such as the frontal, ethmoidal, and sphenoidal sinuses. Asymmetric development of the two sides, pathologic processes on one side, or simultaneous changes in both may easily lead to false impressions. In the lateral view, only segments of the walls of the sinuses are perpendicular to the x-ray film, i.e., only 2 to 3 cm of the bony walls of the frontal sinuses about the midline can be visualized, while the more lateral segments are not easily visible. A similar limitation applies to the visualization of the hard palate, which is convex downward, and the nasal bones, which are tilted laterally.

Submentovertical View (Fig. 11–5). The head is fully extended, and the central plane is perpendicular to the base of the skull. This view gives a good picture of the base of the skull as well as of the paranasal sinuses. The bony walls of the maxillary and sphenoidal sinuses are well visualized. The bony walls of the ethmoids, including the lamina papyracea, are also seen, but the

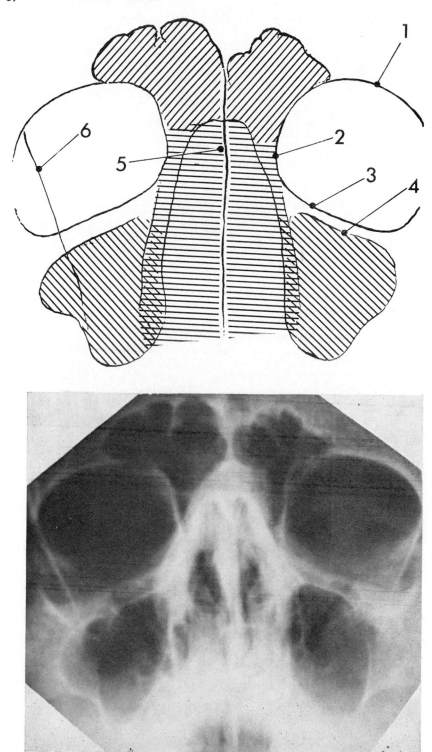

FIG. 11–3. Waters view: (*1*) superior orbital rim; (*2*) lamina papyracea; (*3*) orbital rim; (*4*) orbital floor; (*5*) nasal septum; (*6*) infratemporal line. (The right oblique areas are the frontal sinuses, the left oblique the maxillary sinuses, and the horizontal the ethmoidal cells.)

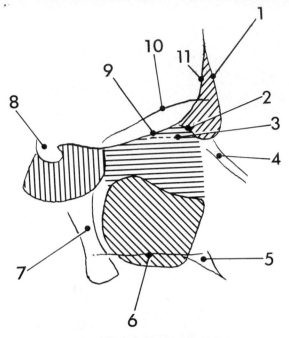

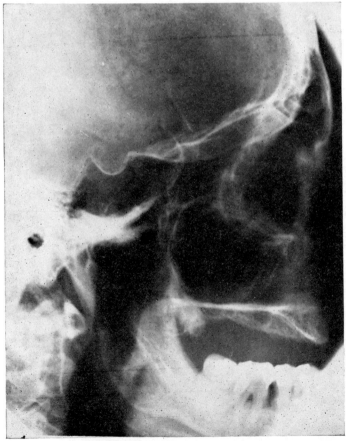

FIG. 11–4.   Lateral view: (*1*) anterior wall of the frontal sinuses; (*2*) infundibular wall of the frontal sinuses; (*3*) cribriform plate; (*4*) nasal bone; (*5*) anterior nasal spine; (*6*) hard palate; (*7*) pterygoid process; (*8*) sella turcica; (*9*) superior wall of the ethmoidal cells; (*10*) superior orbital wall; (*11*) posterior wall of the frontal sinuses. (The right oblique lined areas are the frontal sinuses, the left oblique the maxillary sinuses, the horizontal the ethmoidal sinuses, and the vertical the sphenoidal sinuses.)

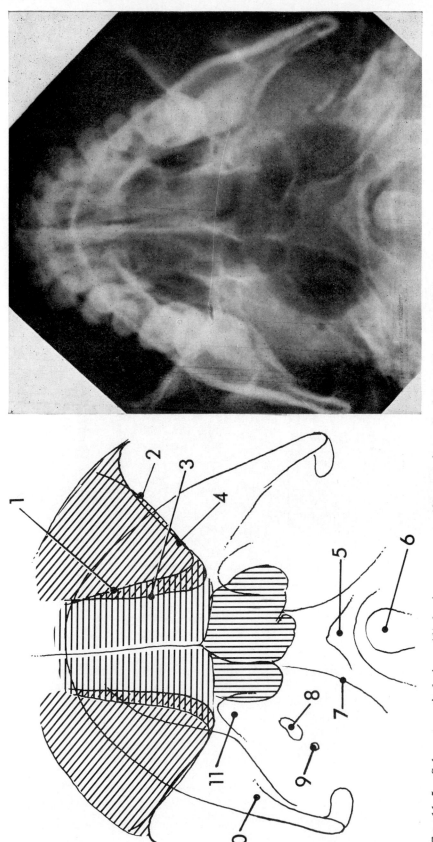

FIG. 11–5. Submentovertical view: (1) lamina papyracea; (2) posterior wall of the maxillary sinus; (3) medial wall of the maxillary sinus; (4) posterior wall of the maxillary sinus; (5) anterior arch of the atlas; (6) odontoid process of the C2; (7) clivus; (8) foramen ovale; (9) foramen spinosum; (10) mandible; (11) pterygoid fossa. (The left oblique lined areas are the maxillary sinuses, the horizontal the ethmoidal cells, and the vertical the sphenoidal sinuses.)

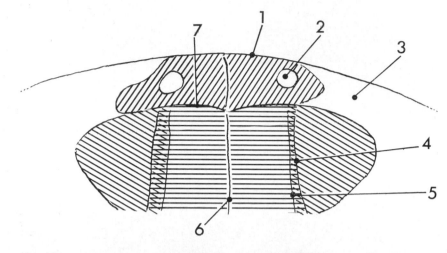

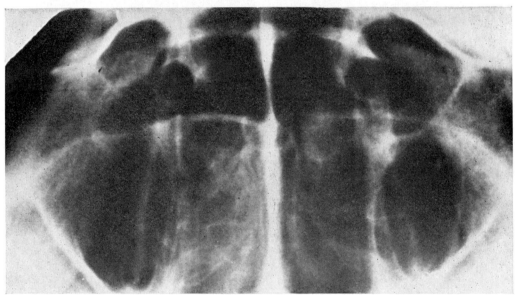

FIG. 11–6. Overextended submentovertical view: (*1*) anterior wall of the frontal sinus; (*2*) bony wall of the nasolacrimal canal; (*3*) frontal bone; (*4*) lamina papyracea; (*5*) medial wall of the maxillary sinus; (*6*) nasal septum; (*7*) posterior wall of the frontal sinus.

ethmoidal cells are superimposed on the nasal structures, i.e., turbinates, hard palate. The bony contours of the orbits, the anterior cranial fossa, and the pterygoid processes are well delineated, offering a good diagnostic evaluation of this area. The frontal sinus is always covered by the shadow of the mandible.

Overextended Submentovertical View (Fig. 11–6). This projection is advantageous for demonstration of the frontal sinuses. The view is obtained by extending the head further than the standard submental vertex view or by angulating the x-ray beam toward the patient's chin rather than perpendicular to the base of the skull. The x-ray beam becomes parallel with both the anterior and posterior walls of the frontal sinus at the level of the suprainfundibular region. Thus, both the depth (AP diameter) and the bony wall of the frontal sinuses, as well as the pathologic processes within the si-

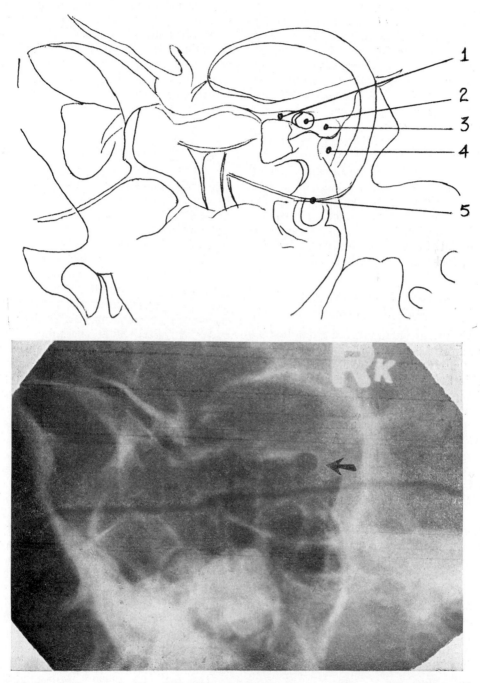

FIG. 11–7. Optic canal view (Rhese projection). Arrow points to the optic canal. (*1*) Planum sphenoidalis; (*2*) optic canal; (*3*) anterior clinoid process; (*4*) superior orbital fissure; (*5*) inferior orbital rim.

nuses, are well demonstrated. The view is the only one in which the bony canal of the nasolacrimal duct can occasionally be seen.

Optic Canal View (Rhese projection) (Fig. 11–7). The head is rotated 45 degrees to the opposite side for visualizing the optic canal and the ethmoidosphenoidal region. This view is not only best for the visualization of the optic canal but also satisfactory for the sphenoidal plane and for the posterior ethmoid cells, which are free from the superimposition of the opposite side.

If conventional x-ray examination does not provide sufficient information, tomography is indicated. Frontal and lateral tomograms are usually satisfactory to demonstrate the facial bones. Axial (basal) sections are useful for the exploration of the sphenoidal bone and the parasphenoidal region, including the optic canals.

RADIOANATOMY AND DEVELOPMENT

Basic radioanatomy and the developmental data of the paranasal sinuses have great importance in the interpretation of the radiographic findings (see Chapter 1).

Compared to the metric data of 40 years ago, a moderate increase in average length and surface of the paranasal sinuses is found today. These figures are consistent with other data indicating an accelerated development of the human body. The first visualization of the paranasal sinuses on x-ray films varies with the age and sex of the youngsters. It was found that, in a large group of children, the development of the sinuses until about age 10 is more prominent in girls than in boys. The average adult size is reached at the age of 13 through 15 in girls and 14 through 16 in boys. Statistical studies have also shown larger paranasal sinuses in adult males than in females. These differences are more significant in the usually asymmetric frontal and sphenoidal sinuses than in the more symmetrical ethmoidal and maxillary sinuses.

The *ethmoidal cells* are the only sinuses demonstrated on x-ray films just after birth. Only one cell is noted bilaterally below the level of the nasofrontal suture. The number and extension of the cells on both sides of the middle line keep increasing and reach the normal adult average at age 13. The lateral wall of the ethmoid is formed by the very thin lamina papyracea, which separates the ethmoidal cells from the soft tissues of the orbit. In the Caldwell and Waters views, the soft tissues of the nose and the turbinates obscure portions of the ethmoidal cells.

It is well known that the two laminae papyraceae are not parallel to each other but rather are oblique, lateralward posteriorly. This cone shape of the orbit accounts for the better visualization of the more posterior ethmoidal cells in the Caldwell view. In contrast, the more anterior cells are recognizable in the Waters view. The ethmoidal cells frequently extend posteriorly into the parasphenoidal area or downward into the maxillary region. Such extensions cannot be well visualized on conventional views. All pathologic processes of the ethmoidal cells and the adjacent structures, such as the optic canals or superior orbital fissures, are better visualized by tomography.

The earliest visualization of the *maxillary antrum* occurs after 6 months of age. Embryologic studies have indicated that the floor of the neonatal antrum lies at the level of the ostium of the sinus in the middle meatus. Later, the antrum develops laterally toward the malar bone and downward in the space occupied earlier by the erupted teeth. Three main recesses are identified in a well-developed maxillary antrum: the lateral zygomatic, the inferior alveolar, and the superior medial ethmoidal recesses.

The volume of the maxillary antrum in adults depends on the size of the maxillary bone and the degree of pneumatization. The pneumatization may not completely fill the maxillary bone, so the bony walls of the antrum may remain quite thick. It is important to differentiate the underdeveloped maxillary antrum, which always presents a sharp inner contour, from the sclerotic bony walls produced by chronic inflammatory diseases.

The maxillary antrum has a quadrangular shape in the lateral view and a triangular shape in the frontal and basal projections. The posterior wall of the antrum is always S-shaped. The medial wall of the antrum is usually straight. Occasionally, it may be slightly curved, creating a double contour in the frontal views. The superior wall of the antrum is formed by the orbital rim and the orbital floor, which appear superimposed in the modified Caldwell views but separated in the Waters view.

Ethmoidal and sphenoidal cells are often projected into the maxillary antrum in the Waters view. The contours of these cells are always well outlined. The technique of tomography will better demonstrate the relationship between the posterior sinus wall and the pterygoid process, as well as the septa of the bi- or tripartite antrum, which is sometimes dehiscent bone or only a mucosal diaphragm.

Anatomically, *the frontal sinus* is located between the outer and inner tables of the vertical portion of the frontal bone, but it may extend posteriorly into the orbital roof. The first radiographic appearance of the frontal sinus usually coincides with the bony closure of the metopic suture. There is, however, no significant correlation between the development of the frontal sinus and the persistence of the metopic suture.

Usually, at the age of 2 to 4, the frontal sinuses are roentgenologically visualized, but occasionally the development may not start until 6 years of age. The frequency of occurrence of frontal sinus aplasia, which may be unilateral or bilateral, varies according to different statistics. However, all frontal sinus developmental anomalies account for 10% of all cases examined.

The well-developed frontal sinus differs considerably in size, shape, and number of recesses. The intraseptal wall may be in the midline or displaced eccentrically and has no pathologic significance. The configuration of the developed frontal sinus is an exclusive characteristic, as is the fingerprint.

The extreme variations in frontal sinus development may render the x-ray diagnosis of certain pathologic conditions difficult, and a combination of the various sinus projections may provide a better evaluation of the frontal sinuses. The difference in radiolucency of the two frontal sinuses is not necessarily indicative of pathology, since it may be due to the difference in the thickness of the anterior and posterior walls or in the depth of one of the sinuses. On the other hand, equal transparency of both frontal sinuses is not necessarily a proof of normalcy.

The first visualization of the *sphenoidal sinus* on x-ray film occurs at age 3 or 4 as a small cavity in the anterior part of the sphenoidal body. For this reason all the sphenoidal sinuses of the younger age group and the underdeveloped sinuses of adults always occupy the anterior portion of the sphenoid bone. The well-developed sinuses extend posteriorly underneath the sella turcica into the dorsum sellae and, after the closure of the sphenooccipital suture, even into the occipital bone. Laterally, the sinuses may extend into the greater wings of the sphenoid and into the pterygoid processes.

The size and shape of the sphenoidal sinuses vary greatly, almost as much as those of the frontal sinuses. The two sphenoidal sinuses are symmetrical only in one sixth of the cases. Three or more partite sinuses are more frequent than a single cavity. The normal anatomic configuration of the sphenoidal sinus, as well as the pathologic conditions of the sinuses, may be inadequately or poorly visualized by conventional views. The Waters and the Caldwell view are not informative. In the lateral view, the two sides are superimposed. The axial view is the only projection which can provide sufficient information about the status of the entire sinus. A more precise examination of the sphenoidal sinus is provided by tomography in the frontal, lateral, and horizontal planes.

TOMOGRAPHY OF THE PARANASAL SINUSES

Tomography of the paranasal sinuses is indicated whenever the extension of the pathologic processes cannot be clearly determined by conventional techniques or when the sinus areas are obscured by the superimposition of other structures. It is evident that tomography is less often requested in acute inflammatory processes than in other pathologic conditions of the paranasal sinuses (see Chapter 41).

Complete tomographic examination of the paranasal sinuses involves sections in the

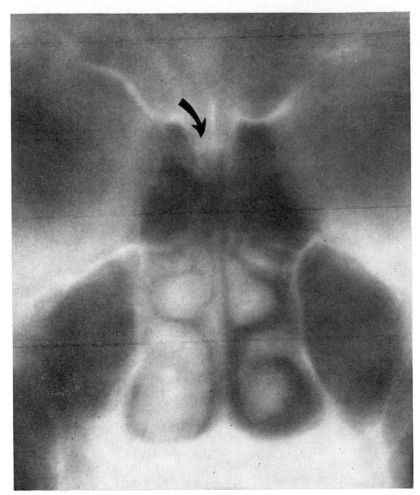

Fɪɢ. 11–8.   Coronal tomogram of the facial bones. Arrow points to the cribriform plate.

coronal, sagittal, and horizontal planes. Sections are usually made 3 mm apart except in the cribriform plate area (Fig. 11-8), where sections 1 mm apart are necessary.

Tomograms in the coronal plane only are capable of visualizing such minute structures as the olfactory groove. The cribriform plate lies in the midline of the floor of the anterior fossa usually about 4 to 7 mm below the upper surface of the ethmoidal capsule and posterior to the crista galli. Tomograms of two different planes are usually necessary for the visualization of the superior orbital fissure, nasolacrimal duct, supraorbital and infraorbital foramina and canals, pterygomaxillary fossa (coronal sections), optic foramina (oblique and horizontal sections),

and foramen lacerum (coronal and axial sections). Malformation of the facial bones and anterior cranial fossa and neoplastic involvement of the paranasal sinuses require tomograms of all three positions.

PATHOLOGIC CONDITIONS OF THE PARANASAL SINUSES

The most important factor in x-ray diagnosis is differentiation between normal and pathologic conditions. Familiarity with the normal anatomy and normal variations of the paranasal sinuses is indispensable for the diagnosis and differentiation of the pathologic processes.

Solitary Densities in the Paranasal Sinuses

A solitary density in the paranasal sinuses may be cast by a foreign body, stone, cyst, polyp, or osteoma.

Conventional views of the paranasal sinuses reveal the presence of radiopaque foreign bodies within the sinuses or facial bones. Among the various foreign bodies, metallic projectiles, impression pastes, and fragments of instruments may be demonstrated. Rhinoliths or antroliths usually require tomographic study for better demonstration.

Cysts are produced by the obstruction of the duct of a mucous gland of the mucosal lining, with consequent accumulation of secretion. The outline of the sinus is unaffected, and a round soft tissue mass is outlined within the lumen of the sinus in different conventional views (Fig. 11-9). Dentigerous, radicular, or primordial cysts of the maxillary sinus usually show no significant difference from the retention cyst, but they occasionally expand the sinus cavity by displacement of its walls.

A solitary polyp in the paranasal sinus presents a radiographic feature identical to a cyst. It is very difficult, almost impossible, to differentiate between the two lesions. The appearance of the nasal cavity may provide some indirect clues. A free nasal cavity with well-outlined turbinates speaks for a cyst, while the presence of soft tissue masses in the nasal cavity or in the choana favors a polypoid process. Occasionally, a cyst or polyp can obliterate the sinus cavity completely, allowing no differentiation even in tomograms.

An osteoma may be symptomatic or merely an accidental finding on x-ray films. Its bony structure is always more radiopaque compared to cysts or polyps. An osteoma is a benign tumor with a slowly progressive growth, causing varying symptoms according to its location. The diagnosis is usually made by conventional x-ray views. Tomograms may be necessary only to detect a pedicle to one of the walls whenever the osteoma fills the sinus cavity as a cast.

Paranasal Sinusitis

The mucosal lining of a healthy sinus is not visualized on x-ray films, but if an in-

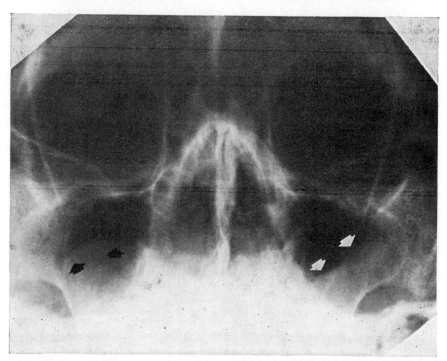

FIG. 11–9.   Retention cyst in the right maxillary sinus (black arrows), early inflammatory process in the left one (white arrow).

fection occurs, it becomes visible through the edema of the mucosal lining. The swollen, edematous mucosal lining appears as a density, parallel with the bony wall of the sinus (Fig. 11-9). In an early stage of infection, this finding may be limited to only one wall. Later, it spreads to other walls, and finally the entire sinus becomes cloudy.

It is not possible to differentiate the homogeneous clouding of the sinus caused by edematous, swollen mucosal lining from accumulated fluid with no drainage. Whenever the fluid does not fill the entire sinus cavity, a fluid level is always seen in the upright views (Fig. 11-10). For demonstration of small fluid accumulations, an additional film with the head tilted to one side may be necessary.

Fluid level without mucosal thickening is found in post-traumatic conditions due to hemorrhage into the sinus. A circumscribed swelling of the mucosal lining in the alveolar recesses of the maxillary antrum is usually produced by infection originating in the teeth or periodontal area.

Single or multiple circumscribed bulgings of the mucosa produced by circumscribed areas of edema are usually characteristic of allergic disease of the upper respiratory system. These changes are reversible, in contrast to the irreversible degenerative changes of the mucosa, such as polyps and cysts.

Chronic inflammatory processes of the paranasal sinuses are characterized by mucoperiosteal thickening along the bony walls. The density of the mucoperiosteal thickening is always more intense than the swollen mucosal lining of the acute infection. When the infection involves the bony wall, the bony contour of the sinus becomes dense owing to marked sclerosis of the surrounding bone (Fig. 11-12).

Views obtained after maxillary sinus surgery performed for inflammatory diseases usually demonstrate homogeneous clouding similar to chronic infection. Starlike striation

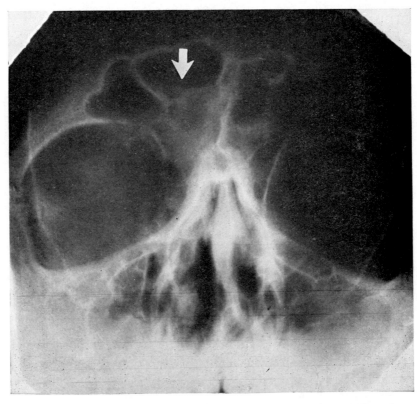

FIG. 11-10.   Acute frontal sinusitis. Fluid level in the right frontal sinus (arrow).

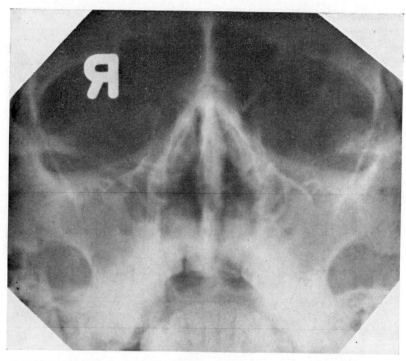

FIG. 11–11.   Chronic maxillary sinusitis. Bilateral homogeneous density of the
maxillary antrums.

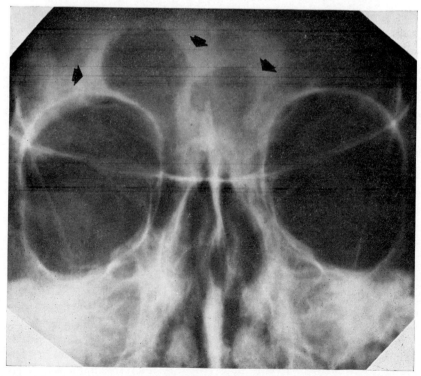

FIG. 11–12.   Sclerosis of the frontal bone around the frontal sinuses (arrows).
(Delayed result of a chronic frontal sinusitis.)

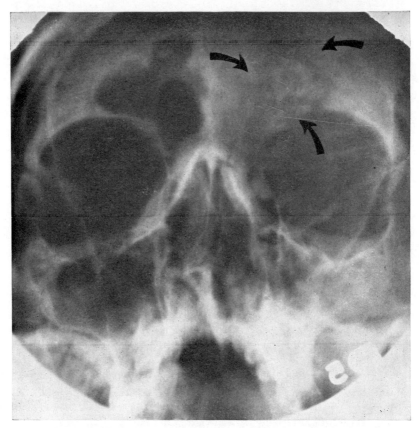

Fig. 11–13. Osteomyelitis of the frontal bone. Arrows show the moth-eaten structure
of the osteomyelitic bone.

directed toward the center of the antrum could be the single differential diagnostic sign indicative of a Caldwell-Luc operation. If reinfection of a sinus should occur after surgery, it may not be recognizable, since no change occurs in the clouding of the sinus unless the sinus walls become eroded by osteomyelitis or neoplasm.

Osteomyelitis of the Paranasal Sinuses

Osteomyelitis may be the consequence of either chronic inflammatory processes of the sinuses or an acute infection following injury to the sinus wall or surrounding soft tissue. The typical x-ray finding in osteomyelitis is a moth-eaten appearance (Fig. 11-13) of the involved bone with or without sequestration or erosion. The frontal bone is most frequently involved. Follow-up films after surgery are very useful in detecting further progression of the osteomyelitic disease.

Mucocele of the Paranasal Sinuses

When a mucocele develops in the paranasal sinus, a well-defined spherical soft tissue mass is noted on the x-ray films. At the early stage of development, no criteria exist for the differentiation of mucocele, polyp, and cyst. Eventually, the enlarged mucocele fills the entire sinus, and the accumulated secretion exerts pressure on the bony wall, causing a gradual expansion of the cavity. The expansive tendency is a pathognomonic x-ray finding of the mucocele.

In the frontal sinus, the pressure is first detected toward the less resistant structures, resulting in early displacement and thinning of the interseptum. Later, there is a displacement or erosion of the floor of the si-

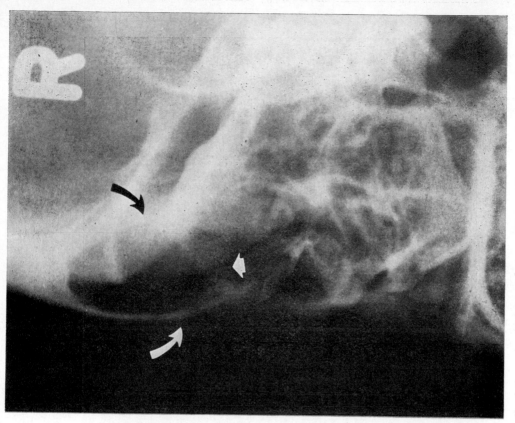

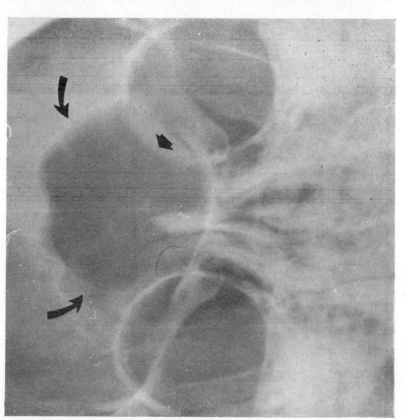

Fig. 11–14. Mucocele of the left frontal sinus. Arrows show the bony wall of the expanded frontal sinus. The small arrows in the Caldwell view (*left*) point to the bony erosion of the superior medial wall of the orbit. The small arrow in the lateral view (*right*) points to the erosion of the infundibular wall of the frontal sinus.

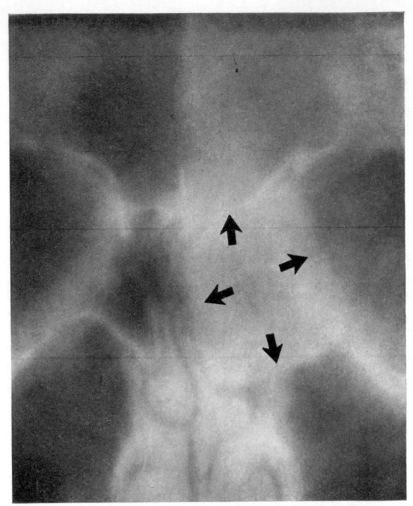

Fig. 11–15.   Legend on facing page.

nus, which is responsible for ophthalmic symptoms. The eventual thinning and displacement of the anterior and posterior walls of the frontal sinus finally account for the classic rounded configuration of the mucocele (Fig. 11–14).

In the sphenoidal sinus, expansion and displacement of the interseptum are followed by similar changes of the inferior lateral and posterior walls. If only the superior wall is eroded, the differential diagnosis between mucocele and pituitary tumors may be difficult. Large mucocele can cause displacement of the carotid artery and narrowing of the chiasmatic cistern.

Mucocele in the ethmoidal sinuses forms a large cavity, first by erosion of the cell septa. In the course of further growth, mu-

cocele displaces and erodes the lamina papyracea, the perpendicular process of the ethmoid bone, and the infundibulum of the frontal sinus (Fig. 11–15). In addition to the thinning or defects of the bony walls, displacement of the nasolacrimal sac and duct and bony erosion of the cribriform plate may occur. Tomograms provide more important details of bony changes of the paranasal sinuses and surrounding structures.

Mucocele of the maxillary antrum is rare.

Fracture of the Facial Bones and Paranasal Sinuses

Fracture of the facial bones is extremely common and may extend into one or several

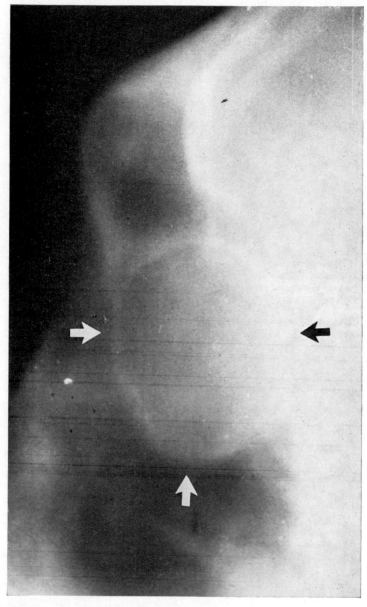

FIG. 11–15.   Mucocele of the left ethmoidal cells in coronal *(top)* and lateral *(bottom)* tomograms (see arrows).

of the paranasal sinuses. Fractures of the facial bones and paranasal sinuses have direct and indirect x-ray findings.

Direct Signs of Fractures. The fracture line is the most important direct sign of any bone injury. Fractures may involve only a single bone—more frequently the nasal bone —or a single wall of one of the paranasal sinuses. A typical example of single wall in-

jury is the blowout fracture of the medial wall or the floor of the orbit.

About one third of patients sustaining injuries have more extensive multiple fractures. Classification of these fractures is given by Le Fort (all these fractures may be unilateral or bilateral) (Fig. 11–16). The Le Fort type I crosses the maxillary bone transversely above the teeth, involving the ante-

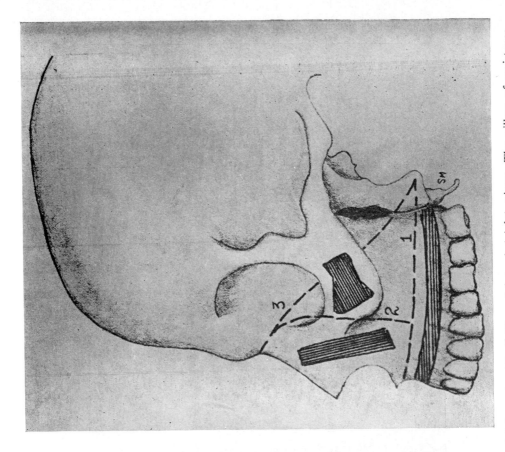

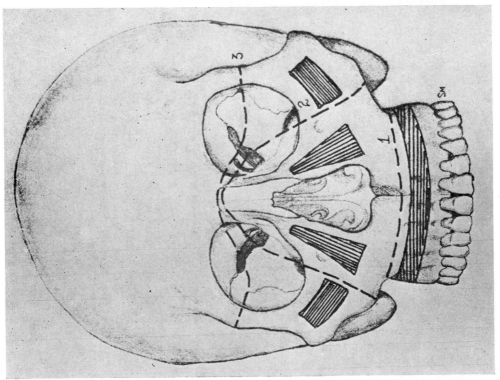

Fig. 11–16. Le Fort I, II, and III types of fractures of the facial bone in AP (*left*) and lateral (*right*) views. The pillars of resistance are indicated by lined areas, and the three classic fractures of Le Fort by broken lines.

rior, lateral, and posterior walls of the maxillary sinus, and may reach the pterygoid processes. The Le Fort type II fracture is generally pyramidal, running through the nasal bone and ethmoidal cells (sometimes also including the frontal sinus), the frontal process of the maxillary bone, the infraorbital floor and rim, and the lateral wall of the maxillary sinus. It may expand to the zygoma and pterygoid processes. The Le Fort type III fracture is a complete disjunction of the facial bones from the cranium by separation of the frontozygomatic, maxillofrontal, and nasofrontal sutures, together with the comminuted multiple fractures of the facial bone.

Of the fractures involving multiple bones, the most common type is the so-called tripod fracture, which disrupts the lateral wall, the floor of the orbit, the lateral wall of the maxillary antrum, and the zygomatic body or the zygomatic arch.

Indirect Signs of Fractures. Clouding of the paranasal sinuses after injury, with or without visible bony fractures, may be partial or complete. Bleeding under the surface of the mucosal lining shows a picture similar to the swelling of the mucosal lining due to inflammatory processes. Hemorrhage within the sinus produces complete clouding or fluid level only if the films are obtained in upright position. A circumscribed soft tissue mass convex toward the sinus cavity represents a hematoma or, in blowout fractures of the infraorbital floor, herniation of the orbital fat and/or muscles (Fig. 11–17).

When communication between the nasal and sinus cavities has been established, the air may easily find its way into the soft tissues. Free air in the orbital soft tissues is usually the result of a fracture or microfracture of the medial orbital wall.

X-ray study of fractures of the paranasal sinuses routinely starts with the four stan-

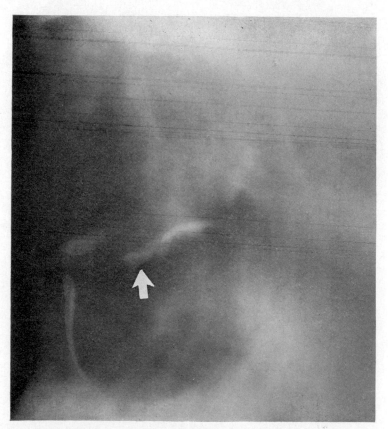

Fig. 11–17.   Blowout fracture of the orbital floor in the lateral tomogram. Arrow points to the fragment depressed into the maxillary antrum.

7

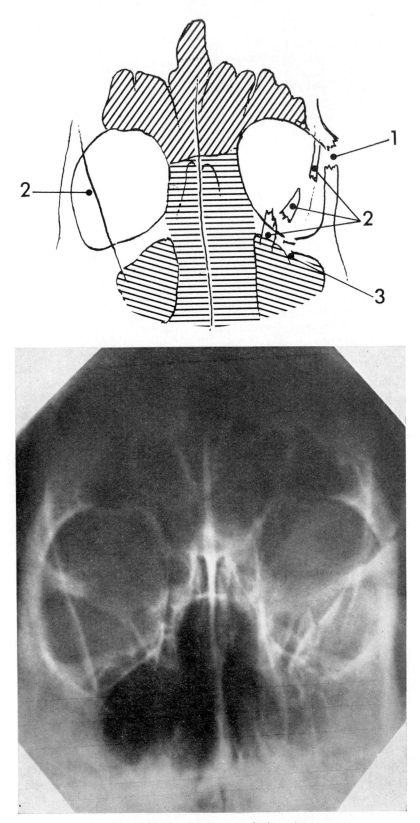

Fig. 11–18.   Legend on facing page.

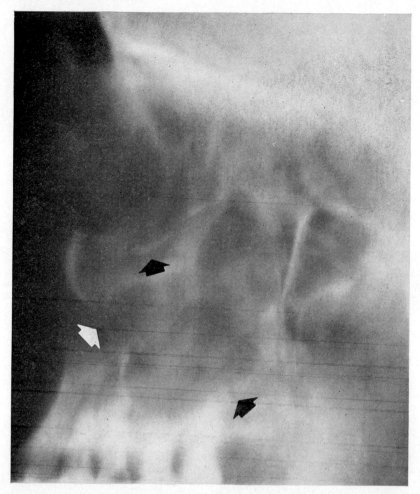

FIG. 11–18. Complex fracture of the facial bones: (*1*) separation of the left zygomatic suture; (*2*) fragmentation of the left temporal line (see normal right side for comparison); (*3*) fracture of the infraorbital rim and floor. In the lateral tomogram of the same case, the arrows point to the multiple fractures.

dard views of the sinuses. Special views and tomograms in two or three planes are necessary in cases with multiple or combined fractures to demonstrate the extent of the involvement accurately (Fig. 11–18).

NASOPHARYNX

The nasopharynx is the portion of the pharynx lying immediately posterior to the nasal choanae and above the level of the soft palate. The superior bony wall is formed by the inferior surface of the sphenoid and occipital bones, the posterior wall by the bodies of the upper cervical vertebrae. The thickness of the submucosal connective tissue anterior to the cervical spine, as demonstrated on lateral views, varies normally with age. Nasopharyngeal lesions originate either from the superior, lateral, or posterior walls and, as they grow into the lumen of the nasopharynx, are demonstrated in the lateral views as a rounded mass.

The mass of adenoid tissue is evident from age 5 or 6, but after puberty the average width of the soft tissue is not more than 5 to 8 mm. Juvenile angioma is the most common tumor during puberty, and it appears as a soft tissue mass in the nasopharynx, protruding into the nasal cavity

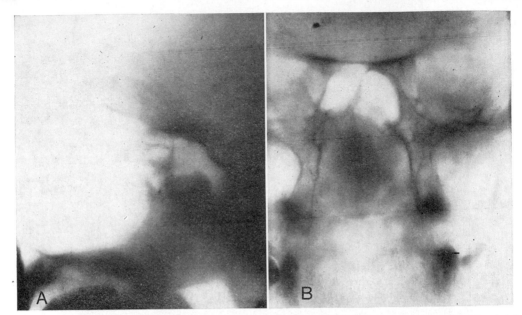

FIG. 11–19.   Carcinoma of the nasopharynx. Conventional (*left*) and tomographic (*right*) views. The mass is well outlined, but no erosion of the base of the skull is seen.

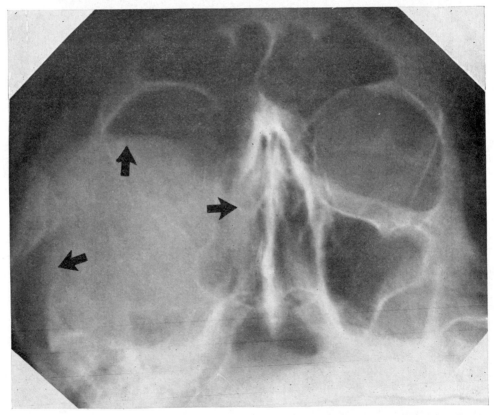

FIG. 11–20.   Carcinoma of the right maxillary sinus extending into the orbit superiorly, into the nasal cavity medially, and into the malar bone laterally (arrows).

and often into the intraosseous spaces of the facial bones.

Anterior bulging of the posterior wall of the maxillary antrum is a diagnostic criterion for involvement of the pterygomaxillary fossa. Tomography in lateral and coronal projections is useful for exact localization of the juvenile angiofibroma.

Malignant tumor of the nasopharynx (Fig. 11–19) may involve the adjacent bony structures, such as the base of the skull superiorly, cervical spine posteriorly, pterygoid process laterally, and nasal cavities anteriorly.

Two different features of bone involvement are also observed radiographically. The most common is erosion or frank destruction; however, reactive new bone formation or sclerosis may also be seen. The submental vertical view is particularly useful for diagnosis of lesions of the base of the skull. However, tomograms in coronal, lateral, and axial projections are necessary for precise evaluation of the extension of the lesion.

MALIGNANT TUMOR OF THE PARANASAL SINUSES

Radiology plays an important role in both the diagnosis and treatment of malignant tumors of the paranasal sinuses. Diagnosis of the malignant tumor becomes radiographically possible only when the bony walls of the involved sinus are eroded. The x-ray findings are not usually characteristic for the different histologic types of tumors. Usually, there is lesser density of the involved sinus in sarcoma than in carcinoma, as a result of the more extensive involvement of the sinus walls in sarcomas. On the other hand, adenocarcinoma shows less bony erosion and therefore more intensive clouding of the involved sinus. In cases of cylindroma, bony sclerosis often is also demonstrated along with the bony erosion.

In addition to showing the site of the tumor, the x-ray examination is extremely important in demonstrating the direction of growth of the lesion and the involvement of the surrounding structures (Fig. 11–20). More detailed information is obtained by tomography of the frontal, lateral, and horizontal planes. The criteria for surgical accessibility of the lesion and the extent of the surgical resection must be established by proper radiographic examination; follow-up radiographic studies offer information about the progression or regression of the tumor.

REFERENCES

1. van Aleya, O. E.: *Nasal Sinus. Anatomic and Clinical Consideration.* Baltimore, Williams and Wilkins, 1951.
2. Etter, L. E.: *Atlas of Roentgen Anatomy of the Skull.* Springfield, Charles C Thomas, 1970.
3. Lundgren, A., and Olin, T.: Muco-pyocele of sphenoidal sinus or posterior ethmoidal cells with special reference to the apex orbital syndrome. Acta Otolaryngol., *53*: 51, 1961.
4. Mayer, E. G.: *Roentgendifferentialdiagnostik des Schadels.* Springer, Wien, 1959.
5. Merrell, R. A., Yanagisawa, E., Smith, H. W., and Thaler, S.: Radiographic anatomy of the paranasal sinuses. Arch. Otolaryngol., 87:184, 1968.
6. Naumann, H. H., Berendes, J., Link, R., Zollner, F.: *Hals-Nasen-Ohrenheilkunde.* Stuttgart, G. Thieme, 1964.
7. Potter, G. D.: *Sectional Anatomy and Tomography of the Head.* New York, Grune and Stratton, 1971.
8. Samuel, E.: *Clinical Radiology of the Ear, Nose and Larynx.* New York, Lewis, 1952.
9. Schinz, H. R.: *Lehrbuck der Rontgendiagnostik.* Stuttgart, G. Thieme, 1956.
10. Valvassori, G. E., and Hord, G. E.: Traumatic sinus disease. Seminars in Roentgenology, Vol. 3. No. 2. 1968.
11. Vandor, F., Laszlo, I., and Kovacs, A.: Ful-orr-gegeszeti rontgendiagnosztika. Medicina, Budapest, 1961.
12. Zizmor, J., and Noyek, A. M.: Inflammatory diseases of the paranasal sinuses. Otolaryngol. Clin. North Am., *6*:459, 1973.

Chapter 12

Nonsurgical Treatment of Sinus Infections

The nonsurgical treatment of sinusitis is frequently the treatment of the viral upper respiratory tract infection of which the sinusitis is a prominent part. This is particularly true of ethmoiditis. Frequently these viral infections are self-limited afflictions of short duration if there are no purulent complications. They respond promptly to good general supportive measures described in the section on treatment of the common cold.

Important among these supportive measures are a constant, clean, humidified environment and bedrest. Ideally the inspired air should have a relative humidity of 45 to 55% at 70°F. Dryness of the nasal mucosa is to be avoided because of the ciliostatic effect. Nasal lysozyme is most active in a slightly acid medium, so alkaline nose drops are unwise.

Pain due to acute sinusitis is treated by decongestion of the nasal mucosa, by salicylates, and by local applications of heat. The latter is effective in part, probably because of its counterirritant effect. Vasoconstrictor medication early in the course of an acute sinusitis is better given systemically by mouth rather than locally as nose drops. A useful combination is ephedrine sulfate 0.015 g, phenobarbital 0.015 g and acetylsalicylic acid (or acetaminophen) 0.300 g, all in one capsule, which is given every 4 hours. Once the acute intumescent inflammation has disappeared, local vasoconstriction (e.g., 1% ephedrine) is useful.

Removal of heavy retained exudate from the nasal spaces by spot suction after thorough vasoconstriction of the nasal mucous membranes gives great relief.

There is little or no place for the local intranasal use of bacteriostatic or bactericidal agents in the treatment of acute sinusitis, because, for one thing, they cannot be brought into contact with a sufficient area of infected mucosal surfaces to be efficient. Also, they irritate or impede ciliary activity, which is the prime cleansing mechanism of the nasal mucosa, the integral functions of which should be rigorously preserved. Sulfonamide drugs are strongly alkaline and must not be used locally in the nose. The various antimicrobial drugs may be instilled into a sinus and accomplish some good. However, their effectiveness in this regard is yet to be determined.

The routine parenteral use of sulfonamide or antimicrobial medication in acute sinusitis is to be condemned because little good is accomplished and there is always the danger of an allergic reaction. If bacterial complications are present, antimicrobial medication given systemically is a most valuable aid. If antimicrobial therapy is decided upon, it is best given specifically (i.e., after appropriate sensitivity tests), continuously over a long period of time, and in doses large enough to eradicate the infecting agent.

The possible complication of an underlying allergic rhinitis must always be kept in mind when treating sinusitis; if it is present, appropriate therapy should be instituted. It is a mistake, however, to use antihistamine therapy routinely in the treatment of sinusitis. Any improvement that apparently is observed stems from the vasoconstrictor medication usually contained along with the antihistamine in the proprietary preparations now on the market.

After the initial inflammation and edema have partially subsided, use may be made of displacement irrigation previously described. By this method nasal secretions can be removed, and bland, gently vasoconstricting solutions (e.g., 0.25% ephedrine in 0.85% saline solution) can be introduced into the sinuses. The evacuation time of the sinus under these circumstances is some hours in duration. During this period prolonged vasoconstriction with increased patency of the ostium is accomplished. The introduction of antibiotics or sulfonamides into the sinuses in this manner probably adds little to the success of the treatment, and the latter, if alkaline, may do harm.

Irrigation of the Frontal Sinus

Irrigation of the frontal sinus is rarely necessary but may be performed through the frontonasal canal, except in those few cases in which it is closed by an enlarged bulla or an enlarged middle turbinate. An understanding of certain anatomic peculiarities of the region of the infundibulum and frontonasal canal will aid materially in the irrigation of the sinuses.

The hiatus semilunaris is a slitlike, crescentic opening in the outer wall of the nose. It is the opening into the infundibulum of the middle meatus, and its inner lip is the upper margin of the uncinate process of the ethmoid bone.

The infundibulum is a deep, narrow groove or gutter in the lateral wall of the nose (see Fig. 12–3, f), the inner wall of which is the uncinate process. The frontonasal canal drains into the infundibulum in about one half of the subjects, whereas in the remainder it drains a little anteriorly directly into the middle meatus.

The frontonasal canal is a closed tubular duct extending upward and forward from the middle meatus or infundibulum, as the case may be, to the frontal sinus. Its opening into the floor of the sinus is known as the ostium frontale. In rare instances the ostium is found on the posterior wall.

The hiatus semilunaris is the key to the insertion of the cannula, since it is the opening into the infundibulum which must be reached prior to entering the sinal canal itself.

The bulla ethmoidalis is situated just above the hiatus, and when large, it encroaches upon the slitlike opening and partially or completely closes it. Occasionally there are accessory cells in the uncinate process which also obstruct the hiatus. In other cases the middle turbinate closely hugs the outer wall of the nose and blocks the hiatus. When any of these anatomic peculi-

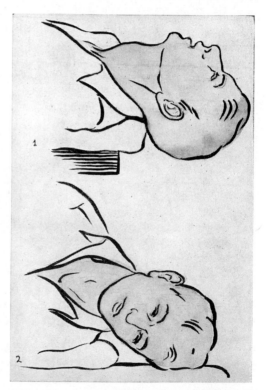

FIG. 12–1. Two "head low" positions for instilling drops in the region of the various sinus ostia: 1, the Proetz position is indicated when the ostia of the posterior group of sinuses are to be reached; 2, the side position will permit the drops to reach the ostia of all the sinuses if the head is rotated slowly back and forth.

arities is present, the introduction of the probe or the cannula is rendered difficult or impossible. If the frontonasal canal opens in front of the infundibulum, the cannula may be passed into it even though the hiatus is closed.

Another difficulty sometimes encountered is that the cannula may enter the ostium of one of the anterior ethmoidal cells instead of the frontal sinus. Some of the anterior cells may open into the infundibulum on its outer wall, while others open into the fronto-nasal canal. The anterior cells are usually located external to the infundibulum and the frontonasal canal, and their ostia open into the infundibulum and frontonasal canal through the outer wall. In inserting the cannula, therefore, the point of the cannula should be kept against the inner or mesial wall of the frontonasal canal in order to avoid the ostia on its outer wall.

Irrigation is generally more difficult in those subjects in whom the frontonasal canal empties into the infundibulum than in those in whom it empties directly into the middle meatus. In the former case the canal is often tortuous and narrow, while in the latter it is usually straighter and of larger caliber.

The middle turbinate is sometimes so close to the hiatus, especially when the turbinate contains an accessory cell, that it is difficult to enter it with a probe or cannula. In this event the removal of the anterior third of the middle turbinate overcomes the difficulty.

Technique. First the part is topically anesthetized. Then a fine silver cannula (Fig. 12–2), bent at its distal end to an angle of about 135 degrees, is introduced between the anterior third of the middle turbinate and the outer wall of the nose. The tip of the cannula should be kept against the outer surface of the turbinate, and it should be passed forward and upward through the hi-

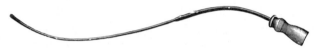

Fig. 12–2.   Frontal sinus cannula.

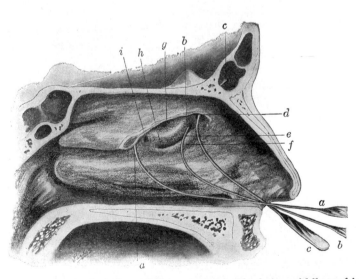

Fig. 12–3.   Irrigating the frontal sinus. The anterior half of the middle turbinate is removed to show the anatomic landmarks: *a, a,* the probe in the first position beneath the middle turbinate and posterior to the bulla ethmoidalis; *b, b,* the probe in the second position beneath the middle turbinate and in front of the bulla ethmoidalis; *c, c,* the probe in the third position introduced through the frontonasal canal into the frontal sinus; *d,* the nasal end of the frontonasal canal; *e,* the lip of the uncinate process; *f,* the inner wall (uncinate process) of the infundibulum; *g,* the ostium bulla ethmoidalis; *h,* the ostium maxillare; *i,* an accessory opening into the maxillary sinus.

atus into the infundibulum, where it readily enters the frontonasal canal even to the frontal ostium (Fig. 12–3). After it is engaged in the middle meatus, it should be passed into the infundibulum and canal for about 6 to 8 cm to reach the frontal sinus.

The syringe is attached to the cannula, and the sinus is gently irrigated with warm normal salt or boric acid solution.

Irrigation of the Maxillary Sinus Through the Ostium

This can be effected through the normal antral opening in most cases by means of Pierce's antrum cannula.

Technique. After the area beneath the middle portion of the middle turbinate is anesthetized, the cannula is introduced upward and backward with the curved tip in a vertical position. When the anesthetized portion of the middle turbinate is reached, the tip of the cannula is inserted beneath the middle turbinate in an upward and outward direction so as to pass over the uncinate process. As this process is passed over, the tip of the cannula is directed downward and outward (sometimes directly outward), when it will usually enter the natural opening. In a few cases it is impossible to irrigate by this method on account of the hidden position in the infundibulum of the nasoantral opening, and on account of its forward and downward direction from the infundibulum to the antrum. The opening into the antrum in these cases is not directly through the lateral wall of the nose, but it is more like a canal extending obliquely downward and forward through the thickness of the wall. In a certain number of cases there are accessory openings into the antrum (Fig. 12–3) which, when present, may be utilized for purposes of irrigation.

Irrigation of the Maxillary Sinus by Puncture Through the Inferior Meatus

If difficulty or an excessive irritation of the tissues is encountered from irrigating through the natural opening, an artificial route should be chosen. The most available one is the inferior meatus. A curved or straight trocar is used for the purpose.

Technique. The mucous membrane of the nasoantral wall of the inferior meatus is anesthetized with a 5% solution of cocaine. The trocar is introduced beneath the inferior turbinate posterior to the anterior antral wall and directed upward and outward, a little above the floor of the nose, in order to avoid the thick wall of bone at this point. In some cases, especially when a maxillary cyst is present, or in infants and children, the floor of the antrum is quite high, and it is not possible to introduce the trocar beneath the inferior turbinate. In this event puncture beneath the middle turbinate through the membranous portion of the nasoantral wall can be done.

The dangers of antrum irrigation by puncture are largely a matter of faulty technique. The trocar should have a very sharp point to avoid pushing the lining membrane before it after the bony wall is pierced. Secondly, any undue force in using the irrigating fluid should be avoided.

After the nasoantral wall has been penetrated, the trocar is removed, the cannula being left in position. The rubber hose of the syringe is attached to the cannula, and normal salt or other solution is used to irrigate.

The irrigations through the artificial opening may be repeated every 3 or 4 days as long as necessary.

Air Embolism

An embolism of air is a rare complication of maxillary sinus irrigation in which insufflation of air is used. The author has never encountered such an incident. Pang, after a review of the literature, found a report of 58 cases of air embolism with 23 deaths, a mortality of about 40%.

The alarming and sudden symptoms are rigidity and unconsciousness with cyanosis and convulsions. An epileptiform type of seizure with trismus has been noted in several cases. The pupils may be dilated or fixed with or without nystagmus, conjugate deviation, or backward rolling of the eyeballs. Death may occur immediately or hours or days later. Survivors may have temporary disturbances of vision, paresis or paralysis, or mental lapses or other mental symp-

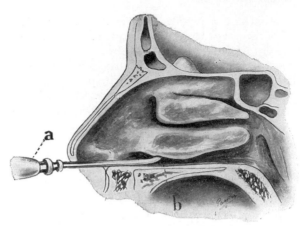

FIG. 12–4. Introducing a trocar (*a*) and cannula into the maxillary antrum beneath the inferior turbinate near the junction (*b*) of the anterior and middle thirds.

toms. The prevention of this mishap would seem to be the avoidance of air insufflation after antrum lavage.

Irrigation of the Maxillary Sinus Through the Alveolar Process

This method is mentioned only to be condemned, unless the alveolar opening is permitted to close before the epithelium has extended into it; otherwise, a chronic fistula results, with constant reinfection of the antrum. It is applicable only to those cases of antrum infection secondary to a root infection of a tooth in which the abscess has eroded a fistula through the floor of the antrum.

Irrigation of the Ethmoidal Cells

This is often impossible except in the case of anterior cells which drain into the frontonasal canal. The bulla ethmoidalis, one of the anterior cells, does not drain into the frontonasal canal but rather directly into the middle meatus, and its ostium is situated at its upper median wall beneath the attachment of the middle turbinate.

The technique for the irrigation of the anterior cells opening into the frontonasal canal is the same as for the frontal sinus, the probe being introduced into the canal only to the second position (Fig. 12–3); indeed, both sets of cells are often irrigated at the same time. Their ostia are bathed with

the irrigating fluid, and the accumulated pus in the canal is removed, thus facilitating drainage of the cells.

Irrigation of the Sphenoidal Sinus Through the Ostium

This is possible when the middle turbinate, or a deflection of the septum, does not prevent the introduction of the sphenoidal cannula into its opening. When such an obstruction is present, it may be necessary to remove it by some surgical procedure before the irrigations can be practiced. A silver eustachian catheter may be used in place of a sphenoidal cannula. The curve used for the inflation of the ear is the correct one for irrigation of the sphenoidal sinus. Myle's cannula may be bent to reach any sinus and is smaller than the eustachian catheter.

When the cannula has been introduced, the patient should be instructed to lean forward and open his mouth; then the hose of the syringe should be attached to the cannula and the sinus irrigated. If the patient's head is inclined forward and the mouth open, the fluid will not enter the eustachian tube.

Irrigation of the Sphenoidal Sinus by Puncture

Puncture of the anterior wall may be done if the natural ostium is not accessible.

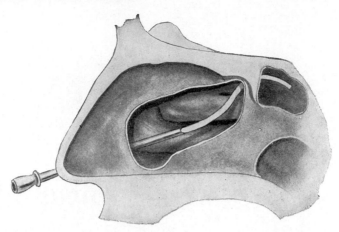

FIG. 12–5.   Irrigation of the sphenoidal sinus with a curved cannula.

After local anesthesia a long-bladed Killian speculum is inserted between the septum and the middle turbinate, separating the two. The anterior wall of the sphenoidal sinus can now be seen. A sphenoidal trocar is introduced backward and upward until the sphenoidal wall is reached. The handle of the trocar is now raised. By pushing it backward the wall is punctured. The opening can be enlarged with a biting forceps or a rasp if necessary.

Minor Surgical Measures

Rarely, if ever, are surgical measures necessary in the treatment of acute sinusitis, and then only after a vigorous trial of the measures previously discussed has been made. If, then, it can be determined that some anatomic feature is obstructing free ventilation and drainage from the sinuses, correction of the obstruction may permit evacuation of the sinus infection. Usually involved in this complication are the anterior group of sinuses, and most commonly a polyp will be found filling or otherwise obstructing the hiatus semilunaris and will require removal. Occasionally a badly deflected nasal septum may do the same thing.

Infracture of the nasal turbinate often improves drainage through the hiatus semilunaris. To accomplish this, local anesthesia is first secured by placing pledgets of cotton moistened with 1 to 2% tetracaine in contact with both the medial and lateral surfaces of the anterior end of the middle turbinate. After 10 minutes the infracture is easily accomplished by placing a flat instrument under the lateral wall of the turbinate and fracturing medially. Bleeding is minimal.

Chapter 13
Surgical Treatment of Sinus Infections

William Montgomery

As a general rule, surgery is indicated in those cases of chronic sinusitis that do not respond to medical therapy. The advent of biochemotherapy and of a better understanding of sinus and intranasal physiology has been instrumental in reducing the frequency with which we must resort to sinus surgery (Fig. 13–1).

Indications for sinus surgery are: (1) intracranial extension of infections such as meningitis, subdural abscess, or brain abscess; (2) persistent pain or discharge that

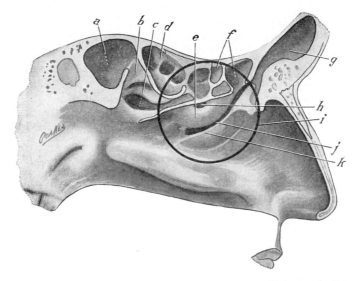

FIG. 13–1.   The circle (*i*) encloses the important structures concerned with the drainage and ventilation of the sinuses of the anterior group: *a*, the sphenoidal sinus; *b*, the sphenoethmoidal fossa; *c*, the superior turbinate; *d*, posterior ethmoidal cells; *e*, bulla ethmoidalis; *f*, anterior ethmoidal cells draining into the frontonasal canal; *g*, frontal sinus; *h*, the ostium of the bulla ethmoidalis; *j*, hiatus semilunaris; *k*, the uncinate process or outer wall of the infundibulum or gutter on the outer wall of the nose into which the frontal, anterior ethmoidal, and maxillary sinuses usually drain. The highlight below and anterior to *j* and *k* indicates the inferior boundary of the infundibulum or gutter into which the sinuses drain. The middle turbinate has been removed to exhibit the anatomic details beneath it.

has not responded to adequate conservative therapy; (3) necrosis of the sinus wall as shown by fistula formation; (4) mucocele or pyocele formation; (5) orbital cellulitis with abscess formation or retrobulbar neuritis.

The purpose of sinus surgery is either (1) to provide free and easy drainage from the sinus into the nose (while at the same time not interfering with intranasal physiology); or (2) to eliminate the sinus (obliteration). Before resorting to any of the radical sinus operations, it is most often preferable to perform simple intranasal procedures in order to establish better drainage. Such procedures as submucous resection of the nasal septum, removal of nasal polyps, resection of the anterior half of the middle turbinate, intranasal antrostomy, and intranasal ethmoidectomy are often sufficient to effect a cure.

THE FRONTAL SINUS

Intranasal Surgery for Chronic Frontal Sinusitis

The establishment of adequate drainage with ultimate resolution of chronic infection in the frontal sinus can often be accomplished by intranasal procedures. The procedures used to accomplish this drainage are careful submucous resection of the nasal septum; removal of intranasal polyps, the anterior portion of the middle turbinate, or both; and anterior ethmoidectomy.

Intranasal probing, attempted enlargement, and cannulation of the nasofrontal orifice are to be condemned. Once the nasofrontal passage is violated, scarring and stenosis are inevitable. If the above-mentioned conservative intranasal surgery is not successful, then radical frontal sinus surgery is contemplated.

External Surgery of the Frontal Sinus

Indications. Complications of chronic frontal sinusitis, such as persistent pain, external fistula, internal fistula, intracranial extension, bone necrosis, orbital complications, and mucocele or pyocele, are positive indications for external frontal sinus surgery. Various benign and malignant tumors of the frontal sinuses are approached externally.

Various Techniques. There are numerous external frontal sinus operations, each having many variations. Those currently popular in the United States are shown in Figure 13–2. These simple box sketches show the resultant anatomic changes effected by each operation.

In the United States, the *Lynch* frontal sinus operation (1920) is probably the most frequently employed procedure for the treatment of chronic frontal sinus disease. Ethmoidectomy, removal of the middle turbinate, and resection of the entire floor of the frontal sinus are accomplished in this operation. A rubber or plastic tube is placed between the frontal sinus and the nasal cavity by way of the ethmoidal labyrinth. This tube remains in place from 1 to 3 months and at times requires considerable postoperative care. As a general rule, the Lynch frontal approach has been a highly effective operation for the control of chronic frontal sinus disease; on the other hand, it is followed by a failure rate sufficient to warrant the search

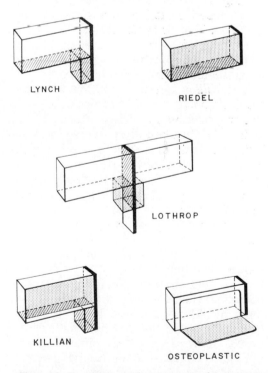

LYNCH

RIEDEL

LOTHROP

KILLIAN

OSTEOPLASTIC

Fig. 13–2. The resultant anatomic changes effected by these frontal sinus operations are indicated and compared to the anterior osteoplastic approach.

for a better operation. Incomplete removal of the sinus mucous membrane may result in mucocele or pyocele formation. Stenosis of the reconstructed nasofrontal passage may lead to recurrent chronic frontal sinusitis.

The *Riedel* operation (1898) consists of removing the anterior wall and floor of the frontal sinus, thus offering wide exposure of the sinus. Complete obliteration of the sinus cannot be executed in many cases—especially when the anteroposterior dimensions of the sinus are large. Mosher modified the Riedel operation by also removing the posterior wall of the sinus. As a general rule, the Riedel procedure is disfiguring and offers a percentage of cure no higher than the Lynch operation.

The *Lothrop* frontal sinus operation (1914) is a unique procedure which entails a unilateral or bilateral anterior ethmoidectomy and middle turbinectomy (Jackson and Jackson). The interfrontal septum is removed. A large opening from the frontal sinuses into the nasal cavity is made by connecting the two nasofrontal ducts. A portion of the superior nasal septum is resected. The operation is at times technically difficult, but it is quite effective when dealing with bilateral frontal sinus disease and a wide anteroposterior frontal sinus dimension.

The *Killian* operation (1904) is another modification of the Riedel operation (Jackson and Jackson). A bridge of bone 10 mm wide is left in place at the supraorbital rim. This functions, of course, to prevent postoperative disfigurement. An anterior ethmoidectomy and middle turbinectomy are also performed. There is much less alteration of the forehead contour; on the other hand, the bridge prevents obliteration of the sinus. Actually, the end result of the Killian operation is quite similar to that of the Lynch operation.

The anterior osteoplastic frontal sinus operation (Goodale and Montgomery) employs an inferiorly hinged bony "trapdoor" fashioned from the anterior wall of the frontal sinus. This affords direct access to the entire contents of the frontal sinus and a view of the nasofrontal orifice from above. The diseased intrasinus tissues can be removed with ease, and if indicated, the sinus is obliterated with adipose tissue.

External Frontoethmoidosphenoidal Operation

The classic incision is made along the inferior margin of the eyebrow extending downward halfway between the inner canthus and the anterior aspect of the nasal bones, well down onto the lateral aspect of the nasal bone (Fig. 13–3). This incision is extended through skin, subcutaneous tissue, and periosteum. Troublesome bleeding is usually encountered from the angular vessels. Before proceeding with the operation it is best to control this bleeding by either ligation or electrodesiccation. The periosteum is elevated from the floor of the frontal sinus inferior to the incision and within the orbit. This elevation is usually most easily begun at the junction of the superior and medial orbital walls. The periosteal dissection is then carried laterally until the floor of the frontal sinus has been completely exposed. By extending this elevation inferiorly, the lacrimal crest and fossa are identified. The lacrimal sac is displaced laterally, thus exposing the cribriform lacrimal bone and more posteriorly the lamina papyracea. The anterior ethmoidal vessels are encountered during the elevation of the periosteum from the lamina papyracea. The bleeding from these vessels is rarely troublesome and can be controlled by a short period of packing. The posterior ethmoidal vessels found posteriorly along the medial orbital wall are

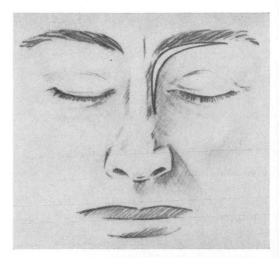

FIG. 13–3.   The incision for the frontoethmoidectomy (Lynch operation).

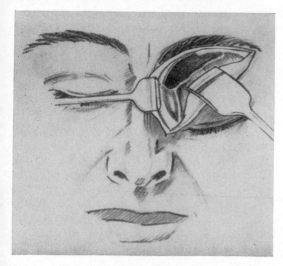

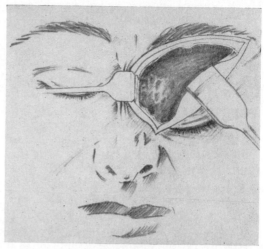

FIG. 13–4. The periosteum has been elevated over the lacrimal bone, lamina papyracea, and orbital plate of the frontal sinus. The floor of the frontal sinus has been partially removed, and the ethmoidal labyrinth has been entered.

FIG. 13–5. A completed frontoethmoidectomy operation. The entire floor of the frontal sinus has been removed. A complete ethmoidectomy has been accomplished.

similarly treated. Some surgeons prefer to ligate these vessels.

The approach to the frontal sinus is by way of the ethmoid (Fig. 13–4). Entrance into the ethmoid sinus is accomplished by removing the thin bone in the posterior aspect of the lacrimal fossa with a sharp curette. It is important not to disturb the underlying nasal mucous membrane. This opening is enlarged with various sized Kerrison forceps and rongeurs. The Smith retractor may be used for exposure. If this is not available, simple orbital retractors are quite adequate. Anterior ethmoidal cells are encountered as this bony opening is enlarged. The anterior ethmoidal cells are removed using Greene or Takahashi forceps. If a mucous membrane flap is to be established, it is well to carry out vertical and horizontal mucous membrane incisions by way of the intranasal approach. A mucosal flap 1 to 2 cm wide and 3 cm long is fashioned by these incisions in the upper lateral nasal wall. This flap is later turned upward for epithelialization of the reconstructed nasofrontal communication.

Using Kerrison forceps, bone is removed from the upper medial orbital wall to the beginning of the osseous frontal sinus floor. At this point the frontal sinus cavity is encountered. The entire floor of the frontal sinus is removed (Fig. 13–5). The entire mucous membrane lining of the frontal sinus is removed by means of periosteal elevators, curettes, and forceps. This is often quite difficult, if there are lateral or superior projections of the frontal sinuses, and is one of the shortcomings of this approach. If the mucous membrane lining is not entirely removed, the procedure may be complicated at a later date by mucocele formation.

The remaining anterior ethmoidal cells and posterior ethmoidal cells are removed, as well as the lamina papyracea and as much of the middle turbinate as is necessary to establish an adequate opening into the nasal cavity. The relative position of the cribriform plate must be kept in mind at all times. A cerebrospinal fluid rhinorrhea is not the complication of a careful surgeon. Lynch marked the position of the cribriform plate by means of a probe inserted through the nostril with the tip of the probe in contact with the roof of the olfactory slit. The anterior wall of the sphenoid is encountered at the posterior limit of the ethmoidal labyrinth. This is entered with a sharp curette, which in turn is enlarged with Kerrison or

Hajek forceps. Polyps and diseased membrane are removed.

The mucous membrane flap which has been fashioned from the upper lateral nasal wall is then turned upward to line the medial wall of the newly formed nasofrontal opening. This is kept in place by petrolatum gauze, a cigarette drain, or a rubber or plastic tube. Boyden advocates removal of the support for this mucosal flap on the fourth postoperative day and states that no further intranasal aftercare is necessary.

Other techniques for maintaining the patency of the reconstructed nasofrontal passage include split-thickness skin graft or Cargile membrane-covered tubes, uncovered plastic or rubber tubing, and tantalum foil. It is necessary that these latter devices remain in place from 1 to 3 months postoperatively.

The success of the external frontoethmoidosphenoidal operation is dependent upon removal of the entire bony floor of the frontal sinus, removal of the entire mucous membrane lining, a complete ethmoidectomy, and the establishment of an adequate opening into the intranasal cavity. Even after these have been accomplished, there is a significant incidence of subsequent stenosis of the nasofrontal passage, recurrent sinusitis, and mucocele formation.

The Osteoplastic Frontal Sinus Operation

The anterior osteoplastic frontal sinus procedure described in the late nineteenth century literature has been revived during the past decade. This operation employs an inferiorly hinged bony "trapdoor" fashioned from the anterior wall of the frontal sinus. Its approach affords direct access to the entire contents of the frontal sinus and an excellent view of the nasofrontal orifice from above. The intranasal disease can be readily removed with ease. Revisions of previously performed sinus surgery can be performed. Adequate drainage from the frontal sinus to the intranasal space can be established, or the frontal sinus can be completely obliterated by the implantation of adipose tissue (Montgomery, 1964).

Preoperative Preparation. Preoperative bacteriologic cultures from the nose should be taken and pathogenic organisms tested for antibiotic sensitivities. This is performed well in advance of surgery so that appropriate antibiotic therapy may be instituted prior to surgery. Pathogenic organisms are often not found by preoperative intranasal cultures, and thus it is important that additional material be taken for culture from the frontal sinus at the time of surgery.

An x-ray cutout (template) is made preoperatively from the Caldwell view of the sinus x-ray pictures. This is done by placing an exposed transparent x-ray film over the Caldwell view and outlining the sinuses with the glass-marking pencil. The cutout may be made slightly smaller than the actual dimensions of the sinus to ensure that the bone cut will lie within the sinus limits. This, however, is not essential, for the beveled bone cut fairly well eliminates this possibility. The cutout is placed in sterilizing solution prior to surgery.

The abdomen should be prepared so that an adipose autograft may be obtained from the subcutaneous layer of the left abdominal wall (a right rectus incision is avoided so that it will not at a later date be interpreted as an appendectomy scar).

Operative Procedure. The forehead and face are prepared and draped in the usual manner as for any frontal sinus procedure.

The patient lies on the table in the supine position with the head slightly raised and inclined forward so that the plane of the forehead is horizontal. The eyelids are sutured together with 5–0 Dermalene to prevent injury to the eyes during the operation.

The eyebrows are not shaved.

Procaine or lidocaine (Xylocaine), 2%, with added epinephrine are infiltrated along the upper margin of the eyebrow, both to reduce the amount of bleeding and to supplement the general anesthesia.

If the procedure is unilateral, the incision is made along the entire length of the upper margin of the eyebrow (Fig. 13–6, A). The incision is carried through the subcutaneous tissues and the frontalis muscle to the periosteum covering the frontal bone. It is essential not to enter this periosteum so that the blood supply to the osteoplastic flap is preserved.

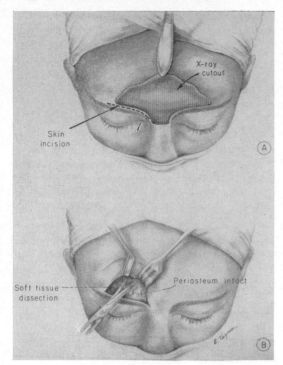

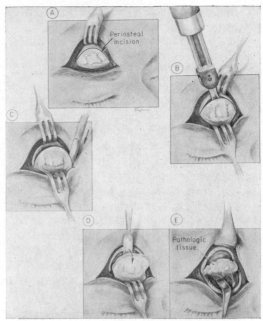

FIG. 13–6. *A*, X-ray pattern used to determine the extent of the frontal sinus. *B*, Soft tissues are elevated superficial to the frontal periosteum.

FIG. 13–7. *A*, The periosteum is incised along the upper margin of the X-ray film template. *B*, The Stryker saw is used to cut a bone flap along the periosteal incision. *C*, The ends of the bone cut are severed by means of a mallet and chisel. *D*, The bone flap is elevated with a chisel. The fracture occurs just below the supraorbital rim. *E*, The bone flap is turned down for inspection of the frontal sinus interior.

A plane of cleavage is easily established between the frontalis muscle and the frontal periosteum by scissors and blunt dissection (Fig. 13–6, *B*). It is important to make this exposure wide enough so that the x-ray cutout may be applied to the periosteum in order to outline the periosteal incision.

The periosteal incision is made around the x-ray cutout (template) to the supraorbital rim medially and laterally (Fig. 13–7, *A*). This should be extended to include the periosteum over the medial and lateral limits of the frontal sinus at the supraorbital rim. The periosteum along the supraorbital rim is not disturbed in order to ensure adequate blood supply for the osteoplastic flap. The periosteum above the incision is then elevated a few millimeters in order to obtain adequate space for a clean bone cut.

The bone incision is made along the outline of the periosteal incision using a Stryker saw blade which has been specially designed

for this purpose. The saw is slightly angulated so that it is directed toward the cavity of the frontal sinus (Fig. 13–7, *B*). Beveling of this bone incision accomplishes two purposes: (1) to ensure that the incision is within the limits of the frontal sinus; (2) to allow for more accurate replacement of the osteoplastic flap. Following the outline of the periosteal incision, the bone incision is extended to include the supraorbital rim medially and laterally. This step is essential to ensure a fracture which hinges the osteoplastic flap along the floor of the frontal sinus just posterior to the supraorbital rim.

A mallet and chisel are used to inspect the completeness of the bone incision (Fig. 13–7, *C*). This is accomplished by inserting the chisel, tapping lightly, and prying around this entire bone incision. The chisel is then placed superiorly, and with a prying maneuver the osteoplastic flap is elevated downward and forward (Fig. 13–7, *D*).

The interior of the frontal sinus can now be inspected. A culture is taken. It is at this point that the surgeon makes his final decision as to the extent of his operation. If a benign tumor, such as an osteoma, is present, this is removed and no further surgery is necessary, provided the mucous membrane lining is not diseased and the nasofrontal orifice is adequate. If the mucous membrane lining of the frontal sinus is so extensively diseased that there is no possibility of its recovery, it is removed and the surgeon should proceed with an obliterative procedure (Fig. 13–7, *E*). The entire inner cortical bony lining of the sinus, including that on either aspect of the osteoplastic flap, is then removed with a rotating cutting burr (Fig. 13–8, *A*). This must be systematically and carefully accomplished. The surgical microscope may be used if necessary. The removal of the inner cortical lining is essen-

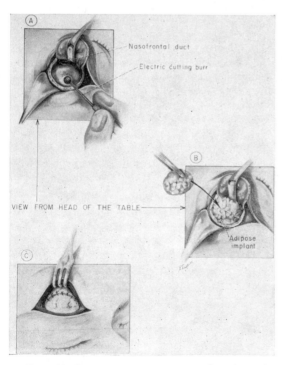

Fig. 13–8.   *A,* An electric cutting burr is used to remove any remaining mucosal lining and the inner cortical lining of the sinuses. *B,* The sinus cavity is filled with the adipose implant. *C,* The bone flap is replaced and the periosteum sutured.

tial both to ensure complete removal of the mucosal sinus and to establish a blood supply to nourish the adipose autograft. The removal of mucous membrane and inner cortical lining is carried to, but not into, the nasofrontal orifice. This is not necessary, for a barrier between the nasofrontal orifice and the sinus cavity is established within a few days. This has been demonstrated by animal experimentation (Montgomery, 1964).

The subcutaneous adipose tissue is obtained from the left abdominal wall by way of a left rectus incision. Subcutaneous catgut sutures are used to eliminate the dead space resulting from this removal. Blood vessels should be carefully ligated to prevent hematoma. A drain is inserted for 48 hours. The adipose tissue autograft is then fashioned so as to completely fill the frontal sinus (Fig. 13–8, *B*). The osteoplastic flap is then returned to its original position. The periosteum is sutured with 4–0 chromic catgut suture (Fig. 13–8, *C*). The wound is then closed with 4–0 chromic catgut suture subcutaneously and 5–0 Dermalene skin sutures.

The forehead dressing consists of Telfa gauze over the incision, an eye pad, fluffed sponges 4 × 4 inches, and three strips of Elastoplast adhesive. An elastic bandage is placed over this dressing.

The elastic bandage is removed at the end of 24 hours. The remainder of the dressing is removed at the end of 48 hours. No further postoperative care is necessary other than institution of antibiotics if necessary and removal of the skin sutures on the fifth or sixth postoperative day.

The Bilateral Procedure. The skin incision for the bilateral osteoplastic frontal sinus operation is shown in Figure 13–9, *A*. The resulting superior flap is easily elevated in a plane between the frontalis muscle and the periosteum. The periosteal and bone incisions should include the supraorbital rims laterally (Fig. 13–9, *B*). A bone incision horizontally across a nasal process of the frontal bone at the supraorbital rims medially is necessary. If there is difficulty in elevating the osteoplastic flap, it indicates that the interfrontal septum is at least partially intact. This can easily be incised by inserting a chisel in the midline superiorly. The remainder of the procedure is carried out

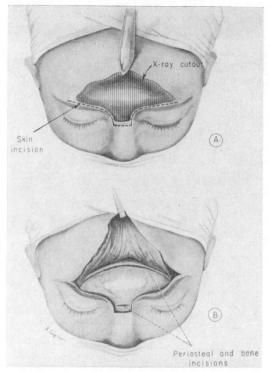

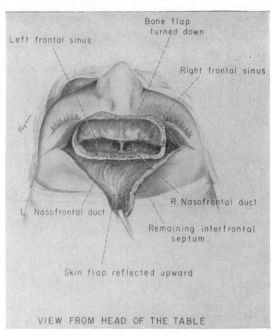

FIG. 13–10. A view of the sinus cavity with the bone flap turned down.

FIG. 13–9. *A,* The incision for the bilateral osteoplastic frontal sinus operation. *B,* The periosteal and bone flap incisions are made so that one large flap will be elevated and reflected inferiorly.

as outlined for the unilateral operation (Fig. 13–10).

THE MAXILLARY SINUS

Intranasal Surgery of the Maxillary Sinuses

An adequate trial of conservative therapy is the treatment of choice for subacute and chronic maxillary sinusitis. Appropriate antibiotics are administered as determined by culture and sensitivity tests. The antibiotics should be continued for at least 10 days. Drainage is established by both local and systemic decongestants. If this therapy is properly instituted, puncture and irrigation of the antrum are rarely indicated. On occasion, however, irrigation of the antrum is indicated to obtain material for a culture or as an attempt to prevent intranasal or external surgery of the maxillary sinus.

If there is a chronic edematous process in the region of the middle meatus and sinus x-ray films demonstrate both thickened membrane and retained exudate, local measures, such as removal of polypoid tissue and middle turbinate tissue or antrum irrigation, are of little value. Biochemotherapy and decongestants have, for the most part, eliminated the necessity for the above local measures. If this conservative medical therapy is not successful, then the surgeon should resort to more definitive procedures, attempting to establish adequate drainage and, if necessary, removing diseased tissue from the sinus.

Nasoantral Irrigation. (See Chapter 12). On occasion a nasoantral irrigation is of value in treating maxillary sinusitis when one is trying to determine whether or not the sinus drainage is adequate and when trying to obtain purulent secretions for culture and antibiotic sensitivity tests. Most otolaryngologists prefer to irrigate the maxillary sinus by way of the inferior meatus. A straight, thin, Lichtwitz needle with a Wolf thumb rest is the instrument of choice. The inferior meatus is anesthetized by packing with cotton strips impregnated with 4% cocaine or 2% tetracaine. Ephedrine solution,

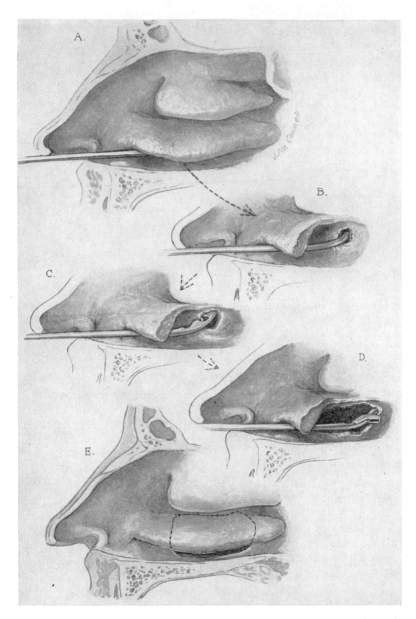

FIG. 13–11.   Removing the nasoantral wall (antrum window) beneath the inferior turbinate. *A*, Puncturing the nasoantral wall with a sharp-pointed rasp or trocar. The hole should be made large enough to admit the bone-cutting forceps. *B*, Enlarging the puncture by means of a curved rasp so as to admit the cutting forceps. *C*, The forward cutting forceps are inserted and the nasoantral wall removed as far forward as possible. *D*, The backward cutting forceps removing the posterior portion of the nasoantral wall. *E*, The nasoantral wall removed beneath the inferior turbinate at the completion of the "antrum window" operation.

1%, may be added to the tetracaine. These cotton strips should remain in place for about 15 minutes. The needle is inserted through the wall of the inferior meatus approximately 1 cm behind the anterior tip. It is well to direct the needle in a slightly upward direction, and it is important not to traverse the cavity completely and enter either the superior or lateral sinus wall. It is essential to aspirate before irrigating. Either pus or air should be obtained if the tip of the needle is in the sinus cavity. If neither air nor pus is obtained, it means that the tip of the needle is not in the antrum or it is filled with solid material, such as a neoplasm or as in polypoid mucositis. The sinus is then irrigated with warm normal saline solution. It is not necessary to inject air following this irrigation. There have been reports of air embolism following the injection of air into the maxillary sinus (see Chapter 12).

Intranasal Fenestration of the Nasoantral Wall

A well-constructed nasoantral window is sufficient to cure a chronic purulent maxillary sinusitis, provided the antrum is not filled with polypoid tissue and there is no bone necrosis or dental complication. It has been repeatedly demonstrated over the years that a small nasoantral window closes quickly and is ineffective. A large window is essential.

Technique of Operation. The intranasal antrostomy should be performed in the hospital where the surgeon can proceed with a radical antral procedure if this is indicated at the time of antrostomy. Many surgeons perform a radical antrum operation in preference to an intranasal antrostomy because the latter procedure effects a cure in less than 90% of cases, thus necessitating an additional hospitalization and operation for those cases which fail.

The inferior meatus is anesthetized with 4% cocaine or 2% tetracaine with 1% impregnated cotton strips. It is wise to leave this packing in place for 10 to 15 minutes, even when administering general anesthesia, for the shrinkage of mucous membrane allows for better visualization of the inferior

meatus and better hemostasis. The topical anesthesia also supplements the general anesthesia.

The inferior turbinate is elevated superiorly with a smooth-edged flat instrument, such as a large periosteal elevator or tonsil dissector. No portion of the inferior turbinates should be removed. The nasoantral wall and the inferior turbinate are broken through with any punch or even a sharp, curved hemostat. The opening is then enlarged in all directions with punches and biting forceps. The diameter should be at least 1.5 to 2 cm. It is obviously important to remove the inferior meatus wall down to the level of the floor of the nasal cavity to permit easier evacuation of the sinus cavity. The sinus cavity may then be inspected by direct vision. If there appears to be disease which is irreversible, then a Caldwell-Luc incision is made and a radical antrum operation carried out.

Usually packing is not necessary following this operation. If bleeding is troublesome, the window may be packed with petrolatum-impregnated, 1-inch iodoform gauze. This is removed at the end of 24 or 48 hours. The patient should be followed closely until there is resolution of his chronic infection (Figs. 13–11 and 13–12).

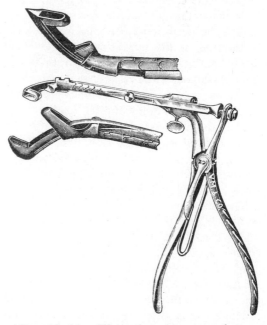

FIG. 13–12.   Wagner's antrum punches.

External Surgery of the Maxillary Sinus

The following are indications for the external approach: (1) failure of the intranasal antrostomy to resolve a chronic infection; (2) polypoid tissue filling the antrum; (3) cystic disease of the antrum; (4) osteonecrosis; (5) a question of maxillary sinus neoplasm; (6) the presence of an oroantral fistula; and (7) complicated fractures of the maxilla.

Technique of the Radical Antrum Operation (Caldwell-Luc). The Caldwell-Luc operation may be performed under either general or local anesthesia. If the operation is to be performed under local anesthesia, the intranasal anesthesia is accomplished by placing cotton pledgets impregnated with 4% cocaine or 2% tetracaine with 1% ephedrine both above and below the inferior turbinate. Procaine or lidocaine, 2%, with added epinephrine is injected in the region of the canine fossa. The injection is continued superiorly to include the infraorbital nerve. Local anesthesia is useful when general anesthesia is employed both to supplement the general anesthesia and to assist with hemostasis. A horizontal incision is made in the gingivobuccal sulcus well above the roots of the teeth. The incision is made between the canine and second molar teeth. It is made through the mucosa and periosteum. The periosteum over the canine fossa is elevated to the infraorbital canal, where the infraorbital nerve is identified and carefully preserved. The best way to avoid injury to this nerve is to make certain of its identification. Gentle retraction throughout the procedure will also reduce the trauma to this nerve as well as to other soft tissues of the cheek. With the use of an osteotome or a rotating cutting burr, the anterior wall of the sinus is fenestrated. This opening is enlarged using Kerrison bone-cutting forceps. It is well to enlarge this opening to a size that will admit the fifth digit. The contents of the antrum can then be visualized. At this point cysts and benign tumors can be removed using various elevators, avoiding injury to the normal mucosa. Removal of the entire mucosal lining of the antrum is rarely necessary. However, when it seems irreversibly diseased, it can be easily removed using elevators, curettes, and tissue forceps.

The nasoantral wall in the inferior meatus is then broken through with a punch trocar or a curved hemostat. This intranasal antrostomy is then enlarged through the external sinus opening with the use of Kerrison forceps and forward bone-cutting forceps. The nasoantral window should be at least 1.5 cm in diameter and should include intranasal mucosa, sinus mucosa, and the bony wall. It is widely agreed that the various mucosal flaps devised for the formation of this nasoantral window are unnecessary.

After the antrum is carefully inspected for retained sponges, the gingivobuccal incision is closely approximated with 00 plain catgut suture. Usually intrasinus and intranasal packing is not necessary. On occasion, with troublesome bleeding, the petrolatum iodoform gauze pack may be inserted into the antrum by way of the nasoantral window. This can be removed at the end of 1 or 2 days. An icepack over the cheek during the first 24 hours postoperatively is essential to prevent edema, hematoma, and discomfort.

OROMAXILLARY FISTULA

Etiology. The number of upper molars in intimate contact with the floor of the maxillary sinus is dependent upon the size of the sinus. The sinus cavity is separated from the apices of these teeth by a thin layer of bone. This is particularly thin, and sometimes absent, in the region of the first molar tooth. On occasion the root may extend into the sinus. An oromaxillary fistula usually occurs following the extraction of a tooth complicated by an apical abscess or cyst.

On occasion an oroantral fistula may occur following the extraction of a nondiseased tooth. These usually heal rapidly following local repair, antibiotic therapy, and instructing the patient not to blow his nose. If a tooth root is broken off during extraction and found to lie within the antrum but submucosally, it is best left alone if there is no infection. If infection is present, antibiotic therapy plus local irrigation may result in resolution of the infection and healing. Otherwise, a more radical procedure is necessary both to remove the foreign body and to close the fistula.

Signs and Symptoms. The symptoms of an oromaxillary fistula, if of recent origin, are blood in the nasal cavity and an escape of air from the fistula's tooth socket; it is usually frothy. Liquids taken into the mouth may escape through the nostril. If infection is present, it usually manifests itself within 1 or 2 days following the extraction of the tooth. Pain over the maxillary sinus and a profuse odoriferous nasal discharge are characteristic. The patient will complain of a foul taste. Purulent discharge can be seen exuding from the extraction site. This discharge may increase when the patient holds his nose and increases the intranasal pressure. Verification of the fistulous tract can be accomplished with a metallic probe.

Treatment. Conservative therapy is worth a try if the oroantral fistula and maxillary sinusitis are detected shortly after their onset. Cultures are taken and sensitivity tests carried out. Antibiotics are administered both systemically and by local irrigation. Nasal decongestants may be necessary to promote drainage. If the patient does not respond to this therapy within 2 weeks, it is useless to continue, and surgery should be performed.

Surgical Therapy. A radical antrum operation is the procedure of choice. A U-shaped incision is made in the canine fossa so as to include the alveolus in the region of the fistula. This flap is elevated, and the surgeon performs a complete radical antrum procedure with a large opening into the inferior meatus. If the fistulous tract is small, it is removed and the buccal flap is sutured in place. Antibiotics are administered postoperatively, and the patient is instructed to discontinue nose blowing. If the fistula is large and there is surrounding osteomyelitis, it is necessary to remove the teeth adjacent to the fistula and also to remove the alveolus in this region up to the level of the palate. The buccal flap described above is sutured in place so that it may be kept in contact with the denuded surface.

Numerous surgical procedures have been devised for the treatment of persistent or large oroantral fistulas. Probably the simplest and most successful involves use of a posteriorly based palatal flap. A more extensive resection of the alveolus is, of course, necessary. A connective tissue flap derived from the area above the buccal flap may be reflected inferiorly into a large oroantral fistula and is sometimes necessary in conjunction with the palatal and buccal flaps to close a large oroantral fistula (Heermann).

INTRANASAL SURGERY OF THE ETHMOIDAL AND SPHENOIDAL SINUSES

Intranasal Ethmoidectomy

Indications. Intranasal surgery of the ethmoid is quite effective when indicated and has been neglected by many otolaryngologists. Chronic ethmoiditis, with or without nasal polypi, is a positive indication for this approach. The eradication of chronic ethmoidal infection is often sufficient to bring about a cure of chronic frontal and sphenoidal infection. Even though the external ethmoidectomy is a safer and a more thorough method of approaching the entire ethmoidal labyrinth, a skillfully performed intranasal ethmoidectomy is perfectly adequate to bring about resolution of the above diseases.

Surgical Anatomy. The ethmoidal labyrinth is pyramidal in shape, being wider posteriorly than anteriorly and wider above than below (Mosher). The anterior width of the ethmoid is 0.5 to 1 cm. The posterior width is approximately 1.5 cm. The anteroposterior diameter or length of the labyrinth is 3 to 4 cm. The height is 2 to 2.5 cm. The medial wall of the ethmoid is made up by the upper half of the lateral nasal wall (Fig. 13–13, A). The lower half is the medial wall of the antrum. Whereas the cribriform plate is the roof of the olfactory slit in the anterior superior nasal cavity, a prolongation of the orbital plate of the frontal bone is the roof of the ethmoidal labyrinth. The attachment of the middle turbinate divides the anterior from the posterior ethmoidal cells and is the most important surgical landmark when an intranasal ethmoidectomy is being performed. The lacrimal bone forms the lateral wall of the anterior ethmoidal cells, and the os planum forms the lateral wall of

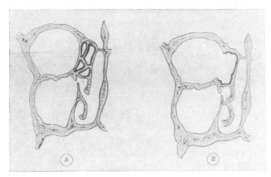

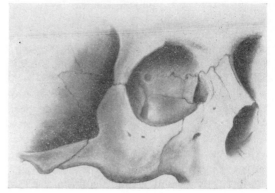

FIG. 13–13. Coronal sections through the orbit, antrum, ethmoid, and nasal cavity. *A,* Relative relationships of the lamina papyracea, roof of the ethmoid, cribriform plate, and medial wall of the ethmoidal labyrinth, which is an upper extension of the attachment of the middle turbinate. *B,* An ethmoidectomy has been completed with the exception of the removal of the middle turbinate and its upper extension, which forms the medial wall of the ethmoid.

FIG. 13–14. A sketch showing the anatomy of the medial wall of the orbit. Note the relationship of the anterior and posterior ethmoidal foramina with the suture line between the orbital plate of the frontal bone and the lamina papyracea. This is in the same plane as the roof of the ethmoid and cribriform plate. The posterior ethmoidal cells are in close proximity to the optic foramen. The lacrimal bone forms the lateral wall of the anterior ethmoidal cells, and the lamina papyracea forms the lateral wall of the posterior ethmoidal cells.

the posterior ethmoidal cells (Fig. 13–14). As a general rule, the outer half of the front face of the sphenoidal sinus is the posterior limit of the ethmoidal labyrinth. The most important relationships of the anterior ethmoidal cells are the lacrimal bone, the floor of the frontal sinus, and the hiatus semilunaris. The most important relationships to the posterior ethmoidal cells are the posterior half of the medial wall of the orbit, the optic nerve, and the lateral half of the front wall of the sphenoidal sinus. The plane of the cribriform plate approximately corresponds to a horizontal line at the level of the pupils. The number of ethmoidal cells varies between four and eight.

Preparation for Surgery. The procedure is facilitated by the use of general anesthesia. An endotracheal tube with a pharyngeal pack is necessary. The entire face is prepared with an antiseptic solution. Cotton saturated with antiseptic solution is introduced into the nasal cavities. The patient is draped so that the nose, eyes, and lower forehead remain exposed. The head is placed on a sponge rubber doughnut so that it may be accurately positioned. The upper face remains exposed so that external landmarks may be used. It is necessary to extend the

patient's head when approaching the anterior ethmoidal cells.

Technique of Operation. A submucous resection of the nasal septum facilitates the intranasal ethmoidectomy and is performed as a routine part of the procedure by many surgeons. This, of course, is not a necessity, provided the septum is straight.

The cotton saturated with antiseptic solution is removed and replaced by cotton impregnated with 1:1000 epinephrine. This remains in place while the patient's head is placed in extension so that the anterior ethmoidal region may be visualized. After about 5 minutes the epinephrine packing is removed. With the patient's head in extension, the area of the bulla can be visualized. A sharp curette is used to enter the anterior ethmoidal cells in this area (i.e., agger nasi and peri-infundibular). Angulated sharp-loop curettes are used to remove the anterior ethmoidal cells. If at this instant the bleeding cannot easily be controlled by suction, the anterior ethmoidal labyrinth is packed with epinephrine-impregnated gauze strips. Since the intranasal ethmoidectomy is most commonly a bilateral procedure, the surgeon may proceed to the anterior ethmoidal cells on the contralateral side. Having accomplished this, he returns to the original side, removes the epinephrine packing, and repositions the head from the extension to the neutral position.

The next step is to remove the anterior one half or two thirds of the middle turbinate. The attachment of the turbinate is cut with turbinate scissors (or, if not available, straight scissors). The body of the turbinate is then cut across with a wire snare or curved scissors. Bleeding at this point is commonly not profuse, but if it is at all troublesome, the packing is reinserted and the surgery continued on the opposite side.

The posterior ethmoidal cells lie behind the attachment of the middle turbinate. This landmark may have been obscured by disease, but its relative position can be fairly well judged, the anterior portion of the turbinate having just been removed. A curette is inserted into the posterior ethmoidal cells. With a knowledge of the approximate dimensions of the area, the surgeon can outline the limits of the posterior ethmoid by gentle curettage. Debris (bone, polyps, etc.) is best removed with cup forceps, such as the Greene or Takahashi forceps. Bleeding may be profuse at any time. It is well to remember that this can be controlled by packing and a little patience.

The posterior limit of the ethmoidal labyrinth is the anterior wall of the sphenoidal sinus. If indicated, the sphenoidal sinus can be entered and a portion of the anterior wall removed for drainage.

Hemorrhage is an occasional complication attending the intranasal ethmoidal sinus operation. A postoperative pack should not be used unless bleeding does ensue; if it is necessary, it should remain in place for only 24 hours. Packing should consist of petrolatum iodoform gauze or gauze impregnated with antibiotic ointment. Systemic antibiotic therapy is usually instituted following an ethmoidectomy operation, and this should be, if possible, specific according to laboratory sensitivity tests. Even though very little local therapy is necessary after the operation, the patient should be carefully scrutinized for 2 weeks. The intranasal spaces are not disturbed during the first week except for a gentle cleansing with suction or forceps. An occasional oily nasal spray may be used to soften the crusts which form. A week or 10 days following the surgery, synechiae may be noted. Excision of these is most important, and if they have a tendency to re-form, a small piece of double-faced Telfa gauze left in place a few days will solve the problem. It also may be necessary to remove small bits of polypoid tissue and spicules of bone during the immediate postoperative period. The patient will complain of dryness and repeated crust formation for a number of weeks following this surgery. If the patient is warned of its possibility, he will more readily accept it as a normal process of healing.

Intranasal Surgery of the Sphenoidal Sinus

Irrigation of the Sphenoidal Sinus. Irrigation of the sphenoidal sinus is indicated for diagnosis and treatment of acute and subacute sphenoidal sinusitis. Cocaine solution, 4%, is used for anesthesia. A sphenoidal cannula 10 cm in length is introduced along the nasal septum toward the end of the middle turbinate. This will make approximately a 30-degree angle with the floor of the nose. On occasion the sphenoidal osteum may be directly visualized. If not, it can be found by gentle manipulation. Aspiration may demonstrate pus. The sphenoidal cavity is then slowly irrigated with warm normal saline solution.

If cannulation of the natural sphenoidal osteum is not feasible, a Hajek sphenoidal hook with a Trumbel guard is introduced into the sphenoidal sinus just lateral to the nasal septum, at the level of the posterior tip of the middle turbinate. This opening is enlarged with a Fletcher or Hajek forceps. The opening should be made as inferior on the anterior wall of the sphenoidal sinus as possible.

The purpose of the sphenoidal sinusotomy is to obtain pus for culture and sensitivity tests and to effect drainage. Followup care, in addition to antibiotic therapy, should include the use of nasal decongestants (see Chapter 10).

External Ethmoidectomy

Indications. External ethmoidectomy is indicated for those cases of ethmoiditis which do not respond to antibiotic therapy and present as a redness, swelling, and fluctuation over the ethmoidal sinuses. Extension of the purulent infection into the orbital cavity with the resultant orbital abscess is indication for this surgery. Mucocele, pyocele, and tumors of the ethmoid must also be approached by way of the external route. The external ethmoidectomy is the route to external frontal sinus surgery, as well as an approach to the sphenoidal sinus and to the pituitary gland.

Technique of Surgery. The patient is prepared and draped as has been outlined for the intranasal ethmoidectomy. The eyelids are sutured together with a single 5–0 silk or plastic suture to protect the cornea from injury. After infiltration with 2% procaine and epinephrine, a 1-inch curved incision is made halfway between the inner canthus and the anterior aspect of the nasal bone (Fig. 13–15). This incision is extended through skin, subcutaneous tissue, and periosteum. Troublesome bleeding is usually encountered from the angular vessels. Before proceeding further with the operation, it is best to control this bleeding by ligation or cauterization. There are a number of retrac-

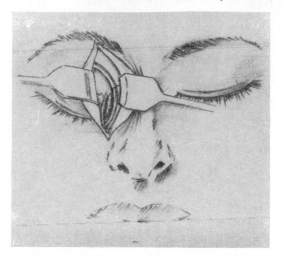

FIG. 13–16. As the periosteum is reflected laterally, the lacrimal fossa, anterior and posterior lacrimal crests, and lamina papyracea are exposed.

tors which have been devised to separate this incision. Two sutures on each skin margin weighted with heavy hemostats usually offer sufficient exposure. By elevating the periosteum laterally, the lacrimal crest and fossa are identified. The lacrimal sac is displaced laterally, exposing the cribriform lacrimal bone and posteriorly the lamina papyracea (Fig. 13–16). The anterior ethmoidal vessels are encountered during the elevation of the periosteum from the lamina papyracea. The bleeding from these vessels is rarely troublesome and can be controlled by a short period of packing. The posterior ethmoidal vessels are found posteriorly along the medial orbital wall. These are similarly treated. The ethmoidal labyrinth is entered by removing the thin bone in the posterior aspect of the lacrimal fossa with a sharp curette. This opening is enlarged with various-sized Kerrison forceps. The anterior ethmoidal cells are readily encountered and removed with Greene or Takahashi forceps (Fig. 13–17). At least the anterior half of the middle turbinate is then removed, using turbinate scissors and a wire snare. At this point it is important to identify the upper limits of the olfactory slit and the roof of the ethmoidal labyrinth. Using these landmarks, the lamina papyracea, and the attach-

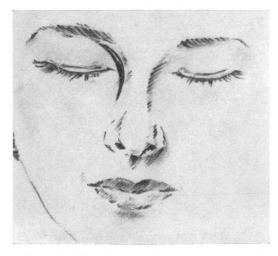

FIG. 13–15. The incision for external ethmoidectomy. This is a 1-inch curved incision made halfway between the inner canthus and the inner aspect of the nasal dorsum.

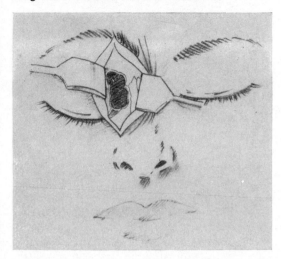

FIG. 13–17. The anterior ethmoidal cells have been removed along with the lacrimal bone.

ment of the middle turbinate, the posterior ethmoidal cells are readily removed with curettes and forceps (Fig. 13–18).

The posterior limit of the ethmoidal labyrinth is the anterior wall of the sphenoidal sinus. This is opened with a sharp curette. The opening is then enlarged with side-biting forceps. If the sphenoidal sinus is found to be diseased, the anterior wall is sufficiently removed to provide adequate drainage. Polyps and diseased membrane are removed from the sphenoidal sinus.

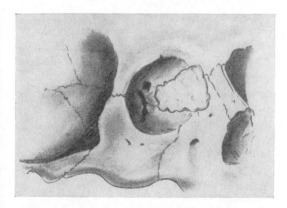

FIG. 13–18. A sketch showing the extent of removal of the medial wall of the orbit during an external ethmoidectomy. Note the close relationship between the posterior ethmoidal cell and the optic foramen.

TRANSETHMOIDOSPHENOIDAL HYPOPHYSECTOMY

During recent years the various rhinologic approaches to the pituitary gland by way of the sphenoidal sinus have offered increasing competition to the anterior craniotomy route. The transsphenoidal technique is popular because it is a more direct route, allowing for a lower morbidity and mortality rate. There is less chance for injury to the optic chiasm. Postoperative complications, such as seizures, extradural hematoma, brain damage, and cerebral edema, are rare. The convalescent period following the transsphenoidal route for hypophysectomy is usually quite short.

There are a number of routes and modifications for the transsphenoidal hypophysectomy.

Transseptosphenoidal Hypophysectomy. This operation was pioneered by Oscar Hirsch in 1910. Cushing later (1912) used a sublabial modification of this route. Heck was the first in this country to use the transseptal approach for the treatment of advanced carcinoma of the breast. The main objection to this route is that it is a long, narrow approach. Two instruments cannot be used simultaneously, and the surgical microscope cannot be employed. It is, however, still used by many surgeons because of its being a direct midline dissection.

Transantroethmoidosphenoidal Hypophysectomy. Hamberger has used this approach in a large series of patients with remarkable success (Hamberger and coworkers). For most surgeons, this is a long, oblique route to the hypophyseal fossa. It also has the disadvantage of increasing the hazard of postoperative infection, for the oral route in some cases is potentially a septic area.

Transnasal Osteoplastic Hypophysectomy. Macbeth has devised a unique direct midline approach using an osteoplastic skin flap based at the root of the nose (Macbeth and Hall). The only disadvantage here is that it leaves undesirable scarring of the nasal bridge. Those who perform this operation indicate that this is not a factor when advanced carcinoma of the breast is being treated.

Transethmoidosphenoidal Hypophysectomy. This technique for hypophysectomy has been used since the turn of the century. Chiari in 1912 described this method for the removal of a pituitary adenoma. A few of the otolaryngologists who deserve credit for improving the techniques for this approach are Nager, Bateman, and James. They have used this operation because it is the shortest route to the hypophysis with a wide field. It permits easy manipulation of instruments. More than one instrument can be used simultaneously. One instrument may be inserted by way of the nasal cavity and another by way of the operative field. The advent of the surgical microscope has also increased the popularity of the transethmoidosphenoidal hypophysectomy.

Radioactive Implants and Cryosurgery. The implantation of radioactive substance by any of the above routes is to be discouraged because of the frequent and numerous complications. Cryosurgery, on the other hand, may become useful, but it has not as yet been thoroughly evaluated.

The *transethmoidosphenoidal* approach for hypophysectomy has been used for solid and cystic pituitary tumors, advanced breast carcinoma (palliative therapy), diabetic retinopathy, and advanced prostatic carcinoma. Cystic tumors can easily be marsupialized. Solid tumors can be resected and/or decompressed. Most authors (Riskaer and coworkers; Bateman) report 60 to 80% transient remissions when generalized metastases from carcinoma of the breast are treated with hypophysectomy. Patients with breast carcinomatosis so weak that they can hardly turn in bed have had dramatic results following hypophysectomy. Similarly good results were obtained after hypophysectomy for diabetic retinopathy.

Preoperative Management. A team consisting of a neurologist, an endocrinologist, and a surgeon is essential for the proper management of the patient during the preoperative and postoperative periods. A rhinologist who attempts a hypophysectomy without the assistance of these two specialists is only inviting disaster. If neurologic and endocrinologic work-ups have not been carried out prior to the patient's admission to the hospital, he should be admitted several days prior to surgery so that this may be accomplished. The neurologist will conduct a careful neurologic survey, which, in the case of pituitary tumors, should include radioactive scanning, pneumoencephalogram, and arteriograms. The endocrinologist will obtain the preoperative endocrine balance and prescribe the necessary hormones during the preoperative, operative, and postoperative periods.

Preoperative X-rays (Sinus Series). *Complete sinus x-rays* are taken to rule out septic or other sinus disease. The lateral view will demonstrate the size and relationship of the sella turcica. This view, however, is misleading as to the exact pneumatization of the sphenoidal sinuses because of the densities cast by the greater wings of the sphenoid bone.

Lateral planograms of the sphenoidal sinus will give a detailed anatomy of the sphenoidal sinuses and their relationship to the sella turcica.

A *submental vertical view* will show the lateral extent of the sphenoidal sinuses and the position of the sphenoidal septum, which is most often not in the midline.

A careful examination of the nasal cavities and the nasopharyngeal space is important to rule out sepsis and other disease and also to orient the surgeon as to the exact anatomy of the nasal septum.

Operative Technique. The objectives of this operation are: (1) to obtain a wide field so that a surgical microscope can be used to illuminate and outline the posterior wall of the sphenoid properly (when this is accomplished, more than one instrument can be used simultaneously); (2) to define the midline with accuracy at all times during the procedure; (3) to control all bleeding and cerebrospinal fluid leakage at the completion of the operation.

An external ethmoidectomy is carried out, as is outlined above. It is most important that the patient's head be secured in a supine position with the aid of sandbags. Any extension or correction of the head during the procedure should be avoided. After the ethmoidectomy has been performed, incision for a septal mucosal flap (Montgomery, 1963) is carried out, as seen in Figures 13–19 and 13–20, *A.* The purpose of this

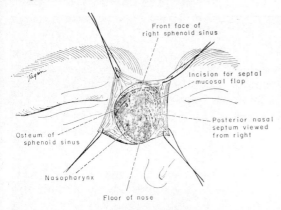

FIG. 13–19. A sketch showing the incision for the septal mucosal flap.

mucosal flap is to reduce the incidence of postoperative hemorrhage, cerebrospinal fluid rhinorrhea, and meningitis. A vertical incision is made through the mucosa of the nasal septum at a point approximately halfway between the nasal orifice and the anterior wall of the sphenoid. Since this incision determines the length of the septal mucosal flap, it may be varied according to the demands of the pneumatization of the sphenoidal sinus. Mucosal incisions are then carried posteriorly from the superior (2) and inferior (3) ends of the vertical incision. The superior incision extends along the nasal septum just inferior to the cribriform plate to the front face of the sphenoidal sinus. It is carried laterally across the superior aspect

(4) of the front face of the sphenoidal sinus and then inferiorly (5). The inferior septal incision is carried posteriorly to the front face of the sphenoidal sinus in the region of the sphenoidal rostrum. The mucosal flap is then carefully elevated and reflected into the nasopharynx until the hypophysectomy has been completed.

The right sphenoidal sinus is entered, and the entire anterior wall is removed. The bony nasal septum is left intact as an accurate guide to the midline. On the other hand, a small portion of the posterior nasal septum may be removed for a wider exposure without destroying its usefulness as a midline guide.

The surgical microscope is employed for the remainder of the operation. The bulge of the sella turcica can be seen on the posterior wall of the sphenoidal sinus. The midline is again checked by using the posterior aspect of the nasal septum as a guide. If the anatomic relationships are doubtful, x-ray films may be taken with a portable machine using metallic probes as pointers (Fig. 13–21). This step becomes decreasingly necessary with the number of cases operated upon. A small opening is made in the posterior wall of the sphenoid (anterior wall of the sella turcica) with a curette or a rotating burr. This is enlarged by using various rongeurs. It is important to remove the entire anterior wall of the sella turcica in order to define accurately the limits of the hypoph-

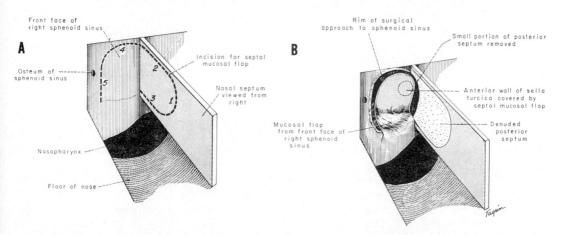

FIG. 13–20. A, Schematic drawing showing the incision for construction of the septal mucosal flap. B, Sketch demonstrating the mucosal flap reflected into the sphenoidal sinus, covering the defect in the posterior wall.

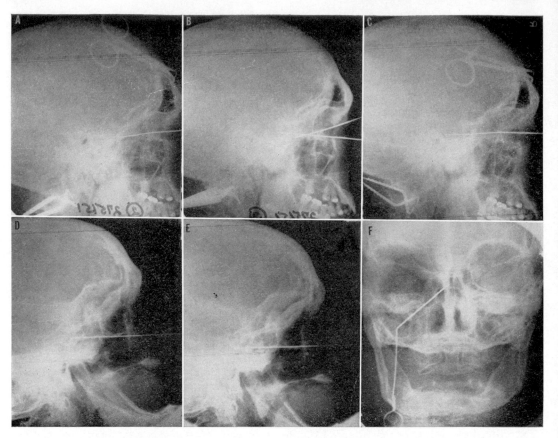

Fig. 13–21.   X-ray films illustrating the use of metallic probes to abet the anatomic relationships. *A,* A probe just inside the sphenoidal sinus. This view demonstrates the inadequate visualization of sphenoid anatomy afforded by the lateral skull or sinus x-ray. Laminograms of the sphenoidal sinus beautifully outline this anatomy. *B,* Anterior wall and floor of the sella turcica. *C,* Probe in the center of a pituitary adenoma. *D,* Anterior wall of the sella turcica. *E,* Floor of the sella turcica. *F,* Probe used to check the midline position.

yseal fossa. Either a vertical or a cruciate incision is made in the dura; the pituitary or tumor thereof is then removed by using suction and various dissectors. Following the completion of the pituitary surgery, the fossa is packed with Gelfoam saturated with thrombin solution if there is any bleeding or spinal fluid leakage. Muscle or adipose tissue may also be used for this same purpose. The septal mucosal flap is elevated from the naso-pharynx and reflected into the sphenoidal sinus. The flap is placed over the defect in the posterior wall of the sphenoidal sinus, covered with a layer of Gelfoam, and then packed in place with petroleum jelly-treated iodoform gauze (Fig. 13–21, *B*). When one is dealing with a cystic pituitary tumor, the septal mucosal flap is reflected into the hypophyseal fossa rather than used to cover the defect. This is done to ensure marsupialization of the cysts. The end of the iodoform gauze is placed in the nasal cavity so that it can be easily removed on the fifth post-operative day. The external ethmoidal incision is closed with 4–0 chromic catgut sub-cutaneously and 5–0 Dermalene as a sub-cuticular suture. A dry external pressure dressing is applied over the eye and lateral nasal bridge.

Postoperative Treatment. Cortisone and other hormonal supportive therapy are pre-scribed by the endocrinologist. Hydrocorti-sone (100 mg) is administered the evening before the operation with the preoperative medication, during surgery, and postoperatively. This amount, however, is variable and must be administered in accordance with the patient's basic hormonal balance. As a general rule, partial or complete removal of the pituitary is not so disturbing to the general glandular metabolism as one would suppose. Symptoms of thyroid insufficiency are not common and usually do not appear until 1 to 3 months postoperatively. Occasionally estrogens or androgens are necessary during a period of the postoperative course.

The use of prophylactic antibiotic therapy is questionable; 600,000 units of procaine penicillin may be administered intramuscularly twice a day. Diabetes insipidus may occur. This is easily controlled by administering vasopressin (Pitressin) in oil. The fluid intake and output chart will demonstrate the onset of this imbalance. Postoperative blood and urine sugar will demonstrate disturbances in the metabolism of glucose.

The pressure dressing over the eye and lateral nasal bridge is removed on the second postoperative day, and the patient is allowed full activity at this time. The iodoform gauze packing and subcuticular sutures are removed on the fifth postoperative day. The patient is discharged from the hospital on the sixth or seventh postoperative day.

Postoperative Complications *Hemorrhage.* The potential hemorrhage hazard from the ethmoidal artery, sphenopalatine artery, and dural sinuses is fairly well eliminated by the use of the septal mucosal flap and the petroleum jelly–treated iodoform gauze pack.

Cerebrospinal Fluid Rhinorrhea. Leakage of spinal fluid may occur in the immediate postoperative period or may occur several weeks postoperatively. The patient complains of lightheadedness, headache, and a soaking of his pillow and clothing from the cerebrospinal fluid rhinorrhea. This, for the most part, is self-limiting but on occasion can be a troublesome complication. The septal mucosal flap, used to cover the posterior wall of the sphenoidal sinus, seems to eliminate this complication.

Meningitis. It would seem that this complication would be fairly common, since the hypophyseal fossa has been exposed to the upper respiratory tract. It is, however, surprisingly rare. Meningitis has been reported in the immediate postoperative period or weeks and months later. The septal mucosal flap may be the necessary barrier to prevent this complication.

Damage to the Eye. Bateman states: "It has been suspected that wide exposure of the sphenoid through an orbital incision would be likely to cause blindness because of stretching of the optical nerve. This has not been reported."

Intracranial Hemorrhage. Subarachnoid hemorrhage has on occasion been reported and has been attributed to anatomic anomalies and misdirected surgery.

REFERENCES

Bateman, G. H.: Trans-sphenoidal Hypophysectomy: A Review of 70 Cases Treated in the Past 2 Years. Trans. Am. Acad. Ophthal. Otolaryng., 66:103, 1962.

Chiari, O.: Zur Kasuistik der Erkrankungen der Unterkieferspeicheldruse. Wien. Klin. Wochenschr., 25:5, 1912.

Cushing, H.: *The Pituitary Body and Its Disorders.* Philadelphia, J. B. Lippincott Co., 1912.

Goodale, R. L., and Montgomery, W. W.: Technical Advances in Osteoplastic Frontal Sinusectomy. Arch. Otolaryng., 79:522, 1964.

Hamberger, C. A., *et al.*: Transantrosphenoidal Hypophysectomy. Arch. Otolaryng., 74:2, 1961.

Hardy, J. M., and Montgomery, W. W.: Osteoplastic Frontal Sinusotomy—An Analysis of 250 Operations. Ann. Otol. Rhinol. and Laryngol., 85:529, 1976.

Heermann, J.: Verchluss des ganzen Fistelkanals alvelarer Kieferhohlen-Mundfistein durch periost-bindegewebe von der Kreferhohle her. Z. Laryngol. Rhinol. Otol., 41:213, 1962.

Hirsch, O.: Uber Methoden der operativen Behandlung von Hypophysentumoren auf endonasalem Wege. Arch. Laryngol. Rhinol., 24:129, 1910.

Jackson, C., and Jackson, C. L.: *Diseases of the Nose, Throat and Ear.* Philadelphia, W. B. Saunders Co., 1959.

Lynch, R. C.: The Technique of a Radical Frontal Sinus Operation Which Has Given Me the Best Results. Laryngoscope, 31:1, 1921.

Macbeth, R., and Hall, M.: Hypophysectomy as a Rhinological Procedure. Arch. Otolaryng., 75:440, 1962.

Montgomery, W. W.: Transethmoidosphenoidal Hypophysectomy with Septal Mucosal Flap. Arch. Otolaryng., *78*:68, 1963.
Montgomery, W. W.: The Fate of Adipose
Implants in a Bony Cavity. Laryngoscope,
74:816, 1964.
Montgomery, W. W.: *Surgery of the Upper
Respiratory System*. Vol. 1, 1971; Vol. 2,
1973. Philadelphia, Lea and Febiger.

Mosher, H. P.: The Surgical Anatomy of the
Ethmoidal Labyrinth. Am. Acad. Oph-
thalmol. Otol., 1929, pp. 376–410.
Riedel, B. M.: Schenke Inaug. Dissertation,
Jena, 1898.
Riskaer, N., *et al.*: Transsphenoidal Hypophys-
ectomy in Metastatic Cancer of the Breast.
Arch. Otolaryng., *74*:483, 1961.
Ritter, F. N.: The Paranasal Sinuses, 2nd ed.
1978. St. Louis, C. V. Mosby Co.

Chapter 14
Complications of Sinus Disease

William Montgomery

ORBITAL MANIFESTATIONS OF SINUS DISEASE

The paranasal sinuses might also be referred to as the paraorbital sinuses, for the orbit is surrounded (except laterally) by these sinuses. The first indication of sinus disease is often an orbital manifestation.

Exophthalmos

Exophthalmos is a protrusion of the eyeball from the orbit, which is usually a manifestation of other disease. Acute and chronic maxillary sinusitis is rarely complicated by exophthalmos unless there is extension of infection by phlebitis into the retrobulbar space. Cystic lesions of the maxillary sinus include mucocele, dentigerous cyst, dermoid cyst, and cystadenoma. Each of these lesions may expand so as to destroy the roof of the antrum and extend into the orbit, thus producing exophthalmos. The pressure exerted in this direction may also cause a ptosis of the upper lid which is produced by a restriction of the upper half of lid elevation. Epiphora may accompany this proptosis. Diplopia results from the upward displacement of the orbital contents. On occasion a mass may be palpated posterior to the infraorbital rim. Malignant lesions of the maxillary sinus which occur high in the sinus will cause early destruction of the roof of the antrum and extend into the orbit, producing exophthal-

mos. Malignant lesions which have their origins elsewhere in the antrum may also extend into the orbit. In these cases the prognosis is poor because as a rule the disease has also spread in other directions, such as through the posterior wall into the pharyngomaxillary fossa. A fracture of the maxilla rarely produces exophthalmos. This, however, is possible with certain tripod fractures.

Acute and chronic ethmoiditis may produce exophthalmos as a result of extension of infection through the lamina papyracea. This will be discussed in the sections on orbital cellulitis, orbital abscess, and lateral sinus thrombosis. Tumors of the ethmoidal sinuses are not common. They extend in the direction of least resistance, which is toward the lamina papyracea, thus causing outward and lateral displacement of the orbital contents. The most common benign lesions are mucoceles, osteomas, papillomas, and fibromas. Carcinomas of the ethmoid are usually not primary. A fracture of the ethmoidal labyrinth and lamina papyracea may cause a degree of proptosis following nose blowing. Subcutaneous emphysema of the lids is diagnostic.

Acute or chronic frontal sinusitis may extend into the orbit by way of the floor of the frontal sinus with resultant cellulitis and orbital abscess, or there may be simple displacement of the orbital contents in an outward and downward direction. The upper

8

lid will be involved in an inflammatory process, or a mass will be palpated between the upper lid and the supraorbital rim. The two most common tumors of the frontal sinus causing displacement of the orbital contents are mucocele and osteoma. The progression of downward and outward displacement of the orbital contents with both of these lesions can be slow and insidious. It can also have a rapid onset if the mucocele becomes infected (pyocele) or if the osteoma becomes complicated by acute frontal sinusitis. Other benign lesions and malignant lesions of the frontal sinuses are rare. They may produce exophthalmos in a similar manner by extension through the floor of the frontal sinus.

Acute and chronic sphenoiditis, cystic (mucocele) and solid benign tumors, and primary or secondary carcinomas of the sphenoidal sinus may extend into the retrobulbar area and produce exophthalmos simply by occupying space or by interfering with the venous return from the orbit. These situations are usually accompanied by interference with the nerves supplying the extraocular muscles and the blood supply entering the orbit, or by visual disturbances. There have been numerous reports of metastatic lesions of the sphenoidal sinuses with orbital complications. These malignancies may arise in the nasal cavity, nasopharynx, other sinuses, intracranial spaces (pituitary), and distant points such as the bowel and kidney.

Orbital Pain

Whereas generalized headache is not a usual manifestation of sinus disease, pain in or above the orbit commonly accompanies sinus disease.

Like a toothache, pain in the eye may be the presenting complaint of acute maxillary sinusitis. Chronic maxillary sinusitis less commonly causes orbital pain. Benign and malignant tumors which extend through the roof of the antrum may cause orbital pain.

Acute frontal sinusitis frequently produces orbital pain. Pain elicited by palpation of the floor of the frontal sinus just posterior to the medial aspect of the supraorbital rim is diagnostic of acute frontal sinusitis. Orbital pain is increased if the infection extends into the orbit through the floor of the frontal sinus or by phlebitis. Chronic frontal sinusitis and benign and malignant tumors may also produce orbital pain if they extend in that direction.

Orbital pain is an early manifestation of acute ethmoiditis. This is, of course, increased with the onset of orbital cellulitis or abscess. Chronic ethmoiditis does not usually produce orbital pain unless the disease extends in that direction. Benign and malignant tumors of the ethmoid may produce orbital pain.

Acute and chronic sphenoiditis produces pain which the patient describes as being behind the eye. Extension of disease beyond the confines of the sphenoidal sinus, whether it be inflammatory or neoplastic, may produce severe retrobulbar pain.

Lid Swelling

Inflammatory edema of the eyelids may occur with acute maxillary, ethmoidal, or frontal sinusitis. This edema is soft with no point of tenderness or localization such as that found in acute meibomian gland infection. Ocular motility and vision are not affected. If the inflammatory process extends into the orbit from the sinuses, this inflammatory edema may become more severe as orbital cellulitis progresses. As a general rule, the upper lid is more swollen with frontal sinusitis. Both lids are swollen with ethmoiditis, and the lower lid may be more swollen with extension of infection from the maxillary sinus.

Enophthalmos

Enophthalmos is a recession of the eyeball into the orbit. It may result from contractures following orbital cellulitis, orbital and sinus operations, orbital injuries, and fractures of the orbital walls. The *blowout fracture* is a relatively common cause of enophthalmos. This is a fracture of the floor of the orbit with prolapse of the orbital contents into the antrum. There may also be a fracture and medial displacement of the lamina papyracea with prolapse of the orbital contents into the ethmoidal labyrinth. Varying degrees of interference with ocular motility may accompany this fracture when the extraocular muscles (especially inferior rectus and inferior oblique) are trapped between the bony fragments. This situation requires immediate surgical intervention. If there is an interference with ocular motility, the procedure should be done in conjunction with an ophthalmologist. Two cases of enophthalmos resulting from mucocele of the maxillary antrum have been reported (Montgomery). The pathogenesis of this is not absolutely clear. It is assumed that the mucocele expands, destroying the roof of the antrum by pressure, and that the enophthalmos occurs with subsequent rupture and partial evacuation of the mucocele.

Mass in the Orbit

A mass palpated in the orbit may be the first sign of sinus disease. A mass in the region of the infraorbital rim may represent extension of disease from the maxillary sinus. The most common diseases of the antrum producing a mass behind the infraorbital rim are carcinoma, mucocele, and osteoma of the maxillary sinus. A mass medial to the inner canthus may indicate a disease in the ethmoidal sinuses, and again carcinoma, mucocele, and osteoma are the most common causes. A mass behind the supraorbital rim may indicate disease extending through the floor of the frontal sinus. The most common causes are mucocele, pyocele, osteoma, chronic inflammatory process, the Lynch frontal sinus procedure (which entails removal of the floor of the frontal sinus), and carcinoma of the frontal sinus.

Epiphora

A prolonged inflammatory process of the nasal mucosa is said to cause epiphora, either by stenosis of the nasolacrimal duct or by obstruction of the orifice in the inferior meatus. It is also within the realm of possibility that an inflammatory process could extend from the ethmoidal sinuses to the lacrimal sac. Epiphora may also accompany exophthalmos of sinus origin.

Orbital Cellulitis and Abscess

An inflammatory process may extend from any of the paranasal sinuses into the orbit by direct extension through the bony wall or by way of the venous circulation. At first there is an inflammatory edema of the lid or lids accompanied by pain. As the disease progresses, there is exophthalmos, chemosis of the conjunctiva, and progressive immobility of the eye. There also may be some interference with the vision. At this point the patient is usually quite ill with a high fever and severe pain. X-ray examination of the sinuses is taken to determine the origin of infection. This is most commonly the ethmoidal sinus but can be any of the other sinuses. This condition should be vigorously treated because of the danger of extension of infection into the intracranial spaces (i.e., meningitis, cavernous sinus thrombosis, etc.). It is often difficult to determine whether or not an orbital abscess is present unless obvious fluctuation can be palpated. As a general rule, if the condition is not responding to intensive therapy, an exploratory operative procedure should be performed.

Cavernous sinus thrombosis can still be a fatal disease even when all modern therapeutic tools are utilized. It is sometimes difficult to differentiate between orbital cellulitis or abscess and cavernous sinus thrombosis. In addition to the above signs of orbital cellulitis, a dilation of the retinal veins and edema of the optic disc may be found with cavernous sinus thrombosis. Intermittent rises of temperature to 104 or 105°F following a chill should make one suspicious of cavernous sinus thrombosis. A blood culture and examination of the spinal fluid are indicated. The examiner should be on the lookout for signs of meningitis.

Optic Nerve

Approximately 15% of retrobulbar neuritis is said to be caused by sinus disease. This is not surprising since the optic nerve may be in close relationship to the sphenoidal, ethmoidal, and maxillary sinuses, depending on their degree of pneumatization. The inflammatory process may spread either directly through the sinus wall or by phlebitis. The loss of vision may be of sudden or gradual onset. The therapy here consists of antibiotics and specific treatment of the involved sinus. Benign and malignant tumors of the sinuses as well as of the pituitary gland can cause blindness or field defects.

Superior Orbital Fissure Syndrome

Involvement of the third, fourth, and sixth cranial nerves, the first division of the fifth cranial nerve, the ophthalmic vein, and sympathetic nerves from the cavernous plexus may occur with disease of the sphenoidal sinus. The lateral wall of the sphenoidal sinus, if well pneumatized, is in close proximity to the superior orbital fissure. An acute or chronic inflammatory process may extend from the sphenoidal sinus to this region. Cystic lesions, such as mucocele or a craniopharyngioma, benign neoplasms, and primary or secondary malignancies of the sphenoidal sinus may be complicated by a superior orbital fissure syndrome. Any or all of these structures passing through the superior orbital fissure may be affected by these disease processes (Reinecke and Montgomery). The sixth cranial nerve is usually involved first, with subsequent involvement of the third, fourth, and fifth nerves. As the disease progresses, the fifth cranial nerve is involved, with resultant pain in the eye and forehead. This is followed by exophthalmos and finally total ophthalmoplegia. X-ray examination of the sinuses should include laminography of the sphenoidal sinuses. Treatment involves immediate exploration by means of the transethmoidal approach to the sphenoidal sinus (see Chapter 13).

Osteomyelitis of the Frontal Bone

Etiology. The organism recovered in the great majority of reported cases is *Staphylococcus aureus*. β hemolytic streptococci, pneumococci, and anaerobic streptococci are found in a few instances. The etiology depends to a certain extent upon the virulence of the organism and the resistance or immunity of the patient to the particular organism present.

In children the origin of osteomyelitis of the frontal bone is almost always hematogenous; in adults the disease is more likely the result of trauma or spread from an adjacent infection.

The majority of patients are under 30 years of age. It is more common in females than in males, and many cases follow swimming. Chronic infection of the sinuses may predispose to osteomyelitis, especially following an acute exacerbation. Trauma in the region of the frontal sinus or operative trauma following surgical procedures on the frontal bone frequently precedes the advent of osteomyelitis. Operating in an infected field, traumatizing the bone, closing the external wound too tightly, rasping the bone, and operating during an acute exacerbation of a chronic infection have been mentioned as possible factors.

Pathology. The infection may be transmitted to the vault by continuity of tissue or, more commonly, by hematogenous metastasis. In the latter event, the inflammatory disease is carried by a thrombophlebitis of the venous system into the bone of the calvarium through the anastomosing diploetic veins through the frontal sinus or on the undersurface of the cranium or the frontal sinus. Isolated foci of osteomyelitis in remote bones of the skull may be accounted for by this method. Furstenberg found the inner plate to be the first affected, while the external plate may remain uninvolved, although the reverse may be true as well. The intracranial extension of the infection is usually by way of the frontal and anterior temporal diploetic veins into the superior sagittal sinus and from there to the cerebral hemisphere of the same or opposite side by way of the connecting veins.

Infection by continuity of tissue is probably the less common form of extension. Direct invasion of the canaliculi and medullary spaces seems to occur, especially in the postoperative cases. The cranial sutures in many instances exercise an inhibiting influence upon the spread of the infection. In rare instances spread of the infection along the perineural sheaths of the olfactory nerve may occur.

In the earliest stage of osteomyelitis of the cranial bones, the diploë show some congestion. Somewhat later marked hyperemia with small drops of pus may be seen. Its consistency is softened, and the diploetic spaces are filled with granulation tissue, bathed in pus. Thrombosed vessels may or may not be found. The bone itself becomes discolored with blood and pus, oozing to the surface through the vascular channels or fistulous openings. Small sequestra occur in the diploetic spaces. The external and internal tables may be broken down, with widespread destruction.

Microscopic examination in the early stage shows edema of the myeloid tissue with a vascular congestion and an infiltration of lymphocytes and polymorphonuclear leukocytes. Some of the vessels may show a septic thrombosis. Later, necrotic areas are found, the result of an obstruction to their blood supply. The myeloid tissue is replaced by granulation tissue and pus. Osteoclasts may surround the sequestra and be seen along the surface of the bone. Evidence of osseous repair and areas of destruction are present at the same time.

The infection may extend along the dura, the periosteum, and the soft tissues of the scalp at about the same rate. If the infection breaks through the inner table, an extradural abscess is formed. Furstenberg believes this abscess is responsible for the further extension of the infection by cutting off the blood supply of the cranial bones.

Symptoms. The clinical course may be acute or chronic. The symptoms depend on the course, the sinus involved, and the extent of involvement.

In the acute fulminating type, fever, headache, and edema of the upper eyelid on the affected side are present. The soft doughy swelling (*Pott's puffy tumor*) or pericranial abscess is pathognomonic of osteomyelitis of the underlying bone. This type frequently follows swimming. It shows a tendency to early spread to the intracranial structures. Death due to severe toxemia or meningitis may occur in a few days or in a week or two. As a rule, however, osteomyelitis is a slow disease even in the acute cases. Cyclic exacerbations are characteristic.

The chronic localized form without perforation of the internal table is characterized by an insidious onset, a low-grade fever, local pain or tenderness, doughy swellings, general malaise, and occasionally chills. In the chronic form of osteomyelitic

fistulas, sequestra and purulent discharge from the bone may be present with cyclic exacerbations.

Diagnosis. The diagnosis is made from the roentgenogram combined with the signs and symptoms of fluctuating swellings, advancing edema, persistent low-grade temperature, leukocytosis, and pain and headache with cyclic exacerbation.

Treatment. High doses of antibiotics should be given, in accordance with bacteriologic study, by the intravenous route. Any localized abscesses should be drained. If x-ray films show the frontal sinuses to contain pus, a trephine operation should be performed. These procedures are important both for surgical drainage and to obtain material for bacteriologic study.

The radical procedures which were most often necessary in the past for the treatment of osteomyelitis of the frontal bone are for the most part no longer necessary, if the proper antibiotics are administered in adequate doses. The operations of Mosher and Judd are procedures of the past. On occasion it is necessary to remove a portion of devitalized bone. The resultant defect can be repaired at a later date using an autogenous osseous autograft. Since regeneration of bone is often a slow process, this plastic procedure should not be attempted for at least one year.

After the osteomyelitis has been controlled using surgical drainage and antibiotic therapy, the surgeon's attention should then more specifically be directed to the frontal sinuses. If there is any question of persistent or chronic frontal sinusitis, a bilateral osteoplastic adipose obliteration operation (Chapter 15) should be carried out. Antibiotic therapy is instituted for at least 10 days following this operation.

OSTEOMYELITIS OF THE SUPERIOR MAXILLA

Acute osteomyelitis of the superior maxilla is usually secondary to an infection of dental origin. In infants, it is occasionally seen secondary to a buccal infection. Involvement of the dental sac follows, with extension of the necrotic process to the walls of the maxillary antrum, creating a pus discharge into the nose and mouth. The infection seems to travel by retrograde thrombosis, which is the cause of the gangrene and sequestration. Lederer believes the associated acute osteomyelitis is the result of the venous infection—not the cause of it. He bases his opinion upon carefully studied serial sections of a case in which a nasal infection and sinusitis were found to be the primary cause of the osteomyelitis of the maxilla in an infant.

Osteomyelitis of the maxilla in nurslings and infants may occur from the first week up to the ninth month. The greatest incidence is during the first three weeks. The portal of entry and the manner of spreading of the primary infection may vary.

As shown by Lederer, a sinusitis may produce a periosteitis and osteitis with a fistulous tract formation which may extend in any one of three ways: (1) to the facial surface with swelling of the soft parts of the cheek, breaking down of Bichat's pad, and abscess formation; (2) to the palatine and alveolar process with a fistula into the roof of the mouth; (3) to the zygomatic process with a necrosis of the zygomatic arch and extension into the pterygoid fossa with abscess formation. Extension along the fascial planes to the mandibular foramen may occur. An ethmoiditis may result in a periosteitis, osteitis, and periorbital cellulitis which may extend in one or both of two ways: (1) thrombophlebitis of the venous channels with extension to the cavernous sinus and the production of a thrombosis; (2) formation of a periorbital abscess with an external fistula.

Symptoms. The signs and symptoms are those of a sinusitis accompanied by marked swelling and edema of the cheek. Exophthalmos with limitation of motion may be present.

The first or septicemic stage may last for about 10 days with the formation of fistulas in the infraorbital regions, palate, and in rare instances in the nose. This is followed by the second or chronic indolent stage with persistence of the fistulas and with sequestration of dead bone. This second stage is not seen if antibiotics, proper drainage, and local therapy are properly instituted early in the disease.

Treatment. Treatment consists of administration of high doses of specific antibiotics, as in osteomyelitis of the frontal bone, free surgical drainage, and local heat. On occasion there is considerable loss of bone as a result of osteomyelitis of the superior maxilla and a resultant large oroantral fistula. This can be repaired using the various flaps outlined under the section on treatment of oroantral fistulas (Chapter 13).

OSTEOMYELITIS OF THE SPHENOID BONE

Osteomyelitis of the sphenoid is quite rare. Many of the reported cases have been associated with osteomyelitis of the base of the skull or have been secondary to an infection of the petrous portion of the temporal bone. Eagleton attributes the rarity of infection of the base of the sphenoid to the preponderance of red cellular bone marrow found in this bone throughout life.

The organisms usually recovered are hemolytic streptococci and beta-hemolytic *Staphylococcus aureus*. The early symptoms are a rather profuse postnasal discharge and a deep-seated headache, described as being either in the center of the head or behind the eyes, which on occasion radiates to the temporal or occipital regions. Infection may spread laterally to the retrobulbar region, producing any of the various manifestations described in the section on superior orbital fissure syndrome.

Later, as the body of the sphenoid becomes more extensively invaded, symptoms of sepsis ensue, although the temperature may be low and the toxemia not marked. The retro-orbital and temporal pain becomes especially severe. There may be, at this time, bacterial invasion of the meninges and bloodstream. Cavernous sinus thrombosis, brain abscess, encephalitis, and intracranial hemorrhage may result.

Treatment. Osteomyelitis of the sphenoid bone is frequently not diagnosed until severe complications which can be fatal have developed. Careful x-ray examination of the sphenoid bone is imperative. This should include laminography. The patient should be followed closely by an ophthalmologist and neurologist. Treatment is essentially that of antibiotics and surgical drainage.

INTRACRANIAL COMPLICATIONS OF SINUS DISEASE

The modern otolaryngologist should still be constantly on the lookout for intracranial complications of sinus disease. Most of these complications are readily apparent by their clinical manifestations. On the other hand, others have a slow insidious onset which makes the diagnosis quite difficult.

The possible intracranial complications from disease of the nasal passages and sinuses are external and internal pachymeningitis, leptomeningitis, extradural and subdural abscess, dural fistula, the various types of brain abscesses, and septic thrombosis of the cavernous or superior longitudinal sinus. The other venous sinuses are rarely involved from infections of the nasal sinuses.

Acute infections of the sinuses are more apt to result in intracranial complications than are chronic infections. These complications are more common in males than in females (4 to 1).

All infected sinuses may give rise to an intracranial complication, but an extension from a maxillary sinusitis is rare. Courville and Rosenvold state that a maxillary sinusitis of dental origin is more apt to provoke intracranial suppurative lesions than any other type.

Meningitis which has its origin in sinusitis is more frequently observed than thrombosis of the venous sinuses.

Infections from the nose or sinuses may invade the intracranial structures after trauma, through congenital dehiscences or nonclosure of fetal defects, by a direct pathway through the sinus wall, along the sheaths of the olfactory nerves, by way of the communicating veins, by means of septic thrombi along the diploetic veins with a retrograde thrombophlebitis or periphlebitis to the cavernous sinus, by way of the angular or ethmoidal veins to the cavernous sinus, and by way of the orbit. There has been some ques-

tion as to the possibility of a direct extension of an infection of the sinuses to the intracranial structures by way of the lymphatic vessels.

Temporal lobe abscesses most commonly originate from infection in the temporal bone and lateral dural sinus. A temporal lobe abscess can originate in the sphenoidal sinus or spread indirectly from the other sinuses by way of the cavernous sinus. Frontal lobe abscesses may accompany acute or chronic frontal sinusitis and tumors of the frontal sinus (such as osteoma) and may follow frontal or ethmoidal surgery or trauma to the forehead.

PNEUMOCELE

A pneumocele (pneumatocele) is a collection of air, under pressure, in the tissues. It usually escapes from a defect in the bony wall of the frontal sinus and collects adjacent to the sinus. If this occurs on the forehead, an external pneumocele results. If the defect is in the posterior wall, an internal or intracranial pneumocele is present.

A pneumocele may follow a fracture, trauma, operation, congenital cleft, dehiscence, or necrosis of the bone. The latter may be due to syphilis, osteomyelitis, sinusitis, etc. Cases have been reported as secondary to or associated with an osteoma.

The mucous membrane or periosteum is intact over the bony defect, so that a ballooning of the mucosa or periosteum occurs, forming an air sac when under pressure from blowing the nose, coughing, etc. A pneumocele may occur in connection with a mucocele if air takes the place of the fluid contents.

In addition to the external and internal pneumoceles, a third type characterized by an excessive dilation of the sinus (*pneumosinus dilatans*) may occur.

The dilation of the sinus is usually associated with acromegaly, localized osteitis, or fractures in the region of the sinuses. The enlargement of the sinus is more apt to result if the initiating bone changes occur before the sinuses are fully developed. Any of the sinuses may be involved either on one or both sides. The exact mechanism by which the dilatation occurs is not understood.

REFERENCES

Courville, C. B., and Rosenvold, L. K.: Intracranial Complications of Infections of Nasal Cavities and Accessory Sinuses. Arch. Otolaryng., *27*:692, 1938.

Eagleton, W. P.: Meningitis—Result of Disease of the Petrous Apex and Sphenoidal Basis. Surg. Gynecol. Obstet., *60*:586, 1935.

Furstenberg, A. C.: Osteomyelitis of the Skull: The Osteogenetic Processes in the Repair of Cranial Defects. Ann. Otol. Rhinol. Laryngol., *40*:996, 1931.

Lederer, F. L.: *Diseases of the Ear, Nose and Throat.* 6th ed. Philadelphia, F. A. Davis Co., 1953.

Montgomery, W.: Mucocele of the Maxillary Sinus Causing Enophthalmos. Eye, Ear, Nose and Throat Monthly, *43*:41, 1964.

Montgomery, W.: Surgery of the Upper Respiratory System. Philadelphia, Lea & Febiger, 1971.

Mosher, H. P., and Judd, D. K.: An Analysis of Seven Cases of Osteomyelitis of the Frontal Bone Complicating Frontal Sinusitis. Laryngoscope, *43*:153, 1933.

Reinecke, R. D., and Montgomery, W. W.: Oculomotor Nerve Palsy Associated With Mucocele of the Sphenoid Sinus. Arch. Ophthalmol., *71*:50, 1964.

Chapter 15

Tumors of the Nose and Paranasal Sinuses

William Montgomery

BENIGN TUMORS

Cystic Tumors

Nonsecreting Cysts. These cysts are lined by loose connective tissue and contain an amber-colored exudate. They are smooth and rounded in appearance and subepithelial in location. Their frequency in routine sinus x-ray examinations tends to indicate a lack of clinical significance. It is, however, important that the otolaryngologist be aware of this lack of pathogenic importance so that he will not be misled into a surgical procedure. The most frequent site of occurrence is the floor of the maxillary sinus.

Retention Cysts. These cysts are formed by enlargement of a gland in the sinus mucosal lining. The blockage of the gland is either inflammatory or allergic in origin. They may either resolve spontaneously or enlarge so as to fill the antrum and produce symptoms requiring their removal.

Mucoceles. Mucoceles are secreting cysts lined by sinus mucous membrane and enlarged by an accumulation of the products of secretion and desquamation. The secretion is usually clear, thick, and tenacious unless the mucocele has been converted to a *pyocele* by the invasion of bacteria. The color and consistency of the contents of the pyocele vary with the pathogenic organism. Mucoceles are most frequently found in the frontal sinuses. They also are found in the other paranasal sinuses, however. Mucoceles will be discussed in more detail as they are related to each sinus.

Frontal sinus mucoceles develop following blockage of the nasofrontal duct, chronic infection, trauma, or surgery of the frontal sinus. The first manifestation of mucocele formation may be intermittent or persistent pain in the supraorbital region as the mucocele expands. As the mucocele enlarges, there is a gradual thinning out of the walls of the frontal sinus. The expansion is in the direction of least resistance, which is usually toward the floor of the frontal sinus. The orbital contents are displaced downward and laterally, producing proptosis and diplopia. Early, there is tenderness elicited by palpation of the roof of the orbit. Later, a palpable mass becomes apparent in this region along with a defect in the roof of the orbit. The mucocele may erode through the interfrontal septum to involve the contralateral sinus. On occasion the mucocele may extend into the ethmoidal labyrinth, through the anterior wall of the frontal sinus causing an external deformity, or through the posterior wall into the anterior cranial fossa. The mucocele may become infected, thus forming a pyocele which can lead to serious intracranial and orbital complications.

The x-ray findings of a mucocele and/or pyocele are rather characteristic. They appear as smooth, globular, punched-out areas of radiotranslucency. Often there are a number of mucoceles or pyoceles in a frontal sinus. The lateral view is valuable for determining extension into the anterior cranial fossa or ethmoidal sinus.

The anterior osteoplastic approach (see Chapter 13) has proved ideal for the treatment of mucoceles and pyoceles of the frontal sinus, as a primary surgical procedure or following other external frontal sinus operations. Usually the entire mucocele lining can be removed. The inner cortical lining of the sinus is then removed and the sinus obliterated with adipose tissue. On occasion a mucocele which develops following the Lynch frontal sinus operation will extend well toward the apex of the orbit and into the ethmoidal labyrinth. In these cases it is impossible to remove the entire mucosal lining, and thus the Lynch frontal sinus operation is revised from the osteoplastic approach.

The etiology of mucoceles and pyoceles of the *ethmoidal sinus* is similar to that outlined for those of the frontal sinus. The direction of expansion is usually through the thin lamina papyracea; the orbital contents are thus displaced laterally or downward. The therapy for mucoceles of the ethmoidal sinus is a complete external ethmoidectomy.

Mucoceles of the *sphenoidal sinus,* by obstructing the sinus ostium, can cause empyema. There may be destruction of the posterior wall and encroachment on the pituitary (Bach and coworkers). An orbital apex syndrome with loss of vision and contraction of the visual fields may occur (Lundgren and Olin). Optic neuritis and enophthalmos may be complications of mucoceles in the sphenoidal sinus. Radiographic planograms of the sinuses are very useful in outlining these mucoceles, as well as the mucoceles of the other paranasal sinuses.

The surgical approach to mucoceles of the sphenoidal sinus is the external ethmosphenoidal approach. Purulent marsupialization may be accomplished by the use of the septal mucosal flap, as described in Chapter 13.

The clinical manifestations of a mucocele in the *maxillary sinus* are produced by slow expansion, which causes pressure atrophy of the mucous membrane lining and also absorption of the bony sinus walls. The clinical signs and symptoms which may result from a mucocele of the maxillary sinus are: (1) upward displacement of the orbital contents, resulting in proptosis of the eye (Ersner and coworkers; Parker; Belal; Maduro and coworkers); (2) ptosis of the upper lid produced by restriction of the upper half of the lid elevation (Parker); epiphora which may accompany the proptosis (Ersner and coworkers; Parker; Belal; Maduro and coworkers; Bromberg and coworkers); (3) enophthalmos caused by a loss of the roof of the antrum (Montgomery, 1964); (4) diplopia resulting from an upward or downward displacement of the orbital contents (Panikkar); (5) a swelling of the cheek over the antrum (Christensen and Houck); (6) a palpable defect occurring in the anterior wall of the antrum or of the infraorbital rim (Bromberg and coworkers); (7) nasal stuffiness or obstruction resulting from a medial displacement of the lateral wall of the nose (Montgomery, 1964); and (8) a defect in the floor of the antrum (Panikkar).

Diplopia caused by an upward displacement of the orbital contents may be cured by simple removal of the mucocele employing the Caldwell-Luc approach. In these cases, the periosteum usually affords sufficient support for the orbital contents. There is usually no subsequent enophthalmos because of the additional support provided by the formation of fibrous tissue and the regeneration of bone. This, however, is not always the case, and later repair of the orbital floor may be necessary.

Ersner, Morse, and Alexander have reported success in reconstruction of the orbital floor using stainless steel wire mesh. They used a horizontal incision following the line of the infraorbital rim and inserted a double-thickness semilunar-shaped piece of No. 60 stainless steel wire mesh. Bromberg, Rubin, and Walden used polyethylene implants which were fashioned to the size and shape of the orbital floor. Multiple holes were made in these implants to allow for an ingrowth of fibrous tissue. Witchell and Vlessing and others have used iliac bone autogenous grafts for restoration of the floor of the orbit.

An Ivalon sponge has been implanted into the antral cavity to support the ptotic orbital contents in two cases of enophthalmos resulting from mucocele of the maxillary sinus (Montgomery, 1964).

Dermoid Cysts. The most common site of onset of the dermoid cyst in relation to the nose and paranasal sinuses is at the suture line between the nasal bones and the nasal process of the frontal bone. This cyst is present at birth but may not manifest itself until adolescence. It may extend into the nasal cavity, frontal sinus, ethmoidal sinus, or maxillary sinus. The dermoid cysts associated with the maxillary sinus usually have their origin in the hard palate. They contain structures of the skin such as glands, hair, and teeth. The treatment is complete surgical excision. The deformities resulting from this excision should be repaired by reconstructive surgery.

Dental Cysts. A dentigerous cyst develops from the enamel margin of an unerupted tooth. It is characterized by an outer bony shell which is separate from the wall of the antrum and is lined by stratified squamous epithelium. A tooth is contained within the cyst along with amber-colored fluid.

Radicular cysts develop at the root of a tooth and do not include the entire tooth as does the dentigerous cyst. It may develop from a granuloma which undergoes cystic degeneration. It may or may not be lined with epithelium and may be covered with a very thin layer of bone as it protrudes into the antrum. The offending teeth involved with the radicular cyst should be removed.

Ameloblastoma (adamantinoma) is a tumor of dental origin that results from an unrestrained proliferation of ameloblasts. It is slow-growing and infiltrative and destroys adjacent tissue. It does not metastasize but has a great tendency to recur after removal. The x-ray film of an ameloblastoma shows a typical cystic defect resembling soap bubbles. A cystadenoma is an ameloadenoma which has undergone cystic degeneration. Ameloblastomas have been encountered in both the antrum and the ethmoidal sinuses.

Treatment. Dentigerous cysts are removed by the Caldwell-Luc route. If adjacent teeth are involved, they should be removed. If the maxillary sinus is involved with the cyst or secondarily infected, a Caldwell-Luc procedure should be carried out. The ameloblastoma should be widely excised because of its tendency to recur.

Solid Tumors

Fibrous Tumors. Fibromas, osteofibromas, neurofibromas, and fibromyxomas may occur in the nose and paranasal sinuses. *Juvenile nasopharyngeal fibroma* is the only one of this group that occurs in significant frequency to warrant special mention. This is a highly vascular angiofibroma which has its origin from a broad base in the vault of the nasopharynx. The attachment may also be high in the posterior wall of the nasopharynx on the posterolateral nasal wall. This tumor almost invariably occurs in boys prior to puberty. The juvenile fibroma is of very firm consistency, round or slightly nodular, and of grayish or purplish red color. It is benign histologically and does not metastasize but is highly destructive locally. It may enlarge to occupy the nasopharynx completely and present in the oropharynx. It may extend anteriorly and protrude through the nares. It is not uncommon for this tumor to invade the paranasal sinuses; the ethmoidal and maxillary sinuses are those most frequently invaded. On occasion it may invade the pterygomaxillary space or the foramina at the base of the skull, or it may extend into the orbit through the ethmoidal or infraorbital fissure.

The first symptoms are severe epistaxis and varying degrees of nasal obstruction. Other symptoms depend upon the size of the tumor and the direction of its extension.

The juvenile angiofibroma has been treated by surgery, radiation therapy, and male hormonal therapy. As a general rule, treatment of these tumors should be carried out only when indicated by complicating symptoms, for they tend to regress spontaneously after puberty. The transpalatal approach is used for those tumors which present posteriorly into the nasopharynx. This is a direct route to the base of the tumor, and a profuse hemorrhage can be more readily controlled. Implantation of radon seeds into the site of origin of the tumor is often useful, and it is certainly indicated after the first recurrence. Those lesions which extend anteriorly into the nasal cavity and paranasal sinuses are best approached by lateral rhinotomy incision. These operations are hazardous because of severe hemorrhage. Adequate blood for replacement should be on hand at the beginning of the operation. In addition to the routine sinus x-rays, planograms are often useful to outline an extensive juvenile angioma prior to surgery. External radiation has been used to reduce the vascularity of these tumors. As a rule this and repeated use of radon seeds are undesirable because of the effect on the growth of the facial bones. The institution of male hormonal therapy has been reported to be successful in reducing the size of these lesions. Cryotherapy may prove to be a much needed tool for the surgical removal of the juvenile nasopharyngeal fibroma.

Giant Cell Tumors. Giant cell granulomas are distinguished by the granulomatous changes in the stroma. These tend to regress spontaneously and thus are treated only by limited surgery. True giant cell tumors have a stroma which is rich in round and spindle-shaped cells of abnormal size and shape. They should be treated by radical excision because of their tendency to undergo malignant degeneration (Leonardelli and coworkers).

Ossifying Fibroma (Osteitis Fibrosa). These tumors are made up of bony trabeculae embedded in fibrous tissue. Spindle-shaped cells with a tendency toward ossification are found in the stroma of these tumors. When this lesion is diagnosed, a skeletal x-ray survey should be carried out because of the incidence of multiple lesions. The superior maxilla is the most frequent site. They most frequently begin in childhood and are manifested only by facial asymmetry. As the disease progresses, it may involve the antrum, orbit, nasal cavity, and other paranasal sinuses. Some authors consider the ossifying fibroma to be a localized manifestation of fibrous dysplasia. This lesion may on occasion undergo malignant change. It is usually impossible to completely excise these lesions. Bleeding is usually profuse during the procedure. There is a tendency for rapid recurrence.

Osteomas of the Paranasal Sinuses. An osteoma of the paranasal sinuses is found in approximately 0.25% of routine roentgenographic sinus examinations. Of the paranasal sinuses, the frontal sinus is the most frequent site of osteoma. In a series of nearly 300 osteomas reported in various early twentieth century literature, 80% were found in the frontal sinus, 16% in the ethmoidal sinus, and 4% in the antrum.

The disease is more common in males and most frequently occurs during puberty (Sasso and Smolcic). No satisfactory pathogenesis has as yet been offered. The most prevalent belief is that the osteoma is a benign mesenchymal neoplasm, developing as a result of metaplasia of connective tissue with the formation of bone by the sinus mucosa acting as periosteum (Brunner and Spiesman).

Osteomas are classified as compact, cancellous, or mixed. The compact osteoma is an ivory-hard tumor, probably formed from periosteal osteoblasts. It is limited to the skull. The cancellous osteoma possesses its own epiphyseal cartilage by virtue of which it grows as long as does the skeleton. The frontal sinus osteoma is the most commonly found of the mixed type, the spongiosa forming the core.

The many suggested sites of origin are as varied as the theories of pathogenesis. In general, the osteoma may arise anywhere in the frontal sinus and is usually covered by mucous membrane. The most frequent site of origin would seem to be between the frontal and ethmoid bones.

Osteomas of the frontal sinus usually are without signs and symptoms. Cases of small osteomas of the frontal sinus with no apparent impingement, but causing local pain or headache, have been published. These symptoms have been relieved by surgical removal of the osteomas.

The direction taken by enlargement governs the character of the symptoms. Increased intrasinus pressure produces frontal neuralgia and sensitiveness over the growth. The most frequent direction of enlargement is toward the orbit, which would be as expected for this is the direction of least resistance. Diplopia results from a downward and outward displacement of the orbital contents. In its abnormal position, the eye becomes prone to secondary infection (Lederer). Proptosis may occur.

The interfrontal septum may be displaced or destroyed by pressure erosion. The opposite frontal sinus is in this manner obstructed, infected, or involved with mucoceles.

Growth in the zygomatic and temporal direction is not common. External deformity is quite apparent here.

Extension of the osteoma downward into the nasal cavity has been reported. Nasal blockage and discharge develop. Advancement of the tumor into the cranial fossa, by way of either the posterior wall of the frontal sinus or the cribriform plate (Jackson and Jackson), can produce a variety of symptoms. Headache, mental dullness, vertigo, nausea, and vomiting are early symptoms of this complication. Papilledema may be found. Hemiplegia, epileptiform seizures, and pneumocephalus have been reported as more serious complications. The pneumocephalus is prone to be followed by cerebrospinal fluid rhinorrhea, meningitis, and brain abscess.

Treatment. Small osteomas not posing immediate surgical problems should have the rate of growth observed by a periodic roentgenographic examination. As soon as there are symptoms secondary to pressure, the treatment should be immediate removal.

Small osteomas have been removed by an external approach through the floor of the frontal sinus without creating a defect. Unfortunately, most osteomas of the frontal sinuses have obtained considerable size before producing the symptoms for their diagnosis. The radical Riedel operation has been most widely used for removal of the frontal sinus osteomas. The resultant deformity is severe enough to warrant subsequent plastic surgical repair. The transcranial route is rejected because it is an unnecessary surgical detour. The anterior osteoplastic approach for removal of osteomas is indeed an ideal

approach (Montgomery, 1960). The osteoplastic flap is reflected, exposing the osteoma, which is then easily removed. If there is no concurrent irreversible chronic sinus infection and the nasofrontal orifice is patent, it is not necessary to obliterate the sinus. If these complications are present, the entire mucosal and inner cortical linings of the sinus should be removed, and the sinus should then be implanted with abdominal adipose tissue (as described in Chapter 13).

Osteoma of the Ethmoidal Sinus. Osteomas of the ethmoidal sinus may enlarge to involve the majority of the ethmoidal cells or extend into the frontal sinus orbit or sphenoidal sinus. There have been reports of osteomas extending into the endocranium (Boenninghaus). Extension of the osteoma in the direction of the frontal sinus may encroach upon the nasofrontal passage and thus be the precursor of chronic frontal sinus infection. Growth in the direction of the orbit results in downward or outward displacement of the orbital contents. Nasal stuffiness may be a complaint if the upper lateral nasal wall is displaced medially.

The external ethmoidectomy approach is the route of choice for removal of osteomas of the ethmoids. If the osteoma is large, a considerable amount of the ascending process of the maxilla and nasal bone may be necessary for adequate exposure.

Osteoma of the Maxillary Sinus. Osteomas of the maxillary sinus are rare and most often symptomless. When complicated, they should be removed by the Caldwell-Luc approach.

Papilloma. Clinically there are two types of papilloma found in the nasal cavity and sinuses, the hard and soft (inverted). The soft papilloma, which is covered by columnar or metaplastic squamous epithelium, is pliable, pink, and tends to bleed quite easily. The hard papilloma is covered by stratified squamous epithelium which shows varying degrees of cornification. It is more cauliflower-like than the soft papilloma and does not bleed easily. The surgeon may not be aware of the diagnosis of papilloma until he receives the pathology report. A single papilloma of the nose may be removed by simple excision. Multiple papillomas of the nose require wide surgical excision by the lateral rhinotomy route. Any recurrence of intranasal papilloma should be treated by wide excision followed by radiation therapy. Some believe the treatment of choice for papillomas of the nose and paranasal sinuses is wide excision followed by radiation therapy. This is justified by the significant potential for malignant degeneration.

Nonneoplastic Tumors. Nasal polyps are an edematous hypertrophy of the nasal mucosa resulting from a chronic edematous inflammatory process. They may occur singly or in numbers and may be pedunculated or sessile. They vary in their glandular component. The polyps may become cystic as a result of glandular degeneration. Polyps may be classified as edematous, fibrous, and vascular. The edematous polyp is that most commonly seen in the nasal cavity and paranasal sinuses. It appears as a smooth, glistening, grayish white, grapelike lesion. The fibrous polyp is more firm, nonglistening, and paler. The vascular polyp by virtue of the high vascularity in the tunica propria layer is distinguished by its pink color.

Cauna and coworkers have recently investigated the ultrastructure of allergic polyps. They found that the polyps were devoid of sensory, vasomotor, and secretomotor innervation. Neutrophilic and eosinophilic leukocytes were present in increased numbers, and plasma cells, single and in clusters, exhibited activity in the cisternae of the endoplasmic reticulum and in the Golgi zones. Mast cells were characterized by partly depleted granules. Most interestingly, the venules of the polyps consistently revealed open endothelial junctions signifying vascular leakage.

The *antrochoanal polyp* deserves special mention because of its clinical difference from the garden variety of nasal polypi. It arises from the mucosa of the maxillary sinus near the ostium or posterior sinus wall. It extends in an hourglass fashion through the ostium and may be found in varying sizes in the nasopharynx. On occasion these antrochoanal polyps obtain such size as to obstruct the entire nasopharynx and present below the level of the soft palate.

Nasal polypi may be removed as an office procedure, using a wire snare and forceps such as the Greene and Takahashi, to obtain an airway. If the polyps frequently recur and the ethmoidal sinuses are found to be filled as shown by x-rays, the patient should be admitted to the hospital, and under general anesthesia a bilateral intranasal ethmoidectomy should be carried out, as outlined in Chapter 13.

There is a special technique for removing the antrochoanal polyp. With the patient under general anesthesia a loop of snare wire is passed into the nasal cavity (from which a polyp arises) and into the nasopharynx. The index finger of the right hand is then placed in the nasopharynx, and the wire is looped over the dome of the polyp, while the left hand pulls the loop back into the nose to the pedicle of the polyp as it exits from the maxillary ostium. The wire is then attached to the snare apparatus. The polyp is grasped by forceps introduced by way of the oropharyngeal route, before the pedicle is sectioned. Usually the sinus x-rays will show a dense antrum on the side of the antrochoanal polyp origin. Unless a Caldwell-Luc procedure is carried out, there is a likely chance that the antrochoanal polyp will recur.

Eosinophilic Granuloma. Eosinophilic granulomas may occur in or around the paranasal sinuses. The punched-out appearance of the x-ray and eosinophilia are suggestive of this diagnosis. The treatment is simple excision. Radiation therapy is rarely necessary but is effective.

Cholesteatoma. Many diagnoses of cholesteatoma of the paranasal sinuses may not be true cholesteatoma but the result of chronic caseous sinusitis with putrefaction. It is conceivable, however, that the sinus epithelium could undergo metaplasia to squamous epithelium, which in turn develops into a cholesteatoma. This situation is usually seen in the maxillary sinus but also may occur in the frontal sinuses. The treatment of choice is the radical antrum procedure or an obliteration of the frontal sinuses.

There are numerous other benign tumors found in the nasal cavities and paranasal sinuses, such as angioma, hemangioma, lymphangioma, chondroma, fibrous dysplasia, amyloid tumor, meningioma, and encephalocele. These tumors are quite rare and do not deserve special mention other than that the procedure of choice is excision.

MALIGNANT TUMORS OF THE NOSE AND PARANASAL SINUSES

In general squamous cell carcinoma is the most common malignant tumor of the nose and paranasal sinuses, accounting for approximately 60% of such tumors involving the sinuses (Jackson and Jackson). This percentage may vary considerably, for it is often difficult to distinguish a Grade IV squamous cell carcinoma from a lymphoepithelioma, transitional cell carcinoma, lymphosarcoma, and reticulum cell sarcoma. Malignant melanomas occur in the nasal fossa and paranasal sinuses. As elsewhere, they are highly malignant and difficult to treat.

Malignant tumors of glandular origin occurring in the nose and paranasal sinuses are adenocarcinomas, mixed tumors, cylindromas, and papillary adenocarcinomas.

Lesions of the sarcoma group include fibrosarcomas, myxosarcomas, rhabdomyosarcomas, fibromyxosarcomas, osteogenic sarcomas, and hemangioendotheliomas. Other minor tumors found in the paranasal sinuses are those of the reticuloendothelial system and lymphoid system and intracranial tumors, such as meningioma, pituitary malignancies, and chordoma. On occasion, metastatic lesions are found in the paranasal sinuses.

Diagnosis. Tumors of the nasal fossa and paranasal sinuses do not produce, for any particular lesion, consistent clinical manifestations. There may be a sensation of pressure or pain, or no pain. A unilateral nasal obstruction should be considered a neoplasm until proven otherwise. Discharge may be serous, serosanguineous, or purulent. There may be paresthesia, anesthesia, or paralysis of cranial nerves. Pain, if present, is apt to be worse at night or when the patient is recumbent. There may be symptoms referable to the upper teeth, or an upper denture may become ill-fitting. External swellings of the upper face, such as the side of the nose and region of the inner canthus, bulging of the cheek, and swelling of the hard palate, soft palate, alveolar ridge, or buccal fold may occur. Orbital manifestations of sinus tumors are relatively common. There may be interruption of the innervation of the extraocular muscles. The orbital contents may be displaced in various directions, resulting in proptosis and enophthalmos. A bulging behind either the infraorbital rim or supraorbital rim may be palpated. Obstructions of the lacrimal apparatus may occur. Trismus is a disturbing symptom, for it usually represents extension of the disease into the pterygoid region. Extension of disease into the nasopharynx may give symptoms of eustachian tube blockage, i.e., earache, tinnitus, and hearing loss.

A careful physical examination should include anterior-posterior rhinoscopy, use of the nasopharyngoscope, palpation for local disease as well as regional lymph node enlargement, and transillumination of the sinuses. The discharge should be carefully evaluated. A foul-smelling discharge may represent tissue necrosis, which is often associated with neoplastic disease. X-rays of the sinuses should include the nasopharynx and base of skull views. Stereoscopic x-rays are of value in determining the extent of disease and amount of bone destruction. Planograms of the involved area are most useful for outlining the disease.

Maxillary Sinus. The maxillary sinus is by far the most frequently involved of the paranasal sinuses with malignant tumors. This amounts to approximately 60% of cases. They also occur many times more frequently in men than in women and most often after the age of 50 years.

Diagnosis. The aforementioned signs and symptoms and x-ray studies may indicate a neoplasm of the maxillary sinus. The interpretation of a biopsy obtained by way of the Caldwell-Luc approach is conclusive. The rate of cure using either x-ray or surgery alone has been discouraging. Most reports indicate this as being below 30%. During recent years reported results using a combination of external radiation followed by surgery have been somewhat more encouraging. Preoperative x-ray therapy tends to shrink the size of the lesion and block the regional lymphatics. The dosage of preoperative radiation therapy must be carefully considered. It should be of sufficient magnitude to effect a shrinkage of the lesion and blockage of the lymphatics but not so great that it results in poor healing, osteoradionecrosis, or subsequent fibrosis of the muscles of mastication. These complications are quite serious, for they can be irreversibly progressive, leading to severe disfigurement and oral crippling. A preoperative dose of approximately 4500 R of cobalt 60 seems to be ideal. Surgery should be carried out 6 weeks after completion of radiation therapy. At this time there has been maximum regression of the tumor, the radiation reaction in the normal tissues is subsiding, and secondary changes in the normal tissue which interfere with healing have not occurred.

Maxillectomy. Endotracheal anesthesia is administered. The intratracheal tube is passed through the nostril on the side opposite the operation. The use of a cuffed endotracheal tube and a carefully placed pharyngeal pack will prevent blood from entering the tracheal bronchial tree. Ligation of the external carotid artery is well worth the extra time, for it considerably reduces the amount of blood lost during the operation. The incision is begun halfway between the inner canthus and the dorsum of the nose. It is continued inferiorly over the nasal bones anterior to the crease between the nose and cheek. If the incision is made in this crease, the scar is apt to become retracted. The incision is then carried around the alar cartilage of the nose to a point beyond the midline under the columella. A Z- or S-shaped incision produces much less scarring than does a vertical incision when the upper lip is split. The incision is then carried laterally from the point of origin of the lateral rhinotomy incision, extending within 2 or 3 mm of the lower lid tarsal plate laterally toward the ear above the zygomatic arch. The incidence of infraorbital edema is markedly reduced by keeping this horizontal incision within a few millimeters of the tarsal plate. Some surgeons prefer to omit the infraorbital incision because of the incidence of infraorbital edema

postoperatively. A cheek flap is elevated laterally. The mucous membrane incision along the buccogingival fold should extend beyond the posterior limit of the upper alveolar ridge. The cheek flap is elevated to expose the anterior aspect of the zygomatic arch and the masseter muscle.

The nasal cavity is entered by incising and reflecting to the opposite side the alar and upper lateral cartilages of the nose. The nasal bone is then incised using either Kerrison forceps or a Stryker saw. It is determined at this time whether or not the nasal septum is resected. The ascending process of the maxillary bone is cut across in like manner to the medial aspect of the infraorbital rim. A Gigli or Stryker saw is used to cut across the zygoma. With the use of an osteotome, the hard palate is split in the midline. A horizontal incision is then made between the hard and soft palates. This extends around the posterior aspect of the superior alveolar tuberosity, where it meets the posterior aspect of the buccogingival incision. The bony attachments of the maxilla have now been completely separated. The specimen can be removed with a heavy curved scissors. There may be considerable bleeding as the maxilla is removed. This is controlled by repeated packing and electrocoagulation of vessels. If there is any question of extension of disease in the direction of the ethmoidal or sphenoidal sinuses, they should be carefully cleaned out.

If there is extension of disease to the orbit, an examination of the orbit must be done in combination with the maxillectomy. The lids are sutured together. An additional incision beginning medial to the inner canthus is extended horizontally above the upper lid margin. This incision joins the lower horizontal incision lateral to the external canthus. The upper lid is dissected in a subcutaneous plane of cleavage to the supraorbital rim. The periosteum along the supraorbital rim is incised, and the upper half of the lateral and medial walls of the orbit and roof is exposed by elevating this periosteum. The operation now proceeds as a maxillectomy. The optic nerve and ophthalmic vessels are transected with curved scissors as the specimen is removed.

A large split-thickness skin graft is then carefully sutured in place so as to completely line the remaining cavity. All incisions are carefully sutured, using both subcutaneous and dermal sutures. The cavity is packed with petrolatum iodoform gauze, Cornish wool placed in a gauze basket, or antibiotic ointment–impregnated gauze packing. It is most important to cover the skin graft with a layer of Gelfoam before packing the cavity. Otherwise the skin graft may be pulled away as the packing is removed.

Postoperatively, the pack remains in place from 7 to 10 days. Prophylactic antibiotic therapy is administered during this time. Intraoral care is also quite important to prevent infection. As soon as healing is complete, impressions can be taken for a dental prosthesis.

Frontal Sinus. Primary carcinoma of the frontal sinus is quite rare and is usually not diagnosed until the time of surgery. If the operator suspects a tumor, a frozen section should be taken. If this reveals carcinoma, the entire sinus should be removed without regard for preservation of normal structures. This should include removal of the anterior-posterior walls, the interfrontal septum, and the floor, and a complete ethmoidectomy. Because of the difficulty of removing this entire complex, the operation should be supplemented by radiation therapy.

Ethmoidal Sinus. Carcinoma of the ethmoidal sinus is usually secondary. Epitheliomas and sarcomas, however, are occasionally primary in the ethmoidal sinuses.

Treatment. Because of the relationships of the ethmoidal sinus, complete removal by surgery of a carcinoma is rarely accomplished. A complete ethmoidectomy is carried out for both diagnosis and adequate drainage (technique in Chapter 13). This is followed by radiation therapy.

Sphenoidal Sinus. Primary malignancies of the sphenoidal sinus are also quite rare. Extension of malignancy from the nasal cavities, nasopharynx, other sinuses, and intracranial spaces is not rare. The cranial nerve involvement and planograms of the sphenoidal sinuses are the most valuable tools in determining the extent of the disease. The sphenoidal sinus is entered by way of the transethmoidal route (technique in Chapter 13) both for the purpose of biopsy and to establish adequate drainage. This is subsequently followed by radiation therapy.

REFERENCES

Bach, A. C., *et al.*: Nasopharyngeal Carcinoma. Arch. Otolaryng., *31*:529, 1940.

Belal, A.: Mucocele of the Maxillary Sinus. J. Laryngol. Otol., *65*:286, 1951.

Boenninghaus, H. G. Von: Siebbunosteom Duradefekt und Intracranielle Pneumatozele. Z. Laryngol. Rhinol. Otol., *39*:229, 1960.

Bromberg, B. E., *et al.*: Implant Reconstruction of the Orbit. Am. J. Surg., *100*:818, 1960.

Brunner, H., and Spiesman, I. C.: Osteoma of the Frontal and Ethmoid Sinuses. Ann. Otol. Rhinol. Laryngol., *57*:714, 1948.

Cauna, N., *et al.*: Fine Structure of Nasal Polyps. Ann. Otol., *81*:41, 1972.

Christensen, Lt. J. R., and Houck, L.: Mucocele of the Maxillary Sinus. Arch. Otolaryng., *59*:147, 1954.

Ersner, M. S., *et al.*: Reconstruction of the Orbital Floor Using Stainless Steel Wire Mesh. Arch. Otolaryng., *53*:658, 1961.

Jackson, C., and Jackson, C. L.: *Disease of the Nose, Throat and Ear.* Philadelphia, W. B. Saunders Co., 1943.

Lederer, F. L.: *Diseases of the Ear, Nose and Throat.* 6th ed. Philadelphia, F. A. Davis Co., 1953.

Leonardelli, G. B., *et al.*: La Pathologie Intraosseuse Gigantocellulaire des Maxillaires. Bibl. Otorhinolar., *6*:27, 1960.

Lundgren, A., and Olin, T.: Muco-pyocele of Sphenoidal Sinus or Posterior Ethmoidal Cells With Special Reference To the Apex Orbital Syndrome. Acta Otolaryng., *53*: 61, 1961.

Maduro, M. R., *et al.*: The Formation of Cysts of the Maxillary Sinus: A Report of 3 Cases. Ann. Otolaryng. (Paris), *78*:301, 1961.

Montgomery, W. W.: Osteoma of the Frontal Sinus. Ann. Otol. Rhinol. Laryngol., *69*: 245, 1960.

Montgomery, W. W.: Mucocele of the Maxillary Sinus Causing Enophthalmos. Eye, Ear, Nose and Throat Monthly, *43*:41, 1964.

Montgomery, W. W.: *Surgery of the Upper Respiratory Tract.* Vol. I, 1972; Vol. II, 1973. Philadelphia, Lea & Febiger.

236

Panikkar, S.: Three Cases of Swelling of the Upper Jaw With Unusual Features. J. Laryngol. Otol., *68*:842, 1954.

Parker, L. S.: Mucocele of the Right Maxillary Sinus With Proptosis of the Right Eye. J. Laryngol. Otol., *75*:527, 1961.

Sasso, B., and Smolcic, V.: Ocnog Odjela Opce Bolnice U Sibeniku T Usnog Odjela Opce Bolnice, Sibeniku. Med. Ark., *9*:113, 1955.

Witchell, I., and Vlessing, E.: Deformity of the Floor of the Orbit; Simulating a Tumor of the Maxillary Antrum. Eye, Ear, Nose and Throat Monthly, *39*:64, 1960.

PART 2
THE PHARYNX AND FAUCES

John J. Ballenger

Chapter 16
Surgical Anatomy of the Pharynx and Tonsil

SURGICAL ANATOMY OF THE PHARYNX

The pharynx is divided into the nasopharynx, or that portion of the pharynx situated above the soft palate, the oropharynx, that portion between the soft palate and the hyoid bone, and the laryngopharynx, which extends from the hyoid bone to the lower border of the cricoid cartilage.

Nasopharynx

The nasopharynx is formed above by the body of the sphenoid and the basilar process of the occipital bone, anteriorly by the choanae and the soft palate, and posteriorly by the cervical vertebrae; inferiorly the nasopharynx is continuous with the oropharynx. Situated on the lateral walls of the nasopharynx, behind the posterior ends of the inferior turbinates, are the orifices of the eustachian tubes. Above and behind the eustachian orifice is an elevation or ridge, formed by the eustachian cartilage, called the eustachian cushion. Extending downward from the posterior end of the ridge is a strong fold of mucous membrane, the salpingopharyngeal membrane. A less prominent fold of mucous membrane, the salpingopalatine membrane, extends downward in front of the eustachian orifice. The deep pocket formed at the angle of the pharynx between the posterior ridge of the eustachian cartilage and the posterior wall is known as the fossa of Rosenmüller. Frequently adenoid tissue is found around the orifice of the tube (tubal tonsil). The roof (fornix pharyngis) and the posterior wall of the nasopharynx form the seat of lymphoid tissue (adenoid, pharyngeal tonsil, Luschka's tonsil), which frequently attains considerable size, especially in children. The nasopharynx is covered with pseudostratified ciliated columnar (respiratory) epithelium. The oropharynx is lined with stratified squamous epithelium.

Adenoid

The pharyngeal tonsil or adenoid is a lobulated, lymphoid mass composed of lymphoid tissue similar to that of the tonsil. Its lobules or segments are arranged in regular order like separated segments of an orange with clefts or pockets between. These lobules are arranged around a central depression, called the *bursa pharyngea*. Many pockets and crevices are thus presented but no compound crypts. Thornwaldt's disease is essentially an infection of the bursa pharyngea.

Adenoid tissue in the nasopharynx is chiefly found on the upper and posterior walls, though it may extend to the fossa of Rosenmüller and to the orifices of the eustachian tubes. An adenoid is composed of lymphoid tissue enmeshed in a definite though comparatively delicate reticulum of fibrous connective tissue. The essential pathologic condition of an adenoid is characterized by hyperplasia of the lymphoid tissue of the nasopharynx.

The adenoid acts as a peripherally placed lymph node, from which efferent ducts pass to the nearest node in the cervical chain.

The adenoid tissue consists of a fibrous connective tissue framework, supporting masses of lymphoid cells. Owing to its peripheral position, however, it differs from the more deeply placed lymphatic nodes in having an epithelial covering upon its free surface. The supporting framework consists of fibrous septa passing through the substance of the gland, from which a very delicate connective tissue network ramifies in all directions toward the surface. It carries in it the blood vessels and the lymphatics, while here and there, lying in clusters in the septa, are many mucous glands whose ducts open on the surface. Mucous glands are frequently found within the adenoid at its base. In the meshes of the delicate network lie masses of leukocytes or lymphoid cells, constituting the lymphoid tissue which forms the main bulk of the adenoid. Groups of these cells are specially differentiated in the form of more or less rounded or oval-shaped areas, having centers of a pale appearance, while their margins are more darkly colored. These areas are the follicles or germ centers of Goodsir.

Epithelium. Completely covering the free surface of the adenoid and dipping down into its recesses and crypts is a layer of pseudostratified ciliated columnar epithelium, continuous with that lining the respiratory part of the interior of the nose and the adjacent mucous membrane of the nasopharynx. The epithelium consists of more than one layer of cells; the superficial ciliated cells are columnar in type, while the deeper cells forming two or three layers are smaller and rest upon a well-defined basement membrane. The epithelium covering the adenoid has no submucosa, as the latter passes directly beneath the base of the adenoid. While preserving its ciliated columnar type, the epithelium varies in thickness in parts, so that the lining of some of the crypts presents an irregular outline and is thinner.

Oropharynx

The oropharynx opens into the oral cavity at the anterior pillar of the fauces.

The soft palate (velum palati) consists of muscle fibers supported by fibrous tissue and an outer covering of mucous membrane. A median ridge or raphe divides it into two halves. The cone-shaped central projection is known as the uvula. The lateral margins of the palate on each side divide into the anterior and posterior pillars of the fauces. The anterior pillar contains the palatoglossus muscle. The posterior pillar contains the palatopharyngeus muscle. Between the two pillars is the recess in which the faucial tonsil is lodged.

The plica triangularis (tonsillaris) is a thin fold of mucous membrane, stretching backward from the anterior pillar and covering a portion of the anterior surface of the tonsil.

The plica semilunaris (supratonsillaris) is the upper fold of mucous membrane which unites the two pillars at their junction.

The supratonsillar fossa is a recess of variable size situated above the tonsil and between the anterior and posterior pillars. It is formed embryologically from the second branchial cleft.

Lingual Tonsil. The lingual tonsil, a sessile structure, is situated on the base of the tongue between the faucial tonsils and extends anteroposteriorly from the circumvallate papillae to the epiglottis. It is separated from the musculature of the tongue by a layer of fibrous tissue. The lingual tonsil is divided in the median line by the median glossoepiglottic ligament. The tonsil consists of numerous rounded or circular craterlike elevations, which are composed of lymphoid tissue and at their circumference are surrounded by connective tissue. In the center of each crater the mouth of the duct of a mucous gland opens. The crater or crypt is lined by stratified pavement epithelium. Branching of the crypts does not occur. They are simple tubes. The veins are part of a venous plexus which lies on the base of the tongue. Varicosities of these veins may occur. The arterial supply is from the external carotid through the dorsal lingual branch of the lingual artery. The lymphatic drainage is to the suprahyoid, submaxillary, and deep cervical lymph nodes. The nerve supply is from the ninth and the superior laryngeal branch of the tenth cranial nerves.

The pharyngeal, faucial, and lingual tonsils and the lateral pharyngeal bands form the so-called *Waldeyer's ring.*

Laryngopharynx

The laryngopharynx is partially separated from the oropharynx by the pharyngoepiglottic fold, which extends from the epiglottis to the side of the pharynx.

The mucous membrane of the laryngopharynx is covered with pseudostratified cilliated columnar epithelium except over the laryngeal surface of the epiglottis, the anterior surface of the arytenoids, and the free edges of the true vocal cords, where stratified squamous epithelium is found. Many mucous glands and much lymphoid tissue are present. The lymphoid tissue is collected into small masses (lymphoid follicles) at numerous points throughout the pharynx.

The muscles of the pharynx consist of the superior, middle, and inferior constrictors of the pharynx; the stylopharyngeus; and the palatopharyngeus.

The muscles of the soft palate are the azygos uvulae, levator palati, tensor palati, palatoglossus, and palatopharyngeus.

PHYSIOLOGY OF THE PHARYNX

Nasopharynx

The chief function of the nasopharynx is to serve as a rigid open tube for respired air. During swallowing, vomiting, belching, and gagging, it is completely separated from the oropharynx by elevation of the soft palate against the posterior wall of the oropharynx.

The nasopharynx also serves as a channel for ventilation of the middle ear through the eustachian tubes and as a channel for drainage from the nose and the eustachian tubes. As a resonating chamber, it is of much importance in the production of the voice.

Oropharynx and Laryngopharynx

This part of the pharynx serves not only as a respiratory passageway but also as a drainage channel from the nasopharynx, as a channel for the passage of food and drink taken into the mouth, and lastly as a resonating chamber in voice production. It is open to the free passage of air at all times except during swallowing or vomiting. The lymphoid tissue found in the nasopharynx, oropharynx, and laryngopharynx also has a protective function; it removes and destroys foreign material entering by way of the mouth or nose and also participates in the formation of antibodies (see discussion of Waldeyer's ring).

The mechanism of *swallowing* consists essentially of three phases. The initial or voluntary phase occurs when the bolus of food or drink introduced into the mouth is forced, after mastication, by the tongue and contraction of the tonsil pillars through the arches of the fauces. As this occurs, the soft palate contracts and closes off the nasopharynx.

The second stage is involuntary and encompasses the passage of food from the fauces to the entrance of the esophagus. A final stage, also involuntary, occurs when the food passes down the esophagus. Contraction of the pharyngeal constrictor muscles presses the food downward to the entrance of the esophagus, which opens to receive it. During the second stage, there is an elevation of the epiglottis and closure of the superior sphincter of the larynx. Food passage down the esophagus is assisted by positive pressure, peristaltic waves of the esophageal walls, and negative pressure within the esophageal lumen.

SURGICAL ANATOMY OF THE TONSIL

Embryology

The tonsil is situated in the sinus tonsillaris between the faucial pillars and has its origin in an invagination of the hypoblasts at this point. Later the depression thus formed is subdivided into several compartments, which become the permanent crypts of the tonsil. Lymphoid tissue is deposited around the crypts, and thus the tonsillar mass is built up. The inner or exposed surface, including the cryptic depressions, is covered with mucous membrane, while the outer or hidden surface is covered by a fibrous sheath called the capsule.

The anlagen of the tonsils appear in early fetal life. They are visible in the fourth month, at first as simple invaginations of the mucous membrane at a point between the second and third branchial arches at the second branchial pouch.

The development of the faucial tonsil is easily studied in the rabbit, in which the single primary crypt generally remains without branches. The tonsil first appears in embryos and is about ⅝ inch long (occipito-sacral measurement), or it appears at about 12 days as a shallow epithelial fold whose apex points directly backward into the connective tissue concentrically condensed around the pharynx. At this stage there is no infiltration of the leukocytes in the connective tissue around the crypt, and it is not until the embryos are about 21 days old (1³⁄₁₆ inches long) that the leukocytic infiltration becomes evident. The crypt has then become much deeper and broader and by its ingrowth has produced a condensation of the connective tissues at right angles to the original peripharyngeal condensation, as well as a great increase in the number of capillary blood vessels. From this stage the elongation of the crypt, the condensation of the connective tissue, the increase in the number of blood vessels, and the amount of leukocytic infiltration go on pari passu until the adult condition is reached. As soon as the leukocytes appear in numbers in the submucous tissue, they proceed to escape through the epithelium.

In the fetus of the pig, the condensation of the connective tissue, especially at the apex of the tonsillar crypts, and the consequent massing of leukocytes, mainly at these points, are particularly well shown.

In the human fetus the process is the same, though complicated by the early ramification of the original epithelial crypt and the appearance of fresh ones. The crypts become so deep that the cells from the surface layers of their epithelium cannot at once be thrown off into the mouth, and they remain as a concentrically arranged mass of degenerated hornified cells filling up the lumen of the crypt; this mass is ultimately forced out by the vis a tergo of the leukocytes emigrating through the epithelium. It will at once be seen how closely this resembles the formation of the concentric corpuscles of the thymus.

The prime factor in the formation of the tonsils is the epithelial ingrowth, which partly mechanically compresses the meshes of the connective tissue and partly causes proliferation of the connective cells and vessels by the slight irritation it produces. This makes it easier for the leukocytes to escape from the thin-walled capillaries and veno-capillaries so formed and, when they have escaped, causes them to be detained in the finely meshed connective tissue longer than in other situations. As the leukocytes are well supplied with nutriment, they divide by mitosis in large numbers, and at a late stage in development (with great variations in individuals), "germ centers" are formed, where a special arrangement of connective tissue and vessels favors the process of division.

The lingual and pharyngeal tonsils develop in the same way as the faucial tonsils. His shows that all the tonsils arise behind the membrana pharyngis; consequently, all these epithelial ingrowths pass into connective tissue already condensed around the primitive alimentary canal.

Anatomy

The faucial tonsils, one on each side of the oropharynx, are almond-shaped masses of lymphoid tissue imbedded in an apparent fibrous capsule. The inner or free surface is covered by a closely adherent stratified squamous epithelial membrane. This epithelium extends into the blind pouches or crypts which have their openings onto the surface of the tonsil. The epithelium lining the crypts is thin and offers poor protection to bacterial infection.

The tonsil does not always completely fill the sinus tonsillaris, the unoccupied space above it being known as the supratonsillar fossa.

The outer aspect of the tonsil is loosely attached to the superior constrictor muscle of the pharynx, thus subjecting it to compression with every act of deglutition. The palatoglossus and palatopharyngeus muscles of the pillars also compress the tonsil.

As viewed under the microscope the tonsil consists of three chief elements: the connective tissue, the germinating follicles, and the interfollicular tissue.

1. The connective tissue, that is, the trabecula or reticulum, acts as a supporting framework for the tonsil substance proper. The trabeculae carry blood vessels, nerves, and lymphatics.

2. The germinating follicles are the centers wherein the large mother cells of the leukocytic group undergo karyokinesis and form young lymphoid cells.

3. The interfollicular tissue is made up of lymphoid cells in various stages of development. These cells differ in size and shape according to their location. They are greater in number around the follicles and show greater difference in their anatomic construction in the immediate neighborhood of the crypts.

Capsule. The tonsil is always described as having a "capsule," but the existence of a definite capsule is denied by certain anatomists. What, for all clinical purposes, serves as a capsule is a white fibrous sheath called the pharyngeal fascia that encloses four-fifths of the tonsil.

Fowler and Todd have found in their dissections a thin, delicate areolar tissue separating the true tonsillar tissue from the muscles of its bed. This areolar tissue can be split into layers, between which are spaces of varying size. This would account for the ease of dissecting the upper pole of the tonsil and also for the tendency of a peritonsillar abscess to burrow around the upper half of the tonsil.

The capsule of the tonsil sends out trabeculae which pass into the parenchyma. These trabeculae carry blood vessels, nerves, and efferent lymphatics. Afferent lymphatics are absent.

Plica Triangularis. The plica triangularis is a normal structure appearing in embryonal life, and in some of the lower animals it develops into the tonsil itself. There is no muscular tissue in the plica triangularis, and it should be removed with the tonsil. When it is left in place, it may form a pocket or pouch where food and other debris collect. It is the source of considerable local irritation, and the lymphoid tissue with which it is thickly studded may be the seat of a future hyperplasia or infection.

Crypts. The crypts, from 8 to 20 in number, are usually tubular and almost invariably extend the entire depth of the tonsil to the capsule on its outer surface. Most are compound, i.e., they divide below the surface into two or more tubules. They are usually comparatively straight, though they may be tortuous in their course. Those opening in the supratonsillar fossa usually extend downward and outward, whereas in the lower portion of the tonsil their direction is outward.

The subepithelial connective tissue which is present in a marked degree beneath the surface epithelium disappears as soon as the epithelium starts to form the crypts. This permits the epithelial cells to come in direct contact with the lymphatic structures of the tonsil, and frequently it is impossible to distinguish a dividing line between the epithelium of the crypt and the interfollicular tissue. The epithelium of the crypt, unlike its progenitor which covers the surface of the tonsil, does not form a compact unbroken barrier of protection. For the greater part of its extent it presents an intact line only one or two, possibly three, cells in thickness. Toward the parenchyma, the epithelial cells show a peculiar condition. They are separated from each other by interposed cells varying in type from slightly changed epithelial cells to well-formed lymphocytes. The epithelial cells may also extend from the crypt into the tonsillar substance, suggesting the ramifications of a malignant epithelioma. The smaller terminal invaginations of the cryptal epithelium are usually solid sprouts, frequently with central keratotic cores. The lumen of the crypt is formed by the subsequent exfoliation of the keratotic cells.

Clinically the crypts seem to be the source of the greatest amount of local and constitutional disturbances, as they often become filled with food, tissue debris, and bacteria.

Tonsillar Fossa (Sinus Tonsillaris)

The anterior pillar contains the palatoglossus muscle (Fig. 16–1) and forms the anterior boundary, whereas the posterior pillar contains the palatopharyngeus muscle and forms the posterior boundary of the sinus.

The palatoglossus has a fan-shaped origin in the oral surface of the soft palate and terminates in the lateral side of the tongue.

The palatopharyngeus is a vertically arranged muscle attached above to the soft palate, the eustachian tube, and the base of the skull. It extends downward to the upper esophageal wall. This muscle is of greater importance than the palatoglossus. Great care should be taken not to injure this muscle during the tonsil operation.

The pillars meet above to unite with the soft palate. Inferiorly they diverge and enter into the tissues at the base of the tongue and the lateral wall of the pharynx. The outer wall of the tonsillar fossa is composed of the superior constrictor muscle of the pharynx.

The superior constrictor muscle has transversely disposed fibers. It forms the circular musculature of the pharynx. It originates

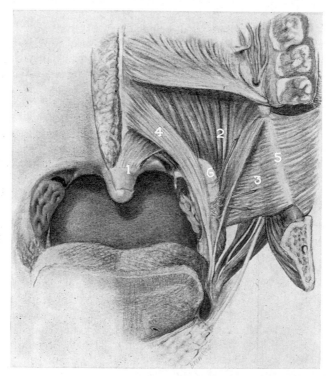

FIG. 16–1.   In front of the raphe is seen the buccinator muscle. The superior constrictor muscle runs back from the raphe. Below this, from without inward, are seen the mandible, internal pterygoid, lingual nerve, styloglossus, glossopharyngeal nerve, stylopharyngeus, and palatopharyngeus, behind which is seen the tonsil capsule (its upper lobe a hood, its lower lobe a pocket). Behind and lateral to these are vertical fibers of the pharynx, running to the soft palate and the hamular process. These are continued posteriorly as coarser fibers—the palatopharyngeus. Vessels and nerves are shown descending from the palate to the tonsil, together with the attachment of the tonsillopharyngeus in the groove between the upper and lower lobes. *1,* Levator palati; *2,* palatopharyngeus; *3,* superior constrictor; *4,* palatoglossus; *5,* pterygomandibular raphe with superior constrictor medially and buccinator laterally; *6,* upper lobe or hood of tonsil. (Fowler, R. H., and Todd, T. W.: J.A.M.A., *90*(2):1613, 1928.)

from the lower portion of the internal pterygoid plate, the hamular process, the pterygomandibular ligament, and the mandible.

Fowler and Todd describe a fourth muscle which they named the tonsillopharyngeus. It is formed by fibers of the lateral part of the palatopharyngeus. It is attached to the capsule of the tonsil at the junction of the upper and lower lobes.

Lymphatics

The lymph nodes are subdivided into groups according to the region occupied (Fig. 16–2). The suboccipital group (2 to 3) usually lies near the insertion of the occipital muscle. These lymph nodes receive afferent vessels from the lower occipital part of the head. The efferent vessels run to the upper substernal mastoid nodes. The mastoid or retroauricular nodes (usually in pairs) are found near the insertion of the sternocleidomastoid muscle. They receive afferent vessels from the temporal portion of the head, the internal surface of the ear, and the posterior part of the auditory canal.

The parotid nodes (3 to 16) are composed of the superficial and deep nodes over the parotid area, under the superior aponeurosis. The afferent vesels are received from the external part of the ear, the skin over the temporal and frontal regions, the eyelids, the outer part of the nose, and the anterior part of the auditory canal.

The submaxillary group (3 to 6) is found along the inferior border of the maxilla lying upon the submaxillary gland. These lymph nodes receive afferent vessels from the nose, cheek, upper lip, external part of the lower lip, gum, and anterior part of the tongue. The efferent vessels empty into the deep cervical chain.

The submental group (1 to 4) has afferent vessels from the skin over the chin, middle of the lower lip, floor of the mouth, and tip of the tongue. Efferent vessels go to the submaxillary nodes and to a node on the external jugular vein.

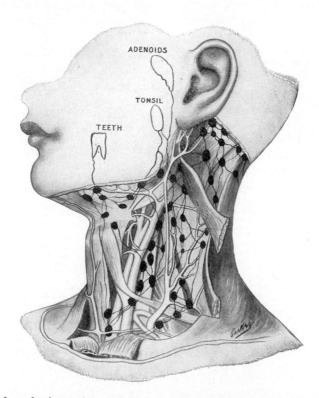

Fig. 16–2. The lymphatic nodes and vessels of the neck which drain the teeth, tonsils, adenoid, pharynx, and mastoid region.

The retropharyngeal nodes (1 to 10) are located on the posterior and lateral pharyngeal walls about the level of the atlas bone. The afferent vessels are from the mucosa of the nasal fossa, sinuses, nasopharynx, eustachian tube, and lymphatics from the internal ear. Efferent vessels empty into the internal jugular chain.

The descending deep cervical chain (carotid group) of nodes accompanies the great vessels of the neck to the chest. These lymph nodes lie beneath the sternocleidomastoid muscle and constitute the most important group of lymph nodes in the body. There are from 15 to 30 nodes in this group. An external jugular group is placed posteriorly and externally to the internal group. The internal nodes lie on and parallel to the internal jugular.

The external group receives efferent vessels from the mastoid nodes, the suboccipital, and some vessels from the nodes about the external jugular, a portion of the occipital region of the scalp, the lobe of the ear, the cutaneous lymphatics from the upper part of the neck, part of the nasal fossae, and the nasopharynx.

The internal group receives efferent vessels from the retropharyngeal, parotid, submaxillary, and submental nodes, a large part of the lymphatics from the tongue and nasopharynx, all the middle and inferior part of the pharynx, the cervical part of the esophagus and trachea, nasal fossa, thyroid gland, tonsils, hard palate, orbit, and larynx.

The tonsillar lymphatic vessels drain into the deep cervical chain underneath the sternocleidomastoid muscle, thence to the thoracic nodes, and finally into the thoracic duct. By this route, infection may be carried to all parts of the body.

Blood Supply

The blood supply to the pharynx comes from many sources and is sometimes irregular. The chief supply is derived from the ascending pharyngeal and faucial branches of the external carotid and from the superior palatine of the internal maxillary.

The tonsillar artery (see Fig. 19–15), a branch of the external maxillary, is the chief vessel to the tonsil, though the ascending palatine, another branch of the external maxillary, sometimes takes its place. The tonsillar artery passes upward on the outer side of the superior constrictor muscle, through which it passes and gives off branches to the tonsil and soft palate. The ascending palatine, another branch of the external maxillary, also sends branches through the superior constrictor muscle to the tonsil. The ascending pharyngeal passes upward outside of the superior constrictor, and when the ascending palatine artery is small, it gives off a tonsillar branch which is correspondingly larger. The dorsalis lingualis, a branch of the lingual artery, ascends to the base of the tongue and sends branches to the tonsil and pillars of the fauces. The descending or posterior palatine artery, a branch of the internal maxillary, supplies the tonsil and soft palate from above, forming anastomoses with the ascending palatine. The small meningeal artery sends more branches to the tonsils, though they are of minor importance.

Chapter 17
Diseases of the Pharynx and Fauces

Many of the diseases of the pharynx and fauces are but another part of a more widespread upper respiratory infection. The etiology and description of these diseases have been covered in Part I, Chapters 8 and 9, and will not be repeated here. Other diseases of particular interest to the pharynx and fauces will be covered here, including those in which a general body ill may be detected by a typical manifestation in the pharynx and fauces.

SIMPLE ACUTE PHARYNGITIS

This form of acute pharyngitis is usually accompanied by acute rhinitis or a "'cold,'" though the pharynx may be involved to a greater extent than the nose or larynx.

Etiology and Pathology. The etiology and pathology are the same as for other acute respiratory infections and will not be repeated.

Symptoms. The onset is characterized by malaise and a slight rise in temperature. The borders of the soft palate and uvula are slightly red, while the adjacent mucous membrane is normal in appearance. As the disease progresses, the uvula becomes slightly edematous and the secretions are increased; it may become markedly edematous and painful, though this is not common. The tonsils are usually congested. Pain on swallowing and stiffness and aching of the muscles of the neck are noted.

Treatment. The general treatment as given for other acute respiratory infections is applicable to this condition.

EDEMA OF THE UVULA

Acute inflammation of the faucial structures is frequently attended by edema of the uvula. It frequently follows acute infections, as well as excessive or faulty use of the voice.

It usually disappears spontaneously. If it becomes troublesome, the edematous portion may be scarified by multiple punctures which allow the excess serum to escape.

CHRONIC PHARYNGITIS; GRANULAR PHARYNGITIS

This disease is a chronic inflammation of the pharynx, usually with granular hypertrophy of the posterior wall.

Etiology. It seems most likely that the cause of this disease lies in allergy, air pollution, or smoking. Mouth breathing, which bypasses the humidifying, tempering, and cleansing function of the nose, certainly would exacerbate the situation. Crusting and dryness of the pharynx accompany atrophic rhinitis.

Pathology. The superficially located lymphoid nodules of the pharyngeal mucosa are the primary site of hypertrophy and impart a granular appearance. In addition, the lateral pharyngeal bands may be much enlarged and the mucosa throughout the pharynx diffusely red.

Symptoms. The most common symptoms are a sense of dryness, soreness, or irritation of the throat. There may be a frequent desire to clear the throat. Secretions are frequently dry, tenacious, or, at a later stage, absent, so that the posterior wall is dry and glazed.

Treatment. Discovery and removal of the etiologic factor is paramount. In general, smoking should be absolutely prohibited and attention then directed to the residual symptoms.

When the superficial lymphoid follicles or lateral bands appear to be the seat of discomfort, they may be treated individually at weekly intervals with 10% silver nitrate. Occasionally surgical removal of the lateral bands is indicated. For the difficult dryness and crusting in the nasopharynx, an irrigating spray consisting of 3% alcohol and 6% glycerine in 0.85% saline solution may be administered via the mouth or nose.

AGRANULOCYTOSIS

Etiology. Agranulocytosis (agranulocytic angina, malignant neutropenia) is an uicerative and gangrenous angina of the oropharynx and other mucosal surfaces accompanied by a profound granulocytopenia and usually by a reduction in the total leukocyte count. The number of drugs and chemical agents capable of depressing leukocytopoiesis is legion. These drugs include derivatives of the benzene ring, amidopyrine, dinitrophenol, some antithyroid drugs, anticonvulsant drugs, some sulfonamides, nitrogen mustard, some tranquilizing drugs, DDT, arsenic, gold, and many others. Irradiation may also be a factor. Whether or not there is a sensitization factor involved is a moot point.

Symptoms and Signs. In the absence of secondary infection, malaise and moderate fever may be the only symptoms. If infection is present, however, the onset may be abrupt, with chills and high fever, marked prostration, and an extreme sore throat. The lesions in the mouth and pharynx vary from a small superficial ulcer to widespread gangrene, frequently beginning as a membrane in the region of the tonsils or along the gingival margins. Later, necrotic ulcers, surrounded by a dearth of inflammatory reaction, appear. Cultures show staphylococci, streptococci, and Vincent's organisms as secondary invaders.

The blood smear demonstrates a remarkable lack of granulocytes. Of the leukocytes that remain, 95% may be lymphocytes. The erythrocytes fail to show diagnostic change, though secondary anemia may be present.

The lesion in the oropharynx may be confused with acute "aleukemic" leukemia, infectious mononucleosis, Hodgkin's disease, acute follicular tonsillitis, Vincent's angina, and diphtheria.

Treatment. Prompt removal of the offending drug is essential. Antibiotics should be administered to control secondary infection, and supportive therapy should be provided. Corticoids and ACTH have been reported to hasten recovery but should be used with caution because they may further depress resistance to infection. If infection can be controlled and the offending drug identified and withdrawn, the prognosis is good for recovery in 5 to 7 days.

LEUKEMIA

Leukemia, a progressive neoplastic disease, is characterized by an abnormal and widespread proliferation of leukocytes, particularly in the bone marrow, spleen, and lymph nodes. Although it is invariably fatal, the course of the disease may run from merely a few weeks to several years. The etiology is obscure, though many workers consider it to be due to an oncogenic virus.

Clinical Manifestations. In chronic myelogenous leukemia, the most common symptoms are anemia, splenic enlargement, and loss of weight. Low-grade fever, usually below 101°F, may be present. Lymph node enlargement, unlike in lymphocytic leukemia, is rarely present. Deafness from infiltration in the middle or inner ears occasionally is noted. In chronic lymphocytic leukemia, the presenting symptoms may be a painless enlargement of the cervical or axillary lymph nodes.

In acute leukemia the onset is much more abrupt and may be indicated by fever, sore throat, and abnormal bleeding from mucous membranes. The gums may be swollen and purplish in color, and ulcerations may be found in the mouth. Lymph node enlargement is less conspicuous than in the chronic forms of the disease.

The most frequent lesion of the throat is the marked enlargement of the tonsils, usually accompanied by considerable pain. Necrotic lesions of the tonsil or pharynx must be differentiated from tonsillitis, diphtheria, tuberculosis, Vincent's angina, and both bacterial and viral afflictions of the pharynx.

LEUKOPLAKIA

Leukoplakia of the mouth and throat is a chronic painless keratinization of the mucous membrane. The milky white patches are usually found on one or more regions of the tongue, palate, buccal mucous membrane, posterior gums, floor of the mouth, angles of the mouth, and at times the larynx.

Etiology. The exact cause is unknown. It is thought to be due to long-continued irritations, such as tobacco or ill-fitting dentures. Chemical or mechanical irritations of any type may be factors in the etiology. It is most common in men past middle age.

Pathology. The keratinization is the result of a proliferation of the superficial layer of the mucous membrane and sometimes of the filiform papillae. It may occur as a smooth area, a raised plaque, or a papillomatous type of lesion. It is considered a precursor of cancer in some instances.

Symptoms. The onset is insidious and without symptoms. In a later stage there may be sensations of burning or irritation. An induration can usually be felt upon palpation.

The differential diagnosis includes syphilis, lichen planus, burns, and various ulcerations. A biopsy may be necessary for differentiation.

Treatment. All possible causes of irritation, including oral sepsis, should be eliminated. Use of tobacco in any form is strictly prohibited, and it is well, too, to eliminate highly seasoned foods and strong alcoholic beverages.

Small lesions may be removed surgically. It does no good and may possibly be harmful to treat leukoplakia with electrocoagulation and radiation therapy. The patient should be examined every 3 to 6 months, and a biopsy should be performed if any change has occurred in the size or nature of the leukoplakic lesion.

Vitamin A therapy, 100,000 to 200,000 units per day for prolonged periods, may be helpful.

PEMPHIGUS

Pemphigus (Fig. 17–1) is a slowly progressive disease of the skin and mucous membrane characterized by the formation of bullae, by remissions, and, if untreated, by death in a year or so.

Etiology. The cause of this disease is not known. It usually occurs in adult life, with a slight prevalence of females over males and perhaps a tendency to occur more frequently in Semitic people.

Symptoms. The first lesions on the mucous membrane of the oropharynx and larynx are small blisters which are not painful. Later the blisters rupture and become secondarily infected and painful. The patient almost invariably is seen in the latter state, so that only tattered remnants of the ruptured bleb are seen. The presence of the epithelial tags at the periphery of eroded painful areas in the mouth is an aid to diagnosis.

Treatment. Secondary infection must be controlled by the use of antibiotics, but this has no effect on the essential problem. Main reliance must be placed on corticosteroid therapy. There is a growing list of patients who have been in remission for several years on this therapy.

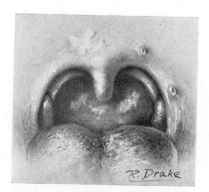

FIG. 17–1 Pemphigus of the pharynx. Note the fibrinous exudate over the palate and pharynx and the two bullae on the left soft palate and anterior pillar. (New, Arch. Otolaryngol.)

CANDIDIASIS AND THRUSH

Occasionally the oral mucous membrane may be the site of infections with *Candida albicans*. In this situation the mucosa, including that of the tonsils, gums, and tongue, is partly covered by white patches. *Candida albicans* is usually culturable from the mucosa of the mouth. It multiplies greatly if the growth of the normal bacterial flora is suppressed by antibiotics or chemotherapy. The presence of inadequately managed diabetes, pregnancy, or debility enhances the growth of the *Candida* as well. A mild form of candidiasis is called "thrush" and is seen commonly in infants. Thrush frequently is related to candidiasis of the birth canal or to contaminated nipples or the bottle.

Symptoms. The stomatitis caused by the *Candida* gives rise to a sore throat, a dry mouth, and to salivation. The infection may persist for years and be relatively refractory to treatment. The lesions resemble somewhat a deposit of coagulated milk but are adherent and when forcibly removed give rise to bleeding from the surfaces of the affected mucosa. Oral candidiasis, if uncontrolled, can eventuate in granulomata of the mucosa and may spread to the trachea and esophagus.

Treatment. Topical applications of nystatin is probably the most effective treatment. Nystatin orally is less useful. Any measures necessary to improve the general health also are in order.

LICHEN PLANUS

Lichen planus in the mouth may consist of gray or dull white dots with a stellate or delicate lacework arrangement (Fig. 17-2). The etiology is obscure, though dental plates of a poor fit or dental disease, as well as smoking, may be factors. Symptoms may consist of no more than a rough or burning sensation in the area.

The treatment consists of removal of all mouth irritants and infections. The general body conditions should be treated as indicated and an adequate intake of vitamins assured.

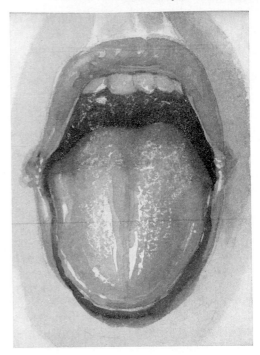

FIG. 17–2. Lichen planus of the tongue and buccal mucosa. Diagnosis of oral lichen planus may be difficult if the characteristic skin lesions are absent.

BLACK HAIRY TONGUE

Black hairy tongue is characterized by an excessive growth of the filiform papillae of the tongue, producing an appearance of hairiness. The pigmentation, varying from brown to black, seems to be due to the superimposed organisms.

Etiology. The exact cause is unknown. It is most frequently found in older men with various types of infections of the upper respiratory tract. The true cases of hairy tongue have been attributed to an anomaly of development, possibly congenital, of the filiform papillae. There is no evidence that fungi or other types of infection are the cause; they merely contribute to the pathology as a superimposed infection. A deficiency of nicotinic acid in the diet has been advanced as an etiologic factor. Excessive use of tobacco, keratosis, and inflammatory changes of the tongue have been mentioned.

Pathology. The tips of the filiform papillae are elongated and usually composed of normally short tufts of cornified cell material which may extend from ⅛ to ½ inch. The papillae are fairly stable and may remain unchanged for an indefinite period. They are usually localized on the posterior portion of the tongue. Hairy black tongue due to the oral use of penicillin usually disappears a week or so after the antibiotic is discontinued.

Treatment. The treatment of the true type of hairy black tongue consists of maintaining proper oral hygiene and clipping off the excessively long papillae. A diet high in vitamins, especially nicotinic acid, may be helpful.

MACROGLOSSIA

Macroglossia or unusual enlargement of the tongue is rare. In congenital cases the overgrowth may be muscular or lymphangiomatous. It has been reported in association with primary systemic amyloidosis, myxedema, acromegaly, tertiary syphilis, and glycogenosis (von Gierke's disease of the muscle).

INFECTIOUS MONONUCLEOSIS

Infectious mononucleosis is a benign infectious disease characterized by irregular fever, pharyngitis, cervical lymph node enlargement, absolute lymphocytosis, and occasionally splenomegaly and hepatomegaly. Evidence has recently accumulated that there is a causal relationship between the Epstein-Barr virus (EBV) and this disease. Antibodies to the EBV can be demonstrated which persist for years. In the past, the time-honored diagnostic test for infectious mononucleosis was a search for heterophile antibodies (Paul-Bunnell), but these are less regularly found and disappear in a matter of weeks. The heterophile antibody test is operationally defined as a sheep agglutinin that gives an antibody titer of 1:28 or greater. This agglutinin is not removed by adsorption with guinea pig kidney antigen but is completely adsorbed by beef erythrocytes.

In the peripheral blood the white blood cell count, after the first week, is 10,000 to 15,000/cu mm, and the lymphocytes constitute 50% or more. In addition to this, many of the lymphocytes demonstrate an "atypical" oval, kidney-shaped, or slightly lobulated nucleus, and the cytoplasm may appear vacuolated.

Symptoms. The incubation period is uncertain, varying from a few days to several

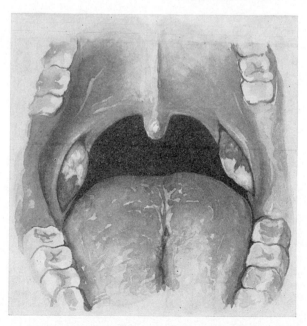

Fɪɢ. 17–3.   Infectious mononucleosis. The white irregular membrane is frequently found in this condition.

weeks. Malaise is followed by fever, sore throat, and headache. Typically the striking feature when the patient presents himself for examination is a diffusely injected and membranous pharyngotonsillitis with cervical lymphadenopathy (Fig. 17-3). Lymphoid hyperplasia within the pharynx itself may be so pronounced as to justify concern about the airway.

Not infrequently fusospirochetal and hemolytic streptococcal organisms may be present as secondary invaders. Less commonly the picture of hepatitis may be seen. Splenic rupture has been reported.

Treatment. No specific treatment is available, and reliance must be placed on symptomatic therapy and bedrest. Secondary bacterial invaders, once identified, should be treated by the appropriate medication. Corticotropin and steroid therapy should be reserved for the most serious situations.

ORAL AND PHARYNGEAL LESIONS ASSOCIATED WITH DERMATOLOGIC CONDITIONS

Oral and pharyngeal lesions associated with dermatologic conditions are varied. They embrace such common conditions as syphilis, tuberculosis, lupus, leukoplakia, neoplasms, the exanthemas, Vincent's angina, and canker sores. Other rare conditions with which they are associated include blastomycosis, coccidioidal granuloma (endemic in certain regions in California), cryptococcosis (due to *Cryptococcus neoformans,* which usually attacks the brain and meninges), sporotrichosis (usually in the form of ulcers), actinomycosis, tularemic ulcers, xanthoma, scleroma (Mikulicz's or foam cells containing Frisch's encapsulated bacillus associated with plasma cells and Russell bodies), lymphoblastomas (mycosis fungoides, Hodgkin's disease, leukemias, and lymphosarcoma), fungal infections (hairy tongue or black tongue, usually actinomycosis), perlèche (due to *Cryptococcus* or *Candida* usually occurring in children as a smooth, grayish white thickening on the mucous side of the commissures of the mouth), thrush (candidiasis), lichen planus, vitamin deficiencies (pellagra and scurvy), acrodynia, allergic gingivitis and stomatitis, and erythema multiforme. Certain drugs may produce eruptions of the mucosa as well as of the skin. These drugs include phenolphthalein, barbiturates, quinine, and arsphenamine.

Pigmentation, gingivitis, and stomatitis may be caused by the heavy metals, such as bismuth, mercury, lead, gold, and silver. Pigmentation of the buccal mucosa may also occur in Addison's disease, acanthosis nigricans, and hemochromatosis.

The mucous membrane may be involved in scleroderma, herpes zoster, impetigo, and granulomatous conditions such as yaws, leprosy, leishmaniasis, lymphogranuloma venereum, granuloma pyogenicum, molluscum contagiosum, and occupational dermatoses.

ERYTHEMA MULTIFORME

Oral lesions are commonly seen in this acute dermatosis of unknown etiology. The onset is abrupt and often accompanied by fever. Initially the lesions are intense red macules which may progress to papules, bullae, wheals, etc. Often in a day or two the lesions show central clearing. Later, overlapping of adjacent lesions produces bizarre shapes. The attack may last 1 to 4 weeks.

This disease may be successfully treated with cortisone drugs. Secondary infections must be controlled with antibiotic medication.

STEVENS-JOHNSON SYNDROME

This syndrome may represent a more severe form of erythema multiforme. It is characterized by a severe stomatitis, frequently a purulent conjunctivitis, and skin eruptions similar to those of erythema multiforme. The onset is abrupt, and prostration is marked. Again the etiology is unknown, and cortisone medication, along with antibiotics to control secondary infection, is the most effective treatment.

ELONGATED UVULA

The cause of elongated uvula is not known; there may be a possible hereditary

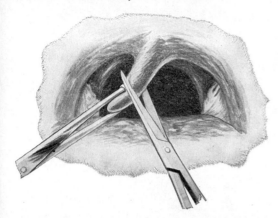

Fig. 17–4. Amputation of the elongated tip of the uvula just below the lower extremity of the muscle. The scissors are so applied that the posterior surface of the uvula will be the wounded surface. This lessens the irritation in swallowing food and in breathing through the mouth.

influence. It has been attributed to a chronic nasopharyngitis.

The uvula may be slender and pendulous, or it may be enlarged and pendulous.

Symptoms. In most subjects it causes slight symptoms or none at all. In sensitive patients it often causes a reflex cough when it touches the epiglottis or base of the tongue. The cough may be spasmodic and is usually dry. Nausea and vomiting, especially early in the morning, are sometimes mentioned.

Treatment. In mild cases astringent lozenges afford relief. The uvula may also be painted with astringent solutions of alum or tannic acid or with epinephrine. In the more severe cases amputation is indicated. In all cases the nasopharynx and the orophayrnx

should be examined and any diseased conditions treated.

Surgical Treatment. The uvula should be painted with a topical anesthetic solution. The tip of the uvula is then seized with forceps and drawn directly forward. While in this position, the tip should be severed with heavy blunt scissors, as shown in Figure 17–4. By cutting the uvula in front while it is drawn anteriorly, the beveled cut surface of the stump faces posteriorly (Fig. 17–5). This is a point of practical importance; thus when solid food is being swallowed, the raw surface is not irritated by it.

CALCULI OF THE SALIVARY GLANDS

Calculi may form in all the salivary glands or their ducts, but the larger proportion, about 70 to 80%, is found in the submaxillary gland or duct. The parotid and sublingual glands furnish from 15 to 20%. They are found more frequently in the ducts than in the glands.

Salivary calculi are largely composed of phosphate and carbonate of calcium. The lesser constituents are calcium fluoride, sodium and calcium chloride, and a small amount of sulfocyanide of potassium. Animal matter and bacteria form a small portion. The salts of the saliva are deposited in the duct or gland.

The causes are thought to be: (1) inflammation of the mucous membrane with an increased precipitation of salts; (2) the deposition of salts around bacterial masses or inorganic particles.

The calculi give symptoms when they grow sufficiently large to block the duct or

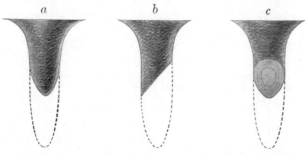

FIG. 17–5.   Three views of the amputated uvula: *a*, anterior view; *b*, lateral view; *c*, posterior view.

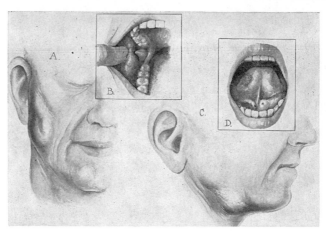

FIG. 17–6. Obstruction of the salivary ducts from stones or infection. *A,* Parotitis from obstruction of Stensen's duct. *B,* Pointing of orifice of Stensen's duct. *C,* Submaxillary swelling from an obstruction of Wharton's duct. *D,* Swelling of the orifice and sublingual course of Wharton's duct from an obstruction.

to cause infection induced by stasis of the gland and duct (Fig. 17-6). When the duct becomes blocked, the affected gland becomes swollen and tender, especially after eating. Partial dryness of the mouth is a common complaint.

Frequently the calculus can be felt by palpation, or a probe may be inserted into the duct, producing a rough, grating sensation when the tip of the probe comes into contact with the calculus. Pressure on the swollen gland may force the saliva or pus around the obstruction and out of the lumen of the duct into the mouth.

Wharton's Duct

The duct of Wharton, after leaving the submaxillary gland, runs forward and upward beneath the mucous membrane of the floor of the mouth over the mylohyoid muscle. It lies between the lingual nerve above and the hypoglossal below until the surface of the genioglossal muscle is reached, where the lingual nerve crosses the inner side. The duct opens on the floor of the mouth through a papilla beside the frenum of the tongue. The duct is 4 to 5 cm in length.

Sialography

In perhaps 75 to 80% of cases, the salivary calculus can be demonstrated by roent-genography. Further information can be obtained by preceding the exposure with the injection of an aqueous iodine-containing solution—e.g., iophendylate (Pantopaque)—into the appropriate duct.

Technique. No anesthesia is necessary. A lacrimal dilator is used to dilate the papilla (that of either the parotid or the submaxillary gland). In the case of the parotid gland particularly, this is more easily done under magnification. Through the dilated papilla a Bowman or similar lacrimal probe is passed for the length of the duct to search for obstruction. If none is found, the probe is withdrawn, and a polyethylene catheter of such a diameter that it will receive a No. 20 or 21 hypodermic needle is passed 2 to 3 cm into the duct. With the catheter taped to his forehead, the patient is positioned in front of the x-ray tube. The radiopaque solution is injected until the patient feels the first evidence of uncomfortable pressure (usually 0.5 to 1.5 ml), and then the picture is taken. The polyethylene catheter stays in place until the roentgenography is completed to prevent leaking of the injected solution back into the mouth.

Treatment. Occasionally a calculus will pass spontaneously. Dilating the duct and probing the stone so as to dislodge it encourages spontaneous passage. The use of sialogogues may also be helpful.

Surgical removal of submaxillary or sublingual gland calculi is usually done under local anesthesia. After the stone is fixed by grasping either the stone itself or the adjacent tissue with a forceps or suture, an incision is made in the long axis of the duct, and dissection is carried downward until the stone is found and removed. Firm digital pressure under the jaw against the gland brings the stone into a higher and more accessible position. Some surgeons find it convenient to localize the stone with the tip of a lacrimal probe and then dissect downward on the tip of the probe and thus find the stone. Care must be exercised to avoid the sublingual artery and the lingual nerve and vein. When calculi are being removed from the submaxillary gland, the close proximity of the hypoglossal nerves should be remembered.

Extirpation of the submaxillary gland may be indicated if multiple calculi occur within the gland in association with a chronic inflammation, if chronic stricture of Wharton's duct occurs, or if recurrences of the calculi are frequent.

If the stone is in the parotid gland or duct, surgical removal is considerably more difficult. If probing is not effective, calculi located near the papilla may be removed intraorally by splitting the duct over a lacrimal probe until the stone is reached. For deeper-lying calculi, particularly those within the gland itself, an external approach is required. Through an incision made just anterior to the auricle, the skin and subcutaneous tissue are reflected anteriorly to expose the lateral surface of the gland. The calculus is located by palpation, and the gland tissue is then incised down to the stone, extreme care being taken to dissect in a parallel direction to the long axis of the branches of the facial nerve so as to avoid injury to them.

After removal, the skin edges are carefully brought together and sutured. Finally, a pressure bandage is applied.

UVEOPAROTID FEVER

Uveoparotid fever is a rare syndrome possibly related to sarcoidosis. The etiology is unknown. It is characterized by an abrupt onset of fever, swelling of the parotid and lacrimal glands, uveitis, and cranial nerve palsies, particularly of the facial nerve. Usually there is spontaneous regression in several weeks.

SJÖGREN'S SYNDROME

This autoimmune disorder is a chronic inflammatory disease characterized by keratoconjunctivitis sicca, xerostomia, and a connective tissue disease. It is generally agreed that only two of the features need be present at one time to make a diagnosis. Rheumatoid arthritis is present in about half the cases, but systemic lupus erythematosus, polyarteritis nodosa, dermatomyositis, and scleroderma have also been reported. When only the keratoconjunctivitis sicca and xerostomia are present, it is spoken of as the "sicca complex." The disease, usually seen in women around the age of 50, often presents with the insidious development of the "sicca complex" in a patient with rheumatoid arthritis. Salivary gland swelling is present about 50% of the time. The disorder occasionally seems to progress from a benign to a malignant lymphoproliferation.

The etiology of Sjögren's syndrome is unknown, but it is considered by many to be a disorder of immunologic behavior Nearly all the patients, especially those exhibiting the "sicca complex" alone, display a hypergammaglobulinemia. On immunoelectrophoresis, it can usually be shown that this consists of an increase of the three major elements—IgG, IgA, and IgM. Recently it has been demonstrated that the lymphoid cells infiltrating the minor salivary glands (see discussion of lower lip biopsy under Diagnosis) actively synthesize significant amounts of IgG and especially IgM.

Histologically the major and minor salivary glands reveal an infiltration with lymphocytes and, to a lesser extent, with plasma cells. There is a decrease or disappearance of the acini, with a hyperplasia of the lining cells of the intraglandular ducts. There are histologic similarities between this disease and Hashimoto's thyroiditis.

Diagnosis. Several diagnostic aids have recently been developed. By use of immunofluorescence it can be shown that the patient's serum may possess an antisalivary duct antibody (IgG). With the sicca complex alone, this is reported as present 10 to 20% of the time, but it is present two-thirds of the time if the complete triad is present.

Scintigraphy has been utilized for evaluation of the xerostomia and accurately measures the salivary gland dysfunction. Salivary flow rates are characteristically depressed. Secretory sialography, in which a radiopaque material is injected directly into the parotid duct by catheter, reveals varying degrees of sialectasia.

A more recent development is the biopsy of the minor salivary glands of the lower lip. After the lip is infiltrated with 2% lidocaine, an ellipse of mucous membrane down to the muscle layer is removed. Histologic analysis reveals the characteristic lymphoproliferation.

Treatment. Treatment revolves around local measures to counteract the dryness of the eyes and mouth. Massage of the salivary glands to encourage flow and to express mucinous plugs may help. If infection has occurred, antibiotic therapy may be useful. A markedly enlarged parotid gland can usually be reduced by x-ray therapy, but this should be used with the greatest caution, if at all, because of the danger of converting a benign lymphoproliferation into a malignant one.

CYTOMEGALIC INCLUSION DISEASE

Cytomegalic inclusion disease (CID) is a virus infection which at one time was thought to be primarily an affliction of the salivary glands of infants. The cytomegalic virus was isolated in 1956 and is now included in the herpesvirus family. Nuclear inclusions are found in all types of normal and neoplastic cells, including white blood cells. Serologic data indicate that the antibody to this virus is present in 15% of the population at age 15 and in about 80% at the age of 35. Localized or systemic CID is frequently associated with prolonged impaired host resistance.

Enlarged cells, with distinctive intranuclear inclusions (10 to 15 nm) are characteristic of the infection. They are found in the lung, gastrointestinal tract, occasionally in the nasal mucosa, salivary glands, liver, adrenal glands, and elsewhere. An infectious mononucleosis–like syndrome has been ascribed to cytomegalic inclusion disease. Absolute and relative lymphocytosis are present in the peripheral blood with some atypical lymphocytes as well, but the heterophile antibody test is negative.

The diagnosis is best established by a rising antibody titer and isolation of the virus. There is no specific therapy, though some success has been reported using interferon and the antiviral agent floxuridine.

BEHÇET'S SYNDROME

Behçet's syndrome is characterized by nonspecific ulcerations of the mucous membrane, particularly of the mouth; by iritis, keratitis, and conjunctivitis; and by inflammation of the genitalia. The etiology is unknown but may be related to viruses, to the autoimmune state, or to collagen diseases.

PLUMMER-VINSON SYNDROME

The Plummer-Vinson syndrome is characterized by anemia, dysphagia, glossitis, and achlorhydria.

Etiology. The exact cause of the syndrome has not been determined. It is nearly always found in women and is frequently associated with achlorhydria and occasionally with a splenic tumor. The achlorhydric anemia is not necessarily related to the syndrome. It has not been determined whether the anemia precedes or is the result of the dysphagia.

Pathology. The anemia is that of an essential hypochromia. The glossitis takes the form of an atrophy of the lingual papillae. The smooth red tongue appears shrunken. Fissures at the corners of the mouth (cheilitis) and spoon nails are frequently observed. Various lesions in the upper portion of the esophagus have been reported, such as cracks, abrasions, hyperkeratosis, adhesions, webs, and bands. The hyperkeratinization of the epithelial lining of the esophagus may be precancerous.

Symptoms. The dysphagia, usually expressed as a tightness or cramping of the throat and referred to the level of the larynx, seems to be the outstanding symptom. The dysphagia may be of sudden onset with subsequent attacks separated by long intervals, or the pain may be of gradually increasing severity. The patient frequently complains of a pain in the atrophic tongue.

Symptoms and signs associated with the anemia, cheilitis, spoon nails, and splenomegaly are found when these conditions are present.

Treatment. The treatment should be directed to any etiologic or pathologic conditions found.

ABSCESS OF THE PAROTID GLAND

Etiology. An inflammatory process (other than mumps) within the parotid gland with or without abscess formation may be due to a blocking of Stensen's duct from inflammation or foreign objects, especially salivary calculi; a direct extension of an infection from neighboring structures, especially the fascial spaces of the neck; or a complication of abdominal or pelvic operations. Furstenberg stresses dehydration as the most important etiologic factor in the latter condition.

Symptoms. The symptoms of an abscess of the parotid gland are pain, tenderness, and swelling of the gland, especially after eating. Symptoms and signs of various degrees of sepsis are present as in any abscess formation.

Treatment. The treatment is adequate hydration, administration of one of the antibiotics or sulfonamides as indicated, application of hot, moist external dressings, suberythemal doses of roentgen rays to the affected part, administration of large doses of the compound solution of iodine, and gentle probing of Stensen's duct.

If definite evidence of suppuration is present and the above measures have failed, the abscess must be incised and drained.

Technique. An incision is begun at the level of the zygoma and extended downward along the ramus of the jaw to the angle, then forward 2 or 3 cm along the inferior margin. The skin and subcutaneous tissues are reflected forward, exposing the lateral surface of the parotid gland. Numer-ous incisions are made into the compartments of the gland as necessary for adequate drainage.

SNORING

Snoring, a symptom, is not considered pathologic unless the etiology is considered abnormal.

Snoring is usually due to vibrations of the soft palate and the thin edges or velum of the posterior faucial pillars. The relative position of the soft palate and tongue influences the noisy breathing. It has been shown that if a reservoir of air fills the nasopharynx, the velum does not vibrate.

Snoring in children is usually due to an enlarged adenoid, although any obstructing lesion in the nose or nasopharynx may produce it.

In the later years of adult life, noisy breathing is quite common, possibly due to lack of tone of the glossopharyngeal structures. Obstructing lesions of the airway are contributing factors. Sleeping in the supine position increases the tendency to snore.

The treatment consists of correcting or removing any nasal or nasopharyngeal obstructions. Other types of treatment have been unsatisfactory except for correction of some known etiologic factor, such as an allergic or infective rhinitis.

REFERENCES

Bloch, K. J. et al.: Sjögren's Syndrome. A clinical, Pathological and Serological Study of Sixty-Two Cases. Medicine, *44*:187, 1965.

Chisholm, D. M., and Mason, D. K.: Labial Salivary Gland Biopsy in Sjögren's Disease. J. Clin. Pathol., *21*:656, 1968.

Cummings, N. A., *et al.*: Sjögren's Syndrome —Newer Aspects of Research, Diagnosis, and Therapy. Ann. Intern. Med., *75*:937, 1971.

Niederman, J. C., *et al.*: Infectious Mononucleosis; Clinical Manifestations in Relation to EB Virus Antibodies. J.A.M.A., *203*: 205, 1968.

Shearn, M. A.: *Sjögren's Syndrome* (Volume II of Major Problems in International Medicine). Philadelphia, W. B. Saunders Co., 1971.

Chapter 18
Diseases of the Tonsils and Adenoid

Waldeyer's Ring. The tonsils and adenoid together constitute the most prominent members of Waldeyer's ring of lymphoid tissue, which encircles the pharynx. The other elements are the lingual tonsil, the lateral pharyngeal bands, and scattered lymphoid nodules located in Rosenmüller's fossa, beneath the mucous membrane of the posterior pharyngeal wall, and near the orifice of the eustachian tubes (Gerlach's tonsil).

Waldeyer's ring (along with Peyer's patches of the gut) is involved in the immune reaction (non–thymus-related or so-called B cells) of the body by mechanisms that are not yet clear. Its importance in this connection is probably greatest in the first few years of life. Veltri and coworkers became concerned that removal of the tonsils and adenoid would be followed by a decrease in the immunoglobulins. On the contrary, following tonsillectomy and adenoidectomy in a group of children, total serum IgA, IgM, and IgD and secretory (parotid) IgA were shown to be present in adequate amounts. Furthermore, the serologic response of these children to numerous human respiratory viruses was unaltered by the surgery. At variance with this report, at least in respect to the poliomyelitis virus in children whose adenoids had been surgically removed, is the adverse effect of the operation on the quantity of secretory IgA found locally in the nasopharynx; this was correlated with the increased incidence of bulbar poliomyelitis in such patients. Even in this instance, however, the amounts of serum IgA were unaltered.

ACUTE CONGESTIVE TONSILLITIS

Acute congestive tonsillitis is almost invariably associated with nasopharyngitis and will not be discussed further here.

ACUTE FOLLICULAR TONSILLITIS AND ADENOIDITIS

Synonyms. Cryptic tonsillitis.

Etiology. The etiologic agent is usually a group A *Streptococcus,* less often a virus. These agents have been discussed separately.

Pathology. In acute follicular tonsillitis, the tonsil is swollen and the crypts contain an accumulation of leukocytic and epithelial debris intermixed with bacteria.

Symptoms. In this as in other acute infectious processes, the onset is sudden and is attended by malaise and fever. Chilly sensations may inaugurate the attack. The temperature gradually rises to 102 or 103°F, until the end of the first to the third day, and in young children it may rise as high as 104 to 105°F. The febrile movement is accompanied by soreness upon swallowing, which as the disease progresses may become quite painful. The inflammation extends to the pharyngeal mucous membrane and even, in exceptional cases, to the eustachian tube and middle ear. There may be pain in the ear through reflex sources without actual inflammation in the tympanum. Tinnitus and slight deafness may also be present. The lymph node under the angle of the jaw is usually swollen and tender. The swollen condition of the tonsil, cervical lymph nodes, and surrounding muscles renders rotary motions of the head somewhat painful. The same condition also renders articulation and phonation imperfect, the voice being thick and indistinct. The tongue is coated with a yellowish-brown "fur," and the breath is fetid and offensive. Transient albuminuria is sometimes present, especially if the attack is severe and prolonged.

The acute symptoms rarely extend beyond the fifth or seventh day. The febrile movement and the swelling and soreness rapidly subside until the temperature is normal and the act of deglutition and rotation of the head may be performed with comfort to the patient. The patient, though convalescent, is often left in a very weakened condition.

Examination of the tonsils during the early acute stage shows them to be red and swollen, with the crypt openings covered with yellow spots of exudate.

The patches are not true membranous products, as found in pseudomembranous and diphtheritic inflammations, but are the secretions and debris which completely fill the crypts. Occasionally a fibrinous exudate is admixed with the debris, which gives it some of the characteristics of an inflammatory membrane. The protruding secretion and debris are easily wiped away, in contradistinction to the diphtheritic membrane, which is closely adherent to the epithelium.

The adenoid and the *lingual tonsil* are usually simultaneously inflamed with the faucial tonsil, and the yellowish exudate or debris peculiar to the faucial tonsil is usually found in the shallow clefts of the adenoid and still more shallow depressions of the lingual tonsil. The debris is similar in composition to that found in the crypts of the faucial tonsils.

Diagnosis. Group A *Streptococcus* follicular tonsillitis must be differentiated from diphtheria, nonbacterial pharyngitis, and infectious mononucleosis.

Treatment. If group A *Streptococcus* is found, immediate therapy with penicillin or erythromycin for a period of 10 days should

be instituted as described under Streptococcal Infections. If a pathogenic or susceptible bacterium is found other than the group A *Streptococcus,* the appropriate therapy must be instituted. Frequently only general measures of therapy plus symptomatic relief can be offered.

HYPERPLASIA OF THE TONSILS AND ADENOID

Etiology. Hyperplasia of the tonsils and adenoid begins early in life and may continue until the age of 10 to 12 years when active development usually ceases and atrophic changes occur. This is particularly true of the adenoid, which is usually of little importance clinically after the age of 10 to 12. Freedom from upper respiratory infections permits a decrease in the size of these structures.

Symptoms. Once the acute symptoms are over, hyperplastic tonsillitis and adenoiditis are characterized by mechanical obstruction of the pharynx, nasopharyngeal airway, and choanae. If these obstructions cause complications to a severe degree, it is best to remove the obstructing tonsil or adenoid or both. The choanae may be so blocked that the patient holds his mouth open, particularly while sleeping at night to obtain an adequate airway. An unrelenting adenoidal nasal or nasopharyngeal blockage may persist following a simple upper respiratory infection or "cold" which in other respects has long since resolved. This unhappy situation—mouth open and upper lip elevated—is spoken of as the "adenoid facies" and may in itself be a pressing problem. With the passage of time and superimposition of a bacterial infection, a distressing and persistent anterior purulent nasal discharge occurs.

Of practical as well as pathologic significance are the recurrent periods of deafness that follow the obstruction of the eustachian tubes. Initially only retraction of the membrana tympani is noted, but this, if unrelieved, is followed by serous or purulent otitis media. The presence of fluid in the middle ear suggests a poorly functioning eustachian tube.

Levy and others have noted that alveolar hypoventilation may follow pronounced adenoidal obstruction to the upper airway, and this in turn can lead to hypertension of the pulmonary artery and to cor pulmonale. Hypercapnia is the key to the diagnosis of these patients with an otherwise unexplained pulmonary hypertension. Establishment of an adequate airway allows for a return toward normal. Occasionally the hyperplasia is present at birth and may continue throughout life.

Pathology. In hyperplastic tonsillitis the enlargement is due to an increase in all the cellular structures composing the tonsil, whereas in a fibrotic tonsil, the connective tissue cells are increased relative to the other cellular elements. The hyperplastic tonsil in children shows great cellular activity with many mitoses in the numerous germinal centers (Fig. 18–1). In a child, the tonsil is soft and smooth in outline, whereas in an adult it is often much harder and is nodular in outline. In children the tonsil is

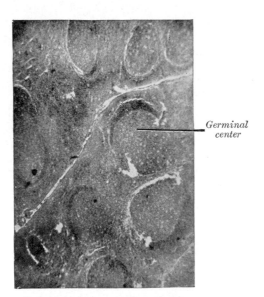

Germinal center

FIG. 18–1. Hyperplasia of the tonsil in a child. Microscopically the hyperplastic tonsil of a child presents a picture of great cellular activity, with many large germinal centers where mitoses are abundant. There is little fibrous tissue. In an adult, hyperplasia of the tonsil does not present such cellular activity. Germinal centers may be numerous but they are small and mitoses are not as numerous. There is an increase in fibrous tissue. × 30.

so loosely attached to the sinus tonsillaris that it can be removed easily without force, with its capsule intact. In many adults the tonsil is loosely attached, though it is ordinarily more firmly attached than in children.

The hyperplastic tonsils may have healthy crypts, but as a rule the reverse is true. The lining epithelium of some of the crypts is usually of low vitality, often hornified, and unable to resist the invasion of pathogenic microorganisms.

Treatment. Palliative treatment directed toward reducing the size of the tonsil in a young child is disappointing. As the patient grows older, there is a tendency toward fibrotic decrease in size, however. Repeated inflammations, whether of bacterial or viral origin, tend to maintain the enlargement. The best advice to anxious parents is to do all they can to prevent upper respiratory infections in the patient and to realize that time will see a regression in the size of the lymphoid structures.

The use of roentgen rays in the treatment of hyperplastic tonsils or adenoid is not recommended because of the possibility that they may ultimately cause a neoplasm in the irradiated area. A surgical approach is preferable. (See also Chapter 19.)

CHRONIC FIBROTIC TONSILLITIS

Definition. Chronic fibrotic tonsillitis is a disease of adults, as a rule. It may be a physiologic atrophy of the tonsil (Fig. 18–2) without symptoms but is frequently characterized by the more or less continued presence of pus in the crypts. Accompanying this pus in many cases are masses of caseous material composed of layers of desquamated epithelial cells enclosing cholesterol crystals, fatty matter, leukocytes, microorganisms, and occasionally calcareous deposits. The masses vary in size from that of a grain of wheat to that of a small bean. The crypts most often involved are those which open into the supratonsillar fossa and those covered by the plica semilunaris (tonsillaris).

Symptoms. Local symptoms may be absent or, if present, are usually not severe in character. The patient may complain of a sticking pain upon swallowing. Some patients have the sensation, lasting perhaps

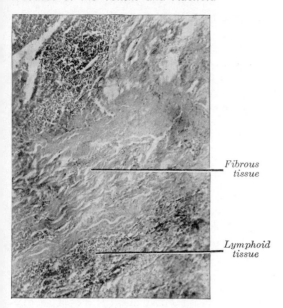

Fibrous
tissue

Lymphoid
tissue

Fig. 18–2. Fibrosis and atrophy of the tonsil. There is a decrease in the size of the germinal centers, which are few and scattered with a much lessened cellular activity. A great increase in fibrous tissue is also present, and a thick trabecula can be seen. × 80.

for only a minute or two, of a foreign body lodged in the tonsil.

The patient frequently coughs up the caseous masses, which have a fetid odor. When pressure is exerted upon the tonsil with a flat instrument, the pus and caseous masses are forced from the crypts, especially from the superior ones.

The repeated removal of the plugs affords some relief, and their tendency to reform is diminished, though a cure by this procedure does not often occur.

The caseous masses in themselves are not necessarily indicative of a great amount of absorption of toxins; however, where these masses are present, fluid pus can usually be demonstrated by pressing on the tonsil. This fluid pus is very significant of a chronic absorption of bacteria or toxins, and in the presence of some condition due to a focus of infection, the advisability of removing the tonsils should be seriously considered.

These infected fibrotic tonsils are subject to acute exacerbations, generally of a mild type, the mucous membrane becoming slightly reddened. There is also some sore-

ness upon swallowing. The temperature is only slightly elevated and may attract no attention.

Occasionally the mouth of a crypt becomes closed by inflammatory adhesions (caseous encystment), and the yellowish color shows through the thin membranous covering over the mouth of the crypt.

Treatment. If the symptoms annoy the patient and recur at frequent intervals, or if the patient has evidence of infection in a remote part of the body which may reasonably be assigned to absorption through the tonsils, they may be removed.

VINCENT'S ANGINA

Synonyms. Ulcerative tonsillitis; pseudomembranous angina; trench mouth.

Etiology. Since Vincent described a spirillum associated with a fusiform bacillus found in certain forms of ulcerative tonsillitis and gingivitis, the condition has been called Vincent's angina. The disease is most frequently found in young persons, though it occurs often in those of middle and later life. A debilitated state of health, local irritative lesions in the mouth, such as decayed teeth, inflamed gums, and oral uncleanliness, favor the development of the disease, which is by no means an uncommon one. A low vitamin C content of the blood seems to be an important factor in the etiology in many individuals. There is a widespread geographic distribution of the disease, but it is more common in the temperate and tropical climates than in the arctic regions. Epidemics have been reported. It is frequently spread from one person to another by kissing, towels, dishes, etc.

Pathology. The lesions commonly involve one tonsil (Fig. 18–3), usually at its upper part, but may spread to the soft palate, the other tonsil, the pharynx, or the gums. They may even spread to the larynx, trachea, and ears. The membrane covering the patches is a pseudomembrane and is formed by the necrosis of the superficial layers of the mucous membrane, not by exudation. The patches are of a grayish white color, surrounded by a red inflamed areola, but separated from each other by healthy tissue. On removal of the pseudomembrane,

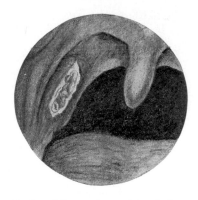

FIG. 18–3.   Vincent's angina of the tonsil.

which is granular and cheesy in consistency, an ulcerative area is exposed, varying in extent and depth. The ulcerated areas bleed freely and are soon covered by a new pseudomembrane. The ulceration at times is very destructive, destroying the whole or a portion of the tonsil, and invades healthy tissue. The spirillum and the fusiform bacillus penetrate the tonsil substance to a considerable depth. They are more numerous in the immediate vicinity of the ulcer.

The microscopic examination of a fresh smear taken directly from the ulcer, or a section of the pseudomembrane, stained with Löffler's methylene blue or fuchsin, shows fusiform bacilli, twice as long as wide and pointed at the ends, together with a spirillum forming a network around the bacilli. The spirillum is 10 to 20 microns in length. Since it is the only fusiform bacillus occurring in the mouth, it is readily recognized when found associated with the spirillum. These bacteria grow best on an acid medium. They will live but not multiply under aerobic conditions. It has been shown that the spirochete precedes the fusiform bacilli in the invasion of the tissues.

Symptoms. The usual symptoms are a subacute or mild tonsillitis, sore mouth and gums, headache, general malaise, chilly sensations, and a temperature varying from normal to 102.5°F. There may be no constitutional disturbances, the patient complaining only of pain on swallowing and tender or bleeding gums, or he may have discovered the yellowish patch on examining his throat or gums with a mirror be-

cause of a slight feeling of discomfort. Occasionally the symptoms are more violent, involving great pain on swallowing or talking, fetid breath, gastric disturbance, and enlarged and tender submaxillary and cervical lymph nodes.

Diagnosis. The diagnosis is made by the recovery of large numbers of fusiform bacilli in conjunction with spirilla. A few of these are sometimes found in normal throats. Differential diagnosis must be made from agranulocytic angina, leukemia, and infectious mononucleosis. Diphtheria, syphilis, tuberculosis, and neoplasms also must be considered but are less likely.

Treatment. The disease usually responds rapidly to penicillin. Concomitant dental care is necessary in the gingival form.

Sodium perborate is effective in Vincent's angina because of its ability to release oxygen. A thick paste is made and spread over the ulcer. Hydrogen peroxide (half strength) as a gargle is also effective for the same reason.

The ingestion of adequate amounts of ascorbic acid should be encouraged. The eating and other personal utensils of the patient should be sterilized and kept separate to prevent spreading of the disease.

HYPERKERATOSIS OF THE TONSIL; MYCOSIS LEPTOTHRICA

Hyperkeratosis of the tonsillar tissue is characterized by the appearance of numerous white projections not only on the cryptic orifices of the tonsils proper but also on the orifices of the lymph follicles, on the posterior and lateral pharyngeal walls, and on the lateral glossoepiglottic folds. This condition does not occur on portions of the throat where there is no lymphoid tissue. The lymphoid tissue of the upper respiratory tract is so ubiquitous, however, that occasionally the little white projections may be seen on almost any part of the mucosa. In the large majority of cases, the condition is limited to the faucial and lingual tonsils. That it reaches its greatest development on the base of the tongue and at a position just behind the lateral glossoepiglottidean folds and the posterior part of the inferior poles of the tonsils is due almost entirely to mechanical reasons. The contractions of the muscles during swallowing prevent food from coming in intimate contact with the surface of these parts and therefore permit the projections to grow undisturbed. Although the horny material is quite resistant to trauma, the bacterial accumulations which form the greater mass of the projection are easily brushed off, so that the size of the growth is much greater where it is protected from mechanical disturbances.

Hyperkeratosis is a condition peculiar to young adults and is self-limited, 2 to 3 years being required for it to run its course.

Symptoms. The symptoms caused by this condition of the throat are either absent or slight and for the most part are due to the local irritation caused by the hard, horny plugs. If they project from the base of the tongue so as to come in contact with the epiglottis, there is an irritating tickling sensation which causes a hacking cough. If they are so placed as to be compressed during the act of swallowing, they may give rise to a slight pricking pain.

Occasionally among the rich and various bacterial flora which grows in such luxuriance on this horny material, there may lurk a germ with pathogenic power, which may set up an accompanying inflammatory reaction in the tonsil or surrounding structures.

Pathology. Some years ago G. B. Wood stated:

In hyperkeratosis the epithelium loses its rarefied condition and becomes ordinary pavement squamous epithelium similar to that covering the surface of the tonsil, except that generally it does not show the connective tissue papillae. The crypt of the tonsil is markedly dilated and filled with a horny mass, which merges at various points into the epithelium. (See Figs. 18–4 and 18–5.)

According to the mechanical circumstances by which the tonsil is surrounded, the horny mass becomes sooner or later broken up into layers, between which multiply and grow organisms of all varieties. This fraying of the cryptal plug may take place within the crypt itself, so that the resulting fissures permit the bacteria at times to penetrate almost but not quite to the living epithelium.

The toxins elaborated by these organisms must be absorbed to a greater or less extent by the tonsillar tissue. It is probably due to the fact that the cryptal epithelium has become an intact protective barrier that a more noticeable reaction is not a common result.

Treatment. Treatment is unnecessary, but if the horny masses cause irritation, they may be removed by cauterization. The electrocautery should be used to destroy

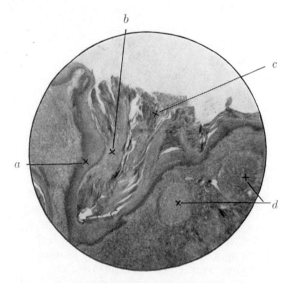

Fig. 18–4. Hyperkeratosis, showing the typical appearance under low power. The horny mass is growing from a comparatively small area of the cryptic epithelium, and the plug shows the ordinary fraying of its edges: a, cryptic epithelium; b, horny material; c, masses of bacteria; d, follicles (Wood).

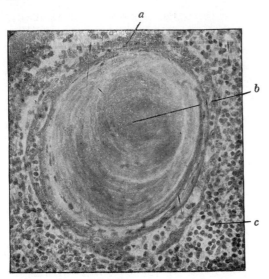

FIG. 18–5. Hyperkeratosis. Cross section of the terminal portion of a crypt showing the concentric arrangement of the layers of horny material and the epithelium, which is still somewhat disintegrated: *a,* epithelium; *b,* horny material in crypts; *c,* lymphoid tissue (Wood).

them, and the surrounding tissues should be penetrated until only healthy tissue remains. From three to four masses may be treated at each sitting at intervals of 1 week.

CALCULUS OF THE TONSIL; TONSILLOLITHS

Small quantities of calcareous or gritty particles are often found in the center of the caseous plugs filling the crypts of the tonsil in chronic follicular tonsillitis. They sometimes become quite large and fill the crypts and are known as calculi of the tonsil or tonsilloliths. They occur much more frequently in adults than in children, and at times they reach an extraordinary size. Such patients usually give a history of repeated attacks of tonsillitis in earlier years.

The calculi are rounded or oval as a rule, but with a somewhat roughened granular surface. They are usually yellow or yellowish gray. A concentrically laminated or radially striated structure may be indistinctly shown in many cases.

Among the group of 80 cases of microscopic tonsillar concretions of the crypts, 47, or about 59% were developing in the

large, so-called "actinomyces-like" colonies of mixed mouth organisms so commonly found in the crypts of the tonsil. This is the most common mode of origin. Such colonies grow peripherally with a more or less clearly rayed or clubbed outer zone. As they become of large size, the central portion dies, and in the dead center lime salts may be laid down. In 33 of the 80 positive cases (41%), the origin of the tonsillar calculi was found to be the accumulated keratohyalin masses in the crypts.

Symptoms. The symptoms are identical to those of chronic follicular tonsillitis with caseous plugs in the crypts; that is, there are recurrent attacks of mild tonsillitis with redness, which is especially marked around the affected crypts. The patient may be aware of a constant sensation as of a forein body in the throat. The breath is often fetid.

Treatment. The treatment consists of removal of the tonsils or of the calculus, as in chronic follicular tonsillitis. If the calculus is not easily disengaged from the crypt, an incision of the wall of the crypt facilitates its removal. Pain may be obviated by injecting a 2% solution of procaine into the substance of the tonsil in the region of the calculus.

CARTILAGE AND BONE IN THE TONSILS

Isolated portions of bone and cartilage found in the tonsils are embryonic "rests" of the branchial arches in many instances. They are found only in the connective-tissue structures of the tonsil.

Bone in the tonsil is frequently caused by an abnormally long styloid process extending into the tonsil.

ELONGATED STYLOID PROCESS

The elongated styloid process may produce two syndromes: (1) the type characterized by painful sensations in the pharynx, painful deglutition, and an otologic pain, occurring after a tonsillectomy which may persist for years; and (2) the styloid process–carotid artery syndrome in which the symptoms are produced by impingement upon the carotid artery. The symptoms and signs are tenderness on palpation over the region of the carotid artery, with parietal headaches and head pains in the area supplied by the ophthalmic artery.

The diagnosis of an elongated styloid process is made by palpation in the tonsillar fossa and by roentgenograms.

The treatment is surgical removal or shortening of the elongated process. Further confirmation of these syndromes is necessary before they can be established as clinical entities.

TONSILLAR ABSCESS (PHLEGMONOUS TONSILLITIS)

Phlegmonous tonsillitis is an abscess within the substance of the tonsil. It is not common. One of the tonsillar crypts usually becomes closed, thereby creating a closed abscess. Injury to the tonsil may produce the condition.

The *symptoms* are similar to peritonsillar abscess except they are not so severe.

The *treatment* is incision and drainage of the abscess with subsequent removal of the tonsils.

PERITONSILLAR ABSCESS (QUINSY)

Peritonsillar abscess is an acute abscess in the peritonsillar tissue.

Etiology. The cause is about the same as that given under acute follicular tonsillitis. Peritonsillitis (quinsy) probably results from an infection of the crypts in the supraton-sillar fossa, which are large, slitlike cavities with irregular outlines, and which are in intimate relationship with the posterior and outer aspect of the tonsil. The disease is common in young adults and rare in children.

Pathology. In the majority of cases of peritonsillar abscess, the pus finds its way into the supratonsillar fossa, which is characterized by marked swelling and edema of the soft palate to the extent that the tonsil is pushed downward and mesially (Fig. 18-6).

In another class of cases, the pus burrows downward and backward, displacing the tonsil forward with little if any swelling in the supratonsillar region. The posterior pillar bulges to a marked extent, with abscess in this location.

If the superior constrictor muscle is penetrated by the abscess, an infection in the parapharyngeal space results. This penetration may take place directly or through the veins. The pus may burrow downward from this locality and enter the mediastinum. The great vessels of the neck may become implicated in rare instances. It is probable that cases terminating fatally belong in this group.

Symptoms. The onset of the peritonsillitis is continuous from a preceding acute follicular tonsillitis as a rule. The temperature rarely exceeds 99 to 100°F, whereas in the early stage of an acute tonsillitis, it often rises to 103°F or higher.

The pain progressively increases with the extension of the purulent accumulation until it is almost unbearable. The muscles of mas-

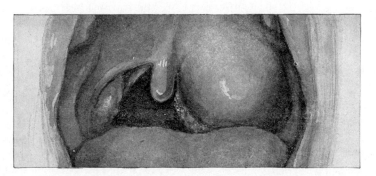

FIG. 18–6.   Peritonsillar abscess. The left anterior pillar and palate are distended. The tonsil is pushed to the center and the uvula to the opposite side.

tication are encroached upon by the abscess; hence, the patient has the greatest difficulty in opening the mouth sufficiently wide to permit an examination of the throat. Swallowing becomes difficult and painful. The disease is usually limited to one side. The saliva dribbles from the mouth and forms one of the characteristic symptoms. Lateral movement of the head produces pain on account of the infiltration of the tissues of the neck in the region of the tonsil.

A thick viscid secretion forms in the throat, and it is with the greatest difficulty that the patient succeeds in removing it. The tongue is heavily coated and the breath fetid. Breathing is interfered with on account of the swollen mucous and submucous tissue of the pharynx. The patient has an anxious expression. During sleep he often has suffocative attacks which awaken him. Laryngeal dyspnea from extension of the edema to the laryngeal tissue is fortunately rare.

Examination reveals a unilateral redness and swelling, as both tonsils are rarely affected at the same time. If both are affected, the second usually begins as the first subsides. If both are affected at once, the suffocative symptoms are more severe and alarming. As the disease progresses, the redness, tenderness, pain, and swelling increase in severity. If the abscess is in the tonsil, the tonsil itself is swollen without much displacement of the palate and uvula. If the abscess is in the peritonsillar tissue, the swelling often appears to be in the region of the upper portion of the anterior pillar. The palate and uvula are pushed over to the opposite side of the throat. This is partly due to the swollen tonsil but largely to the edema, cellulitis, and pressure of the abscess itself upon the tonsil. Incisions in this region often fail to reach the pus cavity for this reason; that is, the incision is carried directly into the tonsil instead of into the pus cavity outside of the tonsil.

The soft palate and uvula, as well as the pharyngeal mucous membrane, are red and edematous. The region of the tonsil is a deep, dusky red color. The crypts are often filled with a pulplike debris, which was probably the original source of infection. The infection does not originate in the peri-

tonsillar tissue but rather in the supratonsillar crypts of the tonsil as a rule.

Digital examination of the tonsillar region shows more or less distinct fluctuation. The focal center of fluctuation is located about ¼ inch external to the free border of the anterior pillar, or at the junction of the upper third with the middle third of the tonsil, posterior to the tonsil.

The disease lasts 5 to 10 days when allowed to run its course, though it may extend over a longer period. The termination is marked by the spontaneous or artificial discharge of fetid pus. When the discharge is spontaneous, it usually takes place through the anterior pillar, though it occasionally occurs through one of the crypts. In some instances there is a spontaneous resorption of the cellulitis without the discharge of pus.

Peritonsillar abscess should be differentiated from infections of the submaxillary space. The latter condition is usually due to caries or infections of the molar teeth. The pus may push the internal muscle against the superior constrictor and hence displace the tonsil toward the median line, as in quinsy.

Complications and Sequelae. Complications and sequelae are rare. Cases are on record, however, in which the following conditions were present: edema of the glottis from the downward extension of the process; strangulation from the spontaneous rupture of the abscess; thrombophlebitis of one of the large veins of the neck; ulceration of one of the large arteries in the submaxillary region; chronic peritonsillitis with an intermittent flow of pus; encysted abscess in the tonsil; and parapharyngeal abscess with or without a mediastinitis.

Treatment. Adequate treatment with antimicrobial drugs should be given until the temperature has reached normal and the pain has disappeared.

Hot (110 to 115°F) 0.85% saline or 5% glucose throat irrigations every 2 to 3 hours will hasten recovery and give relief. Heat to the neck and jaw will reduce the muscle spasm.

Surgical Treatment. *Incision.* If fluctuation is present, incision and drainage are indicated. The local application of a 10%

solution of cocaine or 2% tetracaine solution to the region of the incision is usually sufficient. If marked trismus is present and the patient is unable to open the mouth sufficiently to make the incision, application of cocaine through the nose to the descending palatine nerves in the greater palatine canal may give relief from the muscle spasm.

The point of the incision is determined by the location of pouching or fluctuation. It is usually in front of the anterior pillar on a level with the junction of the upper and middle thirds of the tonsil, though it may be in the posterior pillar or through the tonsil. Many of the failures to evacuate the pus through the anterior incision are due to the fact that the tonsil often extends forward beneath the anterior pillar. The incision as usually made, therefore, penetrates the tonsil instead of the tissue outside of it. If the depth of the incision is carried beyond the outer border of the tonsil, the pus will be found more often. It should be remembered that the anterior third of the tonsil projects forward beneath the anterior pillar; hence, when an incision is made through the anterior pillar to evacuate the pus, it should be made far enough anteriorly to escape the anterior border of the tonsil and should be directed in an outward and a backward direction, outside of the capsule of the tonsil. If these anatomic facts are borne in mind, the anterior incision will nearly always evacuate the pus if present. If a posterior incision is to be made, it should be directed outward through the posterior pillar or in its immediate vicinity, as the pus pocket often extends posteriorly to the tonsil.

THE TONSILS AND TUBERCULOSIS

There is still a divergence of opinion as to whether a primary tuberculosis of the tonsils may occur (Fig. 18-7). Some hold that the tuberculous process in these glands is direct, while others contend that the infection reaches them from the lungs through the lymphatics and the blood vessels, or by the flow of the bronchial secretions over them. Both views are probably correct in selected cases. It is probable, however, that tuberculous infection of the cervical lymphatic nodes is usually due to the entrance of the bacilli and other microorganisms through the tonsils. This is borne out clinically by the fact that suppurating or tuberculous lymph nodes of the neck are rarely found in phthisical patients, whereas if they occurred secondary to pulmonary infection,

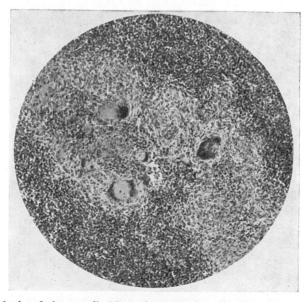

FIG. 18–7.   Tuberculosis of the tonsil. Note the extensive fibrosis with necrosis and giant cells (Evanston Hospital).

they would be found frequently in such patients.

It would seem from a clinical standpoint that a primary latent tuberculous process may exist in the tonsils or adenoid with no clinical pulmonary signs or symptoms of tuberculosis.

THE TONSILS AND RHEUMATIC FEVER

Although at one time it was thought that the removal of the tonsils and adenoid interrupted the direct relation between streptococcal tonsillitis and rheumatic fever, this has been disproved. Tonsillectomy does not prevent infection by streptococci. (See introductory statement under Streptococcal Infections.)

THE TONSILS AND POLIOMYELITIS

In past years evidence has accumulated indicating that recent tonsillectomy and adenoidectomy increase the incidence of bulbar poliomyelitis. A probable explanation of this relationship has been put forth by Ogra, who found deficient secretory IgA in the nasopharynx in children who had been operated on but unaltered serum immunoglobulins, including IgA. Tonsillectomy and adenoidectomy, as well as other elective procedures, should be delayed during periods when poliomyelitis is prevalent.

REFERENCES

Levy, A. M., et al.: Hypertrophied Adenoids Causing Pulmonary Hypertension and Severe Congestive Heart Failure. N. Engl. J. Med., 277:506, 1967.

Ogra, P. L.: Effect of Tonsillectomy and Adenoidectomy on Nasopharyngeal Antibody Response to Poliovirus. N. Engl. J. Med., 284:59, 1971.

Sprinkle, P. M., and Veltri, R. W.: The Tonsil and Adenoid Dilemma: Medical or Surgical Treatment. Otolaryngol. Clin. North Am., 7(3):909, 1974.

Veltri, R. W., et al.: Immunoglobulin Changes in Pediatric Otolaryngologic Patient Sampling Subsequent to T & A. J. Laryngol. Otol., 86:905, 1972.

Chapter 19
Indications for Tonsillectomy and Adenoidectomy

No absolute set of indications for removal of the tonsils and adenoid can be formulated. In each instance an evaluation of the individual case under consideration must be made. As a generalization it might be said that the reasons for removing the adenoid or tonsils or both include importantly the amount of obstruction and interference these structures offer to the normal physiologic function of the eustachian tubes, the choanae, and the pharynx. Obstruction may lead to purulent and other complications, which include conductive deafness, reduced middle ear pressure, middle ear fluid, recurrent suppurative otitis media, nasal obstruction with purulent rhinitis, and difficulty in deglutition. When the ventilatory resistance is marked and longlasting due to the obstructing tonsils and adenoid, cardiorespiratory changes may occur in children. These changes range from moderate cardiac enlargement and right ventricular hypertrophy to cor pulmonale, pulmonary edema, and elevation of the pCO_2. Relief of the obstruction by adenoidectomy or by tonsillectomy and adenoidectomy leads to a return toward normal values.

The evaluation of chronic infection in the tonsils and adenoid is a more difficult problem. Recurrent peritonsillar abscess with its high morbidity and almost certain recurrence is an indication for tonsillectomy. Recurrent pyrexial bacterial pharyngotonsillitis despite adequate antimicrobial therapy is a relative indication. How frequent and severe these must be is a moot point. In general, four such marked infections with cervical adenitis in the previous 6 months in a child under 7 years of age is considered a probable indication for surgery. If the child is over 7, the history of febrile pharyngotonsillitis should be of longer duration. If the infection is repeatedly associated with beta-hemolytic group A streptococci, the indication for surgery is more persuasive.

Persistent low middle ear pressure as measured by tympanometry, the presence of middle ear fluid, and conductive deafness associated with either or both of these causes are relative indications. The advisability of inserting equalizing tubes across the tympanic membrane at the time of surgery is discussed in Part 4.

TONSILLECTOMY

Anesthesia

A general anesthesia is given to all children and is preferable in nervous and uncooperative older patients. In most tractable adults local anesthesia is entirely satisfactory. In both situations preoperative preparation of the patient with a barbiturate and atropine or similar medications is desirable. The local anesthetic solution (e.g., 1% lidocaine with epinephrine 1:200,000)

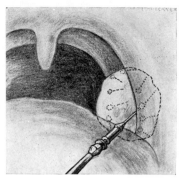

FIG. 19–1. The various points for injecting the anesthetic solution around the tonsil. The injections are made between the tonsil and the pillars, not through the pillars or into the tonsil.

is injected in the several sites illustrated (Fig. 19–1), perhaps using 5 to 7 ml for each tonsil. Additional comfort for the patient may be gained by a preliminary spraying of the tonsil area with 1% tetracaine.

Dissection-Snare Technique

This is the most commonly used method for tonsillectomy. For this description the patient is assumed to be supine in the Rose position.

The tonsil is grasped with vulsellum forceps, one prong placed on the upper pole

and the other on the lower. The incision may be started at the upper pole and carried anteriorly and posteriorly just within the respective tonsil pillars (Fig. 19–2). The aim is to form an inverted U over the upper half of the tonsil, but in so doing to carefully preserve the posterior tonsillar pillar particularly. It is necessary to incise only through the mucosa. If the substance of the tonsil is entered, difficulties may be encountered in finding the dissection plane.

The tonsil is then everted from its bed by traction on the vulsellum forceps in such a way as to cause gaping of the anterior mucosal incision. Through this, curved Metzenbaum scissors or some other dissecting instrument is inserted and used to separate the capsule of the tonsil from its bed (Fig. 19–3). Usually the anterior pillar is separated first and then the upper pole. When the latter can be seen, the vulsellum forceps should be reapplied so as to include the upper pole. The posterior pillar is readily visualized by everting the upper pole, and under direct vision it is dissected free from the tonsil. The finger may also be used as a dissecting instrument.

Once the dissection has progressed to the point where only the inferior pole remains

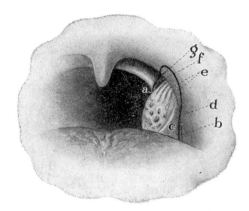

FIG. 19–2. Anatomic landmarks of the fauces: *a, b,* the incision liberating the pillars in the removal of the tonsil; *c,* plica triangularis; *d,* anterior pillar; *e,* supratonsillar slitlike crypts, or hilum of the tonsil; *f,* supratonsillar fossa; *g,* supratonsillar margin.

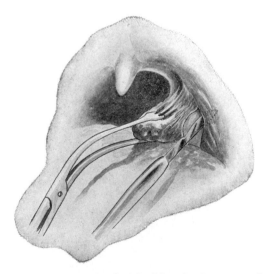

FIG. 19–3. The first incision in the removal of the tonsil with its capsule intact. The tonsil is drawn forward and in a median direction from the tonsillar fossa. The incision is extended upward over the supratonsillar margin to the posterior pillar.

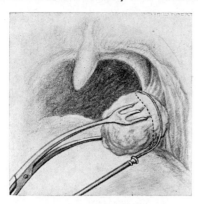

FIG. 19–4. Placing the snare loop over the tonsil after the pillars have been dissected free. The wire loop is tightened, thus severing the remaining attachments.

attached, a snare is usually conveniently used. The forceps are passed through the wire loop of the snare and the tonsil again seized (Fig. 19-4). Then the snare loop is passed over the freed portion of the tonsil and the snare tightened in such a manner as to amputate the inferior pole flush with the tongue. If any tonsil remnant remains at the plica triangularis, it too should be grasped by forceps and removed with a snare or by scissors.

Bleeding points can be controlled by suture (000 plain catgut), ligature, or electrodesiccation. It is frequently convenient when using ligature to pass a slip knot over the hemostat which holds the bleeding point and to tighten it just beyond the tip of the instrument.

The Sluder Guillotine Operation

There are three *fundamental facts* underlying Sluder's technique:

1. The guillotine will remove the tonsil with its capsule intact, provided the tonsil is pushed through the fenestra of the instrument.

2. The tonsillar fossa (bed of the tonsil) is freely movable, allowing the tonsil to be dislocated forward and upward a distance of about 1½ inches.

3. At a distance of 1½ inches anterior and superior to the tonsil, a bony prominence on the mandible, called the eminentia alveolaris, is located. This eminence corresponds to the location of the last molar tooth.

These facts are put to practical use in the Sluder operation (Figs. 19–5 and 19–6). The tonsil is displaced forward and upward over the tubercle, which in turn pushes it through the fenestra of the guillotine; the guillotine blade is then pushed home, removing the tonsil with its investing capsule.

Technique. In the removal of the *right tonsil,* with the patient in the upright position, the Sluder guillotine is grasped by its handle with the operator's *right hand* and introduced through the *left angle of the mouth* until the distal portion of the fenestral margin is in contact with the inferior and posterior portion of the tonsil.

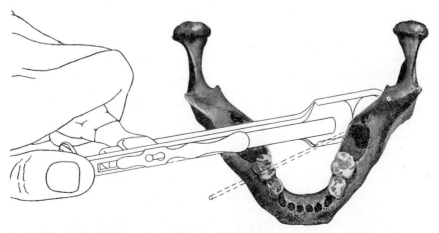

FIG. 19–5. Sluder guillotine in position for removal of the tonsil.

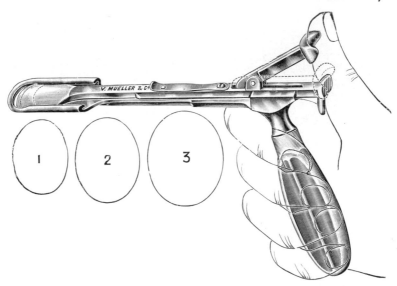

FIG. 19–6.   Sluder's guillotine with thumb lever.

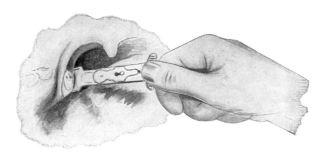

FIG. 19–7.   Sluder's tonsil operation. First step: placing the fenestra behind the tonsil
and in front of the posterior pillar.

The instrument is then pressed firmly against the tissues, which are drawn forward and upward for a distance of about 1 inch. The tonsil then rests over the eminentia alveolaris, which pushes the tonsil through the fenestra of the guillotine (Fig. 19–7), though it may not push it all through the opening. If the blade of the instrument were forced home at this stage of the procedure, the tonsil would not in all probability be removed in its entirety, with its capsule intact. Instead, only the superficial portion of the tonsil would be removed. To prevent this mishap, the tonsil is drawn a little farther forward until the distal margin of the fenestra rests almost upon the apex of the eminence. The handle of the instrument is then slightly depressed, to bring the inferior portion of the margin of the fenestra in firm contact with the inferior portion of the tonsil. This leaves the tonsil exposed to view (Fig. 19–8). The left index finger is then used to push the tonsil through the fenestra (Fig. 19–9). The blade of the guillotine should, however, be gently pressed against the anterior portion of the tonsil to hold it in position while the balance is being pushed through the fenestra with the tip of the left index finger.

In the third step of the operation, the remainder of the tonsil is pushed through the fenestra with the tip of the left index finger. As the tonsil continues to pass through the fenestra, the blade of the instrument is advanced by gentle pressure with the thumb of the right hand.

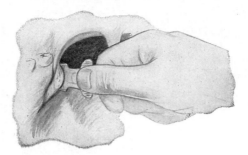

FIG. 19–8. Second step: the tonsil dislocated forward over the alveolar eminence.

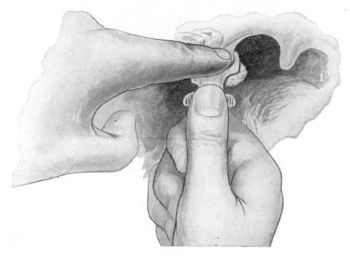

FIG. 19–9. Third step: pushing the tonsil through the fenestra.

The tonsil tissue is readily detected by the sense of touch, as it is firm and nodular, whereas the mucous membrane is soft, thin, and smooth in texture. When the tonsil is completely through the fenestra of the instrument, only the smooth, thin mucous membranes of the anterior and posterior pillars lie between the tip of the finger and the distal margin of the fenestra. The blade is at this time advanced until only the two mucous membranes lie between its cutting edge and the distal margin of the fenestra. The blade is then forced home.

Position of the Surgeon in Relation to the Patient. When the patient is in the upright position, the left tonsil is removed with the guillotine grasped in the left hand, the index finger of the right hand being used to force the tonsil through the fenestra of the guillo-tine. In all other respects the technique is the same.

The Ballenger-Sluder Operation

Sluder's guillotine has been modified by adding a scissors-handle (Fig. 19–10), which greatly facilitates the work and requires much less muscular power to cut through the tissues. The instrument is supplied in three sizes of blades.

The tonsil is pulled against the tip of the finger instead of the alveolar eminence, as suggested by Sluder. This accomplishes the same purpose and simplifies the whole procedure.

Technique of Ballenger-Sluder Tonsillectomy. When the right tonsil is being removed, the guillotine is held in the right

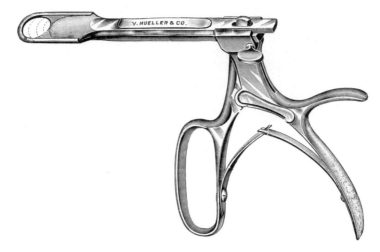

FIG. 19-10.   Ballenger-Sluder tonsillectome with sharp blade and scissors-handle.

hand and inserted through the left side of the patient's mouth until the distal portion of the instrument is in front of the posterior pillar and behind and slightly below the lower pole of the tonsil (Fig. 19–11).

The lower pole of the tonsil is now engaged in the ring of the instrument. The index finger of the left hand is placed over the anterior pillar to furnish counterpressure, and by gently rocking the instrument in an up-and-down motion (upright position), the upper pole will become engaged through the ring. At the same time pressure is made by the index finger of the left hand on the tonsil (through the anterior pillar,

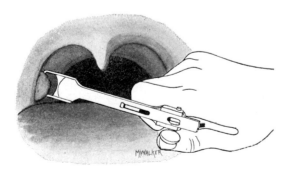

FIG. 19–11.   Tonsillectomy with the Ballenger-Sluder guillotine. The tip of the instrument is placed behind the tonsil and in front of the posterior pillar. The lower pole of the tonsil is engaged first.

Fig. 19–12), until the body of the tonsil is felt to slip through the ring of the instrument. When this occurs the entire rim of the fenestra can be felt by the finger. If a portion of the tonsil is still in the ring, it can be felt as a soft mass, and further manipulating is necessary.

The tonsil having been pushed through the fenestra, the blade of the instrument is pushed down firmly but not so that it severs the tonsil (Fig. 19–13). The handle and shank of the instrument are brought at the same time over to the right side of the throat (Fig. 19–14), and the handle of the instrument is rotated upward to help lift the tonsil out of its bed and to prevent it from falling into the throat, as it might do if the pressure of the blade on the attachments of the severed tonsil were relaxed.

Sufficient pressure should be applied to sever the attachments of the tonsil. If a semisharp blade is used, the pressure from both hands is necessary. If a portion of the tonsillar attachment is still adherent, after full pressure on the blade has been exerted, slight traction on the instrument will finish the severing. It is never necessary to use the finger or knife for "stripping" the tonsil loose. It is desirable to keep the blade of the instrument sharp.

The left tonsil is removed as described for the right, except the instrument should

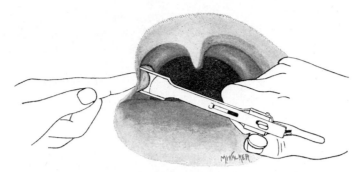

FIG. 19–12.   The tonsil is drawn forward and upward. Counterpressure is furnished by the index finger of the unengaged hand.

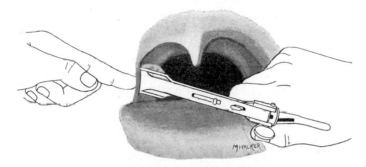

FIG. 19–13.   As the tonsil becomes engaged in the ring of the instrument, the blade is gradually pushed home.

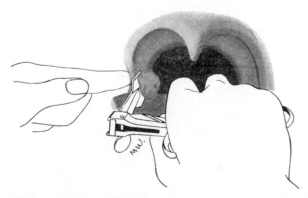

FIG. 19–14.   As the blade is pushed home, the handle of the instrument is brought over to the side of the mouth from which the tonsil is being removed.

be held in the left hand and introduced from the right side of the patient's mouth.

In all types of tonsil operations, including the guillotine technique, it is necessary to remove the plica triangularis and the excess lymphoid tissue in the region of the plica. This may be done by grasping the plica with a forceps or hook and insinuating a snare around the mass. It may be done more quickly and easily and as effectively by means of tonsil scissors of the Metzenbaum type. The plica is grasped with a slender forceps. The convex surface of the scissors hugs the base of the tongue between the inner surfaces of the anterior and posterior pillars, completely separating all the attachments of the lymphoid mass.

The objection made to the guillotine type of instrument is that the anterior pillar is sometimes cut. This objection is not based on experience, as the blade of the instrument may be made to sever the attachment of the pillar as close to the tonsil as desired; indeed, the tendency of the instrument is to hug the capsule of the tonsil.

COMPLICATIONS OF TONSILLECTOMY

Mortality. Pratt reports that the mortality of tonsillectomy and adenoidectomy, when performed by well-trained surgeons and anesthesiologists, is 0.006%. The causes of death are almost equally divided among anesthesia, cardiac arrests, and hemorrhage.

Hemorrhage. Hemorrhage, both minor and severe, is the most common complication. The best preventive measure is to make certain the patient is free of respiratory complications at the time of surgery. When hemorrhage does occur, it is usually within 2 to 4 hours of surgery. There is also an increase in incidence about the fifth to seventh postoperative day, presumably because of the loosening of the sutures at about this time. The arterial blood supply of the tonsil is shown in Figure 19–15. Severe nonfatal bleeding requiring carotid ligation and transfusion of five or more units of blood is reported by Pratt as occurring once in about 2500 operations.

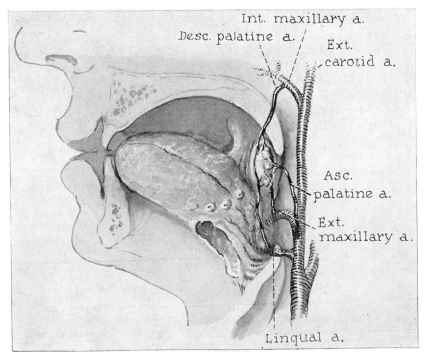

FIG. 19–15. Blood supply of the tonsil.

To control postoperative bleeding it is essential to have good shadow-free illumination, which means a headlight or mirror and not a flashlight. Also it is essential to employ efficient spot suction through a metal cannula. With these advantages the bleeding point can easily be found and controlled by any of several methods of applying pressure. The simplest is to apply sponge-pressure against the bleeding point. If this fails, the surgeon should immediately inject the area around the bleeding point with 5 to 7 ml of a solution containing 1:100,00 epinephrine (e.g., 1% lidocaine with 1:100,000 epinephrine). The localized edema thus produced will exert pressure on the bleeding point for several hours, and the epinephrine will produce vasoconstriction. Saline solution with epinephrine will do as well.

Lastly, if the above fails, the bleeding point can be grasped with a hemostat and ligature or suture-ligature applied in the usual fashion.

Lung Abscess

This is a rare complication of tonsillectomy, though pneumonitis is more frequent. Both are due to aspiration of blood and debris or to a preexisting infection which became manifest postoperatively. Operating in the Rose position enables the blood to collect in the nasopharynx and prevents such aspiration. An operation under local anesthesia is also safer in this regard, because the patient retains his cough reflex.

Rarely, bacteria may be carried into deeper neck tissues by the anesthetic or suturing needle. In this way a pharyngomaxillary space infection occurs.

HYPERPLASIA OF THE THYMUS GLAND; STATUS THYMICO-LYMPHATICUS

The thymus is a ductless gland located in the anterior-superior mediastinum and composed largely of lymphoid cells and fat. Here and there, scattered in the lymphoid tissue, are so-called Hassall's corpuscles, characteristic whorls presumably of epithelial origin. The gland is well-developed in fetal life and reaches its highest development about the end of the second year, although it occasionally remains large in the adult. After the second year it usually reduces in size and is, for the greater part, changed to adipose tissue.

The thymus functions in relation to the "thymus-dependent" lymphoid cells in developing immunologic competence for the delayed or cellular type of immunity. At one time so-called "status thymicolymphaticus," in which an enlarged thymus gland was found, was thought to be responsible for sudden unexplained deaths in infants undergoing surgery. This idea has been abandoned.

REFERENCES

Ogra, P. L.: Effect of Tonsillectomy and Adenoidectomy of Nasopharyngeal Antibody Response to Poliovirus. N. Engl. J. Med., *284*:59, 1971.

Pratt, L. W.: Tonsillectomy and Adenoidectomy: Mortality and Morbidity. Trans. Am. Acad. Ophthalm. Otolaryngol., *74*:1114, 1970.

Sprinkle, P. M., and Veltri, R. W.: The Tonsil and Adenoid Dilemma: Medical or Surgical Treatment. Otolaryngol. Clin. North Am., *7*(3):909, 1974.

Chapter 20
Diseases of the Adenoid and Lingual Tonsil

ACUTE FOLLICULAR INFLAMMATION OF THE ADENOID

Etiology. The general etiologic factors of acute infections of the adenoid are the same as those for inflammatory diseases of the upper respiratory tract (Ch. 8) and will not be repeated here. Adenoidal inflammation is usually associated with an acute tonsillitis.

Symptoms. The disease is usually accompanied by an initial chill, a rise in temperature, swelling of the cervical lymph nodes, and a somewhat prolonged convalescence similar to that of follicular tonsillitis. The inflammation has a strong tendency to recur. The nose becomes obstructed and the voice quite nasal or void of resonance. There may be an indefinite pain in the nasopharynx.

Treatment. The treatment as given for acute respiratory infections is used and will not be repeated.

CHRONIC HYPERPLASTIC ADENOID

Etiology. The chief causes of enlargement of the adenoid are the irritation and inflammation which occur in the nasopharynx during recurrent upper respiratory infections. The same stimulation in adults does not cause lymphoid hyperplasia to a corresponding degree. Chronic hyperplasia of the adenoid may at times be a familial characteristic, perhaps because of a similar environment or anatomic conformation which predisposes to infection.

Symptoms. The symptoms of an enlarged adenoid are largely those resulting from obstruction of the nose at the posterior choanae and obstruction at the pharyngeal end of the eustachian tubes. The mouth is held open, particularly at night, to obtain an adequate airway, and thus snoring results. Also, the patient may develop the habit of elevating the upper lip (the so-called *adenoid facies*) to improve the ease of ingress of air.

More important are the recurrent periods of deafness that follow obstruction of the eustachian tubes. In the beginning the deafness is due to retraction of the membrana tympani, but if unrelieved, the obstruction leads first to serous otitis media and second (with superimposed infection) to otitis media. A pronounced obstruction in the nasopharynx can lead to cardiorespiratory changes (see Ch. 19).

Treatment. A recurrently obstructing hypertrophic adenoid should be surgically removed during a period of health. X-irradiation should be used only when surgery is contraindicated.

ADENOIDECTOMY

An adenoid may be removed with the curette alone (Fig. 20–1), though this

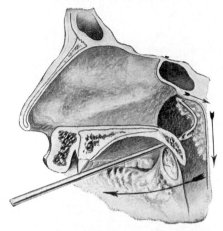

FIG. 20–1. Removal of adenoid remnants with a curette. The arrows indicate the three movements necessary in a normal nasopharynx.

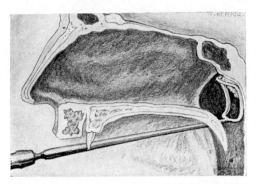

FIG. 20–3. Removing the remaining fringe of adenoid tissue by means of the Barnhill curette, after the mass of adenoid growth has been removed by means of an adenotome.

method does not do as thorough a job as other methods. A more rational and effective method involves use of a La Force or Collum adenotome, or some modification thereof, followed by use of a curette of the Barnhill type.

Technique. General anesthesia is required. When a La Force adenotome is being used, the blade is withdrawn, leaving the fenestra open. The instrument is introduced into the nasopharynx (Fig. 20–2), and the adenoid is engaged by a lifting-depressing sequence.

The curette is introduced in the same manner, and any remaining fringe of adenoid tissue is removed by a wiping motion (Fig. 20–3). Using the finger, one should make certain that all palpable adenoid tissue

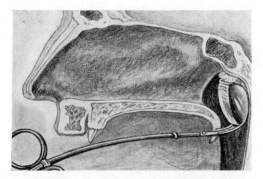

FIG. 20–2. Removing an adenoid by means of an adenotome. A curette removes the remaining fringe.

has been removed from the orifices of the eustachian tubes and choanae. Also, the tip of the finger should be used to explore Rosenmüller's fossa.

NASOPHARYNGEAL BURSA; NASOPHARYNGEAL CYST OR ABSCESS; THORNWALDT'S DISEASE

Etiology. A nasopharyngeal bursa or sac seems to develop from an embryonic pouch. The pharyngeal segment of the notochord is thought to remain united with the pharyngeal entoderm.

Pathology. The sac and its canal, extending to the pharyngeal mucosa, are situated beneath the adenoid or its remnants. The sac extends backward and upward to the periosteum of the occipital bone.

If the canal becomes occluded a cyst forms, or if infection is present an abscess may develop. An infection with an open canal would result in postnasal discharge and crusting. The crusts usually have a conical shape that fits into the conical depression of the discharging canal.

Symptoms. The symptoms usually presented are postnasal discharge, crusting, frequent colds, sneezing, hoarseness, bad taste or odor, hawking, and coughing. Other symptoms may be headache or pains in various parts of the head and neck, especially in the back of the head just below the occipital bone, nasal obstruction, sore throat, nasal speech, and cervical adenitis. Symptoms relating to the ear, such as vertigo, tinnitus, earache, and deafness, may be present.

The canal may be seen by the use of a throat mirror or Yankauer's direct speculum. If an abscess is present, a small dimple may be seen on the surface of the swelling. A probe may be passed upward into it.

Treatment. One blade of the curved pharyngeal scissors (Fig. 20–4) is introduced into the canal, and half of the adenoid mass is cut. The opposite blade of the scissors is then inserted in a similar manner for the other half and that portion cut. The remaining portions of the adenoid are then removed in the usual manner. The posterior and remaining portion of the canal wall or cyst should be thoroughly curetted to remove any remaining membrane.

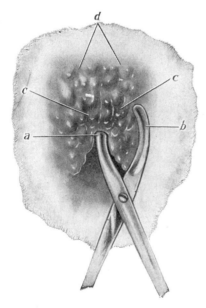

FIG. 20–4. Operative treatment of Thornwaldt's disease: *a,* the left blade of the pharyngeal scissors introduced into the suppurating sinus between the lateral halves of the adenoid; *b,* the right blade of the scissors at the border of the adenoid tissue. When the blades are closed, the lateral half of the adenoid upon this side is severed. The scissors are then transferred to the other lateral half of the adenoid tissue and closed. This completely severs the lower portion of the adenoid tissue and obliterates the suppurating sinus. The remaining upper portion of the adenoid—*c, c, d*—is then removed with the adenotome and curette.

THE LINGUAL TONSIL

The lingual tonsil may be the site of acute or chronic infections, abscesses, hypertrophy, lingual varix, hyperkeratosis, syphilis, tuberculosis, leprosy, benign or malignant neoplasms, cysts from occlusion of the foramen cecum, accessory thyroid, and pointed foreign objects.

Acute Follicular Lingual Tonsillitis

Acute follicular inflammation of the lingual tonsil is characterized by no rise or a moderate rise of temperature, painful deglutition, and a burning, pricking sensation in the throat. There may be some tenderness on pressure in the region of the great cornu of the hyoid bone. Upon inspection, the pharynx and the pillars of the fauces may be slightly reddened, while the faucial tonsils may appear normal. The laryngeal mirror shows the masses on the lingual tonsil to be reddened and swollen.

Abscess of the Lingual Tonsil

This process is usually characterized by a purulent accumulation beneath the lymph nodules at the base of the tongue and is usually limited to one side. The temperature is elevated, and the pain upon deglutition is severe. The patient complains of soreness and great tenderness upon pressure in the region of the great cornu of the hyoid bone upon the affected side. Inspection with the throat mirror shows great swelling and redness at the base of the tongue upon the affected side. Palpation with the finger may or may not elicit fluctuation.

Phlegmonous inflammation here, as in the faucial tonsil, may undergo resolution without the formation of an abscess. Extension beyond the boundary of the lingual tonsil is rare. If the suppuration extends to the floor of the mouth, it may be mistaken for or constitute Ludwig's angina.

Hypertrophy of the Lingual Tonsil

Hypertrophy of the lingual tonsil is rare in children. It is probably caused by repeated or continued infection of the lymph structures of the pharynx and fauces.

Symptoms. The symptoms are sometimes absent, though the sensation of a foreign body in the throat is usually mentioned. There is a pricking sensation, as though a splinter had lodged in the fauces, or the patient complains of the sensation of a lump, a hair, or other foreign body in the throat. Troublesome fits of coughing are often present.

During meals the symptoms frequently disappear. Pain is rarely complained of, but the disagreeable sensation already referred to is present. The use of the voice increases the symptoms and often gives rise to the pricking sensation and the cough.

Upon examination with the throat mirror, a few enlarged masses are seen upon the base of the tongue. The involvement is usually on both sides but may be limited to one. The masses may be so large as to push the epiglottis backward or even to overhang it.

Chapter 21
Deep Neck Infections

Surgical Anatomy

The cervical fascia (Fig. 21–1) consists of the superficial fascia and the deep cervical fascia. There are three subdivisions of the latter: (1) the enveloping layer; (2) the pretracheal layer; and (3) the prevertebral layer.

Superficial Cervical Fascia. This fascial layer lies just below the skin of the neck. It carries the superficial vessels and nerves and is separated from the deep cervical fascia by the thin platysma muscle which extends anteriorly over the neck. This muscle arises inferiorly from the deep cervical fascia and clavicle and extends superiorly to become attached to the inferior border of the mandible. At places the platysma blends with the muscles of the face.

Deep Cervical Fascia. The three subdivisions of the deep cervical fascia, as mentioned above, provide a complete envelope for all the cervical structures except the platysma muscle and the superficial blood vessels and nerves. Passing inward from the superficial cervical fascia, one encounters the investing or enveloping layer of the deep cervical fascia and then successively the pretracheal and prevertebral layers.

The investing or enveloping layer of fascia arises inferiorly from the anterior and posterior borders of the sternum to form the suprasternal space of Burns (Gruber). These two lamellae are then attached to the hyoid bone. Laterally the investing layer is attached to the spinous processes of the cer-

vical vertebrae and encases the trapezius muscle. Anterior to the border of the trapezius, it ensheathes the sternocleidomastoid muscle, and then it unites with its fellow on the opposite side above the hyoid bone as a single layer, and below the hyoid with the two lamellae that form the space of Burns. Superiorly the investing fascia is attached to the inferior margin of the mandible, the posterior angle of the jaw, the zygomatic arch (encasing the parotid gland), the mastoid process, the superior nuchal line, and the external occipital protuberance. As the single layer of fascia above the hyoid bone passes superiorly, it fuses with the fascial coverings of the anterior and posterior bellies of the digastric muscles, so that the submaxillary and submental areas are largely shut off from one another and from the rest of the neck.

The pretracheal layer splits off from the investing layer deep to the sternocleidomastoid muscle. It passes anterior to the trachea, larynx, and hypopharynx. It descends into the root of the neck and mediastinum to blend with the aorta and pericardium. Laterally it ensheathes the omohyoid, thyrohyoid, sternohyoid, and sternothyroid muscles and forms the carotid sheath.

The pretracheal fascia lies posterior to the esophagus and the great vessels of the neck and over the prevertebral musculature.

Fascial Spaces in the Neck. Three fascial spaces (Fig. 21–1) are delineated by three layers of deep cervical fascia. The visceral space lies between the pretracheal and prevertebral fascias and contains the lower pharynx, larynx, trachea, cervical esophagus, thyroid gland, and great vessels of the neck. Infections here are serious because they produce pressure on these structures and because they can extend downward into the mediastinum, laterally along the subclavian vessels into the axillary space, or upward into the retromandibular space. The prevertebral space lies between the prevertebral musculature and the prevertebral fascia. Infections here could burrow laterally or inferiorly into the posterior mediastinum. The suprahyoid space lies above the hyoid bone between the investing fascia and the covering of the mylohyoid muscles. Infections here could break into the submental or submaxillary subdivisions of the space as described below, or they could work downward into the visceral space.

The parapharyngeal space, a large triangular compartment filled with loose fatty tissue, is lateral to the pharynx (Fig. 21–2). The parapharyngeal space, also known as the pharyngomaxillary, the peripharyngeal, and the lateral pharyngeal space, is composed of two compartments—anterior (prestyloid) and posterior (retrostyloid).

The posterior compartment is formed by the carotid sheath. It extends from the base of the skull to the visceral cervical space and contains the internal carotid artery, the internal jugular vein, the ascending pharyngeal artery, and the hypoglossal, vagus, cervical sympathetic, glossopharyngeal, and spinal accessory nerves.

The anterior compartment, a potential space unless infected, contains connective tissue, occasionally the external maxillary arteries, and usually a few lymph nodes. It extends from the base of the skull to the angle of the jaw. Anteromedially the anterior space is bound by the buccopharyngeal fascia covering the superior constrictor; this becomes thickened anteriorly at the pterygomandibular ligament and is reflected onto the fascial covering of the internal pterygoid muscle, which forms the anterolateral boundary. This in turn is continuous with the stylomandibular ligament (medial parotid fascia), which forms the posterolateral wall. The posterior boundary is formed by the fascial covering of the styloid and its muscles and the anterior wall of the carotid sheath. Posteriomedially the alar fascia (stylopharyngeal aponeurosis) is found. All these fascias form a complete fascia-lined

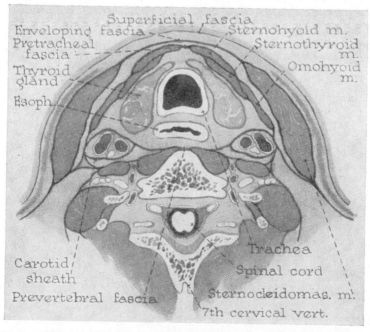

FIG. 21–1.   The cervical fascia of the neck at the seventh cervical vertebra.

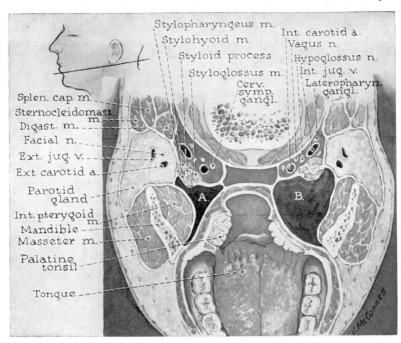

FIG. 21–2. The fascial planes of the neck at the level of the palatine tonsil: *A*, the anterior (prestyloid) space; *B*, an abscess in the anterior compartment of the parapharyngeal space pushing the superior pharyngeal constrictor muscle and tonsil to the median position.

space except superiorly where the medial parotid layer is absent.

Etiology

Deep neck infections may be caused by infections in or about the tonsils, pharynx, teeth, sinuses, thyroid gland (or its fascia), middle ear, mastoid (Bezold's abscess), petrous temporal bone, base of the tongue, floor of the mouth, cervical vertebrae, or esophagus (perforation), or by suppurating cysts, injuries of the jaw, infections of the cervical lymph nodes, thrombosis of the pterygoid plexus of veins, and trauma. The tonsils are the most common portals of entry, usually by way of a phlebitis or a thrombophlebitis of the tonsillar veins. The cervical lymph nodes may be infected without involvement of the fascial neck spaces; however, any cervical lymph node infection may result in a deep neck infection.

The principal bacteria recovered when the teeth are the source of the infection are the spirilla of Vincent. When the source is elsewhere, streptococci are usually found.

Pathology

Once the infection has a start in the soft tissues of the neck, it extends, if unchecked, usually by the line of least resistance into one of the fascial neck spaces. From there it may travel upward, downward, or laterally, following the fascial spaces as described above.

PHARYNGEAL ABSCESS

Etiology. The parapharyngeal space may become infected (1) by direct implantation from an operating needle; (2) through the vascular channels, as would occur with an endophlebitis or thrombosis; and (3) through the lymphatics from suppuration of the deep cervical nodes or lymphangitis.

Infections of this space are especially prone to follow tonsil surgery when it is preceded by local anesthesia. They frequently arise as an extension from a neighboring compartment. The parapharyngeal space may become infected by way of the vascular or lymph channels from the tonsil, pharynx, nose, sinuses, adenoid, pharyngeal lymph nodes, cervical vertebrae, mastoid, or petrous bone.

Pathology. Deep cervical infection usually occurs as a phlegmonous type in which signs of local inflammation are predominant. A vascular form in which the local signs are subordinate but in which the symptoms are suggestive of systemic or bloodstream infection is much less common.

The phlegmonous form is primarily a cellulitis within the prestyloid compartment. A later abscess formation occurs in the majority of cases. It is frequently accompanied by an unrecognized thrombosis of the internal jugular vein, which may produce a fatal septicemia.

The pathogenic bacteria recovered are similar to those usually found in the tonsils and pharynx. Hemolytic and nonhemolytic streptococci, fusiform bacilli, pneumococci, and *Staphylococcus aureus* are the more common ones reported.

Infection may spread from the anterior compartment to the posterior compartment, with extension downward along the sheath of the great vessels, accompanied by a thrombosis of the jugular veins or a mediastinitis or both; or the infection of the posterior compartment may extend upward along the vessel sheath, resulting in an intracranial infection or erosion of the internal carotid artery. Infection of the anterior compartment may extend along the styloglossal muscle, producing an abscess of the floor of the mouth (Brunner).

Symptoms. The symptoms of an abscess in the parapharyngeal space usually develop within 4 to 7 days after the infection has been introduced. A high continuous temperature is frequently present, especially if a lymphatic involvement occurs. Marked drops and elevations of temperature with chills are present with a bloodstream complication. As a rule, however, the temperature is moderate, not exceeding 101 or 102°F.

Trismus due to a splinting of the internal pterygoid muscle is a prominent symptom. It gets increasingly worse until attempts to open the mouth are very painful. Trismus may be absent if the infection is deep to the styloid process and its attached structures, thereby missing the internal pterygoid muscle.

A tender swelling in the submaxillary region of the affected side, especially at the angle of the mandible, usually occurs before the end of the first week.

Pain in the affected area, occasionally referred to the ears, is a constant complaint. Dysphagia is a characteristic symptom that gets increasingly worse. Edema of the uvula, pillars, and palate occurs early. Leukocytosis is usually 20,000 or more. Adenitis of the lymph nodes is almost always present but is usually overshadowed by the swelling in that region.

A displacement of the lateral pharyngeal wall usually occurs without swelling or enlargement of the tonsil. This helps to differentiate this condition from a peritonsillar abscess, in which inflammatory swelling of the tonsil is present. Swelling over the region of the parotid glands is present at times. Infection lower in the neck below the level of the angle of the jaw would not give these signs.

A lateral roentgenogram of the neck shows a displacement of the trachea anteriorly, especially due to infections from the hypopharynx.

If the jugular vein is involved, there is usually a history of a preceding sore throat with later signs of sepsis, chills, and positive blood cultures. A small, deep, tender, nonfluctuating swelling may be located along its course. Emboli are not uncommon.

Treatment. Once pus has formed, there is no alternative to surgical evacuation as described below. Prior to that, bedrest and hot moist dressings to encourage localization of the abscess are necessary. Antimicrobial therapy in large doses, directed whenever possible by sensitivity tests, is necessary. Surgical intervention is indicated by signs of abscess formation and the symptoms of increasing sepsis.

10

Intraoral Incision. If bulging into the pharynx occurs, a preliminary cocainization is done. A curved tonsillar hemostat is inserted about ½ inch through the superior constrictor muscle into the anterior compartment and is spread. The incision should be kept open until drainage stops.

External Incision. If the abscess points externally or shows marked swelling, drainage may be established by making a small incision over the fluctuant area or over the most prominent portion of the swelling. A curved forceps is thrust into the cavity of the abscess, and the opening is enlarged by spreading the forceps. A counteropening to secure dependent drainage may be advisable. A cigarette drain extending to the bottom of the abscess is sutured in place. If a large cavity is found, it should be packed loosely with iodoform gauze around a cigarette drain. The gauze is removed in 1 to 2 days; however, the cigarette drain is usually left in place for about a week.

Daily irrigations of the abscess cavity with solutions of an appropriate antibiotic can be accomplished through a soft rubber tube which may be used as a drain.

Mosher's Operation. In many instances the exact location of the pus may not be known, or symptoms of sepsis may be so marked that delay in surgical intervention is not advisable. If the carotid sheath and its contents are involved, a more extensive dissection, such as that proposed by Mosher, should be done.

The landmarks to be kept in mind when doing the various surgical procedures on the neck are the cricoid cartilage, the tip of the great horn of the hyoid bone, the styloid process, the inner edge of the sternocleidomastoid muscle, and, as dissection proceeds, the posterior belly of the digastric muscle.

Technique. A T-shaped incision is made which gives a wide exposure. The crossbar of the T runs parallel with and close to the border of the jaw. The submaxillary salivary gland is exposed. After the facial vein is tied and cut, the lower border of the gland is elevated. The finger is inserted beneath the gland and carried backward and upward until the stylomandibular ligament is felt beneath the angle of the jaw. The finger is carried upward along this ligament until the styloid process is felt. The parapharyngeal space is located by inserting the finger upward and external to the styloid process to the base of the skull. When there is pus in the floor of the mouth or at the base of the tongue, an incision is made in the center of the floor of the submaxillary fossa and carried forward or backward according to indications.

A. L. Beck uses a single incision running parallel to the border of the jaw. The deep fascia is exposed at a point behind the angle of the jaw. A closed, blunt, artery forceps is inserted through the deep fascia, and the opening is enlarged sufficiently to give room for the introduction of a finger. The finger is passed beneath the angle of the jaw to the stylomandibular ligament, where the fascial spaces are entered as indicated.

The carotid sheath lies beneath the styloid process and may be drained at this point if necessary.

MEDIASTINITIS

The most serious complication of deep neck infections is mediastinitis, which as a rule is accompanied by visible extension of the cervical swelling.

The paths of infection to the mediastinum pass along the deep fascial planes of the neck by way of the sheath of the great vessels, by extension to the retropharyngeal space (rare), and then descending by way of the prevertebral space to the posterior mediastinum, along the esophagus (visceral space) to enter the mediastinum posterior to the sternum.

The signs and symptoms of mediastinitis are high fever, restlessness, rapid pulse, tenderness along the course of the great vessels, and stiffness of the neck. Spasmodic alternations of the pulse and respiration are suggestive.

Jugular thrombosis has been reported in a few cases. Edema of the larynx may occur, requiring a tracheotomy. Ludwig's angina, hemorrhage, osteomyelitis of the cervical vertebra and mandible, pneumonia, erysipelas, vagus involvement, meningitis, parotid abscess, and septicopyemia have all been reported as complications.

LUDWIG'S ANGINA—INFECTIONS OF THE SUBLINGUAL SPACE, SUBMAXILLARY SPACE, AND SUBMENTAL SPACE

Surgical Anatomy of the Floor of the Mouth

In the floor of the mouth there are three important spaces (Fig. 21–3): the submental and submaxillary spaces below the mylohyoid muscle and the sublingual space above it. Any infection in the floor of the mouth may, by edema, encroach seriously on the airway in the pharynx; however, infections below the mylohyoid are less likely to do this, because this firm, unyielding muscle limits the upward spread of the edema.

Submental Space. The lateral borders of this space are formed by the anterior bellies of the digastric muscles, the inferior border by a line through the hyoid bone, the roof by the mylohyoid muscle, and the floor by the investing fascia and skin of the chin. Infections in this space are usually confined by the firm union of the investing deep cervical fascia with the anterior digastric muscles and the hyoid bone. A considerable edema of the chin may occur, and the exploring probe may not find the pus until 2 to 3 cm have been traversed.

Submaxillary Space. The superior border of this space is demarcated by a line along the ramus of the mandible, extending posteriorly until the mastoid process is met. The posterior margin is formed by the stylohyoid and posterior belly of the digastric muscle. The anterior border is composed of the anterior belly of the digastric muscle. The roof is formed by the mylohyoid and hyoglossal muscles and the floor by the investing deep cervical fascia and skin of the

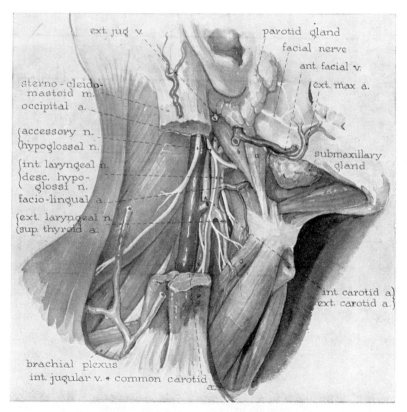

Fig. 21–3. The anterior triangle of the neck. The superficial blood vessels, the lymph nodes, and a portion of the sternocleidomastoid muscle have been removed. The stylohyoid muscle (*a*) and posterior belly of the digastric muscle (*b*) separate the submaxillary space (digastric triangle) from the carotid triangle. The superior belly of the omohyoid muscle (*c*) separates the carotid triangle from the muscular triangle.

neck and chin. Within the space is found the submaxillary gland with its duct passing posteriorly to the posterior margin of the mylohyoid muscle to enter the sublingual space. Infection of the submaxillary space is usually confined to the space itself, but it may work its way along the submaxillary duct (Wharton's) and accompanying gland structure into the sublingual space, or it may extend downward along the hyoglossal muscle to the fascial spaces of the neck.

Sublingual Space. This space is inclosed laterally and anteriorly by the body of the mandible. The posterior boundary of the sublingual space is formed by the tongue, the palatoglossus and styloglossus muscles, and the hyoid bone. The upper boundary is the tongue itself, and the floor is made up of the firm, unyielding mylohyoid muscles. A potential weak spot, where infections in this area may reach the submaxillary space, exists at the point of entrance of the styloglossus and hyoglossus muscles, near the angle filled by a portion of the submaxillary gland with its duct, the glossopharyngeal and hypoglossal nerves, and lingual artery and vein. In an infection of the sublingual space, the edema finds the line of least resistance superiorly and posteriorly, with consequent reduction of the airway.

Ludwig's Angina

Ludwig's angina is a rare, virulent, and often fatal septic inflammation of the soft tissues of primarily the sublingual space with later extension to the submaxillary space or to the tissues of the neck.

Etiology. The etiology of Ludwig's angina has been attributed to trauma of the interior of the mouth, local mouth infections, dental caries, especially of the molar and premolar teeth, tonsillitis and peritonsillitis, trauma of dental extraction, Vincent's angina, facial erysipelas, otitis media and externa, and ulcers of the lip and nose. However, infections of the tonsils and front teeth are not likely to be causative factors. If the infection is from the teeth, gas-producing organisms of the anaerobic type are usually predominant. If the infection has a nondental origin, streptococci are usually found. Most investigators have found that streptococci associated with the spirillum of Vincent predominate in many cases. In other words, a mixed infection is frequently observed.

Ludwig's angina is most frequent in children and young adults. However, no age is immune. Males are more often attacked.

Pathology. The condition has been attributed to a lymphadenitis and a perilymphadenitis, but it is essentially a cellulitis which spreads by continuity of tissue. The accompanying edema usually finds its easiest route of exit superiorly and posteriorly. As a result, the tongue is usually edematous and displaced superiorly and posteriorly, encroaching on the airway. Pus, if it forms, usually points within the mouth. Both the edema and the pointing of the pus tend to be directed toward the mouth by the mylohyoid muscle. The infection may spread to the submaxillary space and from there to the neck by direct extension along the hyoglossus muscle.

Symptoms. The duration of the infection may vary from a few days to 3 or 4 weeks. The temperature is elevated as a rule from 100 to 106°F. Leukocytosis ranges from 10,000 to 35,000 or more.

A hard, boardlike swelling of the submaxillary and submental regions is characteristic. Swelling and induration of the floor of the mouth, gums, and tongue are also present. The tongue is pushed upward and backward. In severe cases the hard, boardlike swelling may extend downward to the clavicle. Suppuration may not occur in these cases.

Trismus is present if the infection or cellulitis invades the parapharyngeal space, causing an irritative spasm of the internal pterygoid muscle.

If it is not treated early, an abscess forms in the majority of cases. Thomas reports that pus was found in 66 of his 106 collected cases.

The first complaints are usually a pain in the floor of the mouth, stiffness in movements of the tongue, pain in efforts to clear the throat, and salivation. Fever is not always present in this stage.

The displaced tongue and pharyngeal swelling may interfere with the breathing and in later stages may produce asphyxia.

There is a grave danger of loss of life from suffocation or later from exhaustion.

The infection usually extends into the submaxillary, the parotid, or the pharyngomaxillary space. Frequently all of them are involved. If the carotid sheath is invaded, a jugular thrombosis may occur. Mediastinitis is common. Osteomyelitis of the mandible is a rare complication.

A type of infection resembling Ludwig's angina, which is due to an abscess in the root of the tongue rather than under, is characterized by a tedious course with severe dysphagia and a marked systemic reaction.

Treatment. An attempt should be made to localize the infection while signs of respiratory obstruction are watched for. A tracheotomy to relieve respiratory obstruction should not be delayed until the patient has exhausted himself by a struggle for air.

Antimicrobial therapy should be given early and vigorously. Heat, both externally in the form of hot packs and internally as hot mouth irrigations, may help localize the infection.

If pus forms, incision and drainage are imperative.

Incisions should be made below and parallel to the body of the mandible through the deep fascia to the depth of the submaxillary gland. The deeper exploration should be carried out with blunt forceps. An additional vertical incision should be made above the hyoid bone to the lower border of the chin. Some operators have passed the median raphe of the mylohyoids and split the geniohyoglossus muscles apart. The object of the incision is not only to evacuate pus but also to relieve tension.

An incision along the anterior border of the sternocleidomastoid muscle, carrying the dissection by blunt or, if necessary, sharp instruments well into the depth of the neck, even to the mucous membrane of the pharynx, may be elected in suitable cases.

CERVICAL LYMPH NODE ABSCESSES

Suppuration of localized groups of lymph nodes is not common. The superficial or deep nodes may be involved.

In inflammation of the superficial nodes with abscess formation, incision should be delayed until fluctuation is present, provided sepsis or evidence of deep neck involvement is absent.

In inflammation of the deep nodes, suppuration, if present, takes place late. If a definite sepsis is present, surgical drainage is indicated. Distant metastasis and thrombosis of the internal jugular vein may occur.

THROMBOSIS OF THE JUGULAR VEIN FROM THROAT INFECTION

Etiology. Infection of the carotid sheath may be secondary to infection of any of the other compartments of the neck or the lymph nodes, especially those located on the vessel sheath itself.

The routes of infection from the pharynx to thrombosis of the jugular vein may be (1) thrombophlebitis of the tonsillar veins into the pterygoid plexus or through the facial veins into the jugular vein; (2) lymphangitis with a secondary periphlebitis and endophlebitis and an associated thrombosis; (3) direct extension by continuity of tissue.

The two principal hematogenous avenues are by way of the tonsillar veins into the pterygoid plexus and through the facial veins into the internal jugular vein.

Symptoms. Signs and symptoms of sepsis are present. Tenderness or swelling over the sheath may be found. Torticollis on the opposite side is significant of inflammation under the sternocleidomastoid muscle. Torticollis from infection along the paravertebral and trapezius muscles occurs on the same side. Metastatic abscesses are common.

Inflamed lymph nodes should be ruled out.

Treatment. Adequate doses of antimicrobial drugs should be given throughout the period of sepsis. If these agents fail, some form of surgical drainage should be instituted. If the carotid sheath and visceral space are involved, an incision along the anterior border of the sternocleidomastoid muscle is made as for a jugular resection. The sheath is opened and the jugular vein ligated and severed. A gauze drain is placed in the wound.

RETROPHARYNGEAL ABSCESS; PREVERTEBRAL SPACE ABSCESS

Clinical Anatomy. The retropharyngeal space extends from the anterior face of the basiocciput downward through the prevertebral space into the posterior mediastinum; however, the prevertebral fascia and the fascia of the superior constrictor muscle become firmly attached, with the prevertebral muscles, to the occiput at about the level of the prominence of the second cervical vertebra. This tends to confine the abscess to the upper portion.

Laterally the retropharyngeal space is continuous with the parapharyngeal space.

The retropharyngeal lymph nodes generally consist of two to five nodes, behind the posterior pharyngeal wall near the outer edge and in close relation externally with the great vessels of the neck. The retropharyngeal lymph nodes drain the adjacent muscles and bones, the accessory sinuses, the pharynx, the middle and internal ears, and the eustachian tube.

Etiology. An abscess of the retropharyngeal space is not common. Among the various factors leading to such an infection are the following:

1. Suppuration in the retropharyngeal lymph nodes, perhaps following an acute bacterial infection.

2. Injuries of the posterior wall due to foreign bodies.

3. Rarely, in neglected cases, a retropharyngeal abscess may follow an ear infection by direct extension.

4. Tuberculosis.

5. Secondary to suppuration of the parotid gland.

Symptoms. There is usually a preceding or concurrent acute infection of the throat.

The patient, if old enough, complains of painful deglutition, and if the swelling is marked or in the lower portion of the pharynx, obstructive symptoms such as snoring, choking respiration, or even dyspnea and stertorous breathing may occur. Cyanosis, if observed, is rarely serious.

A unilateral or predominantly unilateral cervical adenitis on the affected side is al-

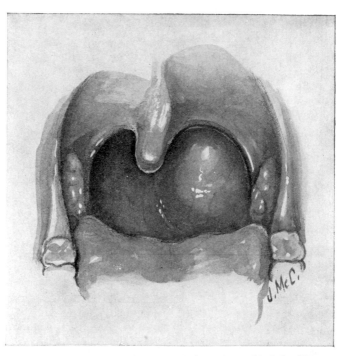

FIG. 21-4.   Retropharyngeal abscess on the left side.

most always observed. Cough is usually present. The voice is much the same as in quinsy. In acute cases the temperature may be elevated from 1 to 2°F, whereas in the chronic tuberculous cases, little or no temperature elevation may be present. A tuberculous retropharyngeal abscess may rupture into the pharynx, producing a granuloma at the site of the rupture. A lateral roentgenogram of the neck usually shows an anterior bulging of the posterior pharyngeal wall.

Aneurysm of an artery in this region has been mistakenly diagnosed as retropharyngeal abscess, a fatal hemorrhage following the incision. The pulsation and bruit present in aneurysm should be sought in all cases of suspected abscesses of the pharynx. The pulsation may be noted with the eye or finger, while the bruit may be distinguished with the stethoscope introduced through the mouth.

Malformation of the posterior wall of the pharynx, causing bulging of one side, is occasionally found. The hard, firm character of the mass readily distinguishes it from the soft, boggy mass which is present in abscess formation (Fig. 21–4).

Acute infectious inflammations of the pharyngeal mucous membrane sometimes simulate retropharyngeal abscess. The difference in the resistance upon digital examination will determine which of the processes is present.

Prognosis. The dangers in young subjects are chiefly suffocation and strangulation upon the spontaneous rupture of the abscess. In older patients these dangers are not so great, as their reflexes enable them to ward it off or to anticipate it. Under treatment, the prognosis is nearly always good except when the disease is due to tuberculous caries of the vertebrae.

The possible but less common results, if the abscess is left to itself, are burrowing into the parapharyngeal space with or without external pointing; traveling downward behind the esophagus into the posterior mediastinum; spreading by the blood and lymph streams into the meningeal area with a general septicemia; hemorrhage by erosion of the great vessels in the neck; pressure on the epiglottis and larynx with edema; rupture and aspiration of infected contents with pneumonia; lung abscess; sudden asphyxia; and rupture into the esophagus.

Treatment. Most cases, if seen early, are successfully treated with antibiotics or sulfonamides. If the case is neglected, suppuration with fluctuation may occur and demand surgical intervention. Obstruction to the airway necessitates immediate evacuation of the abscess.

Surgical treatment consists of immediate evacuation of the pus. This is sufficient in acute cases. In chronic cases secondary to tuberculosis of the cervical vertebrae, this is usually done by the external operation.

Internal Operation. The patient is placed upon a table with his head lowered to prevent the larynx being bathed in pus. With children this precaution is especially urgent, because their reflexes are not sufficiently trained to prevent aspiration of the infected secretion into the trachea and lungs, where it might cause pneumonia.

The left index finger is introduced into the mouth, and the tip is placed against the soft fluctuating tumor.

A short-bladed scalpel or a longer one, the proximal end of which is wrapped with

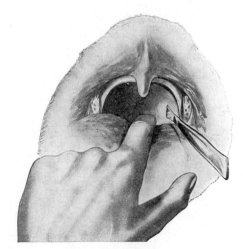

FIG. 21–5. The oral operation for retropharyngeal abscess. The finger is used as a guide to the fluctuating area and as a tongue depressor, while a short-bladed scalpel is used to open the abscess.

a strip of adhesive plaster or cotton, is introduced into the mouth, the finger being used as a guide (Fig. 21–5). If the abscess is pointing, a forceps may be used to puncture the wall.

The abscess wall by the side of the finger is incised. The pus then flows through the incision into the pharyngeal cavity, from which it may be removed with suction or gauze sponges or by expectoration by the patient. In the acute forms of abscess, recovery is rapid, and little further attention is necessary. In the chronic forms, further attention is advisable.

Chapter 22
Chronic Granulomas of the Nose, Throat, and Ear

TUBERCULOSIS OF THE NOSE

Etiology. Tuberculous infection of the nose is rare. When present, it is usually a smooth tumor (tuberculoma) consisting of granulation tissue and giant cells. The tumor is usually attached to the septum, though shallow ulcerations of the septum or floor may be present in which tubercle bacilli may be found. An immediate search for pulmonary disease shoud be made.

Pathology. Granulations, superficial ulcerations, and wartlike or sessile tumors are found. Complications include perforation of the nasal septum, occasionally with extension to the upper lip. With the advent of improved treatment of tuberculosis, both the incidence and severity of tuberculosis of the nose have decreased.

TUBERCULOSIS OF THE PHARYNX AND FAUCES

Primary tuberculosis of the pharynx and fauces (with the exception of the tonsils) is rare and is probably always secondary to pulmonary or laryngeal forms of the disease. Numerous cases are on record in which the faucial tonsils were the seat of tuberculous infiltration.

Symptoms. The symptoms vary with the anatomic location and extent of the lesion. If the soft palate is involved, fluids may enter the nose during the act of swallowing.

LUPUS OF THE NOSE, THROAT, AND AURICLE

Lupus vulgaris probably is an attenuated form of tuberculosis and is characterized by nodules of granulation tissue which may ulcerate. It attacks both sexes equally.

Pathology. Lupus of the nose generally begins on the anterior portion of the cartilaginous septum or on the skin around the nasal orifice. It may spread from the septum to the inner wall of the ala. Four types of lesions may be recognized: (1) granulations; (2) vegetations or proliferations; (3) tumors; and (4) ulcerations. It appears as small nodules which coalesce and ulcerate and may disappear by absorption. The reparative process takes place feebly at the margins of the ulcer, thus forming a smooth pale bluish cicatrix. The ulcers reappear and then disappear. This process may continue for years without spreading to other regions. The nodules are firm and well marked. The disease rarely attacks the cartilage and never the bones.

Lupus of the auricle is similar to that of the nose.

Symptoms. While lupus may be due to the tubercle bacillus, there is a clinical distinction between it and tuberculous ulceration. Lupus is slow and insidious in its development and is not necessarily associated with pulmonary tuberculosis. It has a tendency to heal, cicatrize, and recur and does not often result in death from pulmonary involvement. One or both nostrils may be affected, and there may or may not be stenosis. The discharge varies with the stage of ulceration. At the onset it is thin and watery and later becomes thick and even fetid, especially after crusts appear. Pain and tenderness may be present but are usually absent. Itching is sometimes noted.

Deformity may be present if the alae are involved; when the disease is limited to the septum, deformity is rarely present.

Treatment. Since the disease is self-limited, treatment is often unnecessary. Antituberculosis medication may be tried.

SYPHILIS

Syphilis is a general infection of the blood and lymph streams due to *Treponema pallidum*. It is the presence of the spirochetes in the perivascular spaces that excites the reaction, consisting of an accumulation of mononuclear cells, chiefly lymphocytes and plasma cells. For treatment, penicillin is the drug of choice, usually in large doses.

SYPHILIS OF THE NOSE

A *primary lesion* in the nose is rare. When diagnosed, it may be found just within the alae, at the line of mucous membrane, on the line of the vomer junction with the cartilaginous septum, at the edge of the vertical plate, or in even more obscure locations.

Because of the exposed position, the appearance of the primary lesion may be modified greatly; it may be erosive, neoplastic, scabbed, or impetiginous. In the erosive form, the carmine red ulcer is round or oval with a flattened surface. It may be up to a centimeter or more in diameter.

In the neoplastic form, the surface erosion, 1 to 2 cm in diameter, is convex with the center elevated 2 to 3 mm. It is uniformly red or dotted with gray points, giving it a papular appearance. It has a firm feeling when touched.

The scabbed form is difficult to diagnose. The surface is irregular and partly or completely covered by scabs. It is variable in color.

Secondary syphilis of the nose may manifest itself by a syphilitic rhinitis. It is not always recognized, usually being regarded as a simple obstinate cold in the head. The scanty thick discharge with stenosis of the nose should, however, excite suspicion of the true nature of the disease. It may occur alone or with a syphilitic pharyngitis or laryngitis.

Secondary lesions appear in the nose and throat in the form of erythema or mucous patches. Being superficial ulcerations, they are often overlooked.

Tertiary lesions of the nose are not common occurrences at the present time.

Seen early, the gumma of the septum over the vomer usually appears as a smooth circumscribed swelling, covered by a generally inflamed mucosa. It may appear anywhere along the upper respiratory tract, from the vestibule of the nose down to the subglottic space, in the early form as a gumma or a chondritis and later as an ulcer, circumscribed, deep, and destructive or superficial and serpiginous. The favorite seat of gummas is the bony septum, although they are also found on the hard and soft palates, the posterior wall of the pharynx, and the epiglottis. Usually there is no sharp outline to the infiltration, but a gradual fading into normal tissue. Gummatous infiltrations involve the mucous membrane, cartilage, and bone. Infiltration of the perichondrium and periosteum may become extensive. Necrosis may follow, with loss of the bony and cartilaginous portions of the septum and in some cases suppuration of the accessory sinuses.

SYPHILIS OF THE PHARYNX, FAUCES, AND TONSILS

The fauces and pharynx are second only to the skin as sites for the manifestation of syphilis, particularly in the secondary stage. This may be accounted for in part by the presence of a large number of lymphoid glands, the excessive friction, and the complex embryologic union of tissues in this region.

Congenital syphilis is more common in the pharynx than in the nose. About 50% of the congenital cases become evident here

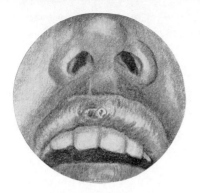

FIG. 22-1. Chancre of the lip.

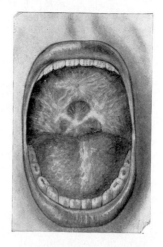

FIG. 22-3. Syphilitic scars of the fauces and pharynx causing a partial constriction of the isthmus between the nasopharynx and mesopharynx.

in the first year of life, 33⅓% within the first 6 months.

Primary. The primary sore of syphilis occurring about the mouth is found most frequently on the lips (Fig. 22-1), tonsils, and tongue, respectively. The tongue is usually involved on its tip or lateral edges and rarely on the posterior two-thirds. Primary syphilis on the lingual tonsil is rare.

Secondary. The secondary lesions consist of the usual erythema of the face and body and mucous membranes (Fig. 22-2). They may appear from 6 to 8 weeks after the initial lesion or even as late as several months.

The erythema of secondary syphilis may be confounded with acute pharyngitis. The differential points are the darker or dusky color (in syphilis) of the mucous membrane; the more marked involvement of the tonsils and soft palate; the diminished secretion; the line of demarcation between the inflamed area and the hard palate; the dusky

symmetrical patches on the anterior pillars; the opalescent appearance of the mucous membrane of the tonsils; and the persistence of the disease, as contrasted with evanescence of acute pharyngitis.

Tertiary. The tertiary lesions appear from 3 to 25 years after the primary manifestation and may be ulcerative, gangrenous, or gummatous; they are very destructive to both soft and bony tissues. The characteristic gummatous formations break down, forming deep, indurated ulcers. The palate may be partly destroyed. After healing takes place, marked cicatrization occurs (Fig. 22-3). A frequent site for the gumma or ulcers is at the base of the tongue.

Symptoms. The primary lesion may have no symptoms other than the soreness or discomfort associated with an ulcer. The cervical lymph nodes are enlarged. The chancre has a hard indurated feel.

There may be no symptoms of the secondary stage other than a slight sore throat. Pain in the ear may be noticed if the arch of the fauces is affected. If the inflammation extends to the pharyngeal orifice of the eustachian tube, there is some deafness and tinnitus. The lymph nodes of the neck are usually enlarged. There may be cough or a tickling sensation in the throat. In some cases pain or a dull aching is mentioned. Dysphagia and a pseudomembranous an-

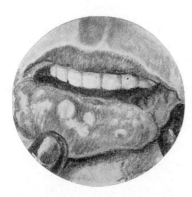

FIG. 22-2. Mucous patches.

gina, accompanied by a slight elevation of temperature, may be present. There may also be erythematous patches on the skin and in the throat, those in the throat often being mistaken for superficial ulcerations. Upon close examination they are found to be mere abrasions or elevations of the superficial epithelium.

In the tertiary stage the characteristic gummatous formations, which break down, forming deep indurated ulcers, may be seen. The palate may be partly destroyed. The odor is characteristic and is known as syphilitic ozena. There is some pain, especially upon swallowing, but it is not as severe as the lesion seems to warrant.

LEPROSY

Etiology. Leprosy is a communicable disease caused by the bacillus of Hansen (*Mycobacterium leprae*) and is characterized by the presence of nodules in the skin and mucous membranes, by destructive granulomas in and about the face, and in some situations by changes in the nerves that lead to anesthesia of the skin. The *Mycobacterium leprae* has many points of resemblance to the tubercle bacillus but can be differentiated. It is cultured with difficulty.

Symptoms. Leprosy symptomatically can be divided into two forms with many gradations between. Lepromatous leprosy, which is one of these forms, is characterized by extensive skin lesions in the form of macules, nodules, and papules. The sites of predilection include the cheeks, nose, brows, and ears. Eventually the skin of the face and forehead may become thickened and corrugated and the ear lobes pendulous to produce the so-called leonine facies. Nasal obstruction, epistaxis, laryngitis, and hoarseness all may be present. Destruction of the nasal septum leads to a saddle nose. The soft palate, epiglottis, and tongue may contain nodules. Neurologic involvement is usually not prominent unless the disease is well advanced.

Tuberculous leprosy, the second type, is characterized by skin macules and plaques. The nerves are involved early and become enlarged, producing areas of anesthetic skin.

Destructive lesions of the nose are rare in the tuberculous leprosy.

Prognosis. Lepromatous leprosy, if untreated, leads to a fatal outcome in 10 to 20 years, but when well treated there is a slow regression of symptoms over a 5 to 8 year period. Tuberculous leprosy is a less severe form of the disease, and spontaneous recovery may be achieved in 1 to 3 years.

Treatment. The sulfones (diaminodiphenylsulfone, dapsone) are the drugs of choice in the treatment of this disease.

SARCOIDOSIS

Sarcoidosis is a systemic granulomatous disease of undetermined etiology and pathogenesis. Immunologically it has been shown to belong to a group of disorders characterized, on the one hand, by a relative depression of cell-mediated, thymus-dependent immunity (delayed hypersensitivity) and, on the other, by a virtually intact, humoral, thymus-independent, antibody immune apparatus. Mediastinal as well as peripheral lymph nodes in many locations are frequently involved. In addition, lesions are found in the parotid glands, bronchi, spleen, skin, and bones. The Kveim reaction is frequently depressed. Hypercalcemia and increased serum globulins are usually noted. The characteristic histologic appearance is one of epithelioid tubercles with little or no caseation. The disease is further discussed in Part 3.

Treatment. Spontaneous remissions occur in about 70% of cases. Corticosteroid treatment is usually employed in cases with recurrence.

GLANDERS

Synonyms. Equinia; maliasmus; malleus; malleus humidus; farcy; morve; farcin; rotz.

Glanders is a contagious disease affecting horses and asses. It is communicable to man. It is caused by *Pseudomonas mallei*. When it affects the mucous membrane, it is called glanders, and when it affects the skin and lymph nodes, it is called farcy.

Etiology. Glanders originates in horses and asses, but it is communicable to man and from man to man. Though the bacillus may gain entrance through the follicles of the skin, it more often does so through an abraded or a wounded surface. Cases are reported of surgeons being infected while operating upon patients who had the disease.

Pathology. There are numerous closely associated nodules of granulation tissue which readily break down and suppurate. The ulcers thus formed have undermined edges, which are the remnants of the wall of the preceding abscess. The process spreads by continuity, though later it may be carried to distant parts. It usually appears first in the skin and then extends to the mucous membrane of the nose, though it may have its origin in the mucosa.

The nasal lesions are usually in the form of numerous closely grouped granulations and nodules in the submucous tissue. There is a profuse proliferation of leukocytes and connective tissue cells, with which are admixed numerous bacilli of glanders. The proliferation continues until the pressure diminishes the nutrition of the mass, especially at its center; liquefaction necrosis then ensues, and the nodules become abscesses. The outer wall soon breaks down, and the contents are discharged into the nasal cavities. The abscesses are thus converted into open ulcers with undermined edges. Cross sections of the masses before breaking down show them to be composed almost entirely of leukocytes, connective tissue cells, and fibrous tissue. Many *Pseudomonas mallei* organisms are imbedded in the masses of proliferated cells. In the acute form there are numerous polymorphonuclear leukocytes in the adjoining tissue. In the chronic form the bone and deeper structures may be destroyed. Gangrene of the softer tissues may occur.

Symptoms. In the acute form the period of incubation is from 3 to 4 days. The acute symptoms in the initial stage often simulate rheumatism or typhoid fever. A little later the nodules appear on either the skin or the nasal mucosa, according to the point of infection. They rapidly increase in size until (in nasal glanders) the purulent contents empty into the nose. The upper air passages are not often involved primarily in man. The progress of the disease is rapid and usually leads to a fatal result in a few days or 2 or 3 weeks.

The chronic form is fatal in about 50% of the cases after 2 months to 2 years. This type bears a close resemblance to syphilis and tuberculosis. The lymph nodes of the neck are often much enlarged in the acute form. Chronic glanders often presents the symptoms of a persistent coryza. The diagnosis is difficult.

ACTINOMYCOSIS OF THE NOSE

Definition. Actinomycosis is a noncontagious suppurative infection characterized by chronic granulation tumors and sinus formation about the jaws, neck, and elsewhere.

Etiology. This disease is caused by the fungus *Actinomyces bovis,* which differs from other actinomycetes by its anaerobic nature and failure to grow on Sabouraud's medium. They may be found as apparently noninjurious "normal" inhabitants of the mouth.

Pathology. The diseased mass is made up of granulation tissue, which, except for the ray fungus, would be mistaken for round cell sarcoma. Epithelioid elements and giant cells are sometimes present. In the granular mass or in the pus, the fungus itself appears in the form of small yellow, brown, or green masses, about the size of a pinhead, which upon microscopic examination are found to be composed of a central interwoven mass of threads, from which radiate club-shaped rays. In man the clubbed bodies are frequently absent (Senn). Water or a weak solution of sodium chloride causes the rays to swell enormously and lose their shape; ether and chloroform have no action upon them. The gross pathologic anatomy of the disease is everywhere associated with chronic indurations, with softening and liquefaction, and with resulting sinuses and cysts. The head, neck, especially the jaw, and the cervical fascia are the sites of the disease. In the cervical fascia the disease gives the neck a brawny hardness. The lymph nodes are not, as a rule, extensively involved. The disease must be differentiated from sarcoma, tuberculosis, carcinoma of tongue, syphilis, epulis (jaw), and lupus.

ACTINOMYCOSIS OF THE PHARYNX AND TONSILS

Symptoms. The frequency of occurrence in different parts of the body in 500 cases, as collected by Poucet and Berard, is as follows: head and lungs, 55%; thorax and lungs, 20%; abdomen, 20%; other parts, 5%. In France the face and neck were affected in 85% of the 66 cases reported.

The symptoms may be grouped in two classes: (1) those referable to local tumefaction and purulent discharge; and (2) those referable to the general intoxication of the system by the suppuration products or their metastatic spread.

The local symptoms develop slowly and are largely those of gradual mechanical interference of the pharyngeal function. At the site or sites of inoculation, a small rounded and reddish elevation appears and is accompanied by the usual attending pharyngitis. The adjacent tissue becomes swollen and tumid, and the evidences of an acute inflammation soon change to the more permanent engorgement and solidity of a chronic condition. The swelling is irregular but well-outlined, firm to probe palpation, and not oversensitive, but it slowly increases in size. Suppuration and the formation of angry-looking sinuses follow, from which issue a purulent discharge, in which are the small yellowish pellets or masses composed largely of the typical ray fungus. The discharge is persistent, and the sinuses extend deeply and produce extensive destruction of tissue. The spread of the process does not, as a rule, occur, and it shows a tendency, if it occurs elsewhere, to do so as an isolated swelling rather than as a connected overgrowth from the original pharyngeal focus. Pain is a variable quantity and depends largely upon the seat and extent of the peculiar swelling. Fetor of the breath and gastric disturbances from the purulent discharge are often present. The appearance of the disease elsewhere, especially in the lungs or the alimentary tract, because of metastasis is to be expected; no portion of the body is free from possible invasion.

The systemic symptoms may be severe or slight and do not differ in their character from those usually observed in other suppurative conditions. Death occurs from slow exhaustion or through some intercurrent complication.

Treatment. Penicillin and the tetracycline antibiotics are effective in controlling the disease and should be used for a long period of time. If fluctuation occurs, surgical drainage should be accomplished. At times the entire infected granuloma can be excised.

BRUCELLOSIS

Synonyms. Malta fever; undulant fever.

Brucellosis is an infection due to *Brucella melitensis* and *Brucella abortus*. It is transmitted by milk contaminated with *Brucella* or by contact with infected animals.

It is of significance to the otolaryngologist because of the occasional impaired hearing or involvement of the pharynx or larynx. Impairment of hearing has been reported in as high as 20% of all cases of brucellosis.

The lesions in the mucosa of the pharynx and larynx are somewhat similar to those of tuberculosis, syphilis, and certain pyogenic infections. At times the disease simulates acute septic infections.

The diagnosis of brucellosis is made from cultural, serologic, and allergic tests. The finding of *Brucella* in cultures of the blood or excreta proves the diagnosis.

The disease is usually self-limited. About 80% of patients recover within a year. The antibiotics seem to hasten recovery.

RHINOSPORIDIOSIS

Rhinosporidiosis, caused by the yeast *Rhinosporidium seeberi,* has a wide geographic distribution. Boles and Maiden state that in the United States 18 cases have been reported in which the nose was involved in 12 and the conjunctiva in 6. Involvement of the pharynx, larynx, ear, and penis have been reported. Young males are affected more frequently than females.

The characteristic lesion is a bleeding polyp from the anterior portion of the nose. Symptoms of an acute rhinitis may be present with partial or complete nasal stenosis on one or both sides. Pain is usually absent.

The diagnosis is made from the finding of characteristic organisms in a smear of the secretions or from a biopsy section.

The treatment is surgical excision followed by electrocoagulation. Recurrence from other portions of the nasal mucosa may take place.

HISTOPLASMOSIS

Histoplasmosis, a fungous disease, is characterized by a tubercle-like granulomatous lesion or calcification of the lungs with frequent primary ulcerations of the mucous membranes of the nose, pharynx, tongue, and larynx.

Etiology. The disease is caused by a small yeastlike fungus, *Histoplasma capsulatum,* probably emanating from infected animals and fowls.

Symptoms. Toxic symptoms such as low-grade fever, night sweats, weakness, and malaise are usually present during some phase of the disease. Painful ulcerations of the mucosa of the mouth, pharynx, or larynx are early manifestations.

The diagnosis is made from the history, blood smears and cultures, biopsy of the infected tissue, positive complement-fixation tests, and positive histoplasmin skin tests.

Treatment. Administration of intravenous amphotericin B, usually in conjunction with sulfadiazene by mouth, is effective in controlling this disease.

COCCIDIOIDOMYCOSIS

Coccidioidomycosis, caused by *Coccidioides immitis,* is characterized by fever, cough, and pulmonary findings similar to those of tuberculosis. Granulomas of the oral and nasal mucosa may be present in the later stages of the disease.

LEISHMANIASIS

Leishmaniasis, also called oriental sore, is caused by the protozoan *Leishmania* and may involve the oral and nasal mucous membranes in granulomatous lesions, particularly those of the nasal septum and less often those of the pharynx and larynx.

WEGENER'S GRANULOMATOSIS

Wegener's granulomatosis is a syndrome of unknown etiology characterized by necrotizing granulomatous lesions, generalized arteritis, and glomerulitis. It is most common in the fourth and fifth decades and is usually fatal within 6 to 8 months, though a more benign form involving the lungs may exist.

Symptoms. The disease frequently first involves an intractable rhinosinusitis with nasal obstruction, ulcerated gums, epistaxis and hemoptysis, cough, and pneumonitis. The relentless progress leads to erosion of the nasal bones and cartilages. The eye may become involved, and the lungs display necrotizing granulomas, which often appear as round opacities with central cavitation. Ulcers may also be found in the mouth, tongue, pharynx, and larynx, and a subglottic granuloma may require a tracheostomy. Blood eosinophilia is usually a feature.

Skin rashes, similar to those observed in polyarteritis, are common, and typical changes consist of papules with necrotic centers or of papulovesicular lesions. Pyoderma gangrenosum, petechiae, or multiform bullae and hemorrhagic exanthemas also occur.

In time renal involvement occurs, and renal failure is sometimes rapid. The terminal phase may be dominated by uremia.

Pathology. The principal histologic alterations consist of the necrotizing granulomas, the focal necrotizing vasculitis of both arteries and veins, and the focal glomerulitis. Wegener's granuloma is distinguished from lethal midline granuloma by the absence of generalized vasculitis in the latter.

Treatment. The use of corticosteroid medication has not been uniformly successful, though some success has followed immunosuppressive therapy.

The successful long-term use of the cytotoxic alkylating agent cyclophosphamide in Wegener's granulomatosis has been reported. It is combined with prednisolone.

LETHAL MIDLINE GRANULOMA

This disease, often referred to as Mikulicz's disease, is sometimes considered synonymous with Wegener's granulomatosis but should be distinguished from it. Lethal midline granuloma clinically implies a rapidly progressive, destructive lesion of the nose (characteristically the septum) and the facial structures. Initially it usually involves the nasal cavity, but spreading by infiltration occurs to the paranasal sinuses, orbit, and even the brain itself. There is a tendency toward development of vascular thrombosis in the affected areas, which may lead to necrosis and destruction of bone and soft tissues. Eventually widespread and distant dissemination may occur.

Kassel believes that careful histologic examination of these cases will place them in one of three categories. Some of these cases will be classified as malignant lymphoma which happened to present in the nasal cavity, and others will be classified as a true Wegener's granulomatosis. A larger group possesses the histologic features of a lymphoproliferative process but yet is separate from the accepted lymphoma types. Kassel terms this type polymorphic reticulosis or midline malignant reticulosis. There is a polymorphic infiltration in this case of mature and immature lymphocytes with a sprinkling of bizarre reticulum cells. There is an *absence* of necrotizing vasculitis, granulomas, prominent inflammatory cell component to the cellular infiltrate, and eosinophilia in polymorphic reticulosis. All of these characteristics are present in varying degrees in Wegener's granulomatosis.

The treatment of lethal midline granuloma varies according to the histologic classification. Wegener's granulomatosis is best treated with corticosteroid immunosuppressive medication. Malignant reticulosis is best treated by tumoricidal doses of roentgen rays.

HISTIOCYTIC GRANULOMA; EOSINOPHILIC GRANULOMA

Goodhill and others have given some evidence that three diseases of nonspecific granulomas—Letterer-Siwe disease, Hand-Schüller-Christian disease, and eosinophilic granuloma—are probably different phases or stages of the same disease process. Goodhill gave the name of histiocytic granuloma to the proposed basic entity which includes the three phases.

This disease is characterized by frequent attacks of otorrhea, erosions and destruction of the temporal bone and portions of the skull, proptosis, and diabetes insipidus.

Etiology. The etiology is unknown. It has been attributed to a virus and to an increased absorption or poor excretion of cholesterol, but little evidence has been produced.

The disease occurs in childhood and early adult life. Males are affected more frequently than females. The lesions respond dramatically to irradiation.

Pathology. The essential pathologic process is a dysplasia and hyperplasia of the histiocytic (reticuloendothelial) system with the production of granulomas. The lesions may affect the skull, long bones, ribs, vertebrae, various organs, or even the brain, meninges, and spinal cord.

The early or acute stage (Letterer-Siwe disease) occurs in infants with rapid involvement of the skull and other skeletal regions. The tubercles are composed of epithelioid cells with few or no lymphocytes. Giant cells may be observed in the tubercles of the epithelial cell nests. Lesions of the nasal mucosa or tonsil may appear before any skin manifestation.

Symptoms. The course of the disease is chronic with little or no constitutional symptoms. At times malaise or slight fever may be present. Nasal involvement may result in partial obstruction to breathing, dryness, crusting epistaxis, or a thick nasal discharge. Laryngeal lesions may cause some obstruction to respiration or hoarseness. Cervical adenopathy or salivary gland swellings frequently occur.

Diagnosis. The diagnosis is made from a microscopic study of the affected tissue of the upper respiratory tract, a negative reaction to the tuberculin test, and a roentgenogram of the chest which may show the frequent lymphomatous masses. Differential diagnosis should be made from lupus and leprosy.

Treatment. Many of the patients need no treatment. The use of adrenal steroid therapy symptomatically improves the patient.

RHINOSCLEROMA

Definition. Rhinoscleroma, or scleroma, is a chronic, slowly progressing granulomatous disease involving the upper respiratory tract, especially the nasal vestibules, choanae, pharynx, and larynx.

Etiology. Almost certainly the causative agent is *Klebsiella rhinoscleromatis* (von Frisch's bacillus). The disease is rarely seen in America and occurs more frequently in southern Europe and in Egypt. A family predisposition is present, probably due to infection on intimate contact. No sex difference exists.

Pathology. The skin and mucous membrane of the nose assume a smooth, nodular appearance of cartilage-like consistency, which pits little, if at all, upon probe pressure. The lesions have been likened in external appearance to keloids. The parts are sensitive to the touch but are otherwise free from pain. The substance of the swelling is composed of large plasma cells, irregularly distributed in all layers of the mucous membrane and in the submucous tissue. They accompany the blood vessels in the new portions of the growth. The plasma cells do not contribute directly to the hypertrophy, but it is possible that they become changed partly into spindle cells and then give rise to the formation of new fibrillary tissue. Two forms of retrograde metamorphosis occur in the plasma cells. These may be transformed into swollen, hydropic, so-called Mikulicz's cells or into hyaline degenerated cells, probably identical with the so-called Russell's fuchsinophils. The hydropic cells lie close together and have a distinct contour and spongy cytoplasm dilated into large masses, in which there is a smaller mass within a faceted nucleus. In this stage one often sees from six to eight bacilli in the cells near the nucleus which lie always at regular distances. This stage appears, however, to be rapidly finished, and when the cell membrane breaks, the fluid contents, together with some of the bacilli, find an exit and fill some of the nearest lymph spaces. These cells are, however, intimately related to the direct action of the bacilli.

Symptoms. The changes in the external appearance of the nose, while presenting many of the characteristics of keloids, are, nevertheless, rather easily differentiated from them by the whole symptom complex. The tissue at the tip of the nose becomes infiltrated, hard, and nodular. The nose broadens and becomes firmly fixed to the face. The tissues become more and more thickened, until the breathing is more or less occluded. The color of the skin varies from a red to a bluish or brownish red. The skin is traversed by small blood vessels and is usually shiny, though it may be finely wrinkled. The extension of the growth is rather slow, requiring months to reach the nasopharynx. The infiltration often interferes with the movements of the lips, fauces, and larynx but rarely with that of the eyes and ears. There is no tendency to ulceration and discharge or to edema and inflammation of contiguous parts.

Diagnosis. Rhinoscleroma should be differentiated from syphilis, tuberculosis, leprosy, epithelioma, and keloid. Rhinoscleroma presents a hard, nodular growth, which usually begins at the anterior end of the nose and spreads gradually to the deeper recesses of the respiratory tract, without pain but with some tenderness upon pressure and without tendency to ulceration or inflammation of the surrounding tissues. In syphilis there is inflammation, while in epithelioma there is pain, ulceration, and discharge. In keloid the similarity is often so striking that it may be necessary to demonstrate the absence or presence of the bacilli of rhinoscleroma in order to make a differential diagnosis.

Treatment. Over the past years many forms of treatment have been ineffective in this disease. Recently the sulfonamides and antibiotics have been used with success, though insufficient time has elapsed to indicate the drug of choice. Surgical therapy is usually reserved for removal of obstructing cicatrixes. In the event of airway obstruction (e.g., laryngeal scleroma), tracheostomy may be required.

REFERENCES

Arvanitakis, C.: Remission in Wegener's Granulomatosis. J. Laryngol., *87*:289, 1973.

Boles, R. J., and Maiden, S. D.: A Case of Rhinosporidiosis. Ann. Otol., Rhinol., Laryngol., *60*:429, 1951.

Eichel, B. S., and Mayberry, T. E.: The Enigma of Lethal Midline Granuloma. Laryngoscope, *78*:1367, 1968.

Goodhill, V.: Histiocytic Granuloma of Skull. Laryngoscope, *60*:1, 1950.

Kassel, S. H., *et al.*: Midline Malignant Reticulosis (So-called Lethal Malignant Granuloma). Cancer, *23*:920, 1969.

Sampter, M. (Ed.): *Immunological Diseases.* Boston, Little, Brown and Co., 1971, p. 581.

Chapter 23

Tumors of the Face, Nasopharynx, and Pharynx; Cysts of the Mouth; Tumors of the Salivary Glands

PAPILLOMA OF THE PHARYNX

Papilloma rarely occurs on the walls of the pharynx but is more common in the faucial region. It is most frequently found on the uvula, the free borders of the tonsillar pillars, and the tonsils themselves. The lesions may be single or multiple, sessile or pedunculated. The elevations vary in size from that of a pinhead to much larger lesions and frequently have a delicate mulberry appearance.

Papilloma of the tonsils is more often multiple than single and presents the general outline of a bunch of grapes. The growths usually give rise to no marked symptoms but do tend to recur. They vary in size from that of a small pea to that of a large walnut.

Treatment. The tumors should be removed surgically.

CRANIOPHARYNGIOMA

The craniopharyngioma or Rathke's pouch tumor arises from the cells of Rathke's pouch, a remnant of the buccal mucosa which extends upward to form the anterior lobe of the pituitary body. It occurs during adolescence, usually between 10 and 20 years of age. In the beginning it is char-

acterized by the syndrome of failing vision, primary optic atrophy, bitemporal hemianopsia, endocrine disturbances (hypopituitarism), enlargement of the sella turcica, suppression of sexual development, and calcification of the suprasellar portion of the tumor. As the tumor extends beyond the sella, signs and symptoms of increased intracranial pressure develop.

FIBROMA

Nasopharyngeal Fibroma

Etiology. Nasopharyngeal fibromas usually occur between 10 and 25 years of age; they occur more commonly in males. The lesion is usually single, although multiple growths have been reported. Softer varieties are called "polypoid fibromas" or "fibromatous polyps." As age advances there is a tendency for the growths to recede or undergo spontaneous cure. The true fibroma usually arises from the nasopharyngeal recess, less frequently from the anterior sphenoidal wall, base of the sphenoid, nasal process of the occipital bone, nasal choanae, first cervical vertebrae, mouth of the eustachian tube, posterior palatine surface, and pterygomaxillary recess. The softer fibromatous myxoma or "polyp" usually arises in the nasal cavity and extends into the naso-pharynx.

Pathology. The surface of the tumor is covered by mucous membrane under which are found large ramifying blood vessels. The mass is made up of dense fibrous tissue and agglomerated cells and contains large venous channels which are most abundant in the peripheral portions. In rare instances a myxomatous tumor may have the tendencies and aspects of a fibroma, just as primary fibromas may become mucoid in character.

Fibromas may be sessile but are more often pedunculated. They often attain large size. Large fibromas are frequently accompanied by inflammatory processes; hence, adhesions to the adjacent structures are common. Additional blood supply is derived through the adhesions.

They do not metastasize but grow by extension. They may invade the orbit, accessory sinuses, pterygoid and temporal fossae, or the intracranial cavity.

Symptoms. The early symptoms are those of nasal congestion and obstruction with hemorrhage. The bleeding sometimes becomes an alarming complication. The voice becomes "flat" or "dead" in quality, and respiration and deglutition are impeded as the process advances. At a later stage, there is pain and mucopurulent discharge. When the growth has attained considerable size, the "frog face" becomes well marked; the maxillary bones are separated, and exophthalmos becomes a prominent symptom. Aprosexia and drowsiness are often present.

The foregoing symptoms increase in severity as the growth extends, until the absorption of bony tissue is considerable, unless the tumor extends beyond the nasal and pharyngeal chambers, such as into the cranial cavity. In this event the pressure necrosis of the bony tissue is not so great.

Examination shows the tumor to be a rounded mass of pinkish or dark purple color. The veins are frequently varicosed; thus, the examination by digital or instrumental aids should be done carefully to avoid injuring them. The growth may project into the posterior nares, or its direction may be toward the antrum and other sinuses. Under finger pressure it is firm and elastic, and if small, its base may be outlined. If pedunculated, it is movable, unless it has become fixed by inflammatory adhesions. If it extends through the sphenomaxillary fissure, it may be felt under the zygoma. As adhesions are usually present, its outline is difficult to distinguish.

Diagnosis. The histologic resemblance to sarcoma is often so close that differentiation is difficult, unless the age, sex, and origin are such as to point to its fibrous nature. Sarcoma is rarely or never pedunculated, whereas soft fibroma is frequently so. Hard fibromas are usually sessile.

Prognosis. The prognosis is favorable in proportion to early recognition and extirpation. It is also favorable when the age of the patient exceeds 25 years. In other words, small fibromas which do not fill the nasopharyngeal space are more easily removed than those which completely fill it. After the age of 25, the growth tends to regress.

Treatment. Various forms of treatment have been used: caustics, electrolysis, galvanocautery, snare and avulsion, external operations, and palate-splitting operations. The latter provides the best approach and has been described in connection with congenital occlusion of the nasopharynx. The use of cryosurgery, perhaps in conjunction with palate splitting, may prove to be the technique of choice. Success in removing a juvenile fibroma depends to a large extent on success in controlling the bleeding. Preoperative irradiation with radium or roentgen rays has been useful.

Fibroma of the Tonsil

Etiology. Fibroma of the tonsil occurs equally often in both sexes and perhaps more often in childhood than in middle and advanced life. It is a benign neoplasm next in frequency of occurrence to papilloma. It rarely becomes malignant. Its growth is slow and is usually limited to one tonsil.

Pathology. The fibroma is usually somewhat pedunculated, though it may be sessile. The larger the fibroma, the larger the pedicle. It is more often single than multiple. Being of connective tissue origin, it must of necessity have its origin in the trabeculae of the tonsil. Occasionally it undergoes cys-

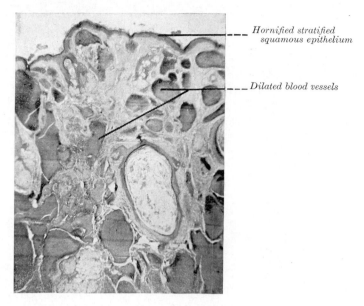

Hornified stratified
squamous epithelium

Dilated blood vessels

FIG. 23–1.   Hemangioma.   Angiomas of the nose, pharynx, and larynx
are rare and are usually congenital. × 30.

tic degeneration. Usually it is firm and scantily supplied with blood vessels. It is composed of white fibrous tissue, the cells often being matted together, closely simulating embryonic connective tissue cells.

Symptoms. Annoying symptoms are seldom present except in the large pedunculated type, which produces mechanical obstruction. Its presence is not accompanied by discharge. It is characterized by symptoms similar to those of enlarged hypertrophic tonsils.

Diagnosis. The diagnosis is usually easily made, and in case of doubt a portion should be excised and submitted to microscopic examination.

Treatment. The treatment is purely surgical and consists of its removal, a procedure easily accomplished if the growth is pedunculated. Occasionally it may be adherent to the tonsil or to the neighboring structures as a result of repeated inflammations of the tonsil.

ANGIOMA

Etiology. Angiomas of the nose, pharynx, and larynx are rare. They are usually congenital.

The growths may not manifest themselves for years. The reported cases range in age from a few months to 60 years.

Angiomas of the external and middle ear are rare. They usually begin as a benign, slow-growing lesion but may produce pressure changes in the surrounding structures.

Pathology. Angiomas are divided into hemangiomas (Figs. 23–1 to 23–3) and lymphangiomas (Fig. 23–4).

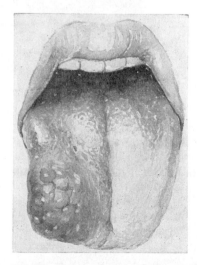

FIG. 23–2.   Hemangioma of the tongue.

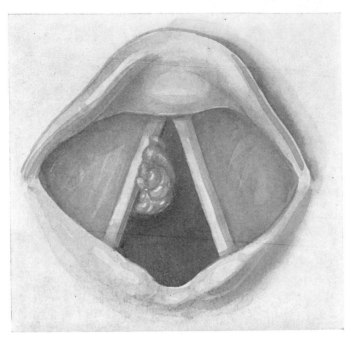

FIG. 23–3.   Hemangioma of the larynx. Simple hemangioma of the larynx may be nodular, polypoid, pedunculated, or in rare instances papillary. Lymphangiomas of the larynx usually have a smooth or papillary surface.

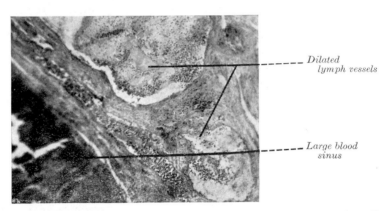

_Dilated
lymph vessels_

_Large blood
sinus_

FIG. 23–4.   Lymphangioma. A lymphangioma is an angioma formed by dilated lymph vessels. It is rarely found in the ear, nose, or throat. × 80.

The hemangiomas are divided into four types: the capillary or simple (telangiectatic angioma, nevi, etc.); the cavernous; the hypertrophic; and the pseudoangiomatous (bleeding polyps, fibroangiomas, cirsoid aneurysms, etc.).

Capillary hemangioma consists of loosely arranged tissue containing numerous thin-walled blood vessels showing, at times, areas of thromboses, hyaline degeneration,

and hemosiderin. The tumor is covered with normal stratified epithelium. Varices are usually found on the posterior wall of the pharynx or on the base of the tongue. They frequently occur in association with chronic pulmonary or circulatory disturbances. Slight hemoptysis may occur at times.

Cavernous hemangiomas are thin-walled, with an afferent artery and efferent veins which do not communicate with the neighboring capillaries. They may occur singly or in groups. Distended veins project above the surface and into the tissue beneath. They may be compressed but refill at once when the pressure is removed. Tumors of this type are usually slightly lobulated and dark purplish in color.

Four types of lymphangiomas have been described: the simple, the cavernous, the hypertrophic, and the cystic.

The simple type (lymphangioma simplex) is characterized by a new growth of lymphatic vessels having a comparatively narrow lumen and more or less parallel walls.

The cavernous type (lymphangioma cavernosum) is characterized by irregularly shaped, intercommunicating lymph spaces of varying sizes.

In the hypertrophic type (lymphangioma hypertrophicum) the lymphatic vessels are lined with several layers of endothelium with at times a nodular or valvular growth of endothelium into the lumen of the vessels.

The cystic type (lymphangioma cysticum) is characterized by one or more large lymphatic cysts in a new growth of lymph vessels.

Angiomas are sessile and nonulcerating with a nodular serpentine outline; they are usually of a soft consistency. Hemangiomas have a purplish blue color. The lymphangiomas are smoother and pale pink.

A hemangioma may be associated with a similar process involving the skin. It is frequently found at the base of the tonsil or tongue arising from a venous plexus.

Cavernous hemangioendothelioma of the nose is rare. It arises from the ethmoidal region in the lateral wall. It grows slowly by infiltration and is destructive to surrounding tissues. It has a tendency to invade the sinuses, especially in the region of the ethmoid, eventually filling the nose, sinuses, or nasopharynx, producing in extreme cases exophthalmos, nasal obstruction, or facial disfigurement.

Hemangioma of the nasal septum arises from the cartilage or cartilaginous vomer junction. It probably has its origin in embryonic rests.

Angiomas of the larynx, when associated with similar conditions elsewhere, may involve the extrinsic structures as well as the intrinsic. When localized in the larynx they are most frequently found in the true and false cords. Hemangiomas in the infant are rare, but when present the reported cases have been subglottic.

Symptoms. The symptoms are variable, depending on the location and the size of the tumor. In some cases no symptoms are present until the tumor reaches a comparatively large size; in vocal cord lesions attention is directed to the larynx by voice changes, such as hoarseness or aphonia.

If the tumor is large, slight or severe respiratory obstruction may be present. Hemoptysis may occur without warning and may be severe. Pain is usually absent. The lesions may be pedunculated or, more frequently, attached by a broad base. They may be single or multiple. Lymphangiomas are usually smoother and paler than the hemangiomas.

The symptoms of angioma of the nose are those of nasal obstruction, epistaxis, and a reducible and pulsating tumor. The nasal obstruction is proportionate to the size of the growth. Pressure upon the growth materially reduces its size. The pulsation is greater when the tumor is attached to a large artery than when it is attached to a vein. In the latter event, the pulsation is much less and the color is blue, whereas if the tumor is connected to both vein and artery, the color will be dark red.

A microscopic examination is essential to an accurate diagnosis. There is no definite association with other general pathologic conditions.

Treatment. The treatment of angiomas is by roentgen ray, radium, cauterization, fulguration, strangulation, and excision.

HEREDITARY HEMORRHAGIC TELANGIECTASIA (OSLER-WEBER-RENDU DISEASE)

The type of angioma known as hereditary hemorrhagic telangiectasia is an inherited abnormality characterized by a marked tendency to bleed.

Etiology. The disease is transmitted as a dominant characteristic and is not sex bound.

The disease is usually considered a simple ectasia or dilatation of the blood vessels but is regarded by some as consisting of acquired multiple angiomas arising from embryonal endothelial rests.

The lesions may appear in various portions of the body but are most frequently found in the nasal or oral mucous membrane, especially in the cartilaginous portion of the nasal septum, tongue, buccal regions, lips, and floor of the mouth. They are commonly observed in the skin of the face, scalp, tips of the fingers, eyelids, ear drums, palate, pharynx, larynx, and trachea.

The angiomas vary in size from a small pinhead to large vascular networks and in color from red to purple. The tissue covering of the dilated vessels is extremely thin, permitting frequent hemorrhages.

Symptoms. Epistaxis or bleeding from other involved areas is the most common symptom. The bleeding varies from a mild loss of blood to a severe hemorrhage. It may occur at long intervals or several times a day. Secondary anemia is common.

Hereditary hemorrhagic telangiectasia should be differentiated from the various bleeding diseases and from telangiectases associated with other conditions, such as syphilis, lead poisoning, senility, and pregnancy.

Treatment. Various means of controlling an epistaxis have been discussed on pages 94–97. Recently full-thickness mucosal or split-thickness skin grafts (septal dermoplasty) have been applied to the involved area. Usually under local anesthesia, the dermal graft is obtained from the anterior thigh or other suitable location. The thickness should be about 14/1000 inch. The nasal bed is prepared by using a sharp ring curette to remove only the mucosa (and not the perichondrium) from the septum from top to the bottom and as far posteriorly as necessary, usually to the anterior end of the middle turbinate. The mucosa is similarly removed from the floor of the nose and medial surface of the inferior turbinate. Both sides of the nose are thus prepared.

The graft is placed over the denuded area of the septum, floor, and turbinates and held in place by carefully placed packs which have been impregnated with an antibiotic ointment. Before the packs are placed, it is well to secure the graft anteriorly by suturing it to a freshly cut margin of the skin located at the mucovestibular junction. The grafts are trimmed if necessary in 1 to 2 weeks.

NEVUS

Traub classifies the pigmented nevi (Figs. 23–5 and 23–6) into five classes:

1. Intraepithelial or intraepidermal nevi lie entirely within the epidermis. Nevus cells are absent. This benign type includes the benign pigmented epithelioma (Block) and

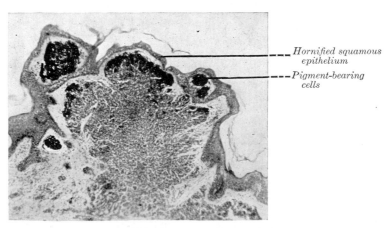

Hornified squamous epithelium

Pigment-bearing cells

Fig. 23–5.   Pigmented nevus of the face. Under the squamous epithelium of the skin, collections of heavily staining pigment-bearing cells are seen.

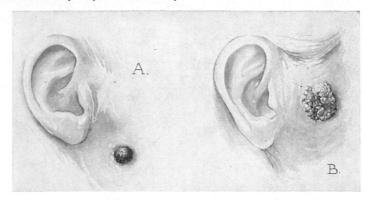

FIG. 23–6. *A*, Melanoma. These growths are usually located on the cheek near the mouth or nose. *B*, Pigmented nevus. Certain types of pigmented nevi, in rare instances, may be the fore-runners of a malignant melanoma or a nevocarcinoma.

the warty or senile pigmented seborrheic verruca.

2. The junction-type nevus originates at the junction of the epidermal and dermal layers. This and the succeeding classes contain the characteristic nevus cells. The junction type, while rarely becoming malignant, may be the forerunner of a malignant melanoma or a nevocarcinoma. A change in color, especially to a darker shade, is significant. The small, brown lesions are frequently found on the face and extremities. They are smooth, soft, and slightly elevated.

3. The intradermal nevus or common or fleshy mole, frequently located on the face, is benign.

4. The blue nevus is located deep in the skin. The color varies from black and blue-black to brown. It is classified as benign, but in rare instances a change to melanosarcoma has been reported.

5. A mixed type of nevus, which may be a mixture of any of the above groups, may be observed at times. A biopsy is frequently necessary for an exact diagnosis.

CYSTS

Cysts of the Mouth and Maxilla

Common cysts of the oral cavity and maxilla include radicular or root cysts, follicular or dentigerous cysts, ranulas (retention cysts), hygromas, and at times dermoid and other cysts. Some of these have been mentioned under Benign Neoplasms of the Nose and Throat.

Root or Radicular Cyst. The root or periosteal cyst arises from an inflammatory change in the tooth root membrane due to injury or disease. It follows the death of the pulp, with subsequent development of a granuloma and a cyst. Roentgenograms show an absence of a tooth in these cysts.

They comprise about 80% of all dental cysts. They are found in the upper jaw more frequently than in the lower.

Dentigerous Cyst. *Etiology.* The follicular or dentigerous cyst comprises about 20% of all dental cysts. It involves, as a rule, the lower jaw but may occur in the maxilla or even in the gums or orbit. It usually occurs between 20 and 30 years of age but is occasionally seen in children or in old people. Most authorities are of the opinion that it represents an expanded tooth follicle. Dentigerous cysts are usually single but may be multiple.

Pathology. A dentigerous cyst should not be confused with a pathologic resorption of bone from an infection. An infection may spread by way of the root canal to the cyst. It is lined with pavement epithelium. The cysts may vary in size from that of a small pea to that of a large walnut. The contents are sterile unless secondary infection occurs. They contain cholesterol crystals at times.

The cyst expands progressively, with displacement and absorption of the bone, so that the cortex may have the consistency of an eggshell.

Symptoms. Symptoms may be absent until the walls of the maxillary sinus are beginning to be displaced. This displacement may be anteriorly into the palate or into the nasal passage. Destruction or perforation of the wall is a late development. Pain is absent as a rule.

An asymmetry of the face may occur, consisting of a dilation of the anterior sinus wall or an inner displacement of the lateral nasal wall. The palate may be depressed at times by the expanding cyst. A fistula into the mouth or nose may occur if the cyst has ruptured. Transillumination may not show cloudiness of the antrum.

Examination may reveal a rounded swelling in the region of the canine fossa. A fistula in the mucous membrane of the oral or nasal cavities usually means an infection of the cyst. The cyst usually has a thin bony shell surrounding the contents, which is easily stripped away from the wall of the antrum. The cysts may contain a fully or partially developed tooth or teeth in a thin or gelatinous fluid which usually contains cholesterol crystals. In some instances multilocular dentigerous cysts are encountered.

Diagnosis. The diagnosis is made from the history, roentgenographic examination, and clinical findings. If a slow-growing, painless tumor of the lower jaw is found associated with an unerupted tooth, a dentigerous cyst should be suspected. The roentgenogram reveals a large radiolucent area containing a tooth crown or an anomalous tooth.

Dentigerous cysts of the maxillary sinus should be differentiated from abscesses; radicular or root cysts; osteomyelitis; maxillary sinusitis; benign tumors, such as odontoma, fibroma, and myxoma; and malignant growths.

Treatment. Aspiration or incision and drainage of the contents are usually followed by a re-formation or an infection of the cyst. The treatment of choice is complete extirpation of the cyst and its bony wall by means of a Caldwell-Luc type of operation. If the cyst is infected, the bony shell may not separate from the antral wall easily. Following complete removal of the cyst, the prognosis is good.

Ranula. Ranula is a degenerative cyst formation of the salivary glands in the sublingual region (Fig. 23–7, *A*). It is the result of a degenerative process of the salivary glands. A mechanical obstruction of the orifices of the duct is absent. It is usually located on one side of the frenum and has a tendency to recur.

Treatment. Aspiration or incision and drainage may not prevent a recurrence. A complete extirpation of the cyst is preferable, either through the mouth or, if the cyst is large and has burrowed inferiorly, through the neck.

Hygromas. Hygromas result from occlusion of the ducts or orifices of mucous glands.

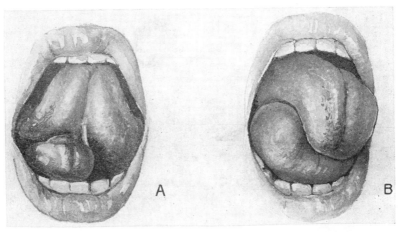

Fig. 23–7.   Cysts of the mouth. *A,* Ranula. *B,* Sublingual dermoid cyst.

They are located in the mucous membrane while ranulas are beneath. Hygromas are true retention cysts, lined with epithelium and containing lymph structures. As a rule they are single, but they may be multiple and about the size of a pea. They may be located in any part of the mucosa of the mouth.

Treatment. Treatment consists of enucleation of the cyst membrane, though thorough cauterization of the lining of the sac is usually followed by obliteration of the tumor.

Multilocular Cyst (Cystic Adenoma or Adamantinoma). The multilocular cyst of the jawbone is rare. According to Malassez, it originates from epithelial rests of fetal life either from the mucous membrane of the jaw or from the epithelial cord or membrane of the enamel organ. It extends inward to the floor of the mouth from the lower jaw.

Dermoid Cyst. A dermoid cyst in the floor of the mouth develops from a misplaced fetal inclusion that takes on activity and forms a cyst (Fig. 23–7, *B*).

Dermoids commence shortly after birth, but on account of their slow and painless growth, they attract little attention until their size gives annoyance. They project into the floor of the mouth or into the neck behind the chin, or both. At times they attain the size of an orange.

The round or oval dermoid cyst has a thick wall lined with stratified epithelium. It usually contains hair or other skin appendages and certain fatty bodies and fatty acid crystals.

Treatment is complete surgical removal of the cyst and its stalk.

Epidermoid Cyst. Epidermoid cysts are similar to dermoids, as they both come from the same embryonic structures. However, the epidermoids do not contain hair, glands, or skin appendages. The epidermoids are lined with an epithelial layer of a mucous type and sometimes with ciliated epithelium.

Mucous Gland Cysts. These retention cysts may form in any mucous gland in the mouth except the gingiva and superior surface of the tongue. The duct or its orifice becomes occluded, causing formation of the pseudocyst. They may be mistaken for a ranula.

Echinococcus Cyst. The *Echinococcus* cysts are rarely found in the mouth. When present, they are usually located on the tongue. Pain is absent, as a rule, unless a secondary infection occurs. A mechanical inconvenience due to the presence of the cyst may be noticed.

Cysts of the Tonsil

Cysts of the tonsil are rare. They may be situated either superficially or deeply. They vary in size and may contain a quantity of fluid or a mass of inspissated secretions and epithelial debris. Cysts usually result from an inflammatory occlusion of the mouth of the crypt.

Cysts of the Tongue

Cysts of the tongue occur in infants or very young children. These cysts may be due to a retention of mucous gland secretion, a cystic crypt of the lingual tonsil, a cystic development of a fetal cell remnant, or a dermoid cyst at the fusion line.

Symptoms, depending upon the size and location, might be inspiratory stridor and respiratory obstruction, with or without cyanosis.

The treatment is incision and drainage.

Cysts of the Nasopharynx

Cysts of the nasopharynx may be inflammatory, degenerative, or developmental in origin. It is possible that many of the larger cysts of the nasopharynx lined with ciliated epithelium originate as cysts of the pharyngeal bursa.

Subjective symptoms referable to the nose or throat may be absent. Postnasal discharge is a common symptom. Chronic pharyngitis and enlargement of the posterior cervical lymph nodes are frequently present. Occipital headaches are mentioned by some patients.

Diagnosis is made by direct inspection and palpation of the nasopharynx. A smooth bulging in the vault of the nasopharynx, usually central but occasionally lateral, is usually seen.

Treatment. The treatment is destruction with the cautery or surgical removal. The technique is similar to that followed in the removal of an adenoid.

Cystadenoma

Cystadenoma of the palate is rare. It is thought to be embryonic or to originate in the germinative layer of the epithelium of the palate. The tumors are usually discovered accidentally. As a rule the hard palate is involved, but the soft palate and the gums may be the seat of the cystic tumor.

The cysts are irregular oval or rounded sessile growths, grayish or pinkish gray in color and soft or firm in consistency. They are usually encapsulated but may break through the capsule. A glutinous colloid material, glandular epithelium, and at times cartilage, bone, and lymphoid tissue may be found within the capsule. The cystic formation is due to the dilated acini.

Treatment. Treatment is excision with the knife or cautery, followed by cauterization of the base.

BENIGN NEOPLASMS OF THE NOSE AND THROAT

Cysts of the Nasal Vestibule (Fig. 23–8) and Hard Palate. Cysts encroaching on the nasal vestibule or the anterior portion of the hard palate are rare. They are usually uni-

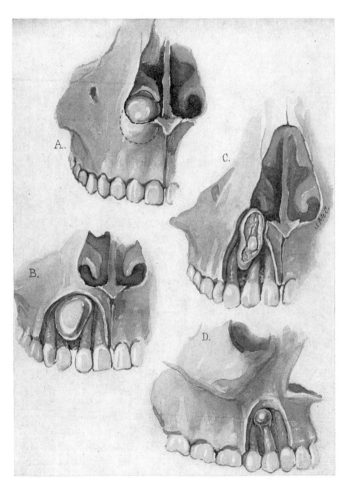

FIG. 23–8.   Nasoalveolar cysts. *A,* A nasoalveolar (anterior) cyst situated anterior to the lateral incisor and canine teeth. *B,* A globulomaxillary cyst situated between the lateral incisor and canine teeth. *C,* A dentigerous cyst containing an anomalous tooth. *D,* A dental root cyst, also known as a dentoperiosteal or radicular cyst, may be found at the apex of any tooth root.

lateral and are assumed to be persistent epithelial remnants in the line of closure of the premaxilla and maxilla or in the line of fusion of the palatal processes (incisive canal cyst, nasopalatine duct cyst).

Globulomaxillary Cyst. These cysts are located between the canine and lateral incisor teeth and usually produce their separation. The roentgenogram reveals an oval or heart-shaped area between the apices of these teeth. Large cysts may result in sufficient thinning of the maxillary cortex to produce crepitation.

Treatment varies from simple incision and drainage to radical removal of the cyst from the palatal side with or without the adjacent teeth.

Branchial and Thyroglossal Cysts and Fistulas. Included among the various developmental anomalies of the neck are branchial and thyroglossal cysts and fistulas.

Branchial cysts or fistulas, especially the lateral ones below the level of the hyoid, are thought to be due in most instances to remains of the thymic duct which descends from the third pharyngeal pouch. True branchial cysts or fistulas are above this level. From a clinical standpoint the two types may be considered the same. These lateral defects of the branchial or thyroglossal system may be located at any level of the neck. The tract extends below the anterior portion of the sternocleidomastoid muscle and anterior to the carotid sheath to the posterior belly of the digastric muscle, arches behind the stylopharyngeus muscle, and ends in the tonsillar fossa. The tract is lined with ciliated epithelium and some layers of squamous epithelium.

Defects of the branchial tract are usually found in young people and predominantly in females.

The usual symptoms are a tumor in the lateral portion of the neck or a fistula with an intermittent or continuous discharge of secretion. Recurrent attacks of inflammation are common. An unexplained cough may be present at times. Symptoms may be noticed for only a few days or for many years.

Thyroglossal cysts may form anywhere in the midline of the neck along the tract of the vestigial thyroglossal duct from the base of the tongue to the region between the hyoid bone and the thyroid gland. Most of these retention cysts occur below the level of the hyoid bone. They may vary in size from a barely perceptible tumor to a lesion the size of a grapefruit.

Thyroglossal fistulas open onto the surface of the neck in the midline or more rarely in the foramen cecum above the dorsum of the tongue. They usually develop from an infection or inflammation of a cyst or of the duct itself. The fistulas discharge a glairy mucus, either clear or milky in color. If the tract is infected, the discharge is purulent.

Symptoms are those of a midline tumor or discharging fistula which moves upon swallowing. Difficulty in swallowing and a choking sensation may be present but are rare. A secondary infection of the cyst or thyroglossal tract is common.

The diagnosis of branchial or thyroglossal cysts or fistulas is facilitated by injecting a radiopaque oil in the suspected tract and then after the opening is closed with a purse-string suture, having a roentgenogram taken.

Treatment of the fistulas or cysts by injection of sclerosing solutions has been very unsatisfactory.

Complete surgical extirpation of the cyst or fistula gives the best assurance of a certain cure. The tract of the fistula can be followed more easily when a preliminary injection of methylene blue solution is used. The entire tract from the neck to the foramen cecum (thyroglossal) or from the neck to the pharynx (branchial) must be removed. In the former case, it may be necessary to resect the central portion of the hyoid bone.

ADAMANTINOMA; ODONTOMA; MULTILOCULAR CYST

An adamantinoma is a tumor which arises from the paradental epithelial debris. It is solid or cystic and located most commonly in the mandible in the molar and bicuspid region and at times in the maxilla. It excavates a cavity and destroys the tissue until the tumor is surrounded by only a thin capsule which crepitates on pressure.

Adamantinomas in the early stage are solid, but cystic degeneration appears later and gives them a softer consistency. They are composed of epithelium growing in masses or cords resembling embryonic enamel organs. Microscopically, ameloblasts are usually visible at some stage of development, most often lining the cavities in the bone.

The slow-growing tumor has a tendency to grow uninterruptedly, to recur if incompletely removed and to metastasize. The most outstanding symptom is the slowly enlarging growth of the jaw. Slight pain may be mentioned in advanced cases.

Included in this group of tumors, in addition to the odontomas, are the dentigerous cysts, which are described separately. The hard odontoma, a tumor of dental origin, is composed of enamel, cement, or dentin. Two or more of these tissues may be included in the same tumor. The hard odontomas grow by direct expansion, while the adamantinomas grow by expansion and infiltration.

These tumors should be differentiated from dentigerous cysts and osteosarcomas. The dentigerous cyst is slow-growing and painless. The roentgenogram shows round, smooth shadows with definite outlines. The odontoma is dense and hard. Osteosarcoma will show signs of malignancy. Bone cysts in the early stage may be mistaken for odontomas. Treatment is radical resection by surgery.

MULTIPLE MYELOMA

Multiple myeloma is a malignant neoplastic disease originating in the bone marrow and characterized by the proliferation of abnormal plasma cells. There is frequently an invasive destruction of the skeleton, including the skull, leading to bone pain, pathologic fractures, hematopoietic destruction, and hypercalcemia. Occasionally the tonsil, cheek, pharynx, and bone of the jaw are involved. Abnormal bleeding is a notable factor.

The myeloma cell varies from a small cell with scant cytoplasm and eccentric nucleus, which closely resembles a normal plasma cell, to a large anaplastic cell with an abundant and vacuolated cytoplasm and an eccentric nucleus. The myeloma cells produce abnormal proteins. Bence Jones proteins are found in the urine in half the cases. Occasionally, amyloid deposits are seen in the larynx.

Treatment. General supportive measures are indicated. Radiotherapy or chemotherapy (e.g., ethyl carbamate) may yield remissions. Steroids may also be useful.

PLASMACYTOMA

Synonyms. Myeloma; plasmasarcoma; malignant plasmoma.

Etiology. Plasmacytoma occurring in the upper respiratory tract is a comparatively rare form of myeloma resembling histologically the multiple myelomas commonly found in the long bones.

The etiology of the tumors is unknown. Their degree of malignancy varies, some reported cases being highly malignant while others follow a relatively benign course.

Pathology. The growths occur chiefly in the nasopharynx, alveolar borders, tongue, lips, and cervical lymph nodes. The plasma cell granuloma usually shows a plasma cell infiltration or proliferation, a marked response of the reticulum cells, and at times the presence of eosinophils.

Symptoms. The prominent symptoms are nasal obstruction, difficulty in deglutition, epistaxis, and hoarseness.

Prognosis. Plasmacytoma is eventually fatal.

Treatment. A combination of surgery and irradiation seems to give the best results.

MENINGOCELE;
MENINGOENCEPHALOCELE

A meningocele is a hernial protrusion of the meninges. If brain substance is enclosed within the meningocele, the hernial formation is called a meningoencephalocele or an encephalocele. It results from a faulty development of the fetal skull. Termination of the meninges near the base of the nose, known as the *sincipital type,* is rare. This variety has three forms: (1) nasofrontal, in which the sac extends between the nasal and frontal bones, resulting in a midline swelling at the nasal root; (2) nasoethmoid, with the defect between the nasal, frontal, and ethmoid bones producing a swelling beneath the skin at the junction of the bony and cartilaginous structures of the nose; and (3) naso-orbital, in which the sac protrudes through the suture line between the lacrimal, frontal, and ethmoid bones, extending into the orbit and producing a swelling near the inner canthus of the eye.

The *basal type,* in which the hernia extends into the nose, orbit, or pharynx, is less common than the sincipital. Herniation occurs through the orbital roof, cribriform plate, or foramen cecum. Three varieties have been described: (1) sphenopharyngeal, in which extension occurs by way of the ethmoid or sphenoid bones or through their suture line to the nasal or nasopharyngeal cavity (according to Anderson, after review of the literature, this is the most common basic type); (2) spheno-orbital, in which the sac passes through the spheno-orbital fissure into the posterior portion of the orbit, resulting in a pulsating exophthalmos; and (3) sphenomaxillary, with passage of the hernia through the spheno-orbital fissure into the orbit and extending downward through the inferior orbital fissure into the pterygopalatine fossa, at times resulting in an external bulge of the cheek below the zygoma or a swelling in the oropharynx medial to the ramus of the jaw.

Treatment. The anterior sincipital type without extension into the nasal cavity is probably best treated by the direct or external approach, that is, by an incision over the swelling, freeing of the mass, and ligation of the pedicle.

Anterior basal hernias extending into the nasal cavity may be removed by the snare or ligation method. However, this has the objection of creating a possible communication between the arachnoid and the nasal cavity, resulting in cerebrospinal fluid rhinorrhea or meningitis. With effective antimicrobial therapy, the latter complication is greatly lessened.

The intracranial approach, using a unilateral or bilateral frontal bone flap, may be advisable in many instances. A plate of bone or tantalum may be necessary to cover any bone defect.

TERATOMA

Tumors and cysts of teratologic origin, the result of congenital disturbances of development or misplacement of embryonic cells, have been observed in the nose, pharynx, mouth, and neck.

These tumors and cysts can be classified into (1) those due to disturbances of the single individual embryo, and (2) those due to disturbances of the twin embryo. The classification would include disturbances of dentition, branchiogenic disorders, craniopharyngeal duct anomalies, irregularities of the thyroglossal duct, and neurogenic disturbances.

Those which involve the twin embryo are:

1. Cysts in the floor of the mouth, submaxillary glands, and mucous glands in the mucous membrane of the floor of the mouth and those involving some irregularity in closure of the second branchial cleft. For all these cysts, the term "ranula" is used. Some of them, however, are acquired; that is, they are due to closure of the ducts of mucous glands.

2. Lingual goiter or aberrant thyroid tissue.

3. Tumors involving the deep peripheral nerves, called perineural fibroblastoma, perineural fibroma, solitary neurofibroma, peripheral glioma, and schwannoma.

4. Tumors derived from the brain due to some disturbance in embryonic development, such as (1) a pinching off within the nasal cavity of a part of the primitive bud, forming a glioma in the nose, or (2) the formation of a meningocele or meningoencephalocele from a dehiscence in the region of the cribriform plate.

5. A chondroma developing from cartilaginous cells which fail to undergo ossification. A chondrosarcoma may develop from these cartilaginous cell rests. It has been found in the nose, septum, and various other parts of the head.

6. Mixed salivary tumors.

7. The large embryoma affecting two or more layers of the body. It is prone to occur in the pharynx and neck. It contains a

profusion of connective tissue elements from the different germinal layers of the body.

These various tumors are described separately elsewhere; therefore, further consideration will not be given here.

NEURINOMA; NEUROFIBROMA; SCHWANNOMA

Neurogenic tumors involving the upper respiratory tract would include all tumors originating from nerve tissue or its covering. Two groups have been recognized: (1) developmental defects, such as meningocele and encephalocele, which are considered elsewhere; and (2) neoplasms of neurogenic origin, such as neurinoma or neurofibroma (Fig. 23–9), ganglioneuroma, and meningioma. Neuromas, in addition to being called neurofibromas, have been termed schwannomas, perineural fibroblastomas, and perineural fibromas. Meningiomas have

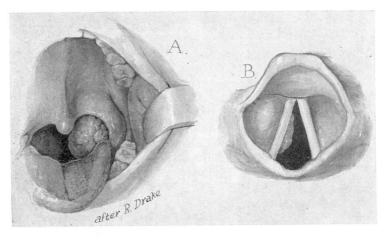

FIG. 23–9.   *A*, Neurofibroma of the pharynx.   *B*, Neurofibroma of the larynx.

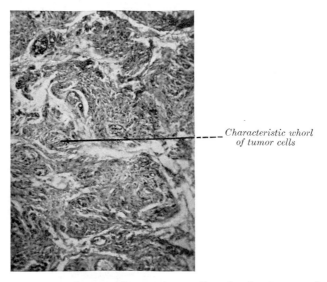

_____ *Characteristic whorl of tumor cells*

FIG. 23–10.   Neurofibroma. A neurofibroma is usually a benign tumor of rather complicated origin. In most instances an overgrowth of both the connective tissue elements of the nerve (epineurium, perineurium, and endoneurium) and the specialized nerve structures is seen. × 30.

been described as psammomas, neuroepithe-liomas, endotheliomas, and meningeal fi-broblastomas.

Etiology. Neurinomas (neurofibromas) originate from the connective tissue sheath of a nerve (Fig. 23–10). They have been attributed to the sheath of Schwann (schwannoma), in which case they would be of ectodermal origin. If multiple tumors originate from the cutaneous, visceral, and cranial nerves, the condition is known as von Recklinghausen's disease, which as a rule does not involve the nose or throat.

Pathology. Neurinomas involving the nose, throat, and larynx are usually solitary lesions. They appear to be encapsulated but may have invasive tendencies and may recur after removal.

Microscopic sections show the typical elongated or spindle-shaped cell with an oval or flattened nucleus, usually with a pal-isading effect. A small amount of eosino-philic cytoplasm may be observed. At times a myxomatous, jellylike material is present in which the palisading appearance is di-minished. Occasionally, degenerative defects such as cysts or hemorrhages may be evi-dent.

The *ganglioneuroma* is characterized by ganglion and glial cells and nerve fibers. These growths are seldom found in the nose and throat.

The *meningioma,* usually a benign tumor, is thought to arise from an arachnoid em-bryonal rest. It may appear extracranially at the root of the nose or in the sinuses. Microscopic sections reveal long fibroblastic nuclei in the form of a whorl. Frequently hyaline formations, producing a sandlike appearance (psammona), are present.

Schwannoma of the pharynx is extremely rare. It may occur at any age and occurs in both sexes about equally. The tumors are encapsualted, smooth, rounded, firm, and usually a yellowish color. The size of the slowly developing growth varies with its length of development.

Symptoms. Symptoms would depend upon the location and size of the slow-grow-ing neoplasms.

A brownish coloration of the skin (café au lait spots) may be present and is usually considered most significant from a diagnos-tic standpoint.

Growths in the oropharynx, if large, may cause some difficulty in swallowing or talk-ing but seldom produce an obstruction to respiration. Bleeding is uncommon.

Tumors of the larynx may produce symp-toms of hoarseness, cough, slight discom-fort, and at times dyspnea.

Examination usually reveals a gray or yellowish red firm, somewhat round, en-capsulated growth. The usual location is in the ventricular bands and aryepiglottic folds.

Neurinomas of the nose or sinuses would produce the symptoms of any slow-growing tumor, such as partial or complete nasal stenosis. Bleeding or pain is seldom present. A roentgenogram may demonstrate an opac-ity of the invaded area.

Neurinomas of the pharynx and tonsils are usually accessible through the mouth. Tumors of the nasopharynx, nasal cavity, or sinuses, where removal is difficult, may re-quire destruction by surgical diathermy or cryosurgery.

CHORDOMA

The chordoma, a neoplasm of the noto-chord, arises from the embryonic remains of the chorda dorsalis. Chordomas may be produced at any point along the axial skele-ton where the notochordal cells are found. They are classified as cranial, vertebral, and sacrococcygeal.

They occur with greater frequency in males, especially in the third, fourth, and fifth decades. The symptoms of chordoma in this region are due to disturbed function of the cranial nerves or to compression of the brain stem or spinal cord. They are slow-growing as a rule.

Chordomas projecting into the nasophar-ynx may be seen by the nasopharyngoscope and may be palpated. They may be mis-taken for sarcomas or fibromas or other smooth, round, firm growths which erode the skull into the nasopharynx and involve the cranial nerves.

Chordomas have extended to the maxil-lary sinus and by metastasis to the cervical lymph nodes.

Roentgenograms may show an erosive lesion or destruction of the sella turcica or cranial floor.

The prognosis is poor, depending on the involvement of the brain and spinal cord.

Surgical intervention may occasionally be successful but is usually followed by a recurrence. Roentgen or radium therapy is sometimes palliative. The diagnosis is made by biopsy.

LINGUAL THYROID; ABERRANT THYROID

Etiology. A lingual thyroid may result from an arrested descent of the thyroid anlage (heterotopic). In this form the cervical thyroid would be absent. Another form develops from aberrant rests (accessory thyroid, aberrant thyroid). The thyroid tissue is located in the great majority of cases in or on the base of the tongue between the epiglottis and the circumvallate papillae or at the site of the foramen cecum (Fig. 23–11). In a small number of cases it extends into the tongue above the frenum. It has its origin in the suprahyoid region. A sublin-

gual type may be seen in the submental region as a rounded swelling beneath the skin.

It is found much more commonly in women, especially during periods of endocrine activity.

Pathology. The lesions vary in size from small tumors to those the size of a hen's egg. They are usually about 2 by 2 cm in width and length and 2 or 2 cm above the base of the tongue.

Symptoms. Symptoms, if present, of a lingual thyroid are due to the enlargement of the tongue. A sense of foreign body, dysphagia, or dysarthria are usually mentioned. If the tumor is large, dyspnea and asphyxia may be present. Hemorrhage due to ulceration or rupture of a vein may occur.

On examination, a circumscribed red swelling on the base of the tongue, sessile or pedunculated, at times with dilated vessels, can be seen. The color is usually reddish or bluish. It may be semisoft or firm. It is painless and does not blanch with pressure.

Histologic examination usually reveals normal thyroid tissue with at times some changes of a colloid or parenchymatous nature.

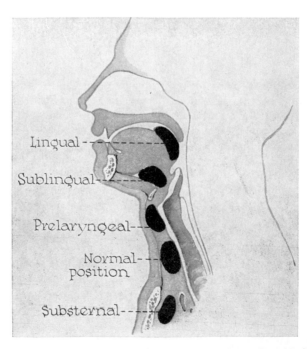

FIG. 23–11.   Most common locations of aberrant thyroid tissue.

Differential Diagnosis. Lingual thyroid tumors should be differentiated from other benign tumors, such as angiomas, amyloid tumors, cysts, fibromas, papillomas, gummas, hyperplasias of the lingual tonsil, lipomas, epitheliomas, and lymphosarcomas. The diagnosis is proved by histologic examination of an incised portion.

Treatment. Symptomless intralingual thyroid tumors do not need to be removed. The presence or absence of other thyroid tissue in the normal location should be determined before the lingual growth is removed, as removal of the lingual thyroid has been followed by myxedema and tetany.

Surgical intervention should be reserved for those cases presenting dysphagia and dyspnea. Surgical diathermy with an electrocoagulating current has been used in recent years for removing enough of the gland to relieve the mechanical obstruction.

External operations, such as a lateral pharyngotomy by either the suprahyoid or subhyoid route, have been employed in extreme cases.

BENIGN GIANT CELL TUMOR

The benign giant cell tumor is a low-grade neoplastic growth, usually single, affecting the epiphysis of the long bones as a rule, but cases have been reported in which the maxilla, ethmoid, sphenoid, temporal, and frontal bones have been involved in that order of frequency.

The cause of a giant cell tumor is unknown. It has been attributed to trauma or inflammation of the bone. It is more common in females and usually appears in the second or third decade of life.

The course is progressive; however, spontaneous cures are sometimes observed. Metastasis does not occur. Death is usually from hemorrhage or secondary infection. Most cases can be controlled by irradiation therapy.

MALIGNANT LYMPHOMA

Objections can be raised to the term malignant lymphoma because it is insufficiently specific. For the purposes of this section, it will include lymphosarcoma and reticulum cell sarcoma, follicular lymphoma, and Hodgkin's disease.

Lymphosarcoma and Reticulum Cell Sarcoma

In both these sarcomas there is an abnormal neoplastic proliferation of the cells of the lymph nodes, the lymphocytes in the former and the reticulum cell in the latter. The sites of origin may be single or multiple.

Pathology. The enlarged lymph nodes display a thickened capsule and may be discrete or matted. Mitotic figures are numerous, and the predominant feature is either the lymphocytic or reticulum cell.

Clinical Manifestations. Symptoms are largely determined, early in the disease at least, by the sites at which lymph node enlargement occurs and by the structures whose normal physiology is deranged. Most commonly the first nodes enlarged are in the cervical, axillary, or inguinal regions; usually they are nontender and painless. It is not unusual for the primary site to be extranodal—the tonsils, nasopharynx, or elsewhere. Rarely, enlarged mediastinal nodes cause a Horner's syndrome or vocal cord paralysis.

Treatment. Irradiation, chemotherapy, steroids, and less frequently surgical removal of isolated single nodes are the modalities of treatment used.

Follicular Lymphoma

It is questionable whether follicular lymphoma deserves a separate classification, but because of its relatively benign course, it will be considered separately.

The enlarged nodes may reach a diameter of 5 cm or more, are not tender, and are usually discrete. Most commonly the enlarged nodes are found in the cervical, inguinal, and axillary chains and rarely in the nasopharynx. Architecturally, follicles, sometimes visible with the unaided eye, are the prominent feature. Constitutional manifestations are infrequent, though hepatomegaly and splenomegaly are frequent. In most instances the disease eventuates in lymphosarcoma or reticulum cell sarcoma.

Treatment is best managed by x-ray therapy.

Hodgkin's Disease

Definition. Hodgkin's disease is an abnormality of lymphatic tissue, both nodal and extranodal. Reticulum cells are more affected than lymphocytes. The etiology is unknown, though many consider it to be a true malignant neoplasm. The possibility of it being an infectious granuloma (of viral etiology) cannot be excluded.

Pathology. The Reed-Sternberg cell is the characteristic feature of lymph nodes in Hodgkin's disease. It is a large cell, 10 to 40 μmm in diameter, with a multilobulated nucleus, coarse chromatin, prominent nucleoli, and abundant cytoplasm.

Clinical Manifestations. Most commonly the presenting complaint is painless enlargement of lymph nodes in the cervical, axillary, and inguinal regions. Later the mediastinal and other nodes enlarge. Tonsillar involvement is unusual. The spleen becomes enlarged in about 50% of cases, and hepatic enlargement is common.

Anorexia, weight loss, fatigue, night sweats, fever, and chills are common systemic manifestations. The fever frequently is of the intermittent (Pel-Ebstein) type. Petechiae and bleeding from mucous membranes may occur, particularly if the platelet count falls to low levels. Anemia may be pronounced.

FREY'S SYNDROME

Also called Baillaiger's syndrome and auriculotemporal syndrome, Frey's syndrome consists of gustatory sweating, flushing, and a feeling of warmth in the area of sensory distribution of the auriculotemporal nerve. Symptoms are triggered by eating foods that produce a strong salivary stimulation. Misdirected nerve fiber regeneration following an injury is considered to be the cause.

TUMORS OF THE SALIVARY GLANDS

The salivary gland that is the most frequent site of tumors, both benign and malignant, is the parotid. The submaxillary and sublingual glands are afflicted less commonly. Tumors are also occasionally found in widely dispersed glandlike accumulations in the mucosa of the pharynx, palate, and larynx, as well as in aberrant accumulations of parotid tissue adjacent to the parotid itself. Perhaps 10 to 20% of parotid tumors are malignant, whereas a much higher percentage of submaxillary tumors are malignant.

Anatomy

The parotid gland, which lies just anterior and inferior to the auricle in the pterygomandibular (retromandibular) space, is a racemose gland of the serous type. It is best described as consisting of a superficial and deep portion. The latter lies on the masseter muscle and extends superiorly to the zygoma. A portion of the deep lobe may extend medial to the styloid process and thus encroach on the tonsil region. An extension of the superficial cervical fascia envelops the parotid gland and also the masseter and sternocleidomastoid muscles. This capsule varies in thickness. (See p. 280.)

The submaxillary gland is located within the submaxillary triangle under the floor of the mouth and just within and below the posterior portion of the body of the mandible. The sublingual gland is found in the floor of the mouth too, but more anteriorly and between the tongue and the body of the mandible. Both the submaxillary and sublingual glands are of the serous and mucous types.

Mixed Tumor of Parotid

The most common benign tumor of the salivary glands is the mixed tumor of the parotid (Fig. 23–12, *A*). Occurring less frequently are Warthin's tumors (papillary adenocystoma, lymphomatosum), sebaceous gland tumors, and adenomas.

Pathology. The neoplasm as a rule is a smooth, hard, circumscribed, and somewhat movable growth with a nonulcerated surface. Tumors with much cartilage are of firmer consistency than those containing mucus, which may be semisolid or cystic.

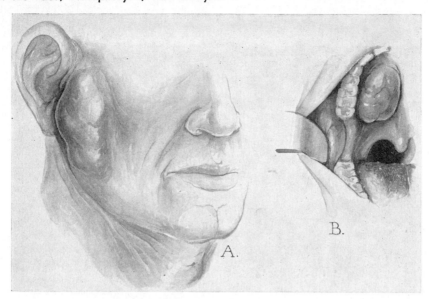

FIG. 23–12. *A*, Mixed tumor of the parotid gland. *B*, Mixed tumor of the palate.

The tumors may fill the pharynx or naso-pharynx, pushing the palate forward. Tumors of the hard palate may extend into the nose or antrum and produce a hard swelling of the cheek.

Microscopically the tumor is thought to consist only of ectodermal elements and in one place or another the following usually are found: (1) masses of epithelial cells, often showing glandular arrangement; (2) mucoid "connective" tissue with evident production of mucin; (3) "cartilage"; and (4) lymphoid tissue. The epithelial cells produce mucin, and this constitutes the mucinous "connective tissue." A cartilage-like appearance is produced by the more homogeneous myxomatous connective tissue. From this point of view, the mixed tumor is more correctly called a "benign epithelial growth with mucoid degeneration which results in the production of a hyaline material like cartilage."

Symptoms and Signs. A smooth, painless, slow-growing mass is readily palpable if the tumor is located in the superficial lobe of the parotid gland, which is usually the case. Deep-lying tumors are palpated externally with much difficulty and occasionally present intraorally in the tonsil region. The tumor is freely movable, though again this is difficult to demonstrate if the tumor lies deep in the gland. If there is a paralysis of the facial nerve, a malignant tumor is to be strongly suspected. Metastases are rare. It is thought that in 10% of cases, mixed tumors may undergo malignant change, and then perhaps metastases may occur.

Diagnosis. Sialography is an important step in determining the exact location of the tumor. The tumor itself contains no salivary ducts, but by noting the area from which the ducts are displaced, one can determine the site of the lesion.

Aspiration and incisional biopsy may be helpful for diagnosis, but it is probably best not to perform them because of the fear of spreading tumor cells. Any procedure, including the surgery itself, must avoid rupturing the capsule to avoid this possibility.

Treatment

Mixed Tumors of Parotid. The only treatment for mixed tumors of the parotid is exposure of the gland and complete removal of the growth. Incompletely removed mixed tumors tend to recur.

Most tumors of the superficial lobe are best removed through a Y incision, the upper arms of which surround the lower portion of the auricle and the vertical arm of which passes just posterior to the ramus of the mandible. After the skin is reflected forward, dissection is carefully carried downward at the junction of the bony external auditory canal and the anterior margin of the mastoid process until the trunk of the facial nerve is clearly in view. An additional aid in locating the nerve is to determine the position of the posterior belly of the digastric muscle. The trunk of the facial nerve lies just superior to the origin of the posterior belly. If the location of the tumor is such that the above is difficult, a peripheral branch of the nerve may be found and traced posteriorly until the trunk itself is isolated.

Once the nerve trunk is found, dissection is carried forward just superficial to the trunk and its branches until the tumor and a wide margin of the parotid gland are included. Amputation of the parotid duct is rarely followed by a salivary fistula or other complication.

Tumors lying in the deep lobe of the parotid are removed with more difficulty. After the facial nerve is exposed and its branches mobilized, the nerve can usually be retracted to one side, so that the tumor can be delivered and removed. Placing a finger in the mouth to exert outward pressure on the tumor is frequently of great help. Tumors which present near the tonsil or in the palate are best removed per os.

Extraparotid Mixed Tumors. The treatment of benign mixed tumors of the salivary glands is excision. In the case of the submaxillary and sublingual glands, the gland itself is removed along with the tumor in order to achieve as low a recurrence rate as possible.

Since removal of the submaxillary gland entails no cosmetic or physiologic disturbance, this should be accomplished when necessary without hesitation. In so doing, care should be taken to preserve the supermandibular branch of the facial nerve and to avoid injury to the lingual and hypoglossal nerves.

Tumors of the palate and elsewhere in the oral cavity and pharynx are removed by extirpation, great care being taken to avoid rupture of the capsule. A less desirable method is to destroy the growth by electrodesiccation.

Warthin's Tumor. A papillary adenocystoma lymphomatosum (of Warthin) is a benign tumor, usually found in the parotid gland. It resembles a mixed tumor. Treatment is complete surgical excision.

Other Benign Salivary Gland Tumors. These include benign adenomas, sebaceous gland tumors, and various miscellaneous forms. Treatment is usually surgical excision.

Malignant Tumors of the Salivary Gland

A useful classification of these malignant tumors follows:

1. Mucoepidermoid carcinomas (mixed carcinoma)
2. Squamous cell carcinomas
3. Adenocarcinomas
   a. Adenoid cystic
   b. Acinic cell
   c. Miscellaneous
4. Unclassified

Mucoepidermoid Tumors. These tumors resemble benign mixed cell tumors and are usually found in the parotid. Facial paralysis may be present. Treatment is radical parotidectomy, the facial nerve being sacrificed when necessary. The prognosis is poor if an early presenting complaint is facial paralysis.

Squamous Cell Carcinoma. The ducts of the salivary glands are believed to give rise to these tumors. On palpation they are found to be hard and adherent to the adjacent structures. Facial nerve paralysis and metastases to regional nodes occur in about one third of cases. Treatment is radical excision. The prognosis is poor.

Adenocarcinoma. The cystic variety is slow-growing; nevertheless, unless radically excised, it carries a poor prognosis. Clinically it is often associated with pain. The acinic cell carcinoma, on the other hand, is of relatively low-grade malignancy and carries a fairly good prognosis if it is completely excised.

EPITHELIOMA OF THE SKIN

Skin cancer is usually a basal cell epithelioma, involving the face, neck, or lower

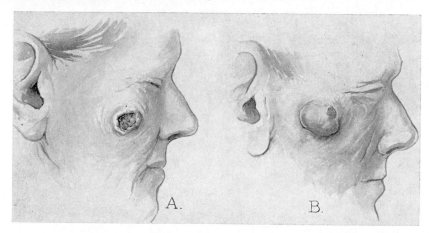

FIG. 23–13.   *A*, Basal cell carcinoma of the face with the characteristic rolled border and punched-out ulceration in the center.   *B*, A papillomatous squamous or prickle cell epithelioma in an area exposed to sunlight.

lip. It most often attacks the fair-skinned, blue-eyed, outdoor type of person, such as the farmer.

Etiology. People, especially men, who are subjected to more sunlight than the light-complexioned skin can tolerate over a long period of time are particularly susceptible to skin cancer. Frequently a premature aging of the skin or a senile keratosis is present. Workers in contact with tars, pitch, and so forth, have shown an added susceptibility. Other predisposing causes are scars of old burns, cutaneous horns, roentgen dermatitis, leukoplakia, chronic ulcers, and lupus vulgaris. Cutaneous cancer may occur at any age, but the great majority of patients are past 50 years of age.

Pathology. The epithelioma may be of the squamous cell or basal cell type (Fig. 23–13) or of the mixed (transitional) form. The squamous cell cancer is more virulent, has a tendency to metastasize, and tends to occur on the mucocutaneous junction of the lower lip. The growth originating from the mucosal border tends to grow rapidly.

The basal cell tumor, sometimes called a *rodent ulcer,* is slow to ulcerate and may even regress or disappear. However, the tumors do spread by local extension in most instances. They may remain stationary for many months or years, but eventually they become active.

The lesions may extend above or below the skin surface or grow in a lateral direction. The pedunculated or upward-growing growths are more amenable to treatment than the downward-growing type. Infiltration and ulceration with a rapid rate of growth denote a later and more ominous stage.

Sarcomas of the skin of the face are rare.

Diagnosis. Suspicion of malignancy should be aroused by any enlarging nodule about the face which forms a plaque with a pearly border, especially if an ulcer forms in the later stage. The characteristic features are the hard, waxy, pearl-like border with a nodular-type base and, if present, the free bleeding ulcer. A biopsy would determine the type of lesion.

Treatment. The treatment of skin cancers about the face consists of either wide surgical excision or roentgen irradiation. Both methods provide 5-year successes in 90% or better of the cases.

CARCINOMA OF THE LIP

Primary carcinoma of the lip originates on the vermilion border, although it may be secondarily involved from a basal cell carcinoma beginning on the adjacent skin.

Etiology. As in skin cancer, undue exposure to the sun in the fair-skinned person seems to be the greatest etiologic factor.

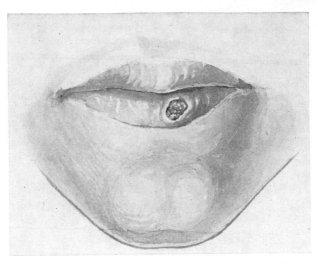

FIG. 23–14.   Early squamous cell carcinoma of the lip. The early lesion may be
similar to a persistent "cold sore."

Tobacco chewing and pipe and cigar smoking are thought to be factors in many instances. The disease occurs in men from middle age on in the great majority of cases.

Diagnosis. The early lesion may be a persistent "cold sore" (Fig. 23–14). Crusting, peeling, or mild ulceration may appear early. Leukoplakia is present at times. A painless induration of the lesion is a characteristic finding. A biopsy will establish the diagnosis.

Treatment. Both surgical and radiologic modes of treatment are successful. In the former case, a V-shaped incision is made so as to include all of the growth plus a generous margin of normal tissue.

MALIGNANT NEOPLASMS OF THE NASOPHARYNX

Malignant neoplasms in the nasopharynx comprise about 2% of all malignant growths in the head and neck. Lederman reports that out of 1727 patients suffering from neoplasms in the nasopharynx, oropharynx, and laryngopharynx, 14% had lesions that were located in the nasopharynx. The average age of the patients in Lederman's series of 248 cases was 54.3 years for men and 49.7 for women. The neoplasms occur more frequently in males. In children and adults below the age of 30,

they occur more frequently than any other malignant tumor of the upper respiratory tract.

Anatomy of the Nasopharynx. The nasopharynx is a cavity with rigid walls superiorly, posteriorly, and laterally. Anteriorly it communicates via the choanae with the nasal cavity, so that obstruction of the nasal airway is often the case. Likewise, spread laterally commonly leads to blockage of the eustachian orifice and subsequently to fluid in the middle ear. Posteriorly the wall slopes superiorly and anteriorly and lies beneath the bodies of the sphenoid and basilar portions of the occipital bone. Pressure necrosis may occur in either place. On the lateral walls are found the eminences of the torus tubarius, which partly encloses the eustachian tubes. Behind and superior to the torus is the pharyngeal recess or fossa of Rosenmüller, and directly above the posterior end of this is the foramen lacerum.

The neoplasms may spread in two directions, each leading to distinct neurologic signs. Direct extension through the foramen lacerum into the cavernous sinus and middle fossa of the skull leads to involvement of cranial nerves III, IV, VI, and more rarely II. By contrast, spread to the lateral pharyngeal nodes in and about the carotid jugular sheath in the retroparotidean space results in infiltration of cranial nerves IX, X, XI, and XII. Cranial nerves VII and VIII are usually spared.

Incidence. The incidence of carcinoma of the nasopharynx is high in southern China, and wherever the Chinese migrate (such migrants are usually from southern China), they carry with them their high incidence. This cancer, however, is rare among the Japanese. Reliable evidence concerning other mongoloid groups is wanting. The above suggests a genetic factor in combination with ethnic environmental factors (e.g., incense smoke).

Etiology. The Epstein-Barr virus (considered a member of the herpesvirus group) has been associated etiologically with nasopharyngeal carcinoma by several investigators. High titers to the virus have been reported in patients of Chinese origin in Hong Kong and in those of African origin in Nairobi, Kenya, as well as in patients of Japanese and Chinese origin in Tokyo and Taiwan. Recently a report on United States citizens appeared in which 71 per cent of patients with nasopharyngeal carcinoma had high serum antibodies to the EB virus (1:160), whereas only 6 of 140 (4.3%) had such titers in the control group. By contrast, the patients with a diagnosis of lymphoma presented a low titer.

Pathology. The lateral walls containing the fossa of Rosenmüller are the most common locations of nasopharyngeal cancer, and the posterior wall of the pharynx is only slightly less so. Less commonly a tumor is found on the roof and only rarely on the floor. To begin with, the neoplasm may be so small as to be unrecognizable, or it may be located in an area where symptoms are not generated, e.g., Rosenmüller's fossa. Later, symptoms arise as a result of the direction of the spread. It may extend through an orifice adjacent to the site of origin, or it may erode the bone by pressure necrosis.

Histologic classification of nasopharyngeal tumors is difficult. Epithelial tumors comprise about 85% of the malignant tumors, and maligant lymphomas are present in 7.5% of cases. Connective tissue tumors are found in less than 2%, and very rarely neuroblastoma and malignant mixed tumor

are found. The following table is a usable one for most epithelial tumors.

1. Epidermoid carcinoma
   a. Keratinizing
   b. Nonkeratinizing (includes those tumors that have been termed "transitional cell" carcinoma and "lympho-epithelioma")
2. Adenocarcinoma
3. Adenoid cystic carcinoma
4. Mucoepidermoid carcinoma
5. Anaplastic carcinoma

Symptoms. In more than 50% of the cases, the presenting symptom is a metastatic gland in the neck. This illustrates the silent nature of nasopharyngeal neoplasms and the need for routine examination of this structure. The next most common symptom is usually homolateral head pain followed by nasal obstruction. It frequently has been observed that a delay of more than 3 months occurs from the time of the first symptom until medical attention is sought, when a further delay may occur before a diagnosis is established. Other early symptoms may include nasal obstruction, vague headache, or sore throat. Defective hearing due to obstruction of the eustachian tube, with or without earache, frequently brings the patient to the otolaryngologist. In 1911 Trotter described a triad of symptoms resulting from nasopharyngeal neoplasms: impaired hearing due to obstruction of the eustachian tube, neuralgia of the second branch of the fifth cranial nerve, and asymmetry of the soft palate.

The next chain of symptoms results from the spread of the tumor extradurally into the cranial cavity. Most commonly the sixth cranial nerve is the first one affected, followed by the fifth, fourth, and third. All of the cranial nerves may be involved. Invasion of the orbit produces proptosis and blindness. Not infrequently a Horner's syndrome is seen.

Pain resulting from nasopharyngeal neoplasia may be referred to any of the three divisions of the trigeminal nerve. Unexplained head or face pain always requires a diagnostic examination of the nasopharynx. Lederman states that, under irradiation, a favorable result is suggested by the disappearance of head pain within 10 to 14 days, and persistent pain well beyond this period suggests an unfavorable response.

Upon admission to the hospital, as many as 85% of patients may demonstrate cervical metastases. Generalized metastases occur in as many as 24%.

Diagnosis. Lesions of the nasopharynx can be diagnosed with certainty only by biopsy; because of the technical difficulty in obtaining this, a negative report may mean only that the previous attempt missed the lesion. Biopsies are usually best taken with a straight biopsy forceps through the nose or with a curved one through the mouth. In either case the tip of the forceps is directed by mirror visualization of the nasopharynx or by a finger inserted simultaneously into the nasopharynx. Frequently, manipulation in the nasopharynx is greatly facilitated by retraction of the soft palate with a catheter inserted through the nose and brought out through the mouth.

Treatment. The nasopharynx is comparatively inaccessible to surgical exposure, so that treatment of malignant neoplasms of this region to date has involved almost exclusively external irradiation and intracavity radiation. The former is usually accomplished through molar portals and the latter by radium or radon utilizing special holders (Hayes Martin) to secure the radiating material in the proper location.

Wilson has suggested several ingenious surgical approaches to the nasopharynx which may enlarge the surgical indications. (See Treatment of Choanal Atresia.)

The use of chemotherapy, either alone or in combination with irradiation and/or surgery, likely will improve the success rate in the future. (See Chapters 38, 38A.)

Prognosis. Lederman reports that radiotherapy yields a 5-year survival rate of 15.7%, though others report individual series of 25 to 30%. The squamous and undifferentiated carcinomas are the most deadly.

Treatment of Cervical Metastases. No general agreement has been reached to date on the treatment of cervical metastases. Formerly irradiation, particularly in highly malignant, anaplastic, radiosensitive bilateral metastases, was almost universally advised. With slow-growing, well-differentiated tumors, the decision of whether surgery is preferable or not is more difficult to make. In recent years radical neck dissection has been elected more and more frequently.

REFERENCES*

Boyd, W.: *Textbook of Pathology.* 7th ed. Philadelphia, Lea & Febiger, 1961, pp. 711–712.

Bunim, J. J., *et al.*: Clinical, Pathologic and Serologic Studies in Sjögren's Syndrome. Ann. Intern. Med., *61*:509, 1964.

Chang, T.: Nasopharyngeal Carcinoma. Surg. Clin. North Am., *53*:121, 1973.

Choa, G.: Nasopharyngeal Carcinoma. J. Laryngol. Otol., *88*:145, 1974.

Henderson, E.: Nasopharyngeal Carcinoma—Present Status of Knowledge. Cancer Res., *34*:1187, 1974.

Kitamura, T., *et al.*: Parotid Gland of Sjögren's Syndrome. Arch. Otolaryngol., *91*:64, 1970.

Saunders, W. H.: Septal Dermoplasty—Ten Years' Experience. Trans. Am. Acad. Ophthalmol. Otolaryngol., *72*:156, 1968.

Snow, J.: Carcinoma of the Nasopharynx in Children. Ann. Otol. Rhinol. Laryngol., *84*:817, 1975.

Wara, W.: Immunosuppression Following Radiation Therapy for Carcinoma of the Nasopharynx. Am. J. Roentgenol. Radium Ther. Nucl. Med., *123*:482, 1975.

*Additional references are found at the end of Chapter 37.

PART 3
DISEASES OF THE LARYNX

Joseph H. Ogura and Richard W. Mallen

Chapter 24
Developmental Anatomy of the Larynx

Embryology

The primordium of the larynx, trachea, bronchi, and lungs arises as a keel-shaped outgrowth from the floor of the pharynx during the third embryonic week. The pharyngeal site of this outgrowth is a depression which elongates posteriorly, forming the laryngotracheal groove. The anterior end of the groove, which is immediately posterior to the hypobranchial eminence, becomes the primitive laryngeal aditus. The aditus lies between the bases of the sixth branchial arch. The margins of the laryngotracheal groove begin to fuse in a caudocranial direction, about the fourth embryonic week, to form the tracheoesophageal septum which separates the trachea from the esophagus and hypopharynx (Fig. 24–1). Closure to the level of the cricoid cartilage is completed by the fifth week, leaving the small pharyngotracheal canal connecting the pharynx and trachea.

The sagittal slit of the primitive laryngeal aditus is altered by the growth of three tissue masses around it. Anteriorly, the posterior portion of the hypobranchial eminence separates to become the furcula, a mound of mesoderm which is the primitive epiglottis. Lateral to the slit, the ventral ends of the sixth branchial arches grow and form two raised mounds, the arytenoid eminences, on the floor of the pharynx. These approximate each other medially, the furcula form-

ing a T-shaped sulcus anteriorly. The pharyngotracheal canal lies between the bases of the arytenoid eminences. The vestibule of the larynx develops from the T-shaped sulcus, which is largely part of the floor of the pharynx and lies anterior to the pharyngotracheal canal. Later, the pharyngotracheal canal moves anteriorly into the posterior part of the vestibule. At this time (eighth week), the analogue of the vocal cords is formed by an epithelial and mesodermal mass separating the floor of the vestibule from the upper trachea, with the pharyngotracheal canal posterior to it. By the

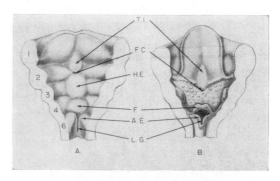

FIG. 24–1. Developmental anatomy of the floor of the pharynx. *A*, The pharynx in the 5-week-old fetus. *B*, The pharynx in the 5-month-old fetus. *T.I.*, tuberculum impar; *F.C.*, foramen caecum; *H.E.*, hypobranchial eminence; *F*, furcula; *A.E.*, arytenoid eminence; *L.G.*, laryngotracheal groove.

tenth week, this mass splits sagittally, giving rise to both pairs of vocal cords.

During the seventh week, a fissure appears on the medial surface of each arytenoid eminence and extends anteriorly and laterally into the floor of the primitive vestibule. This is the laryngeal ventricle, the extremity of which extends laterally past the margins of the primitive vestibule to form the sacculus or appendix of the ventricle. The sacculus is intimately related to the fourth branchial arch and cleft. As the ventricles develop, the true and false vocal cords are separated.

The hyaline cartilages of the larynx develop from branchial arch mesoderm, but the elastic cartilages are derivatives of the mesoderm of the floor of the pharynx. The hyaline cartilages first appear during the fourth week. The arytenoids develop in the arytenoid eminences, and at first they are fused to the two halves of the cricoid inferiorly. They are gradually separated from the cricoid by the development of the cricothyroid joint and by the twelfth embryonic week are well developed. The vocal processes are developed separately in association with the vocal cords, and as a result, consist of elastic cartilage.

The cricoid cartilage is also a sixth arch derivative which initially develops as two mesodermal masses which fuse anterior to the pharyngotracheal canal by the sixth week. Fusion of the posterior lamina is delayed until the eighth or ninth week. The cricoid fuses as the pharyngotracheal canal shifts forward to become a part of the laryngeal lumen. The last portion of the laryngotracheal groove to be obliterated is the interarytenoid sulcus, which is present until the eleventh week.

The thyroid cartilage develops from the ventral portions of the fourth branchial arches, which fuse anterior to the pharyngotracheal canal. Development is fairly complete by the tenth week with the formation of the cricothyroid joint. The fifth branchial arch is vestigial in humans and does not contribute to laryngeal development.

The epiglottis and cuneiform cartilages of Wrisberg are derivatives of the furcula, which is part of the floor of the pharynx, although the fourth arch, which forms the lateral glossoepiglottic fold, may contribute to formation of the epiglottis.

The hyoid bone is derived from the second and third branchial arch cartilages; the second arch forms the lesser cornu and part of the body, and the third arch is the origin of the greater cornu and remainder of the body. The major portion of the supraglottic larynx derives its nerve supply from the fourth arch nerve (the superior laryngeal), which must enter the larynx inferior to the hyoid through the thyrohyoid membrane. Remnants of the fourth branchial groove will be attached to the thyrohyoid membrane posterior to the point of nerve entry.

The intrinsic muscles, with the exception of the cricothyroid, are derived from the mesoderm of the sixth branchial arches, which invades the epithelial and mesodermal primordium of the vocal cords. The cricothyroid muscle is derived separately from the anterior portion of the pharyngeal sphincter at the level of the fourth arch and is supplied by the fourth arch nerve, the superior laryngeal. The extrinsic muscles are derived from the epicardial ridge, as is the sternomastoid muscle, and are therefore supplied by the hypoglossal nerve.

DEVELOPMENTAL DIFFERENCES FROM THE INFANT TO THE ADULT LARYNX

Size. The infantile larynx is of equal size in both sexes. However, it is smaller in relation to body size than the adult larynx and therefore forms a relatively smaller isthmus to the respiratory tract. The infraglottic area is the narrowest area of the larynx in the infant, whereas the glottic area is the narrowest in the adult. The relative laryngeal dimensions are found in Table 24–1. The larynx grows fairly rapidly until the child is 6 years of age; then growth proceeds slowly until adolescence. At this time, there is rapid growth of the male larynx, and by the time growth is complete, the male larynx is considerably larger, as well as having much greater internal dimensions, than the female larynx. The female larynx enlarges slightly after puberty.

Table 24–1.   Dimensions of the Larynx

| | | Infancy | Puberty | Adult | |
				Male	Female
Vocal Cord—Length		6–8 mm	12–15 mm	17 –23 mm	12.5–17 mm
	Membranous portion	3–4 mm	7– 8 mm	11.5–16 mm	8 –11.5 mm
	Cartilaginous portion	3–4 mm	5– 7 mm	5.5– 7 mm	4.5– 5.5 mm
Glottis	—Width at rest	3 mm	5 mm	8 mm	6 mm
	Maximum	6 mm	12 mm	19 mm	13 mm
Infraglottis —Sagittal		5–7 mm	15 mm	25 mm	18 mm
	Transverse	5–7 mm	15 mm	24 mm	17 mm

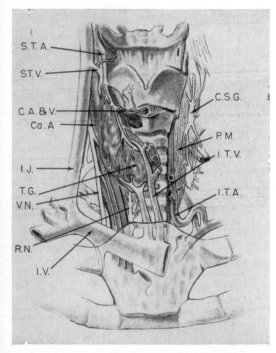

Fig. 24–2.   Relationships of the larynx to adjacent structures in the neck. *C.S.G.*, cervical sympathetic ganglion; *P.M.*, prevertebral muscle; *I.T.V.*, inferior thyroid vein; *I.T.A.*, inferior thyroid artery; *S.T.A.*, superior thyroid artery; *S.T.V.*, superior thyroid vein; *C.A. & V.*, cricothyroid artery and vein; *Ca. A.*, carotid artery; *I.J.*, internal jugular vein; *T.G.*, thyroid gland; *V.N.*, vagus nerve; *R.N.*, recurrent nerve; *I.V.*, innominate vein.

Position. At birth, the inferior margin of the cricoid cartilage is at the level of the upper border of the fourth cervical vertebra, and the tip of the epiglottis is opposite the first cervical vertebra. Thus, the epiglottis may be seen easily over the dorsum of the tongue in most infants. The larynx descends slightly in the neck between birth and age 2 years, but then the position is relatively stationary until age 11 to 12 years. During this period, the cricoid is opposite the intervertebral disc between the fourth and fifth vertebrae, and the epiglottis is at the level of the second intervertebral disc. After puberty, the larynx lengthens rapidly and the cricoid descends to the level of the seventh cervical vertebra in males and to the level of the sixth vertebra in females. The tip of the epiglottis remains almost stationary opposite the third cervical vertebra (Figs. 24–2 and 24–3).

Consistency. In infants, the cartilaginous framework of the larynx is softer and the supporting ligaments more lax, making the larynx more susceptible to collapse when an internal negative pressure is exerted on it.

The subepithelial tissues are less dense as well as more abundant and vascular in infants, which predisposes to accumulation of tissue fluids. This is an important factor contributing to the frequency of obstruction

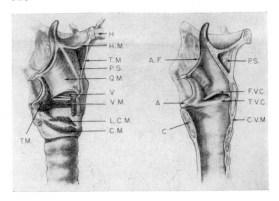

A   B

Fig. 24–3. *A*, Lateral view of the larynx with the thyroid ala removed. *H*, hyoid; *H.M.*, hyoepiglottic membrane; *T.M.*, thyrohyoid membrane; *P.S.*, pre-epiglottic space; *Q.M.*, quadrangular membrane; *V*, ventricular orifice; *V.M.*, vocalis muscles; *L.C.M.*, lateral crico-arytenoid muscle; *C.M.*, cricothyroid muscle; *T.M.*, thyroarytenoid muscle.

B, View depicting the structures of the lateral wall of the laryngeal lumen from within the lumen. *P.S.*, pre-epiglottic space; *F.V.C.*, false vocal cord; *T.V.C.*, true vocal cord; *C.V.M.*, cricothyroid membrane; *A.F.*, aryepiglottic fold; *A*, arytenoid; *C*, cricoid.

of the infraglottic and supraglottic areas by inflammatory edema in small children.

Shape. Several laryngeal structures differ in shape in infants. The epiglottis tends toward an omega shape; therefore, there is a greater tendency for it to obliterate the vestibule should it become edematous. Also, the margins of an omega-shaped epiglottis provide less support for the aryepiglottic folds than do the margins of the flat adult epiglottis which help to hold the folds in a lateral position.

In neonates, the vocal cords are half membranous and half cartilaginous, but the membranous portion becomes relatively longer with growth, forming two thirds of the vocal cord in the adult.

The angle of the thyroid cartilage is relatively constant at 110 to 120 degrees until puberty, when it becomes much narrower in the male (90 degrees) and widens slightly in the female (120 degrees).

The peculiarities of the infantile larynx are important factors in the predisposition of infants to particular laryngeal diseases and to aspiration of foreign bodies.

Ossification of Laryngeal Skeleton

The laryngeal cartilages are irregularly ossified, but the presence of calcium in the cartilages may create confusion in the roentgenographic diagnosis of foreign bodies in the hypopharynx. Also, calcification may be helpful in determining the presence of fractures and neoplastic invasion of the laryngeal skeleton.

The hyoid bone is ossified from six centers beginning shortly after birth. The process is completed by the second year.

Ossification of the thyroid cartilage commences between the twentieth and twenty-third year. It tends to be inconsistent, and there are frequently one or two circular areas in the center of each ala which remain unossified and may be confused with neoplastic invasion and destruction. The calcium appears first along the inferior margins of the cartilage and later extends up the posterior margin of each ala. The superior margin of the cartilage is often never ossified.

The ossification of cricoid cartilage begins somewhat later than that of the thyroid, and again the inferior portions of the cartilage are usually the initial sites of calcium deposits. However, the superior margin of the quadrate lamina may be an early site of ossification.

About the same time, the arytenoids begin to ossify, and in the third decade they may appear as isolated areas of calcification frequently confused with foreign bodies in the hypopharynx. Later, when the lamina of the cricoid is better ossified, the situation is less confusing.

Only the hyaline cartilages undergo ossification, and by age 65 the process is complete.

REFERENCES

Davies, J.: *Human Developmental Anatomy.* New York, The Ronald Press, 1963.

Fraser, J. E.: The Development of the Larynx. J. Anat. Physiol., **44**:156, 1910.

Grasser, O.: The Development of the Respiratory Apparatus. *In* Kiebel, F., and Mott,

E. P. (Eds.): *Manual of Human Embryology*. Vol. 2. Philadelphia, J. B. Lippincott Co., 1912, pp. 473–493.

Hamilton, W. J., *et al.*: *Human Embryology*. 3rd ed. Cambridge, W. Heffer and Sons, 1962.

Hart, M. H.: Early Development of the Human Laryngeal Muscles. Ann. Otol. Rhinol. Laryngol., *81*:524, 1972.

Hatley, W., *et al.*: The Pattern of Ossification in the Laryngeal Cartilages. Br. J. Radiol., *38*:585, 1965.

Negus, V.: *The Comparative Anatomy and Physiology of the Larynx*. New York, Grune & Stratton, 1949.

Noback, G. J.: The Developmental Topography of the Larynx, Trachea and Lungs in Fetus, Newborn, Infant and Child. Am. J. Dis. Child., *26*:515, 1923.

Roche, A. F., and Barkla, D. H.: The Level of the Larynx During Childhood. Ann. Otol. Rhinol. Laryngol., *74*:655, 1965.

Seiter, G.: L'embryologic Comparée des Cordes Vocales, Congrès Internationale sur La Voix, Paris, 1955. *In* Revue de Laryngologie, May, 1956.

Soulie, A., and Bardier, E.: Recherches sur le Développement Anatomique du Larynx Chez L'homme. J. Anat. Physiol., *43*:137, 1907.

Streeter, G. L.: Developmental Horizons in Human Embryos. Contrib. Embryol., *32*: 133, 1948.

Terracol, J.: La Calcification du Larynx et de la Voix. Revue Francais de Phoniatrie, 1935, p. 4.

Terracol, J., *et al.*: Le Sphincter Glottique; Etudé Anatomoclinique. Ann. Otol. (Paris), *13*:451, 1956.

Tucker, G.: The Infant Larynx: Direct Laryngoscopic Observations. J.A.M.A., *99*:1899, 1932.

Tucker, J. A., and O'Rahilly, R.: Embryology of the Human Larynx. Ann. Otol. Rhinol. Laryngol., *81*:52, 1972.

Walander, A.: Prenatal Development of the Epithelial Primordium of the Larynx in the Rat. Acta Anat., *10* (Suppl. 2), 1950.

Wilson, T. G.: The Infantile Larynx. Acta Otolaryng., *43*:95, 1953.

Wind, J.: *On the Phylogeny and Ontogeny of the Human Larynx*. Groningen, Wolters Noordhoff, 1970.

Chapter 25
Anatomy of the Larynx

SKELETAL STRUCTURES OF THE LARYNX

Hyoid Bone. The hyoid bone is not ordinarily included as a part of the larynx, but because of its relationship to the pre-epiglottic space and its attachments to the pre-laryngeal muscles, it is clinically important. The bone consists of a central body, two greater cornua, and two lesser cornua.

The posterior superior surface of the hyoid serves as the attachment for the hyo-epiglottic and thyrohyoid membranes; thus the hyoid forms the anterosuperior boundary of the pre-epiglottic space with the valleculae immediately above. Between the thyrohyoid membrane and the posterior inferior surface of the body, a small bursa or remnant of the thyroglossal duct is occasionally found.

The attachments of the hyoid bone to the mandible and skull by the stylohyoid ligament and the digastric, stylohyoid, mylohyoid, hyoglossus, and geniohyoid muscles serve to maintain the larynx in position in the neck and to raise the larynx during deglutition and phonation. The attachments of the sternohyoid and omohyoid muscles to the hyoid are important in inferior movement of the larynx.

Thyroid Cartilage. The thyroid cartilage is a hyaline cartilage and is the largest in the larynx. It consists of two alae or wings which meet anteriorly at an acute angle. The angle varies between sexes, being 90 degrees in the adult male and 120 degrees

in the female. In the male, the superior portion of the angle forms a subcutaneous prominence, the Adam's apple. The upper portions of the alae are separated by a deep notch, the superior thyroid notch. Each ala is quadrangular in shape, and at each posterior "corner" is a process or cornu. The superior cornua serve as attachments for the lateral thyrohyoid ligaments. The inferior cornua articulate with a facet on the posterolateral surface of the cricoid to form the cricothyroid joint.

Each surface of the cartilage is covered by thick perichondrium. The external surface of each ala is marked by an oblique ridge or line running in an anterior inferior direction from the base of the superior cornu to the inferior tubercle at the midpoint of the inferior margin. This ridge serves as the attachment for the sternothyroid, thyrohyoid, and inferior pharyngeal constrictor muscles.

The inner surface is fairly smooth, but about half the distance between the thyroid notch and the inferior margin is a small prominence which is deficient in perichondrium and serves as the attachment for the anterior commissure tendon (ligament of Broyles). The petiole of the epiglottis is attached by the thyroepiglottic ligament approximately 1 cm above this point.

Cricoid Cartilage. The cricoid cartilage is an unpaired, ring-shaped, hyaline cartilage. It is formed by a narrow anterior arch and a wide quadrate lamina posteriorly. The arch is 5 to 7 mm in height, while the lamina is 20 to 30 mm in vertical length. On the posterolateral aspect of each side is a small, slightly raised facet which articulates with an inferior thyroid cornu. On the anterosuperior surface of the quadrate lamina are two facets with the long axes parallel to the line of the lamina. These are the sites of articulation with the arytenoid cartilages. The posterior surface of the quadrate lamina is marked by a vertical ridge to which are attached the longitudinal esophageal muscle fibers; also, the ridge separates the posterior cricoarytenoid muscles. The inner superior margin of the arch forms the inferior attachment of the cricothyroid membrane and conus elasticus.

Epiglottis. The epiglottis is a thin, flexible, leaf-shaped, fibroelastic cartilage. The narrow inferior portion, the petiole, is attached to the thyroid cartilage just superior to the anterior commissure. Near the inferior end of the petiole is a prominence, the tuberculum epiglotticum, which often obscures the anterior commissure when the larynx is examined indirectly. The cartilage is perforated by several foramina below the attachment of the hyoepiglottic ligament. This portion of the epiglottis forms the posterior wall of the pre-epiglottic space, an important area in the spread of laryngeal carcinoma. Unlike the perichondrium of the hyaline cartilages, the epiglottic perichondrium is tightly adherent. As a result, infections tend to remain localized when involving the epiglottis, whereas they cause widespread destruction of the hyaline cartilages elsewhere because of the perichondrial elevation.

Arytenoid Cartilages. The arytenoid cartilages are paired, pyramidal-shaped, hyaline cartilages which articulate with the cricoid cartilage. The articular surface is saddle-shaped and lies at right angles to the cricoid joint surface. The base of the pyramid gives rise to two processes. The muscular process for the attachment of the cricoarytenoid muscles is directed in a posterolateral direction. The vocal process is directed anteriorly and differs from the body in that it is formed by elastic cartilage. The posterior superior margin of the conus elasticus is attached to the vocal process.

The corniculate cartilages of Santorini are small fibroelastic nodules attached to the apices of the arytenoid cartilages. They are nonfunctional in humans.

The cuneiform cartilages of Wrisberg are rodlike structures of elastic cartilage imbedded in the margin of the aryepiglottic folds. They may be absent.

The triticeous cartilages are small elastic nodules which are variably present in the lateral thyrohyoid ligaments; occasionally they become calcified and are mistaken for a foreign body.

Ligaments and Membranes. The thyrohyoid membrane joins the superior margin of the thyroid cartilage on the posterior superior margin of the hyoid bone. It may be separated from the inferior margin of the hyoid by a bursa. Portions of the membrane are thickened to form the medial and lateral thyrohyoid ligaments. The membrane forms much of the anterior wall of the pre-epiglottic space. The superior laryngeal artery, the internal branch of the superior laryngeal nerve, and the supraglottic lymphatic pedicle pierce the membrane at a point approximately 1 cm above and anterior to the junction of the superior cornu and the ala of the thyroid cartilage.

The hyoepiglottic ligament joins the anterior surface of the epiglottis and the posterior surface of the hyoid to form the roof of the pre-epiglottic space and the floor of the valleculae.

The conus elasticus is a fibroelastic membrane arising from the superior margin of the arch of the cricoid cartilage. Anteriorly, it is attached to the inferior margin of the thyroid cartilage, and it is thickened to form the medial cricothyroid ligament or cricothyroid membrane. The membrane is also attached anteriorly to the inner surface of the thyroid cartilage up to the vocal tubercle. Posteriorly, the conus extends from the cricoid to the vocal process of the arytenoid. The superior free margin is thickened and forms the vocal ligament. The conus elasticus is separated from the alae of the thyroid cartilage by the intrinsic muscles of the larynx.

The quadrangular membrane of loose elastic tissue extends from the lateral margins of the epiglottis to the arytenoid and corniculate cartilages; inferiorly the membrane extends into the false cord. The membrane forms part of the party wall between the upper piriform fossa and the laryngeal vestibule. The quadrangular membrane and the conus elasticus are separated by the elliptical orifice of the ventricle of Morgagni.

MUSCLES

Extrinsic. These muscles are concerned with the movement and fixation of the larynx as a whole. They consist of elevator and depressor groups. The depressor group consists of the thyrohyoid, sternohyoid, and omohyoid muscles and is supplied by the ansa hypoglossi from C2 and C3. The elevator group includes anterior and posterior digastric, stylohyoid, geniohyoid, and mylohyoid muscles supplied by cranial nerves V and VII. These muscle groups are important in the laryngeal functions of deglutition and phonation.

The middle and inferior constrictor muscles of the pharynx are also important extrinsic laryngeal muscles. The middle constrictor is attached to the greater cornua of the hyoid bone. The inferior constrictor is attached to the oblique lines of the thyroid cartilage, to a fibrous band bridging the cricothyroid space laterally, to the cricothyroid muscle, and to the cricoid cartilage. These muscles influence the position of the larynx during deglutition.

Intrinsic. The intrinsic laryngeal muscles are all paired except for the interarytenoid muscle. These muscles are responsible for the function of the vocal cords.

Cricothyroid. The cricothyroid muscle arises from the anterior and lateral surface of the arch of the cricoid cartilage and inserts in two portions, a pars recta and pars obliqua, on the inferior border of the thyroid cartilage and the inferior cornu. It is supplied by the external branch of the superior laryngeal nerve. It serves to narrow the cricothyroid space anteriorly by tilting the thyroid and cricoid cartilages around the fulcrum of the cricothyroid joint, thus lengthening and tensing the vocal cords.

Posterior Cricoarytenoid. The posterior cricoarytenoid muscle arises from a large fossa on the posterior surface of the quadrate lamina of cricoid cartilage. The fibers

are directed in a laterosuperior direction to insert on the posterior surface of the muscular process of the arytenoid cartilage. This muscle is the main abductor of the vocal cord and also helps to support the arytenoid cartilage in its erect relationship with the cricoid.

Lateral Cricothyroid. The lateral cricoarytenoid muscle arises from the superior and lateral border of the posterior part of the cricoid arch lateral to the attachment of the conus elasticus. It inserts on the anterior surface of the muscular process of the arytenoid and adducts the vocal cord.

Thyroarytenoid. This muscle arises from the internal surface of the thyroid ala and

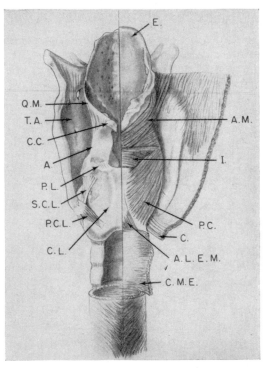

FIG. 25–1. Posterior view of the larynx showing the cartilaginous and muscular structures. *E.*, epiglottis; *A.M.*, aryepiglottic muscle; *I.*, interarytenoid muscle; *P.C.*, posterior cricoarytenoid muscle; *C.*, cricopharyngeus; *A.L.E.M.*, attachment of longitudinal esophageal muscle; *C.M.E.*, circular esophageal muscle; *Q.M.*, quadrangular membrane; *T.A.*, left thyroid ala; *C.C.*, corniculate cartilage; *A.*, arytenoid; *P.L.*, posterior cricoarytenoid ligament; *S.C.L.*, superior cricothyroid ligament; *P.C.L.*, posterior cricothyroid ligament; *C.L.*, cricoid lamina.

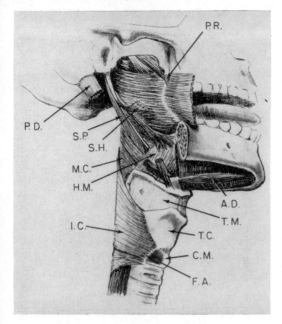

FIG. 25–2. Lateral view of the larynx and its supporting muscular attachments. *P.R.*, pterygomandibular raphe; *A.D.*, anterior belly of the digastric; *T.C.*, thyroid cartilage; *T.M.*, thyrohyoid membrane; *C.M.*, cricothyroid muscle; *F.A.*, fibrous arch; *I.C.*, inferior constrictor; *M.C.*, middle constrictor; *H.M.*, hyoglossus muscle; *S.H.*, stylohyoid muscle; *S.P.*, stylopharyngeus; *P.D.*, posterior belly of the digastric.

the conus elasticus. It is arbitrarily divided into two parts. The vocalis muscle or thyroarytenoid internus inserts on the free margin of the conus elasticus and on the vocal process. The thyroarytenoid externus inserts on the arytenoid between the vocal process and the attachment of the lateral cricoarytenoid. This muscle adducts the vocal cord, as well as altering the tension and bulk of the free edge of the vocal cord.

Interarytenoid. This muscle is unpaired and consists of transverse and oblique fibers connecting the bodies of two arytenoid cartilages. It serves to adduct the vocal cords. The muscle is innervated bilaterally by the recurrent laryngeal nerve and therefore is not paralyzed by unilateral recurrent nerve disease. Also, the muscle may receive motor supply from the superior laryngeal nerves.

Aryepiglottic Muscle. The aryepiglottic muscle is a continuation of the oblique portion of the interarytenoid muscle into the false vocal cord and inserts into the quadrangular membrane and the margin of the epiglottis. It acts to close the superior laryngeal sphincter but is small and often almost absent. It may become hypertrophied when false vocal cord function supervenes that of the true vocal cords.

JOINTS OF THE LARYNX

Cricothyroid. The cricothyroid articulations are small synovial joints between the inferior cornua of the thyroid cartilage and the posterior portions of the cricoid cartilage. Each cricoid joint surface is a slightly raised area with a central depression which fits the slightly convex surface of the thyroid portion of the joint. Each joint is supported by three ligaments—an anterior, inferior, and posterior cricothyroid ligament.

Joint motion is a rotatory motion in the sagittal plane only. The joint is the fulcrum on which the cricothyroid muscle functions. Therefore, destruction or fixation of the joint will lessen the effect of the cricothyroid muscle on the tension of the vocal cords.

Cricoarytenoid. Each arytenoid cartilage articulates with an elliptical facet on the posterosuperior margin of the cricoid ring. The cricoid facet is approximately 6 mm long, with the long axis parallel to a tangent to the cricoid. The articular facet of the arytenoid is saddle-shaped and positioned at right angles to the cricoid facet. The joint is supported by a joint capsule lined with synovium, and the capsule is strengthened posteriorly by a strong cricoarytenoid ligament. The joint structure permits two main types of motion: (1) a rocking motion around the axis of the joint, and (2) a gliding motion parallel to the long axis of the cricoid facet.

Since the axis of the joint is at an angle of 45 degrees from the sagittal plane and 40 degrees from the horizontal plane, abduction and adduction are accomplished by these movements. There is no gross rotation around a vertical plane, as often depicted, although a slight rotatory motion pivoting around the posterior cricoarytenoid ligament does occur.

INTERIOR OF THE LARYNX

The superior boundary of the larynx is marked by the free edge of the epiglottis, the aryepiglottic folds, the corniculate cartilages, and the superior margin of the interarytenoid area. The inferior margin is the inferior border of the cricoid cartilage.

The vestibule of the larynx is that part above the true vocal cords. For surgical purposes, the area superior to the inferior margins of the false vocal cords is referred to as the supraglottis. The anterior wall of the supraglottis is formed by the epiglottis, which tapers inferiorly; the lower end is marked by a prominence, the tuberculum epiglotticum, which is about 1 to 1.5 cm superior to the anterior commissure. The inferior two thirds of the epiglottis separate the vestibule from the pre-epiglottic space. Laterally, the aryepiglottic folds separate the laryngeal vestibule from the piriform fossae, and posteriorly the arytenoid cartilages and the interarytenoid muscle form the partition between the vestibule and hypopharynx.

Bulging into the vestibule are two fleshy masses—the ventricular bands or false vocal cords—which are attached anteriorly to the epiglottis near the petiole and posteriorly blend into the mucosa over the arytenoids.

The rima glottidis refers to the space between the free margins of the true vocal cords. The true vocal cords, however, extend from the floor of the ventricle of Morgagni inferiorly to the cricoid cartilage, a distance of 1.5 to 2 cm, although the bulk of the cord is above the inferior margin of the thyroid cartilage. The term glottis is used to denote an area of larynx between the superior surface of the vocal cord and an arbitrary line about 3 mm below. The area below this is the infraglottis. This division is made because of the different lymphatic supply of the two areas.

The true vocal cords are formed by a membranous anterior two thirds and a cartilaginous posterior one third. The membranous portion of the vocal cords is formed by the conus elasticus and the laterally placed thyroarytenoid muscles. The vocal ligaments are merely the thickened superior margins of the conus elasticus. Anteriorly, the membranous cords meet to form a V-shaped commissure and are attached to the thyroid cartilage by the vocal tendon (of Broyles). Posteriorly, the membranous cords are attached to the vocal processes, which, along with the inferior body of the arytenoid, form the cartilaginous vocal cord. The cartilaginous vocal cords are separated by a variable posterior commissure. The true vocal cords are a maximum 2.4 cm in length in the adult male and 1.7 cm in length in the adult female. The distance between the vocal processes when the cords are widely abducted is about 1.9 cm in males and 1.2 cm in females.

Laryngeal Ventricle (Ventricle of Morgagni). The true and false vocal cords are separated by a laterally directed sulcus called the ventricle. The structure is approximately 2 cm long in the adult male. It extends laterally almost to the thyroid ala, from which it is separated by mucosa and muscle fibers. The floor is formed by the flat superior surface of the true vocal cord. As the ventricle extends laterally, it also extends vertically lateral to the quadrangular membrane. Near the anterior end of the roof of the ventricle is an opening to a vertical extension, the sacculus or appendix, which extends further into the aryepiglottic fold. The opening of the appendix is about 8 mm in length and the height is about 6 mm. The ventricle is lined by ciliated epithelium with numerous seromucous glands emptying into it.

Piriform Fossa. The piriform fossae are usually considered part of the hypopharynx for clinical purposes, but they are also an anatomic part of the larynx. Each fossa lies lateral to the vestibule of the larynx. It lies between the thyrohyoid membrane and the thyroid ala laterally and among the aryepiglottic fold, arytenoid, and superior cricoid cartilage medially. The superior boundary is marked by the lateral glossoepiglottic fold; the inferior margin is less well defined because of the manner in which the fossa blends into the upper esophagus. The apex is usually at the level of the upper border of the cricoid, although there is considerable individual variation. The posterior boundary is marked medially by the arytenoid cartilage and laterally by a line drawn parallel to the vocal cord in the abducted position and projected to the lateral pharyngeal wall.

A ridge may be noted crossing the anterior wall of the piriform fossa transversely. This is the outline of the internal laryngeal nerve lying submucosally and is the site for obtaining topical anesthesia of the larynx.

Histology. The epithelial covering of the larynx consists of either nonkeratinizing squamous epithelium or pseudostratified ciliated epithelium. The upper portion of the epiglottis, the aryepiglottic folds, and the piriform fossae are covered by squamous epithelium. The inferior portions of the false cords and the ventricles and the infraglottic area are covered with pseudostratified ciliated epithelium. The free margin of the vocal cords is covered by stratified epithelium 8 to 10 cell layers thick, although this epithelium tends to be thinner over the vocal processes.

The laryngeal mucosa contains many seromucous glands; these are particularly numerous in the ventricles and may be the site of retention cysts. However, the margins of the true vocal cords are entirely devoid of glands.

The submucosal tissues consist of loose, fibrous stroma except over the epiglottis and true vocal cords; thus there is a propensity for accumulation of inflammatory exudates or edema fluid. The epithelium of the epiglottis is fairly tightly adherent; therefore, edema tends to occur more slowly, especially in adults.

The true vocal cords do not contain a large amount of subepithelial tissue, but at the margin of the true vocal cord there is a potential subepithelial space (Rienke's space). The area is situated between the epithelium and the conus elasticus. The space runs the length of the vocal cord but is limited above and below by the lineae arcuatae, which appear as small linear indentations in the epithelial covering of the vocal cords. Each linea arcuata is about 2 to 3 mm from the free margin of the vocal cord and marks the margins of the squamous epithelium covering the true vocal cords. Thus, inflammatory and neoplastic processes tend to spread in the space along the vocal cord but are limited in their spread beyond the vocal cord.

Blood Supply. The arterial supply of the larynx is derived from the branches of the superior and inferior thyroid arteries. The superior thyroid artery arises from low on the external carotid artery or from the common carotid artery (15%). It arises deep to the strap muscles and branches into the superior laryngeal artery near its origin. The superior laryngeal artery divides into two branches, the infrahyoid and cricothyroid arteries, before entering the larynx through the thyrohyoid membrane with the internal laryngeal nerve.

The cricothyroid artery passes inferiorly in association with the external branch of the superior laryngeal nerve. The artery goes deep to the strap muscles while lying on the inferior constrictor muscle and finally enters the larynx through the cricothyroid membrane just lateral to the midline.

The inferior thyroid artery gives rise to the inferior laryngeal artery as it is crossing the recurrent laryngeal nerve. The artery then travels with the nerve to enter the larynx through the space of Killian-Jamieson posterior to the cricothyroid joint.

The venous return from the larynx is carried by the superior laryngeal vein and the superior and middle thyroid veins, all of which enter the internal jugular vein.

LYMPHATICS OF THE LARYNX

A knowledge of the lymphatic drainage of the larynx is of the utmost importance in determining proper and adequate treatment of carcinoma of the larynx. Most has described the anatomy in considerable detail.

The lymphatics in the region of the free borders of the vocal cord are small and sparse due to a paucity of subepithelial tissue in this area. The laryngeal lymphatic system is divided into two parts by this area, one draining superiorly and the other inferiorly. The lymphatic system is much better developed in infants and children, in whom the channels are longer and more numerous, but regression takes place with increasing age.

The lymphatic network of the supraglottic structures is extensive, especially in areas with abundant submucosa. The channels collect in a pedicle at the anterior end of the aryepiglottic fold, pass laterally, anterior to the anterior wall of the piriform fossa, and leave the larynx with the neurovascular bundle through the thyrohyoid membrane. Almost all (98%) of the channels end in the upper deep cervical nodes between the digastric tendon and the omohyoid muscle. The remainder pass to the lower cervical drain or the spinal accessory chain.

The lymphatics of the infraglottic area have a more variable drainage pattern than those of the supraglottic network. The channels leave the area in three pedicles. The anterior pedicle passes through the cricothyroid membrane, and many vessels end in the prelaryngeal (Delphian) nodes in the region of the thyroid isthmus. Channels then leave these nodes with the remaining anterior channels to travel to the deep inferior cervical nodes. The two posterolateral pedicles leave the larynx through the cricotracheal membrane, with some channels going to the paratracheal chain of nodes while others pass to the inferior jugular chain. The superficial lymph node systems of the neck are of secondary importance with regard to laryngeal drainage. Generally, lymphatic drainage from each half of the larynx is quite separate, and little crossover or mixing occurs.

There is evidence that lymphatic channels do cross the midline in the supra- and infraglottic areas. Lymph flow through these areas is normally negligible, but this is altered when drainage is obstructed on either side of the neck. Contralateral drainage is more likely to occur spontaneously from the infraglottic areas; thus lesions of this area may be associated with less consistent patterns of metastases. The presence of direct lymphaticovenous communications has been demonstrated in dogs and may also account for abnormalities in drainage patterns in humans.

REFERENCES

Arnold, G. E.: Physiology and Pathology of the Cricothyroid Muscle. Laryngoscope, 71:687, 1961.

Broyles, E.: The Anterior Commissure Tendon. Ann. Otol. Rhinol. Laryngol., 52:342, 1943.

Grant, J. C. B.: *Grant's Atlas of Anatomy*. 5th ed. Baltimore, The Williams & Wilkins Co., 1972.

Mayet, A.: Bau und Funktion des M. Vocalis und seine Bezeihunge zu lig. vocale und Conus elasticus. Acta Anat., 24:1, 15–26, 1955.

Most, A.: Uber das Lymphgefacssapparat von Kehlkopf und Trachea und scine Beziehungen zur Verbrietung Krankhofter Prozesse. Dtsch. Z. Chir., 57:199, 1900.

Pernkopf, E.: *Atlas of Topographic and Applied Anatomy*. Vol. 1. Philadelphia, W. B. Saunders Co., 1963.

Rossi, G., and Cortesina, G.: Morphological Study of the Laryngeal Muscles in Man. Acta Otolaryng., 59:575, 1965.

Rouviere, H.: *Anatomy of the Human Lymphatic System*. Ann Arbor, Edwards Brothers, Inc., 1938.

Schugt, H. P.: The Pyriform Sinus: Anatomic and Clinical Observations, with a Review of the Literature. Arch. Otolaryng., 31:326, 1940.

Sonnesson, B.: Die Functionelle Anatomie des Crico-Arytenoidglelenkes. Z. Anat. Entvickliengs Giesch., 12:292, 1952.

Sonnesson, B.: The Anatomy of the Human Vocal Folds. Acta Otolaryng. (Suppl.), 156:11, 1960.

Terracol, J., and Guerrier, Y.: La Vascularization de La Corde Vocale. Ann. Otol. (Paris), 73:6, 1956.

Tucker, G. F., Jr., and Smith, H. R., Jr.: A Histological Demonstration of the Development of Laryngeal Connective Tissue Compartments. Trans. Am. Acad. Ophthal. Otolaryng., 66:308, 1962.

von Leden, H., and Moore, P.: The Mechanics of the Cricoarytenoid Joint. Arch. Otolaryng., 73:541, 1961.

Welsh, L. W.: The Normal Human Laryngeal Lymphatics. Ann. Otol., 73:569, 1964.

Welsh, L. W., et al.: Surgical Alterations of the Laryngeal Lymphatics. Trans. Am. Acad. Ophthal. Otolaryng., 65:539, 1960.

Chapter 26

Respiratory Insufficiency and Tracheostomy

Respiratory insufficiency is defined as a failure of the respiratory system to provide adequate oxygen for metabolic needs and/or to remove carbon dioxide adequately from the body. This may be due to a variety of causes, the most common being alveolar hypoventilation, the management of which may necessitate the services of an otolaryngologist.

ETIOLOGY OF ALVEOLAR HYPO-VENTILATION

There are many important prerequisites for the function and maintenance of a normal ventilating system:
1. Patency of the tracheobronchial tree.
2. Normal function of the thoracic cage and respiratory musculature.
3. Normal resiliency or compliance of the lungs.
4. Adequate function of the stimulating mechanisms.
5. Adequate function of the protective reflexes including:
   (a) Cough reflex.
   (b) Sphincteric action of the larynx.
   (c) Ciliary action of the respiratory mucosa.
   (d) Intact swallowing reflex.

Deficiency or inadequacy of any of these factors may result in respiratory insufficiency due to inadequate ventilation of the alveoli with enough fresh inspired air for immediate metabolic needs.

The causes of alveolar hypoventilation are outlined in Table 26–1. Although these are divided into fairly distinct groups, deficiency of more than one functional prerequisite is usually present in each group.

Depression of the respiratory centers of the medulla may be due to any of the causes listed. In addition to inadequate respiratory drive, central depression is often associated with loss of the protective reflexes. Therefore, secretional airway obstruction will further complicate the situation unless manual methods are used to remove secretions. Inadequate respiratory drive will result in failure of adequate alveolar ventilation, and respiration must be assisted until normal function returns.

Increased resistance to the passage of air from the pharynx to the alveoli is the most common cause of alveolar hypoventilation. Mechanical obstruction of the airway by a space-occupying process may occur anywhere in the respiratory tract, but it is most frequent and serious in the larynx. Laryngeal obstruction is most frequently due to congenital abnormalities, inflammatory edema, neoplasms and other space-occupying lesions, spasm or paralysis of both vocal cords, crusting of the larynx, and foreign bodies. Mechanical obstruction of the larynx is important because it is often

Table 26-1.   Causes of Alveolar Hypoventilation for which Tracheostomy
May Be Indicated

1. Depression of respiratory centers due to general anesthesia, excessive sedation, cerebral trauma, increased intracranial pressure, prolonged hypoxia or cerebral ischemia, hypercapnia.
2. Increased resistance to air flow.
    a. Mechanical obstruction of the upper respiratory tract.
    b. Secretional obstruction of the lower respiratory tract, as with bronchitis, bronchiolitis, bronchiectasis, pneumonia, and any condition causing accumulation of tracheobronchial secretions.
3. Disturbances of the mechanical factors of respiration.
    a. Interference with neuromuscular transmission to the respiratory muscles due to diseases or agents causing neural paralysis, myopathic paralysis, or neuromuscular block.
    b. Disease resulting in restriction of function of the thoracic cage, such as thoracic surgery and trauma, thoracic deformity (kyphoscoliosis), arthritis, pulmonary emphysema, obesity, and elevation of the diaphragm.
    c. Intrinsic pulmonary disease.
        i. Diseases altering compliance or distensibility of the lung tissue, such as pulmonary fibrosis and pulmonary emphysema.
        ii. Diseases altering compliance by inactivation of pulmonary surfactant, which occurs with pulmonary edema, pneumonia, secretion accumulation, and the respiratory distress syndrome of the newborn.
        iii. Pulmonary vascular diseases, such as thromboembolism, vasculitis, and vasoconstriction.

abrupt, producing complete loss of ventilatory function and necessitating emergency treatment. Less often, it may develop slowly.

On the other hand, mechanical obstruction of the lower respiratory tract is usually less severe and is most significant when the process is diffuse. Edema associated with diffuse bronchiolitis, pneumonia, and asthma is the usual cause. Localized lower tract obstruction by neoplasm or foreign body produces a much less severe clinical picture of respiratory insufficiency than higher obstruction.

Secretional obstruction of the lower respiratory tract is a common and often unrecognized cause of hypoventilation. Unlike mechanical obstruction of the larynx, it may progress in seemingly innocuous fashion for some time before the symptoms of severe respiratory failure are present. Under normal circumstances, the combined amount of nasal, oral, pharyngeal, and tracheobronchial secretion is in excess of 3000 ml per day, and any which is not evaporated must be swallowed. Swallowing of these secretions is an unconscious reflex, and failure of this mechanism will result in aspiration and accumulation of secretions in the pharynx and tracheobronchial tree. Inability to swallow secretions may be secondary to esophageal or hypopharyngeal obstruction or pharyngeal paralysis. Incompetence of the laryngeal sphincters due to paralysis or surgical alteration may be associated with aspiration during deglutition. Loss of effective cough due to depression of the central nervous system, disturbance in the function of the thoracic cage, altered pulmonary compliance, and/or incompetence of the glottis prevents effective clearance of the tracheobronchial tree, producing secretion accumulation. The excessive production of secretions associated with inflammatory disease of the bronchi and bronchioles and the production of thick, viscid secretions with cystic fibrosis, dehydration, and the dysgammaglobulinemias are also important causes of secretional obstruction of the respiratory tract.

Alveolar hypoventilation may be secondary to failure of mechanical function of the ventilatory mechanism. Paralysis of respiratory muscles by poliomyelitis, polyneuritis, demyelinating diseases, excess doses of muscle relaxants, myasthenia gravis, botulism, reptile bites, and various poisons may be responsible for inability to overcome airway resistance as well as to prevent accumulation of secretions. Restriction of function of the thoracic cage which produces decreased thoracic compliance and hypoventilation may be due to the pain of an operative procedure, crushed or flail chest, and obesity (Pickwickian syndrome). Thoracic deformities causing fixation of skeletal structures, such as kyphoscoliosis and the barrel chest of chronic emphysema, may be responsible for hypoventilation. Elevation of the diaphragm by abdominal masses can also contribute to alveolar hypoventilation.

Intrinsic pulmonary disease is the most common cause of chronic alveolar hypoventilation. An increase or decrease in the distensibility of the lung (compliance) may be associated with hypoventilation.

Increased pulmonary compliance may be present in patients with pulmonary emphysema with minimal fibrosis. Alveolar hypoventilation in this condition is due to trapping of air secondary to expiratory collapse of the bronchi, because the elastic pull of the lung on the bronchi is lost. Coughing in these patients is often ineffective, and secretional obstruction may develop with minor respiratory infections, producing an exacerbation of pulmonary insufficiency.

Decreased pulmonary compliance occurs with pulmonary and pleural fibrosis. Because of decreased pulmonary distensibility, increased respiratory effort is necessary to maintain adequate ventilation. The necessary increase in oxygen consumption may further compound the alveolar hypoventilation caused by the basic disease.

Pulmonary compliance may be decreased by the absence or loss of surfactant. Surfactant is the active factor at the surface of the alveolar fluid lining which is responsible for a reduction of surface tension as the alveoli constrict with expiration. In its absence, the alveoli completely collapse and are not ventilated. Disturbance of surfactant function will occur when there is pulmonary congestion secondary to cardiac edema, infection, or secretion accumulation. Prolonged inhalation of 100% O_2 has the same effect. The respiratory distress syndrome of infants is associated with absence of surfactant function.

PATHOPHYSIOLOGY

Alveolar hypoventilation causes two basic biochemical alterations, i.e., arterial hypoxia (hypoxemia), and retention of CO_2 (hypercapnia). Hypoxia precipitates the excessive production of metabolic acids (lactic acid), and excess CO_2 leads to an accumulation of carbonic acid; both processes together produce respiratory acidosis. The resulting triad constitutes asphyxia (Fig. 26–1).

The degree of hypoxemia, hypercapnia, and acidosis in each individual with alveolar hypoventilation is quite variable and is determined by the cause and rapidity of onset, oxygen administration, and renal compensation. Hypoxemia and hypercapnia will occur in any patient with respiratory insufficiency breathing air. However, if the onset is acute and severe, the effects of acute hypoxemia are most marked. When the onset is slowly progressive the converse is true and hypercapnia is most important.

Effects of Hypoxemia. The clinical manifestations of hypoxemia are due, in part, to interference with cellular function and, in part, to the effects of the body's efforts to correct the situation. The cells of the central nervous system are the most sensitive to oxygen deprivation, and neurologic symptoms are usually the earliest signs of hypoxemia. When oxygen is totally deprived, cortical cells die in 5 to 8 minutes, and medullary cells may live 12 to 13 minutes. Lesser degrees of hypoxemia may produce nervous system injuries having a transient effect or resulting in permanent deficiencies.

Unfortunately, the body mechanisms for detecting O_2 deficiency are relatively insensitive. The main sites of hypoxemic stimulation are the carotid and aortic bodies (chemoreceptors). The chemoreceptor cells are stimulated by decreased levels of O_2 in solution in the blood as well as by local increases of CO_2 and hydrogen ion (H^+). However, because of the extremely high blood flow through the chemoreceptor organs, pO_2 must fall from 100 mm Hg to approximately 40 mm Hg before a marked physiologic effect occurs. Marked decreases

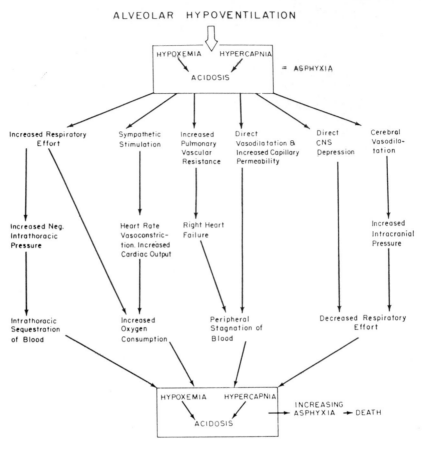

FIG. 26–1.   Schematic diagram depicting the progression of alveolar hypoventilation to asphyxia, circulatory and respiratory collapse, and death.

in blood flow will have a similar effect. Local hypercapnia or acidosis secondary to tissue hypoxia will stimulate the chemoreceptors, but tissue hypoxia is minimized by the O_2 dissociation curve of hemoglobin. Because of the affinity of hemoglobin for O_2, pO_2 must fall to approximately 40 mm Hg before hemoglobin O_2 saturation falls below 70% and significant tissue hypoxia develops. Therefore, a marked decrease in alveolar pO_2 (below 50 mm Hg) or blood O_2 saturation (below 70%) is necessary to produce a physiologic effect. Significant degrees of hypoxemia will cause increased respiratory effort, tachycardia, peripheral vasoconstriction and hypertension, increased pulmonary vascular resistance, increased adrenal activity, and increased cerebral cortical activity due to stimulation of the chemoreceptors and sympathetic nervous system.

These effects are potentiated by acidosis and hypercapnia, which usually accompany hypoxemia due to alveolar hypoventilation.

The clinical reactions to hypoxemia may be divided into three groups on the basis of rapidity of onset and duration of hypoxia. Fulminating hypoxia or anoxia is due to sudden complete airway obstruction and is associated with rapidly developing anoxemia producing unconsciousness and respiratory and circulatory collapse. Death follows in a few minutes.

Acute hypoxia and hypoxemia occur when moderate to severe oxygen deprivation develops over a period of minutes or hours. This may lead to dyspnea, hyperpnea, tachycardia, hypertension, and neurologic signs similar to acute alcoholism, including headaches, restlessness, mental confusion, disorientation, depression, and irrationality. Muscular weakness and incoordination, nausea and vomiting, and disturbances of vision and audition are also symptoms of hypoxemia. The symptoms vary with the severity of hypoxemia, and it should be remembered that hypercapnia may produce the same disturbances. Chronic hypoxemia resulting from chronic pulmonary insufficiency is characterized by similar symptoms but of much milder degree.

When hypoxemia first develops, the body responds to minimize its effects and to improve the pO_2 of blood and tissues. Respiration is augmented to increase alveolar ventilation. Cardiac output and the initial peripheral vasoconstriction caused by stimulation of vasomotor centers are increased. Later, as a result of local tissue hypoxia, peripheral arteriolar dilatation and increased capillary permeability develop, which contribute to circulatory hypovolemia and shock because of peripheral sequestration of blood and body fluids. Hypoxemia also leads to increased pulmonary vascular resistance, pulmonary hypertension, and right heart strain. The eventual result is a vicious circle of hypoxemia, increasing tissue hypoxia, acidosis and hypercapnia, and circulatory collapse.

If hypoxia persists over a few days, physiologic adjustments occur and the symptoms improve. Increased blood flow and polycythemia improve tissue oxygenation, although some degree of hyperpnea usually persists to maintain an adequate alveolar pO_2. Acidosis is lessened by renal compensation, thus improving oxygen dissociation and delivery of oxygen to the tissues. Therefore, hypoxemia is a less serious problem in chronic alveolar hypoventilation because the body becomes conditioned to the decreased availability of oxygen.

Effects of Hypercapnia. Accumulation of CO_2 always accompanies hypoxemia secondary to alveolar hypoventilation. The clinical manifestations of hypercapnia are due to a direct effect of CO_2 on the central nervous system and include respiratory stimulation, circulatory alterations, and the production of acidosis.

The central nervous system reacts to hypercapnia by stimulation of some centers and depression of others. Lesser degrees of hypercapnia cause headache, irritability, mental confusion, tingling, weakness, and lassitude, but as hypercapnia becomes more severe, unconsciousness, depressed reflexes, and flaccidity occur along with muscular tremors and convulsions. Severe hypercapnia causes a coma termed CO_2 narcosis.

CO_2 is a specific respiratory stimulant. While it does produce stimulation via the peripheral chemoreceptors (carotid and aortic bodies), its effects are mainly due to excitation of central chemoreceptors.

The central chemoreceptors are probably separate from the respiratory centers and are on the lateral surfaces of the medulla. They are stimulated by a rising H^+ level in the cerebrospinal fluid (CSF). CO_2 acts as a specific respiratory stimulant because blood H^+ ions do not cross the blood-brain barrier, whereas CO_2 diffuses across rapidly. The increased levels of CO_2 produce CSF acidosis and respiratory stimulation. Because CO_2 must diffuse into CSF, which lacks buffering systems, abnormalities in H^+ ion concentration in the CSF will develop gradually but will persist longer and be greater than the peripheral blood abnormalities. Gradual adjustment of H^+ levels in the CSF is accomplished by HCO_3^- and Cl^- exchange across the capillary walls, and eventually the central chemoreceptors are no longer stimulated by the excess CO_2 levels. Therefore, a considerable degree of chronic hypercapnia may be tolerated without severe symptoms because a normal pH is maintained in the CSF. When this situation develops with chronic alveolar hypoventilation, the sole respiratory stimulus is derived from peripheral chemoreceptors stimulated by hypoxemia. O_2 therapy in such cases will physiologically denervate these organs with resultant loss of all respiratory stimuli, leading to apnea and CO_2 narcosis. The central chemoreceptors are sensitive to the depressive effects of sedatives, narcotics, increased intracranial pressure, and hypoxia, all of which predispose to CO_2 narcosis.

Cardiovascular effects of CO_2 are produced by stimulation of the peripheral chemoreceptors and sympathetic stimulation, as well as by a direct vascular effect. Mild degrees of hypercapnia will be accompanied by an increased cardiac rate and generalized vasoconstriction secondary to sympathetic activity. More severe hypercapnia is marked by vasodilatation produced directly by the excess CO_2. CO_2 is the only true dilator of cerebral vessels; therefore, excess CO_2 may cause increased intracranial pressure and cerebral edema, which produce headache, somnolence, tremors, and papilledema.

Acidosis secondary to CO_2 retention is due to carbonic acid accumulation and in the acute phase produces low blood pH and high pCO_2 and HCO_3^- levels. Renal compensation will take place over a few hours, with the result that the pH reverts to near normal, pCO_2 remains elevated, HCO_3^- is further increased, and Cl^- is decreased.

CLINICAL MANIFESTATIONS OF ALVEOLAR HYPOVENTILATION

The symptoms will vary according to the cause, the rapidity of onset, and the duration of the alveolar hypoventilation.

Mechanical Obstruction. The patients always complain of dyspnea of variable degree. Stridor is usually present and is usually inspiratory when the obstruction is laryngeal, but an expiratory component appears with lower tract obstruction. There is obvious increased respiratory effort with indrawing in the supraclavicular spaces, intercostal spaces, and subcostal area. Cyanosis is often present but may be absent if the patient is anemic or receiving oxygen. Severe obstruction in children may result in an ashen-gray appearance rather than frank cyanosis.

In the earlier stages of obstruction, restlessness, disorientation, headache, and uncooperativeness are evidence of hypoxemia and hypercapnia. Adult patients may seem inebriated. Later, cerebral depression develops, causing lassitude, decreasing respiratory effort, unresponsiveness, and finally coma.

The pulse is usually rapid and hypertension is present initially, but continued obstruction is associated with a weak, thready pulse, hypotension, and evidence of circulatory collapse. Auscultation of the chest discloses decreased air entry, as well as rales and rhonchi. Although many patients have

some degree of fever, a marked rise in temperature often occurs at this stage.

Secretional Obstruction. The symptoms of secretional obstruction vary with the level of consciousness. Generally, symptoms are slow to develop, compared with those of mechanical obstruction. In many instances, the situation is obvious because of the precipitating mechanisms, such as neuromuscular paralysis, aspiration, and conditions depressing the cough.

In most instances, respirations are shallow with a small tidal volume. These may assume a jerky "cogwheel" sequence when the conscious patient's fear of aspiration causes him to terminate inspiration abruptly after a small volume of air is inspired. Rales and rhonchi may be heard throughout the chest, and the cough has a weak, "wet" quality.

The neurologic manifestations are important and helpful in arousing suspicion of this condition. Abrupt changes in personality associated with disorientation, confusion, and rebelliousness are frequent. Some patients become depressed, apathetic, and weak, which contributes further to the secretional accumulation.

As the situation progresses, tachycardia, hypotension, and loss of consciousness are noted. Cyanosis is quite variable and is often not present. Also, many of these patients are given oxygen inhalations, which will provide an adequate alveolar O_2 saturation to prevent cyanosis. However, oxygen inhalation does not relieve the symptoms, which are mainly due to hypercapnia. In fact, it may result in clinical deterioration and CO_2 narcosis because of the elimination of respiratory drive. Therefore, when any patient with chronic alveolar hypoventilation is given O_2 therapy, preparation should be made to maintain and assist respiration.

DIAGNOSIS

The cause of alveolar hypoventilation is usually evident, but in a few cases laboratory aids will be helpful. Determination of blood pH, pCO_2 levels, O_2 saturation, pO_2, and chloride levels is helpful in ascertaining the degree of hypoxemia and hypercapnia present and the amount of renal compensation which has taken place. These factors are of importance in determining future therapy in selected cases of chronic alveolar hypoventilation.

MANAGEMENT OF THE AIRWAY IN RESPIRATORY INSUFFICIENCY

Disturbances of respiratory function have become much more important in patient management because of increased recognition and improvements in respiratory care. The well-recognized problems of acute respiratory obstruction still occur but are now the least common indications for respiratory assistance. Respiratory insufficiency and failure associated with major surgery, trauma, pulmonary disease, and severe systemic disease are the major indications for artificial maintenance of ventilation.

The increasing use of assisted ventilation and recognition of the importance of intensive respiratory care have led to the development of inhalation or respiratory care departments in most hospitals. Therefore, the clinician involved in the care of these patients can no longer confine his knowledge to a narrow aspect of respiratory care. He should view himself as a member of a team involved in respiratory management. The place of the otolaryngologist on such a team is, naturally, most related to the establishment and management of a patent airway, either by endolaryngeal means or by tracheostomy. However, as part of the team, he should be cognizant of the overall aspects of respiratory care.

Control of the airway in order to provide oxygenation and toilet of the tracheobronchial tree and/or to maintain and assist respiration is the basis of all treatment of respiratory insufficiency. This is obtained by intubation or tracheostomy. There has been some controversy as to the relative merits of each procedure.

Endotracheal Intubation

Endotracheal intubation is the most rapid method of establishing the airway. It may be performed transnasally or transorally. Intubation is indicated as a prelude to tracheostomy or to maintain the airway when it is felt the respiratory problem is likely to be temporary. Whenever possible, the procedure should precede tracheostomy, especially in infants and children. The advantages of intubation are:

1. It provides immediate control of the airway.
2. A hasty and traumatic tracheostomy is avoided.
3. A general anesthetic may be given for the tracheostomy.
4. The complication of pneumothorax, occurring during tracheostomy performed on a patient exerting marked ventilatory effort, is avoided.

There are several specific disadvantages to prolonged intubation which will be discussed later.

Technique. The larynx is exposed with a laryngoscope, and a cuffed endotracheal tube or bronchoscope is inserted. Under emergency conditions the tube should be inserted orally. Many patients requiring intubation are unconscious or semicomatose and require no anesthesia. Although there is no evidence that lack of anesthesia increases the incidence of vasovagal reflex and cardiac arrest, when possible, it is wise to attempt improving oxygenation prior to intubation.

If the patient is conscious, local anesthesia may be obtained by topical application via the pharynx and piriform sinus or injection of the internal laryngeal nerves.

Complications. The presence of a tube in the larynx for a long period of time may produce mucosal ulceration, granulation tissue formation, subglottic edema, and, finally, laryngeal and tracheal stenosis. These complications are more common in the conscious or hyperactive patient with an active swallowing reflex. Generally, when it appears that intubation over a period of 48 to 72 hours will be necessary, a tracheostomy should be performed. This is particularly true when secretions are a problem, as tracheobronchial toilet is more difficult and the endotracheal tube is more prone to obstruction.

An endotracheal tube may be of more value in infants and small children in whom the high incidence of acute complications associated with tracheostomy outweighs the disadvantages of intubation. Here again, however, the tube obstruction is a major problem; the nasotracheal tube may require frequent replacement.

Cricothyrotomy (Coniotomy)

In certain situations, an airway may be obtained by opening the trachea through the cricothyroid membrane. The procedure was described by Vicq d'Azur in 1805. The advantage of this procedure is that the cricothyroid membrane is directly under the skin and subcutaneous tissue, and a minimum amount of equipment and dissection is necessary to establish an airway rapidly.

There are numerous disadvantages to the procedure which limit its usefulness. The cricothyroid space is relatively narrow and often is not wide enough to allow insertion of a tracheostomy tube of adequate caliber without damage to the cricoid cartilage. Any injury to the cricoid may be followed by perichondritis and subsequent laryngeal stenosis. Incision of the cricothyroid membrane may damage the conus elasticus, producing permanent voice changes. The cricothyroid arteries enter the cricothyroid space near the midline and may be the source of considerable bleeding during the procedure.

The major complication of cricothyrotomy is laryngeal stenosis. The longer a tube is left in place in the cricothyroid membrane, the greater the chance of perichondritis, granulation tissue formation, and eventual stenosis of the laryngeal lumen.

Indications. When endotracheal intubation is not possible, either tracheostomy or cricothyrotomy may be necessary for respiratory obstruction. Generally, tracheostomy is the better procedure, but under certain emergency circumstances, cricothyrotomy may be the most expedient method of establishing an airway to avoid asphyxia and death of the patient. The indications for cricothyrotomy include:

1. Lack of equipment and instruments to perform endotracheal intubation or tracheostomy for relief of severe respiratory obstruction.

2. The need to establish an airway by nonmedically trained personnel.

3. The need to establish an airway in the presence of an obstructing neoplasm of the larynx, so that the entire site of the cricothyrotomy may be excised at the time of definitive surgery.

Technique. The cricothyroid space is identified by extending the patient's head and palpating the prominent arch of the cricoid cartilage, which is 2 to 3 cm below the prominent V-notch of the thyroid cartilage in the average adult. A small horizontal incision is made with any sharp instrument just above the upper border of the cricoid cartilage. This will expose the cricothyroid membrane, which is punctured in the midline. The puncture wound is enlarged laterally by inserting a thin, blunt instrument into the wound and using blunt force in order to avoid hemorrhage from the cricothyroid artery. If a tube is not available, the airway is maintained by spreading the cricoid and thyroid cartilages apart, using a knife handle or other thin instrument. By placing the incision through the cricothyroid membrane nearer to the cricoid cartilage, hemorrhage from the cricothyroid arteries can usually be avoided.

Puncturing the cricothyroid space using a large hypodermic needle (No. 15) may be attempted in extreme situations, but the airway is inadequate unless more than one needle is used.

Postoperative Care. An ordinary tracheostomy tube should be inserted through the cricothyrotomy as soon as it is available. As soon as the patient's condition is stabilized, the cricothyrotomy should be converted to a tracheostomy through a separate lower incision. If at all possible, conversion should be performed within 24 hours or, at the most, 48 hours.

Tracheostomy

Tracheostomy consists of making an opening in the anterior wall of the trachea for purposes of establishing an airway. The first mention of the operation is in the writings of Aretaeus and Galen in the first and second centuries A.D. Although the procedure was intermittently described thereafter, the first person known actually to perform it was Antonio Brasavola in 1546. The operation was variously termed laryngotomy and bronchotomy until the term tracheotomy was introduced by Heister in 1718. In recent years, the more correct term tracheostomy has been used. The first tracheostomy tube with an inner cannula was introduced by George Martine in Britain about 1730 to avoid the postoperative problem of tubal obstruction.

Indications. Tracheostomy may be necessary for therapeutic purposes or may be performed as an elective procedure. Elective tracheostomy may be necessary when respiratory problems are anticipated in the postoperative period in patients being subjected to major head, neck, or thoracic operations or in patients with chronic pulmonary insufficiency. Rarely, it may be indicated in patients in whom orotracheal intubation is difficult or impossible for purposes of inducing general anesthesia. Tracheostomy should also be performed as a preliminary measure in operations for oropharyngeal or laryngeal neoplasms to avoid unnecessary manipulation of the tumor.

Therapeutic tracheostomy is indicated in any case of respiratory insufficiency due to alveolar hypoventilation in order to bypass obstruction, to remove secretions, or to provide for the use of mechanical artificial respiration.

Whenever possible, therapeutic tracheostomy should be preceded by endotracheal intubation. Although endotracheal intubation will provide relief of the immediate airway problem, tracheostomy should be performed secondarily when airway care for more than 48 hours is anticipated because:

1. Secretion removal is much easier through a tracheostomy tube, and there is less tendency for tubal obstruction to occur.

2. It is extremely difficult for a patient to swallow around an endotracheal tube.

3. An endotracheal tube is difficult to clean in situ, and tube replacement necessitates repeated laryngoscopy.

4. Prolonged endolaryngeal intubation produces mucosal ulceration, which may eventually lead to the development of granulomas, adhesions, and laryngeal stenosis.

5. A tracheostomy causes less stimulation of the cough reflex, which may be impor-

tant in some neurologic and postoperative patients.

6. A tracheostomy will allow speech in conscious patients.

The sole contraindication to tracheostomy is in patients with obstructing carcinoma of the larynx, since there is some evidence that tracheostomy performed more than 48 hours prior to a definitive surgical procedure leads to an increased incidence of stomal recurrence. It is extremely difficult to excise widely a low tracheostomy site at the time of laryngectomy. Therefore, a temporary airway should be provided by endoscopic removal of sufficient tumor or cricothyrotomy.

Timing of Tracheostomy. The conscious patient with upper respiratory obstruction will usually manifest fairly obvious signs of acute hypoxemia. These signs include rising pulse and respiratory rates, restlessness, confusion, and decreased air entry. Under such circumstances the patient will exhaust himself in maintaining adequate blood gas levels before arterial oxygen desaturation occurs, i.e., pO_2 falls to 40 mm Hg. When desaturation occurs, rapid circulatory and respiratory decompensation develops and death is imminent. Therefore, the signs of desaturation, including cyanosis, coma, and hypotension, are late indications of insufficiency and may preclude resuscitation. Generally, when a patient presents with respiratory obstruction with signs of increasing hypoxemia, a tracheostomy is warranted.

In the unconscious patient with respiratory insufficiency, the clinical signs of hypoxemia may be less obvious, but because of the loss of protective mechanisms, a tracheostomy is indicated considerably earlier.

When the onset of respiratory insufficiency is slow, the signs of hypoxemia are minimal, and the manifestations of hypercapnia are more obvious. Headache, dizziness, sweating, and flushing are early signs. Later twitching, confusion, and coma may develop. In many instances these patients are given oxygen, which may produce transient improvement but worsen the CO_2 retention. Therefore, in this situation serial blood gas studies are of great help in determining a need for assisted ventilation. Generally if a patient is unable to maintain an

O_2 saturation of 85% or reduce pCO_2 below 50 mm Hg when breathing 50% O_2, a tracheostomy is indicated.

Function of a Tracheostomy. In addition to bypassing an upper airway obstruction, a tracheostomy has several other physiologic functions which include:

1. Decreasing the amount of dead space in the tracheobronchial tree, usually 70 to 100 ml. The decrease in dead space may vary from 10 to 50%, depending on the individual's physiologic dead space.

2. Reducing resistance to airflow, which in turn reduces the force required to move air. This will result in increased total compliance and more effective alveolar ventilation, provided the tracheostomy opening is large enough (at least a No. 7 tube).

3. Providing protection against aspiration.

4. Enabling the patient to swallow without reflex apnea, which is important in respiratory patients.

5. Providing access to the trachea for cleaning.

6. Providing a pathway to deliver medication and humidification to the tracheobronchial tree, with or without intermittent positive pressure breathing.

7. Decreasing the power of the cough and thereby preventing peripheral displacement of secretions by the high negative intrathoracic pressure associated with the inspiratory phase normal cough.

Technique. The technique of tracheostomy is dictated to some extent by the circumstances necessitating the operation. The important point is to obtain an airway as rapidly and efficiently as possible while avoiding injury to the larynx, trachea, and adjacent structures.

Whenever possible, endotracheal intubation should be performed prior to therapeutic tracheostomy. This is particularly essential in children. Intubation may be accomplished without any anesthesia, if necessary. If intubation is not possible, ventilation and oxygenation via a bag and mask are a valuable adjunct to the procedure. If the airway is under control, a more orderly and less traumatic tracheostomy can be performed.

The patient should be positioned on his back with a pillow well under the shoulders to allow maximal extension of the neck. This is a difficult position for conscious patients with respiratory distress to maintain, and it may be necessary to hold them in position.

Anesthesia for tracheostomy is unnecessary in unconscious patients. A local anesthetic is usually all that is necessary in conscious patients, including children. A general anesthetic may be used if an endotracheal tube is in position but is contraindicated if intubation has not been performed. Local anesthesia is obtained by infiltrating the skin in the line of the incision and depositing the agent in the deeper midline tissues to the level of the anterior tracheal wall. Lidocaine (Xylocaine), 1%, with epinephrine 1:150,000 is a satisfactory agent.

The skin incision is determined by the circumstances. When the tracheostomy is combined with a head and neck procedure, the incision is placed in accordance with the dictates of the proposed procedure. When tracheostomy is performed as an individual procedure, a horizontal skin incision should be used whenever possible. The incision is made 5 cm long, approximately two fingerbreadths above the sternal notch. There is little doubt that the cosmetic results of a horizontal incision are superior to those of a vertical incision. However, when the situation is urgent and help is unavailable, a 4-cm vertical midline incision may be used to obtain rapid access with a minimum of dissection and bleeding.

The skin incision is deepened until the strap muscles (Fig. 26–2) are encountered. At this point, the trachea should be palpated in order to ascertain its location and to avoid dissecting lateral to it. The strap muscles are separated vertically in the midline and retracted laterally. This will expose the pretracheal fascia which covers the trachea and the thyroid isthmus. Numerous veins descend in the fascia from the thyroid, but by staying in a midline vertical plane, most of the veins can be avoided. The thyroid isthmus is almost always above the level of the third tracheal ring. It is usually possible to retract the isthmus superiorly with a small blunt retractor to expose the trachea. It is seldom necessary to transect the thyroid isthmus; thus the bleeding and

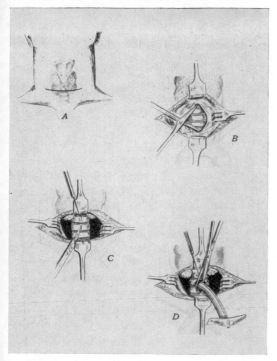

FIG. 26–2. Tracheostomy. *A,* A horizontal skin incision is made about 3 cm above the sternum. *B,* Blunt midline dissection is used to expose the anterior tracheal wall. *C,* The thyroid isthmus is retracted superiorly and a hook is inserted into the second tracheal ring. A vertical incision is made through the third and fourth rings. *D,* A hemostat is inserted into the trachea to spread the incision and permit insertion of the tracheostomy tube.

delay so often encountered when this is done are avoided. An exceptionally wide isthmus must be divided between clamps, and a suture ligature is used to ligate the cut margins. A few drops of 10% cocaine injected into the trachea at this point will help to lessen the severe coughing initiated by insertion of the tracheostomy tube.

The trachea should be fixed by inserting a hook in the anterior wall between the first and second ring, pulling the trachea in an upward and outward direction. The anterior wall of the trachea is incised vertically, dividing two to three rings. The tracheal incision should never extend above the second tracheal ring in order to prevent the tracheostomy tube from impinging on the cricoid cartilage and producing perichondritis. Car-

tilage should not be removed from the anterior tracheal wall because an unnecessarily large tracheal defect is left after extubation, which is often the site of bothersome granulations and delayed healing. In small patients, tracheal stenosis may develop secondary to cartilage excision. It has been shown that a simple vertical incision will heal much more rapidly than when cartilage is excised or a horizontal tracheal incision is used. The tracheal incision is spread with a large hemostat and a tube of appropriate size is inserted immediately. The Trousseau dilator, often used at this point, is usually too large to allow a tube to slip easily into the trachea and is a source of needless fumbling and delay; a Kelly clamp will open the incision adequately.

As soon as the tube is inserted, there is frequently a bout of violent coughing, and some patients may become apneic due to loss of hypoxic respiratory drive. This should be anticipated and artificial respiration instituted if necessary.

Care should be used in the selection of the tracheostomy tube. In recent years the use of the standard silver tube of the Holinger and Jackson type has largely been abandoned in favor of the silicone or Portex type of tube. The reasons for this are reduction of trauma to tracheal walls, elimination of an inner cannula, and economy. The length of the tracheostomy tube is also important, and it is often necessary to adjust the length for an individual. This is easily accomplished by trimming a silicone tube but is impossible with a metal tube. The diameter of the tube is selected so that the largest tube which fits comfortably is used, which is approximately three quarters of the diameter of the trachea. In the average adult female, size No. 6 (30 French) or No. 7 (33 French) suffices, and in the male No. 7 or No. 8 (36 French) is used. A cuffed tube may be necessary when aspiration is a problem or a positive pressure respirator is required. The low-pressure cuffed tubes which are now available should be used, but the cuffs should still be deflated at regular intervals.

The skin incision should not be sutured or dressed tightly, as this leads to the development of subcutaneous emphysema, pneumomediastinum, and pneumothorax. A small gauze pad may be placed between the flange of the tube and the skin of the neck.

Tracheostomy in Infants and Small Children. Because of the size and consistency of the trachea in these patients, there are some special points to be noted. Tracheostomy in all cases should only be done after a bronchoscope, endotracheal tube, or catheter has been inserted to provide an airway and some rigidity to the trachea. This will facilitate dissection and identification of the trachea. It is easy, in these small patients, to carry dissection too deeply and lateral to the trachea, with resulting damage to the recurrent laryngeal nerve, the common carotid artery, or apex of the pleura. Caution must be used when the tracheal wall is being incised not to insert the knife too deeply and lacerate the posterior wall. A bronchoscope in the trachea will help to avoid this complication.

The other source of difficulty in children is the tracheostomy tube. Because of the short, often fat, necks of infants, there is a tendency for the tube to slip out of the trachea, especially when the neck is flexed. It is sometimes wise to insert silk marking sutures in each margin of the tracheal incision and to tape these to the neck to prevent loss of the tracheal opening if the tube becomes displaced. The trachea should be inspected after the tube is inserted to guard against infolding of the cut ends of the tracheal rings, which may contribute to tube displacement and obstruction at the time of decannulation.

Difficulty may be encountered in obtaining a proper fit of the tracheostomy tube. The tube which is too long may ride on the carina or slip into one bronchus, causing atelectasis of the opposite lung. If the curvature is too sharp, the tube may compress the trachea at the upper margin of the tracheal incision, while the lower end of the tube rides on the anterior tracheal wall, whereas an excessively obtuse curve may cause ulceration of the posterior tracheal wall and esophagus. Because of these difficulties in infants, roentgenograms of the neck and chest should be obtained postoperatively.

A Silastic tube of the Aberdeen design is the most preferable for use in infants and children. It is flexible, can be cut to appropriate length, and allows a greater movement of air because of the absence of an inner cannula. A 4.5-mm tube (outer diameter) is used in newborns. A 7-mm tube is used from 3 to 6 months; thereafter, the tube should be increased in size approximately 2 mm per year up to age 5.

Postoperative Care. The most important part of the tracheostomy operation is the postoperative care, which requires diligence and patience. Many patients, especially children, are still lost because of inadequate postoperative care.

A tracheostomy tube in a fresh tracheostomy should be left in place 2 to 3 days before it is changed. By this time a permanent tract exists, and there is little danger of being unable to reinsert the tube. Changing a tube before this time may result in loss of the tracheal opening into the neck wound with disastrous consequences. A tracheostomy tube in an infant should not be changed for the first time without a bronchoscope being on hand.

Special humidification of inspired air is necessary to prevent tracheitis and crust formation. A room with Walton humidifiers or a tracheal collar with nebulized moisture will provide adequate humidification. In addition to atmospheric humidification, 3 or 4 drops of hypotonic saline solution or Ringer's lactate solution should be dropped into the tube every 3 to 4 hours. After several days, the necessity for additional humidity decreases, and it may eventually be discontinued. Patients with thick, copious secretions may require intratracheal instillation of a mucolytic agent, such as 1-acetylcysteine (Mucomyst) to help liquefy secretions for suction removal.

A suction machine is an absolute necessity for tracheostomy care. Sterile rubber catheters with two distal openings with Y-connectors should be available and should only be used in the trachea. Two openings are necessary to prevent the catheter from being sucked against the tracheal wall. A Y-connector will allow the catheter to be inserted into the trachea without suction being exerted, and it is only during withdrawal that the open end of the Y is occluded and suction applied. Suction should only be maintained for 15 seconds or less, since it is possible to precipitate hypoxia and cardiac arrest by prolonged suctioning. Suctioning must be done often, especially during the first few days after tracheostomy, because of the increase in tracheobronchial secretions secondary to tracheal irritation.

Decannulation

A tracheostomy tube should be left in place no longer than necessary, especially in children. Removal as soon as it is expedient will help reduce the incidence of tracheobronchitis, tracheal ulceration, tracheal stenosis, tracheomalacia, and persistent tracheocutaneous fistula.

As soon as the patient's condition permits, the size of the tracheostomy tube should be reduced to a size which allows air to bypass the tube and pass into the upper respiratory tract. This will help avoid physiologic dependence on a large tube due to decreased respiratory resistance. The tube is then plugged, and the adequacy of the airway, as well as the ability to swallow and handle secretions, is determined. When tubal occlusion has been tolerated for 8 to 12 hours, the tube is removed and the tracheocutaneous fistula is taped shut. Immediately after decannulation, the patient must be closely observed and means for reestablishing the airway must be at hand.

Complications. The complications of tracheostomy are numerous, but most can be avoided if the operation is carefully performed and if diligent postoperative care is carried out. They may occur at any time postoperatively but can be roughly divided into immediate, intermediate, and late complications, as outlined in Table 26-2.

Immediate Complications. Immediate complications of tracheostomy include those present at the termination of the operation. When tracheostomy is performed on a patient with a history of chronic hypoxia, the first one or two breaths after the tube is inserted may be followed by cessation of respiration. This is due to physiologic denervation of the peripheral chemoreceptors by the sudden increase of pO_2; because hy-

Table 26-2. Complications of Tracheostomy

Immediate

1. Apnea due to loss of hypoxic stimulation of respiration
2. Hemorrhage
3. Surgical injury of neighboring structures, i.e., esophagus, recurrent laryngeal nerve, and cupula of the pleura
4. Pneumothorax and pneumomediastinum
5. Injury of the cricoid cartilage (high tracheostomy)

Intermediate

1. Tracheitis and tracheobronchitis
2. Tracheal erosion and hemorrhage
3. Hypercapnia
4. Atelectasis
5. Displacement of the tracheostomy tube
6. Obstruction of the tracheostomy tube
7. Subcutaneous emphysema
8. Aspiration and lung abscess

Late

1. Persistent tracheocutaneous fistula
2. Stenosis of the larynx or trachea
3. Tracheal granulations
4. Tracheomalacia
5. Difficult decannulation
6. Tracheoesophageal fistula
7. Problems with the tracheostomy scar

poxia may be largely responsible for respiratory drive in these patients, apnea results. Some form of respiratory assistance is necessary until enough CO_2 is removed to allow a return of sensitivity of central chemoreceptors.

Hemorrhage is a frequent postoperative problem because patients requiring tracheostomy are often hypotensive, and bleeding does not occur until arterial blood pressure is restored or until venous pressure is increased by the coughing associated with insertion of the tube.

Patients, notably children, with sudden respiratory obstruction will manifest markedly increased respiratory effort. If tracheostomy is performed in this situation before a temporary endotracheal airway is inserted, air may be sucked into the mediastinum. This may produce circulatory embarrassment, or the air may rupture into a pleural space to produce a simple or tension pneumothorax. Pneumothorax also occurs secondary to laceration of the apex of the pleural space. This injury is most common in children due to the relatively higher position of the pleura in relation to the trachea. A roentgenogram of the chest should be obtained after any difficult tracheostomy and after tracheostomy in a child for early diagnosis of this complication.

Surgical injury of adjacent structures during tracheostomy is usually due to carrying dissection lateral and deep to the trachea. The trachea can be easily recognized by palpation in the adult, but difficulty may be encountered in children. This can be avoided by inserting a rigid endotracheal airway. Injury to the cricoid cartilage is due to performance of high tracheostomy, which is an operation for which there is no clinical justification. Inadvertent performance of high tracheostomy can be avoided if the tracheostomy tube is inserted below the level of the thyroid isthmus.

Intermediate Complications. Intermediate complications develop during the first few hours or days after tracheostomy. Some degree of tracheitis and tracheobronchitis occurs in all patients due to bypassing of the upper respiratory tract air-conditioning. This is particularly severe in infants, and necrotizing tracheobronchitis is a frequent

cause of death after tracheostomy in these small patients. Careful attention to humidification, humidifiers, nebulizers with a tracheal collar or a croup tent, and endotracheal instillation of fluid being employed, will prevent this complication. The use of high concentrations of O_2 has a drying effect on the tracheal mucosa and is best avoided; when it is necessary, a nebulizer must always be used.

Improper fit of a tracheostomy tube is a source of many complications, but careful preoperative selection of a tube followed by postoperative roentgenographic evaluation is necessary for prevention. Tubes of excessive length may impinge on the anterior wall of the trachea or the carina, producing partial tracheal obstruction, as well as ulceration and possible rupture of the innominate artery. The tube may extend down one bronchus with resultant atelectasis of the opposite lung (Figs. 26–3 and 26–4). Too

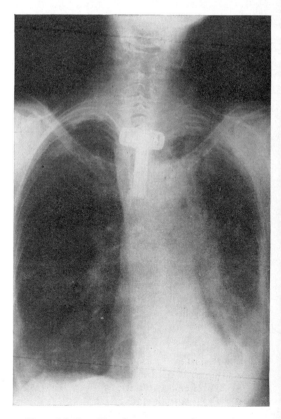

FIG. 26–3. Tracheostomy tube that is too long, causing obstructive atelectasis of the left lung.

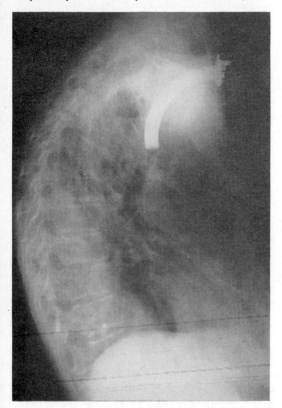

FIG. 26–4. Tracheostomy tube that is too long, impinging on the anterior tracheal wall.

short a tube may predispose to displacement of the tube out of the trachea, especially when the neck is flexed in obese individuals or in small children.

Obstruction of the tracheostomy tube by a mucous plug or blood clot is due to lack of care. If suctioning does not relieve obstructive symptoms, changing of the tube is indicated. Equipment to reestablish an airway should be kept in the room of a patient with a fresh tracheostomy.

Subcutaneous emphysema is caused by suturing the incision tightly or packing the wound around the tracheostomy tube. It may also follow insertion of the tube through a small hole in the pretracheal fascia, which then fits snugly around the tube. The emphysema is usually localized in the neck and upper chest but may involve the whole body. If allowed to progress, it may lead to pneumomediastinum and pneumothorax. Any constricting force around the

tube between the skin and trachea must be removed to prevent progression. Insertion of a chest tube with an underwater seal may be necessary if pneumothorax develops.

When tracheostomy is performed on patients with alveolar hypoventilation secondary to decreased respiratory effort, secretional obstruction, or chronic pulmonary insufficiency, the improvement in alveolar oxygenation may be enough to relieve hypoxemia, especially if oxygen is administered. However, there may be no associated improvement in the respiratory minute volume, and hypercapnia will persist. In fact, because the hypoxic stimulus of respiration has been removed, hypoventilation may worsen and hypercapnia increase, producing clinical deterioration. Ventilation must be assisted until enough CO_2 is blown off to restore normal respiratory stimulation.

Late Complications. Late complications of tracheostomy are most frequent when the tube has been left in place for a prolonged period. Persistent tracheocutaneous fistula is due to epithelialization of the cannula tract. The epithelium must be removed and the wound closed in layers to obtain permanent closure.

Stenosis of the larynx follows injury and perichondritis of the cricoid cartilage. Tracheal stenosis is most common in children and most often follows excision of cartilage from the anterior tracheal wall. Exuberant granulations may develop on the anterior tracheal wall as a result of delayed epithelialization when there is a large defect in the anterior tracheal wall and may cause obstruction and bleeding.

Localized tracheomalacia following tracheostomy usually involves the area immediately superior to the tracheal opening. It may be associated with the use of a tracheostomy tube which is too large and which is sharply angled, causing the tube to impinge on the tracheal ring above the tracheostomy, pushing posteriorly and causing loss of its rigidity. This may be avoided by using a more flexible tube of Teflon or Silastic when necessary. Tracheomalacia may delay decannulation in children.

The use of a vertical skin incision is the most frequent cause of unsightly scar formation. The duration of tracheostomy is also

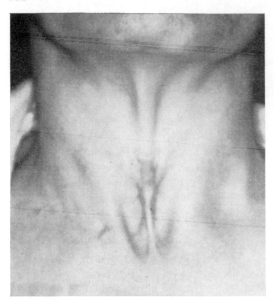

FIG. 26–5. Hypertrophy and contracture following vertical incision for tracheostomy.

important in scarring, which is lessened by early removal of the tube. Vertical contracture and widening of a hypertrophic scar will require a Z-plasty for repair. Other scar problems may occur, including adherence of the skin to the trachea, which may affect swallowing, or formation of a depressed scar. In these cases, the old tracheostomy wound must be taken down and reclosed with careful approximation of tissue layers (Fig. 26–5).

Tracheoesophageal fistula may be a complication of inadvertent incision of the posterior tracheal wall or ulceration secondary to tubal trauma. Tracheal ulceration is most frequent when cuffed tracheostomy tubes are used for prolonged periods. When the use of a cuffed tube is necessary, the cuff should be inspected for symmetry of inflation, since uneven inflation may cause the end of the tube to press on one of the tracheal walls, causing an ulcer and perhaps a fistula. The balloon should be deflated at least once an hour to help prevent mucosal necrosis. Once a fistula is present, spontaneous closure is unlikely, and operative obliteration of the tract is necessary.

Difficult Decannulation. Difficulty with decannulation is a frequent problem in chil-

dren and may be secondary to both psychic and organic factors. Children have poorly developed respiratory habits which are readily altered by tracheostomy. Children become rapidly accustomed to the reduction in airway resistance associated with the operation, and they are loath to resume the increased respiratory effort required for the use of the normal airway. Tracheostomy also causes a breakdown in the apneic reflex associated with deglutition, and this may cause aspiration by some small children when the tube is first removed, thus instilling a fear of choking.

The tracheal lumen of small children may measure 10 mm in diameter, but because of the membranous posterior wall, collapse to a diameter of 5 mm or less during expiration is frequent. Therefore, the mucosal edema which is always present with the tracheostomy may result in considerable compromise of the lumen, producing anatomic obstruction.

In addition to the unavoidable problems of tracheostomy in children, errors in procedure and care may be a source of further difficulty in decannulation. These include use of too large or too sharply curved tubes, excision of tracheal cartilage, recurrent nerve paralysis, and unnecessary prolongation of intubation, which are causes of tracheomalacia, granulation tissue formation, and edema.

Treatment. Provided an uncomplicated surgical procedure has been performed, decannulation problems are rare if tube removal is accomplished in less than 5 days. When symptoms of respiratory obstruction develop after tubal removal, the patient must be carefully investigated to elicit the cause. Investigation should include inspiratory and expiratory roentgenograms of the larynx and trachea to note collapse, the presence of granulations, or stenosis. Direct laryngoscopy and tracheoscopy are indicated to determine vocal cord mobility and to inspect the tracheal lumen for granulations, infractured cartilage, or collapse of the lumen.

Treatment is directed at the cause, if one is present. Surgical removal of granulations and bits of loose cartilage is accomplished by direct laryngoscopy. Stenosis must also be corrected surgically. Tracheomalacia involving the area immediately above the tracheostomy site may be improved by utilizing a better-fitting metal tube or by constructing an individual flexible tube of synthetic material to relieve pressure on the cartilage and permit return of rigidity. In some cases, it may be necessary to wait for tracheal growth and increased rigidity before decannulation is accomplished.

When no organic cause of obstructive symptoms is obvious, decannulation may be carried out by gradual reduction of cannula size, although this is possible only in larger children. In small children, reduction in tube size is carried as far as possible, and final decannulation may be accomplished during sleep, with sedation, or during a light general anesthetic. The use of an indwelling, pliable, plastic nasotracheal tube is often helpful in the more difficult cases to approximate more closely the normal airway resistance and to provide support for the healing trachea. The tube may be left in place for several days if it is adequately fixed to prevent displacement. This helps the child readjust to the increased respiratory effort required to resume use of the normal respiratory tract while still allowing normal deglutition. Finally, waiting may be the only answer in decannulating some children, and the use of a valved or fenestrated tube will permit the use and development of normal speech mechanisms.

TRACHEAL FENESTRATION

When the problem of handling of secretions is likely to be permanent, due either to the nature of the secretions or to irreversible changes in pulmonary function, creation of a permanent tracheal fenestra may be indicated. This will allow the use of a tracheostomy tube to be discontinued, thus avoiding the problems associated with continuous wearing of an intratracheal tube. The disadvantages of a tube are that it requires changing, irritates the trachea, and may result in ulceration or squamous metaplasia of the epithelium with loss of ciliary function. In addition, an open tube permits air escape during phonation unless it is occluded each time, whereas a valved tube

must be removed every time tracheal suctioning is required.

The fenestra may be constructed so that it is covered by an operculum which, when fixed with a piece of adhesive, will obliterate the opening when it is not in use. Also, normal speech is possible without the necessity of occluding a tube.

Indications. The main indication for this procedure is removal of secretions from the tracheobronchial tree. The procedure is most useful in patients with cystic fibrosis, chronic pulmonary insufficiency, and chronic suppurative disease of the lungs who have persistent or recurrent difficulty with secretions. Patients with cystic fibrosis are often bothered by the collection of thick viscid secretions which they are unable to cough up, thus precipitating recurrent pulmonary infections and the development of progressive bronchiectasis. Creation of a permanent fenestra will facilitate the introduction of mucolytic agents into the tracheobronchial tree, as well as removal of secretions.

Tracheal fenestration has been advocated in the treatment of chronic pulmonary insufficiency because of an anticipated improvement in alveolar ventilation. However, this is not borne out by clinical experience. The operation is of value, nevertheless, for patients with pulmonary insufficiency who are subject to recurrent attacks of bronchitis with secretion accumulation, which induce respiratory crises. In this situation, the fenestra provides for tracheobronchial toilet and facilitates the use of intermittent positive pressure breathing or other types of assisted respiration when they are indicated.

Technique. The patient is placed in the usual tracheostomy position with the neck extended. Local anesthesia is used. A collar incision with a small central flap is made about 3 cm above the clavicle (Fig. 26–6). A skin flap is mobilized superiorly. The anterior wall of the trachea is identified as in a tracheostomy, but in this procedure it is necessary to remove subcutaneous fat, fascia, and strap muscles from around the proposed opening in the trachea. The thyroid isthmus should be excised if it is in the way. A square section of the anterior wall of the trachea 1.5 by 1.5 cm is removed, including

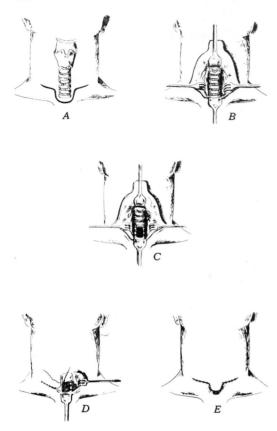

FIG. 26–6. Tracheal fenestration. *A,* Skin incision includes a small flap based superiorly. *B,* The anterior wall of the trachea is widely exposed, removing portions of the thyroid isthmus and strap muscles. *C,* A square section is removed from the anterior tracheal wall at the level of the third to fifth rings. *D,* The inferior margin of the superior skin flap is sutured to the superior margin of the tracheal opening to create an operculum. Skin is advanced and approximated to the other margins. *E,* Completed tracheal fenestration covered by the superior skin flap.

parts of the third and fourth rings. The skin flaps are approximated to the margins of the trachea using nylon or stainless steel wire suture. The superior flap is intentionally redundant in order to construct an operculum. A tracheostomy tube should not be inserted. When wound healing is complete, the patient is able to occlude the fenestra by slight flexion of the neck or by taping the operculum down, permitting relatively normal

speech and avoiding the problems associated with bypass of the humidifying mechanism of the upper respiratory tract.

REFERENCES

Aber, G. M., *et al.*: The Effect of Acute Changes in Inspired Oxygen Concentrations on Cardiac, Respiratory and Renal Function in Patients with Chronic Obstructive Airway Disease. Clin. Sci., *26*:133, 1964.

Aldrete, J. A.: Nasotracheal Intubation. Surg. Clin. North Am., *49*:1209, 1969.

Andrews, M. J., and Pearson, F. G.: Incidence and Pathogenesis of Tracheal Injury Following Cuffed Tube Tracheostomy with Assisted Ventilation: Analysis of a 2-year Prospective Study. Ann. Surg., *173*:249, 1971.

Atkins, J. P.: Current Utilization of Tracheostomy as a Therapeutic Measure. Laryngoscope, *70*:1672, 1960.

Bendixen, H. H., *et al.*: *Respiratory Care*. St. Louis, Mo., C. V. Mosby Co., 1965.

Bergstrom, O., and Diamant, H.: Mediastinal Emphysema Complicating Tracheotomy. Arch. Otolaryng., *71*:628, 1960.

Bilger, J. D., *et al.*: Tracheotomy in Infancy. Pediatrics, *13*:476, 1954.

Canby, J. P., and Redd, H. J., Jr.: Tracheotomy in Severe Bronchiolitis. Pediatrics, *36*: 406, 1965.

Comroe, J. H., Jr.: The Peripheral Chemoreceptors. *In* Fenn W. O., and Rahn, H. (Eds.): *Handbook of Physiology*. Vol. 1, Section 3, Respiration. American Physiological Society. Baltimore, The Williams & Wilkins Co., 1964.

Comroe, J. H.. Jr.: In *Physiology of Respiration*. Chicago, Year Book Medical Publishers, 1965.

Diamant, H., *et al.*: Decannulation in Children. Laryngoscope, *71*:404, 1961.

Ferguson, C. F.: Respiratory Obstruction and the Role of Tracheostomy. In Changing Concepts of Otolaryngology for the Pediatrician. Pediatrics, *25*:1043, 1960.

Ferris, B. G., Jr., and Pollard, D. S.: Effect of Tracheotomy Tubes on the Resistance of Breathing and Pulmonary Resistance in Patients with Poliomyelitis. New Engl. J. Med., *263*:103, 1960.

Froeb, H. F., and Kim, B. M.: Tracheostomy and Respiratory Dead Space. J. Appl. Physiol., *19*:92, 1964.

Gilbert, R., *et al.*: Mechanisms of Chronic Carbon Dioxide Retention in Patients with Obstructive Pulmonary Disease. Am. J. Med., *38*:217, 1965.

Goodall, E. W.: The Story of Tracheotomy. Br. J. Child. Dis., *31*:167, 1934.

Gray, J. S.: Physiology of Respiratory Obstruction. Ann. Otol. Rhinol. Laryngol., *59*:72, 1950.

Gray, L. P.: Infant Tracheostomy. J. Laryngol. Otol., *74*:145, 1960.

Greenberg, L. M., *et al.*: Method for Difficult Decannulation in Children. Arch. Otolaryng., *81*:72, 1965.

Grillo, H. C., *et al.*: A Low Pressure Cuff for Tracheostomy Tubes to Minimize Tracheal Injury. J. Thorac. Cardiovasc. Surg., *62*:898, 1971.

Hardy, K. L.: Tracheostomy: Indications, Technics and Tubes. Am. J. Surg., *126*:300, 1973.

Harley, H. R. S.: Laryngotracheal Obstruction Complicating Tracheostomy or Endotracheal Intubation with Assisted Respiration. Thorax, *26*:493, 1971.

Lewis, R. S., and Ludman, H.: Decannulation After Tracheostomy in Infants and Young Children. J. Laryngol. Otol., *79*:435, 1965.

McDonald, I. H., and Stacks, J. G.: Prolonged Nasotracheal Intubation. Br. J. Anaesth., *37*:161, 1965.

Meade, J. W.: Tracheotomy—Its Complications and Their Management. New Engl. J. Med., *265*:519, 1961.

Mulder, D. S., and Rubush, J. L.: Complications of Tracheostomy: Relationship to Long Term Ventilatory Assistance. J. Trauma, *9*:389, 1969.

Nelson, T. G.: *Tracheotomy: A Clinical and Experimental Study*. Baltimore, The Williams & Wilkins Co., 1958.

Nylen, B., and Fluur, E.: Post-tracheostomy Scar. Acta Otolaryng., *60*:90, 1965.

Oliver, P., *et al.*: Tracheostomy in Children. New Engl. J. Med., *267*:631, 1962.

Pressman, J. J.: Repair of Depressed Tracheotomy Scars. Arch. Otolaryng., *74*:150, 1961.

Rocky, E. E., *et al.*: Tracheal Fenestration for the Treatment of Respiratory Insufficiency. Geriatrics, *21*:174, 1966.

Safar, P., *et al.*: Cuffed Tracheotomy Tube vs. Tank Respirator for Prolonged Artificial Ventilation. Arch. Phys. Med., *43*:487, 1962.

Safar, P. (Ed.): *Respiratory Therapy*. Philadelphia, F. A. Davis Co., 1965.

Stahlman, M. T., *et al.*: The Management of Respiratory Failure in the Idiopathic Respiratory Distress Syndrome of Prematurity. Ann. N.Y. Acad. Sci., *121*:930, 1965.

Talbert, J. L., and Haller, J. A.: Improved Silastic Tracheostomy Tubes for Infants and Young Children. J. Pediatr. Surg., *3*:408, 1968.

Teplitz, C., *et al.*: Pathology of Low Tracheostomy in Children. Am. J. Clin. Pathol., *42*:58, 1964.

Utley, J. R., *et al.*: Definitive Management of Innominate Artery Hemorrhage Complicating Tracheostomy. J.A.M.A., *222*:577, 1972.

Weiss, E. B., *et al.*: Acute Respiratory Failure in Chronic Obstructive Pulmonary Disease. Disease-a-Month, October, 1969.

Chapter 27
Congenital Malformations of the Larynx

Congenital anomalies of the larynx are not common. They are generally a result of abnormal growth and maturation of the soft tissues lining the larynx of the fetus. The most frequent source of abnormality is a failure of canalization of the occluded larynx between the eighth and tenth weeks of fetal life.

Congenital abnormalities of the larynx produce two groups of symptoms:

1. Respiratory stridor is the most noteworthy symptom and, with obstruction at the laryngeal level, is almost always inspiratory. Cyanosis, indrawing, and restlessness are other common symptoms in this group. No symptoms may be present until an upper respiratory tract infection is superimposed on the anomaly.

2. Abnormalities of phonation occur with most laryngeal malformations. The cry may be completely absent (aphonia), but weakness of cry or hoarseness is more common.

These symptoms are common to all types of respiratory obstruction from the external nares to the trachea, although dysphonia is usually indicative of a laryngeal lesion. Therefore, in evaluating an infant with these symptoms, a systematic examination beginning at the anterior nares and ending with direct laryngoscopy and bronchoscopy must be performed.

The diagnosis of a laryngeal anomaly is confirmed by direct laryngoscopy, which can be safely done without anesthesia in infants. Roentgenograms of the neck and chest are of value in locating the site of abnormality. Both inspiratory and expiratory films should be taken, as there may be significant alterations in the configuration of the tracheobronchial tree with the respiratory cycle.

ATRESIA OF THE LARYNX

Complete occlusion of the larynx is rare as far as the clinical otolaryngologist is concerned, since most of the afflicted infants are classified as stillborn or die before tracheostomy can be performed. The condition is due to a failure of the epithelial primordium of the vocal cords to split in a sagittal plane. Therefore, atresia may be limited to the supraglottic, glottic, or infraglottic level or may involve all levels of the endolarynx. The pharyngotracheal canal is the residuum of the laryngotracheal groove, and it is only secondarily incorporated into the laryngeal lumen. Therefore, when atresia is present, the pinhole-sized pharyngotracheal canal can often be found in the posterior part of the larynx between the arytenoids.

The treatment of laryngeal atresia is tracheostomy or cricothyrotomy followed by a definitive procedure on the larynx at a later date.

BIFID EPIGLOTTIS

This rare abnormality is characterized by a division of the epiglottis into two equal and symmetrical halves, which tend to be flaccid and may prolapse into the glottis. The diagnosis is made by direct laryngoscopy, and treatment may require amputation of the flaccid portions by a transoral approach.

CONGENITAL WEBS OF THE LARYNX

Congenital webs are the result of failure of normal splitting of the vocal cord primordium. Therefore, the patency of the laryngeal lumen is deficient because of persistent attachment between the two halves of the larynx. The morphology of the webs varies widely; some are paper thin, while others are quite thick. Also, they may occur at various sites in the larynx. Congenital webs are most commonly found at the level of the glottis between the anterior portions of the vocal cords. Less commonly, they occur in the infraglottic area, in the supraglottic area between the ventricular bands, or in the posterior commissure. Infraglottic webs may be associated with cricoid cartilage abnormalities.

Clinical Manifestations. Symptoms will vary with the site and degree of webbing. Glottic webs produce dysphonia of varying degree, which is marked by a weak, hoarse cry in infants. Frequently this may be the sole symptom and, when minimal, may not be noted until speech is developing. The presence of a web tends to delay the development of speech. Inspiratory stridor and other signs of laryngeal obstruction, which are made worse by respiratory infections, are common symptoms. More extensive webs cause obstruction which may be so severe that emergency tracheostomy is necessary immediately after birth. Webs in the infraglottic area tend to produce little voice change, but they produce stridor which may have an expiratory component. The smaller webs may produce symptoms only when there is superimposed respiratory tract in-

fection. When obstruction is fairly severe, there is usually some feeding difficulty.

Diagnosis. Diagnosis of a laryngeal web is made by direct laryngoscopy, which may be performed without anesthesia in newborn infants. The site and thickness of the webs should be noted in order to plan treatment. Soft tissue roentgenograms and laryngograms are helpful in determining the configuration of the web.

Treatment. Extensive webs of the larynx will require emergency treatment at birth because of obstruction. Tracheostomy is indicated in such instances. Once tracheostomy has been necessary, definitive repair should be carried out as soon as it is feasible so that normal development of the larynx, laryngeal reflexes, and speech is permitted. Surgical correction can usually be carried out by 1 year of age.

Small laryngeal webs causing dysphonia only may be left untreated until the larynx is of more substantial size. Repair, in such instances, is done at age 5 to 6 years when voice and speech become more important.

Methods of Surgical Treatment. *Bougienage.* Thin, friable webs, particularly at the glottic level, may be treated by bougienage and dilatation of the larynx, which will often cure the problem. Laryngeal dilators of appropriate size are passed by direct laryngoscopy. However, if there is any question of traumatizing the larynx by having to use unnecessary force for dilatation, the procedure should be abandoned. Repeated attempts to dilate a thick, resistant web will only worsen the stenosis.

Montgomery Umbrella Keel. After surgical division of a laryngeal web, the opposite sides of the larynx must be separated to prevent reattachment. The use of a silicone keel for this purpose, inserted through a thyrotomy, will usually produce a good result.

Technique. If a tracheostomy tube is already in place, it may be used to give a general anesthetic. In the absence of a tracheostomy tube, one should be placed electively in children under age 5 for anesthesia purposes and postoperative care. Children over the age of 5 or 6 may have the procedure done without tracheostomy, provided the operation is performed with a minimum of trauma. In such cases, a general anesthetic is given, using a Steven-Slater bag to maintain respiration without the use of an endotracheal tube. The thin plate does not cause any postoperative problems in these older patients, and a tracheostomy is avoided.

A small horizontal incision is made over the thyroid cartilage, and a vertical midline thyrotomy is done. The larynx is entered carefully in the midline and the web divided. A flanged silicone plate is then inserted in the thyrotomy, and the flanges are sutured in place between the thyroid cartilage and the perichondrium. The plate is cut to size at the operating table, so that it does not impinge on the posterior laryngeal wall and is of sufficient length to separate all the raw surfaces in the larynx.

The keel is left in place for 2 to 3 weeks, depending on the appearance of the larynx. It should not be removed if there are granulations present in the larynx. If granulations do develop, they may be removed by direct laryngoscopy with the keel in place. The silicone plate is removed by reopening the neck wound. Tantalum or polyethylene keels may be inserted via direct suspension laryngoscopy, but this is difficult, as well as being traumatic to the remainder of the larynx.

Inglauer described the treatment of glottic webs by inserting a polyethylene tube through the anterior commissure and fixing it in place for 6 weeks. The tract around the tube becomes epithelialized, and the web is then divided by connecting the epithelialized tract and the normal laryngeal lumen. Re-formation of the webs, especially the larger ones, is common.

The method of dividing the attachments of the web on each cord in stages has been advocated, but again results are not consistent, and frequent re-formation of the web is a problem.

CONGENITAL INFRAGLOTTIC STENOSIS

This condition may be due to an excess of tissue in the infraglottic portion of the conus elasticus or to an anomaly of the cricoid cartilage. This produces further narrowing of the already narrow infantile infraglottic lumen.

Clinical Manifestations. These infants may not have any symptoms at rest. However, with any upper respiratory infection, they develop inspiratory stridor and dyspnea due to further narrowing of the infraglottic lumen by edema. Exercise may also precipitate stridor and dyspnea. Patients with inspiratory stridor at rest may develop expiratory stridor in addition during an infection. The voice or cry is often near normal.

Direct laryngoscopy will disclose a fullness in the infraglottic area. This must be distinguished from the sharp margin of an infraglottic web. Soft tissue roentgenograms of the neck will show a smooth density indenting the translucency of the laryngeal airway. This condition must be differentiated from benign neoplasms, such as hemangioma and chondroma, by inspection and palpation of the mass with a spatula at the time of direct laryngoscopy.

Treatment. Except for performance of a tracheostomy for obstruction when necessary, the treatment is expectant. As the larynx grows, there is usually a relative lessening of the infraglottic narrowing and symptoms disappear. In cases in which tracheostomy has been necessary, the nonfunctioning larynx does not grow as rapidly, and the symptoms tend to persist much longer. The use of a valved tracheostomy tube may be helpful for speech development during the waiting period before decannulation. Rarely, surgical resection of the stenotic area may be necessary.

CONGENITAL HEMANGIOMA OF THE LARYNX

Hemangiomas, usually of the cavernous type, tend to occur anteriorly in the infraglottic region of the larynx. They occur most commonly in females, and half of the patients will have cutaneous hemangiomas.

Clinical Manifestations. The symptoms are those of laryngeal obstruction, including stridor (which may be biphasic), dyspnea, cyanosis, and indrawing. Symptoms may be absent at birth and may first appear in association with an upper respiratory infection; they then persist after the infection resolves. They are made worse by placing the infant in a Trendelenburg position and are often improved when the infant is held erect.

The presence of cutaneous hemangiomas and the absence of symptoms in the early postnatal period may be clues to the diagnosis. Direct laryngoscopy discloses a red or purple mass covered by normal epithelium in the area beneath the vocal cords. A helpful diagnostic maneuver is the subcutaneous injection of 1 or 2 minims of 1:1000 epinephrine, which will cause blanching and shrinking of the hemangioma and transient relief of symptoms. This procedure should be done at the time of direct laryngoscopy when the changes may be visualized. Biopsy of the lesion is dangerous if a tracheostomy has not been done. After tracheostomy and evaluation of the lesion, a small biopsy may be accomplished with reasonable safety if it is felt to be necessary, although it is perhaps best avoided. Soft tissue roentgenograms of the larynx are of help in delineating the size and extent of the lesion; also, calcium may be noted in lesions present for some time.

Treatment. If symptoms are intermittent and there is no severe respiratory embarrassment, the child may be watched. Often the hemangioma will regress spontaneously, as many cutaneous lesions do, within the first year or 2 of life. Spontaneous regression will usually begin within 8 to 10 months, but if involution is not evident within a reasonable length of time, definitive treatment is indicated.

Irradiation. These lesions usually respond fairly well to small doses of irradiation, from 500 to 750 R. There is, however, the possibility that irradiation in children is a factor in the etiology of carcinomas of the head and neck, as well as the possibility that it damages growth centers. Therefore, most radiotherapists are reluctant to use irradiation for benign lesions in this age group.

Surgery. These lesions may be approached through a vertical tracheal incision. Lesions of the anterior wall may be dissected out submucosally without the tracheal lumen being entered. If the hemangioma is on the posterior wall, a vertical mucosal incision is made and dissection is performed, taking care to preserve the mucosa. The cricoid cartilage should not be injured.

A stent of polyethylene tubing or Ivalon sponge must be left in the infraglottic area for 3 to 4 weeks postoperatively to prevent stenosis. Careful approximation of the tracheal rings is imperative to prevent formation of granulation tissue in the tracheal lumen.

Sclerosing Agents. Sclerosing agents, such as sodium morrhuate, have been used in the treatment of hemangiomas in other areas of the body. The difficulty of controlling the injection of these materials in a tiny larynx, the resulting fibrosis, and the possibility of inducing laryngeal stenosis preclude their use.

Recently the use of systemic corticosteroids in the treatment of hemangiomas has come into vogue. They have been shown to produce considerable regression of cavernous hemangiomas, both of skin and larynx, thus avoiding tracheostomy or surgery.

TRACHEOESOPHAGEAL FISTULAS AND LARYNGEAL CLEFTS

The esophagus and tracheobronchial tree arise from a common tube; initially they are connected by a long laryngotracheal groove, which progressively closes in a caudocranial direction to leave the pharyngotracheal canal. Deficiencies in the closure of this groove give rise to a variety of defects in about 1 out of every 2500 births.

Clinical Manifestations. These anomalies usually give rise to symptoms immediately after birth. The afflicted infants will have persistent barking cough with episodes of choking and cyanosis which are markedly increased by feeding. Aspiration eventually leads to severe bronchopneumonia and death unless the abnormality is corrected.

Diagnosis. A laryngeal cleft consists of a vertical defect in the posterior wall of the larynx extending between the arytenoids and into the quadrate lamina of the cricoid cartilage. This represents a failure of the cranial portion of the laryngeal tracheal groove to close. The laryngeal sphincters are ineffective, and aspiration occurs through the cleft. A Dionosil swallow will show spillage into the trachea on swallowing, which may lead to confusion with a fistula. Generally, the use of radiopaque dye should be avoided in these tiny infants because of aspiration and pneumonia. The defect may easily be seen at direct laryngoscopy with a minimum of risk to the patient.

Tracheoesophageal fistula may be associated with other abnormalities of the trachea and esophagus; four types occur. Three varieties are associated with esophageal atresia. The diagnosis may be easily established by passing a small nasogastric tube and demonstrating its failure to enter the stomach. A lateral roentgenogram of the chest may demonstrate a blind upper esophageal pouch with air in the stomach, indicating an inferior tracheoesophageal connection, or there may be a complete absence of air in the abdomen, which would suggest the opposite defect. The use of a radiopaque dye is not necessary and invites aspiration pneumonia; also, the use of barium sulfate is contraindicated in such patients.

The difficulty in diagnosis is with the H-type fistula not associated with atresia. The fistula may occur at any level in the posterior wall of the larynx or trachea. Esophagoscopy is of little value because the loose esophageal mucosa hides the tract; however, tracheoscopy may disclose the fistula. Frequently, a dye contrast examination using cineradiography is diagnostic. In a small number of cases, it may be necessary to inject methylene blue into the trachea through an endotracheal tube and watch for the appearance of the dye in the esophagus with an esophagoscope in order to determine the site of the fistula.

Treatment. As soon as the presence of an abnormal laryngotracheal connection is suspected, all feeding by mouth must be stopped (Fig. 27–1). Dehydration is treated by intravenous fluids. Antibiotics are given for pneumonia, which must be controlled before surgical repair of the defect is attempted.

When atresia is present, the upper esophageal pouch should be kept empty by a soft catheter inserted into the pouch transnasally and attached to gentle suction. Elevation of the head will help prevent regurgitation into the trachea, and all these infants should be nursed in this position. Gastrostomy is of value for feeding and prevention of regurgitation and is necessary for most patients.

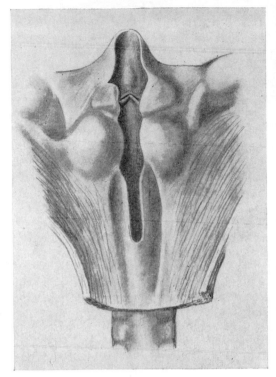

FIG. 27–1.   Posterior view of a laryngeal cleft extending into the posterior tracheal wall.

Definitive surgery should not be attempted until dehydration, nutrition, and pneumonia have been controlled. Surgical repair of laryngotracheal cleft is often difficult, especially if the cleft extends through the cricoid cartilage. Lesser degrees of cleft may be closed by layered approximation. Tracheostomy should always precede surgery because some degree of dysphagia and aspiration is present postoperatively.

Surgical repair of most tracheoesophageal fistulas with atresia must be done through a thoracotomy. However, high H-type fistulas may be repaired by an approach through the neck, followed by isolation and division of the fistula tract and layered closure. A small local muscle flap should be interposed between the trachea and esophagus at the closure site.

LARYNGOCELE VENTRICULARIS

Laryngocele ventricularis is an air-filled dilatation of the sacculus or appendix of the laryngeal ventricle. The appendix of the ventricle was described by Morgagni in 1761. The first laryngocele was described by Abulcasim in the eleventh century, and the lesion was named by Virchow in 1867.

Etiology. The ventricles of the larynx develop from an evagination into the primordium of the endolaryngeal structures beginning during the second month. The primitive ventricles extend quite far laterally under the floor of the pharynx, and the distal extension, the appendix, may be related in origin to the fourth branchial cleft. At birth, the appendix is relatively large, but at about the age of 6 years it begins to regress in size, relative to the remainder of the larynx and ventricle. Members of the Caucasian race tend to have larger appendices. The opening to the appendix in the adult is found at the anterior end of the roof of the ventricle and is an orifice about 8 mm long. The ventricle is lined with ciliated respiratory epithelium, and many seromucous glands empty into the cavity.

Although there is a belief that laryngoceles occur in persons with congenitally large ventricular appendices, the deformity is rare in children. The most common predisposing factor is activity which produces a recurrent, persistent increase in intralaryngeal pressure, such as straining, coughing, playing wind instruments, and excessive straining with voice use. Laryngeal air pressure is increased by the trapping of air beneath the concave lower surface of the false vocal cords, which will increase the air pressure in the laryngeal ventricle. Since the ventricle is outside the thorax, the increased pressure is not compensated for by the simultaneous increase in intrathoracic pressure and dilatation occurs. Less commonly, a lesion causing a ball valve obstruction of the opening of the ventricle or appendix may be a cause of air trapping and dilatation of the appendix.

Clinical Manifestations. Three types of laryngocele are recognized: internal, external, and mixed (Fig. 27–2). The internal

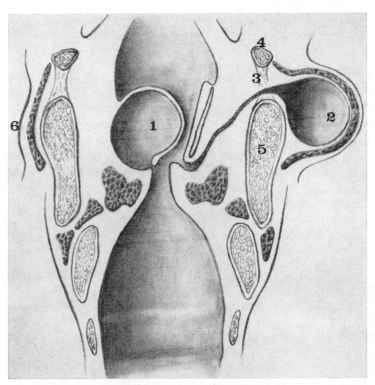

Fig. 27–2.   Schematic drawing showing laryngoceles of the larynx: *1,* internal laryngocele; *2,* external laryngocele; *3,* false vocal cord and quadrangular membrane; *4,* hyoid bone; *5,* thyroid cartilage; *6,* thyrohyoid muscle.

form consists of an air-containing sac confined to the area of the false cord and aryepiglottic fold and within the thyrohyoid membrane. The external form presents as a cystic mass on the lateral surface of the thyrohyoid membrane which is connected to the ventricle by a narrow patent tube. The tube passes through the thyrohyoid membrane in the region of the neurovascular bundle, although it is usually situated inferior to the bundle. The mixed type consists of connected air-containing cavities on both sides of the thyrohyoid membrane.

Laryngoceles are a rather uncommon condition occurring almost exclusively in males who are usually in their fifties. They may be bilateral.

The symptoms tend to fluctuate, increasing with straining and disappearing at rest. The internal and mixed forms will cause hoarseness, stridor, and dyspnea which worsens with continued voice use. The external type may present only as a compressible, spherical mass over the thyrohyoid membrane which moves with the larynx on swallowing (Fig. 27–3). *Bryce's sign* may be present and is characterized by a gurgling and hissing in the throat when the neck mass is compressed. The mass may vary widely in size from time to time and may be absent at times. The patient may have a persistent productive cough, especially if infection is present.

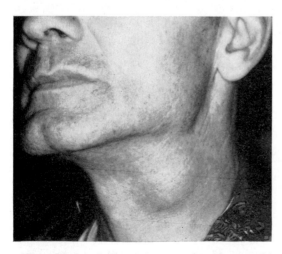

FIG. 27–3. Left neck mass in 40-year-old male. Later demonstrated to be an external laryngocele.

Occasionally, the opening to the laryngocele may become obstructed and filled with mucus, becoming a secondary mucocele; this may become infected, producing a laryngopyocele. In the latter instance, fever, pain, tenderness, and odynophagia appear.

Diagnosis. The masses in the false cord and in the lateral neck are obvious on clinical examination when the patient strains. A soft tissue roentgenogram of the neck during the Valsalva maneuver will disclose the presence of the air-containing cystic structures. If infection is present, an air-fluid level may be noted on the roentgenogram. Direct laryngoscopy and inspection of the ventricle are indicated to rule out an underlying neoplasm.

Laryngoceles are generally lined with ciliated pseudostratified columnar epithelium, although areas of stratified squamous epithelium may be present. The walls do not usually contain collections of lymphoid tissue, which are typical of the usual branchiogenic cysts.

Treatment. Not all laryngoceles need be treated. Small asymptomatic laryngoceles require no therapy and will seldom cause any difficulty if causative factors are removed. Symptomatic laryngoceles and laryngopyoceles should be excised. External and mixed laryngoceles are best excised by a lateral approach through the neck.

The internal laryngocele should be excised via a lateral pharyngotomy. Excision may be carried out through a thyrotomy, but this approach carries the risk of permanent voice impairment and stenosis. The use of sclerosing agents and unroofing of the laryngocele have not been uniformly successful, and recurrence is frequent.

The acute inflammatory stage of a laryngocele may necessitate immediate incision and drainage and later excision during a quiescent period.

CYSTS OF THE LARYNX

Etiology. The appendix and ventricle are lined with respiratory epithelium which contains many goblet cells as well as numerous seromucous glands in the submucosa. A mucous-filled cyst or mucocele may arise either from obstruction of the neck of the

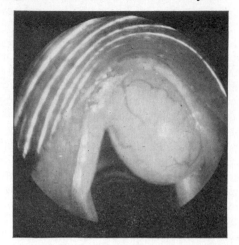

FIG. 27–4. Endoscopic view of a mucocele of the ventricle of Morgagni.

appendix or from obstruction of the duct of the individual gland. Inflammation or a neoplasm may cause obstruction of the appendix. Cysts, unlike laryngoceles, are often present at birth and are much more common (Figs. 27–4 and 27–5). Some of these cystic lesions are called branchial cleft cysts by the pathologist and may, in fact, represent remnants of the fourth branchial cleft. Cysts are most commonly found in the false cord and aryepiglottic fold of the larynx. The other common site of origin is on the thyrohyoid membrane deep to the strap muscles, near the entrance of the internal branch of the superior laryngeal nerve and artery. Frequently, there is a fibrous pedicle extending through the thyrohyoid membrane from the external cyst. Less commonly, a mucocele may be present in both locations, with the parts connected through the thyrohyoid membrane, giving it a "dumbbell" configuration. A laryngocele becomes a mucocele if its laryngeal opening becomes obstructed and it fills with mucus.

Clinical Manifestations. The usual symptom is hoarseness, which is not the raspy hoarseness of a lesion of the true cord. It is often described as a change in the voice by the patient. With larger lesions, the patient may have a "hot potato" voice, similar to that seen in a child with epiglottitis. Inspiratory stridor is common, especially in infants. A cystic mass attached to the thyrohyoid membrane, which moves on swallowing, may be palpable in the neck.

Diagnosis. Laryngeal examination discloses a unilateral mass of the false cord and aryepiglottic fold which bulges into the laryngeal aditus and the piriform fossa (Fig. 27–6). The true vocal cord on the side of the lesion is obscured from view. The entire glottis may be obscured by a large cyst.

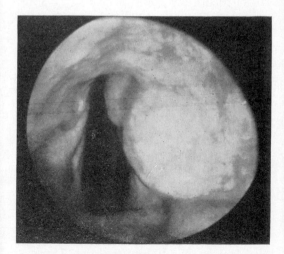

FIG. 27–5. Cyst of the right false vocal cord and ventricle of Morgagni later removed by a lateral pharyngotomy approach.

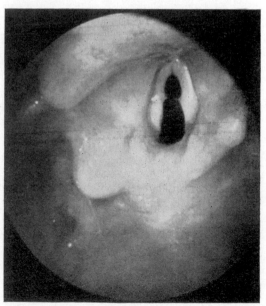

FIG. 27–6. Cyst of the larynx attached to the medial wall of the left piriform fossa.

Soft tissue roentgenograms of the larynx, as well as a laryngogram, will usually differentiate this lesion from an air-filled laryngocele. Direct laryngoscopy is always indicated, and a spatula may be used to palpate the mass and push it laterally to view the true vocal cords. It is imperative to rule out carcinoma in the laryngeal ventricle, and a biopsy should be taken from this area when the patient is in the older age group.

Treatment. The usual method of treatment is excision. This is generally done through an external approach using a horizontal skin incision.

The external type of mucocele is usually easily excised by tracing the pedicle to the thyrohyoid membrane and transecting it. Recurrence is rare.

In the case of the internal type, a lateral pharyngotomy or an anterior thyrotomy may be used. The disadvantage of the thyrotomy is the change in voice produced and possible web formation. It is preferable to approach this through a lateral pharyngotomy and excise the false cord and aryepiglottic fold with the lesion. The arytenoid cartilage should not be disturbed.

In some cases, the mucocele becomes infected and actually presents as a pyocele. In this event, it must be treated as an abscess and may require drainage. This is especially true of the lesions in the false cord. In these cases, it is better to drain the mass early under conditions in which the airway can be controlled to avoid the catastrophe of intralaryngeal rupture of an abscess. The pyocele may be excised when the infection has been controlled.

When a cyst presents in an infant or an elderly debilitated individual, repeated needle aspiration may be used to relieve the symptoms until such time that a definitive surgical procedure can be performed with a minimum of danger to the larynx or the patient.

CONGENITAL VOCAL CORD PARALYSIS

This problem will be discussed more fully in the chapter on neurology of the larynx. However, it should be noted that the congenital paralysis of one or both vocal cords is not uncommon.

The cause is obscure in many cases. In the case of unilateral paralysis, the right cord is most frequently involved. When the left cord is paralyzed, there may be associated cardiac abnormalities, such as patent ductus arteriosus. Bilateral cord paralysis is usually associated with other central nervous system abnormalities, such as Arnold-Chiari syndrome. In these cases, the onset of paralysis is probably related to increasing hydrocephalus, since the cord paralysis is not manifest until 4 to 6 weeks after birth when hydrocephalus becomes marked. When cord paralysis is present, it will often disappear after ventricular tap and insertion of a Holter valve.

Clinical Manifestations. The infant has a weak or hoarse cry, inspiratory stridor, and difficulty with feeding. Stridor is most marked during activity and crying and often disappears at rest if paralysis is unilateral. Bilateral paralysis causes more severe obstructive symptoms.

Diagnosis is made by direct laryngoscopy with the blade of the laryngoscope inserted in the vallecula. If the laryngoscope is inserted in the larynx, it may tense the vocal cord and give a false impression of paralysis.

Treatment. In most cases of unilateral paralysis, spontaneous regression occurs within 6 months. However, a search should be made for any etiologic factor. Persistent unilateral paralysis usually does not require definitive therapy since it is well compensated for by infants.

Bilateral cord paralysis frequently requires insertion of a tracheostomy tube, which must be left in place until regression of cord paralysis or surgical widening of the glottis occurs.

CRI DU CHAT SYNDROME

First described in 1963, the syndrome is recognized by a weak mewing cry in infancy and early childhood. This may be associated with respiratory stridor, mental retardation, hypertelorism, antimongoloid palpebral fissures, and failure to thrive. However, the syndrome is usually first detected because of a very abnormal cry. The syndrome is caused by a deletion of the short arm of chromosome 5.

The laryngeal findings consist of a flaccid epiglottis and a diamond-shaped glottic chunk on inspiration, with persistent air leak in the posterior commissure on phonation. There is no specific treatment.

LARYNGOMALACIA

Laryngomalacia is a specific entity referring to excessive flaccidity of the supraglottic portions of the larynx and is only one of the causes of congenital laryngeal stridor.

Clinical Manifestations. The symptoms of inspiratory stridor and suprasternal indrawing may be present at birth or may arise several weeks later. The stridor is often inconstant, being absent one moment and extremely marked a short while later. It tends to be worse with the child supine and is usually better with the infant in the prone position; also, it is often absent when the infant is asleep. Usually, cyanosis and severe dyspnea are not present. However, in situations of unusual stimulus or during respiratory infection, the symptoms may be marked, with severe respiratory embarrassment requiring urgent therapy. In some cases the stridor interferes with feeding, the child fails to thrive, and the respiratory difficulty increases. The voice and cry are usually relatively normal.

Etiology. The cause of the excessive flaccidity of the structures surrounding the laryngeal vestibule is unknown, but the disorder is probably the result of several factors.

The infant epiglottis is typically "omega-shaped," the lateral margins being parallel to the aryepiglottic folds. The result is that the aryepiglottic folds are poorly supported. Exaggeration of the omega shape of the epiglottis, bulky aryepiglottic folds, and excessive tissue flaccidity are probably present to some degree in each case. The syndrome appears to be more common in lower socioeconomic groups, and poor nutrition may be an etiologic factor.

Diagnosis. It is important to rule out other causes of stridor in the infant. Direct laryngoscopy is always indicated. The laryngoscope blade must be inserted in the vallec-ula to make the diagnosis. On inspiration, the structures around the vestibule, particularly the aryepiglottic folds, will be seen to invaginate with the synchronous production of the stridulous sound. The stridor can be relieved by inserting the laryngoscope into the vestibule of the larynx.

After the diagnosis of laryngomalacia is made, care must be taken to rule out an associated tracheomalacia or bronchomalacia. This may be done by examination of expiratory and inspiratory roentgenograms of the chest.

Treatment. In most cases, active treatment is not necessary, and the condition usually subsides spontaneously by the age of 2 years. At times, these infants may have severe respiratory difficulty, but this usually occurs in association with an upper respiratory infection. In such a situation, tracheostomy may be necessary.

Surgical procedures, such as partial epiglottectomy or denuding the surface of the base of tongue and epiglottis to cause adhesions and increase the rigidity of the supraglottis, have been described but are rarely necessary. Most patients are from lower socioeconomic groups, and attention should be given to assuring an adequate diet. Immunization programs must be completed and careful treatment of any respiratory infection instituted.

MICROGNATHIA, GLOSSOPTOSIS, AND RESPIRATORY OBSTRUCTION (PIERRE ROBIN SYNDROME)

Micrognathia with glossoptosis is responsible for respiratory obstruction in some newborn infants. When these deformities are associated with a cleft palate, the entity is termed the Pierre Robin syndrome. Although cleft palate is frequently associated with these abnormalities, the association of cleft lip is rare. The cause of the deformity is unknown, although it is familial in some instances.

Since the hyoid bone, base of the tongue, and epiglottis are dependent upon their attachments to the mandible to hold them forward, a deficiency in the size of the mandible results in loss of support. The base of the tongue, therefore, falls posteriorly and approximates the posterior pharyngeal wall, occluding the airway. The tongue itself is probably of normal size, and macroglossia is not an important factor. When cleft palate is present, the tip of the tongue may be trapped in the cleft, which will hold the tongue in a posterior position. Tongue-tie (ankyloglossia) is often present and prevents normal forward movement of the tongue.

Diagnosis. The infant presents a typical appearance characterized by a small recessed chin with the lower alveolus 1 cm or more posterior to the upper alveolus. The term "Andy Gump" has been applied to this picture (Fig. 27–7).

Respiratory obstruction results from a ball valve obstruction of the pharynx secondary to glossoptosis. The obstruction may not be marked at birth but becomes much worse during the next few days as the infant becomes weaker because of feeding difficulties. Frequently the obstruction is episodic, attacks of cyanosis, stridor, and indrawing occurring when the infant is su-

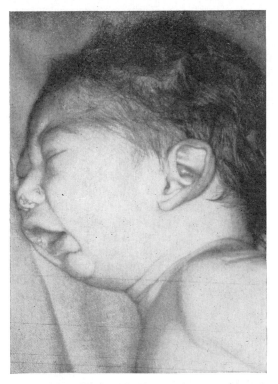

FIG. 27–7. Pierre Robin syndrome with micrognathia, glossoptosis, and cleft palate.

pine, being fed, or asleep. The airway can be improved by placing the infant in a prone position.

Feeding problems are marked. Because of glossoptosis, deglutition is altered, and these infants eat only small amounts, while aspirating frequently. Failure to thrive and repeated respiratory infections result in a worsening of the obstructive symptoms, producing a syndrome of respiratory cachexia.

Treatment. The treatment will vary with the degree of respiratory obstruction, and keeping an infant in a prone position will overcome minor degrees of obstruction. However, if an infant is having difficulty with feeding, the obstructive symptoms will usually get worse before improvement can be expected, and surgical treatment should be instituted early. In the meantime, feeding should be done by gavage. In severely debilitated infants, a feeding gastrostomy may be advantageous.

Tracheostomy will relieve the respiratory obstruction but it does not alter the problems of deglutition and aspiration, which create a difficult nursing problem. Also, the complications, especially with decannulation, are greatly increased in these small, feeble infants. Therefore, tracheostomy is best avoided.

The tongue must be fixed in an anterior position; when this is done, the obstruction and feeding difficulties are usually relieved. Some form of temporary glossopexy is imperative when a history of cyanotic attacks and aspiration is elicited, because the symptoms of glossoptosis will increase in severity before spontaneous improvement occurs. In the majority of cases, the growth of the micrognathic mandible "catches up" with the remainder of the facial structures by the end of the first year. Therefore, glossopexy is a temporary requirement.

The mortality of infants with this syndrome treated conservatively has been variously reported between 30 and 65%. Douglas has reported, on the other hand, only one death in a series of 30 patients treated surgically. Several procedures have been described for glossopexy.

Douglas Operation. This entails denuding an area on the undersurface of the tongue and posterior surface of the lower lip and approximating these surfaces in order to obtain an adhesion to hold the tongue forward. Modifications of this procedure have been proposed by Routledge and Ryan which avoid removal of mucosa from the undersurface of the tongue and floor of the mouth. The disadvantages of these procedures include bleeding, infection, and possible damage to Wharton's ducts. There is no guarantee, even with good healing, that the tongue will be far enough forward to give relief of dyspnea, principally because of the short anterior tongue in these infants. Also, the glossolabial attachment must be taken down at a later second operation (Fig. 27–8).

Kirschner Wire. The insertion of a Kirschner wire through the angles of the mandible and the base of the tongue with the tongue pulled forward has been advocated. The main disadvantage of this procedure is the increasing possibility of infection and osteomyelitis the longer the wire is in place. In some cases, dyspnea will persist for several weeks, and it is not possible to leave the wire in place long enough. The procedure may be of value when the tongue has been badly torn by previous attempts at glossopexy.

Duhamel Suture. We have found this method of treatment consistent in giving adequate relief of dyspnea and avoiding tracheostomy. The advantages are that it is simple, can be done at bedside, and gives immediate results.

A 2–0 silk suture is passed through each side of the base of the tongue as far posteriorly as possible. A small piece of silicon

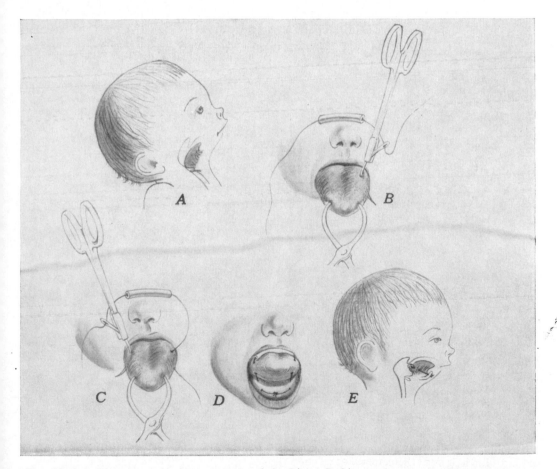

Fig. 27–8. Glossopexy in the treatment of the Pierre Robin syndrome. *A*, Glossoptosis causing obstruction of the larynx. *B*, *C*, Insertion of the suture to pull the tongue anteriorly. *D*, Suture inserted through the mandible and tied. *E*, Result of glossopexy.

tubing may be threaded on the suture exposed at the base of the tongue, to prevent it from pulling through. Each end of the suture is brought out through the floor of the mouth on each side of the tongue; then, using a cutting needle, the end of the suture is passed through the mandible anteriorly. The ends of the suture are tied snugly across the front of the mandible with the tongue held in the desired position. The suture may be left in place for several weeks without danger to the tooth buds.

DYSPLASTIC DYSPHONIA

A form of dysphonia may result from minor congenital abnormalities of one or both vocal cords.

Etiology. The basis of the disorder is a bowing of one or both true cords, which results in an elliptical glottis. Hypoplasia of one or both vocal cords or congenital vocal cord sulcus are the most common causes. The elliptical glottic shape is the same as that necessary to produce the male falsetto voice; therefore, when phonation is attempted, an abnormal unpleasant voice is produced.

Some patients, in an effort to compensate for the disorder, will develop a secondary hyperkinetic dysphonia, such as dysphonia plicae ventricularis.

Clinical Manifestations. The abnormal voice is noted soon after speech begins. The hoarseness has a peculiar, dead, nonresonating quality. The pitch tends to be ele-

Table 27–1.   Classification of Common Causes of Inspiratory Stridor in Newborn Infants (Congenital Laryngeal Stridor)

I. Endolaryngeal Causes	II. Extralaryngeal Causes

A. Congenital
  1. Laryngomalacia
  2. Congenital stenosis (webs, etc.)
  3. Bifid epiglottis
	A. Congenital
	  1. Tracheomalacia and bronchomalacia
	  2. Micrognathia and glossoptosis
	  3. Tracheoesophageal fistula
	  4. Lingual thyroid
	  5. Vascular rings formed by the great vessels

B. Tumors and cysts
  1. Papilloma of the larynx
  2. Cysts (mucoceles)
  3. Hemangioma
  4. Chondroma
	B. Tumors and cysts
	  1. Enlargement of the thymus
	  2. Cystic hygroma
	  3. Thyroglossal duct cysts
	  4. Branchial cleft cysts
	  5. Enlargement of the thyroid gland (congenital goiter)

C. Foreign bodies
  1. In the larynx
	C. Foreign bodies
	  1. In the trachea or bronchi
	  2. In the esophagus

D. Inflammatory
  1. Acute nonspecific laryngitis
  2. Allergic edema
  3. Acute membranous laryngitis	

E. Neurologic
  1. Vocal cord paralysis, unilateral or bilateral
  2. Neonatal tetany (laryngismus stridulus)	

F. Trauma
  1. Birth injury (hematoma or edema)
  2. Endotracheal intubation
  3. Nasogastric intubation	

vated, since high tones are less affected by the glottic configuration. The voice is breathy and weak, and phonation time is decreased.

Examination of the larynx may disclose an obvious hypoplasia of a vocal cord, which results in poor approximation of the vocal cords. A congenital vocal cord sulcus may be noted, which consists of a fine longitudinal furrow on the medial margin of the vocal cord. The furrow may involve all or part of any or both true vocal cords. When the sulcus is complete, the condition is called a double vocal cord. In the presence of sulcus vocalis, vocal cord approximation is poor, and an abnormally high-pitched or falsetto voice is the result.

Treatment. Since the basic cause of this problem is hypoplasia of the vocalis muscle, treatment is directed at correcting this by increasing the vocal cord bulk. This may be done by injecting silicone or Teflon paste into the true vocal cord. Voice therapy may be helpful and should be given to avoid secondary hyperkinetic dysphonia.

CONGENITAL LARYNGEAL STRIDOR

Congenital laryngeal stridor is a term which appears often in the literature and is used by some physicians interchangeably with laryngomalacia. However, it is a term describing a symptom only; therefore, it is defined as laryngeal stridor that is present at birth, or within 1 to 2 days after birth. The stridor is usually confined to the inspiratory phase of respiration.

Stridor in the newborn infant is a frequent problem confronting the laryngologist and requires a rapid, logical, organized assessment of the respiratory tract. Examination should always include direct laryngoscopy. The causes of congenital laryngeal stridor in newborn infants are outlined in Table 27–1.

REFERENCES

Alonso, J. M.: Treatment of Membranes and Synechiae of the Anterior Part of the Glottis. Arch. Otolaryng., *65*:111, 1957.

Arnold, G. E.: Dysplastic Dysphonia: Minor Abnormalities of the Vocal Cords Causing Persistent Hoarseness. Laryngoscope, *68*: 142, 1958.

Blumberg, J. B., *et al.*: Laryngotrachealoesophageal Cleft, The Embryologic Implications: Review of the Literature. Surgery, *57*:559, 1965.

Cavanaugh, F.: Vocal Palsies in Children. J. Laryngol., *69*:399, 1955.

DeSonto, L. W., *et al.*: Cysts of the Larynx: Classification. Laryngoscope, *80*:145, 1970.

Douglas, B.: A Further Report on the Treatment of Micrognathia with Obstruction by a Plastic Procedure. Plast. Reconstr. Surg., *5*:113, 1950.

Ferguson, C. F., and Flake, C. G.: Subglottic Hemangioma as a Cause of Respiratory Obstruction in Infants. Ann. Otol., *70*:1095, 1961.

Fredrickson, J. M., and Ward, P. H.: Laryngocele Ventricularis. Arch. Otolaryng., *76*:568, 1962.

Handley, R. C., and Johnson, J. B.: Utilization of the Kirschner Wire in Pierre Robin Syndrome. Plast. Reconstr. Surg., *31*:587, 1963.

Herwig, J. C., and Ogura, J. H.: Congenital Tracheo-esophageal Fistula Without Atresia. J. Pediatr., *47*:293, 1955.

Holinger, P. H.: Clinical Aspects of Congenital Anomalies of the Larynx, Trachea, Bronchi and Esophagus. J. Laryngol., *75*:1, 1961.

Holinger, P. H., and Steinmann, E. P.: Congenital Cysts of the Larynx. Pract. Otolaryng,. *9*:129, 1947.

Inglauer, S.: A New Procedure for the Treatment of Webs of the Larynx. Arch. Otolaryng., *22*:597, 1935.

Jensen, A. M., and Samuelsen, J.: On Laryngocele. Acta Otolaryng., *57*:475, 1964.

Lindsay, J. R.: Laryngocele Ventricularis. Ann. Otol., *49*:661, 1940.

McHugh, H. E., and Lock, W. E.: Congenital Webs of the Larynx. Laryngoscope, *52*:43, 1942.

McNaught, T. C.: Surgical Correction of Anterior Webs of the Larynx. Laryngoscope, *60*:264, 1950.

Martin, J. A. M.: Congenital Laryngeal Stridor (Laryngomalacia). J. Laryngol., *77*:290, 1963.

Montgomery, W. W., and Gamble, J. E.: Anterior Glottic Stenosis; Experimental and Clinical Management. Arch. Otolaryng., *92*:560, 1970.

Oeconomopoulas, C. T.: The Value of Glossopexy in the Pierre Robin Syndrome. New Engl. J. Med., *262*:1267, 1960.

Pierce, M. K.: Subglottic Hemangiomas in
  Infants. A Presumptive Clinical Test for
  Diagnosis. Ann. Otol., *71*:1057, 1962.
Robin, P.: Glossoptosis Due to Atresia and
  Hypotrophy of the Mandible. Am. J. Dis.
  Child., *48*:541, 1934.
Routledge, R. T.: The Pierre Robin Syndrome:
  A Surgical Emergency in the Neonatal
  Period. Br. J. Plast. Surg., *13*:204, 1960.
Ryan, R. F., *et al.*: Anterior Fixation of the
  Tongue. Plast. Reconstr. Surg., *32*:318,
  1963.
Schwartz, L.: Congenital Laryngeal Stridor.
  Arch. Otolaryng., *39*:403, 1944.
Smith, I. I., and Bain, A. D.: Congenital
  Atresia of the Larynx. Ann. Otol., *74*:338,
  1965.
Ward, P. H., *et al.*: The Larynx in the Cri Du
  Chat (Cat Cry) Syndrome. Trans. Am.
  Acad. Ophthal. Otolaryng., *72*:90, 1968.

Chapter 28
Trauma to the Larynx

Etiology. The causes of trauma to the larynx are listed in Table 28–1. The most frequent cause of injury to the larynx is the blunt trauma associated with smashing of the neck on the steering wheel or instrument panel during an automobile accident. The incidence of injury following endoscopic procedures and indwelling nasogastric tubes is decreasing because of improved techniques, instrumentation, and awareness of the possibility of injury. Irradiation injuries to the larynx are still frequent despite improved techniques, possibly because of the increased willingness of the therapist to deliver larger doses of irradiation in the treatment of carcinoma. Autogenous trauma to the larynx results chiefly from vocal misuse. It is occurring with increasing frequency in America because of increasing pressures and demands on the individual in present-day life.

The pathogenesis and therefore the treatment of any laryngeal injury may be divided into two stages. The first is the acute stage, and the second is the chronic stage or stage of sequelae. This chapter will deal with acute laryngeal trauma. Treatment of the chronic stage of laryngeal trauma becomes treatment of chronic laryngeal stenosis, which will be discussed in a subsequent chapter.

Pathophysiology of Acute Laryngeal Injury. The structure and location of the larynx are such that injury to the organ is followed by the development of lesions producing distinctive signs and symptoms.

The distensibility of the submucosal tissue of the larynx, particularly in the supraglottic portions, permits the rapid accumulation of fluid or blood; therefore, laryngeal edema or hematoma typically involves the aryepiglottic folds and false vocal cords. Since fluid or blood accumulation may be rapid, symptoms of laryngeal obstruction may appear abruptly.

The mucosal lining of the larynx and pharynx is easily torn by traumatic forces,

Table 28–1. Causes of Laryngeal Trauma

I. Mechanical Injury
  1. External
    a. Auto accidents
    b. Other blunt neck injuries
    c. Complication of tracheostomy
    d. Cricothyrotomy
  2. Internal
    a. Endoscopic procedures
    b. Endotracheal intubation
    c. Indwelling nasogastric tubes

II. Burns of Larynx
  1. Thermal burns
    a. Ingestion of hot food or liquid
    b. Inhalation of hot air or gas
  2. Chemical burns
    a. Lye (NaOH, KOH)
    b. Ammonia
    c. Sodium hypochlorite (Clorox)
    d. Orthophenylphenol (Lysol)

III. Irradiation Injury

IV. Autogenous Trauma (voice abuse)

---

and this may be followed by the rapid appearance of subcutaneous emphysema. Also, the dehiscence of the mucosal barrier permits contamination of the deep tissues of the neck, followed by the development of cellulitis, abscess, and, perhaps, fistulous tracts.

Fractures and dislocations of the laryngeal cartilages and joints of a wide variety occur, and they tend to be more severe in the less resilient, calcified cartilages of older individuals. Perichondrial injury is often associated with and may lead to subperichondrial hematoma and devascularization and necrosis of hyaline cartilage. If the area is contaminated by connection with the laryngeal lumen, perichondritis and chondritis may follow.

Healing of laryngeal injuries is by granulation and eventual fibrosis. Since the wounds are usually secondarily infected, epithelization is often delayed, with the result that excessive granulation and fibrous tissue are laid down. Cicatrization is followed by deformity and considerable permanent alteration in laryngeal function, and patency may develop secondary to relatively minor injuries.

Clinical Manifestations. In any patient who has sustained a possible laryngeal injury, the following symptoms are indicative of some derangement of laryngeal structure: (1) increasing airway obstruction with dyspnea and stridor; (2) dysphonia or aphonia; (3) cough; (4) hemoptysis and hematemesis; (5) neck pain; (6) dysphagia and odynophagia.

The preceding symptoms may be accompanied by the following distinctive clinical signs: (1) deformities of the neck, including alterations in contour and swelling; (2) subcutaneous emphysema; (3) laryngeal tenderness; (4) bony crepitus. The presence of airway obstruction and subcutaneous emphysema is diagnostic of a severe disruption of laryngeal or tracheal structure.

Diagnosis. The presence of any of the preceding clinical manifestations is a basis for assuming a severe injury and is an indication for indirect and direct laryngoscopy and bronchoscopy to determine the presence of edema, hematoma, mucosal tears, cartilage displacement, and vocal cord paralysis. Roentgenograms of the neck and chest must be obtained to detect laryngeal fractures, tracheal injuries, and pneumothorax.

Early Treatment. The initial treatment of any acute laryngeal injury requires the establishment of an adequate airway, which may necessitate tracheostomy. This is followed by an assessment of the injury and determination of the necessity for further definitive treatment, which may be carried out immediately or may be delayed as dictated by the clinical situation.

Frequently, a laryngeal injury is only one of multiple injuries resulting from an automobile accident. Unfortunately, in many such situations, a tracheostomy is performed but no further thought is given to the larynx until the time arrives for decannulation, when the presence of dysphonia, aphonia, or persistent obstruction is noted. By this time, it is usually too late to perform a definitive, simple repair, and it is necessary to accept the less desirable results of delayed repair. Therefore, laryngeal trauma must be considered in any patient requiring tracheostomy who has a history of possible neck trauma.

SPECIFIC MECHANICAL LARYNGEAL INJURIES AND THEIR TREATMENT

Edema and Hematoma

Edema and hematoma formation in the loose supraglottic and subglottic tissues are common to almost all laryngeal injuries. They may constitute the sole pathologic findings in some injuries, but care must be taken to rule out the presence of any underlying cartilaginous injury (Fig. 28–1).

Usually, edema and hematoma will resolve spontaneously and completely in the absence of any other injury. Treatment should include absolute voice rest and humidification of inspired air. The use of corticosteroid preparations is of value in reducing inflammatory response and preventing progression of edema. Sometimes temporary tracheostomy is necessary to relieve obstruction.

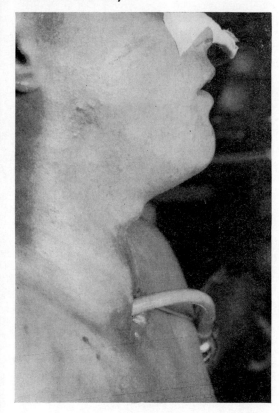

FIG. 28–1. Deformity of the neck following a crushing injury to the larynx.

Dislocation or Luxation of the Cricothyroid Joints

Disturbance of the cricothyroid articulation may follow any trauma to the anterior neck and may be unilateral or bilateral. The injury may result in temporary or permanent disarticulation. Cricothyroid dislocation may follow very minor trauma, and the presence of the deformity is often undetected. The inferior cornu of the thyroid cartilage is usually displaced posteriorly in relation to the cricoid cartilage. This may produce a deficiency in the tensor mechanism of the vocal cord on the side of the injury; also, the recurrent laryngeal nerve may be injured in its position just behind the joint, causing vocal cord paralysis.

In some instances, only a temporary luxation, noted by the patient as a snapping sensation in the neck, may occur. The luxa-tion may become recurrent, in which case it occurs with swallowing and yawning.

Clinical Manifestations. At the time of injury, there is usually pain in the neck, which may radiate to the ear. A snapping sensation may be felt in the neck. In patients without vocal cord paralysis, some change in voice is noted, but with vocal cord paralysis, hoarseness, weakness of the voice, and aspiration on swallowing may be present. Usually aspiration is temporary, and the voice will undergo considerable spontaneous improvement.

Diagnosis. Diagnosis is difficult, but dislocation may be suspected when the patient can voluntarily dislocate the joint or when there is vocal cord paralysis associated with minor neck trauma. Examination of the larynx may disclose some bowing and lack of tension of the cord on the affected side or evidence of acute paralysis of a vocal cord. Soft tissue roentgenograms of the larynx may demonstrate a fracture through the inferior cornu of the thyroid cartilage or dislocation of the joint, if the cartilages are well calcified.

Treatment. Only patients with persistent vocal cord paralysis, persistent dysphonia, or recurrent dislocation require treatment. Paralysis of the vocal cord, with this injury, is often temporary, and spontaneous return of function usually occurs in 3 to 4 weeks. Paralysis lasting more than 6 to 8 weeks is unlikely to resolve spontaneously. The patients should be observed for this period of time, and then consideration should be given to decompression of the recurrent laryngeal nerve if no return of function is evident. Electromyographic studies of the paralyzed cord may be helpful in determining the need for decompression.

Patients with persistent vocal cord paralysis or bothersome, habitual dislocation may be benefited by resection of the inferior cornu of the thyroid cartilage. Many patients with persistent cord paralysis have only physiologic block (neuropraxia) to nerve conduction, and decompression of the nerve by excision of the cornu permits a rapid return of function. The prognosis for return of function of a vocal cord paralyzed more than 4 months is poor.

When dysphonia is a serious complaint and decompression is not feasible, improvement in voice may be obtained by the intrachordal injection of silicone or Teflon paste.

Dislocation of the Cricoarytenoid Joint

Etiology. Dislocation of the cricoarytenoid joint may be due to internal or external trauma. A direct blow to the neck forcing the cricoid cartilage posteriorly against the cervical vertebrae may precipitate anterior dislocation of the arytenoid. In such cases, injury to other parts of the larynx is often present. Endoscopic procedures are also a cause of this injury. Dislocation may result if the end of the esophagoscope catches on and dislocates an arytenoid cartilage, or if extreme force is exerted on the vocal cord while a bronchoscope or endotracheal tube is being passed, which pulls the arytenoid into a dislocated position. The arytenoid may be dislocated anteriorly or posteriorly, but anterior dislocation is most frequent and is usually accompanied by some lateral displacement of the cartilage. Rarely, dislocation may be bilateral.

Clinical Manifestations. The symptoms include hoarseness, pain, and, if edema is severe, dyspnea and stridor. Difficulties with deglutition occur, causing dysphagia, odynophagia, and aspiration. Examination may disclose edema involving the arytenoid area and aryepiglottic fold, which obscures the vocal process and vocal cord. In the absence of edema or after it subsides, the arytenoid will be seen to be tipped forward and rotated medially, while the vocal cord is bowed, flaccid, and immobilized in an intermediate position. The posterior portion of the vocal cord may be hidden by the arytenoid and corniculate cartilages, which are tipped forward. This deformity may permit the superior surface of the cricoid lamina to be seen as a small shelf posterior to the mound of the arytenoid. When the patient is asked to phonate, the vocal cords do not completely approximate, and the displaced arytenoid may move further anteriorly unless it is fixed by scar tissue.

Diagnosis. Direct laryngoscopy should be performed, and in addition to visual inspection, the dislocated arytenoid should be palpated with a laryngeal spatula to test its mobility. A dislocated arytenoid will not have the same mobility as an arytenoid in normal position. However, in long-standing cases of arytenoid dislocation, the arytenoid becomes fixed by cicatricial tissue, and since this also occurs in long-standing cases of paralysis of neurogenic origin, passive mobility tests will be of little diagnostic value in older injuries. Electromyographic studies may be used to demonstrate the existence of normal innervation of the muscles.

Treatment. At the time of acute injury, tracheostomy may be necessary because of edema. After the edema has subsided, it may be possible to reduce the arytenoid by direct manual manipulation with a laryngeal spatula. Pressure is exerted on the lateral surface of the vocal process and body of the arytenoid to lift and push the cartilage in a medioposterior direction into its normal relation to the cricoid cartilage. In some cases, it is possible to effect reduction by inserting an anterior commissure laryngoscope well into the larynx and exerting pressure in an anterior direction while depending on the tension of the vocal cord to pull the arytenoid into position. The posterior surface of the laryngoscope forces the superior tip of the arytenoid posteriorly to aid in the reduction. Usually, reduction is only possible when the patient is seen within 14 days of injury.

When reduction is not possible, disability may persist due to severe dysphonia and dysphagia caused by an incompetent glottis. These problems may be eliminated by the performance of a "reverse King operation" or the intrachordal injection of Teflon paste or silicone.

Fractures of the Hyoid Bone

This injury may occur as an isolated result of neck trauma or in association with fractures of the other laryngeal cartilages.

Clinical Manifestations. The fracture may involve any part of the hyoid bone, but generally it occurs in the central body area because of the resiliency of the cornua.

Isolated fracture of the hyoid is more common in women. At the time of acute injury, there is pain and swelling over the upper anterior neck, and bony crepitus may be noted on palpation of the neck and on swallowing. The patient usually has odynophagia and may complain of the grating of the fracture fragments.

Diagnosis. The fracture can usually be seen on soft tissue roentgenograms of the larynx.

Indirect and direct laryngoscopic examinations are necessary to rule out an associated avulsion of the epiglottis.

Treatment. At the time of injury, there may be supraglottic edema and hematoma formation of sufficient degree to produce airway obstruction and require tracheostomy.

Because of the intimate relation of the hyoid bone with the muscles of deglutition, delayed union or nonunion of fractures is common. This may result in persistent discomfort associated with deglutition.

Fractures of the body of the hyoid should be immobilized and approximated by direct interosseous wiring using No. 28 stainless steel wire. The wire may be left in place indefinitely. In cases of symptomatic nonunion, the area of the fracture may be excised to separate the fragments.

Fractures of the Thyroid and Cricoid Cartilages

Fractures of these cartilages may be divided into three groups: supraglottic, glottic, and infraglottic. Combinations of these injuries may occur, but most often they are present as isolated entities.

Supraglottic Injury. The front seat passengers are more commonly injured in automobile accidents. The higher incidence of injury among women is probably a result of their relatively longer, slimmer necks and shorter statures, so that it is the upper neck that comes into contact with the instrument panel or steering wheel. Also, females are more often passengers than males.

Pathology. The upper part of one or both thyroid alae is often fractured, although no displacement fracture may be present. The important injury is an avulsion of the attachments of the epiglottis and one or both false cords from the thyroid cartilage. This allows posterior displacement of the epiglottis, which may obliterate the vestibular lumen

(Fig. 28–2). As a result of rupture of the hyoepiglottic ligament, a false passage may be created anterior to the epiglottis; this may empty into the laryngeal cavity at a lower level or pass anterior to the thyroid cartilage into the lower neck. Occasionally, an associated unilateral or bilateral vocal cord paralysis may be present at the time of the acute injury. In addition to the laryngeal injury, vertical tears of the posterior pharyngeal wall are common.

Supraglottic injuries are associated with contamination and infection, and healing begins with production of granulation tissue and ends with fibrosis and scar contracture. The epiglottis becomes fixed in a posterior position by scarring. Also, fixation of the arytenoids may occur secondary to the healing process. The end result in an untreated injury is supraglottic laryngeal stenosis.

Clinical Manifestations. Cervical emphysema and airway obstruction are common. Any of the manifestations of acute laryngeal injury may be present, but some are peculiar to supraglottic injury: (1) a normal, but muffled, voice in the face of increasing airway obstruction; (2) signs of coughing and aspiration on attempting to eat or swallow liquids; (3) appearance of food or liquid at the tracheostomy opening without coughing or choking, indicating an extralaryngeal fistula; (4) flattening of the upper neck contour and failure to palpate the thyroid notch.

Diagnosis. Any patient with a neck injury, cervical emphysema, and airway obstruction must have a direct laryngoscopy performed. Direct laryngoscopy will demonstrate soft tissue swelling, cartilage displacement, and vocal cord paralysis. Fistula tracts into the pre-epiglottic space may be difficult to demonstrate, and the vallecula must be carefully inspected with the vestibule at direct laryngoscopy. Laryngograms and cineradiography studies are often necessary to detect the presence and site of a sinus or fistula. Aqueous Dionosil should be used for such studies, and barium should never be given to these patients for obvious reasons. These studies should be carried out as soon as the patient's condition is stabilized after the acute injury.

Glottic Injuries. *Pathology.* With this injury, the thyroid cartilage is fractured in the

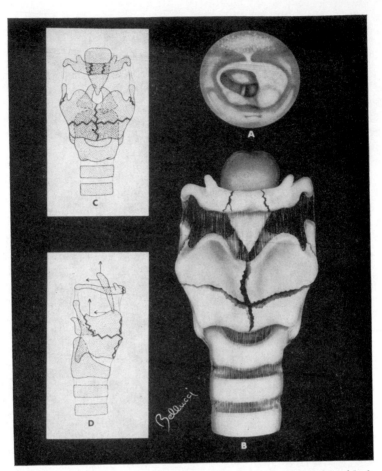

Fig. 28–2. Supraglottic type of laryngeal injury with fracture of the thyroid alae and posterior displacement of the epiglottis. This may be followed by supraglottic stenosis (*A*) in untreated cases. *B, C,* Cartilage injury. *D,* Displacement of epiglottis and arytenoid.

region of attachment of the true vocal cords. The fractures may be vertical or transverse. There is frequently displacement of the fragments in their relation to each other. At the same time, the vocal cords are displaced or actually disrupted by the cartilage displacement. Mucosal tears are common (Fig. 28–3). Vocal cord paralysis secondary to nerve damage or disruption of the cricoarytenoid joint may be present primarily.

Healing in the untreated case frequently results in glottic stenosis.

Clinical Manifestations. Subcutaneous emphysema is present. Marked alteration of the voice and laryngeal obstruction are usually noted. The cartilage deformity may be palpated through the skin of the anterior neck.

Edema and mucosal tears in the endolarynx are common in the acute injury. Foreshortening of the anteroposterior diameter of the glottic chink may be observed, although this may become apparent only after edema subsides. Laceration or avulsion of a vocal cord, with the exposure of pieces of fractured cartilage, may be seen. Displacement of one or both arytenoids or simple vocal cord paralysis due to nerve injury are often observed. The vocal cords may be paralyzed in the median or paramedian position.

Laryngograms are often more consistent

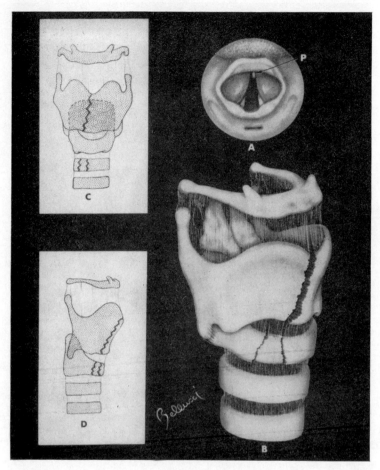

FIG. 28–3. Glottic type of laryngeal injury with vertical fracture of the thyroid ala and displacement of cartilage into the laryngeal lumen (*A*). *B, C, D*, Cartilages fractured and displaced.

in outlining alterations in the endolaryngeal configuration and in demonstrating fistula or sinus formation than direct laryngoscopy.

Infraglottic Injuries. This injury is seen most frequently in males who have experienced blunt trauma in an auto accident.

Pathology. There is a crushing injury of the cricoid cartilage and upper tracheal rings. The anterior part of the cricoid may have one or two simple fractures or may be fragmented. In many cases, the cricoid injury is associated with crushing and separation of the upper tracheal rings. Occasionally, the injury is limited to the upper trachea, which may be completely avulsed from its attachment to the cricoid cartilage

and retract into the upper mediastinum (Fig. 28–4).

Devascularized pieces of cartilage are produced, and, as a result, perichondritis of the cricoid cartilage is a common complication. Because of infection, healing is delayed, and excessive granulation and fibrous tissues are produced. Since the cricoid is a circular cartilage and is located at the level of the narrowest point of the laryngeal lumen, minor injuries, if untreated, frequently cause stenosis.

Vocal cord paralysis, often bilateral, frequently accompanies this injury as a result of disturbance of the cricothyroid joints and injury to the recurrent laryngeal nerves.

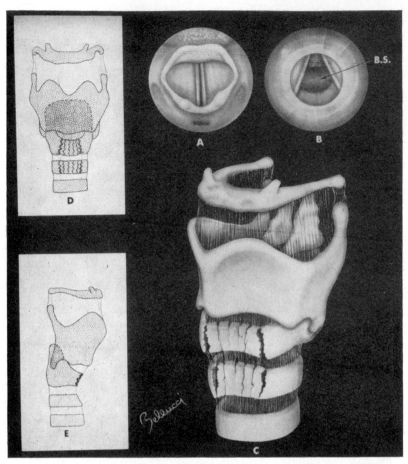

FIG. 28–4. Crushing injury of the larynx with fracture of the cricoid cartilage and upper tracheal ring, accompanied by bilateral vocal cord paralysis (*A*) and infraglottic stenosis (**B**). *C, D, E,* Cartilages fractured and displaced. *B.S.,* Blind sac.

Principles of Treatment of Acute Laryngeal Fractures

Most of these patients arrive in the emergency room with signs of laryngeal obstruction, and tracheostomy is indicated immediately. At this time, care should be taken to perform the tracheostomy in the proper place below the second tracheal ring. If a cricothyrotomy has been done of necessity, steps should be taken to move the tracheostomy as soon as the patient's condition is stabilized. It is disconcerting to see the number of these patients who must suffer the consequences of laryngeal stenosis because of poorly placed or inept tracheostomy.

Suspicion and recognition of the acute laryngeal injury are imperative. Many of these patients have multiple injuries and may be unconscious at the time of admission; a tracheostomy is performed, and the possibility of laryngeal injury is not considered until the time for decannulation, when it is discovered that the patient is still obstructed, but by this time fibrosis and stenosis are well developed. Therefore, direct and indirect laryngoscopy are indicated whenever a laryngeal fracture is suspected.

Surgical exploration of the larynx is indicated in any neck injury with symptoms of stridor, voice change, cartilage disruption, and cervical emphysema. Exploration of laryngeal fracture is best performed through a horizontal incision at the level of the previous tracheostomy incision to minimize scarring of the anterior neck. A skin flap is elevated superiorly to expose the desired portion of the larynx, and the presence of a fracture is confirmed by direct palpation.

Most of these injuries are compound by virtue of a mucosal tear into the larynx or pharynx. Some injuries may be compound with an opening on the external surface of the neck. Patients seen within 48 hours of injury may be treated for acute injuries by immediate reduction of fractures and closure of the wound with adequate drainage. After this time it is best to debride the wound, splint the fracture, and leave the wound open before closing it secondarily.

Laryngeal cartilage fractures, like any other fracture, must be reduced and immobilized. To be effective in avoiding chronic stenosis, reduction and fixation must be carried out within 7 to 10 days of the time of injury. A laryngeal fracture is splinted principally by means of a mold or stent in the laryngeal lumen. A rubber finger-cot, filled with Ivalon sponge, or a silicone laryngeal mold may be used. These molds do not cause as much epithelial injury as do more firm stents. The stent is usually inserted through a thyrotomy or infrahyoid laryngotomy and is fixed above and below by Mersiline sutures passed through the skin. In a few cases in which cartilage damage is minimal, the stent may be inserted through the mouth by direct laryngoscopy.

The stent is fixed in a position so that the upper end is at the level of the aryepiglottic folds and the lower end is just above the tracheostomy site. It should be left in place for 4 to 8 weeks depending on the site or type of injury. Internal splinting of the larynx should be done in most external laryngeal injuries, since the disadvantages of a stent are far outweighed by the problems of a chronic stenosis; also, some amazingly minimal injuries may end with stenosis.

Avulsion of the Epiglottis. When the epiglottis has been completely avulsed from its attachments to the thyroid cartilage and the aryepiglottic folds, it is best to excise it rather than to attempt to reposition it. If there is no associated fracture of thyroid cartilage, the endolarynx may be approached through the thyrohyoid membrane. The remaining attachments of the epiglottis to the tongue are severed, and the epiglottis is removed. Any lacerations of the pharynx should be closed at this time.

A stent is placed in the larynx to extend above the level of the suture line and is fixed in place. The pharyngotomy is closed by approximating the base of the tongue and the hyoid bone to the thyroid cartilage. The use of stainless steel wire sutures between the hyoid and thyroid cartilages is helpful in maintaining the closure.

The patient is fed by nasogastric tube for 8 to 10 days to avoid laryngeal motion, and then oral feedings are started. The stent is left in for 4 weeks; its removal through the mouth is easily accomplished as a minor office procedure.

Fractures of the Thyroid Cartilage. In the presence of such an injury, a thyrotomy should be done carefully in the midline so that the interior of the larynx may be explored. Mucosal tears should be carefully sutured with fine chromic catgut. The epiglottis may be sutured forward to the hyoid bone and thyroid cartilage if it has been only slightly avulsed; otherwise, it should be excised. Dislocated arytenoid cartilages should be replaced in their correct relation to the cricoid cartilage. If bilateral vocal cord paralysis secondary to nerve injury is present, nothing is done to correct it unless there is an obvious dislocation of the cricothyroid joint. Frequently, there will be a return of function of one or both paralyzed vocal cords in 3 to 4 weeks.

A silicone stent is placed in the larynx, and the thyrotomy is closed. Fractures of the thyroid cartilage should also be approximated with fine No. 32 stainless steel wire. Loose pieces of cartilage should be removed, since they will only act as foreign bodies in an already contaminated wound. The wound is closed with Penrose drains in place.

If bilateral vocal cord paralysis persists over 4 weeks postinjury, a decompression of the recurrent laryngeal nerve or an arytenoidopexy may be performed.

Fractures of the Cricoid Cartilage. In many such cases, there is no obvious injury to the thyroid cartilage, and thyrotomy may not be necessary if the site of injury can be adequately examined and reduced through the cricothyroid space or the tracheostomy wound. The use of a right-angled telescope may be helpful. A stent should always be inserted in patients with this injury. If a thyrotomy has not been done, then a stent is best inserted through the mouth and pulled into the larynx from below. Sometimes the cricoid is so badly smashed that it is beyond repair and must be removed; then the uppermost tracheal ring is approximated to the thyroid cartilage. Bilateral cord paralysis is usually present with the severe cricoid injuries because of severe recurrent nerve injury; when there appears to be little possibility of neural recovery, unilateral arytenoidopexy should be preformed when the cricoid is repaired.

Separation of the trachea from the cricoid cartilage or separation between the upper tracheal rings occurs frequently with this injury, and care must be taken to reapproximate these structures. The mucosa should be approximated with fine catgut, and No. 32 wire sutures should be used to approximate the cartilages. It is wise in these cases to keep the head flexed, using a head halter, for 2 weeks postoperatively.

The stent is left in place for approximately 8 weeks in the more severe type of injury.

Antibiotic therapy is probably indicated in most cases because the fractures are compound and there is a high incidence of local infection and perichondritis, which contributes to delayed healing, formation of excessive granulation tissue, and stenosis. In the absence of obvious infection, corticosteroid preparations may be of value in retarding granulation tissue formation and later fibrosis.

Laryngeal Injury Secondary to High Tracheostomy

This iatrogenic injury is the most common cause of chronic laryngeal stenosis at the present time. The tracheostomy tube is inserted through the cricothyroid membrane or through the cricoid cartilage. The injury is most common in children because the cricoid is often difficult to distinguish from a tracheal ring. The injury itself would not be harmful if the tracheostomy tube were removed in 24 hours. However, in the rush of an emergency tracheostomy, the tube position is often ignored until too late.

Pathology. If the tracheostomy has been especially traumatic, there may be fragmentation of the arch of the cricoid. However, the major source of trouble is secondary perichondritis of the cricoid, which begins about 48 hours after the operation. This is associated with the appearance of infected granulation tissue and, later, healing by fibrosis and circumferential scarring of the infraglottic airway.

Clinical Manifestations. Signs and symptoms of laryngeal obstruction are not usually evident until the time for decannulation arrives. Even then, symptoms of laryngeal obstruction may not appear for several weeks. In many instances, the voice may be quite good.

Indirect and direct laryngoscopy may disclose exuberant granulations in the infraglottic area in an injury 10 to 14 days old. Later, these are replaced by firm scar tissue, which may completely occlude the laryngeal lumen.

Diagnosis. Diagnosis of a high tracheostomy in the immediate postoperative period is highly important. If the flange of a tracheostomy tube, after a new tracheostomy, rests in the region of the center of the neck, suspicion of a misplaced tracheostomy should be aroused. If a tracheostomy tube can be easily seen just below the vocal cords by mirror examination, it is too high. A lateral roentgenogram of the neck may indicate a high tracheostomy, and one should be taken postoperatively in all cases of tracheostomy in children.

Treatment. The primary treatment is removal and replacement of the tube at a lower level. If this is done within 24 to 48 hours, no further treatment is necessary unless the cricoid has been badly damaged. In injuries over 10 days old, chronic stenosis will usually develop despite use of a stent because of the diffuse perichondritis at this time.

If the diagnosis is made more than 48 hours and less than 10 days after injury, repair, without residual deformity, can still be performed by insertion of an intralaryngeal stent. The stent can be placed by pulling it down into the larynx from the lowered tracheostomy site under laryngoscopic guidance. If granulations are present, they should be removed before the silicone stent is inserted. The stent should be left in place for 4 weeks. During this time, any perichondritis should be treated vigorously with antibiotics. Corticosteroid preparations may be used in selected patients to retard granulations.

Thermal Burns of the Larynx

Etiology. Burns of the laryngeal mucosa occur after inhalation of hot gases or smoke and are a common injury of firemen. They may also be secondary to the ingestion of excessively hot food or liquid.

Pathology. As with external burns, there may be first, second, and third degree burns. Third degree burns are uncommon, since the period of contact is usually short. First and second degree burns cause supraglottic edema with respiratory obstruction.

Clinical Manifestations. Hoarseness, pain, stridor, and respiratory obstruction may be present. Indirect laryngoscopy reveals the false cords to be red, swollen, and edematous. There may be patches of grayish exudate covering the areas of second degree burns. The true cords, if involved, are usually burned over the anterior two thirds, with redness and swelling occurring in this area.

Treatment. Emergency tracheostomy may be necessary for edematous obstruction of the larynx. However, the edema usually subsides rapidly. Adequate humidification and complete voice rest are indicated. Healing is usually prompt, and the complication of chronic stenosis is rare with this type of burn.

Chemical Burns of the Larynx

Etiology. There are many corrosive chemicals which may cause burns by ingestion or inhalation, but sodium hydroxide is the most common offender. Potassium hydroxide, Lysol, and Clorox are other commonly ingested corrosive agents; however, burns secondary to the latter two are usually not severe. Burns of the larynx are most often secondary to lye ingestion and are associated with hypopharyngeal and esophageal burns.

Pathology. Burns may be first, second, or third degree. The burned areas of the larynx include the epiglottis, the aryepiglottic folds, the arytenoids, and the postcricoid area. Third degree burns are not uncommon and are associated with full-thickness loss of mucosa. Ulceration and infection develop secondary to the burns and are followed by granulation and fibrosis. Cicatricial stenosis of the supraglottic portion of the larynx may be the end result due to adhesions between the false vocal cords or adherence of the epiglottis to the posterior pharyngeal wall. Postcricoid burns may be associated with perichondritis and destruction of the cricoid cartilage.

Clinical Manifestations. There is usually a history of chemical ingestion, and burns will be seen in the mouth and oropharynx. It is uncommon to have a burn of the larynx or hypopharynx without burns in the mouth. With severe burns, respiratory obstruction may develop secondary to edema and will appear within an hour after the burn.

Indirect laryngoscopy may disclose only redness and edema of the supraglottic structures. However, with severe burns there may be actual charring, with a gray-black membranous exudate covering the involved areas. The epiglottis may be denuded of epithelium and may appear quite white in contrast to the surrounding black areas. Cervical esophagoscopy is necessary to detect postcricoid burns.

Treatment. These burns are treated in association with hypopharyngeal and esophageal burns. Attempts to neutralize the caustic substance are usually a waste of time by the time the child is seen. The introduction of substances such as vinegar, lemon juice, and sodium bicarbonate invites aspiration and the risk of aspiration pneumonia because of alteration in sphincter function. Vomiting should not be induced, as this may subject the esophagus to a second exposure to the corrosive agent. After the airway is controlled, by tracheostomy if necessary, every effort must be made to prevent laryngeal stenosis. Broad-spectrum antibiotics and steroid preparations are given in adequate doses to retard infection and fibrosis. Insertion of a silicone stent in the supraglottic area may be of value in preventing stenosis, since most of the burning is usually around the superior margins of the laryngeal vestibule.

Patients with postcricoid burns must be watched for the development of perichondritis. The use of nasogastric tubes for feeding such patients is contraindicated, and a gastrostomy should be inserted for this purpose. Chronic supraglottic laryngeal stenosis may be the end result despite preventive efforts.

Irradiation Injury of the Larynx

Etiology. The diagnosis of carcinoma of the larynx has improved in recent years, with the result that more early lesions of the true cord are being treated by irradiation. Also, there is now a greater effort on the part of radiotherapists to deliver a cancericidal dose. Since therapy must be delivered through overlapping ports on each side of the neck, the possibility of a "hot spot" near the anterior commissure exists. This area may receive a dose far in excess of the estimated tumor dose. Also, the Ca^{++} ions in the thyroid cartilage have the effect of increasing the effective dose in the cartilage itself. The result of gamma irradiation overdose is avascular necrosis of cartilage, which may be complicated by perichondritis if the cartilage becomes secondarily infected. Other etiologic factors in addition to overdose include therapy by insufficiently trained personnel, errors in dosimetry, and poor calibration of machines. Individual tissue response to therapy is also quite variable, and some patients will develop severe complications with relatively small doses of gamma irradiation.

Laryngeal biopsy in the postirradiation larynx may precipitate perichondritis. Therefore, biopsy must be performed with extreme discrimination and care to avoid exposure of cartilage. Since the vascular supply to the cartilage is precarious, exposure of the cartilage to infection will often lead to perichondritis and chondral necrosis.

In view of the possible complications and long-term tissue alterations invoked by irradiation, there is no excuse for the treatment of benign laryngeal lesions, such as keratosis, with cancericidal doses, or in fact any dose, of irradiation therapy.

Pathology. The initial effects of irradiation involve epithelium. The ciliated epithelium ceases to function, and there is a loss of epithelial glands. The result is a mucositis with a dry, granular mucosa, areas of epithelial loss, and patches of exudate.

Edema of subepithelial tissue develops secondary to venous and lymphatic obstruction.

When a tissue dose exceeds 1000 to 1400 R, irreversible vascular injury occurs owing to endothelial proliferation and subintimal fibrosis. These changes cause obstruction of arterioles, small veins, and lymphatics, which tends to progress over several years.

Injury to cartilage is secondary to vascular impairment and is slowly progressive unless secondary infection develops. Secondary infection causes perichondritis, cartilage necrosis, and chronic laryngeal stenosis.

Clinical Manifestations. *Acute Irradiation Injury.* Most patients receiving irradiation to the area of the larynx will experience difficulty with hoarseness, sore throat, dryness, and coughing due to mucositis developing toward the end of the course of therapy. These symptoms usually subside after termination of therapy. Some patients may develop considerable edema of the larynx, which may precipitate obstruction; generally, the edema disappears, but it may persist for months or years.

In the most acute phase, the laryngeal mucosa is bright red and granular; a variable amount of translucent edema may be present in the arytenoid region. Thick, tenacious, greenish secretions are seen lying on the mucosa.

Chronic Radiation Injury of the Larynx. Cancericidal doses of irradiation destroy the seromucous glands, and many patients will complain of cough, dryness, hoarseness, and difficulty clearing secretions.

Irradiation also alters the blood and lymphatic supply of the larynx. Obstruction of

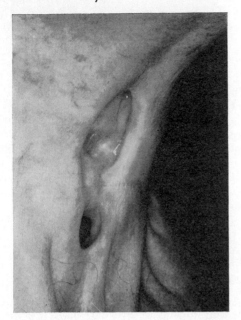

FIG. 28–5. Perichondritis and chondral necrosis following irradiation of the larynx for carcinoma.

arterioles causes a decrease in the blood supply to the already poorly supplied cartilage; thus, chondral necrosis and secondary infection may develop (Fig. 28–5). The onset of cartilage necrosis may be spontaneous and may be delayed for years after the termination of therapy, or additional trauma may be a precipitating factor. The onset of perichondritis and chondral necrosis is marked by fever, pain, tenderness, dysphonia, and increasing laryngeal obstruction. Examination of the larynx discloses redness, edema, purulent secretion, and usually impaired mobility of the true vocal cords.

Persistent laryngeal edema may be a problem after irradiation therapy. This may be worsened by lymphatic obstruction secondary to radical neck dissection. Dysphonia is the usual symptom, although obstructive symptoms are frequent. The visible portions of the larynx are involved by a pale translucent edema, and the overlying mucosa is thin, dry, and atrophic.

Diagnosis. The diagnosis of acute irradiation laryngitis is usually obvious. However, chronic irradiation injuries must be differentiated from recrudescent malignancy. This differentiation may be difficult, and indiscriminate biopsy may worsen the situation. If perichondritis is suspected, a trial of conservative therapy is indicated before direct laryngoscopy and biopsy are performed. Soft tissue roentgenograms may indicate cartilage destruction, in which case a biopsy may be performed, since some surgical procedure will be necessary whatever the diagnosis. When direct laryngoscopy is performed, the tissues should be palpated with a spatula for induration or fluctuation, and any purulent material expressed should be cultured. Biopsies should be small and precise to avoid complications and to obtain maximum assurance as to the presence or absence of recrudescent carcinoma.

Treatment. Acute radiation injury does not necessitate specific therapy, but empirical treatment for subjective complaints, such as the use of bland gargles, humidification, analgesics, and cough suppressants, is helpful.

Treatment of chronic injuries should be as conservative as possible. No surgical procedure should be attempted until infection is brought under control by antibiotic therapy. Cultures should be obtained and the appropriate antibiotic given in large doses. Mouth and pharyngeal care is important, and frequent saline irrigations in addition to the use of weak solutions of sodium perborate or hydrogen peroxide as a mouthwash and gargle three times a day are indicated. Absolute voice rest is a necessity. A tracheostomy is useful for treating obstruction, as well as for putting the larynx at rest.

In the presence of noninfective obstructive edema, administration of a steroid such as prednisone, 5 mg q.i.d., may be helpful. Steroids should not be used in the presence of an acute infection.

When the diagnosis of perichondritis and chondral necrosis is made and the presence of carcinoma has been ruled out, preservation of the larynx should be attempted. Loose, dead pieces of cartilage may be removed endoscopically when they present in the laryngeal lumen or in a laryngeal-cutaneous fistula. Abscesses must be drained to prevent endolaryngeal rupture and aspiration of pus.

When acute infection is controlled, surgical debridement may be indicated. However, surgery on the neck of such a patient practically always leads to sloughing of soft tissues and poor healing, which should be anticipated. At surgery, skin and soft tissue exhibiting marked radiation changes and poor vitality should be excised. Any necrotic cartilage must be removed, but perichondrium and mucosa should be preserved if laryngeal function is to be retained. During this period, it may be necessary to support the larynx with an endolaryngeal stent. The wounds should be left open until healthy granulations appear, unless it is felt that further necrosis is unlikely and that additional blood supply from a transposed tissue flap would be more advantageous. In most of these cases, definitive surgery is followed by a tissue defect which must be repaired by transposed pedicle flaps. Repair by pedicle flaps may be immediate or delayed. The pedicle flaps will bring additional blood supply to the involved areas.

Injury Associated with Indwelling Nasogastric Tubes

More and more patients having radical head and neck surgery require prolonged feeding through an indwelling nasogastric tube. The tube must pass posterior to the cricoid lamina, and with constant swallowing and phonatory movements, trauma to the postcricoid mucosa is a frequent complication. Generally, polyethylene tubes cause less difficulty than rubber nasogastric tubes.

Pathology. Mucosal ulceration in the postcricoid area is the most common lesion, and if it persists, infection of the cricoid cartilage and perichondrium may develop. This may progress to diffuse perichondritis and chondral necrosis, with possible stenosis of the infraglottic area and hypopharynx.

Clinical Manifestations. The patient complains of a sharp pain localized to the lower neck and made much worse by swallowing. Pain may radiate to the ear. If perichondritis should develop, cough and symptoms of laryngeal destruction will be present, as well as pain and tenderness over the larynx.

Diagnosis. Indirect laryngoscopy may reveal the superior margin of the ulcer in the postarytenoid area, or an area of erythema and edema is visible at this point. The presence of an ulcer is confirmed by hypopharyngoscopy.

Treatment. Removal of the nasogastric tube is mandatory. All oral feedings should be withheld until the ulcer is healed. Antibiotics are indicated for infection. Mouth care is important, and frequent use of astringent and antiseptic mouthwashes is helpful. Bismuth subnitrate powder insufflated directly on the ulcer or taken orally will aid in healing if perichondritis is not present.

If a prolonged delay in the reestablishment of oral feeding is anticipated, a cervical esophagostomy or gastrostomy should be performed. When delayed healing or prolonged reconstructive procedures are anticipated following a head and neck operation which precludes normal deglutition, the performance of an elective gastrostomy preoperatively is advisable.

AUTOGENOUS LARYNGEAL INJURIES

Traumatic Laryngitis

Traumatic laryngitis is an acute noninfective inflammatory response to laryngeal trauma.

Etiology. Vocal abuse, such as excessive voice use at a sports event, is the most common cause. Persistent cough, direct endolaryngeal trauma, and irritating inhalants are other causes. Traumatic laryngitis may occur in persons with vocal training after a period of prolonged or strained voice use.

Pathology. The laryngeal mucosa tends to be hyperemic, particularly in the area of the true vocal cords. There may be slight edema involving the true cords and, in particular, Rienke's space (Fig. 28–6). Dilated vessels running parallel to the axis of the true cord are present on the superior surface of the cords, and rupture of such a vessel may be the source of a submucosal hematoma.

Clinical Manifestations. Dysphonia and sometimes aphonia following an episode of unusual voice use is the usual complaint.

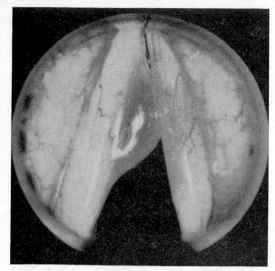

FIG. 28–6. Acute traumatic edema of the vocal cord involving Rienke's space. Note the vasodilatation on the superior surfaces of the vocal cords.

Some patients will note odynophonia and dry throat associated with persistent, irritative, nonproductive cough. These symptoms usually subside spontaneously in a few days unless trauma is repeated.

At indirect laryngoscopy, the true vocal cords appear diffusely red or discrete; dilated vessels may be seen running the length of the membranous cords. Subepithelial hemorrhages on the superior surface of the cords and edema of the cord margins (Rienke's space) may be noted in addition to sluggish movements of the cord. Occasionally, the edema is severe enough to produce obstructive symptoms such as stridor, especially in children.

Treatment. This condition is usually self-limited if normal voice use is resumed; however, absolute vocal silence will markedly decrease the period of hoarseness and aphonia. A true hematoma of the true vocal cord should be evacuated by removing a small piece of mucosa with biopsy forceps and suctioning the clotted blood. Hematoma that is allowed to persist often resorbs spontaneously, but the development of a vocal polyp occurs often enough to warrant more active treatment. If vocal abuse is allowed to persist, one of the forms of chronic laryngitis may develop.

Contact Ulcer and Granuloma of the Larynx

Contact ulcer refers to a small, superficial ulceration which develops on the medial surface of the arytenoid in response to excessively forceful apposition of the two arytenoid cartilages during phonation. The ulceration may be unilateral or bilateral. Two areas of the arytenoid may be involved; the most common site is at the tip of the vocal process, but the area of the colliculus, a small projection on the medial surface below the apex of the arytenoid, may be a site of involvement.

Etiology. Contact ulcer is an uncommon lesion occurring almost exclusively in adult males, most frequently during the fourth decade. Vocal abuse is undoubtedly the most important etiologic factor. The disease is usually seen in preachers, salesmen, managers, and lawyers who use forceful speech. Smoking and persistent coughing may also be etiologic factors. Frequently, the onset of symptoms is related to an acute upper respiratory infection.

Pathology. The tips of the vocal processes are traumatically approximated during forceful speech, with the result that the thin overlying mucosa is damaged, and an area of cartilage is exposed. As trauma continues, an inflammatory response develops, with hyperemia and the production of granulation tissue, causing the ulcer margins to become raised and inflamed. The ulcer crater becomes filled with necrotic debris. If granulation tissue is excessively produced, a sessile granulomatous polyp composed of fibrous tissue and inflammatory cells and covered by a necrotic, dull white membrane may appear. This form of granuloma tends to remain sessile and is usually not epithelized. Perichondritis of the vocal process may be noted (Fig. 28–7).

Contact granuloma should be differentiated from traumatic granuloma, which is usually solitary, pedunculated, vascular, and epithelized. Traumatic granuloma may disappear spontaneously, whereas it is uncommon for a contact granuloma to regress.

Clinical Manifestations. The symptoms vary widely in incidence and type. The voice may be quite normal, although mild dys-

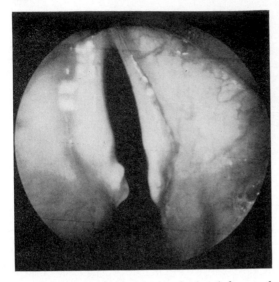

FIG. 28–7. Contact ulcer of the left vocal cord in a 45-year-old male school teacher.

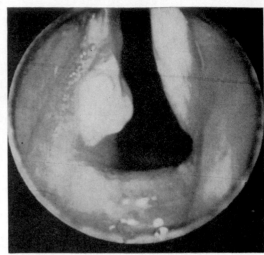

FIG. 28–8. Contact granuloma of the right vocal cord. The lesion is sessile and is covered by exudate lying on the nonepithelized surface.

phonia, which increases with voice use, is usually present and may be accompanied by odynophonia. Other voice alterations include syllabic aphonia, monotone voice, and narrow pitch range. Pain, originating deep in the neck and radiating to the lateral neck area or ear is typical of the condition. Persistent throat tickle, irritative nonproductive cough, a persistent urge to clear the throat, hemoptysis, a sensation of a lump in the throat, aching throat, and dryness may occur in any patient.

The appearance of the larynx will vary, depending on the stage of the development of the ulcers. Initially, small, pale ulcers are noted on the medial surface of the vocal process, and bare cartilage may be seen in the center. Later, the ulcer becomes covered by a necrotic membrane. In a more active phase, the ulcer margins become hyperemic, giving a red halo appearance to the lesion. Still later, a raised, sessile, pale granuloma may appear at the site of the ulcer (Fig. 28–8); this is usually unilateral and may fit a cup-shaped depression in the opposite arytenoid, producing the typical cup-and-saucer deformity. Other laryngoscopic changes include edema of the arytenoid eminences, formation of mucous strands between the vocal processes, and persistence of a chink, during phonation, between the

arytenoid bodies posterior to the vocal processes. The diagnosis is based on the unique appearance and location of the lesions.

Treatment. When the ulcers are in the acute phase, absolute voice rest is imperative. Ideally, this should be continued for several weeks until the ulcers are healed and the patient is asymptomatic, but this is rarely economically feasible. Therefore, a shorter period of voice rest should be followed by a program of gradual voice re-education. Antibiotics may be helpful in the acute stage, and the patient should abstain from smoking.

Since the appearance of contact ulcers and granulomas is quite typical, biopsy or trimming of ulcers is rarely necessary and is unwarranted, since delayed healing and excessive cicatrix formation may follow. However, removal of a large granulomatous mass may be necessary. Biopsy should be performed to rule out carcinoma or an infective granulomatous disease if the clinical appearance is at all unusual. Rarely, an ulcer may persist despite therapy because of perichondritis of the vocal process, and this will require conservative trimming with a small biopsy forceps. Occasionally, persistent, severe odynophonia and odynophagia may be relieved by a small dose (75 to 100 R) of irradiation, although the use of irradiation therapy for benign lesions is open to question. The value of voice rest and vocal re-education is emphasized, as they form the basis of treatment of this disease.

Traumatic Granuloma of the Larynx

Etiology. Traumatic granuloma of the larynx is a localized inflammatory response to mucosal loss caused by endolaryngeal trauma. The lesion may occur following endotracheal intubation, bronchoscopy, stripping of the vocal cords, or excessive vocal abuse. Mucosal loss is followed by ulceration and infection and then by an overproduction of reactive granulation tissue. Granuloma formation is most frequent on the medial surfaces of the vocal processes because of the increased susceptibility to trauma of the thin mucosa overlying rigid cartilage at this point. The lesion is not restricted to this area and does occur on the membranous cord and in other areas of the larynx when the trauma is secondary to vocal cord stripping or bronchoscopy.

Endotracheal intubation is the most common cause of traumatic granuloma. This does not always imply prolonged intubation as the cause, although this is important, since the lesion may occur after short intubations. The lesion occurs most frequently in women, in contrast to contact granuloma, because the endotracheal tube tends to lie more posteriorly in the larynx owing to the size and configuration of the female larynx. Also, the epithelium is thinner in females. The use of too large a tube, traumatic intubation, and excessive movement of the vocal cords against the indwelling tube are other etiologic factors.

Pathology. The lesion begins as a mucosal ulceration which becomes secondarily infected. Re-epithelization is prevented by irritation from continued laryngeal function and infection. Granulation tissue is formed but becomes excessive, producing a sessile polypoid mass. The mass at this point consists of large numbers of vessels, with the larger vessels located at the base and small capillaries occupying the peripheral areas. In addition, some fibroblastic tissue and polymorphonuclear exudate are present.

Epithelium is absent from large areas. As the lesion matures, epithelization is completed and fibrosis occurs, obliterating many vessels and causing the mass to shrink and become pedunculated. Eventually, the lesion may atrophy and disappear completely. The histologic appearance is the same as that of pyogenic granuloma in other areas.

Clinical Manifestations. The history of possible endolaryngeal trauma is always apparent. Hoarseness of some degree is often present immediately postoperatively, and a small ulcer may be seen on the vocal cords. The granuloma does not usually appear for 3 or more weeks and is accompanied by hoarseness, a feeling of discomfort in the larynx, and occasionally ear pain. The laryngeal lesion is a dark red, edematous, sessile mass partially covered by exudate. The mass is usually unilateral and is most frequent in the region of the vocal process (Fig. 28–9). As the lesion matures, it becomes more pedunculated and assumes a lighter color. The symptoms tend to fluctuate more, and periods of slight hoarseness may be interrupted by episodes of aphonia when the polyp prolapses between the vocal cords. As time passes, the mass shrinks in size,

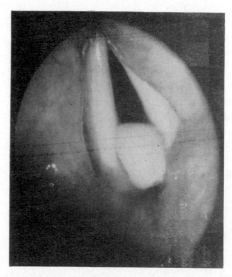

FIG. 28–9. Traumatic granuloma of the larynx in a 42-year-old female 4 weeks after bronchoscopy. The lesion is pedunculated, smooth, and pale pink; it did not recur after removal.

becomes pale and fibrotic, and may disappear spontaneously.

Traumatic granuloma must be distinguished from contact granuloma. The latter occurs mainly in males and the lesion is sessile, often pale from the beginning, and associated with an ulcer on the opposite vocal process. The contact granuloma tends to recur after surgical removal and rarely undergoes spontaneous involution.

Treatment. Conservative therapy is indicated in the early stages; complete voice rest may result in regression and healing in this stage, whereas surgical removal may result in recurrence. Surgical removal for symptomatic relief is indicated when the mature pedunculated granuloma is present, and it is usually curative. The patient should be placed on complete voice rest before and after surgery. If circumstances warrant, nothing may be done, and in most cases the lesion will disappear over a period of several weeks. In the event that the lesion could possibly be confused with a specific infection or neoplasm, immediate biopsy is indicated.

REFERENCES

Alexander, F. W.: Micropathology of Radiation Reaction in the Larynx. Ann. Otol., 72:831, 1963.

Bennett, T.: Laryngeal Trauma. Laryngoscope, 70:793, 1960.

Bergström, J.: Post-intubation Granuloma of the Larynx. Acta Otolaryng., 57:113, 1964.

Bergström, J., et al.: On the Pathogenesis of Laryngeal Injuries Following Prolonged Intubation. Acta Otolaryng., 55:342, 1962.

Brewer, D. W.: Contact Ulcer of the Larynx. N. Y. State J. Med., 63:3100, 1963.

Brodnitz, F. S.: Contact Ulcer of the Larynx. Arch. Otolaryng., 74:70, 1961.

Fitz-Hugh, G. S., et al.: Injuries of the Larynx and Cervical Trauma. Ann. Otol., 71:419, 1962.

Gard, M. A., and Cruikshank, L. F.: Factors Influenceing the Incidence of Sore Throat Following Endotracheal Intubation. Canad. Med. Assoc. J., 84:662, 1961.

Holinger, P. H., and Johnston, K. C.: Contact Ulcer of the Larynx. J.A.M.A., 172:511, 1960.

Holinger, P. H., and Loeb, W. J.: Feeding Tube Stenosis of the Larynx. Surg. Gynecol. Obstet., 83:253, 1946.

Inglauer, S., and Molt, W. F.: Severe Injury to the Larynx Resulting from Indwelling Duodenal Tube. Ann. Otol., 48:886, 1939.

Jackson, C.: Contact Ulcer of Larynx. Ann. Otol., 37:227, 1928.

Jackson, C.: High Tracheostomy and Other Errors, The Chief Causes of Chronic Laryngeal Stenosis. Surg. Gynecol. Obstet., 32:392, 1921.

Knight, J. S.: Cricothyroid Dislocation. Laryngoscope, 70:1256, 1960.

Lu, A. T., et al.: The Pathology of Laryngotracheal Complications. Lesions of the Larynx and Trachea after Intubation Anesthesia. Arch. Otolaryng., 74:323, 1961.

Miles, W. K., et al.: Acute Treatment of Experimental Laryngeal Fractures. Ann. Otol. Rhinol. Laryngol., 80:710, 1971.

Myerson, M. C.: Granulomatous Polyp of the Larynx Following Intratracheal Intubation. Arch. Otolaryng., 62:182, 1955.

Ogura, J. H., and Powers, W. E.: Surgical Correction of Traumatic Stenosis of the Larynx and Pharynx. Laryngoscope, 72:468, 1962.

Pennington, J.: Glottic and Supraglottic Laryngeal Injury and Stenosis from External Trauma. Laryngoscope, 74:317, 1964.

Rush, B. F., Jr.: Repair of the Injured Larynx Following Destruction of the Cricoid Cartilage. Surg. Gynecol., Obstet., 112:507, 1961.

Shaw, R., et al.: Traumatic Tracheal Rupture. J. Thorac. Cardiovasc. Surg., 42:281, 1961.

Warren, S.: Histopathology of Lesions Due to Irradiation. Physiol. Rev., 24:225, 1944.

Chapter 29

Acute Inflammatory Diseases of the Larynx

ACUTE INFLAMMATORY NONSPECIFIC LARYNGITIS

Acute infectious laryngitis is usually a mild, self-limited inflammatory condition which is often a manifestation of a more diffuse upper respiratory infection.

Etiology. The cause of this infection is almost always a virus (see Ch. 8). Bacterial invasion may be secondary. The laryngitis is almost always associated with acute rhinitis (coryza) or nasopharyngitis. The onset of infection may be associated with exposure to sudden temperature changes, dietary deficiencies, malnutrition, and lack of immunity. The disease is more common in winter and is readily transmitted.

Pathology. There is capillary dilatation and hyperemia associated with generalized extracellular edema. A submucosal leukocytic infiltrate, mostly of mononuclear cells, is present initially; later polymorphonuclear cells appear if a secondary bacterial infection develops. The superficial mucosal layers usually slough, and shallow ulcerations covered by pseudomembranes may develop.

Clinical Manifestations. The usual symptoms are those of a common cold with associated hoarseness. The first symptoms involving the throat are dryness, rawness, and a change in voice pitch. Cough is common. If cordal edema is marked, aphonia ensues, and mild inspiratory stridor may be evident.

Fever is usually low-grade (38.5°C). Early in the course of the disease, laryngeal secretions are scanty; later they may become abundant but viscid and may be blood-tinged.

The laryngeal mucosa is variably inflamed and edematous. The mucosa may be granular, with patchy superficial ulceration and areas of grey pseudomembrane formation. Vocal cord motion is normal, although the margins of the cords may be red and edematous and may actually appear polypoid because of edema of Rienke's space.

Diagnosis. Diagnosis is made by the history and laryngeal appearance. Throat cultures are indicated in prolonged or resistant illness. Isolation of the causative viral agent from throat washing is only necessary in the face of a possible epidemic.

Treatment. Treatment should include bedrest and medication for symptomatic relief of fever, cough, and sore throat. Voice rest must be complete. Humidification in a cool room and the use of expectorants help to relieve dryness and tickle and to liquefy the secretions. If laryngitis is severe and stridor is present, a cold steam tent is indicated. A special effort should be made to maintain systemic hydration to avoid further inspissation of secretions. Broad-spectrum antibiotics may be helpful in preventing secondary bacterial infection of the mucosa in the more severe cases. The majority of patients will recover with simple conservative treatment; however, the disease tends to be more severe in elderly patients and may be complicated by pneumonia. Therefore, patients in the older age group should be observed closely for progression of the infection.

ACUTE SPASMODIC CROUP (ACUTE LARYNGITIS OF CHILDHOOD, MILLAR'S ASTHMA)

Acute spasmodic croup is a mild inflammatory disease of children which is significant because of associated laryngeal spasm and attacks of severe dyspnea. It is differentiated from laryngismus stridulus by the fact that there is no abnormality of calcium metabolism.

Etiology. The condition typically occurs in children, mainly boys, between 1 and 4 years of age but may occur up to age 6. There is no specific organism or disease which causes the condition, but it does tend to occur in association with mild upper respiratory infections. There is undoubtedly a psychogenic factor associated with the recurrent form of the disease which occurs in some children.

Pathology. The disease is not a true infection, and there are only minor tissue changes in the larynx. Some patients manifest a redness and swelling on both sides of the infraglottic area. These changes are present only after an attack and are transient. Edema of the supraglottic and infraglottic areas may be present.

Clinical Manifestations. Typically, the child goes to bed feeling well and soon is asleep. A few hours later, he awakes with a croupy cough, stridor, and dyspnea. Because of fear and panic, the respiratory effort is increased, which in turn causes worsening of the stridor and dyspnea. Thus laryngeal spasm is precipitated. Supraclavicular and subcostal indrawing occur, and eventually a dusky to cyanotic tinge of the skin develops. At this point, the child may become unconscious or may vomit and terminate the attack. The child then falls asleep and awakens in the morning with nothing but slight hoarseness and cough.

The attacks may be solitary or may recur for 2 or 3 nights and then disappear completely. In other children, because it is an attention-getting mechanism and because of psychogenic factors, the disorders may recur for some time. Occasionally an attack may not subside spontaneously and obstructive symptoms persist, necessitating more active therapy.

Treatment. Therapy is directed at abortion of the attack. Humidification is important, and it is frequently noted that there is a rapid disappearance of stridor when the child is placed in the bathroom with the hot shower going. An emetic dose of ipecac (½ to 1 tsp.) will induce vomiting and often terminate the attack. Oxygen therapy and tracheostomy are seldom required. Mild sedation at bedtime will often prevent recurrent attacks. Antibiotic therapy is rarely indicated unless evidence of the bacterial infection is found. The parents must be reassured in order to prevent the situation from becoming a means of household control by the child when the attacks are recurrent.

ACUTE SUPRAGLOTTIC LARYNGITIS

Inflammation of the supraglottic structures is a condition that tends to affect small children between the ages of 3 and 6 years, but it occurs quite frequently in adults and is as potentially lethal as in children.

Etiology. *Hemophilus influenzae* type B has been the bacteria cultured most consistently from afflicted individuals. However, staphylococci, streptococci, and pneumococci have also been implicated (see Ch. 8). It is probable that some viruses may also cause the disease. The disease is of most significance in children because of the configuration of the supraglottic larynx, which predisposes to obstruction by a small amount of swelling of structures around the laryngeal vestibule.

Pathology. There is a severe cellulitis of the tissues of the epiglottis and aryepiglottic folds. The mucous membrane is bright red and edematous. Excretions on or in the larynx tend to be thick and inspissated. Obstruction of the laryngeal vestibule prevents effective cough and removal of secretions, creating a second obstructive problem.

Clinical Manifestations. The course of this disease is, in most instances, rapid, progressing from the symptoms of mild upper respiratory infection to almost complete respiratory obstruction over a period of 6 to 12 hours. The disease begins with fever which is often high (40°C). Both adults and children are extremely ill, appearing pale and lethargic. They tend to sit or lie quietly, concentrating only on breathing. It is common to see the child sitting or standing in bed leaning slightly forward with the mandible projected to facilitate respiration. The mouth may be held open with the tongue protruding. The voice is not usually hoarse but has a muffled quality, and the patient has the appearance of having a "hot potato" in his mouth.

The respirations are variable but may change markedly over the space of a few moments. Initially, the patients are amazingly quiet, compared to those with laryngotracheitis, because maximum ventilation is obtained by slow, steady, inspiration, whereas vigorous inspiration will cause the swollen epiglottis to obstruct the vestibule. Stridor is not an outstanding feature, and it is variably present as an inspiratory and/or expiratory rattle. From this point, any increase in respiratory effort causes the swollen epiglottis to act as a ball valve completely obstructing the larynx at each inspiration. The signs of marked indrawing, increasing restlessness, and cyanosis will appear rapidly. As distress continues, the children develop a peculiar ashen-gray color, which is a significant sign of impending respiratory arrest. As respiratory distress increases, they becomes restless and disoriented.

Dysphagia is an important symptom. Early in the course of the disease there may be complaints of sore throat and pain on swallowing. However, with progression, the patient will have difficulty swallowing liquids and secretions and will refuse oral feedings.

General reactions to increasing obstruction and dysphagia include dehydration, hyperpyrexia, tachycardia, anxious facies, and restlessness. Finally, exhaustion with respiratory and circulatory collapse develops.

Oral examination will show the oropharynx to be somewhat injected with pooling of secretions in this area. With a tongue depressor, the cherry-red edematous epiglottis may be seen in most children projecting above the posterior tongue. Caution must be used during examination, as acute obstruction may be precipitated. If direct laryngoscopy is done to insert an airway, the true vocal cords may be seen to be slightly injected but otherwise normal. Auscultation of the chest will often disclose a remarkable paucity of breath sounds, denoting decreased air exchange.

Diagnosis. The diagnosis is usually made on the basis of clinical findings. Direct laryngoscopy is rarely necessary for diagnostic reasons and is contraindicated unless a bronchoscope or an endotracheal tube is immediately available, since respiratory obstruction may be precipitated. Soft tissue roentgenograms of the neck will indicate the characteristic supraglottic swelling impinging on the airway when it is not possible to see it over the base of the tongue. Radiologic examination of the chest is always indicated, since atelectasis and pneumonia may accompany this disease.

Smears and cultures of the pharyngeal secretions should be taken to determine the causative organism. They are of little importance in planning early therapy but are useful if the organism is resistant to initial treatment. If *H. influenzae* type B infection is suspected, the specimen should be cultured on Levinthal agar as well as blood agar, since this will allow identification in 24 hours. *H. influenzae* type B may also be identified by the "quellung test" or capsular swelling in response to specific antiserum.

Treatment. These patients, whether adults or children, should be hospitalized immediately and placed in an intensive care unit with bronchoscope, laryngoscope, endotracheal tubes, and tracheostomy set at the bedside. Many physicians advocate, with complete justification, tracheostomy as soon as the diagnosis of supraglottic laryngitis is made. Tracheostomy should be performed in any case in which there is any degree of obstruction and whenever experienced personnel are not available to observe the patient continuously. Increasing dysphagia and decreased air entry to the lungs are also

and bronchopneumonia are frequent complications. The drugs may be changed if culture results indicate an alteration in the flora or development of bacterial resistance.

Corticosteroids seem to be of particular benefit in this disease in reducing the inflammatory response and the edema of the infraglottic tissues. Hydrocortisone derivatives, such as prednisolone or methylprednisolone, produce the best anti-inflammatory response. Solu-Cortef, 100 mg, or Solu-medrol, 40 mg, is given intravenously in the acute phase of the disease, and the patient should be started on a regular oral or intramuscular regime of steroid therapy. The steroid therapy is maintained until obstructive symptoms regress; then the patient is tapered off the medication.

Mild sedation is occasionally useful in early cases to reduce anxiety and oxygen consumption. However, it must be used with care and should be avoided entirely when respiratory difficulty is present to any degree.

Tracheostomy is indicated when obstruction with cyanosis, tachycardia, ashen-gray pallor, marked decrease in pulmonary ventilation, inability to cough, or collapse is present. However, a large number of patients will respond to conservative measures and will not require tracheostomy if therapy is instituted early enough. Judgment must be used in determining the need for tracheostomy. It is far better to perform the operation early rather than in the stage of exhaustion when it may not save the child. Also, complications such as cardiac arrest are more likely when surgical procedures are performed when hypoxia is present. These children are usually hypercapnic as well as hypoxic and must be watched closely for post-tracheostomy apnea. It may be necessary to assist respirations with a respirator until the excess CO_2 is blown off.

Acute laryngotracheobronchitis is a serious disease of small children requiring close observation and vigorous therapy. Patients are often lost because of sudden rapid respiratory failure when judicious tracheostomy may have been lifesaving. Correct timing of tracheostomy is important in order to avoid the complications of an unnecessary tracheostomy as well as the complications of delayed tracheostomy. When available, serial arterial O_2 saturation levels, O_2 tensions, and arterial blood pH are helpful in determining the need for tracheostomy. Arterial O_2 saturation of less than 70 to 75% and any decrease in serum pH are indications of the need for tracheostomy. Also, a decreasing O_2 saturation and acidosis in the face of increased respiratory effort with acute obstructive disease indicate a need for tracheostomy.

NONSPECIFIC MEMBRANOUS LARYNGITIS

Membranous laryngitis is common but it is usually associated with other disease processes, such as infectious mononucleosis, viral diseases, and Vincent's infection.

Membranous laryngitis of nonspecific etiology may occur in adults but is most frequent in children. It may occur in infants. In small children, it may represent a form of acute laryngotracheobronchitis. It tends to occur during epidemics of respiratory infections both in children and in adults. Recently, we have observed the disease in two neonates born after premature rupture of placental membranes.

Etiology. Various organisms have been cultured from these cases, including pneumococci, streptococci, and staphylococci. However, a significant number of patients have had gram-negative organisms, such as *Pseudomonas aeruginosa, Proteus vulgaris,* and *Proteus mirabilis,* isolated from the membrane. Other predisposing factors appear to be upper respiratory infections, depressed immune responses, debilitation, and diabetes mellitus.

Clinical Manifestations. The symptoms are hoarseness, croupy cough, and dyspnea with inspiratory stridor. There is loss of appetite, and the older patients complain of thirst and odynophagia. As cough becomes worse, post-tussive laryngeal spasm occurs, which increases the respiratory difficulty. Sudden episodes of obstruction may occur, especially in small children, secondary to glottic obstruction by a loose piece of membrane. During such episodes, the patient is aphonic, and crowing inspiratory stridor is evident.

Examination discloses the surfaces of the aryepiglottic folds, arytenoids, and false cords to be covered with discrete patches of loosely attached yellow-white membrane. The membrane is friable and easily detached, while the underlying mucosa is red and granular but does not bleed. In contrast to specific forms of membranous laryngitis, in the nonspecific form the membrane formation is often confined to the larynx.

In addition to the laryngeal symptoms, episodes of gram-negative septicemia may occur, marked by high fever, prostration, and shock. A blood culture should be obtained in such instances.

Treatment. Initial treatment is directed toward airway maintenance. Tracheostomy is often necessary. Loose pieces of membrane should be removed if possible. This is easily accomplished by direct laryngoscopy without an anesthesia in infants and small children. The membrane should be submitted for culture and determination of antibiotic sensitivities.

Large doses of antibiotics are indicated and in the acute phase should be given intravenously. Gentamicin or Tobramycin in combination with Carbenacillin are the drugs of choice.

The patient should be placed in a wet, cool atmosphere. Intravenous fluid maintenance is usually necessary in small patients. It may be necessary to give large amounts of fluids to overcome the initial dehydration. Despite chemotherapy and tracheostomy, this disease is frequently lethal in infants because of pneumonia, septicemia, shock, and respiratory failure.

SPECIFIC ACUTE INFECTIONS OF THE LARYNX

Diphtheria

Diphtheria is an acute infective disease which may involve a part or all of the upper respiratory tract. The disease occurs in children over 6 years of age, but adults may be affected. This disease is uncommon in most areas in the United States because of active immunization in infancy.

Etiology. The disease is caused by *Corynebacterium diphtheriae,* a gram-positive organism of which there are three types: gravis, intermedius, and mitis. Disease caused by the gravis type is rare in North America. The types are separated by colony morphology on the tellurite medium and by their ability to ferment sugars.

The disease is usually spread by droplet and by fomites. It has been noted that this organism may change from a nonvirulent form to a toxin-producing virulent form, which may account for the occurrence of isolated cases. Since the advent of widespread immunization, the disease is uncommon, but it may occur in a mild form in immunized persons.

Pathology. The infection is superficial, involving the mucous membranes of the nose, pharynx, and larynx, producing epithelial necrosis. There is an outpouring of serum, and this agglutinates into a firmly attached membrane of necrotic epithelium, bacteria, fibrin, and phagocytes. The membrane may be present anywhere in the nose, oropharynx, larynx, and trachea.

The bacteria elaborates on exotoxin which specifically attacks heart muscle and peripheral nerves. Death results from airway obstruction or heart failure.

Clinical Manifestations. The incubation period is 1 to 7 days. The onset is insidious, with slight sore throat, malaise, and low-grade fever. There may be a mild tachycardia. Inspection of the pharynx will usually reveal the presence of a grayish white membrane on a tonsil, the pharyngeal wall, or the larynx. Laryngeal involvement is indicated by hoarseness first, followed by cough, stridor, and progressive signs of respiratory obstruction. The membrane is firmly attached and leaves a bleeding bed when removed. Cervical lymphadenitis is usually present and may be marked, giving the characteristic "bull-necked" appearance.

Diagnosis. The diagnosis must be suspected in any form of membranous pharyngitis or laryngitis. The diagnosis can usually be made by microscopic examination of the membrane, which will disclose the organisms. This is confirmed by culture of the organism on Loeffler's and tellurite media.

Treatment. Prophylaxis is the most important and successful method of therapy. Every child should be actively immunized as an infant and then receive periodic boosters until age 10.

Antitoxin should be given empirically if there is a reasonable suspicion of disease, rather than awaiting a positive culture report, since it is the only specific treatment. It should be given in one dose of 20,000 to 100,000 units, one half intramuscularly and one half intravenously.

Penicillin will kill the causative organism but it will not alter the course of the disease. It is used to eliminate the carrier state; 125 mg q.i.d. is given for 10 days.

If the symptoms of respiratory obstruction are marked and there is evidence of tachycardia, tracheostomy is indicated. Bronchoscopy should be done first so that any membrane in the trachea or bronchi may be removed and so that an airway is provided during the performance of the tracheostomy. The indirect insertion of O'Dwyer tubes is seldom indicated and is of historical interest now. (See 10th edition of this textbook.)

Herpes of the Larynx

Etiology. This virus is peculiar in that it has developed a successful host-parasite relationship with man. Most people harbor the virus from infancy. Since most adults develop circulating antibodies to the virus, manifestations of infection are most common in small children between 6 months and 3 years (see Ch. 8).

Pathology. This virus probably resides in the cells of the mucous membranes. Usually there is an initiating factor in the onset of an acute infection, such as an upper respiratory infection or trauma to the mouth. The lesions begin as punctate vesicles surrounded by a red areola. The vesicles rupture, leaving a small ulcer covered by a whitish exudate. The infection usually involves the mouth and pharynx, as well as the larynx.

Clinical Manifestations. Acute herpetic laryngitis usually occurs in association with herpetic gingivostomatitis. This is a severe febrile disease of infants and small children. The lesions in the oral cavity are usually obvious. Symptoms of laryngeal involvement include hoarseness, croupy cough, and stridor. Enlargement of the cervical lymph nodes is usually present. In rare instances, isolated involvement of the larynx may occur.

Diagnosis. The diagnosis may be confirmed by identification of the virus by culture. Biopsy of the lesion will disclose typical intranuclear inclusion bodies. Antibodies appear in the blood within 4 to 5 days after the onset of infection, and a rising antibody titer is a significant indication of the causative organism.

Treatment. The disease is usually self-limited to 1 to 2 weeks, and treatment is supportive. In severe cases, antibiotics may be necessary to control secondary infection of the mucosal ulcers. Laryngeal involvement is seldom severe enough to warrant tracheostomy. Some patients may be subject to recurrent infections, and in such instances repeated small pox vaccinations may possibly be of value. *Lactobacillus* organisms given orally may also have a beneficial effect.

NONINFLAMMATORY EDEMA OF THE LARYNX

Etiology. Edema of the larynx is present to some degree in all infective processes involving the larynx. However, laryngeal edema may also be due to fluid transudation secondary to noninflammatory processes, such as venous obstruction, lymphatic obstruction, alteration in capillary permeability, or disturbance in oncotic pressure of plasma. Causes of noninflammatory edema of the larynx include:

1. Venous obstruction or increased venous pressure
   a. Superior vena cava syndrome
   b. Post–radical neck dissection
   c. Heart failure
2. Lymphatic obstruction
   a. Neoplastic infiltration
   b. Post–radical neck dissection
   c. Irradiation
3. Altered capillary permeability
   a. Allergic edema (angioneurotic edema, Quincke's edema)
   b. Acute glomerulonephritis
4. Decreased plasma oncotic pressure (hypoalbuminemia)

a. Nutritional
b. Hepatic cirrhosis
c. Nephrotic syndrome

Laryngeal edema may occur as part of the superior vena cava syndrome, which is due to obstruction of the great veins in the upper mediastinum. This may be the result of metastatic carcinoma, thyroid tumors, sclerosing mediastinitis, or pericardial effusion. Obstruction of the jugular veins may cause edema and is most frequently secondary to bilateral radical neck dissection. Unilateral neck dissection rarely causes this problem.

Lymphatic obstruction in the neck will cause more persistent edema of the larynx than venous obstruction. Edema following radical neck dissection may be due to both venous and lymphatic obstruction. However, the accumulation of lymph is gradual, and therefore edema is most marked about the fifth to sixth postoperative day. Malignant neoplasms permeating the lymph channels or replacing cervical lymph nodes are a cause of edema. A persistent form of edema may follow irradiation therapy of the neck and is mainly due to endothelial obstruction of lymphatics.

Various systemic diseases associated with decrease of serum albumin may be complicated by slowly progressive laryngeal edema.

Allergic edema involving the larynx (angioneurotic edema) may be due to drug allergy (penicillin, iodides), transfusion reactions, serum injections, insect bites, food, or inhalants.

Pathology. The subepithelial tissues of the supraglottic and infraglottic areas are marked by local fibrotic stroma with low tissue tension. As a result, these areas are the first sites of collection of excess tissue fluid.

Clinical Manifestations. The rapidity of onset of laryngeal edema varies considerably; the clinical picture is therefore variable. Edema of other than allergic origin is usually slow in onset and will rarely be confined to the larynx. Laryngeal symptoms in such instances are progressive, beginning with hoarseness, muffled voice, and altered pitch and leading to signs of increasing obstruction, with stridor, indrawing, tachypnea, and cyanosis.

Laryngeal edema of allergic origin or angioneurotic edema is usually of acute onset, with a history of recent exposure to an allergen. The edema may be confined to the larynx, but there is usually evidence of urticaria or angioedema elsewhere on the body. Angioedema tends to involve the face, lips, hands, feet, and larynx. Symptoms and signs of laryngeal obstruction appear rapidly. The process may arrest spontaneously at any point, or it may progress to complete obstruction, asphyxia, and death.

Treatment. Edema secondary to systemic disease can be controlled by treatment of these conditions, which includes control of serum protein and electrolyte levels.

Persistent laryngeal edema due to mechanical obstruction of veins and lymphatics will often regress spontaneously as collateral circulation develops. When edema is due to malignant disease in the superior mediastinum, considerable relief may be obtained with radiotherapy and chemotherapy. Tracheostomy may be necessary in some instances.

Angioneurotic edema of the larynx is a medical emergency. The process may be arrested by drug therapy, but tracheostomy or intubation may be necessary if the drugs are not immediately available. As soon as the diagnosis is made, epinephrine 1:1000 (0.3 to 0.5 ml) should be given intramuscularly. This should be followed by 100 mg of hydrocortisone intravenously. An antihistamine, such as Benadryl, 50 mg, or Chlor-Trimeton, 8 mg, should also be given intravenously. Benefit may also be obtained by spraying the larynx with a solution of epinephrine 1:1000. After the acute phase of the illness is controlled, the patient should be given maintenance doses of antihistamines and steroids until the edema has subsided.

ABSCESS OF THE LARYNX

Etiology. Abscess of the larynx occurs most commonly as a complication of perichondritis due to irradiation or mechanical trauma. Tuberculosis and syphilitic perichondritis are rare causes. Infections of the mouth and oropharynx may occasionally lead to abscess formation; rarely, metastatic abscess formation may occur. Secondary infection of a mucocele or laryngocele is a relatively frequent cause of abscess formation. Typhoid fever, once the most common cause of laryngeal abscess, is now almost nonexistent in the United States.

The organisms commonly involved are *Staphylococcus* and the gram-negative *Pseudomonas* and *Proteus* organisms. This may be partly due to the indiscriminate use of antibiotics for treatment and prophylaxis of infections, leaving resistant organisms to cause secondary infections.

Pathology. Two types of abscesses occur —those involving soft tissues and those associated with chondral necrosis and perichondritis. Abscesses of the soft tissues usually involve the false cords and aryepiglottic folds. These may be secondary to infection of a mucocele or laryngocele or to septic metastases via blood or lymphatic channels. Abscesses secondary to perichondritis may develop on either the external or internal surfaces of the cartilage. The thyroid and cricoid cartilages may be involved singly or together.

Clinical Manifestations. The general symptoms of infection are present, such as fever, malaise, and anorexia. Local symptoms include hoarseness, muffled voice, croupy cough, pain on swallowing and phonation, stridor, and signs of laryngeal obstruction. Cough may be associated with expectoration of purulent material if the abscess ruptures or drains intermittently.

Palpation of the larynx will disclose local tenderness whether the abscess is external or endolaryngeal. Fluctuation may be noted if the abscess is external to the cartilage. A thickening of the tissues over the larynx on the side of the abscess may be noted when the neck is palpated.

If the abscess is in the supraglottic area, a red bulging mass involving one of the aryepiglottic folds is seen. If the abscess is secondary to perichondritis of the cricoid, the mass may be noted in the infraglottic area and may be associated with impaired function of the vocal cords. Purulent material may be noted in the larynx, and frequently it appears to be coming from the ventricle. External laryngeal abscess is usually associated with an inflammatory reaction of the endolaryngeal tissues, as well as the obvious external inflammatory reaction.

Palpation of the endolaryngeal mass at direct laryngoscopy may suggest fluctuation. Also, bits of necrotic cartilage may be noted along with purulent drainage.

Diagnosis. The diagnosis can usually be made on clinical grounds. Roentgenograms of the larynx may be of help in detecting cartilage necrosis or the presence of air-fluid levels in the infected mass.

Treatment. Tracheostomy is necessary as a preliminary procedure in most cases. The treatment of any abscess is incision and drainage. Abscesses of the laryngeal soft tissues can be drained through a laryngoscope. The procedure should be done under general endotracheal anesthesia with the patient in deep Trendelenburg position to prevent aspiration.

Abscesses associated with chondral necrosis are best approached externally. All pus must be drained and the dead cartilage removed. Any necrotic cartilage left in place will only lead to progression and chronicity of the disease and a greater incidence of chronic laryngeal stenosis. The internal perichondrium should be preserved if possible. The wound should be left open until it is granulating well; then it may be closed secondarily.

Administration of antibiotics in large doses is indicated. The patient should be started on broad-spectrum coverage until the results of a culture are obtained; then drug selection may be altered if necessary.

If there has been extensive cartilage necrosis and infection is controlled and drained, a stent should be inserted by direct laryngoscopy and left in place several weeks in an effort to prevent stenosis. Secondary repair of stenosis may be necessary.

ACUTE PERICHONDRITIS OF THE LARYNX

Etiology. Primary infection of the perichondrium and subperichondral spaces is rare. Most often, perichondritis develops secondary to trauma. The most common sources of trauma are mechanical injury due to high tracheostomy, auto accidents, and irradiation. Neoplastic invasion of the cartilage may be associated with perichondritis. Perichondritis secondary to systemic infection, such as typhoid fever, is rare. Any acute infection of the mouth or pharynx may be associated with perichondritis of the laryngeal cartilages.

Pathology. Pyogenic infection of the perichondrium of the hyaline cartilages results in subperichondral collection of purulent material. The progressive elevation of the perichondrium separates it from the cartilage and decreases the already tenuous blood supply of the cartilage, producing necrosis. Involvement of the thyroid cartilage is most frequent, followed by that of the cricoid and arytenoid cartilages. The elastic cartilages are seldom affected because the perichondrium is tightly adherent.

Perichondritis and chondral necrosis secondary to irradiation are precipitated by the decreased vascularity following irradiation. The process may be sterile initially, but infection often develops after a laryngeal biopsy, which causes cartilage contamination and the development of purulent perichondritis. Therefore, biopsy in a previously irradiated larynx must be done precisely and carefully to avoid this complication.

Ankylosis of the cricoarytenoid joint may occur secondary to infection of the cricoid and arytenoid cartilages. A fibrous fixation of the joint develops, which may immobilize one or both vocal cords.

Clinical Manifestation. Pain is the most outstanding symptom. It is present constantly but is aggravated by swallowing and talking. As a result, these patients may have almost no oral intake, and vocalization is minimized. Hoarseness or aphonia is present. Inspiratory stridor and dyspnea are also common. An irritating, frequently nonproductive cough is persistently present.

Palpation of the neck is associated with marked tenderness over the larynx. The larynx does not move normally during swallowing and may seem fixed in the neck.

The mucosal lining of the larynx is usually red, granular, and edematous with considerable decrease in size of the laryngeal lumen. Pus may be present in the larynx, and this may contain pieces of necrotic cartilage. Frequently, the vocal cords and arytenoids fail to move through their normal excursions because of cricoarytenoid joint disease or soft tissue swelling. As the disease progresses, laryngeal obstruction increases, and sudden, complete obstruction may ensue.

As with any infection, the patient may manifest symptoms of systemic toxicity, such as fever, tachycardia, anorexia, nausea, and dehydration.

Complications. Perichondritis may be associated with early and late complications. Aspiration pneumonia, atelectasis, and lung abscess may occur secondary to inhalation of purulent material. Mediastinitis can develop as a result of inferior extension of the infective process. Late complications include chronic laryngeal stenosis and ankylosis of the cricoarytenoid joints.

Treatment. Treatment is directed toward prevention of asphyxia and the complications. Tracheostomy is required for aspiration of the trachea, to bypass obstruction, and to allow the larynx to rest. If perichondritis is secondary to high tracheostomy, the tube must be placed in the proper lower position immediately.

Since swallowing is usually impossible, parenteral fluid therapy must be used until the acute inflammatory phase has subsided. Nasogastric tube feeding during the acute phase is unwise and will possibly result in progression of the disease. Gastrostomy for feeding is advisable for some patients. The larynx should be at complete rest, and there should be absolutely no speaking. Tracheostomy and gastrostomy aid in minimizing laryngeal function.

Antibiotics should be used in large doses, with selection being guided by bacterial sensitivity tests, if possible. Parenteral routes of administration must be used unless a gastrostomy is in place.

The infected, dead cartilage in the larynx should be removed as soon as possible, and any purulent collections must be drained. Generally, except for the simple drainage of abscesses, surgical debridement should be delayed until the systemic signs of infection have been controlled and there has been improvement in the local signs of infection. As soon as there is evidence that the acute infection has been controlled, the larynx should be explored by an external route.

Dead, infected cartilage must be identified and removed completely; at the same time, involvement of other apparently healthy cartilage by too vigorous exploration should be avoided. An early effort should be made to preserve the internal perichondrium during cartilage debridement. If a considerable amount of cartilage must be removed, a stent should be inserted in the larynx and the wound carefully drained externally. Packing the wound open is necessary, and frequent irrigations with 3% hydrogen peroxide will clean away necrotic debris.

Insertion of the stent will help to prevent stenosis. The stent should be left in place until healing is well advanced, usually for a period of 5 to 6 weeks. However, when marked cricoid cartilage destruction has occurred, stenosis may be present already, and secondary repair is necessary at a later date.

In some cases, bilateral fixation of the cricoarytenoid joint may develop and be permanent. This situation must be relieved by an arytenoidopexy or an arytenoidectomy, if there is an inadequate airway after control of active infection and fixation is demonstrated by palpation.

Special mention should be made of the care of perichondritis secondary to irradiation. In addition to laryngeal changes, the extralaryngeal soft tissues are involved by late irradiation changes, and necrosis of skin with development of draining sinuses or fistulas is a common complication. Care must be used in the placement of incisions in such irradiated areas to avoid further necrosis and skin loss; horizontal incisions should be used when possible. When the necrotic cartilage is debrided, necrotic skin and subcutaneous tissue should also be excised. The remaining defect must be repaired using nonirradiated tissue transposed from the anterior chest or other nonirradiated area. Attempts to conserve laryngeal function should be reserved for situations in which perichondritis is limited and there is assurance that there is no persistence of carcinoma.

When perichondritis and necrosis are extensive and the possibility of persistent carcinoma exists, total laryngectomy is indicated. This procedure is often complicated by the persistence of an extensive pharyngeal and cutaneous defect due to postoperative wound necrosis and poor healing. Repair of this defect may be effected by rotation of bilateral, nondelayed, acromiopectoral pedicle flaps, which will obliterate the defect and reconstitute the pharynx in a two-stage operation.

REFERENCES

Biller, H. F., et al.: Laryngeal Edema: Experimental Study. Ann. Otol. Rhinol. Laryngol., *79*:1084, 1970.

Fearon, B.: Acute Laryngotracheobronchitis in Infancy and Childhood. Pediatr. Clin. North Am., *9*:1095, 1962.

Hawkins, D. B.: Acute Laryngotracheobronchitis in Children. Laryngoscope, *73*:583, 1963.

Jones, H. M.: Acute Epiglottitis and Supraglottitis. J. Laryngol., *72*:932, 1958.

Jordon, W. S., et al.: New Therapy for Postintubation Laryngeal Edema and Tracheitis. J.A.M.A., *212*:585, 1970.

Leegaard, T.: Pseudocroup. Acta Otolaryng. (Suppl.), *158*:10, 1960.

McGovern, F. H., et al.: Post-radiation Perichondritis and Cartilage Necrosis of the Larynx. Laryngoscope, *83*:808, 1973.

McLean, D. M., et al.: Myxoviruses Associated with Acute Laryngotracheobronchitis in Toronto, 1962-63. Canad. Med. Assoc. J., *89*:1257, 1963.

Martensson, B., et al.: The Effect of Corticosteroids in the Treatment of Pseudocroup. Acta Otolaryng. (Suppl.), *158*:62, 1960.

Matteson, A. R.: Acute Epiglottitis. Arch. Otolaryng., *76*:465, 1962.

Miller, M. V.: Edema of the Larynx: A Study of the Loose Areolar Tissues of the Larynx. Arch. Otolaryng., *31*:256, 1940.

Neffson, A. H.: *Acute Laryngotrachealbronchitis.* New York, Grune & Stratton, 1948.

Novik, A.: Corticosteroid Treatment in Nondiphtheritic Croup. Acta Otolaryng. (Suppl.), *158*:20, 1960.

Ogura, J. H., and Dedo, H. H.: Repair of Large Pharyngostoma Utilizing Bilateral Non-delayed Regional Pedicle Flaps. Laryngoscope, *75*:588, 1965.

Rabe, E. F.: Infectious Croup: II Virus Croup. Pediatrics, *2*:415, 1948.

Spielman, A. D.: Urticaria and Angioedema. *In* Prigal, S. J. (Ed.): *Modern Allergy.* New York, McGraw-Hill Book Co., 1960.

Strannegard, O., and Axelsson, R.: Pseudocroup Associated with Viral Infections. Acta Otolaryng., *58*:432, 1964.

Vetto, R. R.: Epiglottitis. J.A.M.A., *173*:990, 1960.

Chapter 30

Chronic Nonspecific Diseases of the Larynx

CHRONIC NONSPECIFIC LARYNGITIS

Chronic inflammatory changes frequently involve the laryngeal mucosa, producing a variety of clinical manifestations. Confusion has arisen because of the large number of terms used to describe the clinical and pathologic appearances. Actually, chronic nonspecific laryngitis exhibits basic pathologic alterations which may have a variable distribution in the larynx.

Etiology. The exact etiology is unknown, but one or more sources of persistent laryngeal irritation may be significant in any single case. Infections of the respiratory tract which produce purulent material that comes in contact with the larynx, such as bronchiectasis and purulent sinusitis, may be a cause. Vocal abuse is an important source of chronic laryngeal irritation. Most people using their voices in their vocations have some evidence of laryngeal mucosal changes. Inhalants, particularly cigarette smoke and industrial fumes, are laryngeal irritants. Persistent mouth breathing secondary to nasal obstruction, with resulting inadequate humidification of inhaled air, will cause laryngeal mucosal alterations. Any kind of vasodilatation may cause submucosal hemorrhage and edema with resulting inflammatory changes. Alcohol is a vasodilating agent which, in addition, acts to reduce social inhibitions, thus predisposing to vocal abuse.

Pathophysiology and Pathology. The basic effect of laryngeal irritants is to produce vasodilatation and hyperemia. This may, in turn, precipitate submucosal hemorrhages, interstitial edema, and production of an inflammatory exudate consisting mainly of mononuclear cells. Eventually, the injured area is invaded by fibroblasts, resulting in fibrosis and hyalinization with thickening and deformity of structure. The pathophysiologic cycle may be arrested at any point, with a resulting clinical entity.

The pathologic changes in the larynx may be diffuse or localized. Most commonly, they are localized to the true vocal cords, the false cords, interarytenoid space, and posterior surface of the epiglottis being involved less frequently. Epithelial changes are generally the most diffuse. The ciliated respiratory epithelium of the supraglottic areas undergoes squamous metaplasia. The areas of normal stratified squamous epithelium may show thickening due to acanthosis, keratosis, and parakeratosis. Glandular structures undergo hypertrophy early in the course of the disease, but later they may undergo complete atrophy, resulting in the sicca syndrome. The subepithelial tissues may exhibit varying degrees of vasodilatation, hemorrhage, interstitial edema, and mononuclear cell infiltration. In the long-standing cases, fibrosis and hyaline degeneration are evident in these tissues.

Types of chronic laryngitis include: (1) chronic simple laryngitis (hypertrophic laryngitis and subglottic laryngitis); (2) hemorrhagic laryngitis; (3) laryngitis sicca; (4) vocal nodules; (5) vocal polyps.

Chronic Simple Laryngitis

Clinical Manifestations. Hoarseness is the most notable complaint. The patient complains of roughening of his voice with variations in pitch (usually lower) and breaks in tone. He may note the hoarseness is worse early in the day and that the voice improves as the day progresses. Vocal fatigue, laryngeal discomfort, and soreness are present in advanced cases. There may be a constant urge to clear the throat, which is usually nonproductive except for small amounts of sticky mucus. This habit may precede each effort to speak.

The laryngeal mucosa is diffusely reddened. The true vocal cords lose their pearly sheen and appear pink to dull red. Small dilated blood vessels may be seen on the superior surfaces of the true cords running parallel to the margins. The margins of the true cords appear rounded, and when the patient phonates, the pattern of vibration is obviously asynchronous and the cords appear flabby (Fig. 30–1). Increased amounts of thick mucus may be evident on the mucosal surfaces, and it is common to see a strand of clear mucus suspended across the glottis.

In more advanced cases, the mucosa takes on a granular appearance and may exhibit polypoid changes. The granules are small elevations produced by glandular hypertrophy and are seen on the false cords and arytenoid eminences. There may be areas of mucosal erosion. As fibrosis progresses, polypoid deformities of the true and false cords appear. In case of diffuse change, the terms hyperplastic or hypertrophic laryngitis have been applied. In a small number of patients, the chronic mucosal changes may be complicated by submucosal hemorrhages, and in such an instance, the term hemorrhagic laryngitis has been applied. This is to be distinguished from laryngeal hemorrhages due to blood dyscrasias, typhoid fever, diabetes, and trauma.

Rarely the pathologic changes may be localized to the subglottic area. In such instances, there is marked fibrous thickening of the conus elasticus which may impinge on the airway.

Treatment. The main efforts in therapy are directed at elimination of irritative factors. This includes elimination of cigarettes and excessive alcohol. Any sinus or pulmonary infection must be treated, and steps should be taken to eliminate any upper respiratory obstruction. Singers and professional voice users will frequently have a hoarseness which is often an exacerbation of a chronic laryngitis. In such patients, complete voice rest is indicated during the acute episode. Many of the patients also benefit from vocal re-education.

Endolaryngeal applications of silver nitrate, silver protein salts, and resorcinol are best avoided, since the applications are often traumatic and the medications irritating. This is especially true in the case of professional voice users, who are frequently nervous, high-strung individuals in whom attempted laryngeal manipulations may be difficult and may result in injury. If it seems necessary, mono-p-chlorophenol, which is aromatic, soothing, and nontoxic, may be

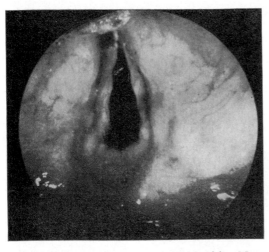

Fig. 30–1. Chronic simple laryngitis. Note the loss of the white color of the true vocal cords and the irregular hypertrophic changes.

dropped into the larynx at intervals of 4 to 8 hours. However, it is doubtful that any local medication is of real benefit in this disease.

A well-humidified atmosphere is important, and in drier climates a humidifier by the bed at night is helpful.

Expectorant drugs, such as saturated solutions of potassium iodide (5 ml every 4 hours) or ammonium chloride (5 g every 2 hours), may be helpful in stimulating or thinning the laryngeal secretions during exacerbations. A high fluid intake is also necessary to thin secretions.

Direct laryngoscopy and biopsy are indicated in any patient in whom there may be a question of malignancy or specific laryngeal disease such as tuberculosis. Chronic laryngitis is often associated with epidermoid carcinoma, but a cause-and-effect relationship has not been proved. Laryngoscopy may also be indicated in patients who have fibrosis and polypoid changes in the larynx in order to remove redundant tissue.

Laryngitis Sicca (Chronic Atrophic Laryngitis)

Etiology. This form of chronic laryngitis is characterized by marked atrophy of the mucosa and mucosal appendages of the larynx. It occurs most frequently in patients who have been subjected to irradiation therapy in which the larynx was included in the field. In other cases, the disease may follow prolonged chronic simple laryngitis. However, in a large group, there is no obvious etiology. This group consists mainly of females; in addition to laryngeal disease, they frequently suffer from atrophic rhinitis. Laryngitis sicca may also occur as part of Sjögren's syndrome and in association with pregnancy.

Pathology. As in atrophic rhinitis, there is a marked decrease in mucosal vascularity due to intimal proliferation and fibrosis of the walls of the small vessels. There is a complete absence of the glandular structures. The ciliated surface epithelium of the layrnx undergoes squamous metaplasia and becomes thin and atrophic, and mucosal erosions are often present. Fibrosis is marked

in the subepithelial areas which also contain a mononuclear inflammatory exudate.

Clinical Manifestations. The main physiologic abnormality is a lack of glandular secretions and mucosal lubrication. The patients will complain of a dry, "tickly" throat. There may be persistent cough to remove the thick, viscid secretions. Cough and hoarseness tend to be more severe in the morning. On occasion, laryngeal crusting may cause respiratory embarrassment, and hemoptysis may occur when crusts are dislodged. Finally, almost all patients complain of the foul, offensive odor of the breath.

The laryngeal mucosa has a dry, glazed, and roughened appearance. Crusts are usually present, especially in the interarytenoid area. The crusts may vary from yellow-green to black in color. Small tenacious globs of thick, green mucus may be seen in the larynx. If crusts are removed, a raw, oozing surface will be left, but actual ulceration is uncommon. This disease is usually easily distinguished, although in some cases syphilis must be excluded. Patients in whom there is no obvious etiology for the condition will often exhibit similar findings in the nose.

Treatment. Since the mucosal glands are partly or completely destroyed and regeneration is not possible, treatment is symptomatic. The treatment consists of furnishing lubrication and moisture to the larynx. Humidification of the home atmosphere is important, especially at night. To help prevent crust formation and remove the offensive odor, a nebulized spray consisting of the following may be used:

Glycerine	6%
70% Ethanol	6%
Rosewater	qtts $\bar{X}$
Saline solution	q.s. ad.

The administration of iodides (i.e., potassium iodide, 30 mg t.i.d.) may be of value in stimulation of secretion if any glandular function remains. Treatment of simultaneous nasal involvement is also important. Occasionally, it may be necessary to remove thick, adherent crusts by indirect or direct laryngoscopy.

it may invade the basilar cell layers and produce blurring of the basement membrane, with resulting diagnostic confusion.

Treatment. The problem of possible malignant degeneration or transformation is still unresolved; therefore, there is disagreement as to the aggressiveness of therapy necessary to avoid this complication. Keratosis with and without cellular atypia occurs frequently in association with carcinoma; however, there is no real evidence that the latter is a result of progression of the former. The occurrence of carcinoma in a larynx with isolated keratosis without cellular atypia is rare. When carcinoma develops in a patient in whom keratosis with atypia has been demonstrated previously, the adequacy of the initial biopsy must be questioned, since the two diseases may be coincidental. Care must be taken to submit adequate as well as representative biopsies for diagnosis.

The presence of a keratotic lesion in the larynx is always an indication for biopsy to rule out carcinoma. When the diagnosis of keratosis, with or without cellular atypia, is returned, one must decide if the biopsy is representative. If there is any doubt, another biopsy is indicated.

Since keratosis is benign, conservative therapy is indicated. The situation should be explained to the patient so that he will make every effort to reduce his exposure to laryngeal irritants, particularly smoking and vocal abuse. Many lesions will disappear on this regimen. The patient should then be followed and examined with watchful expectancy, particularly if cellular atypia is present. In the advent of any suspicious clinical change or persistence of the lesion, repeated biopsies are indicated. Without the diagnosis of carcinoma, radiotherapy or more radical surgery is not indicated. Keratosis is not as responsive to irradiation as carcinoma and therefore requires at least a cancericidal dose. Also, there is no evidence that this will prevent a later appearance of carcinoma.

If the diagnosis of pseudoepitheliomatous hyperplasia is returned on more than one routine biopsy and there is no evidence of underlying disease, such as blastomycosis or granular cell myoblastoma, a deep wedge biopsy is indicated to rule out the presence of verrucous carcinoma. The diagnosis of verrucous carcinoma requires the demonstration of invasion of deep tissues, which usually cannot be determined in the usual specimens from laryngeal biopsy.

CHRONIC CICATRICIAL STENOSIS OF THE LARYNX

Occlusion of the laryngeal lumen by granulation and fibrous tissue is still a frequent problem and is still responsible for some patients' having to retain a permanent, but often unnecessary, tracheostomy.

Etiology. In the past, specific infectious diseases were the most frequent cause of stenosis. These included syphilis, tuberculosis, diphtheria, and typhoid fever, but these are almost nonexistent causes today. The most common cause of stenosis is a traumatic injury to the larynx. Laryngeal injuries, complicated by infection and perichondritis, may eventually result in stenosis because of the production of excessive granulation and fibrous tissue. Automobile accidents cause the majority of laryngeal injuries, and because of lack of adequate treatment in the acute state, laryngeal stenosis may be the eventual result. Less common traumatic causes of cicatricial stenosis are high tracheostomy, trauma secondary to endoscopic procedures, radiation injuries, prolonged nasogastric intubation, and caustic burns.

Pathology. Trauma to the larynx is usually associated with laceration or loss of endolaryngeal mucosa, which is an important barrier to bacteria as well as a source of blood supply to the cartilages.

The raw area becomes superficially infected and, in the presence of cartilage fractures, this predisposes to perichondritis. The result is production of inflammatory exudate, formation of granulation tissue, and finally laying down of fibrous tissue. This excess tissue impinges on the laryngeal lumen, and if displaced cartilage is present, the stenosing effect is enhanced.

Laryngeal stenosis can be divided into three groups which are usually isolated but may be combined.

Supraglottic Stenosis. This type of stenosis is caused most often by caustic burns and by untreated automobile injuries in the female. Caustic burns, usually due to lye, cause denudation of the supraglottic structures of epithelium. When healing occurs, the epiglottis becomes adherent to the false cords, and, in some cases, to the posterior pharyngeal wall. Supraglottic traumatic injuries are associated with posterior displacement of the epiglottis into the vestibule, and since there are usually lacerations of the false cords, healing may be accompanied by the development of fibrous stenosis in untreated cases. Usually, the true vocal cords are normal, but occasionally unilateral or bilateral cord fixation may be present.

Glottic Stenosis. Occlusion of the airway at this level is most often due to web formation between the vocal cords. This is rarely secondary to external trauma and is most frequently caused by indiscriminate removal of mucosa from both vocal cords at the anterior commissure during laryngoscopy and vocal cord stripping.

Infraglottic Stenosis. This is the most common site of stenosis because this is the narrowest position of the laryngeal airway and the cricoid cartilage is susceptible to the development of perichondritis. This area

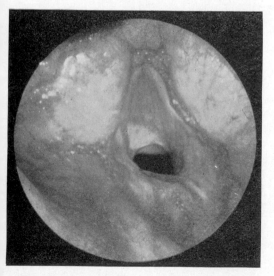

FIG. 30–10. Infraglottic stenosis in a 34-year-old male following a crushing injury to the cricoid cartilage.

is also the most frequent site of crushing laryngeal injuries in males due to automobile accidents.

The performance of a high tracheostomy, which is left in place, through the cricoid or cricothyroid membrane is still a frequent cause of stenosis. In fact, any injury resulting in exposure of the cricoid cartilage to the contaminated pharynx or larynx has a good chance of producing perichondritis of the cricoid and eventual stenosis (Fig. 30–10).

The stenosis is usually circumferential, but when the arch of the cricoid has been crushed, the maximum obstruction may be in the anterior portion of the lumen. Bilateral vocal cord paralysis or fixation is frequently associated with crushing injuries of this part of the larynx because of injury to the recurrent nerves.

Clinical Manifestations. The diagnosis is usually obvious, with a history of injury and symptoms of hoarseness or aphonia, stridor, and dyspnea. Most patients will be seen with a tracheostomy tube already in place. Soft tissue roentgenograms of the larynx as well as laryngograms should be performed to determine the extent and level of the stenosis. These will also confirm the presence of a high tracheostomy if it is present.

Indirect and direct laryngoscopic examination may disclose a confusing picture with supraglottic stenosis. There is usually severe anatomic distortion because of the fixation of the epiglottis to the arytenoids or posterior pharyngeal wall. Often the laryngeal lumen beneath the stenotic area is hidden from view. As a result, laryngograms performed by introducing dye from above the stenosis and from below through the tracheostomy are of extreme diagnostic importance in localizing the stenosis.

Glottic and infraglottic stenosis are more easily assessed by laryngoscopic methods, but again, laryngograms are invaluable in determining the extent of the stenotic area. Xeroradiography is also helpful.

Direct laryngoscopy should always be performed in order to determine the mobility of the arytenoid cartilages by the passive mobility test.

Treatment. Before treatment is planned, the location of the stenosis must be accurately determined. Also, the presence of vocal cord paralysis or ankylosis must be noted. If there is no movement of the vocal cords, if 8 or more weeks have passed since the injury, or if the arytenoids are fixed, arytenoidopexy should be performed at the time of surgical treatment of the stenosis.

Past methods of treatment have included dilatations and the use of core molds, as popularized by Jackson. However, these methods are rarely completely successful except with stenosis of minor degree. Also, the patient may require dilatations at varying intervals for the rest of his life.

Several authors have excised the cicatrix and lined the larynx with a split-thickness skin graft held in place by an intralaryngeal stent. Again, recurrent stenosis is a frequent result, especially if the stenosis is circumferential.

Many patients with cicatricial stenosis are still forced to have a permanent tracheostomy. However, this is an unnecessary and unwarranted hardship to impose on these patients, since many are young and would have 40 to 50 years of life with a tracheostomy. Almost all of these patients may be rehabilitated surgically, with resulting restitution of normal deglutition, respiration, and phonation. The surgical procedure used will vary with the site of stenosis.

Supraglottic Stenosis. It has been found in patients who have had supraglottic resection for carcinoma that the epiglottis is unnecessary for deglutition. Since the scarred, adherent epiglottis is the major factor responsible for the supraglottic stenosis, excision of the epiglottis and adjacent false cords will most consistently produce permanent relief of stenosis.

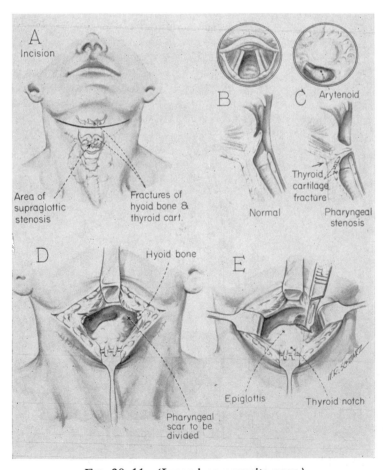

FIG. 30–11. *(Legend on opposite page.)*

A pharyngotomy must be performed to approach the stenotic area of the larynx. The scarred epiglottis and false cords are excised, and the base of the tongue is approximated to the thyroid perichondrium (Fig. 30–11). It is not necessary to approximate all the mucosal edges, as the raw areas will epithelize. A soft silicone stent is then inserted and fixed in place by Mersilene sutures, as in the case of acute laryngeal fractures. The stent is left in place approximately 8 weeks and is then removed by indirect laryngoscopy. In most instances, at least one vocal cord is functioning, and it is rarely necessary to perform an arytenoidopexy in this type of stenosis.

Glottic Stenosis. The treatment of traumatic glottic webs is the same as that described for congenital webs using a McKnaught keel or Montgomery umbrella.

Infraglottic Stenosis. Before reconstruction is attempted, any residual perichondritis must be controlled. When a high tracheostomy is present, it must be replaced in the trachea at a lower level.

Reconstruction is carried out by resection of the stenotic area and reanastomosis of the thyroid cartilage to the upper tracheal

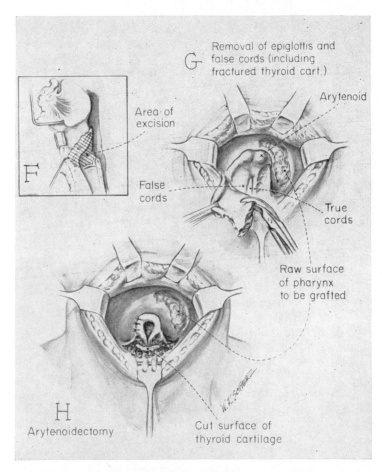

Fig. 30–11. Repair of supraglottic laryngeal stenosis. *A*, Skin incision is made at the level of the thyrohyoid membrane. *B, C,* The level and nature of the stenosis are indicated. *D, E,* The pharynx is entered by an intrahyoid pharyngotomy. *F, G,* The fibrotic structures causing the stenosis are resected, the arytenoid cartilages being preserved. *H,* The procedure may be combined with arytenoidectomy, but this is rarely necessary in supraglottic injury. A stent is inserted in the larynx before the pharynx is closed.

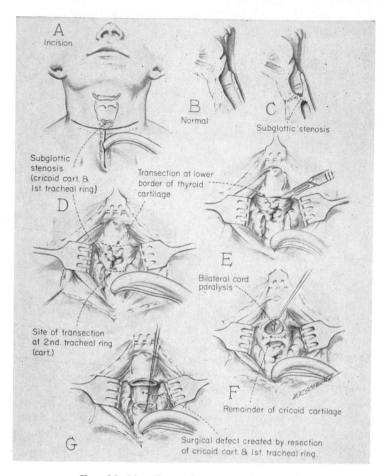

FIG. 30–12. *(Legend on opposite page.)*

rings (Figs. 30–12 and 30–13). When the resulting defect is extensive (i.e., 5 to 6 cm), it may be necessary to mobilize the larynx by incising the thyrohyoid membrane or the hyoglossal muscles in order to "drop" the larynx in the neck and effect reanastomosis. A stent is left in place for 8 to 12 weeks.

Since bilateral vocal cord fixation is frequently associated with this type of stenosis due to external trauma, arytenoidopexy is performed at the same time that the stenosis is repaired. If normal cord mobility exists, the recurrent nerves must be carefully preserved during the surgical repair. Many patients with chronic cicatricial stenosis have had a tracheostomy so long that the tract is well epithelized and may require surgical closure.

ARTHRITIS OF THE CRICOARYTENOID JOINT

Etiology. Rheumatoid arthritis is by far the most common cause. The cricoarytenoid joint is involved in approximately 25% of cases of rheumatoid arthritis. Less common causes of noninfectious cricoarytenoid arthritis are gout, lupus erythematosus, and other collagen diseases. Infectious arthritis, once common, is now rare, and involvement by tuberculosis, syphilis, and gonorrhea has seldom occurred since the advent of chemotherapy. Metastatic infection due to staphylococci or streptococci is rare. Finally, trauma may produce traumatic arthritis of one or both cricoarytenoid joints, which may develop after external or internal laryngeal injury.

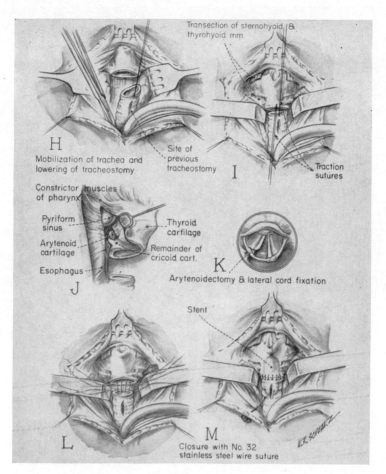

FIG. 30–12. Repair of infraglottic (subglottic) stenosis. *A*, Skin incision is made at the level of the cricoid, or the old tracheostomy incision may be used. *B, C,* The site of the stenosis is indicated. *D, E, F,* The site of the stenosis is resected. *G, H,* The trachea is mobilized and pulled superiorly by separating it from the esophagus. It is usually necessary to lower the tracheostomy site. *I,* The larynx is lowered by dividing the thyrohyoid and sternohyoid muscles. *J, K,* When necessary, arytenoidopexy or arytenoidectomy should be performed at the time of thyrotracheal anastomosis. *L, M,* The thyroid cartilage and remainder of the cricoid cartilage are approximated to the upper tracheal cartilage using stainless steel wires. An endolaryngeal stent should be inserted before the closure is completed.

Clinical Manifestations. The symptomatic manifestation of cricoarytenoid arthritis may be due to acute inflammatory disease of the joint or to fixation or ankylosis of the cricoarytenoid joints. Acute arthritis is almost always a manifestation of rheumatoid arthritis.

The symptoms of acute arthritis include the sensation of a lump in the throat and pain in the throat aggravated by swallowing or speaking. The pain may radiate to the ears. Patients also experience hoarseness, dyspnea, stridor, and occasionally complete laryngeal obstruction. Most patients have other signs of rheumatoid arthritis, but occasionally laryngeal involvement is the initial manifestation of the disease.

Examination of the larynx during the acute stage will disclose a striking, bright red swelling of the arytenoid eminences. The swelling of the posterior larynx may obscure the glottis. The vocal cords may be

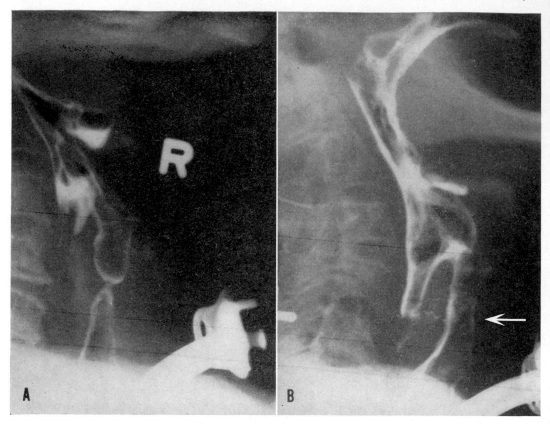

Fig. 30–13. *A*, Preoperative laryngogram of a patient with traumatic infraglottic stenosis. *B*, Postoperative laryngogram after resection of the stenosis and thyrotracheal anastomosis. The arrow shows the previous site of stenosis.

immobilized by the inflammatory process. Manipulation of the arytenoid with a spatula may cause severe pain. As the acute inflammatory reaction subsides, the swollen arytenoid eminences become a translucent gray color, and movement of the arytenoid is resumed.

In the presence of the rheumatoid arthritis, several blood tests, including the sedimentation rate, C-reactive protein level, and gamma globulin levels, are often abnormal. Also, tests for rheumatoid factor are usually positive.

Treatment. Acute cricoarytenoid arthritis is treated by putting the joint at rest; therefore, voice rest is mandatory. Salicylates are of value for analgesia, and steroids may be helpful in reducing the inflammatory response. Severe odynophagia may necessitate intravenous feeding. Tracheostomy may be necessary when obstructive symptoms due to edema and vocal cord immobilization are severe. Patients who have had acute cricoarytenoid arthritis must be observed at intervals because bilateral vocal cord fixation may follow insidiously.

ANKYLOSIS OF THE CRICOARYTENOID JOINTS

Etiology. Any type of cricoarytenoid arthritis may end in ankylosis of the joint and fixation of the vocal cords. Long-standing paralysis of the vocal cords will end in eventual fibrous fixation of the joints. Occasionally, trauma will precipitate insidious fixation of the cricoarytenoid joints without symptoms at the time of injury. In addition to producing joint disease, any of the collagen diseases may cause a paralysis of the vocal cords due to vascular lesions involving the peripheral nerves.

Clinical Manifestations. The symptoms of ankylosis of the cricoarytenoid joints are usually only significant when both joints are involved. Unilateral joint fixation may produce hoarseness but little other difficulty. Bilateral fixation of the cricoarytenoid joints usually causes some degree of laryngeal obstruction manifested by dyspnea and inspiratory stridor. The laryngeal obstruction is made worse by exercise, respiratory infections, sedation, and sleep. Hoarseness is usually present, although the voice may be breathy.

Examination of the larynx discloses the cord fixation. Usually, the vocal cords are in the paramedian or intermediate position. There is a tendency for the membranous portions of the cords to bow outward on inspiration. Direct laryngoscopy and palpation of the arytenoids are necessary to differentiate joint fixation from paralysis. Vocal cord immobilization may be due to either cause in rheumatoid arthritis.

Treatment. Surgical treatment of ankylosis is usually only necessary when both vocal cords are fixed in the midline; then an arytenoidectomy or arytenoidopexy should be performed. Rarely, fixation may occur with both vocal cords in the intermediate position, resulting in glottic incompetence. Treatment may require mediofixation of a vocal cord or the injection of silicone or Teflon into one cord. Unilateral fixation rarely requires therapy except for dysphonia secondary to inadequate approximation of the vocal cords. The voice may be improved considerably by a Teflon injection.

PROLAPSE OF THE VENTRICLE OF MORGAGNI

Etiology. Prolapse of the ventricle refers to a situation in which apparently normal mucosal tissue is seen protruding into the vestibule from the laryngeal ventricle. True eversion of ventricular mucosa is practically impossible because of tissue attachment and is probably rare. Most frequently, this condition is a form of chronic laryngitis, and mucosal protrusion occurs because of inflammatory infiltration and tissue hyper-

trophy. Rarely, traction by a ventricular cyst or tumor may cause mucosal eversion from the ventricle.

Clinical Manifestations. Hoarseness, which may be variable and intermittent, occurs when the mass lies out on the margin of the true vocal cord. An irritative, nonproductive cough is often present.

The appearance of a smooth, pear-shaped pale or purplish mass protruding from the ventricle is quite characteristic. At direct laryngoscopy, the mass can be palpated and moved freely to determine that its attachment lies in the ventricle and not on the true vocal cord. The mass can usually be pushed back into the ventricle. The lesions must be distinguished from cysts or neoplasms of the true cord or ventricle.

Treatment. Direct laryngoscopy and removal with biting forceps are indicated for biopsy as well as eradication of the condition. Once the diagnosis is established, treatment of the associated chronic laryngitis should be instituted.

REFERENCES

Arnold, G.: Vocal Nodules and Polyps: Laryngeal Tissue Reaction to Habitual Hyperkinetic Dysphonia. J. Speech Hearing Disorders, *27*:205, 1962.

Ash, J. E., and Schwartz, L.: The Laryngeal (Vocal Cord) Node. Trans. Am. Acad. Ophthal. Otolaryng., *48*:323, 1943.

Baker, D. C., Jr.: Polypoid Vocal Cord. N. Y. State J. Med., *63*:3098, 1963.

Birck, H. C.: Endoscope Repair of Laryngeal Stenosis. Trans. Am. Acad. Ophthal. Otolaryng., *74*:140, 1970.

Conley, J. J.: Reconstruction of the Subglottic Air Space. Ann. Otol., *62*:477, 1963.

Cracovaner, A. J.: Hyperkeratosis of the Larynx. Arch. Otolaryng., *70*:287, 1959.

Dedo, H. H., and Fishman, N. H.: Laryngeal Release and Sleeve Resection for Tracheal Stenosis. Ann. Otol. Rhinol. Laryngol., *78*:285, 1969.

Epstein, S. S., *et al.*: The Vocal Cord Polyp. J. Laryngol., *71*:673, 1957.

Erich, J. B.: Mechanical Appliances for Cicatricial Stenosis of the Larynx and Upper Trachea. Ann. Otol., *67*:799, 1956.

Gabriel, C. E., and Jones, D. G.: Hyperkeratosis of the Larynx. J. Laryngol. Otol., *87*:129, 1973.

Holinger, P., and Johnston, K. C.: Benign Tumors of the Larynx. Ann. Otol., *64*:469, 1951.

Knight, J. S.: Laryngeal Stenosis: Method of Surgical Correction. Laryngoscope, *74*:564, 1964.

Lederman, M.: Keratosis of the Larynx. J. Laryngol., *77*:651, 1963.

Lowenthal, G.: Treatment of Polypoid Laryngitis. Laryngoscope, *68*:1095, 1958.

McGavran, M. H., *et al.*: Isolated Laryngeal Keratosis. Laryngoscope, *70*:932, 1960.

Montgomery, W. W.: Cricoarytenoid Arthritis. Laryngoscope, *73*:801, 1963.

Montgomery, W. W.: The Surgical Management of Supraglottic and Subglottic Stenosis. Ann. Otol. Rhinol. Laryngol., *77*:534, 1968.

Montgomery, W. W., and Lofgren, R. H.: Usual and Unusual Causes of Laryngeal Arthritis. Arch. Otolaryng., *77*:29, 1963.

Moore, I.: The So-called Prolapse of the Laryngeal Ventricle and Eversion of the Sacculus. J. Laryngol., *37*:265, 333, 381, 1922.

Negus, V. E.: Treatment of Chronic Stenosis of the Larynx with Special Reference to Skin Grafting. Trans. Am. Laryngol. Assoc., *60*:82, 1938.

Norris, C. M., and Peale, A. R.: Keratosis of the Larynx. J. Laryngol., *77*:635, 1963.

Ogura, J. H., and Powers, W. E.: Functional Restitution of Traumatic Stenosis of the Larynx and Pharynx. Laryngoscope, *74*:1081, 1964.

Ogura, J. H., *et al.*: Functional Restoration of the Food Passages in Extensive Stenosing Caustic Burns of the Pharynx and Esophagus. Laryngoscope, *71*:885, 1961.

Pennington, C. L.: Glottic and Supraglottic Injury and Stenosis from External Trauma. Laryngoscope, *7*:317, 1964.

Polisar, I. A.: The Cricoarytenoid Joint. Laryngoscope, *69*:1129, 1959.

Putney, F. J.: Borderline Malignant Lesions of the Larynx. Arch. Otolaryng., *61*:381, 1955.

Reuben, J. J., and Lehrhoff, I.: Pathogenesis and Treatment of Vocal Nodules. J. Speech Hearing Disorders, *27*:150, 1962.

Rienke, F.: Untersuchungen uber Das Menschliche Stimmband. Fortschr. Med., *13*:469, 1895.

Russell, H.: Keratosis of the Larynx. J. Laryngol., *77*:651, 1963.

Schmiegelow, E.: Stenosis of the Larynx. A New Method of Surgical Treatment. Arch. Otolaryng., *9*:347, 1929.

Schmiegelow, E.: The Surgical Treatment of Chronic Cicatricial Stenosis of the Larynx. J. Laryngol., *53*:1, 1938.

Schwartz, A. W., *et al.*: Severe Cicatricial Stenosis of the Larynx Due to Nasogastric Tubes. Plast. Reconstr. Surg., *24*:341, 1959.

Schwartz, L., *et al.*: Hypertrophic Changes in the Interarytenoid Space. Arch. Otolaryng., *82*:287, 1965.

Strong, M. S.: Vocal Cord Nodules and Polyps —The Role of Surgical Therapy. Laryngoscope, *81*:911, 1971.

Waldapfel, R.: Pathology of the Subepithelial (Rienke's) Layer of the Vocal Cords. Ann. Otol., *48*:647, 1940.

Wallner, L. J.: Smokers' Larynx. Laryngoscope, *64*:541, 1960.

Welman, L., *et al.*: The Larynx in Rheumatoid Arthritis. J. Laryngol., *79*:403, 1965.

Chapter 31

Chronic Granulomatous Diseases of the Larynx*

TUBERCULOSIS OF THE LARYNX

Etiology. Infection of the larynx by *Mycobacterium tuberculosis* is almost always a complication of active pulmonary tuberculosis; it is the most common granulomatous disease of the larynx. Clinical laryngeal involvement occurs in approximately 3% of cases of moderately advanced pulmonary tuberculosis, but this incidence approaches 100% in terminal cases.

Previously, it was stated that the disease was most prevalent in the younger age groups, i.e., 20 to 40 years. In the past 20 years, the incidence of disease in people over the age of 60 has increased markedly. At the present time, tuberculosis of all types is twice as common in males as in females. For patients over 50, the ratio of male to female is 4:1. These figures are also reflected in the incidence of laryngeal involvement. Laryngeal tuberculosis is most frequent in older males, particularly those of poor constitution and health, many of whom are alcoholics.

Invasion of the larynx is by direct infection from contaminated sputum. Since sputum and air usually pass through the wider posterior commissure, this may be a factor predisposing to the involvement of the posterior portions of the larynx. Hematogenous

and lymphogenous routes of infection are probably not important in laryngeal infection.

Pathology and Pathologic Anatomy. The posterior structures of the larynx, including the arytenoids and the interarytenoid space, the posterior vocal cords, and, to a lesser extent, the laryngeal surface of the epiglottis, are the most commonly affected. All are sites of impact of sputum upon coughing.

Two types of lesions are produced and recognized clinically:

1. *Exudative Type.* Initially, there is an acute diffuse inflammatory phase, which results in hyperemia, edema, and infiltration of the subepithelial spaces by a nonspecific cellular exudate.

2. *Productive Type.* The exudative phase is followed by the development of the typical tuberculous granuloma in the subepithelial tissues. The avascular tubercle consists of an area of central caseation surrounded by epithelioid cells and a peripheral zone of mononuclear cells. Later, depending on host resistance, the tubercles are surrounded by fibrous tissue, which may eventually replace the tubercles.

The tubercles may coalesce to produce macroscopic yellowish gray nodules. Because of their subepithelial position, the overlying epithelium may be lost, and ulceration with secondary infection frequently occurs. This process tends to involve the

*See Chapter 22 for discussion of allied subjects.

vocal process and epiglottis first because of the thinness of the mucosa covering the avascular cartilage. Ulceration and infection, in turn, cause perichondritis and chondritis, particularly of the arytenoids and epiglottis, producing cartilage destruction and, in the case of arytenoids, destruction of the cricoarytenoid joints.

The presence of the tubercles may also stimulate hyperplasia of epithelium and subepithelial fibrous tissue. This may be manifested in the interarytenoid area as marked thickening resembling pachyderma. The vocal processes and other areas may be covered by morbilliform nodular or papillary masses of granulomatous tissue. In some cases, the mass is large, solitary, and pedunculated and is referred to as a tuberculoma. This is a manifestation of the reparative process, since there is little evidence of caseation in these lesions.

Edema may become quite marked later in the disease and is probably secondary to lymphatic obstruction by the granulomas. The epiglottis and tissue over the arytenoids are the sites of the most marked edema.

Healing of a tuberculous larynx is accompanied by fibrous tissue encapsulation and replacement of the tubercles. The effects of healing may be minimal if the process begins before diffuse tissue infiltration, diffuse ulceration, and perichondritis have occurred. Healing of the advanced lesions may end with fibrous stenosis or fixation of the cricoarytenoid joints.

Clinical Manifestations. The symptoms of laryngeal involvement occur late in the course of the pulmonary disease but may be the first to bring the patient to the physician. The earliest symptom is hoarseness, which is usually mild at first but may progress to extreme dysphonia or aphonia. There may be some dryness and pain in the throat. Pain is usually not severe unless perichondritis is present, in which case there is severe odynophagia and odynophonia which may radiate to the ears. Finally, respiratory obstruction may be secondary to edema, a tuberculoma, or bilateral midline vocal cord fixation.

The systemic symptoms of pulmonary tuberculosis are usually present if the patient is questioned. These include fever, chilly sensations, night sweats, weight loss, and fatigue. Cough with increased mucopurulent sputum and sometimes hemoptysis may occur.

Clinical Appearance. The earliest evidence of laryngeal tuberculosis is redness of the interarytenoid area and posterior vocal cords. This may be accompanied by considerable swelling in the interarytenoid area and the presence of a yellowish exudate. The epiglottis may also be red and swollen, particularly the laryngeal surface. In some instances, the inflammatory infiltration may be localized to one cord, giving it a spindle-shaped appearance. The remaining oropharyngeal mucosa is often pale secondary to general anemia.

Later, yellowish discrete nodules may be visible under intact mucosa in the interarytenoid area and on the epiglottis. These may coalesce and the involved areas become pinkish, swollen, and nodular, which typically occurs in the interarytenoid area.

At this point, there may be some roughening or erosion of one or both true cords. A later stage is manifested by ulceration, which tends at first to be localized to the vocal processes but tends later to spread anteriorly. The ulcers are usually shallow and covered with dirty gray, shaggy exudate,

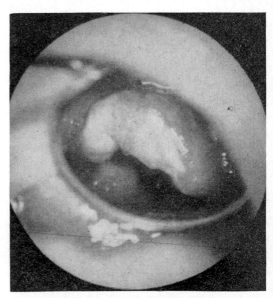

FIG. 31–1. Indirect laryngoscopic view of the turban-shaped epiglottis of tuberculosis of the larynx.

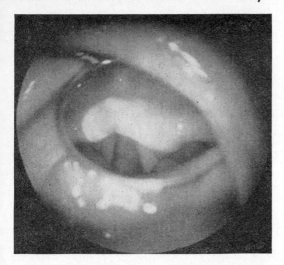

FIG. 31-2. View of the same larynx 3 weeks after institution of systemic antituberculous therapy.

giving the cords a "mouse-eaten" appearance.

The epiglottis and/or the arytenoid areas may be markedly edematous and may appear pinkish and translucent. This picture is characteristic; the epiglottis is often described as turban- or heart-shaped and the arytenoids as piriform or club-shaped (Figs. 31–1 and 31–2). The edema in such cases may entirely obscure the remainder of the larynx and obstruct the airway.

The latest stages of laryngeal involvement may be characterized by any combination of ulceration, edema, exuberant granulations, and tuberculoma formation. Vocal cord paralysis may be present secondary to muscular infiltration or cricoarytenoid joint fixation; also, tuberculous infiltration of pleura or mediastinal lymph nodes may involve the recurrent nerve (usually the left) to produce paralysis. The later stages of the disease are rare since the advent of effective chemotherapy.

When healed, the larynx may appear quite normal, or there may be fibrous adhesions between the vocal cords and residual unilateral or bilateral cord fixation.

Diagnosis. Tuberculosis of the larynx must be distinguished from cancer and other granulomatous diseases which it resembles clinically. The diagnosis is dependent upon finding the acid-fast tubercle bacillus in the patient's sputum, gastric washing, or biopsy specimen. The history and clinical findings are suggestive and are indications for an examination of a sputum or gastric washing specimen stained by the Ziehl-Neelsen method. In some patients, the organisms may be scanty, and several specimens should be examined. The specimen can be improved by digesting with Clorox and centrifuging to concentrate the organisms. Culture on Dubos' media and guinea pig inoculation are indicated in suspicious cases in the absence of positive sputum. Gastric washings are often of more help than sputum specimens in obtaining a positive smear.

A chest x-ray is almost always abnormal and should be done early in the work-up of any suspicious case to avoid needless exposure of personnel.

Direct laryngoscopy and biopsy are indicated in all cases to establish the diagnosis of tuberculosis and rule out the existence or coexistence of carcinoma or other disease. Carcinoma occurs fairly frequently in association with pulmonary tuberculosis and, occasionally, with laryngeal tuberculosis. Therefore, its presence is not ruled out by the finding of an abnormal chest roentgenogram and sputum containing acid-fast bacilli. Some patients may have scanty sputum and a fairly normal chest film, and examination of a specially stained biopsy specimen may be necessary to find the tubercle bacilli.

Treatment. The treatment is essentially that of the pulmonary disease. The antituberculosis drug, isoniazid, in combination with rifampin or ethambutol, is the most used and is given in combination to prevent the emergence of resistant organisms. Combinations containing isoniazid are most effective, and this drug is used with rifampin or ethambutol for initial treatment in the average pulmonary case. The three drugs are utilized in far-advanced disease, at the time of surgery, or when bacterial resistance develops. Patients with laryngeal disease usually have well-advanced pulmonary disease and are placed on triple drug therapy initially. The usual doses are isoniazid, 300 to 400 mg per day; rifampin 10 mg per kg per day; ethambutol 15 to 25 mg per kg per day. The drugs are maintained for at least 6 months after the sputum and gastric washings are negative for acid-fast bacilli.

The response of the laryngeal disease is rapid. Pain, when present, is completely relieved in a few days, and the ulcers are healed in a few weeks. As a result, palliative measures, such as alcohol injection of the superior laryngeal nerve for pain, are seldom necessary. Also, there is seldom any indication for local applications or cautery.

Strict voice rest should be maintained during the active phase of laryngeal disease.

Occasionally, tracheostomy is necessary for laryngeal obstruction. A later definitive surgical procedure may be necessary for bilateral cricoarytenoid joint fixation producing glottic obstruction or glottic incompetence.

Lupus of the Larynx

This is a clinical type of tuberculosis which probably occurs because of increased host resistance or decreased bacterial virulence. The disease is rare in North America.

Etiology. The causative organism is indistinguishable from the tubercle bacillus. The laryngeal disease is usually associated with similar lesions of the facial skin, interior of the nose, or pharynx. Pulmonary tuberculosis is rarely associated with this disease.

Pathology. The histologic lesion is the same as that occurring in tuberculosis. However, there is less tendency for the tubercles to undergo caseation, and they show more fibrosis. Few tubercle bacilli are found to be in the tissue, and the sputum rarely contains acid-fast bacilli. The site of predilection of the pathology in the larynx is the anterior portion of the aryepiglottic folds and the laryngeal surface of the epiglottis; the posterior larynx is not involved. The lesions tend to develop in stages and progress from nodule formation to ulceration and then fibrosis and scarring.

Clinical Manifestations. The patients are remarkably free of symptoms, and in spite of epiglottic ulcerations, the disease is typically painless. There is an anesthesia of the involved areas. The diagnosis may be sus-

pected when the lesions of lupus vulgaris of the face, nose, and pharynx are present.

Scattered yellowish pink discrete nodules on the epiglottis and aryepiglottic folds are characteristic of an early lesion. These later coalesce and develop superficial ulcerations covered by a scanty adherent exudate. Perichondritis and cartilage destruction may involve the epiglottis. There is a tendency toward spontaneous healing, with the result that scarring and deformity appear at the site of healed ulcerations. Ulceration and healing may be present in contiguous areas. In a late case, there may be nothing of the epiglottic margin, and in some cases only a scarred stump of epiglottis remains. Deep infiltration of the false cords may produce a firm, persistent swelling in these areas.

Diagnosis. The finding of the typical laryngeal lesions or deformity in association with similar lesions involving the pharynx, nose, or face is suggestive. The absence of pulmonary disease and the discovery of acid-fast organisms and tubercle formation in a tissue specimen confirm the diagnosis. Laryngoscopy and biopsy are indicated to rule out carcinoma or other granulomatous disease.

Treatment. Since the disease is self-limited and, in fact, may be seen first in the end stage, treatment is often unnecessary. However, the presence of active disease with identification of the causative organism would seem to be an indication for antituberculous therapy.

SYPHILIS OF THE LARYNX

Etiology. Syphilis is due to infection by the spirochete *Treponema pallidum* and is a chronic systemic disease transmitted by sexual contact and pregnancy. Laryngeal involvement may occur in congenital and acquired syphilis. The primary lesion of acquired syphilis, the chancre, is rare in the larynx because of its inaccessibility to primary contact. However, secondary and tertiary manifestations do occur but are now rare, since the disease is usually recognized and treated before it reaches the late stages. Congenital laryngeal syphilis, if present at birth, is similar to the secondary stage of acquired syphilis. The delayed form of congenital syphilis will produce lesions similar to those of tertiary acquired syphilis.

Pathology. The lesions of secondary syphilis appear 4 to 6 weeks after the primary lesion. The histologic change is marked by a perivascular accumulation of plasma cells and lymphocytes, with varying amounts of vascular dilatation and congestion. This infiltration is present in subepithelial tissues and results in a maculopapular rash. The epithelium over the papules may slough, producing superficial ulcerations which coalesce and form mucous patches.

The epithelium may undergo marked hypertrophy and hyperplasia, which may manifest grossly as condylomata. Microscopically, pseudoepitheliomatous hyperplasia is seen and may be confused with carcinoma.

Tertiary lesions develop 3 to 20 years after secondary syphilis. They are marked by localized areas of coagulative gummy necrosis or areas of chronic granulomatous inflammation with gradual tissue destruction and fibrosis. These changes are secondary to endothelial proliferation and obstruction of small arteries. The lesions in the larynx may occur as a diffuse, nodular, gummatous infiltrate. The subepithelial nodules may ulcerate and produce deep necrotic ulcers with undercut margins, or they may coalesce and produce a large, solitary gumma. Perichondritis and chondritis occur secondary to ulceration and syphilitic invasion. Eventually healing occurs, with marked fibrosis and contracture resulting in deformity and loss of function.

Clinical Manifestations. Some alteration in voice is the usual complaint; this may vary from severe hoarseness to aphonia. Cough and hemoptysis are early symptoms. Symptoms of laryngeal obstruction appear when edema, vocal cord paralysis, or inflammatory tissue causes pressure on the glottis. Pain is uncommon except when mucous patches involve the epiglottis, causing odynophagia.

Clinical Appearance. Secondary syphilis is marked by a diffuse laryngeal hyperemia, which may be accompanied by a maculopapular rash. Mucous patches tend to be confined to the epiglottis.

Tertiary lesions vary widely. A patchy, reddish, nodular mucosal infiltration is often associated with discrete, punched-out ulcers. Edema may be present, especially when perichondritis is present. Arytenoid and vocal cord movement may be impaired secondary to perichondritis, fibrosis, or paralysis. The late healing stage of fibrosis is marked by stellate scarring with infraglottic stenosis, adhesions between the vocal cords, and arytenoid fixation.

Diagnosis. A routine serology test for syphilis should be done in all cases of laryngeal disease, whether syphilis is suspected or not. The VDRL is presently in common use. However, the fluorescent treponemal antibody absorption test (FTA-ABS) or the Treponemal Immobilization Test is more reliable.

Direct laryngoscopy and biopsy are indicated to rule out carcinoma. Interpretation of the biopsy specimen must be done with care, as pseudoepitheliomatous hyperplasia which may accompany syphilis may be wrongly diagnosed as carcinoma. The causative spirochete may be seen in specimens of secondary lesions but not in tertiary lesions.

Treatment. The treatment is the same as that for syphilis elsewhere in the body. Penicillin is the drug of choice; a dose of 6 million units given over 10 days is advocated. This is best given as a single intramuscular dose of procaine and benzathine penicillin in view of the unreliability of many syphilitic patients. The patient is then followed with periodic serology tests.

Local treatment is restricted to treatment of complications, such as acute respiratory obstruction, bilateral midline vocal cord paralysis, and chronic cicatricial stenosis.

Neurosyphilis

The nerve supply of the larynx may be involved by the central nervous system manifestations of syphilis. Meningovascular syphilis produces thrombosis of the small vessels of the meninges. The result is the same as a cerebrovascular accident. Laryngeal paralysis secondary to such lesions is usually accompanied by other nerve deficits of medullary origin, although isolated tenth nerve paralysis can occur and may be bilateral. Tabes dorsalis is a form of neurosyphilis in which there is selective degeneration of the posterior columns of the spinal cord and the sensory roots of cranial and spinal nerves. This may result in sudden severe sensory discharges, and in the larynx this tabetic crisis is marked by spasm of the vocal cords with glottic closure. The spasm may be prolonged and may result in asphyxia. Tabes may also cause isolated nuclear degeneration producing laryngeal paralysis.

LEPROSY OF THE LARYNX

Etiology. Leprosy is a specific infectious disease caused by *Mycobacterium leprae* or Hansen's bacillus. The disease is only mildly contagious, and exposure for a prolonged period is necessary to contract the disease. Clinical signs do not appear for 2 to 5 years after exposure. The disease is transmitted to younger patients and is rare after age 40, possibly due to increasing immunity. The disease is rare in temperate climates but does occur in the Southern United States.

Pathology. The disease is divided, on clinicopathologic grounds, into three types: nodular or lepromatous; neural or anesthetic; and tuberculoid. The lepromatous variety is of the most importance to laryngologists. The microscopic picture is characterized by masses of foamy lepra cells containing many organisms. The skin and mucous membranes of the face and upper respiratory tract are insidiously involved by a diffuse or nodular infiltration. The nodules may ulcerate and become secondarily infected. Later the lesions undergo spontaneous healing and cicatrization. The neural and tuberculoid forms of this disease involve nerves and skin, and the microscopic lesions consist of tubercles with a few bacilli or lepra cells present.

Clinical Manifestations. The voice tends to be muffled early in the course of laryngeal involvement due to lesions of the supraglottic structures. Later, hoarseness and dyspnea occur when the vocal cords become affected. The lesions are usually anesthetic; therefore, pain and odynophagia are not a problem. Signs of involvement of the skin, nasal cavity, and oral cavity usually precede those of laryngeal involvement.

In the larynx, the supraglottic structures, particularly the epiglottis, are involved first. Nodular infiltration of these areas causes enlargement which impinges on the airway and obscures the vocal cords. The diseased areas are a dull gray color. Later, the nodules ulcerate and become covered with exudate. There is a tendency toward healing, and in these instances scarring and contractions develop. The vocal cords are usually not invovled until late in the active disease. Cervical lymph node enlargement is frequent and may mimic metastatic cancer.

Diagnosis. The differentiation from syphilis, tuberculosis, and cancer must be made. In spite of the presence of typical cutaneous lesions, laryngeal biopsy is often indicated to rule out coincidental disease. Aspiration and smear of a cervical lymph node will often establish the diagnosis.

Treatment. Spontaneous arrest may occur. The sulfone drugs, such as DDS (diaminodiphenylsulfone), have produced clinical arrest of the disease in many cases, but 20% will show no improvement. The drugs must be given over a long period of time (1 to 4 years) before marked improvement occurs. The corticosteroid preparations will produce temporary improvement and are useful in alleviating impending respiratory obstruction. Tracheostomy may be necessary in rare instances. The lepromatous variety of the disease has the poorest prognosis, with pneumonia, tuberculosis, and amyloidosis being the common causes of death.

GLANDERS

Glanders is a serious infectious disease characterized by the occurrence of multiple granulomatous abscesses throughout the body.

Etiology. The cause is a small gram-negative bacillus, *Malleomyces mallei*. The disease is mainly confined to animals, particularly horses, but man is susceptible and occasionally infected. Transmission is by inhalation, ingestion, or implantation in a mucosal or cutaneous abrasion, particularly around the nose. The disease has been eliminated in horses in the United States and is therefore rare in humans.

Pathology. The site of entry is marked by the appearance of a nodule or nodules of granulation tissue. These nodules undergo caseous necrosis and ulcerate, leaving a painful ulcer with irregular sharp margins. The process spreads by submucous lymphatics and contiguity, and eventually the entire respiratory tract may be involved by the ulcers. Vascular dissemination occurs and results in generalized spread of the disease.

Clinical Manifestations. The disease occurs in acute and chronic forms. The acute form is of most interest to laryngologists. It is marked by the abrupt onset of chills, fever, and prostration accompanied by inflammation and ulceration of mucous membranes, including that of the larynx. Cough, productive of foul, purulent sputum is present. Perichondritis and cartilage destruction may complicate the laryngeal disease, and the resulting edema and granulations may occlude the lumen. The disease progresses over 1 to 3 weeks, and death is a frequent result.

The chronic form of the disease is marked by exacerbations associated with the appearance of abscesses which may involve the larynx.

Diagnosis. The causative organism can be easily isolated from the sputum and exudates. Animal inoculation, serologic testing, and biopsy will establish the diagnosis.

Treatment. Sulfonamide drugs have been effective in humans. Supportive measures such as tracheostomy may be necessary in acute disease. Treatment of laryngeal stenosis or vocal cord fixation resulting from perichondritis should be carried out as indicated.

SCLEROMA OF THE LARYNX (RHINOSCLEROMA)

Scleroma is a chronic granulomatous disease of the upper respiratory tract described by von Hebra in 1870. The disease is endemic in areas of Central Europe and Southern Europe, Egypt, Central and South America, and the East Indies. However, it does occur in nonendemic areas.

Etiology. The disease is attributed to *Klebsiella rhinoscleromatis* (von Frisch bacillus), a gram-negative rod of the coliform group, although this has not been proved. The organism is always present in the lesions, but it is also found in normal noses.

Another etiologic factor may be important in accounting for the geographic distribution and the sporadic invasiveness of the organism. The disease is not highly contagious. There is a tendency for affected patients to be from lower socioeconomic groups.

Pathology. The disease affects only soft tissues, particularly the mucosa and submucosa of the upper respiratory tract. The clinicopathologic picture passes through three stages: (1) exudation, associated with increased discharge of discolored mucous and crusting, particularly in the nose; (2) proliferation, marked by the appearance of masses of granulomatous tissue in involved areas; (3) cicatrization, producing scarring and deformity. The typical microscopic picture is marked by a plasma cell and mononuclear infiltrate, Mikulicz's cells, Russell bodies, proliferating connective tissue, hyalinization of vessels, epithelial atrophy or hypertrophy, and squamous metaplasia. The Mikulicz's cell, a foamy, lacy cell containing the gram-negative organisms, is said to be characteristic. However, these findings do occur in other diseases and are not entirely specific. Also, in the later stages of fibrosis, Mikulicz's cells and plasma cells may be scarce, and the picture is that of nonspecific chronic inflammation.

The infraglottic area of the larynx is specifically attacked and may be the site of a large granulomatous mass or diffuse infiltration. Nodular infiltrations may involve the interarytenoid areas and aryepiglottic folds. Ulceration does not occur.

Clinical Manifestations. Hoarseness and cough are indicative of laryngeal involvement and may even be the initial complaint in patients with nasal involvement. Stridor and dyspnea secondary to proliferating tissue obstructing the larynx are late symptoms. Usually nasal obstruction or deformity of the nose and upper lip is present when the patient is first seen with hoarseness.

In the early stages, the mucosa of the interarytenoid area, aryepiglottic folds, laryngeal surface of the epiglottis, and infraglottic area is hyperemic and has a raw, granular appearance. Crusts and yellow purulent exudate are present. Later a reddish nodular infiltrate is apparent, especially in the infraglottic area. In some cases tissue hypertrophy is marked, leading to the formation of polypoid lesions. Later, the nodules become firm and pale and cartilaginous in consistency.

Diagnosis. Diagnosis is made by isolation of *Klebsiella rhinoscleromatis* from a tissue specimen. The pathologic appearance in the proliferative stage is also diagnostic but is often of little help in the cicatricial stage. Complement filtration tests on patient serum are of questionable value. The laryngeal lesions must be differentiated from syphilis, tuberculosis, leprosy, and neoplasms by laryngeal biopsy.

Treatment. Treatment with a combination of gentamicin or kanamycin with cephalothin is effective in producing arrest and regression of the proliferative lesions. The adjuvant use of corticosteroids may help to reduce cicatricial deformity. In the late stage of scarring, specific therapy is of litle value, and treatment is the same as that for laryngeal obstruction. Surgical removal is necessary for obstructing polypoid masses. There is no indication for irradiation therapy.

SARCOIDOSIS OF THE LARYNX

Sarcoidosis is a chronic granulomatous disease of unknown etiology. It affects individuals in the second and third decades and is especially common in Negroes. The disease follows an unpredictable course with exacerbations and remissions. The clinical manifestations are usually due to the effects of localized lesions, and constitutional symptoms tend to be mild.

Pathology. The basic lesion is the noncaseating epithelioid granuloma, which consists of tubercles containing epithelioid cells, mononuclear inflammatory cells, giant cells, and fibroblastic tissue. There is no caseous necrosis. The tubercles gradually mature and are replaced by fibrous tissue, which hyalinizes, leaving a dense scar.

The laryngeal lesions are composed of the typical noncaseating granulomas and are associated with a diffuse edema. The supra-

glottic structures are the site of maximal involvement.

Clinical Manifestations. Dyspnea and hoarseness, the most frequent laryngeal complaints, are secondary to edematous obstruction of the larynx. Less commonly, dysphagia occurs and is due to mechanical obstruction caused by the enlarged epiglottis.

The appearance of the larynx is quite characteristic. The epiglottis, aryepiglottic folds, false cords, and arytenoids are distorted by a smooth, pale, diffuse swelling. The epiglottis is particularly involved; in addition to the diffuse, edematous thickening, small white or brownish nodules may be seen along the free edge and on the posterior surface. Occasionally, the mucosa may appear granular or roughened.

Sarcoidosis is often accompanied by a polyneuritis which may involve the recurrent nerves, producing a vocal cord paralysis which is usually unilateral.

Diagnosis. Constitutional symptoms, such as fatigue, weight loss, cough, and shortness of breath, are frequent. Less common but more specific manifestations, such as uveitis, erythema nodosum, and salivary gland enlargement, are suggestive of sarcoidosis. The chest x-ray film will almost always show enlarged hilar nodes or a nodular parenchymal infiltrate. Laboratory findings may include eosinophilia, hyperglobulinemia, and hypercalcemia. The sedimentation rate is usually elevated. The Kveim skin test is positive in 75% of cases. Biopsy of the larynx will usually demonstrate the granuloma histologically. Positive biopsies may also be obtained from the tonsils, nasal turbinates, and scalene lymph nodes.

Treatment. Sarcoidosis of the larynx need only be treated if it is obstructive. Corticosteroid drugs will usually produce rapid reduction in the amount of edema. Occasional resistant cases may respond to direct injection of cortisone into the false cords and aryepiglottic folds. In the majority of patients, sarcoidosis eventually undergoes permanent clinical remission.

MYCOTIC DISEASES

Fungous infections of the larynx are uncommon; however, they assume significance because of confusion with more common granulomatous diseases and neoplasms.

Blastomycosis

North American blastomycosis is endemic in North America and is mainly a disease of the skin and lungs; however, primary involvement of the larynx does occur. The causative organism, *Blastomyces dermatitidis,* is a yeastlike fungus with thick, double-contoured walls which invades via skin defects or the respiratory tract.

Pathology. The larynx is involved by a diffuse nodular infiltration and may later ulcerate. Eventually, healing and fibrosis occur, and if ulceration has been extensive, vocal cord fixation and stenosis may occur. The microscopic picture is important. The epithelium undergoes marked hyperplasia of the pseudoepitheliomatous type, which may result in confusion and the erroneous diagnosis of carcinoma. Microabscesses containing the organisms, giant cells, and mononuclear cells occur in the epidermis and dermis and are characteristic of this disease.

Clinical Manifestations. Severe, persistent hoarseness is the most striking initial symptom. Cough with increased sputum or hemoptysis may occur. Pain and dysphagia are uncommon even with laryngeal ulceration. Early in the disease, the laryngeal mucosa is diffusely inflamed and granular, and later, tiny white miliary nodules may be seen on the true and false cords. Superficial mucosal ulcers covered with foul-smelling greenish exudate, under which is a bright red granular bed, appear in the more advanced cases. Later, healing and fibrosis may cause fixation of the arytenoids or cicatricial stenosis.

Diagnosis. The diagnosis is suggested by the presence of skin lesions and pulmonary infiltrates as disclosed by roentgenogram. A skin sensitivity test to blastomycin is of questionable value because of false-negative reactions and cross reactions with other fungous infections. The diagnosis can be made only by identification of the organism in a biopsy specimen.

Treatment. Amphotericin B, which is given intravenously in successive daily doses until 1 g has been given (usually 30 to 40 days), has produced the most successful results. The laryngeal lesions usually disappear very rapidly after treatment is instituted.

South American Blastomycosis (Paracoccidioidomycosis)

This disease is endemic in South America and does not occur in North America. The first signs of the disease are painful mucosal ulcerations in the upper respiratory tract associated with marked cervical lymphadenopathy. The laryngeal lesions resemble clinically and pathologically those of the North American disease, and therefore the differential diagnosis presents similar problems. The South American type differs markedly in that it usually responds well to sulfonamide therapy.

Histoplasmosis

Histoplasmosis is a fungous infection caused by *Histoplasma capsulatum* which attacks the reticuloendothelial system primarily. The basic pathologic process is a multiplication of the fungus in histiocytes, causing histiocytic proliferation. In addition, granulomatous lesions occur in soft tissues. The disease is endemic in the drainage basins of the Mississippi and St. Lawrence Rivers in North America.

Pathology. The disease is manifested by three clinical forms: (1) a mild subclinical pulmonary infection; (2) progressive disseminated infection; and (3) chronic localized disease. The latter two are of importance to laryngologists. Progressive disseminated histoplasmosis tends to occur in children and elderly males. However, localized upper respiratory tract and oral involvement occurs only in the adult patients. Of the adults affected by disseminated histoplasmosis, about 30% will develop mouth, nose, and larynx lesions as the primary manifestation. Chronic localized histoplasmosis is of two main types, pulmonary and mucocutaneous, and it is in the latter type that laryngeal disease is most frequent.

The microscopic appearance of the laryngeal lesions is that of a granuloma made up of epithelioid cells; giant cells; large, pale macrophages containing the fungus; plasma cells; and lymphocytes. Caseous necrosis and fibroblastic proliferation may also be present.

Clinical Manifestations. The adult disseminated disease and the mucocutaneous form of localized disease may show two types of laryngeal lesions. One is a firm, tumorlike, nodular mass of granulomatous tissue, usually brownish in color, which may undergo necrosis and ulcerate. These lesions are most often found in the tongue but do occur on the epiglottis. More often, the true vocal cords are superficially ulcerated, producing a roughened appearance posteriorly. The laryngeal mucosa is no longer pink but becomes a dirty white color. Ulceration is associated with pain and dysphagia in addition to the usual hoarseness. Cervical lymph node enlargement is also common.

Diagnosis. Isolation of the organism is usually easy in the disseminated and chronic localized forms. Cultures of sputum, ulcer, exudate, biopsies, or blood on Sabouraud's medium will usually serve to identify the causative organism. The microscopic examination of a tissue biopsy will also disclose the causative organism.

Treatment. Amphotericin B given intravenously is effective in all forms of the disease. Also, some of the sulfonamide drugs are useful in the adult forms of the disease.

Coccidioidomycosis

This disease caused by *Coccidioides immitis* is endemic in the San Joaquin Valley area of California. The usual form of this disease is a benign, self-limited respiratory infection, but about 0.2% of patients progress to a disseminated form which is frequently fatal, especially in colored races. The lesions consist of nodular masses of granulomatous tissue which may ulcerate. Rarely, the supraglottic laryngeal structures are the site of a lesion. The microscopic picture is almost indistinguishable from that of blastomycosis. Ulcerating skin lesions are frequent. A destructive lymphadenopathy may involve cervical lymph nodes, resulting in enlargement with caseous necrosis. The disease is diagnosed by isolation of the fungus from the sputum, exudate, or tissue biopsy.

Actinomycosis

Actinomycosis is caused by an anaerobic organism (*Actinomyces israelii*) called the ray fungus, although it is not a true fungus. The organism is a natural inhabitant of the mouth and probably invades from this area, which would account for the higher incidence of the craniofacial form of the disease. The craniofacial form is a soft tissue infection involving the jaw and upper neck area. When this infection is extensive, it may spread to paralaryngeal areas and cause perichondritis and laryngeal edema. The infected areas are involved by a chronic granulomatous inflammation, with production of a purulent exudate containing the ray fungus.

Rarely, the larynx is directly involved, and there is a localized area of inflammation in which yellow subepithelial granules may be seen. This type of involvement is marked by hoarseness, productive cough, and fetid breath. The disease responds well to penicillin or tetracycline drugs, but the latter are felt to be superior. The drugs must be given over a considerable length of time. Surgical drainage or excision of accessible lesions is a valuable adjunct to chemotherapy.

Rhinosporidiosis

Rhinosporidiosis is caused by *Rhinosporidium seeberi,* an endosporulating fungus which cannot be cultured and which is associated with characteristic giant sporangia in the tissues. It is characterized by small, pedunculated tissue masses involving the nose and nasopharynx and rarely the larynx.

The disease is endemic in India, although sporadic cases appear elsewhere. It is probably acquired by swimming in contaminated water and for this reason occurs mainly in young people, especially males.

The characteristic lesion is a red, polypoid, sessile mass of hyperplastic epithelium and submucosal tissue containing the fungus. Later the masses tend to become pedunculated. The lesion in the larynx results in hoarseness and occasionally may cause obstruction and dyspnea. The diagnosis is made by tissue biopsy, which discloses the characteristic thick-walled sporangia. Excision of the lesion with cauterization of the base to avoid implantation and recurrence is usually curative.

Candidiasis (Moniliasis)

Etiology. Candidiasis is caused by *Candida albicans,* a normal inhabitant of the gastrointestinal tract of healthy persons. The disease is usually in the form of a mild mucocutaneous infection, but rarely a disseminated visceral infection occurs.

Candidiasis of the mouth and upper respiratory tract is almost always the result of chemotherapeutic suppression of normal bacterial flora. Antibiotics, when used systemically, may cause the infection, especially when administration is prolonged. Another frequent cause is the use of antibiotic lozenges for the treatment of sore throat.

Clinical Manifestations. Laryngeal candidiasis is usually an extension of the oropharyngeal infection known as thrush. Patches of thick, white, membranous exudate are seen in the larynx, and the underlying mucosa is a bright red color. Pain and dysphagia are frequent symptoms. The principal danger of the disease is laryngeal obstruction caused by the sloughing membrane falling into the glottis. This is of particular importance in small children.

Diagnosis. The infection must be differentiated from other forms of membranous laryngitis, but the diagnosis is easily made upon microscopic examination of the membrane, which will disclose the presence of mycelia and yeastlike cells.

Treatment. In many instances, the infection will subside spontaneously soon after antibiotic administration is discontinued.

Local application of 1% gentian violet is helpful for oral lesions but is of little value in the larynx. Nystatin (Mycostatin), 500,000 units t.i.d., is the best drug available. In children, impending laryngeal obstruction may necessitate laryngoscopy and removal of any loose membrane, and occasionally tracheostomy must be performed.

REFERENCES

Bennett, M.: Laryngeal Blastomycosis. Laryngoscope, *74*:498, 1964.

Childs, P.: Paralaryngeal Actinomycosis. Br. J. Surg., *B5*:429, 1948.

Cody, C. C., Jr.: Moniliasis of the Larynx. Ann. Otol., *57*:371, 1948.

Devine, K. D.: Sarcoidosis and Sarcoidosis of the Larynx. Laryngoscope, *75*:533, 1965.

Garson, W.: Recent Developments in the Laboratory Diagnosis of Syphilis. Ann. Intern. Med., *51*:748, 1959.

Kerdel-Vegus, F., *et al.*: *Rhinoscleroma,* Springfield, Ill., Charles C Thomas, Publisher, 1963.

Klassen, D.: Rhinoscleroma Treated with Streptomycin and Dexamethasone. Arch. Otolaryng., *88*:74, 1965.

Lees, J. J.: Moniliasis of the Larynx and Hypopharynx. J. Laryngol., *73*:619, 1959.

Lehman, R. R.: Tuberculosis of the Larynx and Its Treatment with Streptomycin and Hydrazine Derivatives of Isonicotinic Acid. Ann. Otol., *63*:138, 1957.

Lester, C. F., *et al.*: Primary Laryngeal Blastomycosis. Am. J. Med., *24*:305, 1958.

Munoz MacCormack, C. E.: The Larynx in Leprosy. Arch. Otolaryng., *66*:138, 1957.

Mumma, C. S.: Coccidioidomycosis of the Epiglottis. Arch. Otolaryng., *58*:306, 1953.

Rothstein, E.: The Chemotherapy of Tuberculosis. New Engl. J. Med., *263*:588, 1957.

Sobel, N.: Syphilis of the Ear, Nose and Throat. In Coates, G. M., *et al.* (Eds.) *Otolaryngology*: Hagerstown, W. F. Prior Co. Inc., 1960.

Stachowsky, L. N.: Primary Paracoccidioidomycosis of the Larynx. Arch. Otolaryng., *78*:205, 1963.

Steffen, T. N., and Lierle, D. M.: Scleroma in Nonendemic Area. Laryngoscope, *71*:1386, 1961.

Sweany, H. C.: *Histoplasmosis*. Springfield, Ill., Charles C Thomas, Publisher, 1960.

Wilson, G. E., and Stern, W. K.: Tuberculosis of the Larynx. In Coates, G. M., *et al.* (Eds.) *Otolaryngology*: Hagerstown, W. F. Prior Co., Inc., 1960.

Withers, B. T., *et al.*: Histoplasmosis Primary in the Larynx. Arch. Otolaryng., *77*:25, 1963.

Chapter 32

Laryngeal Manifestations of Systemic Diseases

CONGENITAL DISEASES

Cystic Fibrosis (Mucoviscidosis)

This hereditary disease, which mainly affects children, is due to a generalized abnormality of the exocrine glands secreting mucus and sweat. The respiratory tract is almost always involved to some degree, with the result that there is an increased function of goblet cells and seromucous glands, producing a thick, abnormal secretion. At first, the seromucous glands hypertrophy, but eventually the ducts are blocked by inspissated secretions, producing cystic degeneration of the glands. As a result, the gland-bearing structures undergo marked hypertrophy.

Laryngeal involvement in this disease is marked by symptoms of hoarseness and constant efforts to clear the throat. The laryngeal mucosa is dry and granular and may be covered by inspissated mucus and crusts. The true vocal cords appear thick and are often inflamed. The false vocal cords may undergo considerable hypertrophy because of their gland content; also, cysts may occur in the false cords and ventricles.

The problem of utmost interest to the laryngologist with regard to this disease is the difficulty the patients have in clearing the tracheobronchial tree of the thick, tenacious secretions. As a result of secretion retention, these patients are subject to recurrent pulmonary infections and bronchiectasis. Treatment may require repeated bronchoscopy, tracheostomy, or tracheal fenestration for purposes of removing secretions and instilling or insufflating mucolytic agents.

In younger patients with this disease, permanent tracheostomy or tracheal fenestration may be of considerable value in implementing intermittent positive pressure breathing and in nebulizing the humidifying and mucolytic agents. This is particularly true for patients requiring daily nebulization and repeated mechanical removal of secretions.

Lipoid Proteinosis (Lipoidosis Cutis et Mucosae)

This uncommon hereditary disease is initially marked by an altered ability to cry and the presence of hoarseness in infancy. The disease causes hyalinlike infiltrates of skin and mucosa composed of a phospholipid complex. In the larynx, a yellowish-white plaquelike thickening in the interarytenoid area is a constant finding. The yellowish nodules and plaques also occur on the vocal cords and epiglottis. Hoarseness is a constant symptom, even in cases in which the true vocal cords are not actually involved. Occasionally, the larynx becomes obstructed, requiring tracheostomy. In addi-

tion to the laryngeal lesions, similar lesions occur in the mouth and nose and on the face, especially around the eyes. No specific treatment is effective.

ENDOCRINE DISEASES

Myxedema

Myxedema is accompanied by an accumulation in the soft tissues of a viscid fluid, high in protein and mucopolysaccharide content. This material may be deposited in the subepithelial areas of the true vocal cords (Rienke's space) between the anterior commissure and the vocal process. The result is an increase in vocal cord mass, which produces hoarseness and a lowering of voice pitch, which are the symptoms present in almost all cases of myxedema. In some instances, the cord may become frankly polypoid and require stripping. Improvement in the voice usually occurs with thyroid hormone replacement if the myxedema is of relatively short duration.

Hypothyroid myopathy may also contribute to the altered voice because of muscle weakness and stiffness. The tongue may also be involved by this process, causing dysarthria as well as dysphonia.

Acromegaly

This disease is due to an excessive production of growth hormone after puberty, usually caused by a tumor of the pituitary gland. The larynx is one of the organs particularly affected. There is a hypertrophy of the laryngeal cartilages and soft tissues, producing an alteration in voice, including hoarseness and lowering of the pitch. Vocal cord fixation may occur in acromegalics due to arthritis produced by cartilage distortion or to nerve injury caused by stretching as the cartilages hypertrophy. It is always important to inspect the larynx of an acromegalic before surgery to avoid an airway problem postoperatively. If cord fixation is bilateral, surgical correction may be necessary. The laryngeal disorders are not altered by correction of the pituitary dysfunction.

Hypogonadism

Hypogonadism in the prepubertal male, from any cause, leads to persistence of the anatomy of the juvenile larynx. The result is a failure of voice mutation and persistence of an abnormally high-pitched voice. Considerable improvement in voice may occur with male hormone replacement. Common causes of hypogonadism producing this problem include congenital defects, such as Klinefelter's syndrome and Laurence-Moon-Biedl syndrome; mumps; and trauma.

Hypoparathyroidism

Hypoparathyroidism is usually secondary to thyroid surgery, and the resultant tetany and laryngeal spasm are frequent problems in the postoperative patient. Laryngeal spasm can be alleviated by the intravenous administration of calcium gluconate. However, in cases which are difficult to control, tracheostomy may be necessary as an emergency measure.

Diabetes Mellitus

Diabetes mellitus is frequently complicated by diabetic neuropathy. This may involve the laryngeal nerves, producing vocal cord paralysis in poorly nourished and poorly controlled patients. This type of paralysis may respond to improved diet and control of the diabetes. Elderly diabetics may have a chronic neuropathy which is probably secondary to vascular insufficiency of peripheral nerves and is less likely to respond to treatment.

Pregnancy

Pregnancy may be accompanied by the onset of hoarseness due to increased vascularization and enlargement of the true and false vocal cords. Occasionally a disturbance of glandular secretion may occur, producing laryngitis sicca gravidarum. Generally, the laryngeal symptoms disappear after parturition.

The use of some of the present birth control preparations may cause hoarseness in some females. This is mainly associated with agents derived from male hormones.

LARYNGITIS IN SYSTEMIC DISEASES

Acute Laryngitis

Acute simple laryngitis may occur with several specific viral and bacterial infections.

Viral diseases such as mumps, measles, varicella, variola, and influenza may produce laryngeal symptoms. At times, an enanthema may involve the larynx, particularly in adults with varicella. Usually the larynx is diffusely inflamed, with hoarseness and sore throat being the only complaints. Rarely, acute edema of the larynx with obstruction may occur in association with mumps or measles.

Bacterial infections causing secondary laryngitis include streptococcal sore throat, pertussis, and brucellosis. The bacterial infections may produce mucosal ulcerations, which result in odynophagia as well as hoarseness. Occasionally, these infections may produce sudden inflammatory edema and glottic obstruction. Treatment is the same as for acute nonspecific laryngitis (in addition to treatment of the primary disease).

Membranous Laryngitis

Membranous laryngitis may occur as a complication of several diseases producing an alteration in the autoimmune mechanisms. Involvement of the larynx is usually an extension of a similar condition in the pharynx. Infectious mononucleosis, granulocytopenia, leukemia, and hypogammaglobulinemia are four such diseases which may be associated with membranous laryngitis. The laryngeal manifestations include inflammation, mucosal erosion, and formation of a grayish membranous exudate, which is often loosely attached. There is a constant danger of glottic obstruction by a piece of the membrane.

Renal failure and uremia seem to be more frequent causes of death as the elderly live longer and treatment of previously fatal respiratory infections is more successful. One of the manifestations of uremia may be a diffuse membranous laryngotracheal bronchitis. The patients are usually stuporous and hoarse and may have stridor. Examination of the larynx discloses the typical dry, granular, bright red mucous membrane. This may be covered in patches or completely by a loosely adherent white membrane. The mucous membrane is friable and bleeds easily and profusely. The same membranous inflammation occurs in the trachea and bronchi.

Membranous laryngitis secondary to blood diseases and uremia must be differentiated from membranous laryngitis associated with diphtheria, candidiasis, and Vincent's infection. Treatment is directed at the primary disease and prevention of laryngeal obstruction by the membrane. Laryngoscopy and tracheostomy may be necessary.

Hemorrhagic Laryngitis

The larynx may be a common site of submucosal hemorrhage because of the loose stroma in various areas of the organ and its constant function in deglutition and phonation. Any of the blood dyscrasias associated with clotting abnormalities may be associated with submucosal laryngeal hemorrhage. The use of anticoagulant drugs may be complicated by laryngeal hemorrhage.

Submucosal hemorrhage is most frequent in the area of the false vocal cords and arytenoid eminences. The onset of symptoms is usually sudden, beginning with hoarseness and stridor followed by dyspnea and obstruction. Examination of the larynx will disclose one or both aryepiglottic folds to be replaced by a dark red or purple swollen mass which impinges on the vestibular lumen. The formation of the hematoma is followed by an inflammatory reaction and absorption of the sequestrated blood. Specific treatment other than voice rest and correction of the clotting defect is not necessary unless laryngeal obstruction is present.

Laryngeal Abscess

Abscess of the larynx due to specific infection is rare today, principally because it is a late manifestation of various diseases. It once was common in typhoid fever during the third or fourth week of the disease. Streptococcal tonsillitis, gonococcal infections, and typhus may rarely spread to the larynx and produce an abscess.

The manifestations are the same as those

of nonspecific laryngeal abscess. Pain is an early symptom and is aggravated by talking and swallowing. The symptoms are accompanied by the presence of an inflamed, bulging mass, most often in the region of the false vocal cord. Laryngeal obstruction is a late symptom and may require performance of a tracheostomy. Rarely, perichondritis and chondral necrosis are complications which may end in laryngeal stenosis.

Treatment of the abscess is the same as that for nonspecific laryngeal abscess (in addition to treatment of the causative disease).

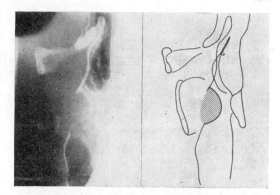

FIG. 32–1. Laryngogram from a patient with amyloidosis of the larynx localized to the infraglottic area.

PARASITIC DISEASE OF THE LARYNX

Trichinosis

Infestation with *Trichinella spiralis* is quite common in America. Along with the eye muscles, tongue, and diaphragm, the laryngeal musculature is a frequent site of encystment of the adult worm. No laryngeal symptoms occur with muscle invasion; however, the cysts are found incidentally during microscopic examination of the larynx for other disease. Although *Trichinella* cysts have been found with laryngeal carcinoma, a causal relationship is unlikely.

Leishmaniasis Americana (Mucocutaneous Leishmaniasis)

This disease, due to the parasite *Leishmania braziliensis,* is transmitted by the sandfly and is endemic in Central and South America. The protozoan usually attacks the nose first, but the larynx may be involved later. The lesion begins as a raised ulcer, which enlarges and becomes destructive. A polypoid type of lesion may also occur. Laryngeal lesions cause hoarseness, cough, dysphagia, and dyspnea.

MISCELLANEOUS DISEASES CAUSING LARYNGEAL MANIFESTATIONS

Amyloidosis

Amyloid, a complex of protein and polysaccharide, may be deposited in the tissues as a primary disorder or secondary to other disease. There are four types of amyloidosis: (1) primary systemic amyloidosis; (2) secondary amyloidosis associated with a chronic destructive disease, such as tuberculosis; (3) amyloidosis secondary to multiple myeloma; and (4) localized tumor-forming amyloidosis.

The larynx may be involved by each form of the disease. Systemic amyloidosis tends to produce a diffuse infiltrative type of involvement, which is differentiated from the localized tumorlike form. The larynx is the commonest site of the latter in the respiratory tract. The infiltrative type of involvement is the most common, and deposition is most marked in the loose stroma of the supraglottic structures. The localized form seems to occur most often in the anterior infraglottic area (Fig. 32–1).

Clinical Manifestations. The symptoms of laryngeal involvement may vary widely from mild hoarseness to stridor, dyspnea, and dysphagia. The infiltrative form may produce marked enlargement of the false cords, thus hiding the true cords and obstructing the laryngeal lumen. The involved structures are covered by smooth mucosa which has a yellowish coloration. The localized form appears as a bulging dark red mass, usually in the infraglottic area.

The diagnosis is made by tissue biopsy and the specific staining reactions of amyloid to Congo red, iodine, and silver. The Congo red test is not of much value in the diagnosis of a laryngeal lesion, especially with the localized form of the disease.

Treatment. There is no specific medical treatment. Surgical removal is the treatment of choice for the localized form of the disease and may be accomplished by suspension laryngoscopy or thyrotomy. If involvement is diffuse and infiltrative, a careful search should be made for a primary disease, such as multiple myeloma or a chronic granulomatous infection. Cortisone preparations may be of value in relieving laryngeal symptoms in these instances.

Pemphigus of the Larynx

Pemphigus is an uncommon disease of unknown etiology which initially affects mucocutaneous surfaces. It is a relapsing disease which is invariably fatal unless adequate therapy is instituted. There are five clinical forms of the disease, but it is pemphigus vulgaris, the most common form, which involves the larynx.

Pathology. The disease is characterized by a disruption of intercellular connections (acantholysis). The first microscopic sign is intercellular edema in the epithelium, with a loss of cellular connections in the prickle cell layers. Clefts then form in this layer and become filled. These bullae rupture and produce superficial ulceration and secondary inflammation. Because there is no keratin formation by the normal laryngeal mucosa, the bullae burst almost immediately; therefore, they are seldom seen. When a biopsy is performed, the epithelium strips off in big sheets, leaving the basal layer behind.

Clinical Manifestations. The usual complaint is a sore throat which may be associated with odynophagia. Dysphonia is uncommon. In some cases, laryngeal involvement may appear as a recurrence several years after the initial attack which involved another organ.

Bullae may be noted in the mouth or on the skin. Examination of the larynx discloses a thickened red epiglottis. Superficial epithelial ulcerations covered with membranous exudate are seen on the epiglottis and false cord. Bullae are rarely seen. The oropharynx may be involved by similar mucosal erosions. Nikolsky's sign, a detachment of sheets of superficial epithelial layers when any traction or abrasive form is applied, may be noted on the palate during laryngoscopy.

Diagnosis. Biopsy of an involved area will usually disclose the typical microscopic picture. Care should be exerted in performing laryngeal biopsy, as it is possible to denude large areas of endolarynx by the trauma of laryngoscopy and biopsy, and adhesions between the false vocal cords develop. If bullae are present on the skin or in the mouth, the Tzanck test may be done, which consists of staining and examining the vesicle fluid for acantholytic cells. In the absence of bullae, cantharides may be injected intradermally to produce a bulla from which the fluid is obtained and examined.

Treatment. It is important to make the diagnosis early so that corticosteroid therapy may begin. The corticosteroids will usually produce a remission within a short space of time. ACTH given intramuscularly or intravenously is used to initiate therapy because of the high dose of cortisone preparations required. After stabilization, the patient may be maintained on an oral steroid preparation.

Wegener's Granulomatosis

Wegener's granulomatosis (see Ch. 22) is a syndrome characterized by necrotizing vasculitis and focal glomerulitis. The etiology is unknown, but hypersensitivity may be a factor. The respiratory tract is the principal site of involvement, although renal disease is frequently the cause of death. Both sexes are affected equally by the disease.

Pathology. The respiratory tract is involved by a granulomatous inflammation which is associated with necrosis and ulceration. Disease in the nose and paranasal sinuses is often the first source of symptoms, but laryngeal and pulmonary symptoms eventually develop.

In addition to granuloma formation, there is a true necrotizing angiitis similar to that which occurs in polyarteritis nodosa. This finding separates this disorder from lethal midline granuloma, which rarely involves the larynx.

Clinical Manifestations. Hoarseness is the initial indication of laryngeal involvement. The onset of the disease is often mistaken for an upper respiratory infection, but the symptoms of rhinitis, sinusitis, and laryngitis persist. Diffuse ulceration and secondary infection may produce crusting and edema, which may cause laryngeal obstruction. Otitis media and recurrent pneumonitis also occur frequently. Eventually, clinical evidence of renal involvement is marked by the appearance of hematuria and signs of renal failure (uremia). Death due to renal failure or diffuse pneumonitis occurs within 2 to 18 months.

Diagnosis. Lesions of the nose and larynx often have a characteristic appearance at biopsy but may be confused with neoplasms or specific granulomas. The occurrence of pansinusitis with roentgenographic evidence of nodular, possibly cavitary, pulmonary infiltrates in association with glomerulitis is suggestive of the disease. Occasionally, pulmonary or renal biopsies are necessary for diagnosis.

Treatment. There is no effective cure. However, various chemotherapeutic agents such as azathioprine have been very helpful. Corticosteroids may have a temporary repressive effect, and antibiotics are indicated for secondary infections. Tracheostomy may be necessary for obstruction at the laryngeal level or for sectional obstruction in the lower respiratory tract.

COLLAGEN DISEASES

In addition to rheumatoid arthritis, the larynx may be involved in other collagen vascular diseases, including systemic lupus erythematosus, polyarteritis nodosa, and scleroderma.

Systemic lupus erythematosus is an inflammatory disease of probable autoimmune origin which tends to affect females. The disease is marked by fibrinoid degeneration of collagen and inflammation which affects the small arteries of the skin, mucous membranes, and viscera. The larynx may be involved during an acute phase of the disease, with the development of mucosal ulcerations and hemorrhagic bullae which cause hoarseness and sore throat. More chronic forms of laryngeal involvement include laryngitis sicca and cricoarytenoid arthritis. Transient cranial nerve paralysis due to vascular lesions may cause a vocal cord paralysis in this disease, which must be differentiated from cricoarytenoid arthritis.

Polyarteritis nodosa is characterized by inflammatory damage to blood vessels, which may be focal or nodular. Nodular lesions may appear in the submucosal tissues of the larynx. They tend to occur in groups which heal and regress rapidly. The larynx may also be involved by nonspecific urticaria and purpura in this disease. Vocal cord paralysis secondary to peripheral neuritis may appear but characteristically regresses within a short period of time.

Scleroderma is a chronic disease marked by fibrosis and sclerosis of connective tissue of the skin and mucous membranes. The larynx may be affected, with increasing stiffness of the laryngeal tissues which may affect vocal cord motion. Vascular lesions may produce mucosal ulcerations and recurrent nerve paralysis which may be persistent or may regress spontaneously.

Relapsing Polychondritis

Relapsing polychondritis is an intermittently progressive disease marked by inflammatory destruction of cartilage. The cause is unknown. Cartilage of the external and internal ears, larynx, trachea, bronchi, and nose may be involved.

Involvement of the larynx and trachea results in a gradual dissolution of the rigid framework of these organs. The cartilage is replaced by connective tissue, with the eventual development of laryngeal and tracheal stenosis.

The symptoms tend to be episodic, and during acute inflammatory episodes, hoarseness and odynophagia denote laryngeal disease. Fever, anemia, and elevated sedimentation rate are general signs. As the disease progresses, symptoms of increasing respiratory obstruction become apparent. In addition to the laryngeal symptoms, pain and tenderness of the nose and ears and labyrinthine disturbances may be present.

The diagnosis of this condition is made on the basis of the clinical finding, supported by the increased sedimentation rate. A roentgenogram of the chest may disclose marked narrowing of the trachea and larynx. If bronchoscopy is attempted, it may be impossible to pass a bronchoscope of appreciable size. Biopsy of any involved cartilage may disclose cartilage necrosis, inflammation, and fibrosis.

Treatment of this disease depends upon the use of corticosteroids. The steroids will usually control the acute inflammatory episodes, and a course of therapy may be followed by remission of symptoms. However, relapse upon the discontinuance of steroid therapy is common. Tracheostomy may be necessary for respiratory obstruction, but as the lower tracheobronchial tree is involved, it is of little value, and the patient's course is progressively downhill to death.

REFERENCES

Beasley, P.: Localized Amyloidosis of the Larynx. J. Laryngol., *85*:83, 1971.

Dickey, R. F., and Davis, S.: Lipoid Proteinosis. Ann. Otol., *73*:287, 1964.

Grotting, J. K., and Pemberton, J.: Vocal Cord Fixation in Acromegaly. Arch. Otolaryng., *52*:608, 1950.

Hilger, J. A.: Otolaryngologic Aspects of Hypometabolism. Ann. Otol., *73*:404, 1964.

Lewy, R. B.: Carcinoma of the Larynx and Trichinosis. Arch. Otolaryng., *80*:320, 1964.

Lineback, M.: Laryngeal Mucoviscidosis. Eye, Ear, Nose and Throat Monthly, *41*: 908, 1962.

McAlpine, J. C., *et al.*: Primary Amyloidosis of the Upper Air Passages. J. Laryngol., *77*:1, 1963.

Maloney, W. H.: Laryngeal Manifestations of Systemic Diseases. Ann. Otol., *73*:404, 1964.

Myerson, M. C.: A Manifestation of Uremia in the Larynx, Trachea and Bronchi. J.A.M.A., *89*:685, 1927.

Nieberding, P. H., *et al.*: Periarteritis Nodosa. Arch. Otolaryng., *77*:513, 1963.

Purcelli, F. M., *et al.*: Relapsing Polychondritis with Tracheal Collapse. Ann. Otol., *71*:1120, 1962.

Richards, S. H., and Ball, P. D.: Lipoid Proteinosis of the Larynx. J. Laryngol., *87*:187, 1973.

Ritter, F. N.: The Effect of Hypothyroidism on the Larynx of the Rat. Ann. Otol., *73*: 404, 1964.

Schechter, G. L., and Kostianovski, M.: Vocal Cord Paralysis and Diabetes Mellitus. Trans. Am. Acad. Ophthal. Otolaryng., *76*:729, 1972.

Segova, D., and Brown, A. L.: Classification and Etiologic Aspects of Necrotizing Angiitides. Proc. Staff Meet. Mayo Clin., *3*:205, 1964.

Thomas, K.: Laryngeal Manifestations of Wegener's Granulomatosis. J. Laryngol., *84*: 101, 1970.

Vieta, L. J., and Guraieb, S. R.: Laryngeal Involvement in Amyloidosis. Arch. Otolaryng., *79*:490, 1964.

Wallner, L. J., and Alexander, R. W.: Pemphigus of the Larynx. Laryngoscope, *74*:575, 1964.

Walton, E. W.: Wegener's Granulomatosis. Br. Med. J., 2:265, 1958.

Chapter 33
Functional Disorders of the Larynx

This group of disorders includes conditions in which there are no organic lesions present in the larynx, but there is a disturbance of voice production or sensation. Most of these conditions occur in individuals who have emotional problems or personality defects. Some of the conditions may be secondary to organic disease involving the central nervous system.

MOTOR DISTURBANCES

Functional Aphonia
(Hysterical Aphonia)

Complete loss of voice in the absence of organic disease may be of psychosomatic origin or a result of malingering. Psychosomatic aphonia is a form of conversion hysteria and is a neurosis.

Etiology. Typically, the condition occurs in young females between 15 and 35 years of age. The patient tends to be a thin, pale, asthenic type of person with a history of emotional lability. The onset of the condition often follows an episode of acute psychic trauma. When the condition occurs in males, it is usually secondary to some occupational hazard, such as warfare, which is a source of mental or physical shock. Malingering may be a cause, especially in male patients.

Clinical Manifestations. The patient complains of a sudden voice loss unaccompanied by other symptoms. In a majority of cases, the ability to whisper is retained. If aphonia includes loss of whisper, the term apsithyria is applied.

The larynx appears normal when examined, except when the patient is asked to phonate. When phonation is attempted, there may be a slight jerky movement or no movement of the true vocal cords, which remain in an abducted position. However, if the patient is asked to cough or laugh or is made to gag, the vocal cords will be seen to be completely approximated. Less commonly, the vocal cords may partially approximate during phonation, but adequate vocalization is prevented by bowing of the cords or persistence of an interarytenoid chink.

Treatment. In most patients, the voice may be reestablished immediately. This may be accomplished by convincing the patient he has an intact vocal mechanism. These patients are managed best by the speech therapist.

No attempt should be made to reestablish voice without awareness of the basic etiology. Elimination of one conversion reaction may lead to development of another and further worsening of mental status. Some form of psychotherapy must begin immediately.

Hypokinetic Dysphonia
(Myasthenia Laryngis)

Dysphonia in this situation is due to inadequate approximation of the vocal cords, with the result that there is air escape and vocal weakness.

Etiology. The problem may be psychological but is more commonly a manifestation of age, characterized by hypotonia of the laryngeal muscles.

Clinical Manifestations. The condition is marked by voice change, which usually consists of reduced volume and air escape. Usually the voice will be improved after a period of rest and tends to worsen with voice use. On indirect laryngoscopy the arytenoids will usually be seen to approximate, but there will be bowing of the membranous cords with asynchronous vibration of the cords.

Treatment. In the young patient in whom psychological problems are a major cause, the emotional problems must be treated. The problem is much more common in elderly females as a result of muscle fatigue. Unfortunately, nothing specific can be done; in fact, vocal exercises will usually increase the problem.

SPASM OF THE LARYNGEAL MUSCULATURE

Conditions causing spasm of the glottic musculature may be of organic or functional origin.

Laryngeal Spasm in Children

Episodic glottic spasm in children is usually of a reflex nature secondary to laryngeal irritation by a foreign body or piece of food. It may also occur in emotionally labile children when crying or during a fit of temper.

The situation usually develops when the child has just forcibly exhaled after crying, yelling, or coughing. There is then a great effort to inspire, but because of the configuration of the true vocal cords, there is a check valve effect which tends to keep the cords in apposition. The harder the child tries to inspire, the worse becomes the spasm. The situation is further aggravated by the excitement of the parents and by slapping the child on the back. Occasionally, the spasm will last so long that cyanosis develops and the child loses consciousness. At this point, relaxation occurs and normal respiration resumes.

Treatment. Almost all cases of acute spasm will end spontaneously. However, in situations in which a foreign body may have triggered the reaction and spasm is prolonged, it may be necessary to turn the child upside down. If there is no improvement, the tongue should be pulled out and the pharynx palpated for a foreign body. A history of possible foreign body or food ingestion followed by an attack of laryngeal spasm and cyanosis makes it mandatory to rule out the presence of an intrabronchial foreign body.

Emotionally labile children who have recurrent episodes of spasm may be helped by mild sedation on the advice of a pediatrician.

Laryngismus Stridulus

Laryngismus stridulus is the term applied to episodic spasms of the larynx in children under 2 to 3 years of age.

Etiology. The condition is a manifestation of tetany, which may have several causes in the infant and small child. Tetany neonatorum is a condition arising in the first week or two of life, which is probably secondary to an abnormality of parathyroid function in the newborn infant, causing hypocalcemia and hyperphosphatemia. Later in infancy, tetany develops as a result of inadequate calcium or vitamin D intake or excessive calcium loss. Hyperventilation causing alkalosis may be a factor in precipitating the attacks of muscular spasm.

Clinical Manifestations. Infants with neonatal tetany manifest increased irritability, muscular twitching, carpopedal spasms, tremors, and convulsions. Episodes of glottic spasm with crowing inspiratory stridor, indrawing, cyanosis, and temporary apnea are part of the syndrome. Stridor may be the first indication of the disease. Serum levels of ionic calcium are usually low.

Tetany of older infants, due to hypocalcemia, does not appear until after 3 to 4 months of age. The symptoms are due to increased irritability of the nervous system.

Muscular spasms, twitching, and convulsions occur, in addition to spastic closure of the glottis. The attacks may occur at any time, often at night, and without warning. Chvostek's and Trousseau's signs are usually present. Affected infants are usually thin and malnourished and from lower socioeconomic groups. This condition should be distinguished from spasmodic croup, which occurs in older children and is unrelated to calcium metabolism.

Treatment. The symptoms of neonatal tetany will respond well to intravenous injections of calcium gluconate. Subsequent control can be maintained by dietary supplements of calcium and vitamin D. The condition is self-limited and will regress as the infant's parathyroid function becomes adequate.

Laryngismus stridulus due to hypocalcemia in older infants can be controlled by similar methods. However, causes of hypocalcemia other than dietary deficiency, such as renal disease, should be considered when malnutrition is not obvious.

Spasmodic Laryngeal Cough (Nervous Cough)

This uncommon form of laryngeal spasm is a purely functional habit secondary to neurosis. It usually occurs in young females at puberty or in times of emotional stress. It has been called the barking cough of puberty.

Clinical Manifestations. The cough usually appears suddenly and is often related to an upper respiratory infection. The cough is unproductive, loud, low-pitched, and barking and occurs at short intervals. The cough may be continuous while the patient is awake but disappears with sleep. It usually causes no interference with eating. The patient is afebrile, and physical examination, including chest x-ray, is normal.

The larynx appears normal, and the vocal cords are seldom edematous or hyperemic, as might be expected. In addition, there is no alteration in the speaking voice.

Treatment. The condition is usually self-limited and often does not recur after one episode. Mild sedation of the patient and reassurance of the parents is all that is necessary. Recurrence of the condition may be an indication of neurosis requiring psychotherapy. Occasionally reflex cough due to irritation of the vagus nerve, as with impacted cerumen, may mimic this condition.

Laryngeal Spasm in Adults

Spasm of organic etiology may be divided into two types: tonic and clonic.

Tonic Spasms. Tonic muscular spasms confined to the larynx may be of reflex origin, as in children. Tabes dorsalis may be a cause of laryngeal crises, producing severe spasm and pain. Syringomyelia, multiple sclerosis, and progressive bulbar palsy may also produce episodic spasm. Irritation of the recurrent laryngeal nerve by thoracic neoplasms, pleural adhesions, or aortic aneurysm is a less common cause. Tonic laryngeal spasms are also caused by tetanus and rabies.

The symptoms are the same as in children, and the diagnosis is made by finding a normal larynx and recognizing the presence of any underlying disease.

Relief of respiratory obstruction is usually unnecessary except in the presence of tetanus or rabies. Tracheostomy should be done electively in most patients with these diseases because of the unpredictable occurrence and duration of spasm.

Clonic Spasms. The presence of rhythmic, involuntary, jerking movements in the larynx and pharynx is usually associated with similar movements in other areas. The tongue, palate, and facial muscles may be involved. The cause is always of central nervous system origin. Cerebrovascular insufficiency or hemorrhage, multiple sclerosis, encephalitis, meningitis, and cerebellar or frontal lobe tumors may cause the clonic spasms. Vascular lesions in the olivary area of the brain stem are the most frequent sources of nuclear irritation.

The movements are usually continuous and may be associated with myoclonic contractions of the diaphragm, trunk, and extremities. The term pharyngolaryngeal nystagmus has been used to describe this condition. This type of spasm seldom causes respiratory distress, so local therapy is rarely necessary.

Dysphonias Due to Laryngeal Hyperkinesis

Spasm of laryngeal musculature due to a breakdown in muscular coordination may occur in nervous, hyperkinetic individuals as a manifestation of neurosis, or it may be secondary to overexertion of intrinsic laryngeal muscles in speaking or singing. This results in a voice produced with too much force, incorrect pitch, or faulty respiratory pattern. A variety of clinical conditions may occur as a result of laryngeal incoordination and hyperactivity.

Hyperkinetic Dysphonia. In this instance, incoordination of the tensors and adductors of the true vocal cords produces phonatory dysfunction. The degree of dysfunction may vary from intermittent, mild hoarseness to almost complete aphonia. Dysphonia of this type is a reaction to stress or anxiety and is usually transient and reversible.

Hoarseness of emotional origin affects individuals who evidence, by history or examination, emotional instability. The usual type of patient is a young adult female with a history of a recent emotional experience. The hoarseness may be of variable degree and is usually intermittent. The patient will have a normal voice when speaking to friends or younger people, but hoarseness occurs when the patient is fatigued, upset, or speaking in stressful situations. Under these circumstances, there may be abrupt pitch changes or cracking. The voice tends to rise in pitch and become rough. Alterations in breathing patterns may be noted, and the patient may bring the neck muscles into play during phonation.

Diagnosis. The larynx is frequently normal, but some hyperemia of the true vocal cords may be present. During phonation, when the patient is symptomatic, the glottis closes tightly; this is followed by jerky, irregular movements of the arytenoids and vocal cords. At the same time, there is an obvious strain to speak, with contraction of neck muscles, facial contortions, and irregular breathing.

Voice therapy and rest are helpful when the condition is mainly due to overuse of the voice. Psychotherapy is often necessary when emotional factors are present.

Spastic Dysphonia (Mogiphonia, Phonic Spasm, Laryngeal Cramp). Individuals such as teachers, salesmen, lecturers, and preachers are all predisposed to vocal overuse and consequent vocal fatigue. Vocal fatigue plus the hyperkinetic personality of the individuals may precipitate sudden episodes of glottic spasm. This condition usually develops after prolonged anxiety and represents a late stage of hyperkinetic dysphonia.

Usually, these individuals have a normal voice for ordinary conversation, but when they are called upon to project, as when lecturing, there is a sudden voice failure. This is manifested by obvious physical effort to initiate speech, associated with a voice that may be extremely hoarse, although only a high-pitched croaking sound is produced by some patients. The term mogiphonia is applied to this condition.

A similar situation may occur in singers. Normal voice is present for conversation, but when singing is commenced, there may be a sudden loss of voice. This is most common when a difficult portion of a song is attempted. The sudden loss of ability to produce sound is termed a phonic spasm. Immediately following the episode, the speaking voice is found to be intact.

Treatment. This is an occupational neurosis occurring in emotionally labile people. Both psychiatric therapy and vocal reeducation are required. Usually, the occupation must be altered, as therapy is rarely successful in reestablishing a normal voice.

Laryngeal Vertigo (Ictus Laryngis, Laryngeal Epilepsy). This uncommon ailment was described by Charcot in 1876. Spasm of the true vocal cords with glottic closure results in vertigo or temporary unconsciousness.

Etiology. The condition is limited mainly to males. In most instances, the attack is preceded by a fit of coughing due to laryngeal paresthesia. Chronic bronchitis or chronic pulmonary disease producing cough may be a contributing factor. Also, impacted cerumen causing a reflex cough may precipitate an episode. Emotional instability or tension exists in most cases.

Clinical Manifestations. The patient may experience a burning sensation in the larynx, which is followed by a paroxysm of violent coughing. Laryngeal spasm occurs and may be accompanied by a high, sharp, inspiratory stridor. The patient is often pale but may become cyanotic. At this point, he may experience dizziness or light headedness or lose consciousness momentarily. Tremors, convulsions, and urinary incontinence do not occur, thus differentiating this condition from epilepsy. Recovery is rapid and complete, with no residual effects. The attacks may never occur again or may recur at frequent intervals.

Pathophysiology. The violent cough almost completely empties the lungs of air. Then an excessive inspiratory effort catches the vocal cords in adducted position and tends to maintain them in this position. The result is an excessive subatmospheric pressure which traps blood in the lungs. There is a sharp decrease in cardiac output and cerebral ischemia develops, causing alteration in consciousness and termination of the episode.

Diagnosis. Epilepsy can be ruled out by the absence of convulsions, tremor, and postictal state. The diagnosis is made in the light of the history and absence of physical findings.

Treatment. The majority of patients have isolated attacks and require no therapy. In the presence of repeated attacks, any source of irritative cough should be eliminated. Also, emotional and personality defects may require psychotherapy.

Dysphonia Plicae Ventricularis. Phonation using the false vocal cords or ventricular bands was first described by Czermak in 1860 and was named by Jackson in 1935.

Etiology. Ventricular band phonation may be due to (1) compensation for inadequate glottic function; (2) central nervous system diseases; or (3) functional incoordination of the laryngeal musculature. Glottic function, particularly phonation, may be impaired by vocal cord paralysis or fixation, surgical excision, and neoplastic diseases. Occasionally, cerebral and cerebellar disease may result in spastic or atactic movements of the true cords. The ventricular folds will assume phonatory function secondary to or-

ganic dysfunction of the vocal cords in these diseases.

Functional laryngeal incoordination producing this condition is a form of hyperkinetic dysphonia. Arnold feels that emotional factors cause subcortical centers to initiate phonation because of inhibition of cerebral function. Since this is a regressive phenomenon, sphincteric laryngeal function is accentuated, and the ventricular bands usurp the phonatory function of the true cords. Functional dysphonia plicae ventricularis occurs in the same types of individuals as do other types of spastic or hyperkinetic dysphonia.

Clinical Manifestations. The only complaint is disturbed phonation. In the compensatory form, the voice may be surprisingly good, with only a minor degree of hoarseness. The pitch tends to be lower, and vocal fatigue occurs easily. The cases of functional origin manifest a more protean group of symptoms. The voice tends to be more rough, is lower pitched, and frequently breaks. Diplophonia, or double voice, is typical; phonation begins normally with the true vocal cords, but immediately a second sound of lower pitch and increased roughness is heard as the false cords assume the vibratory function. The voice is weak, and phonation time is shortened. In severe cases, only a groaning or grunting noise may be produced.

Indirect examination of the larynx must be done with the patient phonating. In some instances, the reddened hypertrophic false cords may completely hide the true vocal cords. Most often, the margins of the true cords may be seen to approximate just before the false cords come into apposition. The margins of the false cords then begin to vibrate with a coarse flapping motion, and alteration of voice pitch is heard. The bulging false cords (Fig. 33–1) may suggest the presence of a mass in the ventricle, and laryngograms may show obliteration of the ventricles by the hypertrophic false vocal cords.

Treatment. Functional dysphonia plicae ventricularis is often improved by voice therapy, but some individuals also require psychiatric help.

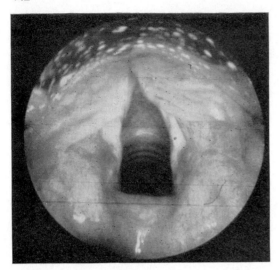

FIG. 33–1. Hypertrophy of the false vocal cords in a patient with dysphonia plicae ventricularis.

In rare instances, hypertrophy of the ventricular bands is so marked that trimming may be required. This may be done endoscopically using biting forceps. Direct laryngoscopy may be necessary to rule out underlying disease of the false vocal cords and ventricles.

Functional Falsetto Voice. Normally, at the time of puberty, the male voice will drop approximately an octave. This usually occurs smoothly over a period of time as the male larynx undergoes a sudden increase in size. In some instances, this mutation does not occur or is not completed. The result is persistence of a high-pitched, abnormal voice, which is actually a variety of hyperkinetic dysphonia.

Etiology. The failure of voice maturation may be secondary to a personality disorder. The typical patients are thin, effeminate, shy, insecure males. Usually, they are completely dominated and protected by their mothers. In fact, it is usually the mothers who bring them for consultation, even though the patients may be in their twenties.

The cricothyroid muscle is the main vocal cord tensor and is therefore responsible for production of a falsetto voice. Because of

an emotional disturbance, there is hyperkinetic function and spasm of the cricothyroid muscle.

Clinical Manifestations. Patients with incomplete voice mutation tend to have a high-pitched, hoarse voice which is subject to frequent "breaks" in pitch. During the breaks, the pitch may range widely from falsetto to low tones. Complete failure of mutation results in the mutational falsetto voice, which is maintained continuously at an abnormally high pitch.

During phonation, the glottis remains open, forming an oval or elliptical slit. In some instances, the cartilaginous glottis partially closes so that there is a triangular defect posteriorly. This is called the mutation triangle; it is normally present in the maturing larynx, but persistence is abnormal. The true cords may be hyperemic and slightly edematous. On x-ray examination, the cricothyroid space may be narrowed to palpation. Also, a pronounced elevation of the larynx during phonation will be noted.

Treatment. Treatment consists of vocal re-education, although psychiatric help may be required.

Hyperkinetic Phonasthenia

Etiology. This disorder is the result of faulty vocal function and is characterized by excessive contraction of all muscles used in phonation.

Clinical Manifestations. The voice problem tends to occur in hyperkinetic individuals who are obviously nervous. Usually they have a very active gag reflex and will frequently gag simply on opening the mouth. It is often difficult to visualize the larynx.

The voice is usually harsh and excessively loud. There is obvious straining to phonate, with elevation of the larynx, contraction of neck muscles, and engorgement of cervical veins. Phonation time is shortened. When the larynx is visualized, there may be accompanying findings of chronic laryngitis, vocal nodules, and hypertrophy of false vocal cords.

Treatment. The only treatment for this problem is vocal re-education, which must usually be accompanied by psychological evaluation and treatment.

FUNCTIONAL SENSORY DISTURBANCES

Hyperesthesia, Paresthesia, and Cancerphobia

Complaints of abnormal sensations relating to the throat area are often secondary to psychoemotional disturbances. Various sensations such as "pins and needles," the feeling of a lump, or the feeling that the breath is being cut off may be experienced.

The patient is most often a female in the third or fourth decade. The symptoms tend to be worse later in the day or during periods of anxiety or fatigue. Frequently, there is a basic fear that cancer is present somewhere in the throat.

Treatment. Treatment consists of careful examination of the larynx, followed by reassurance of the patient, convincing the patient that the larynx and throat are normal. The symptoms usually subside spontaneously when the patient has this knowledge. Psychotherapy may be necessary in the frankly neurotic patient.

REFERENCES

Arnold, G., and Heaver, L.: Spastic Dysphonia. Logos, 2:3, 1959.

Bernstein, L.: A Respiratory Tic: The Barking Cough of Puberty. Laryngoscope, 73:315, 1963.

Freud, E. D.: Functions and Dysfunctions of the Ventricular Folds. J. Speech Hearing Disorders, 27:334, 1962.

Furstenburg, A. C.: Evidence of Laryngeal Participation in Emotional Expression. Its Relation to Hysterical Aphonia. Ann. Otol., 67:516, 1958.

Gardener, L.: Tetany and Parathyroid Hyperplasia in the Newborn Infant. Pediatrics, 9:534, 1952.

Greene, M. C. L.: *The Voice and Its Disorders.* Philadelphia, J. B. Lippincott Co., 1972.

Jackson, C.: Myasthenia Laryngis. Arch. Otolaryng., 32:434, 1940.

Landes, B. A.: Further Study of Spastic Dysphonia. California Med., 97:77, 1962.

Lell, W. A.: Diagnosis and Direct Laryngoscopy Treatment of Functional Aphonia. Arch. Otolaryng., 34:141, 1941.

Levin, N. M. (Ed.): *Voice and Speech Disorders.* Springfield, Ill., Charles C Thomas, Publisher, 1962.

Perelló, J.: Dysphonies Fonctionelles. Folia Phonat. (Basel), 14:150, 1962.

Smurthwaite, H.: War Neurosis of the Larynx and Speech Mechanism. J. Laryngol., 34: 13, 1919.

Chapter 34
Neurologic Diseases of the Larynx

NEUROANATOMY OF THE LARYNX

Motor Supply

The lower portion of the precentral gyrus of the cerebral cortex contains the Betz cells which give origin to the corticobulbar fibers to the lower motor neuron nuclei of the larynx. This area corresponds to Broca's area. In addition, there are other cortical areas in the frontal, parietal, and occipital lobes which, when stimulated experimentally, produce vocalization. The corticobulbar fibers pass in the anterior, inferior portions of the internal capsules to enter the cerebral peduncles. At the upper portion of the pons, some fibers leave the main pyramidal tracts and pass dorsally to the medial lemnisci as aberrant pyramidal fibers. The remaining fibers continue in the pyramidal tracts. At the upper border of the medulla, all fiber tracts undergo partial decussation before terminating in the nuclei ambigui. Because of the decussation of the corticobulbar tracts, a cortical lesion usually must be bilateral and symmetrical to produce laryngeal paralysis. However, there is considerable individual variation in decussation, and superior laryngeal nerve paralysis has been reported with unilateral temporal lobe lesions.

Each nucleus ambiguus is the somatic motor nucleus of the ninth, tenth, and eleventh nerves. Each is continuous caudally with the dorsal lateral nucleus of the anterior horn of the spinal cord. Cranially, they are continuous with the motor nuclei of the seventh and fifth nerves. Each nucleus is approximately 2 cm long and begins at the upper border of the medulla. Experimental evidence in monkeys indicates that the anterior third of the nucleus is responsible for function of the pharynx and esophagus, via the ninth and tenth nerves. Slightly more caudally is the center for the cricothyroid muscle, the next portion is related to function of the abductor muscles, and the most caudal portion is responsible for adduction. Because of the length of the nucleus, it is entirely possible that a localized lesion of the cranial or caudal portion could result in an isolated paralysis of a laryngeal muscle. In addition to supply by the corticobulbar fibers, the nucleus ambiguus is supplied by fibers from cerebellar and extrapyramidal centers. These connections are important in coordinating the tonus, balance, and fine movements required for phonation and deglutition.

The blood supply of this area of the medulla is derived mainly from the vertebral arteries, the most important branches of which are the posterior inferior cerebellar arteries. However, the anterior inferior cerebellar arteries are also important in supplying the area, and the territory they supply varies inversely with that of the posterior inferior cerebellar arteries. In addition, the superior, middle, and inferior lateral medullary arteries, all branches of the vertebrals, supply portions of this area.

The vagus nerve arises from the lateral surface of the medulla, between the inferior cerebellar peduncle and the inferior olive, as a series of discrete roots. The roots contain efferent fibers from the nucleus ambiguus and the dorsal motor nucleus of the vagus, and afferent fibers to the nucleus tractus solitarii and the sensory nucleus of the fifth nerve. The roots containing the motor fibers for the pharyngeal and cricothyroid muscles soon combine to form a single intracranial trunk. The nerve then enters the anterior part of the jugular foramen and turns inferiorly. In the jugular foramen, the nerve enlarges to form the jugular ganglion, which contains the cells of the somatic afferent fibers from the ear canal. Caudal to the vagus roots are the origins of the roots of the spinal accessory nerve, which immediately combine into two separate portions, a cranial (bulbar) accessory and a spinal accessory nerve. The cranial portion contains most of the motor fibers to the intrinsic laryngeal musculature. After a short course of less than a centimeter, the cranial portion or internal ramus enters the jugular foramen and joins the vagus at or just below the jugular ganglion. Immediately inferior to this point lies the nodose or inferior vagal ganglion, which contains the cells of the visceral afferent fibers and a few taste fibers.

At the level of the nodose ganglion, many small branches pass between the ninth, tenth, and eleventh nerves. Also, the vagus receives fibers from the superior sympathetic ganglion, and the numerous motor branches of the pharyngeal plexus arise. Just below the inferior border of the nodose ganglion, the superior laryngeal nerve arises (Fig. 34–1).

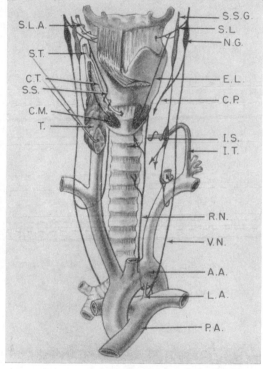

Fig. 34–1. Schematic drawing of the laryngeal nerve supply. S.S.G., Superior sympathetic ganglion; S.L., superior laryngeal nerve; N.G., nodose ganglion; E.L., external laryngeal nerve; C.P., cardiopulmonary branches; I.S., inferior sympathetic ganglion; I.T., inferior thyroid artery; R.N., recurrent nerve; V.N., vagus nerve; A.A., aortic arch; L.A., ligamentum arteriosum; P.A., pulmonary artery; S.L.A., superior laryngeal artery; S.T., superior thyroid artery; C.T., cricothyroid artery; S.S., sympathetic plexus; C.M., cricothyroid muscle; T., thyroid gland.

Superior Laryngeal Nerve

This nerve carries the major portion of the sensory fibers from the larynx, the motor fibers for the cricothyroid muscle, and some autonomic fibers. The superior laryngeal nerve is the nerve of the fourth branchial arch in the embryo.

The nerve leaves the vagus trunk at the inferior border of the nodose ganglion and passes to the medial side of the internal and external carotid arteries. At the same time, it passes inferiorly to reach a point slightly mediosuperior to the superior thyroid artery. At this point (about 2 cm from the nodose ganglion), the nerve divides into internal and external branches.

The internal branch travels medially with the superior laryngeal branch of the superior thyroid artery. They both pass through the thyrohyoid membrane at a point about 1 cm anterior to the superior cornu and 1 cm above the ala of the thyroid cartilage. The nerve then passes anterior to the piriform fossa submucosally and divides over the surface of the supraglottic structures. The sensory supply to the mucosa of the posterior portions of the supraglottis is much greater than that to the anterior portions.

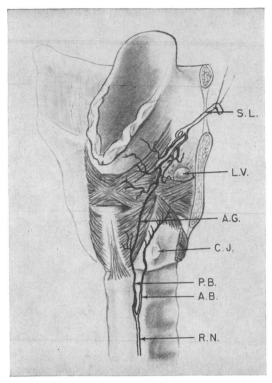

Fig. 34–2. Peripheral ramifications of the laryngeal nerves. *S.L.*, Superior laryngeal nerve; *L.V.*, laryngeal ventricle; *A.G.*, ansa Galeni; *C.J.*, cricoid facet of cricothyroid joint; *P.B.*, posterior branch recurrent nerve (sensory); *A.B.*, anterior branch recurrent nerve; *R.N.*, recurrent nerve.

The internal nerve also sends a small branch inferiorly (nerve of Galen) to anastomose with the posterior branch of the recurrent nerve and form the ansa Galeni, which has a sensory function (Fig. 34–2).

The external branch passes posterior to the superior thyroid artery and proceeds inferiorly following the oblique line of the thyroid cartilage. The nerve lies on the inferior constrictor muscle, to which it sends a branch, and passes deep to the sternothyroid muscle to reach the cricothyroid muscle. In the region of the superior pole of the thyroid gland, the nerve is often just slightly above the superior thyroid artery and is in danger of injury during thyroidectomy.

There is still considerable controversy as to the innervation of the interarytenoid muscle. The present consensus is that the muscle receives its motor supply solely from the recurrent laryngeal nerves. However, several authors have demonstrated motor end plates on the terminal branches of the superior laryngeal nerve in this muscle in man suggesting that the interarytenoid has a double as well as a bilateral innervation. However, the arguments against this are:

1. That the fibers merely pass through the muscle to reach the aryepiglottic folds.

2. That no interarytenoid muscle response has been elicited in man or dogs by stimulating the superior laryngeal nerve.

More recently, Réthi has stated that the superior laryngeal nerve sends motor fibers to all the laryngeal muscles. This may be corroborated by some recent electromyographic studies in dogs, in which it was shown that motor potentials persisting in the thyroarytenoid muscle after recurrent nerve division were ablated by division of the superior laryngeal nerves.

This controversy originally arose because of the possible influence of persistent function of the interarytenoid muscle on the position of a paralyzed vocal cord. In view of other reasonable explanations for vocal cord position, this point is now of less importance. However, the possibility of extensive muscular innervation by the superior laryngeal nerve leaves some doubt as to the validity and reliability of electromyographic studies interpreted in the light of the present, generally accepted, pattern of innervation.

Recurrent Laryngeal Nerve

Most motor fibers eventually ending in the larynx travel with the main trunk of the vagus. The vagus leaves the nodose ganglion to pass inferiorly down the neck lateral to the internal and common carotid arteries. In the lower neck, the nerve gradually assumes a slightly more anterior position in relation to the common carotid artery. The fibers of the vagus nerve innervating the larynx are derivatives of the nerve of the sixth branchial arch and are therefore displaced by the arteries of the preceding arches which descend into the lower neck and thorax. This necessitates a change in direction of the laryngeal nerves so they can reach the larynx, hence the term recurrent.

The right recurrent nerve recurs around the subclavian artery, a fourth arch derivative, which is responsible for nerve position because of atrophy of the fifth and sixth arch arteries. The nerve arises from the main trunk of the vagus on the anterior surface of the subclavian artery slightly lateral to the origin of the right common carotid artery. The right phrenic nerve is about 1 cm lateral to the recurrent nerve at this point. The recurrent nerve then passes inferiorly around the artery to the posterior surface and travels superiorly and medially, crossing the fat-filled space between the common carotid artery and the trachea, to reach the tracheoesophageal groove. At this point, it is usually intimately related to the branches of the inferior thyroid artery. Because of a relatively high origin, the right recurrent nerve lies in a more lateral position than the left nerve at the level of the inferior thyroid arteries. In fact, it may be as much as 1 cm lateral to the trachea; therefore, the right recurrent nerve is more prone to surgical injury because it is assumed to be tucked into the tracheoesophageal groove. The fibers of the right recurrent nerve are more likely to pass between or lateral to the branches of the inferior thyroid artery. Just above this artery, at a point 1 to 2 cm inferior to the cricothyroid joint, the main trunk of the vagus divides into two or more branches in 70 to 80% of the cases. These may lie medial to, lateral to, or within the suspensory ligament of the thyroid gland. The nerve branches enter the larynx through the Killian-Jamieson area, under the cricopharyngeus and immediately posterior to the cricothyroid joint, before further dividing to supply the intrinsic muscles. In some instances, the anterior branches of the nerve may pass anterior to the cricothyroid joint. There is no definite relationship between extra laryngeal branching and the muscles or groups of muscles supplied by each branch; however, the posterior branch is mainly sensory and anastomoses with the nerve of Galen from the superior laryngeal nerve.

An abnormality in the course of the right recurrent nerve may occur when the right subclavian artery is derived from the caudal portion of the right aortic arch and its usual fourth arch component disappears. Because of this abnormality, there is no artery to displace the nerve into the lower neck, and the nerve passes directly from the vagus to the Killian-Jamieson area at the level of the larynx. This abnormality is relatively common in clinical practice and is especially frequent in mongoloids.

The left recurrent nerve travels a course similar to that of the right one except that it is carried further into the thorax. The nerve arises on the anterior surface of the arch of the aorta just inferior to the interspace between the origins of the left common carotid and subclavian arteries. At this point, the recurrent nerve is immediately medial to the phrenic nerve, which is also crossing the aorta. Since the aorta is a fourth arch derivative, the nerve passes inferiorly around it. As the nerve loops under the aorta, it is distal to the ligamentum arteriosum, which is a vestige of the fifth branchial arch. Then the course is similar to that on the right; however, the left nerve is placed more deeply in the tracheoesophageal groove, and it is more likely to be medial to the branches of the inferior thyroid arteries.

Sensory Nerve Supply

Sensory fibers are carried in both the superior and recurrent laryngeal nerves. They end in cells in the nodose ganglion, from which central fibers leave to terminate in the nucleus tractus solitarii in the medulla. The nucleus is richly connected with the visceral centers and cranial nerve nuclei in the medulla, and these connections are important in the generation of the various laryngeal reflexes. There are no proven cortical connections from the nucleus tractus solitarii. The recurrent nerves carry many sensory fibers which are distributed to the inferior larynx, upper trachea, and esophagus by several branches that are more numerous on the left. They also send a branch which anastomoses with the superior laryngeal nerve, forming the ansa Galeni.

Autonomic Nerve Supply

Parasympathetic fibers arise in the medulla from the dorsal motor nucleus of the vagus, synapse in the nodose ganglion, and then travel in both laryngeal nerves to the larynx. Sympathetic fibers enter both nerves via connections with the superior cervical ganglion; also, perivascular fibers reach the larynx with the laryngeal arteries. The autonomic nerves are mainly secretomotor and vasomotor, although the sympathetic fibers are also important in maintenance of muscle tonus in the vocal cords.

LARYNGEAL PARALYSIS

Sensory Paralysis

Anesthesia of the larynx is due to disruption of the internal laryngeal nerves, the superior laryngeal nerves, or their bulbar connections.

Etiology. Isolated sensory paralysis of the larynx is due to a lesion of the internal branch of the superior laryngeal nerve. The lesions are most frequently due to surgical trauma, such as radical neck dissection or operations on the supraglottic portion of the larynx. Laryngeal anesthesia secondary to disease proximal to the bifurcation of the superior laryngeal nerve is always associated with signs of involvement of the external laryngeal nerve to the cricothyroid muscle and in some cases with involvement of other cranial nerves and medullary pathways.

Clinical Manifestations. Sudden interruption of the sensory supply to the larynx may cause difficulty with deglutition and aspiration. When paralysis is unilateral, symptoms are minimal and compensation is rapid. More difficulty may be encountered with bilateral sensory paralysis, but complete compensation eventually develops.

The diagnosis is made by demonstrating anesthesia by direct palpation of the larynx with a probe and noting the absence of reflex responses. Absence of reflex response may be an indication of sensory paralysis but may be present in hysterical individuals. The larynx will appear normal if the nerve to the cricothyroid is intact and functioning and phonatory function is normal.

Treatment. No specific treatment is usually required for isolated unilateral sensory paralysis. Bilateral sensory paralysis may cause considerable dysphagia and aspiration, but most patients will compensate for this deficit, as can be demonstrated in patients who have had both nerves removed in the process of a supraglottic subtotal laryngectomy. More serious problems arise when the sensory deficit is combined with laryngeal motor paralysis. Treatment involves reassuring the patient and reestablishing swallowing habits.

Motor Paralysis

Motor paralysis of the larynx of neural origin may be classified into four groups based on the site of lesion responsible and the neurologic deficits produced. These are cortical, corticobulbar, bulbar, and peripheral. Myopathic disease may also cause paralysis.

Etiology. *Cortical Paralysis.* Lesions of the cerebral cortex are not a common cause of laryngeal paralysis because of the decussation of connections with lower centers. Therefore, lesions must be diffuse and bilaterally symmetrical to produce a complete laryngeal motor paralysis.

The function of the cerebral motor cortex is to initiate voluntary coordinated movements by an overall inhibitory effect on lower centers. Therefore, loss of this function will result in a spastic paralysis. However, since complete destruction of the motor areas is uncommon, a spastic incoordination rather than frank paralysis is most likely. Either of these situations may exist in the larynx. The causes include cerebral concussion, congenital cerebral palsy, encephalitis, kernicterus, and diffuse cerebral arteriosclerosis.

Corticobulbar Paralysis. Lesions producing laryngeal paralysis by interruption of the corticobulbar tracts are rare. Because of the localized decussation of the corticobulbar tracts, a small lesion would have to be in the region of the decussation to produce a supranuclear laryngeal paralysis before the death of the patient. This region is near the cranial end of the medulla. Basilar artery insufficiency and occlusion of both of its paramedian branches are the most common causes of a lesion at this point. Usually, the laryngeal paralysis is not complete, and spastic incoordination is more likely.

Bulbar Paralysis. Laryngeal paralysis of bulbar origin is due to destruction of all or part of the nucleus ambiguus in the medulla. The paralysis is of the flaccid type. The most common cause is vascular insufficiency, which in this area may be due to occlusion of one or any of the following arteries: vertebral; posterior inferior cerebellar; anterior inferior cerebellar; superior, middle, and inferior lateral medullary branches. Other less common causes of bulbar paralysis include progressive bulbar palsy, syringobulbia, multiple sclerosis, cranial trauma, syphilis, rabies, encephalitis, and poliomyelitis. Intramedullary tumors, usually gliomas, may cause destruction of the nucleus ambiguus.

Not all of the nucleus ambiguus is necessarily destroyed in each case, and it is quite possible to have an isolated paralysis of the tensor, abductor, and adductor muscle groups because of segmental localization of the cell groups in the nucleus. Almost all cases of bulbar laryngeal paralysis will show signs of involvement of sensory and motor tracts in the medulla, as well as paralysis of other cranial nerves. They are then classified as associated paralyses.

Peripheral Paralysis. Diseases involving the fibers of the laryngeal nerves in their course from the surface of the medulla to the larynx are, by far, the commonest causes of laryngeal paralysis. They are responsible for paralysis in 90% of cases. The causes are outlined in Table 34–1.

Paralysis of peripheral origin can be generally divided into two groups: high and low vagus paralysis. High vagus paralysis is due to lesions at, or central to, the nodose ganglion. As a result, all the nerves to half of the larynx are likely to be involved, producing a combined paralysis; in addition, other cranial nerves are frequently paralyzed, producing a syndrome of associated paralysis. The most common cause of this type of paralysis is lymphadenopathy high in the cervical chain. The lymph nodes just beneath the jugular foramen, known as the nodes of Krause, may be involved by inflammatory or neoplastic processes emanating from the postauricular area, the ear canal, and the nasopharynx. Carcinoma of the nasopharynx is the usual cause of enlargement producing paralysis. Herpes zoster and other types of neuritis may also produce this type of vagal involvement without associated paralysis.

Low vagal paralysis, in which the nerve to the cricothyroid is intact and only the fibers of the recurrent nerve are damaged, is much more common. It occurs approximately twice as frequently on the left side owing to the course of the left recurrent laryngeal nerve deep into the mediastinum. Neuritis is a frequent cause of isolated recurrent nerve paralysis and is usually related to an upper respiratory infection caused by a virus, particularly influenza A or B. Infectious mononucleosis is a common disease which must be considered when isolated laryngeal paralysis occurs in younger persons. Sarcoidosis is often accompanied by a polyneuritis or mononeuritis and is more frequent in the Negro. Infections of the parapharyngeal spaces may cause neuritis producing a temporary paralysis. Neuritis associated with specific infections, such as syphilis, tuberculosis, and diphtheria, is rare today, especially in North America.

Peripheral neuropathy associated with diabetes mellitus is becoming increasingly common as a result of increasing longevity and better medical care of diabetics. It is estimated that 50% of older diabetics eventually develop some degree of peripheral neuropathy due to nerve ischemia. Laryngeal paralysis is most likely to occur in older, poorly controlled diabetics. Rheumatoid arthritis and other collagen diseases may involve the cricoarytenoid joints but may also produce peripheral neuropathy of ischemic origin.

Neoplasms, particularly carcinoma, are the most common cause of peripheral laryngeal paralysis at the present time. The carcinoma may arise in several sites to produce paralysis (see Table 34–1). Carcinoma of bronchogenic origin with mediastinal metastases is the most frequent cause of left recurrent nerve paralysis, and this is an indication of unresectability. Bronchogenic carcinoma of the right lung may produce laryngeal paralysis, and in such cases the superior sulcus tumor is the cause. Metastatic carcinoma in lymph nodes may produce paralysis by direct invasion of the nerve or

Table 34–1.   Classification of Causes of Peripheral Paralysis of the Laryngeal Nerves

A. Inflammatory (Neuritis)
    1. Meningitis and arachnoiditis
    2. Thrombophlebitis of the jugular bulb
    3. Cervical and mediastinal infections
    4. Diphtheria
    5. Leprosy
    6. Tuberculosis
    7. Sarcoidosis
    8. Infectious mononucleosis
    9. Herpes zoster
   10. Neuritis secondary to viral infections
       (i.e., influenza, mumps, measles, Coxsackie infections)
   11. Acute polyneuritis (Guillain-Barré syndrome)
   12. Radiation neuritis

B. Neuropathy Secondary to:
    1. Diabetes mellitus
    2. Rheumatoid arthritis
    3. Polyarteritis nodosa and lupus erythematosus
    4. Chronic alcoholism and other causes of thiamine lack
    5. Poisons and toxins (lead, mercury, arsenic, botulism, tick paralysis)
    6. Serum sickness

C. Neoplastic Diseases
    1. Meninges
       Metastatic carcinoma
       Meningioma
       Neurilemoma
    2. Middle ear
       Carcinoma
       Glomus jugulare
    3. Nasopharynx
       Carcinoma
       Malignant lymphoma
       Rhabdomyosarcoma
    4. Parotid gland
       Carcinoma of the deep lobe
    5. Neck
       a. Cervical lymph nodes
          Metastatic carcinoma
          Malignant lymphoma
       b. Thyroid
          Simple goiter
          Adenoma
          Carcinoma
       c. Neurogenous tumors
          Neurilemoma
          Neurofibroma
          Ganglioneuroma
       d. Carotid body tumor
       e. Glomus intravagale
       f. Carcinoma of the cervical esophagus and hypopharynx
    6. Mediastinum
       a. Thymus tumors
       b. Malignant lymphoma
       c. Metastatic carcinoma

Table 34–1.   *(Continued)*

7. Lung
Bronchogenic carcinoma
D. Trauma
1. Chronic mechanical trauma (pressure, stretching)
a. Arnold-Chiari malformation
b. Platybasia
c. Cervical lymphadenopathy
d. Mediastinal lymphadenopathy
e. Pleural fibrosis
f. Cardiovascular disease
i. Aneurysm of aorta, subclavian or innominate arteries
ii. Enlargement of left auricle, secondary mitral stenosis and insufficiency
iii. Patent ductus arteriosus
iv. Enlargement of left pulmonary artery
2. Acute external trauma
a. Blunt trauma to neck
b. Stab and bullet wounds
c. Traction on neck
d. Fracture of clavicle
e. Fracture of base of skull
3. Surgical trauma
a. Thyroidectomy
b. Tracheostomy
c. Diverticulectomy
d. Scalene node biopsy
e. Radical neck dissection
f. Removal of neck masses
g. Pneumonectomy
h. Ligature of a patent ductus arteriosus
E. Idiopathic

---

by pressure and stretching effects. However, the nodes usually must attain a substantial size before paralysis ensues. As a result, they are more likely to produce paralysis when situated in confined spaces, such as at the base of the skull or in the root of the neck.

Mechanical pressure or stretching of benign origin exerted on a nerve over a period of time causes paralysis. Displacement of the brain stem, causing stretching of the vagus nerves over the edge of the jugular foramen, is the probable cause of paralysis in the Arnold-Chiari malformation and in platybasia. Benign lymphadenopathy uncommonly produces paralysis secondary to pressure effects. Pleural fibrosis secondary to tuberculosis, pneumoconiosis, and fungous infections may involve the vagus or recurrent nerves to produce paralysis. The left side is usually involved, and signs of paralysis may not occur until long after active pulmonary disease has disappeared.

Cardiovascular lesions almost always involve the left recurrent laryngeal nerve. Aneurysms of syphilitic origin, previously numerous, are now uncommon; however, there is an increase in paralysis due to congenital heart disease, which is most likely a result of increased survival of these patients. Left auricular hypertrophy and dilatation due to mitral stenosis are seldom allowed to reach a sufficient degree to produce paralysis. Generally, dilatation is more marked with mitral insufficiency, and paralysis is noted more often with this disorder. Laryngeal paralysis associated with cardiomegaly is termed Ortner's syndrome.

Acute external trauma to the neck is an increasing cause of laryngeal paralysis because of the increasing number of automobile accidents. In these cases, unilateral or bilateral recurrent nerve paralysis is often associated with crushing injuries of the larynx. Nevertheless, neck trauma of a fairly minor nature may produce isolated laryngeal paralysis. Such injuries may be due to circumferential squeezing of the neck, as in wrestling, light blows to the anterior neck, and lateral flexion of the head during birth. In many of these minor injuries, luxation or dislocation of the cricothyroid joint is probably responsible for producing compression of the laryngeal nerve.

Surgical injury of the recurrent laryngeal nerves is still a frequent complication of operations on the neck and mediastinum. It is often secondary to deliberate sacrifice of the vagus or recurrent nerve but may be the result of inadvertent surgical injury. Thyroidectomy was once the most common cause of all laryngeal nerve paralysis; however, this is not true at present, and the decreased incidence of paralysis after thyroidectomy is a result of routine dissection and isolation of the nerve. Although the incidence of post-thyroidectomy paralysis has decreased, isolated paralysis of the external laryngeal nerve and bilateral recurrent nerve paralysis are still, in the majority of cases, secondary to damage during thyroid procedures. The right recurrent laryngeal nerve is the most likely to be damaged during thyroidectomy because of its more lateral position at the level of the inferior thyroid artery. It is during the ligation of this artery that injury to the nerve usually occurs.

Recurrent nerve paralysis secondary to tracheostomy is uncommon in adults but may occur in infants. Lymph node biopsies in the neck, particularly scalene node biopsy, can be complicated by laryngeal paralysis when either the vagus or recurrent nerve is injured. In recent years, pneumonectomy and increasingly radical attempts to remove mediastinal nodes for bronchogenic carcinoma have resulted in an increased postoperative incidence of left recurrent nerve paralysis. The nerve may be paralyzed by traumatic edema, inclusion in a ligature, or transection; the latter two causes may be avoided by careful dissection of the vagus and recurrent nerves during any surgical procedure involving their locations.

Laryngeal nerve paralysis of unknown etiology still constitutes a substantial group of cases. The incidence varies from 1 to 35% in various series. However, this variation can often be accounted for by patient selection, with the higher incidence occurring in clinics receiving more difficult diagnostic problems. In an average group of patients, the incidence of laryngeal paralysis without obvious cause is probably about 20%. The incidence is considerably higher in males and involves the left cord more often than the right cord.

Positions of the Paralyzed Vocal Cord. Much controversy has arisen, in the past, regarding the explanation of the various positions of the paralyzed vocal cords. At the present time, five positions of the vocal cord are recognized by clinical examination. They are the median, paramedian, intermediate, slightly abducted, and fully abducted positions (Fig. 34–3). Rosenbach in 1880, and Semon in 1881, tried to explain the sequence of positions of the vocal cords, associated with a slowly progressive paralysis of the recurrent nerves, on the basis of increased susceptibility of the abductor nerve fibers to injury. They recognized four stages of paralysis: (1) isolated abductor paralysis; (2) median or paramedian position due to spasm of the abductor muscles; (3) cadaveric position when all the muscles innervated by the recurrent nerve were paralyzed; and (4) stage of compensation of the normal vocal cord. It is now recognized that this sequence of events is rarely associated with isolated recurrent nerve paralysis.

Wagner and Grossman explained the median and paramedian positions of the vocal cord after recurrent nerve paralysis on the basis of continued function of the cricothyroid muscle, which is a tensor of the vocal cord and adductor of the arytenoid. This explanation has been supported experimentally and is generally accepted. The intermediate position of the vocal cord occurs when there is combined paralysis of all the muscles of the hemilarynx. However, Negus has supported Semon's theory on the basis

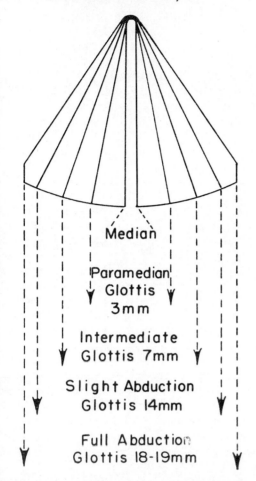

Median

Paramedian
↓ Glottis ↓
3mm

Intermediate
↓ Glottis 7mm ↓

Slight Abduction
Glottis 14mm

Full Abduction
Glottis 18-19mm

FIG. 34–3.   Cord positions and glottic dimensions in the average adult male.

of the phylogenetic development of sphincter and respiratory functions of the larynx. Semon's observation of the greater vulnerability of abductor function is, in fact, a clinical sign of incipient recurrent nerve paralysis. This may be explained by the fact that the posterior cricoarytenoid is the sole abductor of the vocal cord, and it operates at a considerable mechanical disadvantage. Therefore, when paralysis is developing, weakness may produce the clinical picture of abductor paralysis. It should be recognized that abductor paralysis does not result in a paramedian cord position or produce immobility of the vocal cord. The neutral position of the cricoarytenoid joint occurs when the arytenoid is in the intermediate

position, and the adductor and abductor muscles only move it from this position.

King and Gregg explained cord position in post-thyroidectomy paralysis as being the result of damage to the "abductor" or "adductor" branch of the recurrent nerve. This explanation has been discarded, since it has been shown that the posterior branch is often solely sensory. Also, the paramedian position is by far the most common position of the paralyzed cord, while it is the more anterior "adductor" branch which is most likely to be damaged (which would produce an intermediate position). Isolated paralysis of the abductor and adductor branches is seldom recognized clinically; therefore, these terms should be discarded, and for practical purposes, paralysis should be identified by the cord position present on examination.

It is recognized that the paralyzed vocal cord may change position over a period of time. A vocal cord in the intermediate position after recurrent nerve paralysis may gradually shift to a paramedian or median position. Also, a vocal cord in the paramedian position may move to the midline. These changes are due to continued function of the cricoarytenoid muscle and fibrosis and contracture of the thyroarytenoid muscle. Also, the interarytenoid muscle is a factor producing this change in unilateral paralysis.

The shift of a paralyzed cord from the median or paramedian position to a more lateral position is uncommon and is dependent upon a paralysis of the superior laryngeal nerve developing after the recurrent paralysis and while the cricoarytenoid joint is still mobile.

In summary, there can be no fixed laws governing the positions assumed by the paralyzed vocal cord. These positions are determined by a combination of factors:

1. Continued function or paralysis of the cricothyroid muscles.

2. The degree of fibrosis of the denervated musculature.

3. Persistent tonus associated with autonomic nerve supply.

4. Fibrosis and ankylosis of the cricoarytenoid joint.

5. Function of the interarytenoid muscle in unilateral paralysis.

6. Tension of the conus elasticus.

Clinical Aspects of Laryngeal Paralysis. The symptomatology associated with recurrent nerve paralysis and superior laryngeal nerve paralysis, or both, varies widely. The factors altering the degree of dysfunction include (1) the shape of the glottis; (2) differences in the levels of the vocal cords; (3) permanent structural changes; (4) the position of the arytenoid; (5) the degree of compensation accomplished by the patient; (6) whether paralysis is unilateral or bilateral; and (7) position of the vocal cord.

The position of the vocal cord is the most important single factor, and the clinical manifestations of paralysis vary depending on cord position.

Paralysis in the Median and Paramedian Positions. These positions are usually attributed to isolated paralysis of the recurrent laryngeal nerve. Paralysis of a vocal cord exactly in the midline is unusual, and a position with the posterior end of the vocal cord about 1.5 mm lateral to the midline is much more common.

1. Unilateral paralysis in the median position may be present after recurrent laryngeal paralysis of long duration. On examination, the paralyzed vocal cord may appear somewhat atrophic and at a slightly lower level than the normal vocal cord, but on phonation the appearance may be almost normal. The arytenoid on the paralyzed side is tipped forward. The symptoms are usually not marked, and the speaking voice may appear quite normal. However, voice use requiring wide pitch alterations, such as in singing, is disturbed. Dyspnea and mild stridor may occur with extreme exertion.

2. Unilateral paralysis in the paramedian position is the usual result of a recent recurrent nerve paralysis. The degree of dysfunction is most dependent on the degree of compensation attained. Examination of the larynx will disclose the paralyzed cord in the paramedian position. The membranous cord is usually slightly bowed and at a lower level than that of the normal cord. The paralyzed cord may be seen to balloon upward on phonation, and the glottis remains somewhat elliptical. The arytenoid is seen to cross the midline and pass behind or in front of the immobile arytenoid when paralysis has been present for several days.

Symptoms in the uncompensated cases of paramedian paralysis include breathy voice, hoarseness, shortened phonation time, decreased volume and pitch range, and diplophonia. As compensation occurs, the symptoms decrease, and in a few cases the voice will become quite clear. Usually there is some dysphonia, and in some instances the pitch may be abnormally high (falsetto) because of attempted compensation for the elliptical glottis. Generally, elderly patients do not compensate as well for this cord position.

3. Bilateral paralysis in the paramedian position is the usual result of bilateral paralysis of the recurrent nerves of fairly recent onset. The symptoms are subject to considerable individual variation and are manifested as dysphonia and dyspnea. Dysphonia varies inversely with dyspnea and stridor. Dysphonia is marked by a weak, breathy voice which is somewhat hoarse and by impaired volume and pitch alterations. Dyspnea, on the other hand, is usually not significant at rest, but exertion will usually produce some degree of inspiratory stridor and difficult breathing.

Examination of the larynx will disclose the condition. Usually the glottis will be 3 to 4 mm wide at the posterior commissure. The cords are usually slightly bowed and will be seen to bow further on inspiration and to balloon superiorly on expiration.

4. Bilateral paralysis in the median position may occur immediately after injury to both recurrent laryngeal nerves, or it may be delayed for as long as 20 years. Dyspnea is the most marked symptom, and inspiratory stridor is present. The patient tends to limit activity and remain still in order to obtain enough oxygen for his needs. Any upper respiratory infection may precipitate complete laryngeal obstruction, as might stimuli causing a sudden, deep inspiration. The sudden obstruction with inspiration is secondary to vocal cord adduction caused by the aerodynamic effect of the blast of air hitting the superior surfaces of the vocal

cords and forcing them medially. Because of this danger, these patients usually breathe shallowly and slowly and avoid any exertion or stimulus.

The voice is surprisingly good, and many patients will deny any voice change. However, the fine functions of voice, such as singing, are impaired. The larynx may appear quite normal if it is examined during phonation, but the cords do not abduct from the midline position in inspiration, and a thin, elliptical chink is the only airway. In some instances, the airway may be subjectively adequate because of difference in the levels of the vocal cords.

5. Paralysis of the vocal cord in the intermediate position is classically secondary to paralysis of the recurrent and superior laryngeal nerves on one side, which is termed combined paralysis. Bulbar and high vagus paralysis may be responsible, but injury during thyroidectomy is the most common cause of dual nerve damage. Paralysis of the recurrent nerve alone may produce this cord position; this is particularly true in cases of recurrent nerve damage in the thorax. Acute recurrent nerve paralysis of any origin may cause a cord paralysis which is initially in the intermediate position. The intermediate position is usually temporary, and the cord moves toward the midline over a period of days or, in some instances, months or years.

The symptoms are those of an incompetent glottis. The voice is weak, breathy, and hoarse, the phonation time is short, and shortness of breath occurs because of excess air escape during speech. Initially, many of these patients experience some dysphagia with aspiration on swallowing; however, compensation develops in most instances. Some patients, especially the elderly, may have persistent difficulty due to inadequate compensation.

Examination of the larynx will disclose the paralyzed cord to be about 3.5 to 4 mm from the midline. The cord is bowed laterally, and a glottic chink of 1 to 2 mm persists during phonation. In some cases of combined paralysis, anterior prolapse of the arytenoid is not as marked as that occurring with the median and paramedian positions.

Compensation may occur in two ways: (1) the normal cord crosses the midline to approximate its fellow; and (2) the false vocal cords assume the phonatory and sphincteric functions, and dysphonia plicae ventricularis results.

Persistent bilateral paralysis in the intermediate position is rare, since it is usually due to bilateral bulbar or high vagal lesions, which are incompatible with life.

6. Paralysis of the vocal cords in abduction is extremely rare. It does occur in diffuse cortical lesions secondary to trauma but does not represent a flaccid paralysis but rather a spastic paralysis. The paralysis tends to be bilateral, and the symptoms are those of paralysis in the intermediate position but are more marked.

CLINICAL ASPECTS OF SPECIFIC NEUROLOGIC LESIONS

Cortical Lesions

The cerebral cortex is mainly involved in laryngeal function of more phylogenetic development, such as phonation. Therefore, cortical function is concerned mainly with production and coordination of adduction and tension of vocal cords. While the cortex does have an excitatory function, the overall effects are due to inhibition of the tonically discharging bulbar nuclei, which tend to maintain the vocal cords in the respiratory position. Disturbances in cortical function will therefore result in a spastic incoordination of movements of adduction, or if cortical paralysis is complete, the vocal cords may be maintained in a widely abducted position.

Complete loss of cortical function may occur in head injuries accompanied by extensive cerebral concussion. The vocal cords will assume a position which may be intermediate or abducted. This cord position will further contribute to the loss of effective cough and inability to handle secretions which are commonly seen in comatose patients. This type of paralysis is usually temporary, and recovery may be complete; however, if some permanent cortical damage is present, some degree of spastic incoordination will remain, marked by dysarthrophonia.

Dysarthrophonia. The cortical centers for laryngeal function are intimately related to the centers for articulation; thus cortical disease will usually result in some degree of dysarthria as well as dysphonia. Dysarthrophonia suggests a partial loss of cortical function and is a manifestation of partial spastic paralysis of the larynx and organs of articulation.

Cerebral palsy or encephalopathy resulting in spastic motor dysfunction may be of congenital origin or may be acquired after cerebral hypoxia, kernicterus, encephalitis, or cerebral trauma. Widespread cerebral arteriosclerosis may have the same effect.

The speech and voice of a patient with partial cortical paralysis is quite typical. Articulation is slurred and slow. The voice lacks resonance and has a harsh monotone with limited pitch variation. Considerable nasal air escape occurs. The voice may be excessively loud as speech is initiated but soon fades and becomes breathy owing to failure to sustain adduction of the vocal cords. Respiratory incoordination with shallow breathing contributes to the difficulty.

Treatment. Complete paralysis of the vocal cords in abduction occurs in comatose patients and necessitates tracheostomy for removal of secretions.

Incomplete cortical paralysis resulting in dysarthrophonia is helped by intensive speech and voice therapy to develop better coordination of articulation, phonation, and respiration.

PARALYSIS OF THE RECURRENT (INFERIOR) LARYNGEAL NERVES

Isolated paralysis of the muscles supplied by the recurrent laryngeal nerves is usually suggestive of nerve involvement between the nodose ganglion and the laryngeal termination. However, this paralysis may occur as the first evidence of an incipient bulbar lesion, and further bulbar involvement will eventually appear.

Two clinical pictures associated with recurrent nerve paralysis, determined by whether the paralysis is of acute onset or of chronically progressive development, are recognized.

Acute Unilateral Recurrent Nerve Paralysis

Acute paralysis is most often of traumatic origin but may be a result of toxic or infectious processes.

Clinical Manifestations. At the onset, the patient usually experiences a severe voice disturbance, which may include temporary aphonia due to the intermediate position of the newly paralyzed cord and lack of compensatory function by the normal cord. The symptoms are those of paralysis in the abducted position. However, over a period of time varying from weeks to months, the paralyzed vocal cord moves to a paramedian or median position, and the normal cord begins to compensate. As a result, the symptoms improve and the patients are often misled into thinking the condition is regressing spontaneously. In many instances, compensation is marked and a normal speaking voice returns. This is most likely in young people, since elderly individuals tend to compensate less.

The preceding sequence of events is usual, but there are exceptions. The most notable exception occurs in paralysis due to intrathoracic lesions of the nerve. In many instances, the vocal cord may remain in the intermediate position; as a result, complete compensation rarely occurs. This has been explained by Hofer as being the result of retrograde degeneration of the nucleus ambiguus with eventual paralysis of the superior laryngeal nerve, producing a combined laryngeal paralysis.

Diagnosis. The etiology may be quite obvious in many cases, but in others the cause is obscure. A careful search must be made for an etiologic factor. Examination should include a chest roentgenogram and, when indicated, roentgenograms of the skull and jugular foramen. Blood tests should include a blood count, sedimentation rate, serology, and blood sugar level. Serum viral antibody titers may be of academic interest when an infectious neuritis is suspected.

Direct laryngoscopy is not usually indicated in a case of recent acute paralysis. However, it must be remembered that cricoarytenoid arthritis may fix the vocal cord in any position and that a nerve paralysis of long duration will also eventually have some degree of cricoarytenoid fixation superimposed. Therefore, in paralysis of many weeks' duration, direct laryngoscopy and testing of the passive mobility of the arytenoid are indicated for prognostic as well as diagnostic purposes.

Prognosis. An assessment as to the eventual outcome of a unilateral recurrent nerve paralysis is important in planning future therapy as well as allaying anxiety.

Many patients with acute paralysis eventually have complete recovery of function. This is particularly true in cases of inflammatory origin or of unknown etiology. In this group, 80% or more of the paralyzed cords recover.

When paralysis is of traumatic origin, the chances of recovery are variable, particularly following surgical trauma. The surgeon will always insist that he could not possibly have cut the recurrent or vagus nerve. However, unless the possibly involved nerves were completely isolated and identified, it is best to assume that the nerve has been transected or severely injured and that spontaneous recovery is unlikely. When the nerves have been identified and their integrity assured at the end of the procedure, a subsequent paralysis is usually temporary. Paralysis associated with crushing laryngeal injuries is usually permanent, but when the less severe neck trauma causes paralysis, return of function is possible.

Evidence of spontaneous return of function is usually present within 3 months after the onset of paralysis. If function has not returned within 6 months, recovery is unlikely, although it has been reported up to 1 year after paralysis.

Treatment. The initial treatment of acute unilateral recurrent nerve paralysis is conservative, but later therapy will vary depending upon the position assumed by the vocal cord and the severity of persistent symptoms. Voice therapy should be begun early, as it will enhance compensation, especially in patients in whom the paralysis is eventually permanent. The indications for early surgical procedures are few. One exception is when the paralysis is secondary to minor neck trauma, and a dislocation of the cricothyroid joint or a fracture through the

inferior thyroid cornu can be demonstrated. In this instance, surgical resection of the inferior thyroid cornu and decompression of the nerve may result in rapid return of function.

When paralysis is immediately evident in a postoperative surgical patient and the integrity of the nerve is unproved, exploration of the wound is indicated to remove any ties which may be impinging on the nerve. Repair of a transected recurrent or vagus nerve is unlikely to result in return of normal function because of misdirection of the reinnervating axons. In fact, disordered cord movements may make the dysphonia worse than that due to simple paralysis. Postsurgical paralysis of delayed onset is usually due to edema or hematoma, and recovery can be expected without surgical intervention.

When paralysis has been present 3 to 4 months, the chances of spontaneous recovery are small, and maximum compensation has usually occurred. At this time, further consideration should be given to surgical therapy in selected patients with persistent symptoms:

1. When paralysis may have been due to a luxation or dislocation of the cricothyroid joint, decompression of the laryngeal nerve should be done before 4 months.

2. When paralysis is due to a lethal lesion, such as carcinoma of the lung, and severe dysphonia and aspiration occur because of glottic incompetence, surgery is indicated.

3. When the problem of aspiration is severe and persistent, surgical repair of the glottic function is indicated regardless of etiology.

When acute paralysis is due to a benign process and symptoms are fairly mild, the patient should be observed for 1 year, since recovery is theoretically possible during that time; then, if dysphonia persists, surgical treatment may be instituted.

CHRONIC PROGRESSIVE UNILATERAL RECURRENT NERVE PARALYSIS

This type of paralysis is due to a slowly advancing lesion anywhere in the course of the peripheral laryngeal nerves or to advancing bulbar lesions. Since changes in mobility, position, glottic shape, and cord tension are gradual, compensatory changes develop coincidentally, and symptoms are not pronounced.

The initial change is loss of abduction. Isolated paralysis of abduction is rarely recognized clinically, unless it is searched for in a patient with a disease process, such as a thyroid tumor, which requires examination of the larynx. The vocal cord is not immobilized, since adduction from the intermediate position and passive relaxation to this position after phonation still occur. The only abnormality will be glottic asymmetry during deep inspiration. The V-shaped configuration of the vocal cord centered at the tip of the vocal process fails to appear at this time. No symptoms result from paralysis of abduction.

Eventually, some degree of dysphonia develops. This may consist of an inability to sing or produce wide pitch alterations, or there may be considerable hoarseness. The vocal cord is found to be lying in the median or paramedian position, and symptoms will vary with the cord position, the tension, the presence of bowing of the cord margin, and the degree of compensation. The degree of dysphonia is usually greater as the age of the patient increases. The dysphonia may be markedly increased by a mild upper respiratory infection which causes the patient to seek attention, and only careful questioning will reveal a previous history of slight voice alteration.

If the causative lesion is in the medulla or above the level of the nodose ganglion, a superior laryngeal nerve paralysis may become superimposed on the inferior nerve paralysis, giving a combined or complete laryngeal paralysis. If the arytenoid is still mobile, the vocal cord may move laterally to the intermediate position, with the development of symptoms associated with this position.

Diagnosis. The diagnostic problems are the same as those associated with acute recurrent paralysis, but since the paralysis is of unknown duration, it may be more difficult to determine the etiology.

Prognosis. Paralysis with a chronic progressive onset is more likely to be due to an irreversible process, but spontaneous recovery is still possible, especially in patients with idiopathic paralysis. The symptoms are unlikely to change greatly over a period of time unless a superior laryngeal nerve paralysis develops.

Treatment. Many patients with this type of paralysis will not require therapy because spontaneous compensation is adequate. The remainder may acquire voice improvement from voice therapy. Elderly patients with severe dysphonia may require surgical therapy when the paralyzed cord is bowed and in the paramedian position.

Bilateral Paralysis of the Recurrent Laryngeal Nerves

Bilateral paralysis is usually of acute onset, since the most frequent cause is trauma or acute neuritis.

Clinical Manifestations. Initially, the vocal cords lie in a paramedian or intermediate position, producing symptoms of a severe dysphonia with an adequate airway. Aspiration may be a problem in elderly patients. Over a period of time, the vocal cords gradually move toward the midline, with a resulting improvement in voice and increasing dyspnea. Dyspnea and inspiratory stridor are made much worse by exertion. Acute laryngeal obstruction may occur in the later stages when an upper respiratory infection is superimposed on laryngeal paralysis.

Diagnosis. Examination will disclose bilateral immobility of the vocal cords. Cordal position will vary with the length of time from the onset of paralysis. In the cases with paralysis of long duration, the only airway may be an elliptical slit between the membranous vocal cords, which widens on inspiration. Direct laryngoscopy is indicated to establish mobility of the cricoarytenoid joints for prognostic purposes.

Prognosis. Spontaneous recovery of function of one or both vocal cords is possible in many cases of nontraumatic origin. Spontaneous recovery is less likely after surgical trauma or severe neck injuries. Most patients with a bilateral paralysis will eventually progress to a symptomatic stage of glottic obstruction unless one vocal cord recovers. The time required for the appearance of severe dyspnea due to bilateral median position may vary from a few days to 20 years. Generally, patients with post-thyroidectomy paralysis go the longest time before laryngeal obstruction becomes severe.

Treatment. Treatment will vary depending on the symptomatology, but it is mainly directed at relief of dyspnea. Any procedure to improve voice will entail narrowing of the glottis, and this is dangerous because of possible further spontaneous narrowing; therefore, rehabilitation of dysphonia is of secondary importance.

Relief of dyspnea will usually necessitate a tracheostomy as an initial procedure. Further therapy will depend on the duration of the paralysis, the mobility of the cricoarytenoid joints, and the possibility of recovery. Patients who have a possibility of spontaneous recovery should be observed for at least 6 months before any procedure other than tracheostomy is performed. Patients with persistent bilateral paralysis and an inadequate airway have several avenues of treatment open to them:

1. A permanent tracheostomy.
2. A permanent tracheostomy using a valved tube (e.g., Kistner tube).
3. Neurolysis of an external laryngeal nerve.
4. Surgical widening of the glottis, usually by some form of arytenoidopexy or arytenoidectomy.

Maintenance of a permanent tracheostomy without further therapy is indicated in patients with a lethal disease or in elderly, debilitated patients who are unlikely to tolerate the necessarily incompetent glottis produced by surgical correction. A valved tracheostomy is of value in patients who require continued use of a good voice, in patients refusing surgery or, as a temporary measure, when recovery may still be anticipated.

Neurolysis of the external laryngeal nerve has been discussed by Tschiassny. By dividing this nerve, it is hoped that a cord in the median position will move laterally to the intermediate position, since opening of the glottis to this position is a passive move-ment. Paralysis of one cricothyroid muscle will result in widening of the glottis by as much as 3 mm. The advantage of the procedure is that it is simple compared to arytenoidopexy and avoids the complications of that operation, which include excessive widening of the glottis. Prognostic tests should be carried out before neurolysis is performed.

1. The mobility of the cricoarytenoid joint must be established.

2. The cricothyroid muscle may be temporarily paralyzed by infiltrating it with local anesthetic. The position assumed by the cord would indicate the degree of improvement to be expected.

The success of this procedure is limited by the degree of fibrosis of the denervated musculature and the degree of limitation of cricoarytenoid joint movement.

Surgical widening of the glottis for dyspnea due to bilateral recurrent nerve paralysis is indicated when:

1. The paralysis is 6 to 8 months old and no recovery is evident.
2. The cause of paralysis leaves little possibility of recovery.
3. The cricoarytenoid joints are fixed.
4. Temporary paralysis of a cricoarytenoid muscle does not produce an adequate airway.

Many different surgical procedures have been utilized successfully, and these are discussed beginning on page 465.

PARALYSIS OF THE SUPERIOR LARYNGEAL NERVE

The superior laryngeal nerve is responsible for sensory innervation of the supraglottic larynx and motor innervation of the cricothyroid muscle. Paralysis may result from injury to the main nerve trunk or either of the terminal branches. Lesions proximal to the division of the nerve will result in both sensory and motor loss. Above the level of the nodose ganglion, paralysis is usually in the form of an associated paralysis. Bulbar lesions differ from more peripheral lesions in that the sensory loss tends to be less discrete.

Surgical trauma is the most common cause of nerve injury below the nodose ganglion, and the most frequent injury is damage to the motor branch during thyroidectomy. Isolated paralysis of the superior laryngeal nerve may have the same causes as recurrent nerve paralysis. Bilateral paralysis of the superior laryngeal nerves is also most frequently secondary to surgical procedures, such as supraglottic laryngectomy.

Clinical Manifestations. When sensory loss has developed, the patient may have temporary difficulty with aspiration and choking spells. Rapid compensation occurs when the paralysis is unilateral but appears more slowly with bilateral paralysis.

Alterations in voice are the main complaint of the patient. The voice is weak, lacks resonance, and becomes monotonic. Raising the pitch of the voice is almost impossible, and air wasting causes a shortened phonation time. The symptoms are explained by the lack of cord tension, which allows the cord to balloon superiorly during phonation, preventing effective glottic closure and producing a drop in voice pitch which is especially noticeable in females. There may be some spontaneous improvement of symptoms with time, but generally they are persistent.

Diagnosis. Isolated paralysis of one cricothyroid muscle presents a distinct picture when viewed by indirect or direct laryngoscopy. The patient must be asked to phonate, since the muscle is active only at this time. The posterior commissure is seen to deviate toward the paralyzed side owing to the action of the intact cricothyroid muscle, producing an oblique glottis. The vocal cord on the paralyzed side appears bowed, short, and bulky due to the unopposed action of the thyroarytenoid muscle. It should be noted that the wavy cordal margin depicted in older publications does not exist. The intact thyroarytenoid tends to pull the arytenoid forward and increase the prominence of the tip of the vocal process on the side of paralysis. The vocal cord is usually at a lower level than that on the normal side because the tilting of the cricoid and displacement of the hypotonic cord by inspiratory air currents.

When the sensory branch is involved, anesthesia of the hemilarynx may be demonstrated by palpation. Also, the involved hemilarynx may appear injected secondary to vasodilatation resulting from loss of sympathetic nerve supply, but simultaneous destruction of the superior laryngeal artery prevents hyperemia.

These physical findings are less marked or absent when superior laryngeal paralysis is bilateral. The manipulation tests may help in the diagnosis of bilateral as well as unilateral paralysis. Frontal pressure on the thyroid cartilage (Guttmann's test) will normally lower voice pitch by counteracting cricothyroid function, whereas lateral pressure on the thyroid has the opposite effect. Abnormal results suggest cricothyroid paralysis. Failure of the cricothyroid space to narrow on phonation may be noted by palpation or serial roentgenograms. Manual compression of this space will raise the voice pitch when paralysis is present. Electromyography is of value in diagnosis due to the accessibility of the cricothyroid muscle.

Treatment. Correction of the vocal abnormalities is the main aim of therapy. However, unlike unilateral paralysis of the recurrent nerve, which may be compensated for by overaction of the opposite vocal cord, the symptoms of unilateral cricothyroid paralysis are made worse by overaction of the functioning cricothyroid muscle. Therefore, voice therapy is of no avail in these cases and may make the symptoms worse.

A surgical procedure to narrow the cricothyroid space may be of benefit if symptomatology is severe. Arnold has described suturing the thyrohyoid muscle to the cricoid cartilage to elevate the cartilage during phonation. Approximation of the thyroid and cricoid cartilages with a wire suture may also be of value in increasing cord tension.

As a rule, no therapy is necessary once the situation is explained to the patient. Most patients will have a voice satisfactory for everyday needs, and only a few demanding improvement in voice will require surgery.

COMBINED PARALYSIS OF THE LARYNX

Paralysis of both the recurrent and superior laryngeal nerves on one side causes paralysis of all the muscles of the hemi-larynx except the interarytenoideus. The paralysis is usually due to a high vagal lesion in the region of the jugular foramen or a bulbar lesion. However, combined injury of the recurrent nerve and the motor branch of the superior nerve may result from thyroid surgery.

Clinical Manifestations. The symptoms are those of an incompetent glottis due to the intermediate position of the vocal cord. Unlike the symptoms in an acute recurrent nerve paralysis, which tend to improve spontaneously, the symptoms in this situation are persistent.

Diagnosis. Since the clinical pictures of an early recurrent nerve paralysis and a combined paralysis are the same, it is important to differentiate between the two for prognostic and diagnostic purposes. Combined paralysis is usually part of an associated paralysis except in post-thyroidectomy patients or after neuritis.

High vagal lesions caused by neuritis will usually cause sensory changes which can be detected. Therefore, the diagnostic problem is usually presented by the post-thyroidectomy patient. The picture of the oblique glottis due to superior laryngeal paralysis may not be evident, especially if compensation by the functioning cord has developed. The manipulation tests and determination of cricothyroid space alterations may be helpful but not conclusive in unilateral paralysis. Electromyographic analysis of the cricothyroid muscle is easily performed transcutaneously, making a determination of the status of the cricothyroid muscle relatively easy.

Treatment. The initial treatment includes voice therapy and physiotherapy. However, compensation is often less than adequate, and surgery for the abducted vocal cord may be necessary.

ASSOCIATED PARALYSIS OF THE LARYNX

The intimate relationships of the laryngeal bulbar nuclei and the vagus nerve to the nuclei of cranial nerves IX, XI, and XII leads to the association of laryngeal paralysis with paralysis of other bulbar centers and

of the other three posterior cranial nerves. Associated paralyses tend to fall into two groups:

1. Those due to lesions involving the medulla.
2. Those due to lesions of the extramedullary portions of the last four cranial nerves, which can be further divided into four groups:
   (*a*) Paralysis within the posterior cranial fossa.
   (*b*) Paralysis within or adjacent to the jugular foramen.
   (*c*) Paralysis in the lateral pharyngeal space.
   (*d*) Paralysis inferior to the level of the clavicle.

Numerous eponyms have been applied to the various groupings of the associated paralyses; these are of little direct clinical importance but are of historic interest. The main importance of the groupings is the clue they give to the site of the pathologic disorder.

Medulla Syndromes

In the lateral medulla, the nucleus ambiguus is adjacent to the descending nucleus and tract of the fifth nerve, both spinocerebellar tracts, the lateral spinothalamic tract, the descending sympathetic tract, and the restiform body. This area of the medulla is supplied by the superior, middle, and inferior lateral medullary branches of the posterior inferior cerebellar artery, which arises from the vertebral artery. The vertebral artery supplies the medial medullary area of the hypoglossal nucleus, the medial lemniscus, and the pyramidal tract by separate branches. The commonest cause of bulbar-associated syndromes is a cerebrovascular accident. Encephalitis, tabes, syringomyelia, multiple sclerosis, and progressive bulbar palsy may involve the same areas. Bulbar syndromes are often progressive, first involving one nerve and then others. They also may be regressive, with resulting fluctuation of symptoms and signs (see Table 34–2).

Lateral Medullary Syndrome (Wallenberg). This is due to infarction of the medullary area supplied by the posterior infe-

Table 34-2. Neurologic Defects of the Syndromes of Associated Laryngeal Paralyses

Usual Site of Disease	Eponym	Medullary Tracts		Sympathetic Horner's Syndrome	Pharyngeal Plexus Paralysis Soft Palate	IX Nerve Dec. Taste Post. Tongue	X Nerve Dec. Laryngeal Sensation Cricothyroid Paralysis	Vocal Cord Paralysis	XI Nerve Paralysis Sternomastoid and Trapezius M.	XII Nerve Paralysis Tongue	Phrenic N. Paralysis Diaphragm
		Sensory	Motor								
Medulla	Wallenberg	+	−	+	+	+	+	+	+	−	−
	Babinski-Nageotte	+	+	+	+	+	+	+	+	+	−
	Cestan-Chenais	+	+	+	+	+	+	+	−	+	−
	Avellis	±	−	−	+	−	+	+	−	−	−
	Jackson	±	±	−	+	−	+	+	+	+	−
	Schmidt	±	±	−	+	−	+	+	+	−	−
	Mackenzie	±	±	−	+	−	+	+	−	+	−
	Bonnier	−	+	−	+	−	+	+	+	−	−
Posterior cranial fossa	Collet-Sicard	±	−	−	+	+	+	+	+	+	−
Jugular foramen	Vernet	−	−	−	+	+	+	+	+	−	−
Lateral pharyngeal space	Villaret	−	−	+	+	+	+	+	+	+	−
	Tapia	−	−	−	−	−	−	+	−	+	−
	Gard-Gignoux	−	−	−	−	−	−	+	+	−	−
Superior mediastinum	Klinkert	−	−	−	−	−	−	+	−	−	+
	Pancoast	−	−	+	−	−	−	+	−	−	+

rior cerebellar artery, immediately posterior to the inferior olive. The findings include paralysis of half the larynx, pharynx, and palate, contralateral pain and temperature loss below the neck, loss of facial sensation, vestibular dysfunction, ataxia, and Horner's syndrome.

Total Unilateral Medullary Syndrome (Babinski-Nageotte). This syndrome is the same as the previous syndrome except that paralysis of the medial bulbar area is included, causing paralysis of the tongue, contralateral hemiplegia, and loss of position and vibration sense.

Cestan-Chenais Syndrome. This group of neurologic symptoms is caused by obstruction of the vertebral artery below the posterior inferior cerebellar artery. The symptoms and signs are similar to those of the preceding syndrome except that involvement rarely extends proximal to the motor areas of the nucleus ambiguus.

In many instances, the complete medullary syndromes are not present. Eponyms have been applied to the various syndromes of associated paralysis caused by incomplete destruction of bulbar centers. Some confusion exists because the same names are also applied to similar cranial nerve paralyses caused by peripheral lesions. However, the following syndromes are most often due to bulbar lesions.

Avellis' Syndrome. This syndrome is the result of a lesion involving the nucleus ambiguus or the vagus nerve and the cranial portion of the spinal accessory nerve. In addition, there is often contralateral loss of pain and temperature sensation due to spinothalamic tract destruction.

Symptoms include dysphagia and dysphonia due to laryngeal and pharyngeal paralysis and nasal regurgitation and rhinolalia due to paralysis of the soft palate. The symptoms may be progressive in that the palate paralysis may not develop until after the laryngeal paralysis.

The cause is usually a vascular or inflammatory lesion in the medulla, but disease involving the vagus nerve above the level of the nodose ganglion will cause a similar paralysis.

Hughlings Jackson Syndrome. This syndrome is characterized by paralysis of the last three nerves: the vagus, spinal accessory, and hypoglossal. Symptomatology is produced by ipsilateral paralysis of the soft palate, pharynx, larynx, sternomastoid muscle, and tongue. There may be a contralateral spastic hemiplegia due to involvement of the pyramidal tract. The causative lesion is usually intramedullary, but it may be situated high in the lateral pharyngeal space.

Schmidt's Syndrome. This syndrome is characterized by ipsilateral paralysis of the larynx, pharynx, and soft palate, as well as paralysis of the sternomastoid and trapezius muscles. The lesion is located in the caudal portion of the medulla and is usually of vascular origin.

Mackenzie's Syndrome. This syndrome consists of unilateral paralysis of the palate, pharynx, larynx, and tongue. It is similar to Jackson's syndrome and is most often due to a vascular lesion in the medulla.

Bonnier's Syndrome. This condition is due to a lesion of Deiters' nucleus or the associated vestibular tracts. A general sense of apprehension and weakness exists. When vertigo and deafness are present, the condition simulates Meniere's syndrome.

Peripheral Syndromes

These syndromes may be caused by bulbar lesions but are more often due to peripheral causes. Generally, syndromes including paralysis of the ninth nerve and the spinal portion of the eleventh nerve are peripheral in origin. Lesions causing these syndromes arise in four areas.

Posterior Cranial Fossa. Diseases and tumors of the meninges are the main causes. Paralysis of all last four cranial nerves is present without long tract signs or Horner's syndrome.

Jugular Foramen. The ninth, tenth, and eleventh nerves are paralyzed, and the twelfth nerve is not involved because of its separate position in the hypoglossal canal. The cervical sympathetic chain ends below this level; therefore, Horner's syndrome is not a part of this complex. Causes of paralysis include lymphadenopathy, tumors, basal skull fracture, and inflammation in the region of the jugular foramen.

Lateral Pharyngeal Space (Retrostyloid). Associated paralysis in this area usually does not involve the eleventh nerve, but paralysis of the sympathetic may be present. The usual cause is a neoplasm.

Infrahyoid. Paralysis from lesions inferior to the hyoid do not paralyze the superior laryngeal nerve, the hypoglossal nerve, or the glossopharyngeal nerve, but the phrenic nerve may be involved.

Collet-Sicard Syndrome. This syndrome is characterized by paralysis of the last four cranial nerves without sympathetic paralysis. The cause is usually a tumor such as meningioma en plaque, meningitis, or trauma involving the nerves in the posterior cranial fossa.

Vernet's Syndrome (Jugular Foramen Syndrome). This syndrome is due to involvement of the ninth, tenth, and eleventh nerves in the region of the jugular foramen. The features include dysphagia, dysphonia, nasal regurgitation, torticollis, and inability to raise the ipsilateral arm above shoulder level. The syndrome is most often caused by lymphadenopathy of the nodes of Krause in the jugular foramen. Thrombophlebitis, tumors of the jugular bulb, neurogenous tumors, and basal skull fracture are other causes.

Villaret's Syndrome. This syndrome is the same as the preceding one except that sympathetic paralysis and Horner's syndrome are present. Therefore, the causative lesion involves the nerves in the area deep to the parotid gland (retroparotid or lateral pharyngeal space).

Tapia's Syndrome. Characteristically, paralysis of the ipsilateral tongue and vocal cord constitute the syndrome. The soft palate and cricothyroid muscle are not affected. The causative lesion is usually a neoplastic process at the point where the hypoglossal nerve crosses the vagus nerve and internal carotid artery in the lateral pharyngeal space.

Gard-Gignoux Syndrome. This syndrome is characterized by paralysis of the eleventh nerve and the vagus below the nodose ganglion. Therefore, laryngeal sensation and cricothyroid function are intact, and symptoms are due to vocal cord paralysis and

weakness of the trapezius and sternomastoid muscles.

Klinkert Syndrome. This syndrome is marked by paralysis of the recurrent and phrenic nerves by a neoplastic process in the root of the neck or upper mediastinum and occurs most often on the left. Sympathetic paralysis may be associated with the syndrome as part of the superior sulcus syndrome (of Pancoast).

Diagnosis. The presence of laryngeal paralysis in association with paralysis of any of the last four cranial nerves is an indication for careful investigation of the upper neck, base of the skull, and posterior cranial fossa. Complete neurobiologic examination and inspection of the middle ear and nasopharynx are especially important.

Examination of the jugular foramen should include stereoscopic submentovertex views of the base of the skull, as well as laminograms when necessary. In some instances, retrograde jugular venography will demonstrate lesions in the jugular foramen, especially tumors of the glomus jugulare

Space-occupying lesions in the postcranial fossa may be associated with signs of increased intracranial pressure. If the pressure is normal, pneumoencephalogram or dye contrast examination may be of value in isolating the lesion. In some instances, vertebral angiography is also necessary and helpful.

Treatment. Therapy is mainly directed at the causative lesion. Since the laryngeal paralysis is seldom reversible, treatment is only necessary for functional problems of phonation and deglutition.

LARYNGEAL PARALYSIS IN INFANCY

Unilateral or bilateral paralysis of the vocal cord is the second most common cause of stridor in a neonate after laryngomalacia.

Etiology. Some form of trauma is the usual cause. This takes the form of acute trauma at birth or a chronic progressive mechanical trauma.

Acute trauma at birth may be secondary to lateral traction on the neck when the shoulders are being delivered or to the umbilical cord constricting the neck. The right vocal cord is most often paralyzed, possibly because of excessive tension on the right recurrent nerve, which occurs more readily owing to the intimate relationship of the right subclavian artery to the movements of the shoulder and arm. The paralysis is usually unilateral, but bilateral paralysis may occur.

Chronic mechanical trauma is usually secondary to abnormalities of the nervous system or skull which produce traction on the vagoaccessory nerves in the region of the jugular foramen. The Arnold-Chiari syndrome is an example. This syndrome is due to displacement of the cerebellum and medulla into the spinal canal because of fixation of the spinal cord by a myelomeningocele and by progressive internal hydrocephalus which tends to increase the medullary displacement. As the medulla is displaced caudally, the fibers of the vagus and spinal accessory nerves are stretched, causing paralysis. Platybasia is a congenital deformity of the base of the skull which may produce bilateral paralysis secondary to stretching of the vagus at the jugular foramen.

Clinical Manifestations. Symptoms may be present at or shortly after birth, or they may be delayed in onset. The symptoms of unilateral paralysis due to birth injury are usually noted within 24 hours of birth and include a hoarse cry and stridor on deep inspiration. While crying the infant may become cyanotic, but at rest or while sleeping respirations are fairly normal and stridor is absent.

Paralysis associated with the Arnold-Chiari syndrome is often delayed in onset for several weeks. The symptoms are marked by increasing stridor, difficulty in feeding, and finally laryngeal obstruction due to complete bilateral paralysis. Initially, this type of paralysis is reversible and will often disappear when the hydrocephalus is relieved.

Diagnosis. The diagnosis is made by direct laryngoscopy. The laryngoscope should be inserted into the vallecula to inspect the movement of the vocal cords. If the tip of the laryngoscope is inserted into the larynx, it may tense the cords, giving a false impression of paralysis.

The paralyzed cord usually lies in the paramedian position and tends to be bowed. When bilateral paralysis exists, the glottis is elliptical, with the widest opening at the center of the membranous vocal cords during inspiration. Because the soft tissues of the infantile larynx are normally flabby, considerable motion occurs with respiration, which may give the false impression of normal function. The immobility of one or both arytenoids is the most important diagnostic finding.

Treatment. Unilateral right vocal cord paralysis in an infant due to a probable birth injury is followed by recovery in a high percentage of these cases in 6 weeks or less. As a result, treatment is seldom necessary. When the left cord is paralyzed, congenital heart disease should be suspected or ruled out. If unilateral vocal cord paralysis is persistent, any deficiency is usually well compensated for by the normal cord.

Bilateral paralysis may be due to birth trauma, or the cause may be unknown. There is spontaneous recovery of one or both cords in a high percentage of cases. However, respiratory obstruction may develop before recovery, necessitating a temporary tracheostomy.

When bilateral paralysis is associated with a nervous system abnormality, such as in the Arnold-Chiari syndrome, relief of the hydrocephalus by ventricular tap often will result in immediate return of function. This is especially true in early cases. Permanent relief of hydrocephalus is necessary to avoid return of paralysis. This may require insertion of a Holter valve and perhaps high cervical laminectomy.

If bilateral paralysis is persistent, a permanent tracheostomy is necessary until age 4 or 5. The use of a valved tracheostomy tube is helpful for speech development. At age 4 to 5, lateral fixation of the arytenoid may be performed.

SURGICAL TREATMENT OF PARALYSIS OF THE LARYNX

Failure of recovery of normal motion and function or failure of development of complete compensation with persistence of symptoms may necessitate surgical treatment of laryngeal paralysis. Surgery may be indicated for treatment of the incompetent glottis due to paralysis of a cord in a position lateral to the median position or for treatment of a stenotic glottis due to bilateral paralysis in the median position.

Treatment of Paralysis in Abducted Position

Surgical treatment is indicated to improve the voice after maximum spontaneous compensation by the normal vocal cord or to prevent aspiration or both. The timing of surgical intervention is variable; generally, early treatment of aspiration is indicated, especially if a lethal disease is the cause. Treatment of dysphonia should be delayed longer, at least 6 months, to allow for spontaneous recovery, stabilization of cord position, and maximum compensation. Several procedures have been utilized with success.

Intrachordal Injections. Teflon paste injection has been described by Arnold. The material used is a nonabsorbable suspension of Teflon in glycerine which is injected into the cord. The procedure is most useful for alleviation of dysphonia when the vocal cord is permanently in a paramedian or intermediate position. In addition, it is useful in the treatment of dysphonia in selected cases of dysplastic dysphonia, surgical absence of a vocal cord, and fixation of the cricoarytenoid joint. Excessive glottic width after arytenoidectomy may also be treated in this manner. The procedure is also useful for treating the problem of aspiration due to lateral position of a paralyzed vocal cord.

Procedure. A test injection of absorbable gelatin may be carried out before Teflon injection to ascertain the result to be expected. Direct laryngoscopy is performed under local anesthesia. A Bruening syringe and a special 18-gauge or 19-gauge needle is used to inject the Teflon. The injections are performed as indicated in Figure 34–4. The first injection is made at the midpoint of the membranous vocal cord, where 0.3 to 0.4 ml is deposited, and this is repeated at the tip of the vocal process. A small injection (0.1 to 0.2 ml) may be made between the first two sites if necessary. Care must be taken to place the Teflon laterally in the cord and about 2 mm below the sur-

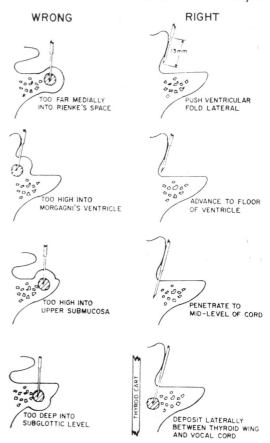

FIG. 34–4. Method of Teflon paste injection (Arnold). A 19-gauge needle is used. The needle is inserted in the lateral portion of the vocal cord to a depth of 2 to 3 mm before injection is made.

face. The injection may be repeated in 3 to 4 weeks if necessary.

Postoperatively, edema may occur, causing considerable hoarseness, but this rapidly disappears, and the voice will improve over 1 to 2 weeks. Voice therapy should be continued.

Liquid silicone or its derivative, Silastic, may be used for intrachordal injection. Silicone is slowly absorbed, and the results of injection are temporary. Silastic RTV 5392, when injected, remains in situ and has the advantage of producing less tissue reaction than Teflon paste. The disadvantage of Silastic is that it is technically more difficult to use than Teflon paste.

Glycerine injection into the vocal cord may be of value for the temporary treatment of vocal cord paralysis. Since glycerine is slowly absorbed, it may be used to alleviate severe dysphonia or aspiration in situations in which there is a good chance that paralysis may be temporary.

Cartilage Implantation. Various procedures have been described in which cartilage is implanted between the thyroid ala and the internal perichondrium, displacing the fixed abducted cord medially, to relieve aspiration and dysphonia.

The Meurman operation is perhaps the oldest such procedure described. This procedure necessitates performing a thyrotomy, through which a piece of autogenous rib cartilage or Silastic is inserted lateral to the internal perichondrium.

More recently autogenous thyroid cartilage has been used in a similar fashion. However, this is inserted from the inferior border of the thyroid ala after the internal perichondrium has been incised and elevated to create an appropriately sized implant pocket. The graft material is obtained from the superior border of the opposite thyroid ala.

Postoperatively, considerable edema may occur, causing laryngeal obstruction. Therefore, performance of an elective tracheostomy is often advisable.

These procedures have been largely supplanted by the intrachordal injection of Teflon when available.

Reverse Arytenoidopexy. Morrison described this procedure for moving an abducted cord to the midline. The approach is the same as that for arytenoidopexy. The cricoarytenoid joint is opened and the capsule completely divided. In some cases of cricoarytenoid arthritis, it may be necessary to use an osteotome to separate the cricoid and arytenoid cartilages. The mobilized arytenoid is then moved to a more medial position and sutured to the cricoid. This procedure has also been supplanted by intrachordal injections.

Treatment of Vocal Cord Paralysis in Adduction

Unilateral paralysis in the median position does not require surgical treatment, but bilateral paralysis does require it for relief of laryngeal obstruction. Many different surgical procedures have been suggested and used, including neurolysis of the external laryngeal nerve, arytenoidectomy, and arytenoidopexy.

The aim of surgical repair is to provide an adequate airway for average everyday physical activity and still retain a usable voice. A glottic chink 5 mm wide is adequate for respiratory purposes, but the voice tends to be poor. This situation may be improved if the chink is made slightly less wide and the vocal cords are placed at different levels to create a baffle effect.

Neurolysis of the External Laryngeal Nerve. It is generally accepted that the median position of the vocal cord after recurrent nerve paralysis is due to continued and possibly excessive function of the cricothyroid muscle; it follows that paralysis of this muscle should result in widening of the glottis. Tschiassny claims that an increase of 3 mm in the glottic width may be obtained.

The results to be expected from division of the superior laryngeal nerve may be tested preoperatively by infiltrating the cricothyroid muscle with a local anesthetic. Generally, a glottic width of 3 mm is inadequate for normal everyday activity, although the voice is quite good. Therefore, the procedure is of most value in a senescent individual who is most interested in the quality of his voice or in the patient whose cords are in the paramedian position.

Failure of neurolysis of the external laryngeal nerve to produce glottic widening may be due to degenerative changes in the vocalis muscle and in the cricoarytenoid joint capsule, which should be ruled out by preoperative paralysis of the cricothyroid muscle.

Arytenoidopexy. The first arytenoidopexy was described by King in 1939. In the original King procedure, the arytenoid was fixed in a lateral position, and the omohyoid muscle was attached to it, supposedly to aid in maintaining the lateral position. Numerous modifications of this operation have been described, but the one described by Clerf has given consistently good, reliable results.

Technique for Arytenoidopexy (Clerf). If a tracheostomy has not been performed, one

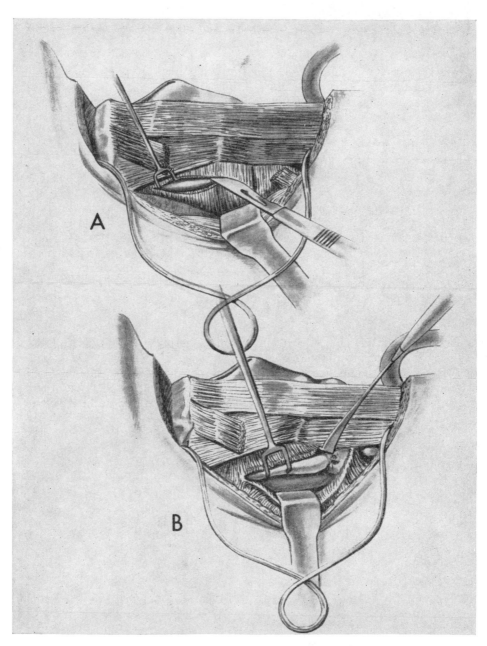

Fig. 34–5.   *(Legend on opposite page.)*

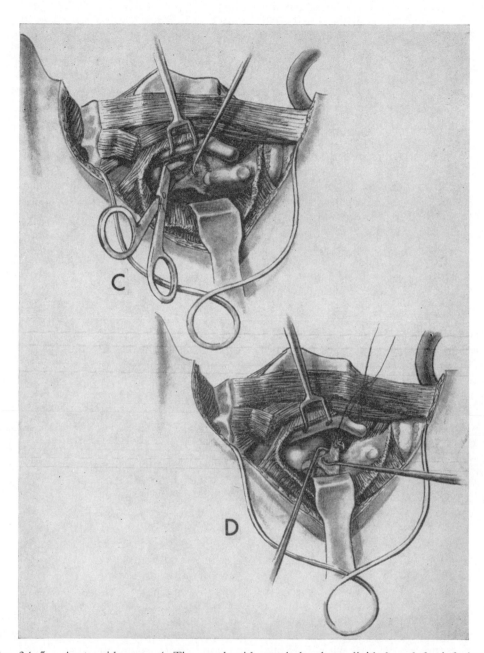

FIG. 34–5.   Arytenoidopexy. *A,* The omohyoid muscle has been divided, and the inferior constrictor has been divided along the posterior margin of the thyroid ala. *B,* The thyroid ala is pulled anteriorly, disclosing the mucosa of the piriform fossa and separating the cricothyroid joint. *C,* The arytenoid is identified and fixed with a hook. Right-angled scissors are used to divide the fibers of the interarytenoid muscle medial to the arytenoid. *D,* After the arytenoid is mobilized, a ligature carrier is used to pass a suture around the vocal process. The suture is tied around the thyroid cornu.

should be done under local anesthesia before general anesthesia is given. The patient without a tracheostomy should never be given preoperative respiratory depressants, as this may precipitate obstruction. After the patient is asleep, a small endotracheal tube may be placed between the vocal cords to push the arytenoid laterally and facilitate its localization.

If thyroidectomy was the cause of paralysis, the larynx is approached by excision of the old incision; otherwise, a horizontal incision is made over the thyroid cartilage. The incision is deepened vertically between the sternomastoid and strap muscles. The omohyoid must be divided to approach the posterior margin of the thyroid ala, which is then pulled forward by a hook. The inferior constrictor muscle is separated from the thyroid ala, which will expose the slightly bulging mucosa of the anterior wall of the piriform fossa. Immediately inferior to this mucosa is the lamina of the cricoid cartilage, which is followed medially in a submucosal plane to the arytenoid cartilage. If exposure is difficult, the inferior thyroid cornu may be detached or resected to facilitate the approach to the arytenoid.

The arytenoid is completely mobilized by dividing the cricoarytenoid joint capsule and separating the attachments of the posterior cricoarytenoid and interarytenoid muscles. Separation of the interarytenoid muscle is facilitated by using right-angled scissors to cut on the medial side of the arytenoid (Fig. 34–5). Care must be taken not to perforate the mucosa into the pharynx or larynx. The arytenoid should be handled with a fine hook, as grasping it with forceps often results in fragmentation of the cartilage.

Using special needles of the aneurysm type, sutures are placed around the body of the arytenoid and the vocal process without perforating the mucosa. Heavy silk is preferable if the mucosa is intact, but a chromic catgut suture may be best if the mucosa has been lacerated. Two holes are made in the posterior margin of the thyroid ala, preferably at a slightly lower level than the vocal cord. This will place the repositioned cord at a slightly lower level than the opposite cord. One suture is passed through each hole and tied. If the inferior cornu of the

thyroid is intact, the suture may be passed around it. When the sutures are tied, the arytenoid is approximated to the thyroid ala, which tenses as well as adducts the vocal cord. In the male, this will usually result in a satisfactory glottis for respiration and speech; however, in the female, the wider angle of the thyroid cartilage may result in the arytenoid being placed too laterally when it is tightly approximated to the ala. Therefore, it is best to inspect the glottis before the wound is closed and to loosen the sutures if necessary. The chinks should be about 5 mm wide between the vocal process. The wound is then closed in layers, with a small drain in place.

Postoperatively, the patient is given oral feedings if the pharyngeal mucosa is intact, but if laceration has occurred, intravenous feedings are necessary for 5 to 6 days. About 1 week postoperatively, the airway is tested; if it is adequate, the tracheostomy tube is reduced in size to a No. 5, corked for 24 hours, and then removed.

The results of this operation are usually satisfactory, but on occasion the healing process may result in some narrowing of the glottis; therefore, it is advisable to leave the glottic chink slightly overcorrected at the time of surgery. In the event that the airway remains inadequate after the first procedure, the same procedure may be repeated on the opposite side.

Arytenoidectomy. Several methods and approaches have been described for arytenoidectomy.

Extralaryngeal Methods. *Woodman Operation.* The approach to the larynx is the same as that for arytenoidopexy. The cricothyroid joint is disarticulated for additional exposure of the cricoarytenoid joint. The arytenoid is dissected subperichondrially and completely mobilized. A suture is passed submucosally around the vocal process and through some of the thyroarytenoid muscle. When this suture is in position, the body of the arytenoid is removed. The vocal process is drawn laterally, and the suture is tied around the inferior cornu. The glottis must be inspected with a laryngoscope before the wound is closed.

The disadvantages of this procedure include the following: (1) there is sometimes considerable difficulty in getting an adequate, firm suture around the vocal process; (2) when the arytenoid is absent, the glottis is often made too wide, especially in females.

The procedure is necessary when the vocal process is inadvertently fractured during arytenoidopexy. When the glottis is apparently too wide, the vocal cord may be injected with Teflon paste to improve the voice.

Kelly Operation. Kelly described this operation in 1939. This approach to arytenoidectomy was developed to avoid the difficulty in approaching the arytenoid around the posterior margin of the thyroid ala. The approach to the larynx is the same as that in the Woodman operation. The thyrohyoid muscle is elevated from the side of the thyroid ala, and a window 1.5 cm square is made in the lower posterior portion of the ala using a Stryker pencil saw. The internal perichondrium is slit, and the arytenoid, approached through the fibers of the thyroarytenoid muscle, is dissected free and removed. A fine silk suture is used to approximate the vocal process to the external perichondrium at the margin of the window, while an assistant observes the glottis by direct laryngoscopy.

The disadvantages of this procedure are that a branch of the laryngeal artery usually traverses the window and that the dissection of the arytenoid is made unnecessarily difficult by the small operative field.

Orton's Operation. Orton's modification of arytenoidectomy includes the use of Trotter's pharyngotomy approach to the arytenoid. After the skin and subcutaneous incision, a vertical incision is made 1 cm anterior to the posterior border of the thyroid ala through muscles and external perichondrium. The perichondrium is dissected from the posterior border of the ala to expose the external surface of the internal perichondrium. An incision is made through the internal perichondrium to approach and remove the arytenoid cartilage. The vocal process is sutured to the thyroid ala. The advantage claimed for this procedure is the wide exposure of the arytenoid.

McCall and Gardener Operation. This operation is similar to the Kelly operation except that a brightly lit laryngoscope is used to press the arytenoid laterally against the ala where it can be identified by transillumination. A window is cut in the thyroid ala, and the mobilized arytenoid is sutured into the window. The method is time-saving compared to the Kelly procedure but is still more difficult than the Clerf arytenoidopexy.

Intralaryngeal Methods *Thornell Operation.* The suspension laryngoscope is used for this procedure. A tracheostomy is done first if one has not already been performed; then a general anesthetic is given and the patient suspended.

A small 1.5-cm incision is made on the superior aspect of the arytenoid eminence and the aryepiglottic fold. A needle is inserted into the incision, and the area is infiltrated with 1 to 2 ml of saline solution containing some epinephrine to facilitate hemostasis and dissection. Injury to the mucous membrane must be avoided. The interarytenoid muscle is detached medially using a fine alligator forceps or scissors. A sharp Lynch elevator is used to separate muscle attachments laterally. The joint capsule and vocal process are divided with a laryngeal knife and scissors, and the cartilage is then cauterized to achieve hemostasis as well as to stimulate fibrosis and contracture in order to pull the vocal cord laterally.

A Silastic mold is inserted in the larynx and left in position 7 to 10 days. At this time, it is removed and the airway tested by reducing the tracheostomy tube size and plugging the tube. If this is well tolerated for 24 hours, the tube is removed.

This procedure is simple and avoids a comparatively extensive external operation, but it requires the special skills and equipment needed for suspension laryngoscopy. The disadvantage of the procedure is that arytenoidectomy alone will usually produce only a 3-mm widening of the glottis; therefore, an adequate glottis is often dependent on scar formation and contracture. Any damage to the laryngeal mucosa may nullify the effects of the operation.

Transthyrotomy Operations. Réthi, Hoover, Loré, and Pearlman are among many authors who have described the thyrotomy approach to simple arytenoidectomy, cordectomy, or a combination of the two procedures. The larynx is approached through the horizontal skin incision, and a vertical midline thyrotomy is done, which divides the anterior commissure. A mucosal incision is made to expose and remove the arytenoid, after which the area is cauterized. A submucosal removal of one vocal cord may be combined with this procedure. The main objection to this procedure is the possibility of damage to the anterior portions of the vocal cords and the arytenoid area, which may result in eventual fibrous stenosis. Also, the voice in many of these patients is very poor, although the airway is adequate.

Anterior Commissuroplasty. In some situations when there is scarring and fibrosis of the posterior commissure or after failure of bilateral cordopexy, an adequate laryngeal airway may be obtained by widening the anterior commissure. A midline thyrotomy is done, preserving the internal perichondrium, which is elevated from the anterior portions of the thyroid ala. A suture is placed in each vocal cord a short distance behind the anterior commissure, and these are tied to the external perichondrium. Next, a piece of autogenous cartilage 5 mm wide is taken from the superior margin of either thyroid ala and placed between the anterior ends of the thyroid ala to keep them separated. The voice, after this procedure, is poor, but the use of a tracheostomy is eliminated.

DECOMPRESSION OF THE RECURRENT LARYNGEAL NERVE

In selected cases of vocal cord paralysis in which there is a history of trauma to the

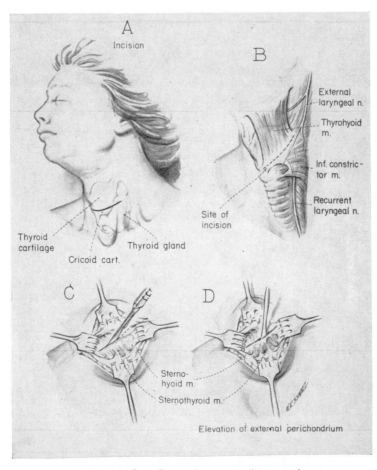

FIG. 34–6. *(Legend on opposite page.)*

neck and spontaneous recovery does not occur, decompression of the laryngeal nerve may be indicated. Any injury to the anterior neck may result in luxation or dislocation of the cricothyroid joint. Because of the close proximity of the recurrent nerve to the joint, the nerve may be injured by acute compression or it may be involved by post-injury cicatrix causing cord paralysis.

In the absence of any demonstrable fracture or dislocation of the inferior thyroid cornu, approximately 3 months is allowed for spontaneous recovery before surgical intervention is considered. If a fracture or dislocation can be demonstrated by clinical or roentgenologic examination, decompression is indicated immediately. When the onset

of vocal cord paralysis is delayed for 6 to 8 days after injury, involvement by the healing process may be suspected and decompression considered.

The principles of decompression of the recurrent laryngeal nerve are similar to those of decompression of the facial nerve, but information as to the exact status of the innervation of the laryngeal muscles is more difficult to obtain. Demonstration of fibrillation potentials in the vocalis muscle by electromyography would be an indication for exploration and decompression of the laryngeal nerve.

Procedure. The procedure may be done under local or general anesthesia. A small horizontal incision is made over the mid-

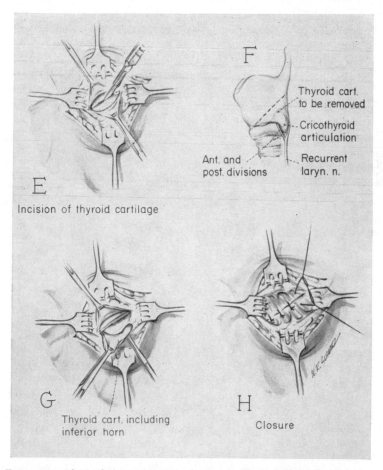

Fig. 34–6. Decompression of the recurrent nerve. *A,* Horizontal skin incision. *B, C, D,* The thyroid perichondrium is divided along the oblique line and elevated inferiorly. *E, F,* The posterior inferior portion of the thyroid ala is divided, the internal perichondrium being preserved. *G,* The inferior cornu is removed by subperichondrial dissection, and the wound is closed.

point of the thyroid ala. The inferior cornu of the thyroid ala is exposed by sharp dissection and the external perichondrium incised as in Figure 34–6. The inferior posterior corner of the thyroid ala, including the cornu, is removed by subperichondral dissection. The recurrent laryngeal nerve should be identified and followed superiorly as far as possible, without trauma, to ensure its integrity and decompression. The wound is closed in layers, with a small Penrose drain in place.

Decompression may result in return of function shortly (within 1 week) after surgery, even when paralysis has been present for 3 months. However, the chances of return diminish greatly when paralysis has been present 6 months or longer. The disadvantage of the procedure is that the fulcrum, around which the cricothyroid muscle functions, is removed, resulting in some loss of tension in the paralyzed cord. However, if recurrent nerve function returns, there is little voice abnormality.

LARYNGEAL PARALYSIS DUE TO MUSCULAR DISEASE

Myotonic Dystrophy (Myotonia Atrophica, Steinert's Disease)

This syndrome involving excessive myotonia and muscular atrophy is a variation of progressive muscular dystrophy. The disease is hereditary and may affect either sex, usually beginning in the first or second decade. In addition to myotonia and muscular wasting, cataracts, frontal baldness, and testicular atrophy occur. Myotonia is present early and is followed by progressive muscular atrophy and weakness. The typical facial and neck involvement produces expressionless facies, severe ptosis, and marked atrophy of the temporalis and sternomastoid muscles.

Involvement of the larynx produces alteration of the voice. The voice is a flat, expressionless monotone which tends to improve as talking continues. Later in the course of the disease when muscular atrophy is marked, the voice becomes weak and breathy. Examination of the larynx early in the disease may not disclose any severe abnormality except after phonation, when there is a delay in the vocal cords' return to the intermediate position for inspiration. As a result, the speech is faltering as well as monotonous. As muscular atrophy progresses, the cords become atrophied and bowed, causing increased air escape and dysphonia. Articulation is also affected, and speech may be difficult to understand.

Treatment. Administration of quinine in doses of 0.3 to 0.6 g every 6 hours will result in improvement during the myotonic phase but is of little value when atrophy is well developed.

Polymyositis and Dermatomyositis

This disease results in a generalized subacute progressive weakness of the striated muscles. If skin lesions are present, the disease is termed dermatomyositis. The disease is insidious in onset and slowly progressive over weeks or months. When the patient is first seen, the muscles of the face, neck, larynx, pharynx, and trunk muscles are usually involved.

Involvement of the pharynx and larynx results in dysphagia, aspiration, choking spells, and dysphonia. Examination of the larynx in the severe stage of the disease may disclose the vocal cords to be in the intermediate position, with the configuration of a combined neural paralysis. The membranous cords are bowed, the arytenoids are tipped anteriorly, and the tips of the vocal processes project into the lumen, producing a keyhole configuration of the glottis.

Diagnosis. The laryngeal symptoms associated with diffuse muscular weakness are suggestive. Laboratory findings include increased creatine urinary excretion and decreased creatinine excretion, elevated transaminases, elevated gamma globulin, and elevated sedimentation rate. The electromyogram and a muscle biopsy will usually confirm the diagnosis.

Treatment. Fatalities are rare, and most patients recover partly or completely. Acetylsalicylic acid and corticosteroids are helpful in the acute phase. If aspiration is a problem, tracheostomy utilizing a cuffed tube may be temporarily necessary.

Polymyositis, as well as occurring idiopathically, may occur with any of the collagen diseases, i.e., scleroderma, lupus erythematosus, rheumatoid arthritis, and rheumatic fever. Approximately 10% of cases are associated with carcinoma, especially in elderly patients. The same laryngeal and pharyngeal symptoms occur in these situations.

Myasthenia Gravis

This disease is characterized by episodic weakness most frequently affecting the facial, ocular, laryngeal, pharyngeal, and respiratory muscles. It is due to failure of transmission of impulses across the neuromyal junction.

Clinical Manifestations. The disease occurs at all ages in both sexes but is most frequent between the ages of 30 and 40. Laryngeal and pharyngeal symptoms of dysphonia, dysphagia, and choking are often the first to appear. Speech is feeble and has a nasal quality. The disease develops over a few weeks, and the first symptoms tend to be episodic, being absent after rest or sleep and worsening with activity and toward nightfall. The voice may seem quite normal, but with continued use it becomes weak and breathy. The same sequence of events affects deglutition.

Because of the weakness of the laryngeal protective mechanisms, these patients are subject to recurrent pulmonary infections. Also, respiratory insufficiency develops abruptly or insidiously due to diaphragmatic and intercostal muscle weakness.

Diagnosis. If the disease is suspected, a therapeutic test using neostigmine intramuscularly or Tensilon intravenously is indicated. When the disease is present, there is a rapid recovery of muscular function if these agents are given.

Examination of the larynx during a period of weakness may show the vocal cords to be immobile or only capable of weak, inadequate movements. Coughing will be ineffective, which will help to differentiate this condition from hysterical paralysis.

Treatment. Myasthenia gravis is subject to exacerbations and remissions; therefore, treatment is divided into the care of acute episodes and long-term maintenance. Anticholinesterase drugs, such as neostigmine, Mestinon (pyridostigmine bromide), or Mytelase (ambenonium chloride), may be used for maintenance or for exacerbations. Tensilon is also useful in severe exacerbations. There are some patients who fail to respond adequately to any therapy.

Severe cases are subject to recurrent respiratory problems, which include pneumonia, secretional obstruction, and respiratory insufficiency. Tracheostomy may be necessary and helpful in many cases. In some situations, a tracheostomy must be permanent, and a valved tube or tracheal fenestration may be used to allow speech. At other times, a severe myasthenic crisis may necessitate respiratory assistance using a respirator, in which case insertion of a cuffed tracheostomy tube will be necessary.

REFERENCES

Arnold, G. E.: Vocal Rehabilitation of Paralytic Dysphonia. III. Present Concepts of Laryngeal Paralysis. Arch. Otolaryng., 65: 317, 1957.

Arnold, G. E.: Vocal Rehabilitation of Paralytic Dysphonia. IV. Paralytic Dysphonia Due to Unilateral Recurrent Nerve Paralysis. Arch. Otolaryng., 68:284, 1958.

Arnold, G. E.: Vocal Rehabilitation of Paralytic Dysphonia. V. Vocal Symptomatology after Bilateral Loss of Abduction. Arch. Otolaryng., 70:444, 1959.

Arnold, G. E.: Vocal Rehabilitation of Paralytic Dysphonia. VII. Paralysis of Superior Laryngeal Nerve. Arch. Otolaryng., 75:549, 1962.

Arnold, G. E.: Vocal Rehabilitation of Paralytic Dysphonia. IX. Technique of Intrachordal Injection. Arch. Otolaryng., 76:358, 1962.

Avellis, G.: Klinische Beitrage zur Lalbseitgen Kehlkopflamungen. Klin. Wochenschr., 40:1, 1891.

Berger, H.: Associated Paralyses of the Vocal Cord. J. Laryngol., 49:1, 1934.

Bernstein, L., and Holt, G. P.: Correction of Vocal Cord Abduction in Unilateral Recurrent Laryngeal Nerve Paralysis by Transposition of the Sternothyroid Muscle. Laryngoscope, 77:876, 1967.

Capps, F. C. W.: The Semon Lecture "Abductor Paralysis" in Theory and Practice Since Semon. J. Laryngol., 72:1, 1958.

Clerf, L. H.: The Surgical Treatment of Bilateral Posticus Paralysis of the Larynx. Laryngoscope, *60*:142, 1950.

Clerf, L. H.: Paralysis of the Larynx of Peripheral Origin. Acta Otolaryng., *43*:108, 1953.

Clerf, L. H.: Unilateral Vocal Cord Paralysis. J.A.M.A., *151*:900, 1955.

Clerf, L. H., and Baltzell, W. H.: Re-evaluation of Semon's Hypothesis. Laryngoscope, *63*:693, 1953.

Cody, C. C., Jr.: Associated Paralyses of the Larynx. Ann. Otol., *55*:549, 1946.

Dedo, H. H., and Ogura, J. H.: Vocal Cord Electromyography in the Dog. Laryngoscope, *75*:201, 1965.

Doyle, P. J., et al.: Results of Surgical Section and Repair of the Recurrent Laryngeal Nerve. Laryngoscope, *77*:1245, 1967.

Evoy, M. H.: Paralysis of the Vocal Cords after Thyroidectomy. Am. J. Surg., *102*:73, 1961.

Faarborg-Anderson, K.: Electromyographic Investigation of Intrinsic Laryngeal Muscles in Humans. Acta Physiol. (Suppl.), *140*:1, 1957.

Faarborg-Anderson, K.: The Position of Paretic Vocal Cords. Acta Otolaryng., *57*: 50, 1964.

Faarborg-Anderson, K.: Unilateral Paralysis of the Superior Laryngeal Nerve. Acta Otolaryng., *57*:155, 1964.

Frazier, C. F.: The Treatment of Nerve Anastomosis of Paralysis of the Recurrent Laryngeal Nerve. Ann. Surg., *79*:161, 1924.

Furstenberg, A. C.: Anatomical and Clinical Study of Central Lesions Producing Paralysis of the Larynx. Ann. Otol., *46*:39, 1937.

Furstenberg, A. C., and Magelski, J. E.: Evidence of Laryngeal Participation in Emotional Expression. Trans. Am. Laryngol. Soc., *79*:60, 1958.

Furstenberg, A. C., and Magelski, J. E.: A Motor Pattern in the Nucleus Ambiguus. Ann. Otol., *64*:788, 1955.

Graham, M. D.: Bilateral Recurrent Laryngeal Nerve Paralysis Associated with Upper Respiratory Infection. J. Laryngol., *76*:535, 1962.

Graham, M. D.: Bilateral Vocal Cord Paralysis Associated with Myelomeningocele and the Arnold-Chiari Malformation. Laryngoscope, *73*:85, 1963.

Gupta, S. K.: The Syndrome of Spontaneous Laryngeal Palsy in Pulmonary Tuberculosis. J. Laryngol., *74*:106, 1960.

Hogan, P. J.: Vocal Cord Paralysis. Ann. Otol., *72*:306, 1963.

Hoover, W. B.: Bilateral Abductor Paralysis. Operative Treatment by Submucous Resection of the Vocal Cords. Arch. Otolaryng., *15*:339, 1932.

Huppler, E. G., et al.: Causes of Vocal Cord Paralysis. Proc. Staff Meet. Mayo Clin., *30*: 518, 1955.

Jeschek, J.: Uber Wechselseitige Funktionsbeziehungen der Kehlkopfmuskulatur. Arch. Ohren. Massenin Kehlkopfh., *163*:372, 1953.

Kamer, F. M., and Som, M. L.: Correction of the Traumatically Abducted Vocal Cord. Arch. Otolaryng., *95*:6, 1972.

Kelly, J. D.: Surgical Treatment of Bilateral Paralysis of the Abductor Muscles. Arch. Otolaryng., *33*:293, 1941.

King, B. T.: New and Function-restoring Operation for Bilateral Abductor Cord Paralysis. J.A.M.A., *112*:814, 1939.

King, B. T., and Gregg, R.: An Anatomical Reason for Various Behaviors of Paralyzed Vocal Cords. Ann. Otol., *57*:925, 1948.

Kirikae, I., et al.: An Experimental Study of Central Motor Innervation of the Laryngeal Muscles in the Cat. Laryngoscope, *71*: 222, 1962.

Koenig, W. F., and von Leden, H.: The Peripheral Nervous System of the Human Larynx. Arch. Otolaryng., *73*:1, 1961.

Koenig, W. F., and von Leden, H.: The Peripheral Nervous System of the Human Larynx. Arch. Otolaryng., *74*:494, 1961.

Kratz, R. C.: The Identification and Protection of the Recurrent Laryngeal Nerve, a New Microsurgical Technique. Laryngoscope, *83*:59, 1973.

Lemere, F.: Innervation of the Larynx. IV. Analysis of Semon's Law. Ann. Otol., *43*: 525, 1934.

Lore, J. M., Jr.: *An Atlas of Head and Neck Surgery*, Vol. 2. Philadelphia, W. B. Saunders Co., 1973, p. 721.

McCall, J. W., and Gardener, F. S.: A Simplified Operation for Bilateral Abductor Paralysis. Laryngoscope, *53*:307, 1943.

Meurman, Y.: Operative Mediofixation of the Vocal Cord in Complete Unilateral Paralysis. Arch. Otolaryng., *55*:544, 1952.

Morrison, L. F.: The "Reverse King Operation." Ann. Otol., *577*:945, 1948.

New, G.: Laryngeal Paralysis Associated with Jugular Foramen Syndrome and Other Syndromes. Am. J. Med. Sci., *165*: 727, 1923.

Ogura, J. H.: Surgical Decompression of the Recurrent Laryngeal Nerve in Idiopathic Unilateral Vocal Cord Paresis. Ann. Otol., *70*: 451, 1961.

Orton, H. B.: Surgical Approach for Arytenoidectomy in Bilateral Abductor Paralysis of the Pharynx. Laryngoscope, 53:709, 1943.

Pearlman, S. J., and Killian, E. W.: Thyrotomy Approach for Arytenoidectomy in Bilateral Abductor Paralysis of the Vocal Cords. Ann. Otol., 63:307, 1953.

Pichler, H., and Gisel, A.: Clinical Significance of Ramification of the Recurrent Laryngeal Nerves. Laryngoscope, 67:105, 1957.

Plotz, M., and Brooks, M. J.: Vocal Cord Paralysis in Heart Disease. Arch. Otolaryng., 54:372, 1951.

Pressman, J. J., and Kelemen, G.: Physiology of the Larynx. Physiol. Rev., 35:506, 1955.

Priest, R. E., et al.: Arytenoidectomy in Children. Ann. Otol., 69:869, 1960.

Réthi, A.: L'innervation du Larynx. Acta Otorinolaryngol. Iber. Am., 13:585, 1962.

Riddell, V. H.: Injury to Recurrent Nerves During Thyroidectomy. Lancet, 2:638, 1956.

Rosenbach, O.: 1st der Satz von der Verschiebeven Vuererabilitatät der Recurrenbasern Berechtigt? Arch. J. Laryngol. u Rhinol., 6:583, 1897.

Ross, D. E., and Chambers, D. C.: Recurrent Laryngeal Nerve Paralysis Occurring in an Infant. Am. J. Surg., 94:513, 1957.

Rullan, A.: Associated Laryngeal Paralysis. Arch. Otolaryng., 64:207, 1956.

Rustad, W.: Recurrent Laryngeal Nerves in Thyroid Surgery. Springfield, Ill., Charles C Thomas, Publisher, 1956.

Semon, F.: On the Position of the Vocal Cords in Quiet Respiration in Man and or the Reflex Tonus of their Abductor Muscles. Proc. R. Soc. London, 48:403, 1890.

Semon, F.: On the Proclivity of Abductor Fibers of the Recurrent Laryngeal Nerve to Become Affected Sooner than the Abductor Fibers. Arch. Laryngol., 2:112, 1965.

Stuart, D. W.: The Otolaryngologic Aspects of Myasthenia Gravis. Laryngoscope, 75:112, 1965.

Svien, H. J., Baker, H. L., and Rivers, M. H.: Jugular Foramen Syndrome and Allied Syndromes. Neurology, 13:797, 1963.

Tschiassny, K.: Therapeutically Induced Paralysis of the Cricothyroid Muscle or Its Removal in Paralytic Laryngeal Stenosis. Arch. Otolaryng., 65:133, 1957.

Thornell, W. C.: Transoral Intralaryngeal Approach for Arytenoidectomy in Bilateral Vocal Cord Paralysis with Inadequate Airway. Ann. Otol., 66:364, 1957.

Vernet, M.: The Classification of Syndromes of Associated Paralysis. J. Laryngol., 33:354, 1918.

Vogel, P. H.: The Innervation of the Larynx in Man and the Dog. Am. J. Anat., 90:427, 1952.

Wagner, R.: Die Medianstellung des Stimmbandes bei Recurrenslahmung. Virchows Arch. Pathol. Anat., 120:437, 1890.

Wicker, J. H., et al.: Long Term Results of Thornell Arytenoidectomy in the Surgical Treatment of Bilateral Vocal Cord Paralysis. Laryngoscope, 82:1331, 1972.

Williams, A. F.: The Nerve Supply of the Laryngeal Muscles. J. Laryngol., 65:343, 1951.

Williams, R. G.: Idiopathic Recurrent Nerve Paralysis. J. Laryngol., 73:161, 1959.

Woodman, D.: Modification of Extralaryngeal Approach to Arytenoidectomy for Bilateral Abductor Paralysis. Arch. Otolaryng., 43:63, 1946.

Work, W. P.: Paralysis and Paresis of Vocal Cords. Statistical Review. Arch. Otolaryng., 34:267, 1941.

Work, W. P.: Unusual Position of the Right Recurrent Laryngeal Nerve. Ann. Otol., 50:769, 1941.

Chapter 35

Tumors of the Larynx and Pharynx

Joseph H. Ogura, Richard Mallen, and Gershon J. Spector

BENIGN TUMORS

The otolaryngologic aspects of benign tumors will be described collectively because of the relative rarity of these tumors when compared to the occurrence of malignant neoplasms in the same areas. They occur in the following order of frequency: papilloma, chondroma, neurofibroma, leiomyoma, angiofibroma, myoma, hemangioma, and chemodectoma. Vocal nodules, cysts, and laryngoceles are not true tumors and will be discussed elsewhere.

The terms "fibroma of the cord," varix, and angioma are often incorrectly applied to lesions of the larynx and are not true neoplasms.

Symptoms and Signs. Hoarseness is by far the commonest complaint when such a tumor is located in the vocal cord. Dyspnea will result if the tumor is large and causes nearly complete obstruction of the glottic airway. A "lump in the throat" usually is a persistent complaint when the tumor is large in size and obstructs the pharyngeal food passage. Cough and hemoptysis result if such a tumor obstructs the airway and is ulcerated.

Diagnosis. In most instances the diagnosis can be made by direct mirror examination. The papillomas appear as single or multiple warty excrescences of the true cord

but may also be located over the supraglottis and less frequently in the infraglottis.

Chondromas appear as a smooth, "firm-appearing," sometimes lobulated surface mass arising from the cricoid or thyroid cartilage.

Myomas are rare, but myoblastomas are more common. These are benign tumors originating over the arytenoid area as red excrescences of the larynx. These should be treated by transoral excision or by a pharyngotomy approach rather than medically.

A myoma appears as a smooth benign mass. The diagnosis is often not made by biopsy, but only after the entire mass is removed transorally (if pedunculated) or by a pharyngotomy approach if it is located deeper in the soft tissues or has a broad base in the larynx or pharynx.

A chemodectoma is a rare tumor having the gross appearance of a cyst of the ventricle or a benign tumor of the false cord or aryepiglottic fold. Essentially it looks like a laryngocele except the laryngograms or planograms show it to be a solid mass. In our cases the diagnosis is made by laryngoscopy, and an exploratory pharyngotomy reveals the true nature of the tumor. The growth is so slow that hoarseness and dyspnea take years to develop. Laryngograms or planograms may lead one to suspect its presence, though such a tumor is rare in

479

adults. The diagnosis may not be made at the time of laryngoscopy because tissue sufficient for diagnosis is difficult to obtain. The diagnosis can only be made at the time of pharyngotomy.

A neurofibroma is a rare tumor arising from the Schwann cells and appears in our experience in the "extrinsic portion" of the larynx. It appears as a smooth mass of the aryepiglottic fold, and diagnosis is difficult unless sufficient material is obtained through a sample of the tumor.

Angiomas appear as simple or cavernous hemangiomas of the pharynx or larynx. The common complaint is bleeding, often severe; generally a biopsy of such a lesion is not indicated. They appear bluish and, when exophytic, as a "bag of blue worms." Because of our experience with profuse bleeding, once the diagnosis is established, excision is best handled by suspension laryngoscopy (if a small angioma) or by lateral pharyngotomy (if a large angioma).

CANCER OF THE LARYNX AND LARYNGOPHARYNX

Introduction. Since the natural histories of cancer of the larynx and laryngopharynx are significantly different and the ultimate outcome for the patient is dependent on the initial therapeutic modality employed, it follows that these patients are best handled by those thoroughly familiar with the accurate assessment of the primary lesion. Cancer of the larynx is a highly curable disease, whereas cancer of the laryngopharynx is less curable because of its aggressive nature. In most instances, the treatment of cancer of the pharynx and larynx should employ therapeutic modes that yield as much physiologic preservation of the organ as possible without compromising cure rates. Today, the idea is no longer valid that treatment is restricted to either x-ray therapy or total laryngectomy.

At present the treatment of cancer of the larynx and pharynx can be divided into three methods. The treatment employed may entail (1) radiotherapy as a curative measure; (2) a primary surgical procedure involving some form of conservation technique or a total laryngectomy; or (3) a combination of preoperative irradiation with either a conservation procedure or a total laryngectomy.

A great deal of new information has been obtained during the past decade by a concentrated study of cancers arising from the pharynx and larynx. Because of certain anatomic, physiologic, and pathologic information obtained from this study, a change of modality of therapy has taken place called conservation surgery. There is a better understanding of the physiology of deglutition and of the latitude of compensation and adaptation in humans with this type of surgery. The continued improvements in surgical technique for restricted tumors in the pharynx and larynx have led to further application of the technique in situations previously considered only to be treated adequately by total laryngectomy.

Five factors have accounted for this change in approach.

1. The addition of routine neck dissection for cancers of the pharynx and certain forms of cancer of the larynx has yielded improved cure rates, compared to those of total laryngectomy and watchful waiting for possible neck nodes.

2. A review of the pathologic material from a homogeneous series of cases treated in one manner has allowed a study of the relationships between nodal metastases and primary lesions.

3. The development of the laryngogram has provided a critical diagnostic tool for separating lesions into various zones, which can then be handled differently.

4. Cure rates in patients on whom conservation of function surgery was performed are as good as those in patients with the same lesion previously treated by total laryngectomy.

5. Present-day improved radiotherapeutic techniques have yielded good results for certain tumors, and the value of radiotherapy as a planned preoperative therapeutic measure, combined with radical surgery, has been reflected in the decreased early failure rate.

Etiology. Some of the factors that have been stated to cause laryngeal cancer are (1) smoking, (2) leukoplakia, (3) alcohol, (4) chronic infection of the upper and lower respiratory tract, (5) dietary deficiencies, (6) air pollution, and (7) viruses. Whether these same causal factors operate for hypopharyngeal cancers is less certain. A discussion of the immunologic aspects of cancer of the head and neck occurs in Chapter 38.

One fact is apparent from studies made by the Public Health Service of morbidity of cancer of the larynx and lung. Between 1930 and 1950, mortality from cancer of the larynx increased only 20% over the previous 20 years, whereas the corresponding rate for cancer of the lung increased 420%. Taking into account a population increase and the fact that nearly one half of the population smokes, if the most important factor was smoke, then its passage to the lung should affect the larynx as well. There is, however, no such increased incidence of cancer of the larynx. Since smoking occupies such a prominent position in the etiology of cancer, one might question this from several aspects. Why is it that cancer of the upper esophagus, previously more common in females, now is more common in males? Certainly more women smoke today, yet if tobacco is indeed an important factor, it should apply to the females also. Tobacco as a factor for gastric cancer is not so important. Its incidence has fallen markedly.

Why is it that tobacco deposits, which accumulate notoriously in the vestibule proper of the nose, are associated with so strikingly low an incidence of cancer in man? Even if the role of the thickened mucous membrane is considered, what about the delicate ciliated respiratory mucosa immediately posterior to this? The incidence of nasal fossa cancer is indeed low and not increasing. Tobacco can only be incriminated as a possible contributing factor, but to state that it is a primary etiologic cause from statistical evidence alone is another matter.

Leukoplakia or hyperkeratosis has been said to be a precancerous state in the larynx. Clerf, Grossman, Jackson, Putney, and O'Keefe have all stated that, at least for carcinoma of the true cords, this lesion eventually leads to cancer in a significant percentage of cases. No one knows the reasons for the development of isolated ker-

atosis, but it is not infrequently associated with invasive cancer at its advancing margin. One cannot assume that keratosis in this instance leads to the development of cancer. Reasonable certainty of some causal relation is evident if, after a time lapse of 6 months or longer, a cancer appears in or from a previously proven isolated keratosis stripping. With this in mind, McGavran, Bauer, and Ogura reviewed 87 successively proven isolated keratoses from the true vocal cord and found that the incidence of cancer was 3.4%, a remarkably low incidence.

Wynder felt that alcohol consumption "increased" the risk of pharyngeal cancer. Actually, one could conclude from his article that alcohol is as important as tobacco consumption. Dietary restrictions with increased alcohol intake appear to be important.

Air pollution has also been said to be a factor. "Smog" or combustion products of gasoline, oil, gas, or coal or other air pollutants are said to have adverse effects on health and are suspected of causing lung cancer.

Heller has proposed a virus as a cause of cancer. His ideas did not specifically relate to laryngeal cancer but to cancer in general: (1) a virus may entwine itself in the normal cell's genetic mechanism and so modify it that the cell begins to reproduce abnormally; (2) a virus may enter a cell, attach itself to some of the cell's genes, and transport them to a second cell, again causing an abnormal malignant change; (3) a dormant virus hidden within a cell may be activated by some external agent, such as x-rays, and thus start the malignant growth.

It is evident that among the many suggested causes for laryngeal and pharyngeal cancer, several factors can be considered, but there appear to be many discrepancies in laryngeal and pharyngeal cancer as compared to lung cancer. The flat incidence of cancers in these areas over several decades, the rarity of tracheal cancers, and the failure to induce cancers with realistic amounts of tobacco condensates are enigmas. At best, tobacco can be considered only a contributing factor in the etiology of cancer of the larynx and pharynx.

Pathology. Ninety-five percent of cancers of the larynx and pharynx are of the squamous cell variety. The incidence of nodal metastases from such a lesion varies according to the primary site. Thus, classification as to site and extent is important before any clinical characteristics of the laryngeal or pharyngeal lesion are anticipated and prognosis given.

Lesions of the pharynx and larynx are separated according to specific anatomic zones (Fig. 35–1). Tumors that involve marginal structures, such as the aryepiglottic fold, are classified as residing in the pharynx (piriform sinus) rather than the larynx.

In squamous cell carcinoma of the larynx there is a progressive increase in metastatic rate in glottic, infraglottic, supraglottic, and transglottic disease of 0, 20, 33, and 52%, respectively. The metastatic rate, therefore, of the transglottic group represents the addition of the infraglottic and supraglottic groups, confirming the expected results derived from the theoretical considerations of the lymphatic drainage of the larynx. The transglottic group yields a higher incidence of clinically apparent and inapparent metastases. The metastatic rates of the inapparent metastases (derived from elective neck dissection) are as follows: glottic, 0%; infraglottic, 20%; supraglottic, 12%; and transglottic, 31%. All of the metastases of the infraglottic cancers were of the nonpalpable type. Supraglottic and infraglottic cancers, of moderate or poor differentiation, larger than 2 cm provide a high incidence of metastases. A low yield of metastasis in these two locations is found, however, if the lesion is well differentiated or of 2 cm or less in size, regardless of the differentiation. Thus size is important in determining the metastatic incidence and is a determining factor in deciding on the neck dissection. In 23 patients with supraglottic or transglottic cancer, of those who had cervical metastases initially, 11 (48%) developed positive nodes on the contralateral side in the follow-up period. Consideration should be given to bilateral neck dissection (one- or two-stage) when ipsilateral palpable nodes are present initially with a lesion that is over 2 cm in diameter. This same concept also applies to pharyngeal tumors. The majority of supraglottic tumors appear to be "pushing" rather than infiltrating in type.

Thus, the majority of tumors can be separated into low or high metastatic grades by using preoperative information about the

CLASSIFICATION

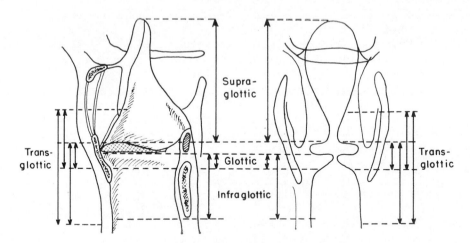

FIG. 35–1.   Classification of cancer of the larynx.

Supraglottic—from tip of epiglottis, free border of epiglottis, including false cords.
Glottic—floor of ventricle, cord to 1 cm infraglottic from free margins.
Infraglottic—to lower border cricoid cartilage.
Transglottic—lesions that cross the ventricle or involve larynx above and below cords.

site, size, biopsy differentiation, and clinical evaluation of the cervical lymph nodes.

Pharyngeal Tumors. Tumors which are on the lingual surface of the epiglottis and invade the vallecula are biologically more aggressive and should be considered superior hypopharyngeal in origin. Likewise, tumors which, although present on the epiglottis, involve the aryepiglottic fold or extend into the piriform fossa should be classified according to the region of higher metastatic incidence. Thus these lesions are considered with the primary pharyngeal tumors. Primary lesions of the aryepiglottic fold or of the arytenoid are considered with the piriform fossa tumors. Tumors which extend behind the arytenoid on the postcricoid surface or in the piriform fossa and extend into the postcricoid area are classified with postcricoid tumors.

The piriform fossa, base of the tongue, and posterior wall of the pharynx are known for their high incidence of cervical metastases. Pharyngeal cancers metastasize in the order of 50 to 90%. Fifty-five percent of tumors of the base of the tongue metastasize, and 90% of those of the piriform fossa metastasize. The larger the size of the tumor, the more probable that metastases are present. Furthermore, by examining the margins of these resected tumors and by follow-up, one frequently can find a second cancer. An important factor in this high incidence of metastasis in pharyngeal cancer is the frequent finding of precancerous epithelium adjacent to the resected specimens. The majority of these tumors are infiltrating in type and only infrequently pushing.

CLASSIFICATION OF LARYNX AND LARYNGOPHARYNX CANCERS

Glottic

Glottic cancer refers to a tumor which is on the cord. It usually begins on the superior surface of the true cord but may extend from the anterior commissure to and including the vocal process. The lower limits of a glottic lesion are 1 cm from the free margin, the superior margin, and the floor of the ventricle. One centimeter represents the lower border of the intrinsic muscles of the vocal cords. Thus, a glottic tumor may be unilateral or bilateral and may extend infraglottically for a distance of 1 cm (Fig. 35–1).

Infraglottic

Infraglottic cancer refers to a tumor which extends to the lower border of the cricoid. When initially seen, the tumor may extend to the undersurface of the true cord and in general is always more than 1 cm in size.

Supraglottic

Supraglottic cancer refers to a tumor which is confined to a zone from the false cord up to the tip of the epiglottis; the margin of the aryepiglottic fold is spared, however. The aryepiglottic fold, which begins on the lateral midsurface of the epiglottis, can be defined as that portion which leaves the cartilaginous surface of the epiglottis and fuses the arytenoid eminence (Fig. 35–2).

Transglottic

Transglottic tumors are those which cross or involve the ventricle. Thus the tumor can

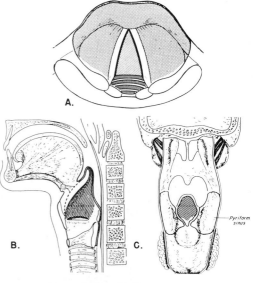

FIG. 35–2. Supraglottic cancer. *A*, Indirect laryngoscopy. *B*, Lateral view. *C*, Posterior view.

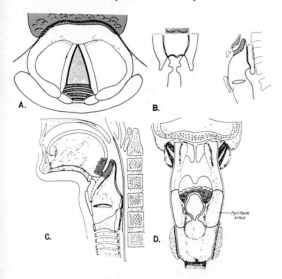

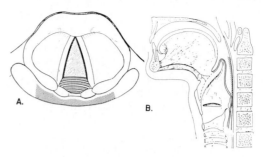

FIG. 35–4. Posterior hypopharyngeal cancer. *A*, Indirect laryngoscopy. *B*, Lateral view.

FIG. 35–3. Superior hypopharyngeal cancer ("base of tongue"). *A*, Indirect laryngoscopy. *B*, Laryngogram. *C*, Lateral view. *D*, Posterior view.

be a glottic cancer which has involved the false cords or a false cord tumor that has crossed the ventricle and involved the true cords. In addition, a tumor which extends subglottically from the level of the cord and crosses the ventricle is a transglottic tumor. The rare primary ventricle tumor is included in this group.

Pharyngeal tumors are divided as follows: *Superior hypopharyngeal* is the anatomic zone (Fig. 35–3) composed of the lingual surface of the epiglottis, vallecula, and "base of the tongue." It includes the lateral glossoepiglottic folds and is confined to an area inferior to the V-ring of the circumvallate papillae of the tongue. This actually is the true superior margin of the base of the tongue. Tumors suitable for this "extended supraglottic subtotal laryngectomy procedure" should not extend to the superior margin of this anatomic zone of the base of the tongue.

Posterior pharyngeal wall tumors (Fig. 35–4) are those in the zone between a posterior projected line from the superior margin of the base of the tongue to the level of the arytenoids and medial to each lateral wall of the piriform sinus. Tumors in this area are rare, and they often involve the

glossoepiglottic fold. Their metastatic behavior pattern is similar to that of the superior hypopharynx tumors, and they are included in this classification for statistical consideration.

Piriform sinus or hypopharyngeal cancers (Fig. 35–5) are defined as those tumors confined to a zone bounded superiorly by the glossoepiglottic fold, inferiorly by the arytenoid and apex of the piriform sinus, laterally by the thyroid cartilage, and medially by the aryepiglottic fold and anterior piriform sinus wall. The medial border of the piriform sinus is lateral to the free border of the epiglottis. Posteriorly, the landmark is an ill-defined vertical line at the level of the arytenoid cartilage which divides

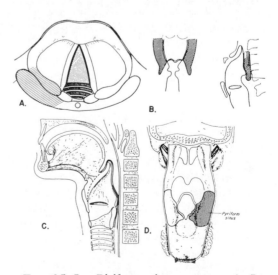

FIG. 35–5. Piriform sinus cancer. *A*, Indirect laryngoscopy. *B*, Laryngogram. *C*, Lateral view. *D*, Posterior view.

the piriform sinus from the posterior pharyngeal wall lesions. Arbitrarily the position of the arytenoid cartilage at midabduction is selected for this vertical line. Since the aryepiglottic fold is the medial wall of the piriform sinus, tumors involving this structure are grouped with the piriform sinus neoplasms.

Tumors which are on the lingual surface of the epiglottis and invade the vallecula are biologically more aggressive and should be considered pharyngeal in origin. Likewise, tumors which, although present on the epiglottis, also involve the aryepiglottic fold or extend into the piriform fossa should be classified according to the region of higher metastatic incidence. Thus, these lesions are considered with the primary pharyngeal tumors.

Tumors which extend behind the arytenoid on the postcricoid surface or which appear in the piriform fossa and extend into the postcricoid area are treated as postcricoid tumors.

SYMPTOMATOLOGY

Hoarseness. The voice may be gravelly; it may change to a lower coarse volume and on to one of near aphonia. This is common with glottic, transglottic, and large exophytic supraglottic tumors that pedunculate into the glottic chink; it is also common with a large infraglottic lesion that infiltrates the glottic margin and a piriform fossa lesion that fixes the arytenoid in the lateral abducted position.

The voice can best be described as a "hot potato" voice when there is a bulky lesion of the epiglottis, superior hypopharynx, or piriform sinus. The quality of the voice and speech may be entirely normal when smaller lesions in any of these locations are present.

Airway Obstruction. Respiratory stridor can result from any of the lesions described if they are of sufficient size to result in luminal encroachment of the airway. Usually involvement of one arytenoid or cord due to fixation and partial paresis or a bilateral position of the lesion above and below the glottis narrows the chink greatly and causes airway obstruction.

Sore Throat. A vague or real complaint of persistent sore throat with tumors of the described areas is associated almost exclusively with tumors of the pharyngeal region, i.e., piriform sinus, aryepiglottis, and base of the tongue. Occasionally this complaint is related to a lesion of the epiglottis. Commonly, the local physician prescribes antibiotics for a period of time before seeking consultation.

Diet and Deglutition. A change can be made in the usual beverages enjoyed by the patient, e.g., warm beer instead of ice cold beer. A pain in the throat on swallowing, a burning sensation, and the feeling of a lump in the throat can all be easily confused with psychoneurosis.

When obvious obstructive complaints develop, at first just with solids, then with liquids, the bulkiness of the tumor is quite apparent to any physician.

Referred Pain. Malignant tumors of the piriform fossa, aryepiglottic fold, and vallecula or any tumor of the larynx with or without cartilage destruction can refer pain to one ear. This is true even when there are no palpable nodes.

Silent Primary Focus. The primary lesion may be located in certain areas without giving rise to symptoms. These areas include the base of the tongue, the piriform fossa, the entire epiglottic area, and the false cords. This is also true of the nasopharynx, which is not discussed in this chapter.

DIAGNOSTIC PROCEDURES

A careful indirect examination of the hypopharynx and larynx is the most important step in diagnosis and evaluation.

Description should include a freehand drawing of the lesion on a previously prepared drawing of the hypopharynx and larynx. The tumor description should include the following: size and extent, margins (distance from vocal cord), topography (ulceration or exophytic), margins about the tumor that appear or feel indurated (palpation or direct examination), fixation of cords.

Further aids in the diagnosis are the presence or absence of nodes, their location, and their number if positive. Some mention should be made about the size and degree of fixation. Palpation of the tongue is an extremely important aid in disclosing a lesion at the base of the tongue and also in evaluating the extent of the tumor when it cannot be directly visualized.

Laryngograms are of definite diagnostic importance. The patient is prepared by topical anesthesia in a manner similar to preparation for laryngoscopy or bronchoscopy. Previous arrangements are made with the radiologist. Aqueous Dionasil is dripped into the hypopharynx under fluoroscopic examination, and the following spot films are taken: inspiration, phonation, Valsalva, and expiration. PA and lateral views are made in all instances. (Most radiologists will need the operative specimens to acquaint themselves with the varying shadows of the complicated folds of the larynx and the various respiratory positions of each structure.)

Biopsy by direct laryngoscopy is essential. However, it should be deferred until after laryngographic examination.

Open biopsy of an enlarged positive node is to be avoided. Incisional biopsy can complicate the surgical management of that case. It is better to leave the direct biopsy and management of the neck to the otolaryngologist best equipped to handle the case.

A word should be said about patient referral with or without an accompanying slide biopsy. If the clinical findings do not match the biopsy, the original diagnosis should be questioned and another biopsy of the primary lesion should be considered, particularly if the first slides are questionable. Tragedies have occurred when a slide diagnosis by a pathologist is accepted without question. Generally, overinterpretation of the presence of cancer on the original slide commits the surgeon to unnecessarily radical surgery.

INDICATIONS FOR SURGERY OR RADIATION

Once the diagnosis of infiltrating cancer is made, a decision as to treatment should be made in close consultation with the referring physician and radiotherapist. Noth-ing is worse for the patient with a large aggressive cancer than for the physician to treat it with irradiation and wait for recrudescence before referral for a surgical procedure.

Those cancers of the larynx curable by irradiation alone are small, restricted lesions of the membranous portion of the vocal cord, and possibly a small lesion of the epiglottis. These are the only lesions for which full therapeutic irradiation should be considered. All other lesions of the larynx, whether treated by a conservation or radical surgical procedure, should have planned, low-dose, preoperative irradiation employed when deemed advisable. This group consists of transglottic and infraglottic lesions in which stomal recurrences are likely. Preoperative irradiation may reduce this incidence significantly. Selected supraglottic lesions with palpable nodes or those close to the glottis are given low-dose irradiation.

Preoperative irradiation is given for all hypopharyngeal cancers because of the low cure rate. Local persistence and lateral neck recurrence are common causes of failure in the nonirradiated surgical group. This mode of therapy is employed whether the biopsy is well-differentiated or anaplastic.

Table 35–1 lists recommendations for therapy in relation to the primary lesion.

SURGICAL TREATMENT

Surgical treatment depends entirely upon an exact localization of the primary lesion, extent of disease, and knowledge of the behavior of such tumors in their primary locations. Two factors are critical in determining operability for conservation surgery: absence of cartilage destruction, and minimum requirement for a functioning simplified larynx. The pathologist and radiotherapist are necessary in the surgical team.

Two types of treatment are still used throughout the world: total laryngectomy and full irradiation irrespective of location of the cancer. Conservation surgery is successful if the surgeon is cognizant of the fact that in selected cases, subtotal removal is just as successful as radical surgery (Fig. 35–6) (see Table 35–1).

Table 35-1

Irradiation

Cancer of the mobile true vocal cord or bilateral superficial carcinoma.

Hemilaryngectomy or frontolateral hemilaryngectomy

1. Cancer of the vocal cord which extends to the vocal process.
2. Cancer of one true cord with extension across anterior commissure.
3. Cancer of the vocal cord which extends 5 mm subglottic.
4. Irradiation persistence of cancer of one cord.

Anterior commissure removal and McNaught Keel

1. Cancer of anterior commissure.

Laryngectomy without neck dissection

1. Cancer of the glottis with fixation of cords.
2. Cancer of the glottis with fixation and "infraglottic extension" (more than 1 cm).
3. Cancer of both true vocal cords.
4. Persistent tumor of the true vocal cord following irradiation and without nodal metastases.
5. Persistent cancer of larynx following full irradiation.

Laryngectomy and neck dissection

1. Cancer of true cord with fixation and palpable nodes.
2. Infraglottic cancer with or without palpable nodes.
3. Supraglottic cancer with extension to the anterior commissure with or without palpable nodes. Neck dissection necessary if nodes are palpable or lesion is larger than 2 cm.
4. Transglottic cancer with or without palpable nodes.
5. Cancer of the piriform sinus with fixation of cord and invasion of endolarynx with or without palpable nodes.
6. Irradiation persistence of cancer of the larynx and pharynx with palpable nodes.

Subtotal supraglottic laryngectomy

1. Epiglottic cancer, tip or free portion (supraglottic). Neck dissection necessary if nodes are palpable.
2. Epiglottic cancer, inferior vestibule, petiole to false cord. Neck dissection with or without palpable nodes.
3. Cancer of lingual epiglottis and base of tongue (superior hypopharyngeal). Neck dissection necessary in all instances.
4. Irradiation persistence if restricted to epiglottis.

Subtotal laryngopharyngectomy

1. Cancer of piriform sinus.
   a. Lateral wall
   b. Lateral and posterior walls
   c. Lateral and medial walls
   d. Lateral and anterior walls
   e. Arytenoid and aryepiglottic fold
   Cords must be mobile. Edema of arytenoid is not a contraindication. There must be no destruction of thyroid cartilage by x-ray examination. Neck dissection necessary in all instances.
2. Cancer of posterior pharyngeal wall with questionable or no esophageal extension. Neck dissection necessary in all instances, except when lesion is very small, when there would be a question concerning the need for neck dissection.
3. Irradiation persistence restricted to above sites.

Extended laryngectomy, pharyngectomy, and partial esophagectomy

1. Annular cancer of cricopharyngeus.
2. Cancer of piriform sinus that extends into the esophagus. Skin graft or laryngotracheal autograft of unilateral or bilateral pedicle flaps. Neck dissection in all instances.

Combined radiotherapy and surgery

Used for tumors listed under *Laryngectomy and neck dissection, Subtotal supraglottic laryngectomy,* and *Subtotal laryngogpharyngectomy.*

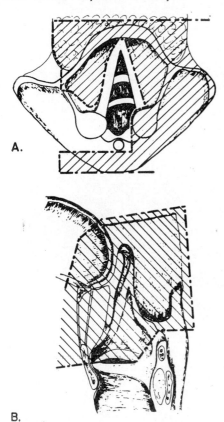

A.

B.

FIG. 35–6. Conservation surgery area of resection. *A,* Indirect laryngoscopy. *B,* Lateral view.

Glottic Lesions

Cordal lesions, because of their sparse lymphatics, rarely metastasize to the cervical lymphatics and usually remain confined to the true cord for a long time. Consequently they behave like cutaneous lesions, and the cure rate by radiotherapy is good for these glottic Stage I tumors. With careful follow-up, salvage of the irradiation failures is possible in half of the cases by hemilaryngectomy and in the remainder by total laryngectomy. While there is little doubt that a small lesion can be cured to nearly the same degree by a hemilaryngectomy, a better functional result is obtained by irradiation. Thus, there should be no question that bilateral superficial cancers of the cord are better treated by irradiation.

These data should not be interpreted to mean that all larynx cases should be treated

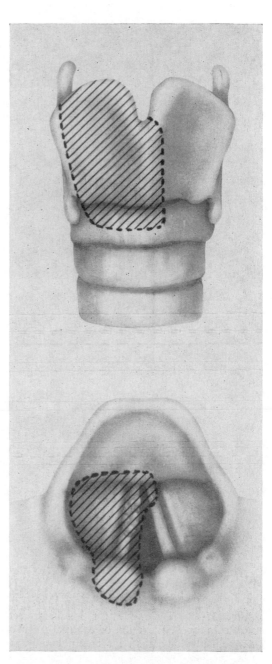

FIG. 35–7. Area of resection in hemilaryngectomy. Part of the anterior cricoid may be removed, but not in its entirety. The vertical cartilage cut is 2 to 3 mm off the midline, depending on how much of the opposite cord one wishes to remove.

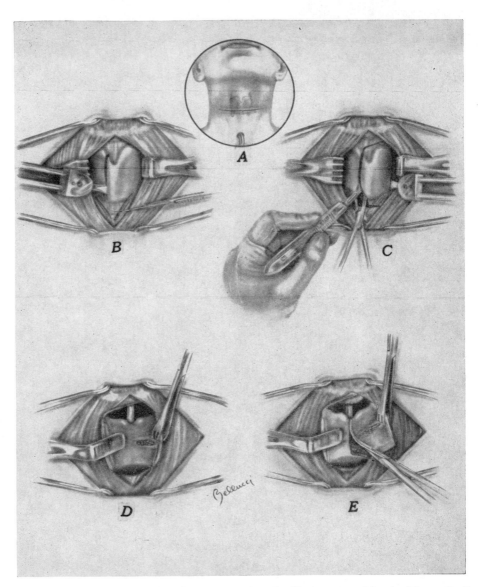

FIG. 35–8. Technique for hemilaryngectomy. *A,* Transverse skin incision. Preliminary tracheostomy. *B,* Elevation of external perichondrium; vertical cut in thyroid cartilage 2 mm off midline and along posterior lateral border. *C,* Transverse cut low on cricothyroid membrane (may include strip of cricoid). A large Kelly clamp is inserted to separate cords, and a vertical cut is made wih a No. 15 BD knife. *D,* Army-navy retractor is inserted, and thyroid cartilage is grasped with tenaculum. *E,* Cut is made along cricoid cartilage, and arytenoid is removed with fine 90-degree curved scissors. All or part of the arytenoid may be cut with this maneuver.

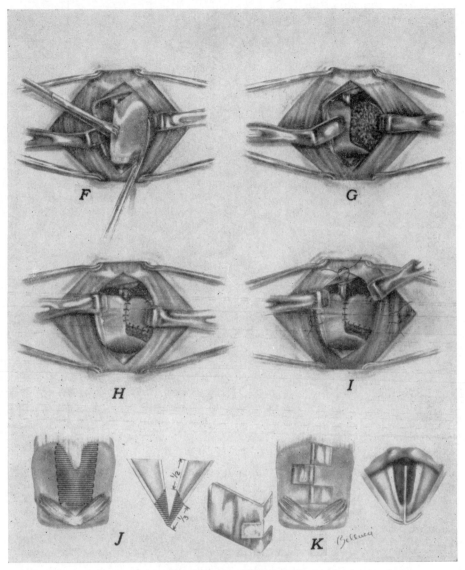

FIG. 35–8.   (Continued)

F, Cut long thyroid cartilage along posterior lateral saw cut. *G*, Raw surface left by hemilaryn-gectomy. *H*, The posterior aryepiglottic fold mucosa thinned and trimmed into larynx to reline interior. *I*, Mucosa sewed to interior and excess mucosa pulled laterally. Anterior commissure of remaining cord lengthened. *J*, Technique for anterior commissure resection. Cartilage cuts are made 3 to 4 mm to each side of midline. *K*, A tantalum McNaught Keel inserted.

by irradiation and recurrence treated expectantly by surgery. For the large lesions of the larynx treated by this method, there is usually a decreased possibility for obtaining as good a cure rate and sparing function.

An ideal candidate for curative irradiation is as follows: over 50 years of age, male or female, with a superficial tumor restricted to the middle third of the true vocal cord. If the tumor is extremely small and an accidental biopsy report of carcinoma in situ is reported, one may elect to follow the patient closely. Considerable thought should be given before using curative radiation. The evolution of carcinoma in situ to invasive carcinoma follows an unknown course.

A glottic lesion less favorable for irradiation therapy and considered a candidate for surgery is characterized by the following: invasion of anterior commissure, subglottic extension more than 5 mm, and vocal process invasion. While these cases can be treated by full irradiation, the study of our failures treated by irradiation indicates that these are the types that are prone to recur. It is for this reason that a hemilaryngectomy is the procedure of choice.

Frontolateral Hemilaryngectomy

(Figs. 35–7 and 35–8)

The choice between frontolateral hemilaryngectomy and total laryngectomy depends upon the experience of the surgeon. The techniques include laryngofissure, hemilaryngectomy, frontolateral hemilaryngectomy, and anterior commissure resection with McNaught Keel. For small, superficial, restricted lesions, a laryngofissure undoubtedly will be successful, but as a general principle, the widest conservation excision with good function is preferred.

Surgical variations of the hemilaryngectomy approach are as follows: the structures that may be removed are the entire arytenoid, one third of the opposite cord, and a partial section of the cricoid cartilage; in the event that more than one third of the remaining cord is removed together with the commissure, the opposite arytenoid should not be removed, and a McNaught Keel must be used (Figs. 35–7 and 35–8).

Total Laryngectomy and Radical Neck Dissection

The concept of en bloc excision of the larynx and the lateral cervical lymphatics is not new, particularly when the primary larynx lesion is large, when no possibility of sparing function exists and palpable nodes are present in the neck. Open biopsy of such nodes prior to radical surgery is not just contraindicated but emphatically discouraged. The value of elective neck dissection is firmly established by improved survival rates (see Results); this procedure should be considered in addition to the treatment of each primary site. Neck dissection is indicated in addition to treatment of the primary lesion in the following cases:

1. Cancer of true cord with fixation and palpable nodes.
2. Subglottic cancer with or without palpable nodes.
3. Supraglottic cancer with extension to the anterior commissure with or without palpable nodes.
4. Transglottic cancer with or without palpable nodes.
5. Cancer of the piriform sinus with fixation of the cord and invasion of the endolarynx with or without palpable nodes.
6. Irradiation persistence of cancer of the larynx or pharynx with palpable nodes.
7. All cancers of the vallecula and epiglottis with any of the above.

Technique. A hockey-stick incision is used (Fig. 35–9). The vertical arm extends from the tip of the mastoid along the posterior border of the sternomastoid, and the horizontal arm extends across the midline 1 inch above the space of Burns to the lateral border of the opposite sternomastoid muscle. A short transverse incision is made into the posterior triangle for better exposure.

Since the tracheostomy is performed under local anesthesia, only a short transverse skin incision is done until the tracheotomy is performed, and the remainder of the skin incision is delayed until general anesthesia is started (Fig. 35–10).

Traction of the specimen at all times is most important to facilitate exposure. Using sharp dissection the sternal and clavicular

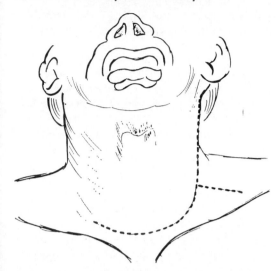

FIG. 35–9.   Incision for laryngectomy and neck dissection.

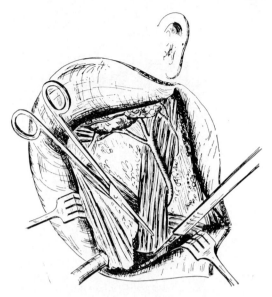

FIG. 35–11. Sternocleidomastoid muscles are sectioned from the clavicle, and dissection is carried into posterior triangle.

heads of the sternocleidomastoid muscle are divided from the clavicle (Fig. 35–11). Dissection is carried out laterally along the clavicle until the anterior border of the trapezius is reached. The large external jugular vein is divided, ligated, and transfixed. Dissection is carried deep until the omohyoid muscle is reached, and it is divided.

The internal jugular vein is isolated, divided, tied, and transfixed (Fig. 35–12). The upper proximal divided vein is sutured. At this point it is easier to complete the transverse section of the lateral strap muscles and to isolate, divide, and suture the inferior thyroid artery. One can separate one inferior pole of the thyroid gland from the trachea and leave it attached to the larynx. Dissection of muscles and fat is carried posteriorly until the prevertebral fascia is reached and the phrenic nerve identified. The transverse scapular artery inferiorly and the superficial cervical artery are seen to cross the phrenic nerve before the phrenic nerve is isolated. As dissection is carried laterally into the posterior triangle, the brachial plexus must be identified. Occasionally the brachial plexus has a more anterior course rather than its usual position posteriorly and can be traumatized.

In the posterior triangle, the fat is dissected upward from the deep pocket along the trapezius muscle, and dissection is carried superiorly along the trapezius and anterior to the prevertebral fascia. No attempt should be made to save the spinal accessory nerve. Great care must be taken not to injure the phrenic nerve. This can occur by

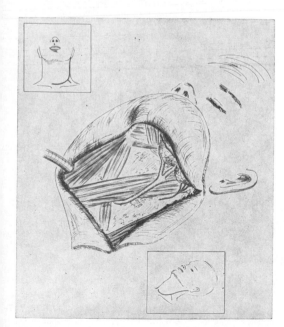

FIG. 35–10.   A hockey-stick incision is made, elevating platysma with skin.

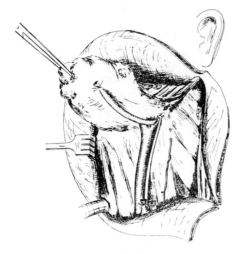

FIG. 35–12. Internal jugular vein isolated, tied, and sutured and dissection carried up along trapezius muscle to bifurcation of carotid artery.

grasping the nerve with forceps or hemostat or in dividing across C4 and C3. Dissection can be carried upward along the carotid artery as far as the bifurcation, the superior thyroid artery being ligated, and then laterally into the neck to the trapezius and mastoid areas.

At this point, unless there are palpable nodes close to the mandibular branch of the facial nerve, this nerve branch should be preserved. The skin flap is raised until the angle of the mandible is reached. The skin flap should be elevated with the platysma muscle. If one is deep to the platysma, it is easier to find this nerve. There are two anatomic zones between which the mandibular branch is found. One zone is from a point over the inferior border of the submaxillary gland to an area where the posterior facial vein enters the parotid gland. The mandibular branch may dip 1 inch below the angle of the mandible lateral to the submaxillary gland in an arc toward the lower lip. The nerve dips over the external facial artery as it traverses across the mandible.

The nerve can be identified by gently pinching it with a forceps. However, if it is pinched more than once, it often fails to respond at any point proximal to this site. The mandibular branch of the facial nerve

is reflected up to the angle of the mandible. The assistant must be repeatedly advised not to place the rake retractor over this nerve. It is easy to avulse the nerve by this maneuver.

The sternomastoid muscle is separated from the mastoid process, and the digastric is likewise severed. The tail of the parotid is divided and carried toward the angle of the mandible, the previously isolated mandibular branch of the facial nerve with the posterior facial vein, which has been reflected superiorly, being noted. Sharp dissection is carried toward the base of the skull and then toward the carotid artery. In this manner the hypoglossal nerve is identified. Superior dissection should be carried as high as possible; this is assisted by the use of deep Richardson retractors and downward traction of the specimen.

The internal jugular vein is isolated and divided, and both ends are sutured and transfixed (Figs. 35–13 and 35–14). The structures lateral and superior to the hypo-

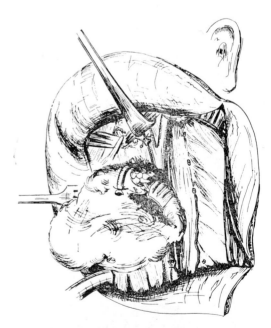

FIG. 35–13. Dissection carried to mastoid; jugular vein isolated, tied, and sutured at upper neck under posterior belly of digastric. Submaxillary gland isolated, and submental space cleared out after mandibular branch of facial nerve is isolated. Usually neck dissection specimen is left attached to thyrohyoid area.

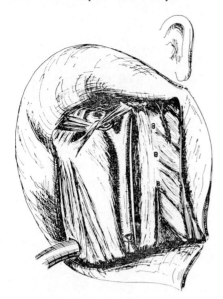

Fig. 35–14.   Completed neck dissection, if no
laryngectomy is done.

glossal nerve are next separated to the point
where it enters the tongue. En route, numerous arteries and veins are ligated. Next,
dissection is carried toward the submaxillary gland, with ligation of the facial artery
and vein at the mandible. The submaxillary
duct is ligated and sutured. The submental
triangle is cleared by dividing the anterior
belly of the digastric muscle close to the
mandible. Dissection of the specimen is carried toward the body of the hyoid bone.

The neck dissection has been completed
except for its attachment to the side of the
larynx.

The trachea is divided transversely beneath the first ring, and this ring is grasped
with a tenaculum. The infraglottis area is
blocked with a large tonsil sponge. The lobe
of the thyroid in the side of the neck dissection is isolated up to the first tracheal ring
and thyroid cartilage by ligating the inferior
thyroid artery. Dissection posterior to the
cricoid is carried upward to the region of
the arytenoid.

The larynx is separated from the contralateral neck structures on the side opposite
the tumor by dissecting along the anterior
border of the sternocleidomastoid muscle
toward the posterior border of the thyroid

cartilage. In so doing the omohyoid muscle
is divided, and the superior thyroid artery
and vein may be ligated, provided the inferior thyroid artery is not disturbed and this
lateral lobe of the thyroid is allowed to remain. The greater cornu of the thyroid cartilage is isolated, separated from its subperichondral bed, and clipped close to the
body of the thyroid cartilage. This demar-
cates the area of the piriform sinus for entrance to the pharynx.

The hyoid bone is grasped with a tenaculum, and the suprahyoid muscle is separated from the lesser cornu to the greater
cornu in the uninvolved side. The greater
cornu is separated from the subperiosteal
bed. Dissection is carried down to the mucous membrane, but not into the vallecula.
In the event the tumor is within the larynx,
the greater cornu of the hyoid on the involved side may be isolated and freed from
its subperichondral bed. This step is not performed when the tumor invades the laryngopharynx.

The cricopharyngeus and inferior constrictor muscles are severed along the posterior border of the thyroid cartilage on the
uninvolved side.

The pharynx is entered at the piriform
sinus, then posterior to the arytenoid. In so
entering the pharynx, the epiglottis is
grasped with a tenaculum to better outline
the vallecula. With sharp dissection the constrictors are divided away from the posterior border of the thyroid cartilage together
with the neck dissection.

By so rotating the neck dissection and
larynx upward, constant suction is maintained in the pharynx to keep blood and
secretion free from the neck wound. At the
same time the landmark of the posterior
thyroid cartilage and hyoid will mound up
with the pharynx. This can be sharply divided and then a cut made across the vallecula until the specimen is freed. In the zeal
of final removal of the specimen, great care
must be taken not to injure the carotid artery.

The pharynx is closed with a running
single line suture of 000 chromic Dulox and
reinforced with two layers of interrupted
silk. A nasogastric feeding tube should be
in place. The constrictor muscle is then im-

bricated, and the skin is approximated with interrupted silk sutures.

LARYNGECTOMY WITHOUT NECK DISSECTION

Five clinical situations are possible in which only total laryngectomy is indicated. These are: (1) cancer restricted to one cord with fixation when the tumor is moderately to completely undifferentiated; (2) cancer of both vocal cords unsuitable for the McNaught Keel and anterior commissure technique; (3) cancer of one cord with or without cord fixation and subglottic extension from 5 to 10 mm; (4) persistent tumor of the true vocal cord following irradiation (absence of nodal metastases); and (5) late persistent cancer of any portion of the larynx following a full course of irradiation.

The latter two groups normally indicate late recrudescence after a full course of therapy and a cancer that is no longer confined to the glottis and often is transglottic. If there are late radiation changes, sacrifice of the overlying skin may be necessary in this situation, and use of nondelayed acromiopectoral flaps are required.

Technique for Wide-field Laryngectomy

It is generally accepted that wide-field laryngectomy rather than "narrow-field laryngectomy" is the method of choice. There are many articles written on this subject. After preoperative medication, a nasogastric feeding tube is placed into position before surgery.

Incision. There are many advantages to the "U" or Sorensen-Glueck incision or "thyroid type" of incision over the midline incision (Fig. 35–15). Not only is the cosmetic result of the scar better, but also midline incision contracture of the scar is eliminated. The method described will involve delivery of the larynx from below in contrast to exposure from above.

Technique. Under local anesthesia, a transverse incision about 3 to 4 inches long is made 1 inch above the space of Burns, and the strap muscles are divided (Fig. 35–16). The isthmus of the thyroid gland is divided and sutured.

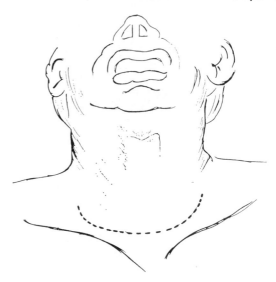

FIG. 35–15.   Incision for wide-field laryngectomy.

The trachea is divided transversely between rings I and II, 10% cocaine is dropped into the trachea, and endotracheal anesthesia is started. The infraglottic area is packed off with a large tonsil sponge to prevent secretions from entering the wound. The skin flaps are now elevated to the base of the hyoid bone. The larynx is mobilized

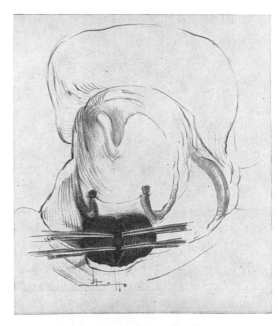

FIG. 35–16.   Transverse skin flap elevated.

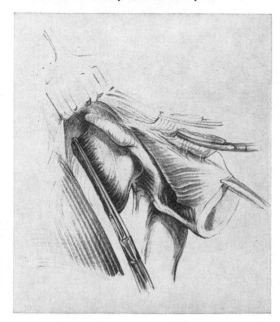

FIG. 35-17. Larynx sutured below first tracheal ring, and constrictor muscles severed at posterior lateral border.

on both lateral aspects of the larynx from along the anterior border of the sternomastoid muscle toward the superior cornu of the thyroid and greater cornu of the hyoid using sharp dissection (Figs. 35-17 to 35-19). The omohyoid muscle is divided at a point where it emerges from the anterior belly of the thyroid cartilage. On the side of the tumor one lobe of the thyroid gland is dissected away from the trachea to be left attached to the larynx. The posterior cricoid area is partially dissected from the esophagus further, but dissection is not carried up to the arytenoid area.

The constrictor muscles are next divided along each posterior lateral border of the thyroid cartilages and allowed to retract posteriorly. The muscles are later used to imbricate the closure of the pharynx.

The hyoid bone is isolated in the midline by separating the suprahyoid muscles from their attachment (Fig. 35-19). The midportion is grasped with a thyroid tenaculum, and the remainder of the supraglottic muscles are separated from the hyoid toward the pharynx. The greater cornu of the hyoid cartilage is separated from its subperiosteal bed to approximately a point where the lesser cornu begins.

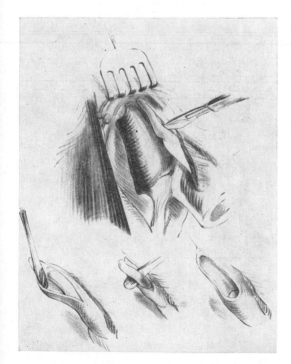

FIG. 35-18. Greater cornu of thyroid cartilage isolated and removed. Piriform sinus is just medial to this.

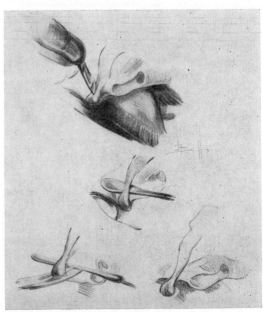

FIG. 35-19. Hyoid bone freed from suprahyoid muscles and dissected subperiosteally.

The greater cornu of the thyroid cartilage opposite the tumor is separated from its perichondral bed, exposing the piriform sinus. Each greater cornu of the hyoid is separated from its periosteal bed. This allows additional pharyngeal mucosa for closure of the pharyngostoma. The pharynx at the piriform sinus opposite the tumor is entered, and the pharyngeal suction is immediately placed into this opening (Fig. 35–20). Dissection is carried inferior to the arytenoid and into the base of the tongue (Figs. 35–21 and 35–22). By placing a tenaculum on the tip of the epiglottis, one can delineate the superior margin under direct examination. (Note: The illustration shows the tenaculum through the infraglottic space on the epiglottis. The tip of the epiglottis is held out of the pharyngostoma.)

Closure of the pharyngostoma is done with a continuous catgut mucosal inverting suture (000 chromic Dulox), and this line is reinforced with two layers of 000 interrupted silk.

Penrose drains are placed, and the subcutaneous layers are approximated with fine silk, and the skin is closed with interrupted sutures. Continuous suction for drainage

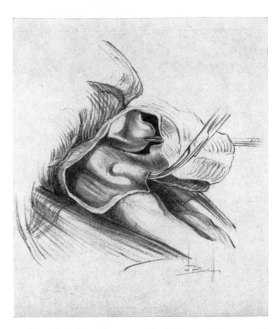

FIG. 35–21.   Larynx (with or without neck dissection) is moved using tenaculum on epiglottis for traction.

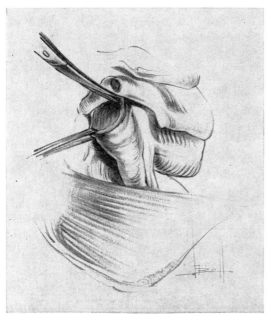

FIG. 35–20.   Piriform sinus opened on side opposite lesion.

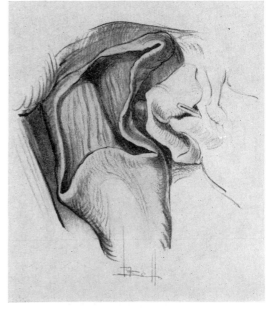

FIG. 35–22.   Larynx separated, and pharyngostoma remains.

using a Gomco suction machine helps to keep the wound dry. Pressure dressings are of great help.

BILATERAL NECK DISSECTIONS

Ordinarily, simultaneous bilateral neck dissection in conjunction with excision of the primary tumor is not performed as a routine procedure in the treatment of cancer of the larynx or pharynx.

Each case must be considered individually. There is no question that the postoperative course is more difficult for the patient with a bilateral as opposed to a unilateral neck dissection. Intracranial edema, increased regional tissue vascularity, and pharyngeal fistula are complications of concern to the surgeon. Thus, such measures are employed only after these factors are taken into account. (The factors to be considered are curability of local disease by resection, difficulties with surgery, general health, risk of surgery, and position and size of palpable nodes.) The indications for bilateral neck dissection include:

1. Moderate-sized primary lesion of the larynx, pharynx, or oral cavity (over 2 cm) with palpable positive nodes on one side and "questionable positive node" on the opposite side.

2. Bilateral palpable nodes. This group of patients should receive low-dose preoperative irradiation with planned bilateral neck dissection.

3. Elective resection of opposite neck because of palpable node on other side.

Technique. A preliminary tracheostomy is done in any case in which bilateral neck dissection is performed. The skin incision utilized depends on the area to be removed. A high H-type incision for a lesion of the hypopharynx or oral cavity is ideal when surgery follows irradiation; a broadly based U-incision is ideal when total laryngectomy is done.

Whether the jugular vein is to be spared or not depends on the clinical situation. Where nodes are not palpable or only questionably palpable (with preoperative irradiation), the internal jugular vein and anterior jugular vein joining the subclavian vein on the contralateral side should be tied. The ipsilateral neck dissection is then completed. At the conclusion of this neck dissection, if there is minimal congestion of the lips and eyes, the contralateral neck dissection can be performed, sacrificing the internal jugular vein. This procedure has been accomplished in 36 cases without undue complications.

When the vein is spared, meticulous care is taken to suspend the sutured vein free from its thoracic inlet to the base of the skull and from all tissue about the vein and to ligate and suture veins entering the jugular vein. While such a procedure is laborious, the end results are gratifying to the surgeon.

CONSERVATION SURGERY

Conservation Surgery. Operations including conservation of laryngeal function can be performed in over half of the laryngeal and pharyngeal cases when they are first seen. The critical decision as to whether the procedure can be done or not is dependent upon the clinical finding of freedom of mobility of the true vocal cords. Even though the tumor is close to the larynx, the procedure can be performed, and one can obtain end survival results comparable to those of total laryngectomy. This implies that the selection of cases is dependent upon accurate assessment of the extent of the primary lesion. The term conservation operation is used for the particular technique which removes the entire supraglottis down to and including the false cord and ventricle and, if necessary, one arytenoid and great portions of the pharynx. The operation can also be extended by removing one vocal cord and subglottis. Reconstruction of one fixed vocal cord is necessary in this instance. This leaves only one cord and, in effect, a simplified larynx which functions adequately. The operation usually includes a routine neck dissection.

Subtotal Supraglottic Laryngectomy and Partial Laryngectomy. The term subtotal supraglottic laryngectomy is reserved for lesions confined to the epiglottis and the term partial laryngectomy for lesions of the piriform sinuses and base of the tongue. Whether or not neck dissection is recommended in the absence of palpable nodes depends on the lesion size and the experience of the surgeon. Because of the low incidence of nonpalpable metastasis (14%), one might not consider a neck dissection for a lesion of the epiglottis less than 2 cm in diameter. The following situations should be noted: (1) A tumor of the epiglottic tip or free portion less than 2 cm probably does not require neck dissection, but if the tumor is greater than 2 cm and extends to the aryepiglottic fold, a neck dissection should be done on the side closest to the richer lymphatic area. (2) Tumor of the inferior vestibule of the epiglottic petiole to and including the false cord requires neck dissection in all instances. Bilateral neck dissection is indicated if nodes are palpably enlarged on one side. (3) Tumors of the lingual surface of the epiglottis require neck dissection.

In the classic example of the epiglottic lesion, the neck dissection operation which removes these structures can be extended to those areas in the anterior piriform sinus or the base of the tongue in continuity with a radical neck dissection. For moderate or small lesions of the piriform sinus, we have routinely resected the piriform sinus with the thyroid cartilage and arytenoid in conjunction with a reconstruction of the pharynx. Elective neck dissection is necessary for lesions of the piriform sinuses and base of the tongue when nodes are clinically absent.

Technique. A tracheostomy is performed under local anesthesia and endotracheal anesthesia induced. The usual Y-incision for neck dissection is made (Fig. 35–23). It starts at the mastoid tip, passes down and forward three fingerbreadths below the angle of the jaw, over the thyrohyoid membrane, and 2.5 cm across the midline. The inferior leg starts at the posterior edge of the sternomastoid at right angles to the first incision and reaches the clavicle with the dogleg to minimize a contracture ridge as shown (Fig. 35–23). The flaps are elevated without entering the tracheostomy wound to avoid an air leak at the end of the procedure.

A radical neck dissection is performed whether metastatic lymph nodes are palpable or not. The only variation from the routine radical neck dissection is that the

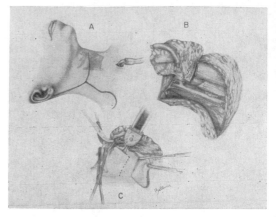

FIG. 35–23. Technique for subtotal supraglottic laryngectomy. *A*, Y-incision after stab local tracheostomy. *B*, Neck dissection completed but left attached to thyrohyoid membrane. *C*, External perichondrium of thyroid cartilage elevated down to its inferior border. Transverse cuts are made into the thyroid cartilage at one-half distance in midline and angle, superiorly on the opposite side and transversely on the side of the dissection.

thyroid lobe and sternohyoid and sternothyroid muscles are preserved (Fig. 35–23, *B*). The superior thyroid lobe is sacrificed if it is adjacent to the area of a piriform fossa. The neck dissection is left attached to the thyrohyoid area (Fig. 35–23, *B*).

The sternohyoid is divided at the upper edge of the thyroid cartilage and reflected inferiorly (Fig. 35–23, *C*). The perichondrium is incised along the same line and elevated to the lower edge of the whole thyroid lamina on the involved side and from the medial portion of the opposite lamina (Fig. 35–23, *C*). The hyoid is freed from the suprahyoid musculature on the involved side to just past the opposite lesser cornu and is divided there with the Lefertz scissors (Fig. 35–23, *C*). The Stryker pencil saw is then used to make the thyroid cartilage cuts (Fig. 35–23, *C*). Note that this transection crosses the anterior midline of the thyroid cartilage exactly half way between the notch and the bottom edge in order to be just above the anterior commissure and then rises steeply to the upper edge of the thyroid lamina on the opposite side of the lesion.

The piriform sinus is entered just posterior to the superior thyroid cornu (Fig. 35–

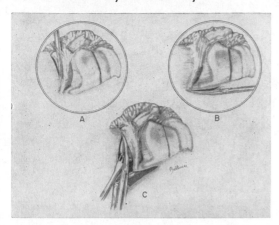

FIG. 35–24. Approaches to the pharynx. *A,* Entry through the vallecula in case of piriform sinus lesion. *B,* Entry through the piriform sinus in case of epiglottic lesion. *C,* Communication of *A* and *B,* depending on location of lesion.

24, *B*) unless there is a question of piriform sinus involvement, in which case it is entered in the opposite vallecula (Fig. 35–24, *A*). The incision is carried around the end of the hyoid and through the vallecula, assisted by downward traction of the tip of the epiglottis. After the incision is carried inferiorly through the hyoid cut, along the opposite edge of the epiglottis, and through the normal aryepiglottic fold and false cord to the anterior commissure, it is possible to see the supraglottic structures quite well (Fig. 35–24, *C*).

Four steps are necessary for adequate exposure of the inferior portion of the supraglottic structures: (1) adequate exposure by incision along the opposite free border of the epiglottis through the false cord to the anterior commissure; (2) constant superior traction (not anteriorly) of the tip of the epiglottis; (3) anterior traction of the free portion of the transected thyroid cartilage with a hook; and (4) lateral traction of the arytenoid with a hook if it is to be removed.

In the usual supraglottic procedure (epiglottic cancer), the next cut is through the aryepiglottic fold just anterior to the arytenoid down the true cord (Fig. 35–25, *A*), the medial arm of the Metzenbaum scissors being used as a "landmark, palpation, and cutting" instrument. With lesions on the aryepiglottic fold and piriform fossa, the scissors cut is posterior and medial to the arytenoid down through the interarytenoid membrane to the cricoid cartilage. The cut is then made anteriorly over the superior surface of the true cord through the body of the arytenoid, leaving only its vocal process (Fig. 35–25, *B, C*). The entire piriform fossa can be excised by a preliminary oblique cartilage incision to a point just superior to the thyrocricoid articulation. The vocal process must be fixed in the midline to the cricoid cartilage by a suture to avoid abduction of the nonfunctioning cord.

However, with the new technique this interarytenoid incision can be extended through the cricoarytenoid joint, under the true cord, and subglottically to the anterior commissure (Fig. 35–25, *D*). This is determined only after exposure of the anterior commissure of the cord involved. To obtain exposure one must cut through the aryepiglottic fold and false cords on the uninvolved side. All these soft tissue incisions are carried through to the adjacent thyroid lamina by Stryker saw incisions. By dissecting immediately under the internal perichondrium, one can excise the entire cord and subglottis for a distance of 8 mm (Fig. 35–26, *A, B*).

If this exposure of the lesion reveals that the tumor is too extensive for a conservation procedure, a total laryngectomy can still be performed without tumor contamination of the operative field.

Reconstruction of the midline cord or pseudocord is necessary for the opposite mobile cord to oppose to prevent aspiration. When the vocal cord is spared but the body of the arytenoid is removed, repair is accomplished by midline fixation of the vocal process to the cricoid cartilage with a heavy silk suture.

When the entire cord and arytenoid are resected, a pseudocord can be created by a triangular cut of the thyroid cartilage (Fig. 35–27). A right-angle infracture of the upper edge of the remaining thyroid lamina can be done and held with mattress stay sutures. A mucosal pedicle graft from the piriform sinus is then sutured over this (Fig. 35–27).

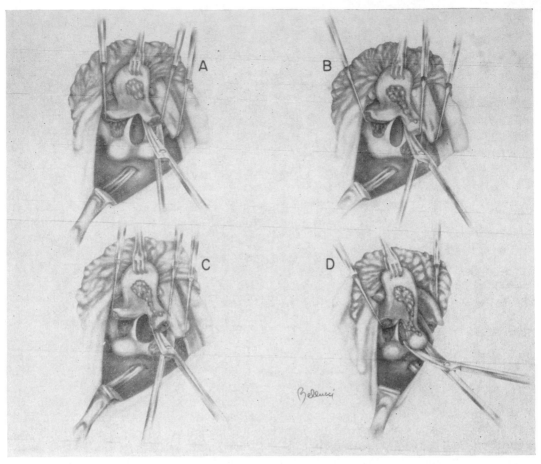

FIG. 35–25.   Technique for removal of local lesion. *A,* The aryepiglottic fold is pulled laterally, and precut thyroid cartilage has been pulled anteriorly. *B,* Arytenoid is cut, but just anterior to vocal process. *C, D,* Arytenoid cord, and subglottis removed subperichondrially.

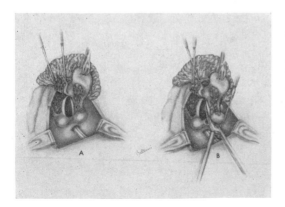

FIG. 35–26.   Technique of excision by approaching the cordal extension of supraglottic carcinoma from the lesser uninvolved side. *A,* Uninvolved side. *B,* Excision of arytenoid and subglottis.

Regardless of method of resection, repair of the pharynx is the same.

A finger is placed through the cricopharyngeus into the upper esophagus, and a cricopharyngeal myotomy is performed behind the thyroid (Fig. 35–28). This is important for reestablishing deglutition.

The pharynx is closed with 2–0 interrupted silk sutures between the perichondrium and the base of the tongue and pharyngeal constrictor (Fig. 35–28, *B*). Since a mucosal closure is not possible and the closure is under some tension even after flexing of the neck, the sutures must go deeply into the base of the tongue for strength and effect a tight seal. Closure is assisted by flexing the head and holding the perichondrium against the tongue by "crossing" the previ-

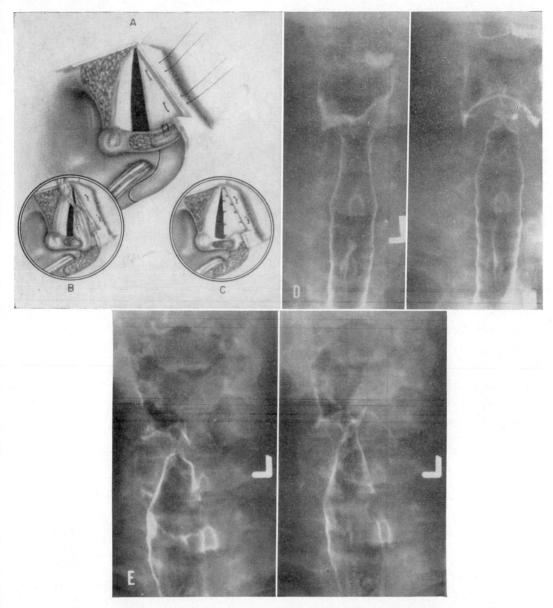

FIG. 35–27. *A*, Right angle cartilage fracture. Fixation of cartilage with mattress stitches. *B*, Pedicle mucosal flap. *C*, Suturing of pedicle flap. *D*, Preoperative laryngogram. *E*, Postoperative laryngogram.

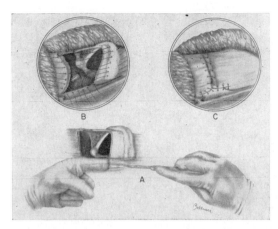

FIG. 35–28. *A*, Cricopharyngeal myotomy. *B*, Closure of external perichondrium to tongue by an inverted T. *C*, Closure.

ous suture adjacent to the one being knotted (Fig. 35–28, *C*). The second layer of closure is made by suturing the strap muscles to the base of the tongue. The hypoglossal nerve needs to be identified and preserved to assist rapid rehabilitation of deglutition.

The skin is closed with subcutaneous gut sutures and skin clips. Hemovac drainage, a full-length tracheotomy tube, and antibiotics are used routinely. The tracheotomy tubes are removed in 1 to 2 weeks when the larynx edema has subsided.

The cricopharyngeal myotomy is one of the most effective measures for rehabilitation of a functioning pharynx. The selection of cases has been based purely on the location and extent of removal of the lesion, which often includes parts of the larynx. This, of course, has been determined by the direct laryngoscopy and laryngogram. Sample cases and results are illustrated in Figures 35–29 to 35–33.

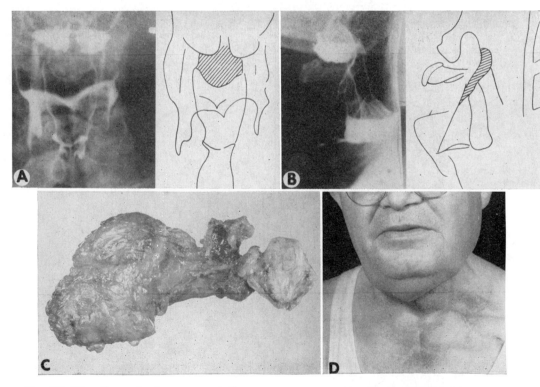

FIG. 35–29. Supraglottic cancer. *A*, Laryngogram—see mass in tip of epiglottis. *B*, Laryngogram lateral view shows normal free margin to cord is great. *C*, Specimen. *D*, Postoperative result (6 years).

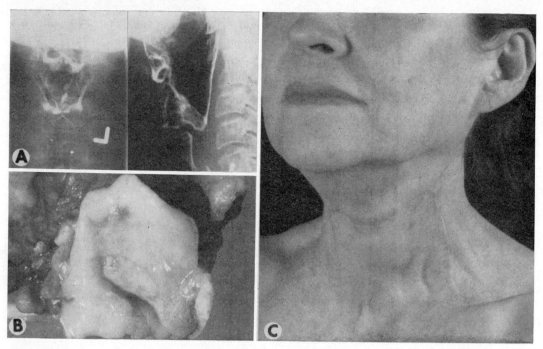

FIG. 35–30.   Supraglottic cancer (inferior vestibule). *A*, Preoperative laryngogram. Note narrow margin of normal tissue. *B*, Specimen. *C*, Postoperative view (4 years).

REHABILITATION AFTER CONSERVATION SURGERY

It is surprising how much can be removed from the larynx without damage to the functions of airway, voice, and deglutition. Occasionally, with extensive resections of the pharynx and supraglottis in which the larynx has been spared, the quality of food that can be swallowed is compromised. This is particularly true when this surgery follows heavy irradiation. For example, the opening of the esophagus can be resected, and some of the patients can only swallow soft foods and must wash down large particles of meats with fluid. When large areas of the posterior pharynx have been resected and the graft placed, there may be some side effects from the accumulation of mucus, which the patient must frequently clear from the throat. In the majority of the conservation operations, swallowing is normal and deviations are extremely minor; in all cases successful tracheotomy tube extubation can be accomplished. Of the 250 conservation operations which have been done to date, only two patients exhibit inability to swallow food in a nutritionally sufficient amount. These two patients eventually underwent total laryngectomy. One had preoperative irradiation and subsequent perichondritis, and the other used a feeding tube and developed postcricoid ulceration and stricture formation.

CONCEPTS OF PLANNED LOW-DOSE PREOPERATIVE IRRADIATION AND SURGERY

The pressing problem following radical or subtotal excisional surgery for cancer of the head and neck is the rather high incidence of local recurrent cancer.

In some instances these recurrences appear to be submucosal in opposition to the surgical margin (e.g., 10% pharyngeal cancer); in other cases the surgical wound is "seeded by cancer cells" (2% upward).

The late appearance of contralateral nodes immediately adjacent to the previous primary lesion is between 12% for supraglottic lesions and 30% for pharyngeal malignancies.

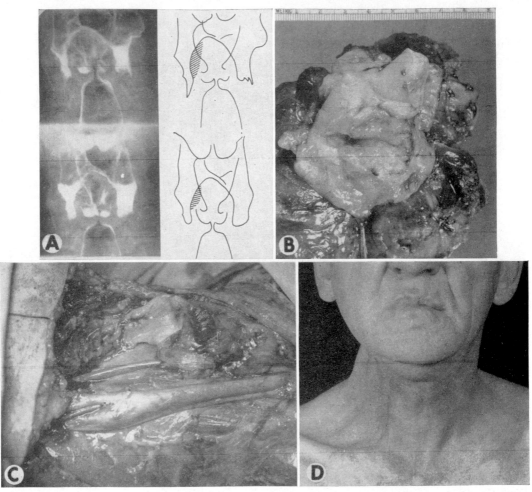

FIG. 35–31. Piriform sinus cancer. *A*, Preoperative laryngogram (lesion of medial wall).
B, Specimen. *C*, Operative view: arytenoid has been removed with epiglottis. *D*, Patient 7
years later.

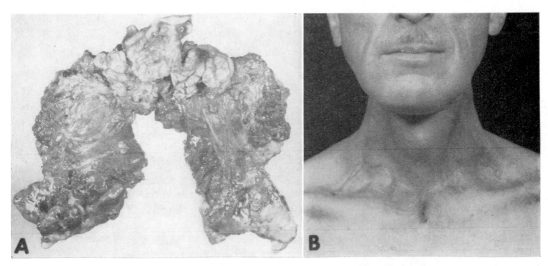

FIG. 35–32. Superior hypopharyngeal cancer. *A*, Resection of base of tongue with bilateral neck
dissection. *B*, Patient 7 years later, free of disease.

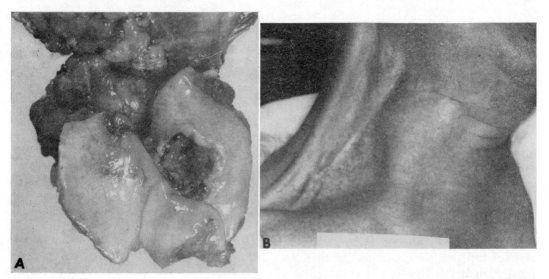

FIG. 35–33. Postirradiation of a persistent piriform sinus cancer. A, Specimen removed after 6000 R and irradiation persistence 15 months later. Partial laryngopharyngectomy done, including epiglottis, arytenoid and piriform sinus. B, Patient 5 years later, free of disease.

Moore reports a 50% postoperative recurrence following surgery for carcinoma of the larynx, pharynx, and base of the tongue. Frazell noted a 39% incidence of recurrent cancer in 277 tongue cancers. Morfit reported a 50% local recurrence rate for mouth cancers and Beahrs noted a 25% local recurrence rate in the primary lesion and 27% in the neck.

The possibility of seeding the operation wound at the time of initial excisional surgery has been reported as varying from 5.7 to 36% by various investigators.

While it would be reasonable to assume that those patients with positive wound washings develop recurrence, a 5-year follow-up study shows no significant correlation between wound washing results and local recurrence. In a selected group of head and neck cancer patients, positive and negative wound washing groups behaved similarly in relation to development of local recurrent cancer (Harris). Thus the prognostic value of positive wound washings and recurrent disease and failure remains to be established.

The high local recurrence rate for aggressive cancer is reflected at least in part by local recurrence following surgery and by the seeding of the wound at the time of surgery. Probably the finding of cancer cells in wound washings signifies a poorer prognosis. Statistical data in this regard are not abundant or clear-cut. Factors other than the presence of free cancer cells in a wound must influence the result, such as the number of cells, the viability of the cells, and the host's resistance to cell implantation.

Experimental studies are now under way at other institutions which demonstrate that the implantability of free cancer cells is influenced by drugs and irradiation. In our own series of 224 patients with head and neck cancer, in 55 patients with cancer of the hypopharynx for over 2 years, only 9 patients developed recurrent disease (14%), compared to a 40% recurrence rate for the same period of time. This follow-up is short. All patients were treated with 3000 R of preoperative irradiation over 3 weeks, followed by a radical surgical procedure.

There was some delay in healing compared to those cases without irradiation; 8 to 9 days is the average time for healing, compared to 7 days without irradiation. Planned preoperative irradiation for moderate-sized lesions is generally included for the pharyngeal cancers. This means that tumors of the base of the tongue, hypopharynx, and piriform fossa should receive preoperative low-dose therapy. When we study the surgical results of tumors in this area, we find that local recurrences are not uncommon in the base of the tongue and are less likely in the piriform fossa. The modality of treating patients with 4000 R is based on the practical consideration of obtaining an adequate margin of safety. Marked regression of the size of the tumor or nearly complete disappearance of the tumor is a frequent finding. Rarely do we find no response to irradiation.

The objective of this method of treatment is to secure an adequate surgical margin based on a preirradiation evaluation without compromising the margin of resection and tumor. Another reason for preoperative irradiation is to avoid the implantation and dissemination of tumor at the time of the surgical procedure. Because stomal recurrences are uncommon but significant, preoperative irradiation should be reserved for infraglottic and transglottic tumors of the larynx. In a completely retrospective study of cases which we have made, stomal recurrences have resulted from tumors in these two sites. It has been our experience that wound healing with 4000 R has been excellent. It is our plan always to deliver 3000 to 4000 R within 3 weeks and to operate on the patient at the end of the first month from the time the patient is initially seen. A full therapeutic dose of irradiation is given for glottic lesions, but it is seldom given for those lesions of the larynx (epiglottis) in which primary surgery can effect good results and not destroy function. It is given in those cases in which nodes are palpable.

Preliminary reports on the effects of low-dose preoperative irradiation to metastatic nodes show that survival is apparently prolonged.

Persistence of the primary tumor a year after a full course of irradiation is a different problem from planned preoperative irradiation to be followed by surgery. In this form of discontinuous, unplanned, therapeutic modality in which there are increased fibrosis and recrudescence or repopulation of tumor, there is a marked increase in the morbidity. Healing is delayed, and the instances of postoperative loss of skin or vascular complications are common. The use

of regional chest flaps has been necessary in our experience in such cases, and the salvage rate is low.

CHEMOTHERAPY

The use of intra-arterial infusions of methotrexate and leucovorin has not been promising. In the experience of Sullivan and Daly, some palliation has been noted. In our limited experience we have noted only temporary regression of the tumor, and in no instance have we observed a cure (see Chap. 38A).

RESULTS

Glottic Carcinoma. The cure rates for glottic epidermoid carcinoma treated by hemilaryngectomy for T_1N_0, T_2N_0, and T_3N_0 lesions were 87%, 82% and 94%, respectively, with an overall cure rate of 86%. The salvage rate from secondary modalities of treatment was 74% (Tables 35–2 to 35–4). The overall cure rate was 91%. This has been improved upon in Bauer's recently reported series of 111 consecutive glottic carcinomas treated by hemilaryngectomy. In this series there were 11 recurrences. There was a 90% primary cure rate for hemilaryngectomy. Five of six local recurrences and two of five neck recurrences were salvaged by combined radiotherapy and surgery, for a salvage rate of 64% and an overall cure rate of 96%.

Ogura's study of glottic carcinomas revealed that one out of five primary glottic tumors had extension greater than 5 mm subglottically. Surgical treatment in this series of patients with primary glottic cancer with subglottic extension included hemilaryngectomy for Stage II (58) and Stage III (5) and total laryngectomy for Stage II (23)

Table 35–2. Glottic Carcinoma:
Modality of Therapy

Hemilaryngectomy	281
Total laryngectomy with/without RND	182
	463

Table 35-3. Glottic Carcinoma: Surgical Treatment and Survival Rates (3 yr. NED)

Lesion	N_0		N_1		N_2		N_3	
	HEMI	TL	HEMI	TL	HEMI	TL	HEMI	TL
T_1	177/205 (87%)	19/20 (95%)	2/2 (100%)	—	0/1 (0%)	—	—	—
T_2	45/55 (82%)	32/47 (68%)	—	4/6 (66%)	—	—	—	—
T_3	17/18 (94%)	49/71 (69%)	—	11/17 (65%)	—	5/6 (83%)	—	0/1 (0%)
T_4	—	5/11 (54%)	—	2/2 (100%)	—	1/1 (100%)	—	—
Total	278	149	2	25	1	7	0	1

and Stage III (23) lesions. Overall absolute survival rates (all patients) for this series were 83% (52/63 patients) for hemilaryngectomy and 63% (29/46 patients) for total laryngectomy (Table 35–5).

A study (Sessions) revealed that one out of four patients with primary glottic carcinoma had secondary extension to the anterior commissure. Surgical treatment in this series of patients with glottic cancers with anterior commissure involvement resulted in overall absolute survival rates of 74% (45/61) for hemilaryngectomy and 62% (51/82) for total laryngectomy (Table 35–6).

In a series of 100 consecutive early carcinomas of the larynx at Washington University Department of Radiation Oncology (1952–1967), Perez reported 5-year determinate survival rates of 82% in T_1 lesions and 77% in T_2 lesions. His conclusion was that irradiation was not effective in T_3 lesions. The overall cure rate was 78%, and the salvage rate was 62%. Horiot, in an analysis of 366 patients with early glottic carcinoma from M.D. Anderson Hospital, reported a 90.5% cure rate for T_1 and an 86% cure rate for T_2 carcinomas. He noted an overall cure rate for invasive carcinoma of 88% for T_1 and 74% for T_2 lesions. Hibbs reported a cumulative survival rate of 76% (35 patients), and Boles and Komorn reported a 74% survival rate (12 patients) with radiation therapy for T_2 glottic lesions. Lederman, in a larger series (137 patients), obtained a 65% cumulative survival rate for T_2 lesions.

The problems involved in comparing the results of treating different patient populations with different therapeutic modalities are obvious. No final answer can be made without a universally accepted staging and classification system, as well as standardized end results reporting. It is apparent to us that, while hemilaryngectomy may be only slightly more advantageous than irradiation in treating T_1 glottic lesions, it is definitely superior in the curing of T_2 and T_3 lesions. The slightly better salvage rate (74%) after hemilaryngectomy also increases the patients' chances for eventual cure.

Supraglottic Carcinoma. The survival rates of supraglottic epidermoid carcinoma treated by subtotal supraglottic laryngec-

Table 35–4.   Glottic Carcinoma: Survival by Stage (3 yr. NED)

Stage	Hemilaryngectomy No. Pts.	%	Total Laryngectomy No. Pts.	%
I	177/205	87	19/20	95
II	45/55	82	32/47	69
III	19/21	90	77/114	68
IV	—	—	0/1	0

Table 35–5.   Glottic Primary with Subglottic Extension: Absolute Survival by Site and Procedure (109 Patients)

Site	Total Laryngectomy	Hemilaryngectomy
TVC-UNI	11/17 (65%)	35/41 (85%)
TVC-BIL	—	0/1 (0%)
Ant. Com. Prim.	0/1 (0%)	—
TVC-UNI with Ant. Com.	7/8 (88%)	9/12 (75%)
TVC-BIL with Ant. Com.	11/19 (58%)	7/8 (88%)
Other	0/1 (0%)	1/1 (100%)
Total	29/46 (63%)	52/63 (83%)

Table 35–6.   Anterior Commissure Tumors: Absolute Survival by Site and Procedure (143 Patients)

Primary Site	Total Laryngectomy	Hemilaryngectomy
Ant. Com. Prim.	0/2 (0%)	1/2 (50%)
TVC-UNI with Ant. Com.	16/22 (73%)	31/42 (74%)
TVC-BIL with Ant. Com.	35/58 (60%)	13/17 (76%)
Total	51/82 (62%)	45/61 (74%)

Table 35-7. Supraglottic Carcinoma:
Survival After SSL

Lesion Stage	No. Pts.	N_0	No. Pts.	N_1-N_3
		Nodes		
T_1	64/78	82%	8/14	58%
T_2	23/34	79%	8/12	61%
T_3	7/10	70%	2/3	66%
T_4	9/12	75%	8/13	73%
Total	134		42	

tomy (SSL) for T_1, T_2, T_3, T_4N_0 lesions are 82%, 79%, 70%, and 75%, respectively, with an overall survival rate of 76% (Tables 35-7 and 35-8). The salvage rate from secondary modalities of treatment is 47%. The overall cure rate is 82%. On the basis of present data, we believe that conservation surgery is the treatment of choice in supraglottic carcinoma. The results (Wang, Goepfert) compare favorably with those of irradiation alone for smaller T_1 and T_2 lesions and are superior for T_3 and T_4 lesions. These results are in accord with those of total laryngectomy (Wang). If a comparison is made on the basis of physiologic restitution of phonation and deglutition, then conservation surgery is superior to irradiation and total laryngectomy as a combined modality of treatment.

One of the limitations of subtotal supraglottic laryngectomy becomes apparent with T_3 lesions which are associated with cordal

Table 35-8. Supraglottic Carcinoma
Treated by SSL: Survival by Stage*

Stage	No. Pts.	%
I	64/78	82
II	28/36	78
III	39/57	69
IV	3/6	50

*Overall determinant survival 76%.

fixation. In such situations a total laryngectomy and radical neck dissection are performed. The 3-year determinate cure rate is 66% (22/35 cases).

Our present observations give some support to Fletcher's recent observations that clinically positive neck nodes have a better prognosis for resection without recurrence if preoperative radiation is given (50% as compared to 64.5%). The survival rate for various "T"-group lesions with positive clinical nodes is influenced less by the size and extent of the tumor than by the clinical size and fixation of the neck nodes. The survival ranges between 57.5 and 66%, the best results being achieved with N_1 neck nodes.

Aryepiglottic Fold (AE) Carcinoma (Marginal Lesions). We have noted that carcinoma of the supraglottis (laryngeal surface of the epiglottis, ventricular bands, and laryngeal ventricles) has a primary surgical cure rate of 76% with a salvage rate of 47%. The overall survival rate is 82%. Lesions of the aryepiglottic fold (marginal lesions) have an overall survival rate of 53% (Tables 35-9 to 35-12). The presence or absence of clinically nonfixed positive nodes does not alter the survival rates to a significant extent (52% versus 54%). However, lesions that are amenable to partial laryngopharyngectomy on a selected basis have a better prognosis, a 65% 3-year NED (with clinical nodes), and a 59% 3-year NED (without clinical nodes). In patients with large tumors that can only be treated by total laryngectomy, the survival drops to a 43% 3-year NED (without clinical nodes) and a 27% 3-year NED (with clinical nodes). In the latter case with large T lesions (T_4), survival is dependent on the tumor extent and the presence of multiple clinical nodes.

When AE fold lesions were staged according to AJC classification based on our T system, survival analysis was significant in Stage III lesions. Those which were treated by partial laryngopharyngectomy (PLP) had a 62% 3-year NED survival rate, as opposed to those treated by total laryngectomy, which had a 28% survival rate. This confirms our previous observation that survival in marginal lesions is de-

Table 35–9. Marginal Carcinoma of Aryepiglottic Fold: Primary Treatment
by PLP and TL (Results—NED)

	PLP	PLP with PREOP	TL	TL with PREOP
T_1 N_0	1/1	1/2	2/3	
N_1	1/1	2/3		
T_2 N_0		1/2	1/1	
N_1	1/2			
N_3		2/2		0/1
T_3 N_0	2/4	11/17	0/1	1/3
N_1	1/1	6/8		1/4
N_3	0/1			
T_4 N_0	4/6	3/7	1/3	1/3
N_1	2/4	3/4	2/6	0/1
N_2		0/2		0/1
N_3		1/1	1/1	
Total	12/20 (57%)	30/48 (63%)	7/15 (40%)	3/13 (23%)

pendent mainly on the extent of the primary lesion and to a lesser degree on the lymph node metastasis. This is also confirmed by the finding of no significant change in overall survival when patients were staged with respect to the T lesions and compared for clinical positive lymph nodes (survival rates of 54% versus 52%). This survival pattern is quite different than that in supraglottic carcinoma and implies greater extensiveness of primary lesions in the marginal zone. Only in extensive T_3 and T_4 lesions does the survival depend on the clinical staging of the cervical lymph nodes (N_0 + N_1 lesion had a 43% and N_2 + N_3 had a 27% 3-year NED survival rate). Thus, with AE fold marginal lesions, survival depends primarily on the lesion size and its immediate local extent.

These results compare favorably with those of combined preoperative irradiation and total laryngectomy (Wang) and are superior to those of irradiation alone (Ennyer, Fletcher, Hendrickson, Lederman). In addition, they confirm the previous observations by Ogura that AE fold lesions behave more as hypopharyngeal lesions than as supraglottic lesions and must be considered separately in any future classification.

Therefore, for small marginal lesions without nodes—T_1N_0 and T_2N_0—partial laryngopharyngectomy with preoperative irradiation is the preferred treatment. For T_3

Table 35–10. Marginal Carcinoma of Aryepiglottic Fold: Survival After PLP and TL (All Patients)

Positive Nodes	PLP	TL	Overall
Present	19/29 (65%)	4/15 (27%)	23/44 (52%)
Absent	23/39 (59%)	6/14 (43%)	29/53 (54%)
Overall Survival			52/97 (53%)

Table 35–11. Marginal Carcinoma of Aryepiglottic Fold: Survival by Stage and Surgical Therapy (N—97)

Stage	PLP* No. Pts.	%	TL* No. Pts.	%
I	2/3	66	2/3	66
II	1/2	50	1/1	100
III	32/53	61	6/22	28
IV	1/1	100	1/2	50

* Three-year NED survival rate.

Table 35–12. Supraglottic and Marginal Carcinoma: Primary Treatment by Conservation Surgery (3-yr. Survival NED)

Lesion	No. Pts. Cured	No. Pts. Treated	%
Supraglottic	134	177	76
Marginal	52	97	53
Total	186	274	67%

and T_4 lesions, preoperative irradiation with partial laryngopharyngectomy or total laryngectomy is the treatment of choice.

Since we have demonstrated that primary AE fold lesions are more extensive than can be visualized by direct laryngoscopy, we have already instituted a higher preoperative irradiation dose (5000 rads to the tumor site) as part of the combined therapy.

Piriform Sinus Carcinoma. Carcinoma involving the inferior hypopharynx was seen in 175 patients. In 97 patients the lesion arose on the aryepiglottic fold or supraglottic area, and in 75 the lesion was in the piriform sinus proper. The overall 3-year absolute survival for the entire group was 34% (surgery, preoperative irradiation, and irradiation alone).

In those patients with piriform sinus cancer, the 3-year absolute survival was 40%. Pathologic evidence of cervical lymph node metastasis was present in 68% of the patients. The occult metastatic rate was 33%. The 3-year absolute survival for these patients was 34%. No clinical or histologic evidence of cervical lymph node metastasis was present in 32% of the patients. Their

3-year absolute survival was 48%. Those patients presenting with bilateral cervical metastasis had a 17% 3-year absolute survival.

Patients presenting with small T_1 and T_2 lesions had a 66% 3-year survival, while those with large T_3 and T_4 lesions had a 35% 3-year survival rate. In the irradiation group, the overall absolute survival was 4%.

Analysis of the most prevalent factors in therapeutic failures indicated that local persistence and cervical metastasis were the main causes. In analysis of the size of cervical metastasis in relation to survival, it was noted that, with small and occult (N_1) lymph node metastasis, the survival was 36%, and with large metastatic masses (N_2 and N_3), it was 30%. It appears, then, that the presence of metastasis and not the size of the lesion is the crucial factor determining survival. The size of the primary lesion is not as critical except when there is extralaryngeal tumor extension (T_4 lesions). The 3-year survival according to the T classification is as follows: T_1, 65%; T_2, 66%; T_3, 40% and T_4, 30%.

Our results indicate that the proper therapeutic approach to these lesions is the use of high-dose preoperative radiation (4500-5000 rads) followed by surgery. If the lesions are amenable to conservation techniques, these should be employed, since there is preservation of normal phonation and deglutition. From a statistical point of view, there is no difference in survival by staging and classification between those patients treated by total laryngectomy and those treated by conservation surgery. Surgery or irradiation when used alone for the treatment of piriform sinus carcinomas has a much inferior therapeutic and survival rate.

CAUSES OF MORBIDITY AND MORTALITY

The causes of morbidity and mortality are not necessarily listed in order of hospital morbidity and refer to the early and late postoperative period. Obviously, the worst complication following the operation is local recrudescence, however delayed this might be in the follow-up of the case. This list of complications includes those occurring in all patients subjected to conservation procedures.

Skin Loss. In a few instances, loss of skin with pharyngocutaneous fistula requires the use of delayed or nondelayed acromiopectoral pedicle flaps. The importance of covering the exposed carotid artery immediately cannot be overstressed. This complication can best be avoided by using a levator scapulae muscle flap at the time of surgery.

Fistula. Wound disruption of the pharyngolaryngeal area is not common; it is best repaired by use of an acromiopectoral flap. Small indirect fistulas are unusual and often close spontaneously. Fistulas have been uncommon since we began using the external perichondrium of the thyroid cartilage to anastomose to the base of the tongue without bothering about mucosal approximation. Pharyngeal stenosis has not occurred.

Hemorrhage. Oozing from the pharynx occurs occasionally postoperatively and can best be controlled by application of an intraoral pharyngeal pack for 1 or 2 days. Carotid artery rupture occurred in one case secondary to wound infection.

Wound Infection. Wound infection is uncommon and is usually due to coliform organisms or occasionally to staphylococci.

Pulmonary Problems. Bronchopneumonia early in the postoperative period is infrequent, but when it does occur, it may be due to aspiration in the postoperative period (3 of 83 patients). Pulmonary embolus occurred in one patient, but the patient survived and has lived for 6 years.

Cardiac Failure. Myocardial infarction occurred in three patients. In two patients it was the direct cause of death in the immediate postoperative period, and one patient died 13 months postoperatively without disease.

Immediate postoperative deaths occurred in 4 of 83 cases, or 4.9%. Death was due to the following causes: coronary thrombosis, myocardial failure, pneumonia, and carotid artery rupture.

Local Recurrences. There was no local recurrence in the epiglottis and false cord group. Three of 28 cases in the piriform fossa group and 3 of 15 cases in the superior hypopharynx group developed local persistence within 18 months of operation.

References—see Chapter 37, pp. 526–528.

Chapter 36

Malignant Tumors of the Tongue

The surgical principle upon which treatment of lingual cancer is based is the anatomic fact that the tongue, being a paired organ, is ideally suited for therapeutic measures. Thus in the usual case, the treatment of malignancies in this area requires either full irradiation for cure or surgical extirpation alone, or a combination of the two modes.

Embryologically the tongue is primarily a pharyngeal derivative, and its growth forward into the mouth is secondary. The body of the tongue is thus ectodermal, whereas the root or base is entodermal. Its embryologic development reflects itself in the fact that tumors arising from the anterior two thirds of the tongue are quite different from those which arise from the base of the tongue.

The mucous membrane which covers the base of the tongue is thick and relatively freely mobile over the adjacent muscle and contains a great deal of lymphoid tissue that forms the lingual tonsils. The mucous membrane of the anterior portion of the tongue is thin and closely adherent to the underlying muscle. In this mucous membrane are numerous papillae, and the mucosa is essentially stratified squamous epithelium; accordingly, the vast majority of lingual cancers are epidermoid in character. The main arteries of the tongue are the linguals; smaller branches from the maxillary and ascending pharyngeal arteries are also present. Because of the minimal cross communication between arteries and veins from one side to the other, loss of both lingual arteries may cause necrosis of the entire tongue.

Incidence. The incidence of cancer of the tongue is between 0.5 and 0.8 per 100,000 population. Many factors have been stated to be important in the development of lingual cancer: alcohol and tobacco, trauma from ill-fitting dentures or carious teeth, syphilis, and poor oral hygiene. Leukoplakia has been stated to be observed in 10 to 40% of all patients with lingual cancer. Since the age incidence of tongue cancer is in the median of 58 years, it is rarely seen in young individuals. It is important to remember that occasionally multiple foci of cancer may be present in the tongue, and for that matter the same may be noted throughout the entire buccal mucosa. There is a preponderance of these cancers in men. However, there is a high incidence of tongue cancer in women in Sweden, which is believed to be associated with the Plummer-Vinson syndrome.

Location of Lingual Cancer. The mobile portion of the tongue is defined as that portion in front of the anterior pillars and the circumvallate papillae in the midline. The most frequent site for cancer is along the lateral borders (approximately 65% of the cases). The dorsum of the tongue accounts for 15% and the base of the tongue for 25%. The undersurface of the lateral aspects of the tongue is included with the lateral borders of the tongue. In our series,

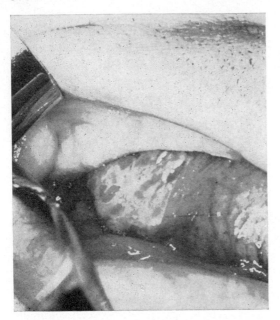

FIG. 36–1.   Cancer of the tongue over 2 cm in size.

fully 50% of cases arose from the base of the tongue (Fig. 36–1).

Symptomatology. A painful ulcer is noted in approximately one fourth of the patients. An asymptomatic mass is found in 40% of the cases. It is remarkable that pain is not more frequent as the initial symptom for cancer of the base of the tongue. Many of the complaints can be attributed to the broad grouping of psychosomatic or hysterical complaints. Such symptoms as gravelly sensation, mild sore throat, preference of warm liquids to cold liquids, or the complaint that "my tongue just does not feel right" should be carefully investigated and distinguished from functional symptoms.

Physical Findings of Lingual Cancer. Tumors of the mobile portion of the tongue or the lateral aspects appear to be either an ulcerative fungating mass or a bulky localized mass. By contrast, tumors of the base of the tongue are frequently overlooked but are readily felt by the palpating finger. Any painless cervical lymph node enlargement in the adult should be considered cancer until proven otherwise, and the diagnosis should not be established by an open exci-

sional biopsy. Every attention should be directed toward finding the primary malignant lesion.

Between 40 to 70% of the nodes are positive when the patient has a primary lesion in the tongue. The incidence of cervical node metastases is higher when the primary lesion is larger than 2 cm. The incidence of nodal involvement with base of the tongue lesions is significantly higher than that with lesions of the mobile portion of the tongue. Cancers of the tip of the tongue tend to be localized for a rather long period of time, and metastases can be suspected when they spill over onto the floor of the mouth. Distant metastases are unusual and only account for approximately 3% of the cases. In this instance, the lung is the most common site of metastases.

Therapy. Small or incipient tumors can be treated adequately when excisional biopsy is necessary to establish the diagnosis. If the surgical margins of the specimen are adequate, no further surgical management is necessary except for frequent observation. For the majority of cases, treatment is dependent upon (1) the size and location of the primary tumor, (2) the presence of bone involvement, and (3) the presence of palpable metastases. If palpable metastases are present in the neck, the size, mobility, and position are important. Lesions that are 1 cm in size and are located on the mobile portion of the tongue can be treated either by excision or by radium needles.

Radium needle implantation yields a better functioning result than hemiglossectomy. Small wedge excisions do not cause much functional impairment, but a full hemiglossectomy causes some derangement. Thus the size of the tumor is important. It has not been our practice to use radon seeds, to use external irradiation alone, or to perform simultaneous dissection procedures, such as neck dissections, electively. If radium is used, complete regression and disappearance of the primary lesion should occur before a decision is made regarding neck dissection. Whether or not neck dissection is indicated for small lesions depends entirely upon the presence or absence of nodes. In general, small lesions do not require radical neck dissection, and lesions larger than 2 cm require neck dissection whether nodes are palpable or not.

Surgical Extirpation. Only *small circumscribed well-differentiated tumors,* particularly those located on the margins of the anterior two thirds of the tongue, can be treated by simple wedge excisions. Tumors which require hemiglossectomy should not be classified as small circumscribed tumors.

Superficial well-differentiated tumors of the dorsum of the tongue, particularly those which arise from leukoplakia, are treated by local extirpation. Large lingual tumors measuring about 2 cm are best treated by radium needles or in combination with external irradiation.

Large and infiltrating tumors located on the anterior two thirds of the tongue require hemiglossectomy, and radical neck dissection should be included. The question as to whether this can be accomplished by a discontinuous procedure or composite resection depends upon the inclination and training of the surgeon.

Large lingual tumors that extend to the mandible by involving the floor of the mouth require a combined modality of therapy. Since most cancers that involve the anterior two thirds of the tongue may invade the mandibular foramen and resection requires hemimandibulectomy, it is best to plan low-dose preoperative therapy along with radical excision. The therapeutic modality should be a planned attack directed at an all-out curative result. Surgery should not be considered as a mode of therapy for inadequate irradiation, nor irradiation therapy as a crutch for inadequate surgery.

Tumors Best Treated by Combined Methods. Large tumors are best treated by combined methods of therapy, namely preoperative irradiation followed by composite resection based purely upon resectability and location of the tumor. If the tumor is large and curability poor with primary extension resection, it has been our practice to give the patient 3000 R preoperatively to the tumor and nodes in the neck, followed by composite resection. Preoperative irradiation is administered 2½ to 3 weeks before surgery.

SURGICAL TECHNIQUES FOR OPERATION OF CANCER OF THE TONGUE

Local Excision. Conservative procedures are seldom indicated and should be utilized only for small well-differentiated tumors. In general, this refers to a lesion about 1 cm with less than 2 cm between the borders. A small lesion suspected of being cancer is best treated by wide local excision. This elliptical excision should be followed by a direct mucosal closure. If the tumor is on the tip of the tongue, excision of the entire tip is followed by approximation of the edges. If a wedge excision is done, direct mucosal suturing of opposing edges gives a good functional result. Thus, preneoplastic lesions and small areas of invasive cancer lend themselves well to this type of therapy. Most of the difficulty involved in conservative management arises from improper selection of treatment in these cases. When a larger lesion is handled in the same manner, quite often the resected margins show a questionable margin of safety when followed for a longer period of time, as evidenced by local recurrence with metastatic nodes in the neck. Thus, small infiltrative lesions should be biopsied rather than managed by local wedge excisions, and the lesion should be implanted with radium.

Treatment of Lingual Cancers by Hemiglossectomy. Basically the techniques for hemiglossectomy have not changed over the past 80 years (Fig. 36–2). When a stay suture is placed into the tip of the tongue, the incision is made along the medial fibrous raphe back to and including the circumvallate papillae with and without part or all of the floor of the mouth. If this amount of tissue needs to be removed, then a hemiglossectomy alone should not be performed without consideration of en bloc radical neck dissection. The only exception to this rule is a cylindroma considered locally malignant, in which lymph node dissection alone is not necessary. Inclusion of neck dissection is considered only in the presence of palpable nodes. In general, the discontinuous procedure of managing tumors of the mobile portion of the tongue was given

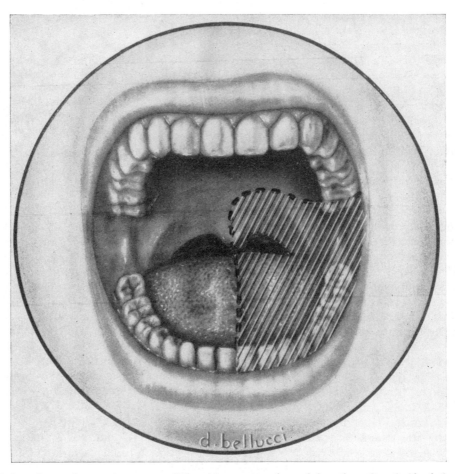

Fig. 36–2.   Area of resection compatible with preservation of function. One half of the tongue may be removed entirely, or one half of the palate with part of the tongue.

up many years ago in favor of the combined resection. This experience is based on the moderate number of local recurrences resulting from such methods of treatment.

Likewise, resection of the floor of the mouth and the mandible is rarely indicated without inclusion of the composite excision of the primary lesion with radical neck dissection.

Hemiglossectomy Associated With Hemimandibulectomy and Radical Neck Dissection. A variation of the operative technique is the mandibular osteotomy without mandibulectomy (Fig. 36–3); access is gained to the floor of the mouth using this technique rather than a pull-through operation (Fig. 36–4). The pull-through operation refers to the radical neck dissection and removal of the intraoral lesion without a mandibular osteotomy. In general, this method is much more difficult, and there is a risk of spilling the tumor in the oral cavity at the time of excision.

Technique. The incision is outlined in the illustration. After preliminary tracheostomy under local anesthesia, the skin flaps are reflected, and a radical neck dissection is started at the sternocleidomastoid muscle at its sternoclavicular attachment. The dissection is carried down into the posterior triangle and along the anterior border of the trapezius muscle. This is done rather than ligation and division of the internal jugular vein at the level of the clavicle. The dissection is then carried up anterior to the prevertebral fascia along the greater vessels of the neck. The sternohyoid and sternothyroid muscles are left intact. Dissection is carried upward beyond the carotid artery to the bifurcation, and the hypoglossal nerve is identified. The sternocleidomastoid muscle is divided from its attachment to the mastoid, and the digastric muscle is identified. The tail and deep lobe of the parotid are transected toward the angle of the mandible. At this point the posterior facial vein is identified, and the facial nerve and the mandibular division are identified right after the anterior facial artery and vein are located and reflected upward in order to preserve the facial nerve. When the digastric muscle is retracted superiorly, the internal jugular vein is identified, ligated, and sutured. The

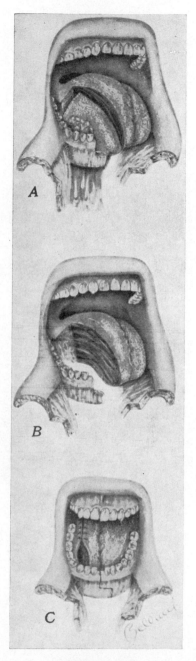

FIG. 36–3. Hemiglossectomy and neck dissection without removal of mandible. *A*, With notched type of mandible osteotomy, composite tongue and neck dissection is done. *B*, After resection. *C*, Closure—the osteotomy is wired together.

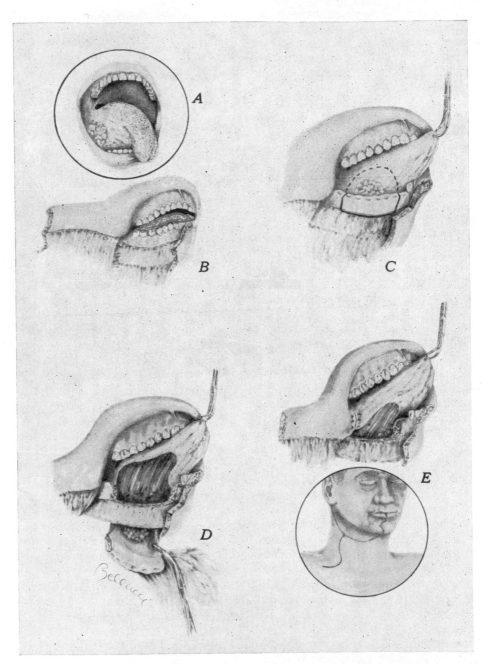

FIG. 36–4. Segmental mandible removal and pull-through with neck dissection. This operation is suitable for selected lesions of the floor of the mouth. *A*, Location of lesion. *B*, Cheek flap reflected laterally. *C*, Segmental bone removal. *D*, Pull-through. *E*, Closure.

nodes are dissected high over the neck dissection, and the mass is left attached to the lower border of the mandible starting from the angle to the anterior portion of the mandible.

No further separation of the tissues is done at this point whether the mandible is

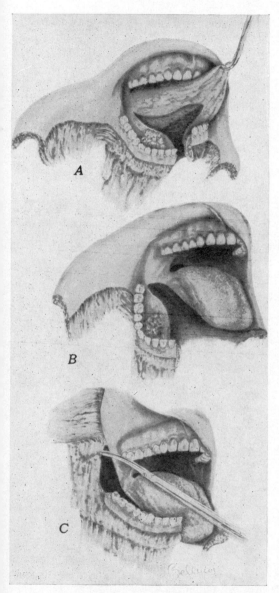

FIG. 36–5. Floor of mouth lesion. Mandible split off midline and part of tongue; mandible removed with neck dissection. *A,* Mandible split off midline. *B,* Floor of mouth resected with the mandible. *C,* Mandible excised by cutting above coronoid process.

sectioned in part marginally, subtotally, or without removal. The specimen is dissected anteriorly and superiorly to include the submental triangle to the zone where the mandible is to be sectioned. A V-notch skin incision is carried along the mandible in order to give a better cosmetic result and to allow primary closure. If the mandible is to be spared, it is divided in the midline using a Gigli saw and notched in order to facilitate suturing of the mandible with wire at the end of the operation. To accomplish preservation of the mandible, the incision of the soft tissue is carried intraorally and down along the midline of the tongue. The floor of the mouth is included with the radical neck dissection, and the incision is made along the mucoperiosteal attachment of the inner aspect of the mandible. In this manner the tonsil and part of the soft palate may be removed if necessary. In the event that the mandible is removed, the external periosteum of the mandible is reflected upward until the neck of the condyle of the mandible is identified (Fig. 36–5). If primary prosthetic repair of the mandible is carried out, a good portion of the neck is left in order to put a Kirschner wire (Fig. 36–6) or vitallium mesh artificial mandible in to preserve the external contours. There are other methods of repairing mandibles, such as the use of premolded, precast portions of the mandible made of wire mesh. The alternative is to use no prosthesis. In either case, whether or not the mandible is removed (Fig. 36–7) or reconstructed, such as in partial resection of the mandible, the remaining portions of the tongue should be attached to the mucoperiosteum or soft tissues of the lateral buccal mucosa. If a wire prosthesis or wire mesh prosthesis is used for resurfacing, this must be completely buried to prevent secretions from getting into the reconstructed portions of the soft tissues of the neck. Delayed bone grafts can be done for restoring mandibular contour if a Kirschner wire is used at a later date.

Treatment of potential metastases to the opposite cervical lymph nodes with a lesion on the ipsilateral portion of the tongue depends on each surgeon's viewpoint. A supraomohyoid neck dissection on the contralateral neck can be employed in the ab-

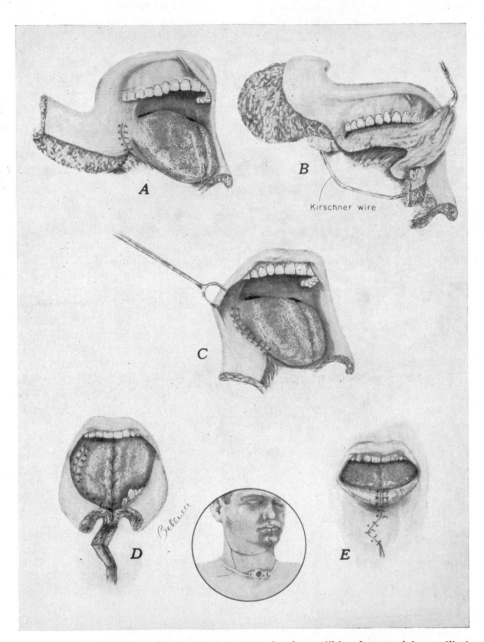

FIG. 36–6.   Tongue or floor of mouth lesion.   Repair of mandible after partial mandibulectomy. *A*, After resection. *B*, Kirschner wire connects condyle with remaining mandible. *C*, Tongue-buccal mucosa closure covers prosthesis. *D*, *E*, V-incision minimizes scar.

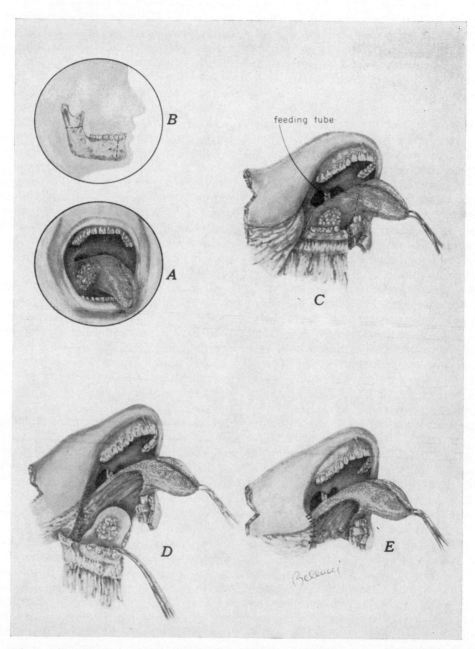

FIG. 36–7.   Composite resection of tongue with neck. A large tumor of the mobile portion of the tongue (no prosthesis). *A,* Location of tumor. *B,* Area of transection through mandible. Decision to remove mandible depends on whether tumor encroaches on mandible. *C,* Mandible removed in continuity with neck dissection. *D,* Excision from tongue. *E,* Partial closure of buccal mucosa with tongue.

sence of nodes, or one may elect to do nothing on this side. If at the first visit nodes are present bilaterally with a unilateral lesion on the tongue, following external irradiation, bilateral neck dissection should be done along with hemiglossectomy in one sitting. Theoretically it is possible to resect the entire tongue as well as half of the mandible and to perform a bilateral neck dissection, but the serious functional impairment would deter any surgeon who has had any experience in managing these cases. The seriousness of the functional impairment is characterized by swallowing by gravity only. These patients can successfully swallow only by lying flat on their backs. The other way to overcome this difficulty is to remove the normal larynx from the tongue and lateral neck structures. This is a handicapping disability, and disfigurement will be great. Functional impairment is greatest if the greater portion of the anterior mandible is resected, together with bilateral neck dissection. Repair is done using a vitallium mesh mandible and a large cervical flap for reconstruction of the floor of the mouth. The temporary orostoma is repaired later. Performance of a total mandibulectomy in any patient is usually out of the question. In addition to the disfigurement, the patient would, of necessity, have to wear a tracheotomy tube, contend with constant salivation, and be unable to maintain his nutrition. If cervical metastases appear late after primary lingual cancer and neck dissection, a secondary neck dissection can be done at any point after 8 weeks.

Surgical Treatment of Cancer of the Base of the Tongue. In essence, the surgical approach is a modification of the supraglottic resection technique. For lesions of the valleculae, it is important to determine that only small lesions of the base of tongue are considered resectable. In every instance, preoperative irradiation is included with the surgical approach. Subtotal resection of the tongue together with the epiglottis can be performed. Only one lingual artery is sacrificed—never both arteries. Another approach following irradiation of the base of the tongue for a limited lesion involves performing a midline osteotomy and splitting the tongue down the midline along the median raphe. This is an excellent approach for certain tumors of the base of the tongue region. Tumors of such size as to extend to the circumvallate papilla ridge are considered inoperable. This method of approach to the base of the tongue is still in the experimental stage; however, the results may justify this method of management for cancer of the base of the tongue. Most of the results have been obtained in terms of 5-year cures and functional impairment. Presently, the results of resection of base of the tongue lesions using a subtotal approach indicate a 40% survival. The subtotal resection of the base of the tongue has not given the patient much difficulty with regard to deglutition. The results are indicated under supraglottic subtotal laryngectomy.

Results. Lesions smaller than 1 cm are most easily treated by local excision, but they may be treated equally well by radium needles. We have had cure rates of 70% in our experience.

Lesions of 2 cm or less are best treated by radium needles and should give nearly the same cure rate, provided the nodes are negative.

Lesions larger than 2 cm, confined to one side of the mobile tongue with and without palpable nodes, yield an overall cure rate of 40%. Fifty percent of the cases prior to the advent of preoperative irradiation failed because of local recurrences.

With the use of low-dose preoperative irradiation, our experience has changed. Of 200 consecutive head and neck cancers treated by irradiation and surgery, 30 were in the mobile tongue and 20 in the base of the tongue. While it is not possible to discuss the results in terms of 5-year survivals, one can discuss the results of short-term experience, i.e., surgical complications and recurrences. Whether a patient is treated with or without irradiation before operation, if that patient survives the first 2 years, his chances for surviving 5 years are about 80% or more.

References—see Chapter 37, pp. 526–528.

Chapter 37

Neoplasms of the Pharynx and Tonsils

BENIGN NEOPLASMS OF THE PHARYNX AND TONSILS

Benign tumors are relatively infrequent in these areas. The most common types of benign neoplasms are papillomas, hemangiomas, angiofibromas, lipomas, cysts, and mixed tumors.

Papillomas. The papilloma is the most common form of benign tumor seen in the area of the tonsil. Papillomas may grow in any part of the mucous membrane of the oral cavity, and they may be seen at the base of the uvula and on the tonsil itself. Many of them are pedunculated with a narrow base; some are more warty, flat, or sessile, with a broad attachment. When they are single, they can be easily eradicated by excision and electrocautery, whereas if they have a broad, irregular base, it may be difficult to remove them entirely. Frequently when they occur in this latter form, they have to be removed from the oral cavity several times, similar to when they occur in the larynx. The use of papilloma vaccines is not of established value.

Angiofibromas. Angiofibromas or fibromas more commonly occur in the hypopharynx as solitary smooth masses arising underneath the mucous membrane. They vary in size considerably, but their removal can be accomplished via the transoral route by suspension laryngoscopy or by the lateral pharyngotomy approach. In general, the presence of a tumor in the hypopharynx is better handled by the external route. In terms of incidence these tumors are relatively uncommon compared to the more frequent form of angiofibroma arising from the rostrum of the sphenoid in the nasopharynx.

Hemangiomas. These tumors appear as bluish masses which may arise in the tonsil fossa or in the soft palate region. They are seen not infrequently in the hypopharynx. They frequently extend up into the base of the skull. A number of these can be removed by the transoral route, but if they extend in any manner into the neck, an external procedure may be necessary. The mandibular osteotomy approach allows for good access and removal.

Cysts can either arise in the tonsil fossa or in the lingual surface of the hypopharynx of the epiglottis, or they may arise as a solitary retention cyst in the aryepiglottic fold, arytenoid, or hypopharyngeal areas. These can be recognized by their smooth shape and the yellow appearance of their surface. One should remove it entirely rather than merely biting into it and marsupializing the cavity. This allows the cystic contents to evacuate.

Perhaps the commonest location for *mixed tumors* seen in the oral cavity is the region of the tonsil and soft palate (Fig.

37–1). They are sometimes mistaken for a peritonsillar abscess, but the clinical history, lack of inflammation, and rubbery sensation upon palpation should lead one to suspect a mixed tumor. The removal in some cases should be planned in conjunction with an external approach. The large intraoral tumors may extend into the pterygomaxillary fossa or may represent extension from the deep lobe of the parotid gland. Frozen

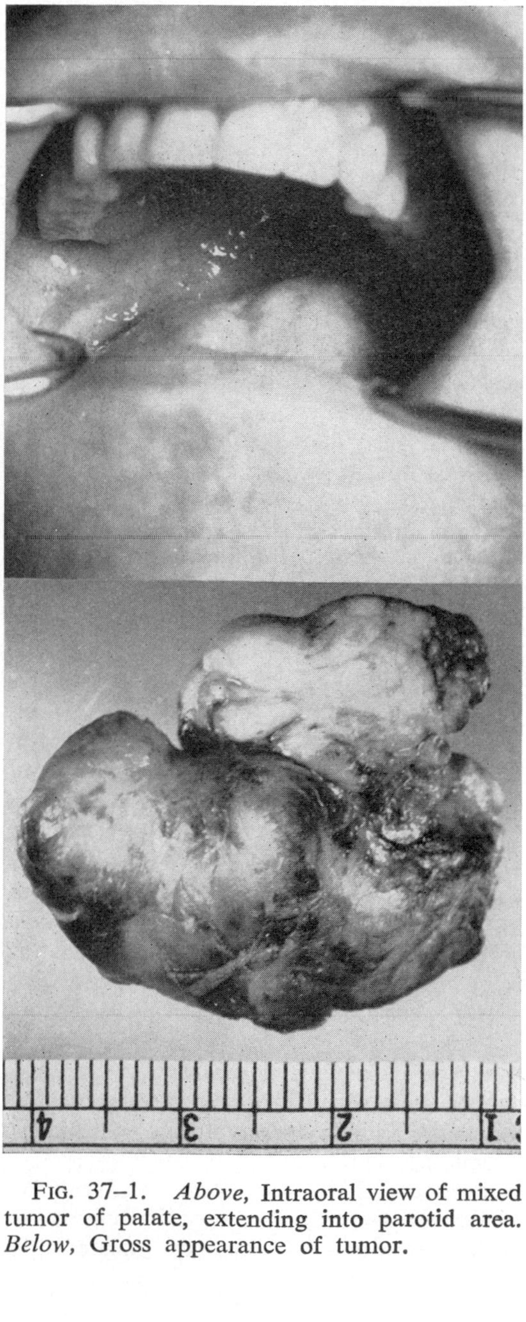

FIG. 37–1. *Above,* Intraoral view of mixed tumor of palate, extending into parotid area. *Below,* Gross appearance of tumor.

section may occasionally be necessary, but an open biopsy is seldom necessary. Since many of these can recur, it is important not to take a biopsy initially. On the other hand, if a biopsy has been taken when the case is first seen, the mucous membrane area should be left with the specimen so as not to contaminate the surgical field. To obtain proper exposure, a mandibular osteotomy approach has been done as a primary surgical attack.

Surgical Treatment. The surgical approach for benign tumors in the area of the tonsil and hypopharynx should be planned with several objectives in mind. Consideration should be given to the ease of resection and the possibility of recurrences. Hypopharyngeal tumors located in the piriform fossa and below the glossoepiglottic fold require a transhyoid pharyngotomy approach. However, tumors in the base of the tongue, off the midline, are better approached by a mandibular osteotomy technique. A tumor that is in the midline of the base of the tongue is best approached by splitting the mandible and incising downward along the median raphe of the tongue. In general, transoral removal should be limited to a large benign tumor or a small carcinoma. Thus clinically the lesion might eventually prove to represent a superficial cancer, and the recurrence rate is minimal. Transoral resection is limited to those types of benign tumors which are not apt to recur if removal is not complete.

MALIGNANT TUMORS OF THE TONSIL AND BASE OF THE TONGUE

Anatomy. The palatine tonsils are two lymphoid structures located on either side of the lateral wall of the oropharynx between the anterior and posterior pillars. The inferior poles of the tonsils form a lingual extension to the base of the tongue. The lymphatics are quite rich from the tonsil draining into the jugulodigastric node area.

Malignancies. Cancer of the tonsil is the second most common form of cancer of the upper air passage superseded only by cancer of the hypopharynx. It is estimated that it accounts for approximately 2% of all forms of cancer.

Pathology. Most malignancies of the tonsils are located at the upper poles, appear ulcerated, and when first seen are thought to be inflammatory in type or are commonly mistaken for Vincent's angina. Occasionally they are bulky. Ninety% of the malignant tumors arising from the tonsils are squamous cell carcinomas, and the remaining are unclassified or undifferentiated to the extent that they may be thought of as lymphoepitheliomas by some pathologists. The second common form is a lymphosarcoma or a variant of this type, e.g., reticulum cell sarcoma.

Clinical Evolution. Generally tumors that are superficial on the tonsil elicit few complaints. However, when they spill past the anterior pillar or extend into the base of the tongue, pain or discomfort is a frequent complaint. Otalgia on the same side is common with ulcerating lesions. Physical examination often shows the presence of an enlarged palpable lymph node in almost 50% of the cases.

Diagnosis. One should be suspicious when such a lesion is seen for the first time. Whereas inflammatory lesions are not indurated, neoplastic tumors are commonly firm to palpation.

A biopsy of the tumor should be performed in order to establish the diagnosis. If the pathologic examination reveals an anaplastic undifferentiated tumor which is not classifiable or a lymphosarcoma, the treatment should consist of a full course of radiotherapy.

The response of squamous cell carcinoma of the tonsil to irradiation in a series at this hospital has shown a 60% (12 of 18) 5-year survival rate by irradiation alone. Only two cases required neck dissection alone. Eight patients had clinically positive nodes which were controlled by irradiation. However, in this series half of them were women. All the failures were due to the fact that the primary lesion initially was quite large and was not controlled by irradiation. The good responses were established in those cases in which the tumor was restricted to the tonsil and was less than 1.25 cm in total size. Until a few years ago it was our practice to wait for recurrence or persistence of tumor following irradiation before surgical management was considered. All these cases (40%) failed in spite of radical surgery after tumor recrudescence.

Surgical Management. Whether a case should be treated by irradiation and surgery depends upon the situation when it is first seen. The area of resection compatible with reasonable deglutition and speech is outlined in the anatomic drawing (see Fig. 36–2). Small superficial lesions of the tonsil without palpable nodes are best treated by a full course of radiotherapy. Nodes are occasionally clinically positive with small lesions and are usually high in the jugular system. Large malignant tumors of the tonsil may extend past the anterior pillar or become attached to the jaw. They may extend inferiorly to involve part of the base of the tongue or may extend into the retromolar trigone and soft palate. Any extension of tumor into these sites is generally considered a poor prognostic sign. Nearly all these cases are associated with palpable nodes. These cases are considered for treatment using planned preoperative irradiation followed by a jaw-neck dissection. In such cases, the tumor should not cross the midline of the soft palate area. When initially seen, it should not encroach on the uvula.

A preoperative dose of 3000 R is delivered by external means to the primary tumor over a 3-week period. Usually moderate regression is noted; persistent ulceration may be noted in the sulcus of the lingual tonsil area, or residual firmness may be noted on palpation. In this situation, therapy is discontinued and the patient is allowed to rest for 1 week. During this time a reevaluation of his medical status is done prior to the jaw-neck dissection.

Whether the mandible should be sacrificed or not depends on the initial examination. If the tumor, when first seen, is not attached to the mandible, a mandibular osteotomy is carried out and the mandible is spared. However, if the tumor still shows residual attachment to the angle of the mandible, segmental resection of the mandible or a greater composite segment of resection is carried out in combination with a neck dissection (Fig. 37–2). There are two things to be stressed. First, if an operative procedure is carried out late after irradiation, a

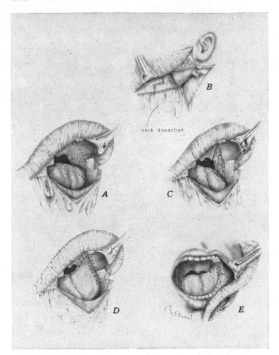

FIG. 37–2. Cancer of the tonsil—composite resection. *A,* Lesion of left tonsil. *B,* Osteotomy without removal of mandible. *C,* After excision. *D,* Repair by tongue rotation to cover raw area. *E,* Operative result.

tremendous effort should be made to preserve the carotid artery system. The carotid arteries and their branches are buried under the scalene muscle flap, and a part of the tongue is mobilized to close the defect in the oropharynx. Second, if a segmental jaw resection is done in order to protect the carotid system and eliminate dysphagia, a forehead flap is used. After reconstruction, the forehead flap is returned. If, however, the jaw should be preserved, then the mucoperiosteal reflection of the alveolus is spared for anastomosing with part of the tongue to obtain closure.

One striking feature is noted in a small series of cases in which we have done this operation, namely that immediate recurrences, in terms of 2 years, have been unusual. The functional results are good, and at present it appears that combined preoperative irradiation and resection of the tonsil and tongue is a worthwhile procedure (Fig. 37–2).

Results. Prior to the advent of preoperative irradiation, experience is limited to two types of cases. In the group treated by external irradiation alone and secondary surgery for persistent nodes, there were 27 patients with 12 5-year survivals. Eight of the 12 were female. Eight of the 12 had positive nodes. This is a 40% survival. In the group (20 patients) treated by composite resection without irradiation during 1952–1957, staged as II and III, only 6 or 30% have survived for 5 years.

REFERENCES

Alonso, J.: Conservation Surgery of Cancer of the Larynx. Trans. Am. Acad. Ophthal. Otolaryng., *51*:633, 1947.

Alonso, J.: *Cancer Laringeo.* Madrid, Paz Montalvo, 1954.

Asherson, N.: Pharyngectomy for Postcricoid Cancer; One Stage Operation with Reconstruction of Pharynx Using Larynx as Autograft. J. Laryngol., *68*:550, 1954.

Bauer, W., *et al.*: Significance of Positive Margins in Hemilaryngectomy. Laryngoscope, *85*:1, 1975.

Boles, R., and Komorn, R.: Carcinoma of the Laryngeal Glottis: A Five-year Review at a University Hospital. Laryngoscope, *79*:909, 1969.

Brown, J. B., and McDowell, F.: *Neck Dissection.* Publication #207, Monograph in Bannerstone Division of American Lectures in Surgery. Springfield, Ill., Charles C Thomas, Publisher, 1954.

Clerf, L. H.: Keratosis of Larynx. J.A.M.A., *132*:823, 1946.

Clerf, L. H., Putney, F. J., and O'Keefe, J. J.: Carcinoma of the Larynx. Laryngoscope, *58*:632, 1948.

Conley, J. J.: Vocal rehabilitation by autogenous vein graft. Ann. Otol., *68*:990, 1959.

Conley, J. J.: One Stage Radical Resection of Cervical Esophagus, Larynx, Pharynx, and Lateral Neck, with Immediate Reconstruction. Arch. Otolaryng., *58*:645, 1953.

Crile, G.: Excision of Cancer of Head and Neck. J.A.M.A., *47*:1780, 1906.

Ennyer, A., and Bataini, P.: Treatment of Supraglottic Carcinoma by Telecobalt Therapy. Br. J. Radiol., *38*:661, 1965.

Fletcher, G. H.: Clinical Dose-response Curves of Human Malignant Epithelial Tumors. Br. J. Radiol., *46*:1, 1973.

Fletcher, G. H., *et al.*: Place of Radiotherapy in Management of Squamous Cell Carcinoma of the Supraglottic Larynx. Am. J. Roentgen., *108*:19, 1970.

Goepfert, H., *et al.*: Optimal Treatment for Technically Resectable Squamous Cell Carcinomas of the Supraglottic Larynx. Laryngoscope, *46*:130, 1975.

Goodyear, H. M.: Hemilaryngectomy; Method of maintaining a Satisfactory Airway and Voice. Ann. Otol., *58*:581, 1949.

Grossman, A. A., and Mathews, W. H.: Keratosis of larynx with Progression to Malignancy. Canad. Med. Assoc. J., *66*:39, 1952.

Heller, J. R.: Director, National Cancer Institute, Washington, D.C. Testimony given before House Appropriation Committee, May, 1960.

Hendrickson, F. R., and Liebner, E.: (No title listed.) Ann. Otol., *77*:222, 1968.

Hibbs, G. G., *et al.*: Radiotherapy for Early Stages of Vocal Cord Cancer. Ann. Otol., *78*: 319, 1969.

Holtz, S., *et al.*: Contrast Examination of the Larynx and Pharynx; Glottic, Infraglottic and Transglottic. Am. J. Roentgen., *89*:10, 1963.

Horiot, J. C., *et al.*: Analysis of Failures in Early Vocal Cord Cancer. Radiology, *103*: 663, 1972.

Huffman, W. C., and Dierle, D. M.: Neck Dissections. Plast. Reconstr. Surg., *11*:115, 1953.

Jackson, C.: Cancer of the Larynx. Ann. Surg., *71*:1, 1923.

Jackson, C., and Jackson, C. L.: *Carcinoma of the Larynx*. Philadelphia, W. B. Saunders Co., 1939.

Jackson, C. L.: Personal Communication and Association with Committee on Classification and Staging of Cancer of the Larynx.

Jackson, C. L., *et al.*: Carcinoma of the Larynx: Survey of Twenty-five Years' Experience in Treatment by Surgery and Irradiation. J.A.M.A. *163*:1567, 1957.

Lederman, M.: Place of Radiotherapy in Treatment of Cancer of the Larynx. Br. Med. J., *1*:1639, 1961.

Lederman, M., and Dalley, V. M.: The Treatment of Glottic Cancer: The Importance of Radiotherapy to the Patient. J. Laryngol., *79*:767, 1965.

LeJune, F. E., and Lynch, M. G.: Value of the Laryngofissure Operation. Ann. Otol., *64*:256, 1955.

McGavran, M. H., *et al.*: Laryngofissure in the Treatment of Laryngeal Carcinoma; a Critical Analysis of Success and Failure. Laryngoscope, *69*:44, 1959.

McGavran, M. H., *et al.*: Isolated Laryngeal Keratosis: Its Relation to Carcinoma of the Larynx Based on a Clinicopathologic Study of Eighty-seven Consecutive Cases with Long Term Follow-up. Laryngoscope, *70*:932, 1960.

McGavran, M. H., *et al.*: The Incidence of Cervical Lymph Node Metastases from Epidermoid Carcinoma of the Larynx and Their Relationship to Certain Characteristics of the Primary Tumor; a Study Based on the Clinical and Pathologic Findings in Ninety-six Patients Treated by En Bloc Laryngectomy and Radical Neck Dissection. Cancer, 14: 55, 1961.

McGavran, M. H., *et al.*: Carcinoma of the piriform sinus. Arch. Otolaryng., *78*:826, 1963.

McGavran, M. H., *et al.*: Small Dose Preoperative Radiation Therapy. Radiology, *83*: 509, 1964.

Martin, H., *et al.*: Neck Dissection. Cancer, *4*:441, 1951.

Meurman, Y.: Operative Mediofixation of the Vocal Cord in Complete Unilateral Paralysis. Arch. Otolaryng., *52*:544, 1952.

Morbidity from Cancer in the United States. Public Health Monograph #56, U.S. Department of Health, Education and Welfare, Jan., 1958.

Ogura, J. H.: Supraglottic Subtotal Laryngectomy and Radical Neck Dissection for Carcinoma of the Epiglottis. Laryngoscope, 68:983, 1958.

Ogura, J. H.: Cancer of Larynx, Pharynx, and Upper Cervical Esophagus; Five Year Results of Laryngectomy and Radical Neck Dissection for Laryngeal Cancer. Arch. Otolaryng., 72:66, 1960.

Ogura, J. H.: Cancer of the Larynx and Hypopharynx. Am. J. Med. Sci., *244*:501, 1962.

Ogura, J. H.: Management of Early Cancer of the Vocal Cord—Laryngofissure, Hemilaryngectomy and Irradiation. Trans. Pacific Coast Ophthal. Otol. Soc., 47th Annual Meeting, Seattle, Washington, May, 1963.

Ogura, J. H., and Bello, J. A.: Laryngectomy and Radical Neck Dissection for Carcinoma of the Larynx. Laryngoscope, *62*:1, 1952.

Ogura, J. H., and Mallen, R. W.: Carcinoma of the Larynx; Diagnosis and Treatment. Postgrad. Med., *34*:493, 1963.

Ogura, J. H., and Mallen, R. W.: Partial Laryngopharyngectomy for Supraglottic and Pharyngeal Carcinoma. Trans. Am. Acad. Ophthal. Otolaryng., *69*:832, 1965.

Ogura, J. H., and Mallen, R. W.: Conservation Surgery for Cancer of the Epiglottis and

Hypopharynx. *In* Conley, J. J. (Ed.) : *Proceedings International Workshop, Cancer of the Head and Neck.* Australia, Butterworths, 1967, pp. 407–422.

Ogura, J. H., *et al.*: Laryngograms: Their Value in the Diagnosis and Treatment of Laryngeal Lesions; a Study Based on Clinical, Radiographic, and Pathologic Findings on Ninety-nine Patients with Cancer of the Larynx. Laryngoscope, *70*:780, 1960.

Ogura, J. H., *et al.*: Partial Laryngopharyngectomy and Neck Dissection for Pyriform Sinus Cancer; Conservation Surgery with Immediate Reconstruction. Laryngoscope, *70*:1399, 1960.

Ogura, J. H., *et al.*: Partial Pharyngectomy and Neck Dissection for Posterior Hypopharyngeal Cancers; Immediate Reconstruction with Preservation of Voice. Laryngoscope, *70*:1523, 1960.

Ogura, J. H., *et al.*: Experiences with Conservative Surgery in Laryngeal and Pharyngeal Carcinoma. Laryngoscope, *71*:258, 1961.

Orton, H. B.: Lateral Transthyroid Pharyngotomy; Trotter's Operation for Malignant Conditions of the Laryngopharynx. Trans. Am. Laryngol. Assoc., *52*:91, 1930.

Orton, H. B.: Treatment of Extensive Cancer of the Larynx. Laryngoscope, *61*:496, 1951.

Perez, C. A., *et al.*: Irradiation of Early Carcinoma of the Larynx. Arch. Otol., *93*:465, 1971.

Pietrantoni, L., and Fior, R.: Clinical and Surgical Problems of Cancer of the Larynx and Hypopharynx. Acta. Otol. (Suppl.), *142*:1, 1958.

Powers, W. E., *et al.*: Contrast Examination of the Larynx and Pharynx. Radiology, *68*: 169, 1957.

Powers, W. E., *et al.*: Contrast Examination of the Larynx and Pharynx; Accuracy and Value in Diagnosis and Therapy. N. Y. State J. Med., *63*:1163, 1963.

Pressman, J. J.: Personal Communication.

Pressman, J. J.: Extended Retrohyoid Radical Neck Dissection for Cancer of Oral Cavity and Neck. Surg. Gynecol. Obstet., *100*:329, 1955.

Putney, F. J.: Preventive Dissection of the Neck in Cancer of the Larynx. Ann. Otol., *67*:136, 1958.

Putney, F. J., and O'Keefe, J. J.: Clinical Significance of Keratosis of Larynx as a Premalignant Lesion. Ann. Otol., *62*:348, 1953.

Reed, G. F.: Neck Dissection; Its Role in Cancer of the Larynx. Laryngoscope, *66*: 237, 1956.

Schall, L. A.: Cancer of the Larynx; Five Year Results. Laryngoscope, *61*:517, 1951.

Sessions, D. G., *et al.*: Laryngeal Carcinoma Involving Anterior Commissure and Subglottis. Can. J. Otolaryngol., *4*(4):666, 1975.

Som, M. L.: Hemilaryngectomy; Modified Technique for Cordal Cancer with Extension Posteriorly. Arch. Otolaryng., *54*: 524, 1951.

Som, M. L.: Laryngoesophagectomy; Primary Closure with Laryngotracheal Autograft. Arch. Otolaryng., *63*:474, 1956.

Spjut, H., *et al.*: Unpublished Data on Clinical and Pathologic Findings of Nodal Metastasis from Cancer of the Piriform Sinus.

Trotter, W.: Method of Lateral Pharyngotomy for Exposure of Large Growths of Epipharyngeal region. J. Laryngol., *35*:289, 1920.

Wang, C. C., *et al.*: Combined Radiation Therapy and Surgery for Carcinoma of the Supraglottic and Pyriform Sinus. Laryngoscope, *82*:1883, 1972.

Wynder, E. L., *et al.*: Study of Environmental Factors in Cancer of the Larynx. Cancer, *9*: 86, 1956.

Chapter 38

Tumor Immunology: An Overview*

H. Bryan Neel III

It has been clearly established that malignant tumors in animals have cell-surface antigens that are different from those of the tissue from which they arise—hence, the term tumor-specific antigens (TSA). By definition TSA exist neither in the normal tissues of the host nor in the tissues of animals isogenic to this host. Their presence has been demonstrated in tumors induced by chemicals and viruses as well as in tumors arising spontaneously. Largely responsible for this discovery was the development and use of syngeneic, or genetically identical, animals for tumor transplantation studies.

Gross first demonstrated that active immunization of mice, using transplants of methylcholanthrene (MCA)-induced tumor of recent origin, provided immunity to subsequent transplants of the same tumor.[26] However, the possibility exists that this tumor may have arisen in a mouse bearing a mutant gene at some histoincompatibility locus because he did not cross-challenge with another syngeneic tumor. Subsequently, Lewis and Aptekman showed immunity to sarcoma and carcinoma in a strain of rats that they considered inbred.[47] Primary tumors were rendered ischemic by temporarily wrapping the base of the tumor with a tourniquet, that is, ligation and release. This

led to atrophy of tumor and presumably to "absorption" of TSA. A second graft of the same tumor was rejected in the animals in which the tumor had been strangled, but not in control animals.

The first clear demonstration of tumor-specific transplantation immunity (TSTI) was made in the classic experiments of Foley.[20] With an established line of inbred mice and tumors recently induced by methylcholanthrene in animals from the same inbred stock, he used the technique of ligation and release of the tumor and subsequent challenge with a graft of the same tumor at various intervals. Animals in which ligation produced tumor regression were challenged with viable tumor introduced by a trocar, and the incidence of subsequent tumor growth at the challenge site was compared with that in untreated syngeneic controls. Unquestionable resistance was demonstrated against the MCA-induced sarcomas, but not against unrelated spontaneous mammary carcinomas.

Foley's results were confirmed by Prehn and Main.[71] They demonstrated conclusively that genetic differences among tumor hosts were not responsible for the findings. This was established by (1) reciprocal skin grafting between animals, (2) pretreatment with normal tissues from the original mouse (which failed to induce resistance to tumor),

*Reproduced in part from Mayo Clinic Proceedings, *49*:118, 1974.[74] By permission.

and (3) the finding that skin from the primary tumor host was not rejected when grafted to syngeneic mice pretreated with the tumor, as noted by Sjögren.[79] Therefore, it was established definitely that the antigens involved were unique to and confined to or within tumor tissue, and not shared with normal tissues. The tumor protected the host against subsequent growth of grafts of the same tumor, but grafts of normal tissues did not confer this immunity.

Using a slightly different approach, Révész confirmed Prehn and Main's experiments and introduced a new technique for producing TSTI.[72] His method of immunization was not by temporary tumor growth, but rather with two separate subcutaneous inocula of tumor cells that had been irradiated. Although these irradiated tumor cells were irreversibly damaged and unable to replicate, they still retained strong isoantigenic activity. In addition, he used quantitated cell inocula instead of trocar transplants for challenge. This technique enabled him to demonstrate that weak host resistance against the growth of the graft of the tumor may be masked easily by the rapid proliferation of large doses of tumor, such as those introduced with the trocar. This masking is a consequence of the rate of tumor-cell replication being quantitatively greater than the primary immunocompetent clonal proliferation, as well as of the relatively weak antigenic stimulus of TSA. The importance of this was apparent to Hammond and associates,[27] who demonstrated TSTI to spontaneous mouse tumors. After amputation of the primary tumor, TSTI was demonstrated in these hosts when appropriate challenge dosages were selected.

Klein and co-workers have shown that autochthonous hosts can also be made resistant to challenge with their own primary tumor by repeated immunizations with irradiated cells of the same tumor.[41] This excluded completely the possibility that genetic differences in animals played a role in the tumor-specific immune reactions against chemically induced tumors. Of additional importance in the studies of Klein and associates was the finding that pretreatment with an unrelated tumor does not result in protection against subsequent transplantation of another tumor induced by the same chemical.

Several important principles have evolved from this series of transplantation experiments. (1) Tumors of recent origin must be used in studies of tumor-specific transplantation immunity because, with serial passage through many generations, the tumor may undergo antigenic change. Tumors may contain isoantigens that were present in the primary host, but are no longer present in the animal strain because of continued inbreeding. (2) Use of single-cell suspensions of graded doses of viable tumor cells is required to detect tumor-specific immunity, because tumor-specific antigens are relatively "weak" and reflect minor immunologic differences. (3) The specificity of the immune response to the tumor must be confirmed by challenge with another tumor, a tumor other than that used initially to immunize the host but originating in the same strain. (4) Syngeneity of the animals must be confirmed by reciprocal skin grafting to determine that the immunity is tumor-specific—that it is conferred neither by normal tissues of the primary host nor by the tissues of animals isogenic to that host.

Given these facts, it became apparent that resistance to subsequent transplantation of grafts of the same tumor could be induced by tumor excision or amputation, by use of sub-take tumor dose, by use of cells that had been irreversibly damaged in their reproductive capacity by irradiation or chemicals, or by necrosis in situ by ligation-release,[47,68,83] cryosurgery,[58-62] or electrocoagulation. A comparison of TSTI after excision, cryosurgery, ligation-release, and electrocoagulation of tumors in a standardized murine tumor-host system is shown in Figure 38–1. Mice from which tumors had been excised showed a reduced rate of growth at the challenge site, compared to controls, indicating existence of immunity after excision. Mice from which tumor had been eradicated in situ by cryosurgery, ligation-release, or electrocoagulation showed a reduced rate of tumor take and growth at the challenge site, compared to controls and to mice subjected to tumor excision, indicating even greater immunity after necrosis of tumor in situ. The *pattern* of differential

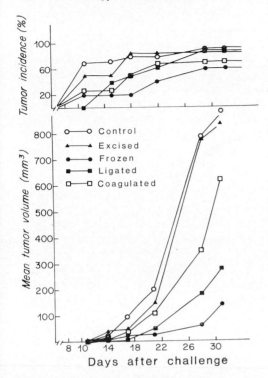

FIG. 38–1. Methylcholanthrene-induced tumors (1.0 ± 0.2 cm in diameter) in $C_{57}BL/6J$ mice were excised, frozen cryosurgically, rendered ischemic by ligation-release, or electrocoagulated; cured mice were challenged with 10^4 viable cells of the same tumor 3 weeks after treatment. Shown are cumulative tumor incidences and mean tumor volumes after challenge.

immunity is consistently seen after challenge with graded doses of tumor cells and in other tumor-host systems (H. B. Neel III, unpublished data).

It has been shown convincingly in syngeneic tumor-host systems that a chemically induced tumor will not cross-react with another chemically induced tumor in most instances, even if the identical carcinogen is used repeatedly in the same animal.[65,66] Although virus-induced tumors have tumor-specific transplantation antigens (TSTA), they also have a common neoantigen that is virus-specific.[33,89] Regardless of the tissue affected or the species of animals used, virus-induced tumors cross-react with a common viral antigen and, therefore, with other tumors induced by that virus. For this

reason, an alternative method of immunization against virus-induced tumors exists: active immunization can be induced by infection with the tumor-inciting virus and will produce resistance to transplants of all tumors induced by that virus.

HUMAN TUMOR ANTIGENS

Considerable effort has been directed toward detecting TSA in human neoplasms.[5,23,24,42,43,51,53–55,86,87,91,92,94] A few of these human tumor antigens exhibit a specificity similar to that of embryonal tissue derived from the same histogenetic origin, provided the tissue had not differentiated or "matured" beyond six months of gestation.[23,24,86] Initially, these findings appeared to be monospecific within one histogenetic organ system (e.g., the colon carcinoma-embryonic antigens [CEA]),[23,24,45,85] but recent clinical evidence indicates that antibody titers to CEA are elevated in bronchogenic carcinoma[78] as well as in non-neoplastic disease. However, higher levels are generally associated with neoplasia. These data reinforce the idea that oncogenesis probably involves a loss of mature, differentiated, "self" surface antigens to an embryonal specificity on the tumor-cell surfaces rather than the generation of a true neoantigen, as is seen in viral-transformed neoplasia.[76] At least two corollary observations in human cancer are consonant with this possibility. In carcinoma of the cervix, normal isoantigens are gradually lost and this loss appears to be temporally related to the increasing severity of malignant transformation, as judged histologically by the degree of metaplasia and of invasiveness.[15] A loss of normal gastric mucosal antigenic substance has been found in patients who have carcinoma of the stomach.[11]

It is clear from several penetrating studies that, in viral-transformed animal tumors, the change in the surface membrane of tumor cells is related to the loss of contact inhibition that "permits" unregulated, disorderly growth.[8,9,70]

The structure of tumor antigens closely resembles that of normal human HL-A or the murine H-2 counterpart. Tumor antigens are glycoproteins with molecular

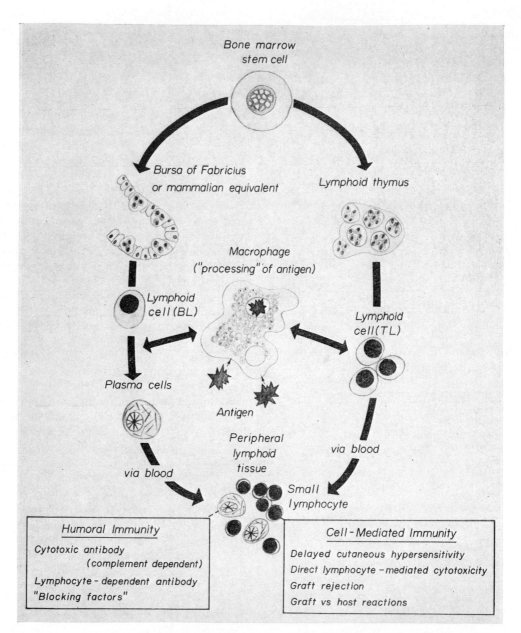

Fig. 38–2. Evolution and regulation of cellular and humoral immune mechanisms. Thymus-dependent lymphocytes (TL) control cell-mediated immunity while bursa-dependent lympho-cytes (BL) and plasma cells produce immunoglobulin (antibodies). Specificity of immune response depends on macrophage "processing" of antigen. (Modified from Neel, H. B., III, and Ritts, R. E., Jr.[62] By permission of the Annals Publishing Company.)

weights of about 50,000 daltons, but all studies to date have failed to identify the precise chemical nature of the immunogenic moiety of a specific cancer antigen. It is apparent that tumor antigens have a significant polysaccharide component, which is thought to be responsible for their specificity.[6,9,28,29,52]

IMMUNE MECHANISMS

A simplified schema of the developmental aspects and cellular components of the immune system is shown in Figure 38–2. Two prominent, functionally different lymphocyte cell lines arise from primordial stem cells of the marrow (Table 38–1). The most numerous of these are the small lymphocytes developing under thymic regulation, T cells or T lymphocytes (TL), which comprise 70 to 80% of the lymphocytes circulating in thoracic duct lymph and blood. These cells retain immunologic memory and are responsible for the immunologic response to cancer, either by direct cytotoxic interaction with the tumor cell or by

Table 38–1.   Characteristics of the Two Major Lymphocyte Populations

Functions	T lymphocytes (70–80%) Cell-mediated immunity (CMI)	B lymphocytes (15–20%) Humoral immunity (HI)
Blastogenesis		
PHA	+	−
Con A	+	−
PWM	−	+
Identification		
Attraction to SRBC	+	−
Electron microscopy	Smooth	Irregular
Surface immunoglobulins	−	+
Memory	Yes	Unknown

Table 38–2.   Putative Mediators of Cellular Immunity Associated with Lymphocytes

Direct toxicity upon interaction with target cells	
Preformed substances in immunocompetent lymphocytes	
Cytophilic antibody	Principally IgM bound antibody
Lymph node permeability factor	
Transfer factor	In vivo transfer of cell-mediated immunity
"Lymphokines" released by antigen stimulation	
Blastogenic factors	Induce lymphocyte blastogenesis
Chemotactic factors	Stimulate monocytic migration
Interferon	Prevents new virus replication
Lymphocyte transforming factor	Sensitizes "normergic" lymphocytes to respond to new antigen
Lymphotoxin	Nonspecific cytotoxicity
Migration inhibitory factor	Activates macrophages and inhibits their migration from antigen-containing areas
Skin-reactive factor	Mimics skin reactivity, in vivo monocytic infiltration

Modified from Neel, H. B., III and Ritts, R. E., Jr.[62]

the elaboration and release of a considerable number of mediators referred to as "lymphokines" (Table 38–2). TL are also responsible for delayed cutaneous hypersensitivity reactions, defense against intracellular organisms, graft rejection, and graft-versus-host reactions. Sensitization of one TL leads to a proliferation of a population of similarly sensitized cells.

Less numerous are the lymphocytes developing under the influence of the bursa of Fabricius in birds and its unidentified equivalent in mammals. These cells—B cells or B lymphocytes (BL)—comprise about 15 to 20% of circulating lymphocytes, and their progeny elaborate antibodies, some of which may be cytotoxic. Antibody may be inimical to host survival because it can combine with antigen and form complexes (blocking factors) that intercede in the tumor cell-TL cytotoxic reaction.

Macrophages are the fundamental phagocytic cells. They migrate to engulf both insoluble or particulate (including cellular) and soluble antigens and, more important, "process" them. Processing involves endogenous ribonucleic acid (RNA), which acts perhaps as an adjuvant or as a constituent in the encoding mechanism. The newly encoded "message" is transmitted to other effector cells—the BL and plasma cells that generate specific antibodies (immunoglobulins) and the TL. TL possess immunologic memory and effect cell-mediated immunity (CMI) or delayed cutaneous hypersensitivity, either directly or indirectly via the "lymphokines" and other preformed substances (Table 38–2). The final pathway of these interactions leads to phagocytosis, release of lysosomal enzymes, and degradation of antigen.

Host Response to Tumor. Cell-mediated immune mechanisms are primarily responsible for rejection of normal tissue grafts in genetically dissimilar individuals, and it appears that the major immunologic defense against cancer is mediated similarly.[74] This observation was based on early studies in which adoptive transfer of sensitized spleen cells or lymph node cells conveyed tumor-specific transplantation immunity. This was first demonstrated in 1962 by Old and associates,[66] and several more recent reports confirm that immunity to tumor-specific transplantation antigens may be transferred passively. Injections of either sensitized spleen cells or lymph node cells by several routes, including intravenous or intraperitoneal injection, can mediate tumor destruction successfully provided the tumor "dose" or "burden" is small. Similarly, admixtures of tumor cells and spleen cells, lymph node cells, or leukocytes (particularly lymphocytes) from a specifically immunized host prevent or retard tumor growth when such mixtures are introduced into syngeneic hosts.[41] This test is referred to as "neutralization," and subsequent studies of adoptive transfer have been used to assay CMI to a variety of chemically, physically, and virally induced tumors.

It has become apparent that humoral antibodies do play a role in the immunobiology of tumor growth. The paradoxic phenomenon of tumor enhancement is well known. It resulted from attempts to immunize animals against a tumor transplant, attempts that resulted not only in successful takes, but also in more rapid tumor growth than in nonimmunized control animals.[39] This was implicitly understood to be caused by a tumor-specific antibody coating the tumor cells in vivo and protecting them against cell-mediated destruction. In contrast, serum from tumor-bearing animals may actually convey a protective effect in vivo, even when the donors have gross metastases.[63] Incubation of sera with tumor suspensions also yields divergent responses. The incidence of tumor take at the site of inoculation and the growth of tumor are suppressed, apparently unaffected, or enhanced, depending upon the quantity of antibody injected.[25,41] Combined with suspensions of tumor cells, serum antibodies are often cytotoxic in the presence of complement, but they may also form antigen-antibody complexes that induce a protective effect by "blocking" or preventing tumor-cell destruction by immune lymphocytes.

The Hellströms have offered impressive evidence, both in animal models and in certain human neoplasia (e.g., neuroblastoma),[30,31] that there is actual enhancement of tumor growth resulting from a humoral blocking factor. Indeed, in neuroblastoma there was an inverse correlation between the amount of blocking factor and the patient's recovery or survival. Further, specific cell-mediated reactivity against this tumor was intact both in survivors and in those who died. Equally interesting was the observation that the lymphocytes of unaffected parents or siblings of the patients frequently were immunologically reactive against neuroblastoma. It does not require much imagination to invoke an infectious-genetic implication from these data.

Immunosurveillance. In 1959, Thomas suggested that the host possessed a normal homeostatic cellular mechanism that was active in preventing establishment of "nonself."[84] Burnet later termed this homeostatic mechanism immunosurveillance.[10] There is considerable support, both clinical and experimental, for this concept. However, animal transplantation experiments, as well as the simple evidence of the occurrence of cancer in humans, indicate that the mechanism is not totally effective or perhaps even operative under certain circumstances. In contrast to some experimental animal data, there is little evidence that the human host's immune system fails to recognize a neoplastic growth; rather, there is a diminishing ability to cope with it. In fact, with respect to the cellular expressions of immune competency in human cancer, any defect appears to be a general one manifest to all antigens, even those formerly recognized at a cellular level, rather than a specific one related to a specific tumor antigen. A possible exception to this generalization occurs in solid-tissue tumors, in which the appearance of a blocking antigen-antibody complex, specific for the tumor antigen, precludes the direct and indirect action of those cells that remain competent.

Among the more impressive indirect evidence establishing the phenomenon of surveillance in cancer are the observations that the frequency of neoplasia ranges from 10 to 15% in patients who have cellular immunodeficiency diseases—10,000 times that of an actuarially matched population[22]—and is 0.7% in patients who have received selective immunosuppressive therapy, primarily at the cellular level, for kidney transplantation.[56] It is interesting that the neo-plasia observed to occur in children with T-cell deficiency syndromes is most often (more than 60%) of the reticuloendothelial system. Spontaneous, complete regression of established tumors is uncommon, but cases are well documented; on the other hand, every physician has observed apparently "cured" patients for many years only to discover metastases as long as 20 years after ablation of the primary neoplasm. Lymphocytic infiltration of solid tumors, including squamous cell carcinoma of the head and neck, is associated with a better prognosis.[12] Surgeons, particularly those working with diseases of the head and neck, know that identification of viable tumor cells in wound washings or in circulation will not reliably predict local recurrence or survival.[2] Finally, immunologic mechanisms are relatively weak at the extremes of age—early childhood and late adulthood—and these are the times when the incidence of malignancy is greatest.

IMMUNODIAGNOSIS: AN IMMUNOLOGIC "PROFILE"

Skin Testing (Delayed Cutaneous Hypersensitivity). To assess CMI, simple recall reactivity to common antigens such as tuberculin (PPD), mumps virus, *Candida albicans,* and streptokinase-streptodornase may be assessed after intradermal injection. The site of injection is inspected at 48 hours and the reaction is considered positive if the diameter of induration is 5 mm or more. De novo sensitization is most commonly done with 2,4-dinitrochlorobenzene (DNCB), a simple chemical compound to which few people have been exposed. DNCB in acetone is applied to the skin. Nonspecific erythema and edema may appear within 12 hours of contact, but sensitization requires 7 to 21 days, at which time the test site is inspected for flare and induration. If there is no sensitization reaction in this period, patients are challenged again with a series of smaller doses of DNCB; the test results are considered positive if induration or bright red erythema, or both, particularly with blister formation, appear within 48 hours. Catalona et al. describe the method in detail.[13]

Skin testing requires participation of the patient, and therefore laboratory correlates of CMI have been developed and are now done in laboratories at many medical centers.

In Vitro T and B Lymphocyte Identification. There are many published reports of nonimmunoglobulin-mediated rosette formation of sheep red blood cells (SRBC) around TL. This attraction between SRBC and TL can be used to quantify TL from samples of peripheral venous blood. Most methods depend on separating the lymphocytes from whole blood and incubating them with the SRBC. Cell suspensions are counted in a hemocytometer well with transmitted light and phase microscopy. An alternative method uses fixed stained cells, which can be stored and examined at a later time.[32] The method also allows for accurate morphologic examination of the cells. Seventy to 80% of lymphocytes in blood are TL, depending on the method of assay.[32]

Lymphocytes with immunoglobulin markers (BL) can be identified specifically by immunofluorescence and phase microscopy. A commercially available polyvalent anti-human immunoglobulin conjugated with fluorescein is added to the lymphocyte pellet. Numerous fluorescent caps, or membrane beadings, are seen at microscopy on the surface of BL due to the presence of immunoglobulin (Table 38–1).

Stimulation of Lymphocytes With Mitogens and Specific Antigens (Blastogenic Transformation of Lymphocytes). In 1960, Nowell demonstrated that an extract of kidney beans (phytohemagglutinin or PHA) produced large blastlike cells in cultures of human blood, and it became apparent that the precursor cell of these blasts was the small lymphocyte.[64] Activators such as PHA, *Concanavalin A* (Con A), and pokeweed mitogen (PWM), which stimulate a sizable proportion of the lymphocytes of all normal individuals, can be classed as nonspecific, and those that stimulate only lymphocytes from sensitized individuals can be classed as specific (e.g., tumor extracts and antigens such as PPD). Although these lectins are polyclonal in their effect, PHA and Con A predominately stimulate TL, and PWM predominately stimulates BL in mixed populations (Table 38–1). Transformation of lymphocytes is commonly quantitated by incorporating tritium-labeled thymidine into the lymphocyte DNA; this is readily done in the laboratory.

Immunoregulators. An apparent humoral blast-transforming inhibitor is found in patients who have cancer.[77,78,90] The cellular defect and the humoral suppressor of lymphocyte reactivity do not occur together in squamous carcinoma, whereas they coexist in sarcoma, suggesting at least two distinct mechanisms acting to impair the cellular response.[13] An α-2-globulin is increased in cancer and suppresses PHA-induced lymphoblastic transformation; presumably it is responsible for regulating the immunoregulatory feedback mechanism.[14] The inhibitors are likely to be glycoproteins known to inhibit antibody synthesis[57] and to suppress graft rejection.[40,49,57] These substances have also been observed in rodents that have MCA-induced tumors.[93] Tumor-specific sera with putative blocking effect may well be another class of immunoregulator,[30] but there is no evidence of direct lymphocytic inhibitory effect.

Macrophage Function. It would seem important to study macrophage function in patients who have solid-tissue cancer because macrophages are important in antigen recognition, processing, and storage and in antibody production. Macrophage inhibition is thought to be another correlate of CMI, although it has recently been suggested that BL may elaborate macrophage inhibitory factor (MIF). By exposure to specific antigen for 24 to 36 hours, macrophages with a few immune lymphocytes from sensitized hosts are inhibited from migrating from capillary tubes in tissue culture. Inhibition of normal macrophage function is effected by MIF, a soluble factor released from immune lymphocytes. The extent of inhibition of migration is taken as a rough measure of the degree of sensitivity of the cells. Inhibition is not observed in patients with defective CMI. The response is highly specific in animal systems, using several different tumors with distinct TSTAs, and in human disease.

Chemotaxis. Mononuclear leukocyte chemotactic responsiveness to various chemoattractants (e.g., culture filtrates of gram-negative organisms or casein) can be assessed in vitro by the use of modified Boyden chambers and polycarbonate filters. Chemotaxis may be an important parameter to measure because macrophages participate in the destruction of neoplastic cells.

The functional capacity of leukocytes to effect intracellular killing after phagocytosis can be measured by nitroblue tetrazolium reduction—the NBT test. Both intracellular killing and phagocytosis can be measured by opsonocytophagic assay and constitute important elements of an "immune profile."

Antibodies. Antibody-producing cells (BL) are readily identified and counted. Although serum immunoglobulin levels (IgG, IgM, IgA, IgE) are assayed by standardized techniques in most laboratories, current approaches to immunodiagnosis generally do not encompass identification of specific antibodies except in patients with nasopharyngeal carcinoma and Burkitt's lymphoma. Complement may indirectly reflect cytotoxic antibody activity because cytotoxic antibody bound to cell-surface determinants activates the complement sequence and leads to lysis of tumor cells in vitro. Lymphocyte-dependent antibody is another class of antibody, quite distinct from complement-dependent cytotoxic antibody. So-called blocking antibodies, or blocking factors, which appear to be antigen-antibody complexes, actually inhibit cytotoxic activity of immune lymphocytes in vitro and may enhance tumor growth.

SOLID-TISSUE NEOPLASIA

There are few well-controlled studies of the immune status of the more common solid-tissue neoplasias.[74] In patients who have solid tumors, no reports have been found that correlate all of several important considerations: type of cancer, clinical findings, staging, the status of skin reactivity, inhibition of macrophage migration, and the functional capacity of leukocytes to effect phagocytosis.

Cellular Immunity. The diminution or absence of delayed cutaneous hypersensitivity or cellular-mediated immunity has been frequently reported with tuberculin,[34,37] skin allografts,[1,4,36,75] cancer cell-line implants,[81] keyhole limpet hemocyanin,[68] and substituted nitrobenzenes[12,13,38,44] (e.g., dinitrochlorobenzene [DNCB]). The diminution of preexisting sensitivity to tuberculin and the diminished ability to respond to new antigen (e.g., DNCB) in patients with cancer, including those patients with squamous cell carcinoma in the head and neck, appear to be related directly to disease progression (Table 38–3). Indeed,

Table 38–3. Immunodiagnostic Test Results in Patients With Squamous Cell Carcinoma of the Head and Neck, by Stage

Stage of cancer*	DNCB negative (% patients)	Depressed blastogenesis (PHA)†(% patients)	Absolute TL levels (mean cells/mm³)
$T_1N_0M_0$	30	15	1,700
$T_2N_0M_0$	30	50	1,400
$T_3N_0M_0$	68	71	1,250
$T_{1-2}N_1M_0$	44	33	1,000
$T_{3-4}N_1M_0$	47	29	1,600
$T_{1-4}N_{2-3}M_0$	50	75	900
Benign head and neck tumors	—	15	1,800
Controls	5	0	1,900

*Two to 38 patients in each group.
†Values 2 SD below mean control level.
Data from Wanebo, H. J., Jun, M. Y., Strong, E. W., et al.[88]

patients who have the capacity to respond in delayed fashion to DNCB seem to have a better short-term prognosis.[18,50,88] The same general pattern of decreased reactivity with disease progression and somewhat better prognosis with intact response has been observed with tuberculin.

A progressive lymphopenia is observed in patients with bronchogenic carcinoma and in patients with squamous cell carcinoma in the head and neck.[44,50,88] Although the degree of lymphopenia has been correlated with survival time, neither a cause nor an effect relationship has been ascribed to this event, nor to the apparently parallel loss of reactivity to DNCB or the elevated IgA levels.

It is becoming increasingly evident that lymphocytic blastogenic transformation induced by phytohemagglutinin and by specific antigens, as an in vitro correlate of delayed-cutaneous hypersensitivity, is impaired in patients with cancer. Because the endpoint of such studies is unrelated to the inflammatory response, it is generally concluded that there is a cellular immune defect or diminution. These studies have given further information that, at least on an operational level, the failure to manifest cellular immunity in cancer is caused by a deficit or a malfunction, or both, of TL[12,16,17,21,67,69,82,88,90] (Table 38–3). In preliminary studies, the impression that failure to manifest cellular immunity is a poor prognostic event has been confirmed.[7,18,46,80] It has also been shown that successful chemotherapy (in terms of length of survival of patients who have bronchogenic carcinoma) is directly correlated with intact cellular immunity.[7]

Humoral Aspects. Elevated complement activity is seen in patients who have untreated malignancies of the bowel, breast, or lung.[35] These increased levels have been ascribed to specific elevations of the C8 and C9 components. This is not an event commonly seen in disease states, but it has been noted occasionally in some children who have immunodeficiency diseases associated with elevated IgA levels.

Primary antibody response to xenogenic erythrocytes and to tetanus toxoid is reported to be depressed.[48] It is of interest that heavy smokers without evidence of neo-plasia have lower hemagglutinin titers to sheep erythrocytes than do nonsmokers.[19] The more pronounced diminution of antibody responses was observed in advanced metastatic or terminal disease, but this fact makes interpretation difficult because of the absence of an appropriate age-matched control group wherein protein synthesis is meager, frequent profound leukopenia is seen, and potent cytotoxic chemotherapy or radiation has been administered. In well-controlled studies,[3,44] no significant alteration in antibody response was found. In a well-designed sequential study, no difference was found between controls and patients with bronchogenic carcinoma in their primary humoral response to diphtheria toxoid or to plague vaccine.[44] With the exception of long-surviving patients who had nonsignificant elevations of IgA, there was no difference in immunoglobulin levels.

Even though these observations give apparent insight into oncogenesis and are useful in clinical application, they require substantial validation, particularly in long-term clinical correlation, cell type of cancer, and staging. Without such information, it is difficult to perceive the exact significance for failure of the immunologic mechanism, much less consider a logical basis for rational immunotherapy. It appears that some patients with cancer die with functioning, intact immune systems. We know little about the significance of these findings. In fact, is cancer really a manifestation of an immune deficiency or are the immunologic perturbations secondary to the process—further evidence of the systemic nature of this disease?

REFERENCES

1. Amos, D. B., Hattler, B. G., and Shingleton, W. W.: Prolonged Survival of Skin-Grafts from Cancer Patients on Normal Recipients. Lancet, 1:414, 1965.
2. Arons, M. S., and Smith, R. R.: Distant Metastases and Local Recurrence in Head and Neck Cancer. Ann. Surg., 154:235, 1961.
3. Ashikawa, K., Motoya, K., Sekiguchi, M., et al.: Immune Response in Tumor-Bearing Patients and Animals. II. Incidence of Tuberculin Anergy in Cancer Patients. Gann, 58:565, 1967.

4. Ben-Hur, N., Wexler, M., Neuman, Z., et al.: Tissues with Antigenic Change in a Patient With Malignant Disease: An Experimental and Clinical Study. Harefuah, 77:41, 1969.

5. Björklund, B., and Björklund, V.: Antigenicity of Pooled Human Malignant and Normal Tissues by Cyto-immunological Technique: Presence of an Insoluble, Heat-Labile Tumor Antigen. Int. Arch. Allergy Appl. Immunol., 10:153, 1957.

6. Bouroncle, B. A., Clausen, K. P., and Aschenbrand, J. F.: Studies of the Delayed Response of Phytohemagglutinin (PHA) Stimulated Lymphocytes in 25 Chronic Lymphatic Leukemia Patients before and during Therapy. Blood, 34:166, 1969.

7. Brugarolas, A., and Takita, H.: Sequential Skin Tests in the Follow-Up of Patients with Carcinoma of the Lung (abstract). Clin. Res., 20:564, 1972.

8. Burger, M. M.: A Difference in the Architecture of the Surface Membrane of Normal and Virally Transformed Cells. Proc. Natl. Acad. Sci. U.S.A., 62:994, 1969.

9. Burger, M. M.: Proteolytic Enzymes Initiating Cell Division and Escape from Contact Inhibition of Growth. Nature (Lond), 227:170, 1970.

10. Burnet, F. M.: Immunological Surveillance. Sydney, Australia, Pergamon Press, Inc., 1970.

11. Burtin, P.: Recherches Immunochimiques sur les Tumeurs Humaines. Acta Unio. Int. Contra. Cancrum., 19:89, 1963.

12. Catalona, W. J., Sample, W. F., and Chretien, P. B.: Lymphocyte Reactivity in Cancer Patients: Correlation with Tumor Histology and Clinical Stage. Cancer, 31:65, 1973.

13. Catalona, W. J., Taylor, P. T., Rabson, A. S., et al.: A Method for Dinitrochlorobenzene Contact Sensitization: A Clinicopathological Study. N. Engl. J. Med., 286:399, 1972.

14. Cooperband, S. R., Davis, R. C., Schmid, K., et al.: Competitive Blockade of Lymphocyte Stimulation by a Serum Immunoregulatory Alpha Globulin (IRA). Transplant. Proc., 1:516, 1969.

15. Davidson, J., and Ni, L. Y.: The Role of Isoantigens A, B and H in the Formation of Cancer Metastasis (abstract). 10th International Cancer Congress, Houston, 1970.

16. Ducos, J., Migueres, J., Colombies, P., et al.: Lymphocyte Response to P.H.A. in Patients with Lung Cancer (letter to the editor). Lancet, 1:1111, 1970.

17. Eastham, R. J., III, Mason, J. M., Jennings, B. R., et al.: T-Cell Rosette Test in Squamous Cell Carcinoma of the Head and Neck. Arch. Otolaryngol., 102:171, 1976.

18. Eilber, F. R., and Morton, D. L.: Impaired Immunologic Reactivity and Recurrence Following Cancer Surgery. Cancer, 25:362, 1970.

19. Fletcher, R. D., Sumney, D. L., Langkamp, H. H., et al.: The Ability of Human Serum to Agglutinate Sheep Erythrocytes and the Effect of Tobacco Mosaic Virus: Comparison Between Smokers and Nonsmokers. Am. Rev. Respir. Dis., 100:92, 1969.

20. Foley, E. J.: Antigenic Properties of Methylcholanthrene-Induced Tumors in Mice of the Strain of Origin. Cancer Res., 13:835, 1953.

21. Garrioch, D. B., Good, R. A., and Gatti, R. A.: Lymphocyte Response to P.H.A. in Patients with Non-Lymphoid Tumours. Lancet, 1:618, 1970.

22. Gatti, R. A., and Good, R. A.: Occurrence of Malignancy in Immunodeficiency Diseases: A Literature Review. Cancer, 28:89, 1971.

23. Gold, P., and Freedman, S. O.: Demonstration of Tumor-Specific Antigens in Human Colonic Carcinomata by Immunological Tolerance and Absorption Techniques. J. Exp. Med., 121:439, 1965.

24. Gold, P., and Freedman, S. O.: Specific Carcinoembryonic Antigens of the Human Digestive System. J. Exp. Med., 122:467, 1965.

25. Gorer, P. A., and Kaliss, N.: The Effect of Isoantibodies In Vivo on Three Different Transplantable Neoplasms in Mice. Cancer Res., 19:824, 1959.

26. Gross, L.: Intradermal Immunization of C3H Mice Against a Sarcoma That Originated in an Animal of the Same Line. Cancer Res., 3:326, 1943.

27. Hammond, W. G., Fisher, J. C., and Rolley, R. T.: Tumor-Specific Transplantation Immunity to Spontaneous Mouse Tumors. Surgery, 62:124, 1967.

28. Harris, H., and Robson, E. B.: Precipitin Reactions Between Extracts of Seeds of Canavalia ensiformis (Jack Bean) and Normal and Pathological Serum Proteins. Vox. Sang., 8:348, 1963.

29. Havemann, K., and Rubin, A. D.: The Delayed Response of Chronic Lymphocytic Leukemia Lymphocytes to Phyto-

hemagglutinin *In Vitro.* Proc. Soc. Exp. Biol. Med., *127*:668, 1968.

30. Hellström, I., and Hellström, K. E.: Cell-Bound Immunity to Autologous and Syngeneic Mouse Tumors Induced by Methylcholanthrene and Plastic Discs. Science, *156*:981, 1967.

31. Hellström, K. E., and Hellström, I.: Immunological Enhancement as Studied by Cell Culture Techniques. Annu. Rev. Microbiol., *24*:373, 1970.

32. Hepburn, B., and Ritts, R. E., Jr.: Human T Lymphocytes: Assay Method Using Permanently Fixed Slides. Mayo Clin. Proc., *49*:866, 1974.

33. Hirsch, H. M., Bittner, J. J., Cole, H., et al.: Can the Inbred Mouse be Immunized Against Its Own Tumor? Cancer Res., *18*:344, 1958.

34. Hughes, L. E., and Mackay, W. D.: Suppression of the Tuberculin Response in Malignant Disease. Brit. Med. J., *2*:1346, 1965.

35. Israël, L.: Personal communication.

36. Israël, L., Mannoni, P., Delobel, J., et al.: Note sur les Résultats des Intradermo-Réactions de Lymphocytes Viables, Homologues et Hétérologues chez des Receveurs Cancéreux et des Témoins. Pathol. Biol., *15*:593, 1967.

37. Israël, L., Mawas, C., Bouvrain, A., et al.: Étude de L'Hypersensibilité Rétardee à la Tuberculine chez 130 Cancére Adultes: Effets du B.C.G. Pathol. Biol., *15*:597, 1967.

38. Johnson, M. W., Maibach, H. I., and Salmon, S. E.: Skin Reactivity in Patients with Cancer: Impaired Delayed Hypersensitivity or Faulty Inflammatory Response? N. Engl. J. Med., *284*:1255, 1971.

39. Kaliss, N.: The Elements of Immunologic Enhancement: A Consideration of Mechanisms. Ann. N.Y. Acad. Sci., *101*:64, 1962.

40. Kamrin, B. B.: Successful Skin Homografts in Mature Non-littermate Rats Treated With Fractions Containing Alpha-Globulins. Proc. Soc. Exp. Biol. Med., *100*:58, 1959.

41. Klein, G., Sjögren, H. O., Klein, E., et al.: Demonstration of Resistance against Methylcholanthrene-Induced Sarcomas in the Primary Autochthonous Host. Cancer Res., *20*:1561, 1960.

42. Kolmykova, V. N., and Eroshkina, A. M.: The Similarity and Difference in the Antigenic Composition of Tumour, Embryonal and Adult Tissues in Man. Probl. Oncol., *5*:1, 1959.

43. Kosyakov, P. N., and Korostelevog, V. S.: The Antigens of Cancerous Tumors in Man. Acta Unio. Int. Contra. Cancrum., *19*:158, 1963.

44. Krant, M. J., Manskopf, G., Brandrup, C. S., et al.: Immunologic Alterations in Bronchogenic Cancer: Sequential Study. Cancer, *21*:623, 1968.

45. Krupey, J., Gold, P., and Freedman, S. O.: Purification and Characterization of Carcinoembryonic Antigens of the Human Digestive System. Nature (Lond), *215*:67, 1967.

46. Levin, A. G., Miller, D. G., and Southam, C. M.: Lymphocyte Transfer Tests in Cancer Patients and Healthy People. Cancer, *22*:500, 1968.

47. Lewis, M. R., and Aptekman, P. M.: Atrophy of Tumors Caused by Strangulation and Accompanied by Development of Tumor Immunity in Rats. Cancer, *5*:411, 1952.

48. Lytton, B., Hughes, L. E., and Fulthorpe, A. J.: Circulating Antibody Response in Malignant Disease. Lancet, *1*:69, 1964.

49. Macbeth, R. A. L., and Bekesi, J. G.: Plasma Glycoproteins in Malignant Disease. Arch. Surg., *88*:633, 1964.

50. Maisel, R. H., and Ogura, J. H.: Abnormal Dinitrochlorobenzene Skin Sensitization: A Prognostic Sign of Survival in Head and Neck Squamous Cell Carcinoma. Laryngoscope, *83*:2012, 1974.

51. Makari, J. G.: The Polysaccharide Behaviour of Cancer Antigens. Br. Med. J., *2*:355, 1958.

52. Markowitz, H., Person, D. A., Gitnick, G. L., et al.: Immunosuppressive Activity of Concanavalin A. Science, *163*:476, 1969.

53. McKenna, J. M., Sanderson, R. P., and Blakemore, W. S.: Extraction of Distinctive Antigens From Neoplastic Tissue. Science, *135*:370, 1962.

54. McKenna, J. M., Sanderson, R. P., and Blakemore, W. S.: Studies of the Antigens of Human Tumors. I. Demonstration of a Soluble Specific Antigen in HeLa Cells and Some Human Tumors. Cancer Res., *24*:754, 1964.

55. McKenna, J. M., Sanderson, R. P., Davis, F. E., et al.: Studies on the Antigens of Human Tumors. II. Demonstration of a Soluble Specific Antigen (G) in Cell Lines Derived From Malignant Human Tissue. Cancer Res., *26*:984, 1966.

56. McKhann, C. F.: Primary Malignancy in Patients Undergoing Immunosuppression for Renal Transplantation: A Request for Information. Transplantation, *8*:209, 1969.

57. Mowbray, J. F.: Ability of Large Doses of an Alpha$_2$ Plasma Protein Fraction to Inhibit Antibody Production. Immunology, 6:217, 1963.

58. Neel, H. B., III., Ketcham, A. S., and Hammond, W. G.: Comparison of Tumor Immunity after Complete Excision, Cryonecrosis, and in the Presence of Persistent Tumor. Surg. Forum, 21:120, 1970.

59. Neel, H. B., III., Ketcham, A. S., and Hammond, W. G.: Cryonecrosis of Normal and Tumor-Bearing Rat Liver Potentiated by Inflow Occlusion. Cancer, 28: 1211, 1971.

60. Neel, H. B., III., Ketcham, A. S., and Hammond, W. G.: Requisites for Successful Cryogenic Surgery of Cancer. Arch. Surg., 102:45, 1971.

61. Neel, H. B., III., Ketcham, A. S., and Hammond, W. G.: Experimental Evaluation of In Situ Oncocide for Primary Tumor Therapy: Comparison of Tumor-Specific Immunity After Complete Excision, Cryonecrosis and Ligation. Laryngoscope, 83:376, 1973.

62. Neel, H. B., III., and Ritts, R. E., Jr.: Tumor-Specific Immunity and the Otolaryngologist, Ann. Otol. Rhinol. Laryngol., 82:323, 1973.

63. Neel, H. B., III., and Ritts, R. E., Jr.: Transfer of Tumor-Specific Immunity with Syngeneic Spleen Cells and Serum from Mice Bearing Large Tumors and Metastases (submitted for publication).

64. Nowell, P. C.: Phytohemagglutinin: An Initiator of Mitosis in Cultures of Normal Human Leukocytes. Cancer Res., 20:462, 1960.

65. Old, L. J., and Boyse, E. A.: Immunology of Experimental Tumors. Ann. Rev. Med., 15:167, 1964.

66. Old, L. J., Boyse, E. A., Clarke, D. A., et al.: Antigenic Properties of Chemically Induced Tumors. Ann. N. Y. Acad. Sci., 101:80, 1962.

67. Olkowski, Z. L., and Wilkins, S. A., Jr.: T-Lymphocyte Levels in the Peripheral Blood of Patients with Cancer of the Head and Neck. Am. J. Surg., 130:440, 1975.

68. Olsson, C. A., Rao, C. N., Menzoian, J. O., et al.: Immunologic Unreactivity in Bladder Cancer Patients. J. Urol., 107: 607, 1972.

69. Pérez Cuadrado, D. S.: Blastogénesis y Cáncer Humano: Depresión del Indice Blastogénico en los Enfermos Canceroso. Rev. Clin. Esp., 103:14, 1966.

70. Pollack, R. E., and Burger, M. M.: Surface-Specific Characteristics of a Contact-Inhibited Cell Line Containing the SV40 Viral Genome. Proc. Natl. Acad. Sci. U.S.A., 62:1074, 1969.

71. Prehn, R. T., and Main, J. M.: Immunity to Methylcholanthrene-Induced Sarcomas. J. Natl. Cancer Inst., 18:769, 1957.

72. Révész, L.: Detection of Antigenic Differences in Isologous Host-Tumor Systems by Pretreatment with Heavily Irradiated Tumor Cells. Cancer Res., 20:443, 1960.

73. Reynoso, G., Chu, T. M., Holyoke, D., et al.: Carcinoembryonic Antigen in Patients with Different Cancers. JAMA, 220:361, 1972.

74. Ritts, R. E., Jr., and Neel, H. B., III.: An Overview of Cancer Immunology. Mayo Clin. Proc., 49:118, 1974.

75. Robinson, E., Ben-Hur, N., Shulman, J., et al.: Comparative Study of Skin Homografts of Normal Donors and Donors with Malignant Neoplasia in a Host with Malignant Disease: A Preliminary Report. J. Natl. Cancer Inst., 34:185, 1965.

76. Rowe, W. S.: Virus-Specific Antigens in Viral Tumors. In Cross-Reacting Antigens and Neoantigens (with Implications for Autoimmunity and Cancer Immunity). Edited by J. J. Trentin. Baltimore, Williams & Wilkins Company, 1967, pp 74–78.

77. Sample, W. F., Gertner, H. R., Jr., and Chretien, P. B.: Inhibition of Phytohemagglutinin-Induced In Vitro Lymphocyte Transformation by Serum from Patients with Carcinoma. J. Natl. Cancer Inst., 46:1291, 1971.

78. Silk, M.: Effect of Plasma from Patients with Carcinoma on In Vitro Lymphocyte Transformation. Cancer, 20:2088, 1967.

79. Sjögren, H. O.: Transplantation Methods as a Tool for Detection of Tumor-Specific Antigens. Prog. Exp. Tumor Res., 6:289, 1965.

80. Solowey, A. C., and Rapaport, F. T.: Immunologic Responses in Cancer Patients. Surg. Gynecol. Obstet., 121:756, 1965.

81. Southam, C. M., Moore, A. E., and Rhoads, C. P.: Homotransplantation of Human Cell Lines. Science, 125:158, 1957.

82. Sutherland, R. M., Inch, W. R., and McCredie, J. A.: Phytohemagglutinin (PHA)-Induced Transformation of Lymphocytes from Patients with Cancer. Cancer, 27: 574, 1971.

83. Takeda, K., Aizawa, M., Kikuchi, Y., et al.: Tumor Autoimmunity against Methylcholanthrene-Induced Sarcomas of the Rat. Gann, 57:221, 1966.

84. Thomas, L.: Discussion. In *Cellular and Humoral Aspects of the Hypersensitive States*. Edited by H. S. Lawrence. New York, Harper & Row, Publishers, 1959, p. 530.

85. Thomson, D. M. P., Krupey, J., Freedman, S. O., et al.: The Radioimmunoassay of Circulating Carcinoembryonic Antigen of the Human Digestive System. Proc. Natl. Acad. Sci. U.S.A., *64*:161, 1969.

86. Von Kleist, S., and Burtin, P.: Isolation of a Fetal Antigen from Human Colonic Tumors. Cancer Res., *29*:1961, 1969.

87. Wadstrom, L., Almgard, L. E., Franzen, S., et al.: Cell Bound Tumor-Distinctive Immunological Reactions in Patients with Renal Carcinomas (abstract). 10th International Cancer Congress, Houston, 1970.

88. Wanebo, H. J., Jun, M. Y., Strong, E. W., et al.: T-Cell Deficiency in Patients with Squamous Cell Cancer of the Head and Neck. Am. J. Surg., *130*:445, 1975.

89. Weiss, D. W., Faulkin, L. J., Jr., and DeOme, K. B.: Acquired Resistance to Spontaneous Mammary Carcinomas in Autochthonous and Isologous Mice (abstract). Proc. Am. Assoc. Cancer Res., *4*:71, 1963.

90. Whittaker, M. G., Rees, K., and Clark, C. G.: Reduced Lymphocyte Transformation in Breast Cancer. Lancet, *1*:892, 1971.

91. Wood, W. C., and Morton, D. L.: Microcytotoxicity Test: Detection in Sarcoma Patients of Antibody Cytotoxic to Human Sarcoma Cells. Science, *170*:1318, 1970.

92. Yachi, A., Matsuura, Y., Carpenter, C. M., et al.: Immunochemical Studies on Human Lung Cancer Antigens Soluble in 50% Saturated Ammonium Sulfate. J. Natl. Cancer. Inst., *40*:663, 1968.

93. Zacharia, T. P., and Pollard, M.: Elevated Levels of α-Globulins in Sera from Germfree Rats with 3-Methylcholanthrene-Induced Tumors. J. Natl. Cancer Inst., *42*:35, 1969.

94. Zilber, L. A.: Study of the Tumor Specificity of Gastric Cancer Tissue. Ann. N.Y. Acad. Sci., *101*:264, 1962.

Chapter 38A

Chemotherapy of Head and Neck Cancer

Janardan D. Khandekar

The ultimate objective of chemotherapy is to cure the patient of his malignant disease. This is now possible in at least ten types of disseminated cancer, occurring largely in children, adolescents, and young adults. In most disseminated solid tumors, cure is not yet possible, although significant palliation and lengthening of survival can be achieved with drugs.

Head and neck cancer accounts for only 5% of malignant conditions in the United States, but the associated pronounced cosmetic and functional deformities and malnutrition heighten their relative importance. These tumors challenge the expertise of surgeons, radiation and medical oncologists, reconstructive surgeons, prosthodontists, pathologists, dieticians, physiatrists, nurses, and social workers.

Traditionally, chemotherapy has been used only after failure of irradiation and/or operation to control head and neck tumors. However, it has become quite apparent that these therapeutic modalities fail to cure a sizable percentage of patients. Drug therapy of cancer began about 30 years ago, but until lately it has had little impact on the practice of cancer medicine. Reasonably favorable results from single-agent chemotherapy are seen in advanced head and neck

tumors. The data on combination chemotherapy in this disease are still preliminary, but encouraging. It is therefore possible that therapy with various combinations of surgery, radiation, chemotherapy and immunotherapy may prove useful in the future. In this section these aspects of therapy are considered in detail. This discussion is preceded by a brief consideration of the principles governing the practice of chemotherapy.

THE CELL CYCLE

Malignant tissues are largely made up of dividing cells, which synthesize DNA at some point in their life cycle, and nondividing cells. The dividing cells pass through four different phases (Fig. 38A–1). Mitosis (M) occupies a discrete phase of the cell life cycle. Following the division, the cell enters G_1 phase. This phase is then followed by DNA synthesis, which is termed the S phase. After completion of the DNA synthesis, the cell then enters a phase of apparent rest (G_2) before the initiation of mitosis.

In most dividing cells the periods for S, G_2, and M phases are of relative constant duration. Variation of the length of the cell

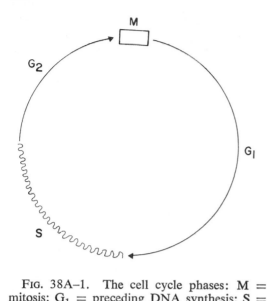

FIG. 38A–1. The cell cycle phases: M = mitosis; G_1 = preceding DNA synthesis; S = DNA synthesis; G_2 = premitotic resting.

cycle generally occurs in the G_1 phase. When the proliferating cells stop dividing, they do so in the G_1 phase. This phase seems to hold the key to the proliferative activity of the tissues. When the cell cycle time (time taken for a proliferating cell to move from one mitosis to another) is short and thus the proliferative activity high, the G_1 phase is of brief duration. When proliferative activity is slow, the G_2 phase is long.

It is not clear at present how a mammalian eukaryotic cell decides to leave the G_1 phase and start DNA synthesis. There is some evidence that this action requires interaction between the nucleus and cytoplasm of the replicating cells. During the S phase, biosynthesis of enzymes essential for purine, pyrimidine, and nucleic acids is accentuated and the DNA content of the cell doubles. The phase of DNA synthesis is then complete and the cell enters G_2 phase. None of the phases is quiescent, and RNA and protein synthesis occurs throughout each of them.

In addition to differences in the biochemical mechanism of action, which are discussed later, antineoplastic agents also differ in the point in the cell cycle at which they act. The drugs can be grouped as follows:

1. *S phase specific*: These are the agents that inhibit only DNA synthesis that occurs in the S phase of the cell cycle. Drugs like methotrexate inhibit not only DNA, but also RNA and protein synthesis and are called S phase specific, self limiting agents.

2. *Non S specific*: Alkylating agents and antitumor antibiotics exert a direct effect on DNA, and thus their activities are not dependent on the phase of the cell cycle.

3. *Antimitotics*: Plant alkaloids like vincristine arrest mitosis during metaphase.

Studies of the cell kinetics indicate that the often held belief that all malignant tumors are rapidly proliferating is not necessarily true. The mean doubling time of human tumors (time taken by a tumor to double its volume) can be as short as one week in Burkitt's tumor or as long as several years in some adenocarcinomas.

Malignant tumor formation occurs when either of the following three events occur together or separately: (1) The growth fraction, defined as proportion of tumor cells in mitotic cycle at a given time, may become large. (2) The cell cycle time may get shorter. On average, the cell cycle time of tumors is two days, which is not faster than normal cells. (3) Renewal of normal cells is accompanied by cell loss. When this cell loss is reduced, tumor formation can occur. This seems to be the major factor in the production of a large majority of tumors.

Epidermoid neoplasms have about 35% growth fraction (dividing cells) as contrasted to 3 to 5% in breast cancer and virtually 100% in embryonal tumors. Since most of the chemotherapeutic agents act on these dividing cells, epidermoid cancers would be intermediate in their response to drugs. A recent work suggests that at metastatic site a tumor may still be proliferating rapidly, while the parent neoplasm has a low growth fraction. This would then suggest that chemotherapy given to these patients may still be useful. However, methods for measurement of cell kinetics parameters in patients are cumbersome. The results of therapy based on these considerations are also at present not much different from the conventional therapy. Nevertheless, newer advances in this field may considerably alter the present practice of chemotherapy.

MODE OF ACTION OF ANTINEO-
PLASTIC AGENTS

The DNA synthesized during the S phase of the life cycle acts as a selective template for the production of specific forms of messenger, ribosomal, or transfer RNA. The specific sequences of the messenger RNA determine which enzymes will be synthesized in the cell. The enzymes in turn are responsible for the structure, function, metabolism, and proliferative rate of the cells.

Most of the clinically useful antineoplastic drugs appear to work by inhibition of synthesis of either enzymes or substrates acted upon by enzyme systems essential for the nucleic acid synthesis or function. Based on the mechanism of drug action, agents that are useful in head and neck tumors can be classified as follows:

1. **Antimetabolites.** These drugs inhibit purine or pyrimidine biosynthesis. Methotrexate, for example, inhibits formation of reduced folates, which are essential for thymidylate synthesis. Arabinosylcytosine inhibits DNA polymerase.

2. **Drugs that Interfere with the Structure or Function of DNA Molecule.** Alkylating agents like cyclophosphamide change the structure of DNA, thereby arresting cell replication. On the other hand, antibiotics like actinomycin D and adriamycin bind and intercalate with nucleotide sequences of the DNA molecule and thereby block messenger RNA production.

3. **Mitotic Inhibitors.** Vinca alkaloids like vincristine and vinblastine, by disrupting the microfilaments of the mitotic spindle, arrest cell division.

A number of other drugs, including L-asparginase and steroids, are not considered here since they are not being used at present in the treatment of head and neck tumors.

GENERAL TOXICITY OF ANTI-
CANCER AGENTS

Most of these agents act on the proliferative fraction of cells. Therefore an undesirable consequence of this drug action is damage inflicted on the normal cells undergoing rapid cell division. These tissues are the cells of the hair follicles and skin, the gastrointestinal mucosa, and the normal bone marrow elements. Clinically then, damage to these tissues is manifested by alopecia, stomatitis, nausea, vomiting, anemia, leukopenia, and thrombocytopenia. In addition to these effects, special problems can occur with each drug, and these are briefly discussed here.

The chemotherapeutic agents generally are immunosuppressive, less so when the drug is given intermittently rather than on a continuous schedule.

ADJUVANT CHEMOTHERAPY

Adjuvant chemotherapy can be defined as the administration of drugs in conjunction with surgery and/or radiation. This type of therapy has already proved effective in osteogenic sarcoma, in Wilms' tumor, probably in Ewing's tumor, and in Stages IIB and IIIB of Hodgkin's disease. It is also currently being evaluated in common malignant disease, such as breast carcinoma, and preliminary results are encouraging. The adjuvant chemotherapy has also been used in patients with head and neck cancers, and the results are summarized later in this section. It might seem unlikely that a treatment program like methotrexate, which produced only partial response (reduction of measurable disease by greater than 50%) in a minority of patients with overt metastatic disease, would prove effective in the eradication of micrometastasis. However, studies in experimental tumor problems provide compelling evidence for such a concept.

Pulmonary metastasis up to 0.3 cm in diameter is barely detectable radiologically, but contain up to 10^8 neoplastic cells. Induction of complete remission (defined as complete disappearance of the measurable tumor) would result in 90 to 99% destruction of tumor cells. Large numbers of viable tumor cells still remain to allow definitive treatment. In contrast, micrometastatic disease is easier to eradicate for a variety of reasons. Large growth fraction of smaller tumors decreases as the tumor enlarges. In the experimental tumor system, when the tumor is perturbed, the noncycling cells reenter the cell cycle. Since most antitumor agents, including methotrexate, have a greater killing effect on proliferating cells, treatment is far more effective in the presence of large growth fraction (microscopic tumor). The second reason for the apparent success of adjuvant chemotherapy is related to the so called log kill hypothesis. It is known that chemotherapeutic agents kill cells by first-order kinetics, i.e., they destroy a certain percentage and not a number. This hypothesis also explains the necessity for repeated prolonged chemotherapy, since the number of tumor cells destroyed decreases as the tumor becomes smaller. This is in contrast to immunotherapy, which kills by zero-order kinetics, i.e., a known number of cells is destroyed. However, a major limitation of immunotherapy is its ineffectiveness in the presence of large bulky disease. Thus, these two modalities may complement each other.

The blood supply of tumors may also be an important factor in the effectiveness of therapy against microscopic disease. The small tumor foci have a greater blood supply than the large bulky tumors. This can be explained by the geometric fact that in a spheroidal tumor, the cell population grows in proportion to the cube of the radius, whereas the surface increases only as the square of the radius. Thus, in small tumors delivery of antineoplastic agents is more efficient. Surgery or radiation usually compromises the blood supply of tumors, and this may explain the high responsiveness of the totally untreated neoplasms. Finally, chronic debilitation caused by advanced disease may interfere with the drug effectiveness.

COMBINATION CHEMOTHERAPY

It has become apparent in recent years that a combination of drugs gives better results than single-agent therapy. These superior results could be explained on the basis of a number of theoretical and practical considerations. It is conceivable that multiple-action agents prevent the emergence of resistant tumor clones, since these drugs may have dissimilar modes of action. Similarly, by acting on different phases of the cell cycle, the drugs may have addictive or synergistic effects. Finally, with the combination of drugs with different spectra of clinical toxicity, administration of full or nearly full doses of each of the active agents is possible. As will be discussed more fully later in this chapter, some of these principles are now being applied in the treatment of head and neck cancer.

In order to appreciate the rational basis of chemotherapy of head and neck cancer, knowledge of the natural history and prognosis of the various types of cancer is essential. These neoplasms originate from the laryngeal, nasopharyngeal, and oropharyngeal tissues, from the paranasal sinuses, and from the salivary glands. The majority of these tumors in this area are squamous cell carcinoma. History of heavy drinking and smoking is often associated with the development of these tumors. In parts of the Orient and Africa, nasopharyngeal cancer is the prevalent lesion, and this is often associated with a high titre of antibodies to Epstein-Barr (EB) virus. It has been proposed that the EB virus may be of etiologic significance in these tumors.

Squamous cell tumors of the head and neck are a heterogeneous group of lesions, and response to chemotherapy depends on the site of origin, histology, and stage of tumor. Ideally, therapeutic results of the cancer of this region should be analyzed in the light of the aforementioned variables. MacComb and Fletcher have reviewed the data that give the determinate three- and five-year survival according to the site of the primary lesion. The TNM classification has been extensively used in this area, and it is known that patients with nodal involvement fare more poorly than those without it.

In addition to squamous cell carcinoma, other types of cancer also occur in the head and neck region. These include lymphoepithelioma, lymphoma, adenocarcinoma, sarcoma, and plasmocytoma. The therapy of these types of cancer is not discussed in this section.

SPECIFIC CHEMOTHERAPEUTIC AGENTS

There have been few systematic studies on the response of head and neck cancer to chemotherapeutic drugs. There is not enough uniformity in reports to allow evaluation of responses in terms of pre-treatment performance status, specific primary sites, or previous therapy. This limitation is further compounded by the poor pre-therapy nutritional status of these patients. This malnutrition caused by local tumor, surgical extirpation, radiation fibrosis, fistulas, and aversion to protein, due to change in taste, is aggravated by systemic toxicity of the antineoplastic agents. These considerations, along with the heterogeneity of the head and neck tumors as discussed previously, make a precise analysis of response rates for particular tumor sites impossible. This review deals primarily with epidermoid carcinomas, since it is mainly patients with these tumors who require chemotherapy and are also cared for by the otolaryngologist.

Systemic Single Agent Chemotherapy

Wasserman, Carter, and their colleagues have extensively reviewed the results of single-agent chemotherapy (Table 38A–1). Methotrexate (MTX) clearly emerges as

Table 38A–1. Activity of Drugs in Head and Neck Cancer

Drugs	No. of responses/ No. of evaluable patients	Response rate (%)
Methotrexate	298/630	47
Bleomycin	24/158	15
Cyclophosphamide	28/77	36
Chlorambucil	5/34	15
5 Fluorouracil	18/118	15
6-Mercaptopurines	6/45	12
Vinblastine	10/35	29
Adriamycin	15/95	16
Methyl CCNU	6/40	15
Hexamethylanine	9/75	12
Dibromodulcitol	11/50	22
Hydroxyurea	7/18	39
Nitrogen mustard	5/66	8
CCNU	4/88	5
cis-Platinum	10/38	26

the most effective single agent, although cyclophosphamide (CTX), hydroxyurea, and vinblastine also have considerable activity. By conservative estimate, at least one third of the patients with advanced carcinoma experience more than 50% regression of their tumor masses.

MTX has been given by multiple schedules, including intermittent weekly or bi-weekly intravenous doses. The intermittent schedule of administration is superior (50% response) to daily low dosage or daily dosage for five consecutive days once a month (29% response). However, complete remissions are unusual and short-lived. Most responding patients experience an exacerbation of their disease within 3½ to 4 months.

The main toxicity of this drug, when given weekly or bi-weekly, includes bone marrow suppression, stomatitis, mucorrhea, and sometimes nausea, vomiting, and diarrhea. Sometimes unexpected and apparently sudden severe toxicity from the drug has been known to occur and the factors underlying this unusual host response are not known. Low serum and red blood folate in some patients may be responsible for these reactions. Since MTX is excreted by the kidneys, dehydration and impaired creatinine clearance may potentiate drug toxicity. MTX, when given orally, is slowly and erratically absorbed.

Impressed with the need to increase the therapeutic index of MTX, several authors have used the drug either by intra-arterial infusion, or with Leucovorin (folinic acid) or thymidine "rescue." It is pertinent here to review the biochemistry and pharmacology of high dose MTX with Leucovorin "rescue," since this form of therapy is currently being widely evaluated in epidermoid cancers.

Biochemical Effects of High-Dose Methotrexate and Leucovorin

As shown in Figure 38A–2, MTX acts primarily by inhibiting activity of the enzyme dihydrofolate reductase, which converts dihydrofolate to tetrahydrofolate. The reduced folates are required for the formation of thymidylate, which then gets incorporated into DNA. Other evidence suggests

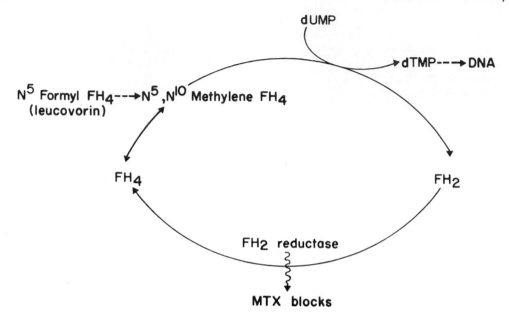

FIG. 38A–2.   Biochemical effects of MTX and leucovorin. FH_2 = dihydrofolate; FH_4 = tetrahydrofolate; dUMP = deoxyuridylate; dTMP = thymidylate.

that the drug also inhibits purine biosynthesis. Leucovorin, which is N^5, N^{10} formyl tetrahydrofolate, supplies the product of the inhibited reaction. Leucovorin should prevent the three major effects of MTX inhibition (DNA, RNA, and protein synthesis). Recently it was shown that thymidine prevents the antithymidine effect of MTX without interfering with the antitumor effects of the drug. Thymidine provides a selective rescue and has already been shown to be useful in patients. Recently combined Leucovorin and thymidine "rescue" programs have been introduced in an attempt to further increase therapeutic effectiveness of MTX.

Rationale for Leucovorin "Rescue"

Why does Leucovorin "rescue" normal cells but not tumor cells? Considerable evidence indicates that a carrier mediated cell membrane transport mechanism exists for folates and MTX. It is postulated that tumor cells lack such a transport mechanism. However, when concentrations of 10^{-3} to 10^{-4} M of MTX are achieved (this is possible only when the drug is given in large amounts), the drug enters the cell by infiltration

through pores or by other passive mechanism. Leucovorin and its metabolite N^5 N^{10} methylene tetrahydrofolate share a common transport mechanism with MTX. Leucovorin can rescue normal host cells, since they contain the carrier transport sites. On the other hand, Leucovorin will not enter and rescue epidermoid cancers of the head and neck, since these tumors lack transport sites. It was shown that following HDMTX administration, bone marrow DNA synthesis was inhibited, but switched on within four days after the administration of Leucovorin. On the other hand, in metastatic epitheliomas, the marked decrease in DNA synthesis persisted for 9 days in spite of Leucovorin administration. While this rationale for Leucovorin is gaining support, other explanations such as unique biochemical effect of high drug concentrations may be of considerable relevance. Clearly, much work remains to be done in this field.

Pharmacology of High-Dose MTX

Pharmacologic studies have indicated that MTX, when administered to children in doses of 50 to 100 mg/kg over a period of 6 hours, has a serum half life of 2 to 3.5

hours. This is comparable to the MTX disappearance on more conventional dosages. In the 24-hour period immediately following termination of MTX infusion, the fall in serum levels of the drug obeys first order kinetics. The studies also indicate that capacity for clearing MTX from the blood may not be overtaxed by these larger doses, and that biliary excretion may become an important factor. Most of the drug is excreted unchanged in urine by glomerular filtration, although a recent study demonstrated that infusions of very high doses (more than 50 mg MTX/kg) in patients and primates resulted in excretion of a significant amount of 7 hydroxy-methotrexate. This metabolite is a weak antifolate and therefore would not contribute significantly as an antitumor agent. However, as discussed below, this hydroxylated compound may contribute to renal toxicity.

Although the combination of MTX and Leucovorin has been used clinically over a decade, the optimal time for MTX infusion and the timing and dose of Leucovorin required to prevent MTX toxicity are poorly defined. Penta has recently reviewed the variables associated with HDMTX regime and summarized the protocols. Some authorities have given four- to six-hour MTX infusion and administered Leucovorin two hours later. Others have extended the infusion up to 36 hours and given Leucovorin six hours after termination of the infusion. Since mice exposed to inhibitory concentration of MTX longer than 48 hours developed fatal gastrointestinal toxicity, Leucovorin should be given within 42 hours of the onset of MTX infusion. We have elected to give 24-hour MTX infusion, since toxic action of MTX on the target organ is primarily a function of the duration of exposure to suprathreshold concentration of the drug, rather than of peak levels of drug achieved. We give Leucovorin six hours after the termination of MTX therapy, but there is no consensus on these issues.

Recent work indicates that vincristine inhibits efflux of intracellular MTX, thereby increasing intracellular concentration of the drug. This then may result in increased amount of free intracellular drug, which is critical for cytodestructive effect. Several investigators are now using vincristine along with HDMTX in order to increase intracellular MTX. However, definitive studies regarding its augmentation of MTX activity are lacking.

Toxicity of High-Dose MTX

Nephrotoxicity is the principal limiting factor of HDMTX therapy. Administration of this therapy often causes a rise in serum creatinine and a decline in creatinine clearance. The pk_a of MTX is 5.4 Therefore, when urine pH is near this value, MTX is present predominantly in insoluble free acid form, and if a patient is dehydrated, MTX will precipitate as a crystalline material in the renal tubules. The recently described 7 hydroxy metabolite of MTX has three- to fivefold less aqueous solubility than that of the parent compound and may be a significant factor in nephrotoxicity. It has been demonstrated that at pH 8.1, the solubility of MTX titrated to saturation is 440 mg/ml, but that at the pH of 5.7, the solubility drops to 48 mg/ml. These considerations dictate that patients receiving HDMTX should be well hydrated and their urine kept alkaline. Similarly, such drugs as aspirin, which interfere with MTX excretion, are best avoided during therapy. Studies by Frei and his colleagues also showed that an elevation of serum creatinine at the end of 48 hours of MTX infusion by more than 50% over the pre-therapy value signals impending toxicity. There is also a good correlation between the rise in serum creatinine and MTX blood levels at various times following MTX infusion. It is seen that MTX levels of more than 10^{-5} M and 10^{-6} M, at 24 and 48 hours respectively, signal possible drug toxicity. These levels then dictate continuation of Leucovorin "rescue" over and above the scheduled times, and it has been suggested that this simple measure, occasionally combined with hemodialysis, may prevent drug toxicity. Since aminopterin, an antifolate, has a higher aqueous solubility than MTX, there is a renewed interest in that compound.

Generally high-dose MTX is not myelosuppressive, a feature that permits its combination with other bone marrow suppressive agents. However, occasionally bone marrow suppression and nephrotoxicity do occur. Other side effects of this therapy include nausea, occasional violent vomiting, diarrhea, and on rare occasion cutaneous vasculitis and pneumonitis. It is important therefore that HDMTX be given in an institution where unlimited quantities of (preferably HL-A matched) platelets, along with other supportive measures, are available. Nevertheless, it seems that HDMTX is becoming safer and, in general, is less toxic than the conventional-dose MTX.

In our fairly large experience, patients tolerate HDMTX therapy very well, and this includes three patients in their eighties. Patients are well hydrated and receive sodium bicarbonate and acetazolamide (Diamox) for alkalinization of urine. It should be pointed out that acetazolamide causes drowsiness and sometimes anorexia.

Therapeutic Efficacy of High-Dose MTX

The earlier results of HDMTX in epidermoid carcinoma were at least comparable to, if not better than, those achieved with conventional MTX therapy. In addition, HDMTX causes a marked decrease in incidence and severity of mucosal and hematologic toxicity. The only large-scale randomized trial that compared conventional-dose MTX with HDMTX had many deficiencies. The dose of MTX in that study was not properly escalated, nor were patients hydrated or their urine kept alkaline. Recent studies, although not randomized, indicate superiority of HDMTX in a number of carcinomas including head and neck tumors. In our consecutive series, 65% of the patients responded with 25% of the remissions being complete. In a few other patients, the disease remained stable for over six months, indicating some beneficial effects of therapy. All these patients had been heavily irradiated and many had undergone extensive operation or were inoperable. In patients having pain, relief was almost universal. Since the toxicity of this program has been minimal, other active drugs such as cyclophosphamide (CTX) and vinblastine are now being added to HDMTX. Induction of complete remission must be the goal of any chemotherapeutic program, since only these patients may have normal life expectancy. I believe that HDMTX, in combination with other chemotherapeutic agents, will become an important arm of the radiation and/or surgical management of the head and neck cancers.

Other Single-Agent Chemotherapy

As shown in Table 38A–1, CTX, vinblastine, and hydroxyurea also have some activity in this tumor, although the data are limited. Cyclophosphamide is an alkylating agent that is widely used in cancer chemotherapy and acts on nonreplicating as well as replicating cells. The drug has no antineoplastic action in vitro. Activation of CTX occurs primarily in the liver. The drug can be given intravenously or by oral route. The common toxic effects of the drug include nausea, alopecia, bone marrow suppression, and hemorrhagic cystitis. This drug has considerable activity in the head and neck tumors, and trials should be undertaken to assess its value in combination chemotherapy.

Vinblastine is derived from vinca alkaloids and it acts on the mitotic phase of the replicating cells. The drug probably combines with tubulin, a protein required for metaphasic spindle formation. Unlike its congener vincristine, vinblastine is myelosuppressive, but not neurotoxic. Hydroxyurea is a radiomimetic agent and its use is discussed later. Adriamycin, which is a broad-based antitumor agent, gave only a 19% response rate. This drug causes bone marrow suppression and has dose-limited cardiotoxicity. Bleomycin, which gave a high response rate in head and neck tumors in Japan, has been disappointing in the United States. Out of 158 evaluable patients, only 15% responded. Whereas bleomycin has minimal bone marrow toxicity, the acute febrile reaction and pulmonary fibrosis which is cumulative and irreversible limits its use. Recently cis-platinum (dichloro-di aminoplatinum), a heavy metal chelating agent, has attracted considerable attention. Although the results are preliminary, some responses have been seen with this agent. This drug is not myelosuppressive and the dose-limiting factor is nephrotoxicity. This precludes its combination with HDMTX, but it could be combined with other myelotoxic active agents. Its renal toxicity to a certain limit can be prevented by continuous mannitol diuresis. The otic toxicity of this metal complex requires audiometric surveillance.

Combination Chemotherapy

In recent years combination chemotherapy has been quite successful in treating hematologic malignant disease and breast cancer. In head and neck cancer also, combination chemotherapy is being used with some success (Table 38A-2).

The last two trials in the table were designed on the principles of biochemical pharmacology and tumor cell kinetics. In the study by Livingstone et al., although the response rate was not particularly high, the duration of response was comparatively long (26 weeks). In the British study, the response rate was high and surprisingly toxic-

ity was moderate. In a more recent study, bleomycin was administered by continuous infusion for 96 hours to synchronize the malignant cells in S phase of the cell cycle. This was followed by HDMTX. Results of the study are preliminary.

It seems that head and neck cancer is responsive to multiple agents with different biochemical mechanisms of action, having quantitative differences and toxicity, and acting on both the cycling and noncycling cells. This situation is not different from that of some of the hematologic malignant diseases more than a dozen years ago.

Intra-arterial (IA) Chemotherapy

It was postulated that administration of anticancer agents by intra-arterial route, resulting in high local concentration and/or long exposure of the tumor to the drug, would improve the rate as well as duration of response. Furthermore, by systemic administration of metabolic products of chem-

Table 38A–2. Results of Combination Chemotherapy

Investigator	Drug Combinations	No. of responding pts./ No. of evaluable pts.
Nervi et al.	Methotrexate + vincristine	15/28
Cortes et al.	Adriamycin + bleomycin	4/8
Hanham et al.	Cyclophosphamide + methotrexate + vincristine + 5 Fluorouracil	8/10*
Jacquillat et al.	Vinblastine, streptenigrin, thiophospheranide, chlorambucil, 6 MP, methotrexate, procarbazine	45/82*
Deconti.	HDMTX, cyclophosphamide and cytosine arabinoside	14/70
Moselley et al.	CCNU, bleomycin	5/14
Moselley et al.	CCNU, bleomycin, methotrexate, vinblastine	3/15
DeWell et al.	Fluorouracil, methotrexate, vincristine, cyclophosphamide	4/13
DeWell et al.	Four drugs as above with Prednisone	14/32
Livingstone et al.	Cyclophosphamide, methyl CCNU, vincristine, bleomycin	11/31
Livingstone et al.	Sequential combined therapy using methotrexate, adriamycin, in addition to above agents	12/28
Price et al.	Kinetically based, vincristine, adriamycin, bleomycin, methotrexate, 5 FU, hydroxyurea and 6 mercaptopurine	19/24

*Definition of response unclear

otherapeutically inhibited reaction, the drug toxicity could be minimized. Use of IA MTX with systemic Leucovorin is based on these conditions. Although these methods have somewhat improved the response rates (overall 53% with MTX), the high complication rate attendant to these procedures has limited their general use. Faulty placement of catheters, major problems of bleeding, embolization, and tumor growth outside the infused area have dampened the enthusiasm for this form of therapy. For example, in the series of 68 patients catheterized by Watkins and Sullivan, eight died of hemorrhage and four had major embolization related to the treatment. The overall improved results of IA MTX could also be related to prior selection of good-risk patients. Freckman, in his series of 311 cannulations in 193 patients, observed 9 catheter-related major complications with 1 death. In addition, in 81 patients (i.e., 13.3% incidence) minor complications were also noted. Using multiple drugs such as 5 Fluorouracil, MTX, CTX, and vinblastine, he observed a 44.9% response rate in 169 evaluable patients. The median duration of response was 14.5 months.

Bertino used agents that, when given IA, are rapidly inactivated as they leave the perfused tumor area and enter systemic circulation. Dichloromethotrexate, which is extensively metabolized by the liver, was used in 12 patients with head and neck cancer. Nine of his patients responded and toxicity was minimal.

In conclusion, at present IA chemotherapy should be given only by the experienced team, preferably as a part of a control trial. Its general use does not seem to be indicated.

Chemotherapy Combined with Surgery

There are sufficient theoretical reasons to combine surgery with chemotherapy. Preoperative chemotherapy would reduce tumor size and facilitate subsequent operation. Postoperative therapy may destroy malignant cells that exist beyond resection margins or have already metastasized to distant sites. Unfortunately there are no published controlled trials on the pre- or postoperative

adjuvant chemotherapy. Some studies have incorporated radiation, surgery, and chemotherapy in their protocols.

Richards and his colleagues combined radiation and hydroxyurea. They reported that the combination resulted in greater antitumor effects on the primary site as well as on nodes affected by metastasis (Table 38A–3). The survival rate increased with the addition of chemotherapy in his uncontrolled series. However, because of the combined use of radiation, the role of chemotherapy in the surgical management cannot be ascertained.

Recently the group at the National Cancer Institute treated 30 consecutive patients with head and neck tumors preoperatively with 36-hour infusion of HDMTX. Twenty-three of these patients responded, and their disease-free survival rate was superior to that of similar patients treated at the institution without preoperative chemotherapy. More recently, the Eastern Cooperative Oncology Group, as well as other workers, have initiated controlled studies testing the efficacy of pre- or postoperative chemotherapy in high-risk patients with head and neck cancer. Others have used IA methotrexate with systemic Leucovorin along with operative treatment. DeSprez et al. treated 103 patients with this approach. These authors gave MTX by the standard 10-day IA infusion technique with systemic Leucovorin. This infusion was followed within three to six weeks by operation. Twenty-eight pa-

Table 38A–3. Effects of Combining Chemotherapy with Operation and Radiation

	Negative at Operation	
	Primary	Nodes
Radiation	2/12	5/12
Radiation + Hydroxyurea	6/11	11/11

	Survival at Time of Report	
	No.	%
Radiation + Operation	118/185	63
Radiation + Operation + Hydroxyurea	57/70	81

(Based on Richards et al.)

tients had complete response following the infusion with no demonstrable residual tumor at operation. These patients had better survival figures. The second group (75 patients) had residual tumor at operation and results no different from those obtained by operation alone. However, closer analysis reveals that of the 28 responders, 19 had T_1 and T_2 lesions and nine had T_3 and T_4 lesions. Only four patients had positive nodes. These patients may have done as well with surgical treatment only. However, the authors believe that even the 75 patients who exhibited residual tumor at operation derived some benefit from the chemotherapy —in the form of pain relief, decreased local inflammation, partial tumor reduction, and occasional conversion of an inoperable to an operable lesion.

DeSprez et al. analyzed the characteristics of the responders and nonresponders. The responders were untreated and had small exophytic tumors limited to lateral surface of the tongue, gingiva, buccal mucosa, and tonsils. The poor responders had had previous radiation, and had large widespread ulcerative lesions of the floor of the mouth, palate, base of tongue, lateral pharynx, and cervical nodes. In most studies the pretherapy status of the patient was not discussed, but undoubtedly played an important role. Ambulatory patients usually respond more favorably to therapy than do semi-ambulatory or bedridden subjects. A large number of other reported studies on the IA infusion of drugs have included a small number of patients, and conclusions are difficult to draw.

Radiotherapy and Chemotherapy

Some of the reasons for combining chemotherapy with radiation are similar to those for integrating operation and drugs. These include: (1) Reduction in the tumor cell mass, thereby facilitating more effective radiation therapy. It is known that the center of the tumor contains hypoxic cells, and conventional radiotherapy is ineffective in the absence of oxygen. Reduction in tumor cell mass would result in a smaller number of hypoxic cells. (2) Control of distant metastasis. (3) Modification of the DNA molecule by drugs resulting in sensitization of the cell to subsequent radiation.

Many drugs can increase radiation-induced damage, but often such effects are accomplished at the expense of greater damage to normal tissues. Besides chemotherapeutic drugs, other agents like metronidazole also increase the sensitivity of the tissues to the radiation. Ideally, these radiosensitizers should distribute themselves in a greater concentration in the tumor cells than in surrounding normal tissues. This would provide the best groundwork for increased selective tumor destruction. A large number of agents have been used in conjunction with radiation, but a detailed analysis of these studies is beyond the scope of this text. However, a brief overview of the results would considerably aid the otolaryngologist in making clinical judgments.

Hydroxyurea. This drug, a radiosensitizer, acts principally on the replicating cells and thereby synchronizes the tumor cells in G_1 phase. Data suggest that biochemically it acts as an inhibitor of nucleotide reductase, an enzyme essential for DNA synthesis.

Richards and Chambers, in a prospective randomized trial, noted the increased antitumor effect of adding hydroxyurea to radiation. A closer look at their series indicates that their control group had a greater number of advanced cases. Subsequently, these authors entered 610 additional patients into a nonrandomized study and concluded that patients receiving hydroxyurea survived longer than did untreated controls.

Lerner et al. reported an 80% complete regression rate and a 55% NED (no evidence of disease) rate. On the other hand, Stefan et al. were unable to demonstrate any advantage of combined radiation and hydroxyurea in controlled double blind study of 114 patients with advanced head and neck cancer. The recent study of Hussey and Abrams re-emphasizes the necessity of controlled clinical trials as well as an analysis of multiple variables known to affect the outcome of treatment in patients with head and neck tumors. Their promising pilot study of combined hydroxyurea and radiation therapy led to a controlled trial. The controlled study showed no better control of head and neck tumors with combined hydroxyurea and radiation.

5 Fluorouracil (5 FU). In a randomized study using 5 FU intravenously in conjunction with radiation, a greater survival was seen in the combined therapy group only in patients with oral cavity and oropharyngeal lesions. The statistically significant difference was seen only in patients with oral cavity lesions in whom survival was doubled with 5 FU.

There have been several other studies using 5 FU administered either as IV or by IA route in combination with radiation. It appears that the drug may add something to survival when given IV to patients with oral tumors, but probably has no role in patients with disease at other sites.

Methotrexate. There are only a few well-designed studies using MTX and radiation. Friedman and colleagues gave MTX to 168 patients prior to radiation. Fifty-six of these had partial response. These authors believed that survival was increased in patients receiving the drug. A number of other workers have used MTX along with radiation, but either the trials are not controlled or they are too small in terms of the number of subjects studied. The radiation therapy oncology group is currently conducting a well-designed controlled trial of radiotherapy alone versus MTX (25 mg IV for 3 days a week for 5 weeks) followed by irradiation. Study results should be available in the near future and may give us definitive answers regarding pre-therapy MTX.

More recently, HDMTX was used prior to radiation. The authors found no difference in disease-free interval or survival in the chemotherapeutically treated group as compared to conventionally treated patients. However, the dose of MTX in this series was small. More recently at our institution a small number of patients with T_4 squamous cell carcinoma of the head and neck were given three doses of HDMTX therapy. This resulted in more than 75% tumor reduction in all but one patient. These patients then received radiation. It is too early to say whether such an approach is warranted; a controlled trial is needed.

In addition to systemic drugs, IA chemo-

therapeutic drugs have also been used along with radiation. These studies are uncontrolled, and at present no definite conclusions can be drawn.

Chemotherapy Combined with Immunotherapy

Cancer immunobiology has been extensively discussed in Chapter 38. The tumor-related host immunodepression is further accentuated by chemotherapeutic drugs. Donaldson treated patients with squamous cell carcinomas of head and neck with a combination of MTX, BCG and Isoniazid. Twenty of his thirty-two patients responded. However, a number of his patients had received no prior therapy, and it is known that a larger percentage of such patients respond to treatment. More recently the group at the M.D. Anderson Hospital conducted a randomized study of patients on chemotherapy versus chemotherapy and BCG. The group given chemo-immunotherapy had a longer median survival. Since a number of patients with head and neck tumors have a defect in their cell-mediated immunity, mitogens such as BCG, C. parvum, levamisole, and autologous tumor cell vaccines are currently being evaluated in conjunction with or without chemotherapy, particularly in early stages of the head and neck cancers.

Concluding Remarks

In patients with head and neck tumors, malnutrition is a significant factor in the outcome of therapy. Chemotherapy may further aggravate this problem. Poor nutrition leads to immunosuppression which may lead to tumor enhancement. Trials are now under way to establish efficacy of intravenous hyperalimentation in these patients. Nevertheless, careful attention to the dietary needs of the individual patient may prevent weight loss and probably aid in the success of chemotherapy.

It is quite apparent that in patients with stage IV carcinoma of the head and neck, significant palliation can be achieved by chemotherapy. However, barring major breakthroughs, a cure for these patients is not on the horizon. The exact place of chemo-immunotherapy in combination with surgery and radiation in the treatment of these tumors has not been delineated. There is some evidence that tumors at certain specific sites (oral cavity—excluding the lip, oropharynx and maxillary sinus) may benefit from adjuvant chemotherapy. Some recent studies with hyperthermia and particulate radiation such as neutron beam suggest that these modalities may achieve a better local control of the head and neck tumors as compared to conventional measures. If this is borne out in future trials, systemic control of the disease would continue to be an ever increasing challenge to us. Chemo-immunotherapy is probably the only answer to this problem.

REFERENCES

General Reading

Aron, B. S., and Lorvidhaya, V.: Combination Therapy in Head and Neck Cancer. JAMA, *233*:177, 1975.

Cline, M. J., and Haskell, C. M.: Cancer Chemotherapy. Philadelphia, W. B. Saunders Co., 1975.

Holland, J. F., and Frei, E.: Cancer Medicine. Philadelphia, Lea & Febiger, 1973.

James, A. G.: Control of Head and Neck Cancer. Amer. J. Surg., *128*:456, 1974.

Rubin, P.: Clinical Oncology. 4th Ed., Rochester, N.Y., University of Rochester School of Medicine and Dentistry, 1974.

Zubrod, C. G.: Present Accomplishments of Cancer Chemotherapy. *In* Progress in Clinical Cancer. Edited by I. M. Ariel. New York, Grune and Stratton, 1975.

Cell Cycle

Anonymous: Cell Cycle and Death in Human Tumors. Brit. Med. J., *1*:177, 1976.

Murphy, W. K., Livingstone, R. B., Ruiz, V. G., et al.: Serial Labeling Index Determination as a Predictor of Response in Human Solid Tumors. Cancer Res., *35*:1438, 1975.

Shields, R.: New View of Cell Cycle. Nature, *260*:193, 1976.

Skipper, H. E., and Schabel, F. M., Jr.: Quantitative and Cytokinetic Studies in Experimental Tumor Models. *In* Cancer Medicine. Edited by J. F. Holland and E. Frei. Philadelphia, Lea & Febiger, 1973.

Steel, G. G.: Cytokinetics of Neoplasia. *In* Cancer Medicine. Edited by J. F. Holland and E. Frei. Philadelphia, Lea & Febiger, 1973.

Zimmerman, A. M., Padilla, G. M., and Carnesal L. L.: Drugs and the Cell Cycle. New York, Academic Press, 1973.

Mechanism of Action and Toxicity of Antineoplastic Agents

Chabner, B. A., Myers, C. E., Coleman, N., et al.: Clinical Pharmacology of Antineoplastic Agents. N. Eng. J. Med., *292*:1107, 1159, 1975.

Gershwin, M. E., Goetzl, E. J., and Steinberg, M.: Cyclophosphamide: Use in Practice. Ann. Int. Med., *80*:531, 1974.

Krakoff, I. H.: Cancer Chemotherapeutic Agents. Ca for Clinicians, *23*:208, 1973.

Weiss, H. D., Walker, M. D., Wiernik, P. H.: Neurotoxicity of Commonly Used Antineoplastic Agents. N. Eng. J. Med., *291*:75, 127, 1974.

Zubrod, C. G.: The Basis for Progress in Chemotherapy. Ca for Clinicians, *23*:202, 1973.

Adjuvant Chemotherapy

Bonadonna, G. et al.: Combination Chemotherapy as an Adjuvant Treatment in Operable Breast Cancer. N. Eng. J. Med., *294*:405, 1976.

Jaffe, N., Frei, E., Traggis, D. et al.: Adjuvant Methotrexate and Citrovorum Factor Treatment of Osteogenic Sarcoma. N. Eng. J. Med., *291*:994, 1974.

Perez, C. A., Stewart, C. C., and Wagner, B.: Experimental Observations on the Significance of Cell Burden in Tumor Control. Cancer, *34*:113, 1974.

Schabel, F. M.: Concepts for Systemic Treatment of Micrometastasis. Cancer, *35*:15, 1975.

Combination Chemotherapy

Carter, S. K., and Soper, W. T.: Integration of Chemotherapy into Combined Modality Treatment of Solid Tumors. I. The Overall Strategy. Cancer Treatment Rev., *1*:11, 1974.

DeVita, V. T., Young, R. C., and Canellos, G. P.: Combination Versus Single Agent Chemotherapy: A Review of the Basis for Selection of Drug Treatment of Cancer. Cancer, *35*:98, 1975.

Frei, E.: Combination Cancer Therapy: Presidential Address. Cancer Res., *32*:2593, 1972.

Biology of Head and Neck Cancer

Epstein, M. A.: Epstein-Barr Virus. Is it Time to Develop a Vaccine Program? J. Nat. Cancer Inst., *56*:697, 1976.

MacComb, W., and Fletcher, G.: Cancer of the Head and Neck. Baltimore, Williams & Wilkins, 1967.

Single Agent Chemotherapy

Goldsmith, M. A., and Carter, S. K.: The Integration of Chemotherapy into a Combined Modality Approach to Cancer Therapy. V. Squamous Cell Cancer of the Head and Neck. Cancer Treatment Rev., *2*:137, 1975.

Johns, D. G., and Bertino, J. R.: Folate Antagonists. *In* Cancer Medicine. Edited by J. F. Holland and E. Frei. Philadelphia, Lea & Febiger, 1973.

Livingstone, R. B., and Carter, S. K.: Single Agents in Cancer Chemotherapy. New York, I. F. I. Plenum, 1970.

Wasserman, T. M., Comis, R. L., Goldsmith, M., et al.: Tabular Analysis of the Chemotherapy of Solid Tumors. Cancer Chemotherapy Rep., Part 3, *6*:399, 1975.

High-Dose Methotrexate Therapy

DeConti, R. C.: Phase III Comparison of Methotrexate with Leucovorin vs. Methotrexate Alone vs. a Combination of Methotrexate Plus Leucovorin, Cyclophosphamide and Cytosine Arabinoside in Head and Neck Cancer. Proceeding Amer. Soc. Clin. Oncol., *17*:46, 1976.

Ensminger, W., Frei, E., Pitman, S., et al.: Prevention of Methotrexate Toxicity by Thymidine in Man. Proc. Amer. Soc. Clin. Oncol., *17*:189, 1976.

Frei, E., Jaffe, N., Tattersall, M. H. N., et al.: New Approaches to Cancer Chemotherapy with Methotrexate. N. Eng. J. Med., *292*: 846, 1975.

Goldman, I. D.: Membrane Transport of Methotrexate and Other Folate Compounds: Relevance to Rescue Protocol. Cancer Chemother. Rep., Part 3, *6*:63, 1975.

Jacobs, S. A., Stoller, R. G., Chabner, B. A., et al.: 7 Hydroxy Methotrexate as a Urinary Metabolite in Human Subjects and Rhesus Monkeys Receiving High Dose Methotrexate. J. Clin. Invest., *57*:534, 1976.

Penta, J. S.: Overview of Protocols on Clinical Studies of High Dose Methotrexate with Citrovorum Factor Rescue. Cancer Chemother. Rep., Part 3, *6*:7, 1975.

Price, L. A., Mill, B. T., Calvert, A. M., et al.: Kinetically Based Multiple Drug Treatment for Advanced Head and Neck Cancer. Brit. Med. J., *3*:10, 1975.

Combination Chemotherapy

Bertino, J. R., Boston, B., and Capizzi, R. L.: The Role of Chemotherapy in the Management of Cancer of the Head and Neck. A Review. Cancer, *36*:752, 1975.

Bertino, J. R., Mosher, M. B., and DeConti, R. C.: Chemotherapy of the Cancer of the Head and Neck. Cancer, *31*:1141, 1973.

Intra-arterial Chemotherapy

Bertino, J. R., Boston, B., and Capizzi, R. L.: The Role of Chemotherapy in the Management of Cancer of the Head and Neck. A Review. Cancer, *36*:752, 1975.

Freckman, H. A.: Results in 169 Patients with Cancer of the Head and Neck Treated by Intraarterial Infusion Therapy. Amer. J. Surg., *124*:501, 1972.

Watkins, E., and Sullivan, R. D.: Cancer Chemotherapy in Prolonged Arterial Infusion. Surg. Gynec. Obstet., *118*:3, 1964.

Surgery with Chemotherapy

DeSprez, J., Kiehn, C. L., Sciotto, C., et al.: Response of All Carcinoma to Preoperative Methotrexate Infusion Therapy. Amer. J. Surg., *120*:461, 1970.

DeWys, W. D.: Current Concepts of Chemotherapy Combined with Other Modalities for Head and Neck Cancer. Canad. J. Otolaryngol., *4*:195, 1975.

Richards, G. J., Jr., and Chambers, R. G.: Hydroxyurea: A Radiosensitizer in the Treatment of Neoplasms of the Head and Neck. Amer. J. Roentgenol., *105*:555, 1969.

Richards, G. J., and Chambers, R. G.: Hydroxyurea in the Treatment of Neoplasms of the Head and Neck. A Resurvey. Amer. J. Surg., *126*:513, 1973.

Tarpley, J. L., Chretien, P. B., Alexander, J. C., et al.: High Dose Methotrexate as a Preoperative Adjuvant in the Treatment of Epidermoid Carcinomas of the Head and Neck. Amer. J. Surg., *130*:481, 1975.

Radiation and Chemotherapy

Fletcher, G. H.: Textbook of Radiotherapy. Philadelphia, Lea & Febiger, 1973.

Hussey, D. H., and Abrams, J. P.: Combined Therapy in Advanced Head and Neck Cancer: Hydroxyurea and Radiotherapy. *In* Progress in Clinical Cancer. Edited by I. M. Ariel. New York, Grune and Stratton, 1975.

Knowlton, A. H., Percarpio, B., Bobrow, S., et al.: Methotrexate and Radiation Therapy in the Treatment of Advanced Head and Neck Tumors. Radiology, *116*:709, 1975.

Lipshutz, H., Lerner, H. J.: Six Year Survivals in the Combined Treatment of Far Advanced Head and Neck Cancer Under a Combined Therapy Program. Amer. J. Surg., *126*:519, 1973.

Richards, G. J., and Chambers, R. G.: Hydroxyurea in the Treatment of Neoplasms of the Head and Neck. A Resurvey. Amer. J. Surg., *126*:513, 1973.

Silverberg, I. J., Phillips, T. L., et al.: Bleomycin with Radiotherapy in the Treatment of Head and Neck Malignancies. Amer. Soc. Clin. Oncol., *17*:170, 1976.

Stefani, S., Eells, R. W., and Abbate, J.: Hydroxyurea and Radiotherapy in Head and Neck Cancer. Radiology, *101*:391, 1971.

Chemo-Immunotherapy

Copeland, E. M., MacFayden, B. A., and Dudrick, S. J.: Effects of Intravenous Hyperalimentation on the Established Immunity in the Cancer Patient. Ann. Surg., *184*:60, 1976.

Donaldson, R. C.: Chemo-Immunotherapy for Cancer of the Head and Neck. Amer. J. Surg., *126*:507, 1973.

Khandekar, J. D., DeWys, W. D.: "Chemoimmunotherapy of Head and Neck Cancer." Amer. J. Surg. *135*:688, 1978.

Penn, I.: Immunosuppression and Cancer. Importance in Head and Neck Surgery. Arch. Otolaryngol., *101*:667, 1975.

Chapter 38B

Cryosurgery for Treatment of Neoplasms of the Head and Neck

Daniel Miller

The therapeutic application of local cold dates back to the use of cold compresses in the treatment of compound skull fractures and infected wounds of the chest as early as 2500 B.C. A reapplication of this method of therapy was brought to the fore at the Saint Barnabas Hospital in New York City by Dr. Irving S. Cooper, who treated Parkinson's disease with cryosurgery of the thalamus and attempted to freeze brain tumors for excision or destruction in situ. Prior to this in 1959, Rowbotham and coworkers had designed a cooling cannula to remove a frozen cylinder of tumor from a patient's brain using circulating 95% alcohol through a freezing mixture of solid carbon dioxide and acetone.

My experience with cryosurgery over the past 10 years includes treatment of more than 1500 patients with various neoplasms of the skin, oral cavity, nasopharynx, middle and external ear, sinuses, larynx, and neck. The technique used involves an open cryospray as well as a closed cryoprobe and liquid nitrogen at −196°C. In order for cryosurgery to be effective as a destructive agent, the tissue to be destroyed must reach a temperature of at least −20°C. An open spray of liquid nitrogen at −196°C. penetrates much deeper and faster than the closed cryoprobe. However, the closed cryoprobe is more precise than the spray.

All tissues can be thought of as heat-sinks, and the application of the cold serves as a heat extractor, with resultant destruction of the tissue in which the temperature level is dropped below −20°C. Originally, the closed probe was used for small tumors or in regions in which the accessibility of the tumor was limited. However, we have applied the direct liquid nitrogen spray in areas of the head, oral cavity, and neck that are exposed or that can be made accessible by surgery.

Freezing represents nothing more than the removal of pure water from solution and its isolation into biologically inert foreign bodies and ice crystals. Thus, the primary event is crystallization. The actual mechanisms of cell death are dehydration and concentration of electrolytes resulting from removal of water from solution, denaturation of protein molecules, rupture of the cell membranes, thermal shock, and vascular stasis. If at all possible, a thermocouple should be placed tangentially at the depth and/or the periphery of the area to be treated in order to ascertain that −20°C. is reached. If it is not reached, destruction of the cells, despite the formation of a good

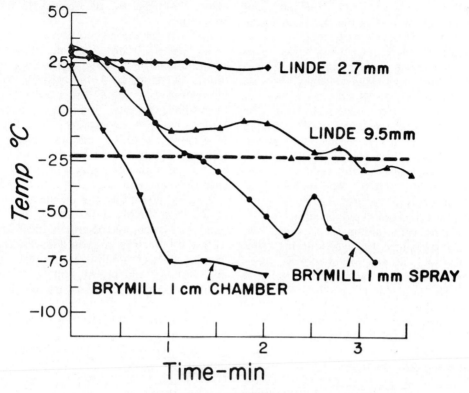

Fig. 38B–1. Muscle, 0.5 cm.

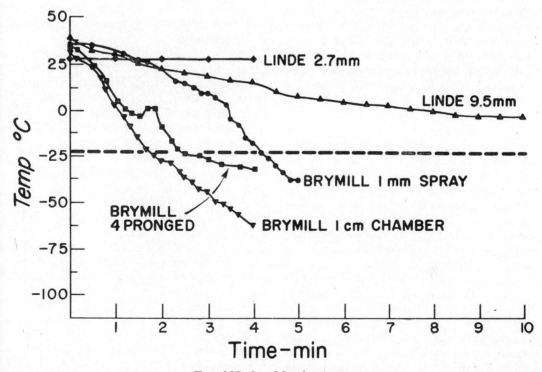

Fig. 38B–2. Muscle, 1 cm.

ice ball, is not a certainty. Neel and De-Santo, in their studies of the effects of freeze rates, tumor temperatures, and ischemia, have rightfully concluded that a rapid freeze and a slow thaw, repeated in two or occasionally three freeze-thaw cycles, provide the most effective destruction. As a result of the thrombosis that takes place in the smaller vessels, the vascular stasis, and the loss of heat in the heat-sink, the second freeze and slow thaw enable one to achieve a 100% destruction of the cells so treated to a level below $-20°C$. The thawing process is probably as destructive as, or more destructive than, the rapid freezing.

In dealing with tumors of the head and neck, one is confronted with varying types of tissue, such as mucous membrane, periosteum, bone, muscle, and often large blood vessels. The large blood vessels are not destroyed by the application of liquid nitrogen spray, mainly because of the warmth of the blood passing through the vessel. However, smaller vessels, such as capillaries, veins, and arteries, are readily destroyed by the spray.

Cryosurgery can be used for extensive tumors that have already received their full course of radiation therapy with or without surgery. Thus, another palliative measure for relief of pain is available. Sensory nerve fibers concerned with pain located adjacent to the tumor are easily destroyed almost on contact with the freezing liquid nitrogen.

When freezing of tissue takes place, an ice ball forms; with subsequent thawing, the resultant necrosis becomes apparent in a few hours and remains for 2 to 4 weeks, depending on the size of the tumor and the tissue destroyed. This gangrenous, edematous area is sharply demarcated from the surrounding tissue. Blebs may form. Grossly, the necrotic area resembles the tissue response of infarct due to vascular ischemia. Histologically, the cells look as though they have been irradiated. When the necrotic mass is removed, a clean granulating base that heals slowly is left. Re-epithelization of the mucosa in the oral cavity or the larynx at the site of the cryosurgery eventually occurs unless residual tumor remains or unless there is secondary infection or lack of blood supply. Frequently a reduced amount of pigment characterizes the regrowth of soft epithelium.

In order for the cell to function properly, many enzymes are essential, some being stable and others being relatively unstable during the freezing. One investigator has discovered that many fast freezes and fast thaws have resulted in injury to some enzymes, but not necessarily their complete breakdown. Without certain enzymes the cell cannot function as before. Therefore, if enough of these enzymes (including DNA and RNA) can be destroyed, another method of disrupting the chemical workings of the cells involved in cancer may be at hand. Goldstein, and Sherman and Kim have shown by electron microscopic studies that freezing causes definitive changes in the mitochondria and chromosomes, as well as definite disruptive changes in the cell membrane.

Most current investigations are directed toward the preservation rather than destruction of tissues by freezing. Audrey Smith has diluted bull semen with a media containing glycerol in a frozen state between $-79°$ and $-196°C$. After thawing, the sperm proved viable and successfully used for artificial insemination of cattle. Sherman and Kim have also been successful in this area of investigation.

Other areas of investigation which are important in this field include the preservation of viruses by freezing. Viruses are characterized by their ultramicroscopic size and their ability to propagate only within living cells. They contain one type of nucleic acid and at least one antigenetically active protein. The maintenance of viruses in the frozen state has become a practical procedure and is used routinely in most virus laboratories. The Registry of Viral and Rickettsial Organisms in Washington, D.C., maintains over 300 viral agents in the frozen state, and these are available for use after thawing. Nevertheless, virus-induced laryngeal papillomas may represent another lesion susceptible to cryosurgery.

It can readily be seen that freezing of tissue, even below $-20°C$, involves more than the simple removal of all available water in the cell and its transformation into inert foreign bodies (ice crystals). Appar-

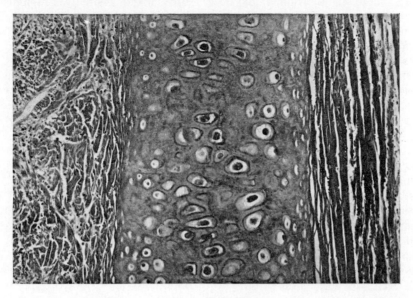

FIG. 38B–3. After cryosurgery of the cartilage in the dog auricle, showing marked destruction of the nuclei.

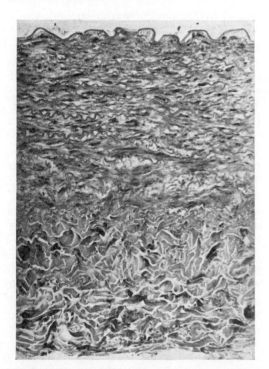

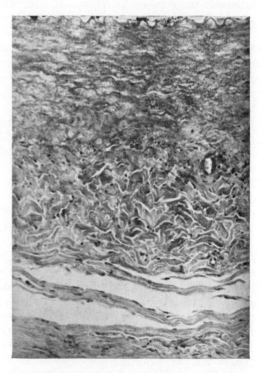

FIG. 38B–5. Dog carotid artery after cryosurgery. Most of the nuclei of the muscle cells beneath the intima are missing, yet the architecture of the vessel wall is preserved.

FIG. 38B–4. Dog carotid artery prior to cryosurgery.

ently much more than isolated physical phenomena are involved. Kline and Trapani have excised mouse tumors and, after slowly freezing them and maintaining the cell blocks in liquid nitrogen, have successfully transplanted them again. This indicates the feasibility of freezing intact tumors and actually preserving their tumorigenic characteristics, which raises many more questions.

Specific studies on cartilage reveal that this tissue is very easily destroyed by cryosurgery in a very short time. This, of course, suggests that cryosurgery should be used cautiously near cartilage. Studies on the effect of liquid nitrogen on the internal, external, or common carotid arteries have shown that the walls of the large vessels, such as the common carotid artery, are not destroyed, even with temperatures of −50° C. However, if the tumor has invaded the wall of the artery, the tumor cells will be destroyed by the cryosurgery and may cause a weakening of the wall. Bone is much more resistant to cryosurgery. However, the destruction of tumor in bone, especially in a previously irradiated area, will allow for sequestration to take place over a period of time. This eventually extrudes itself or can easily be removed, sometimes as long as a year later, with regrowth of either epithelium or mucous membrane.

The author performed studies on the vocal cords of cats, using the Brymill 3.2-mm laryngeal closed probe. The superior surfaces of the true cords were frozen for 2 minutes and were monitored by a thermocouple inserted 4 mm below the cord to measure temperature changes during and following freezing. Sacrifice of the animals 2 months later revealed adequate epithelial regeneration in all sections taken through the epithelial surfaces. In some areas the respiratory epithelium regenerated in an epidermoid fashion. No areas were left uncovered. Some of the skeletal muscle fibers underwent degeneration with migration of the sarcolemmic nuclei to the center of the bundle and with fibrosis and interstitial inflammatory infiltrates. In many areas there was frank fibrous replacement of the muscle cells. Interestingly, Schwann cells were found proliferating in the nerve bundles in

some areas. There was significant destruction of cartilage, probably because of the relatively poor blood supply of chondral tissue compared, for instance, to that of skeletal muscle. Yet there was some active regeneration of cartilage in these animals. The cartilage retained its shape in spite of the ischemic infarct type of necrosis. Studies on the larynx are discussed later in this chapter.

METHOD OF APPLICATION

When cryosurgery is applied in the form of liquid nitrogen spray, the nontarget area of tissue should be carefully protected from the target area by covering it with 8-ply petrolatum-impregnated gauze. If the closed cryoprobe is used, only the area that might be touched by the cryoprobe as it passes to the target needs to be protected. Should the closed or open probe be utilized in a skin carcinoma, whether basal cell or squamous cell, melanoma, or hemangioma, depigmentation of the treated area will occur, although some of this will clear over a period of a year or two. The Brymill apparatus has proved to be a most flexible unit for use in the head and neck. The large Brymill SP5 unit contains a Dewar flask which is filled with liquid nitrogen and to which is attached the delivery arm. Many varied shapes and sizes of probes with open or closed tips can easily be screwed onto the delivery arm. It is a self-pressurizing unit and requires no electrical apparatus. In addition, the spray unit with its varying tips, ranging from 0.1 mm to 1 mm, can be readily used when desired. The cryolaryngeal unit, using a 3.2-mm closed probe or ½-mm open spray tip, can be utilized through direct suspension laryngoscopy with or without a microscope. More recently, an increased size of probe tip has become available and can be utilized through a tracheostomy and directed by direct laryngoscopy from above. Either the Brymill or the Linde temperature monitor and thermocouple should be used in accessible areas to achieve more precision in the application of the destructive freeze.

When the closed probe is used, there is only an additional 20% increase in the size of the ice ball after the first minute. However, this depends a good deal on the water content of the tissue being frozen. When the application of cold is discontinued and the lesion thaws, the previously frozen area becomes red and pulpy, then violaceous and edematous with bleb formation. There is a very thin reactive zone of perhaps a few cells between the outline of the ice ball and the adjacent nontreated tissue. The Brymill SP5 unit must be monitored carefully to make sure it uses between 15 and 20 pounds of pressure. The duration of time should not be counted until the liquid nitrogen spray is applied directly to the target area or, should a closed probe be used, until the liquid nitrogen vents through the side of the delivery arm.

The dura is susceptible to destruction by freezing, so when the cryosurgeon is near this structure, he must proceed with great caution. Therefore, in doing cryosurgery about the ethmoidal region or the mastoid area, an attempt should be made to protect as much of the cribriform plate or tegmen and adjacent dura as possible. If destroyed, the bone will undergo a very slow sequestration over a period of many months.

ORAL CAVITY

Cryosurgery has been used successfully in many lesions of the oral cavity, including lymphomas of the tonsil and alveolar ridge, carcinoma and ameloblastoma of the alveolus, and verrucous carcinoma of the palate, tonsil, and alveolar ridge. It has been particularly successful in the treatment of multicentric lesions of the oral cavity. It is well known that if a patient has a carcinoma of the palatine arch, he has a 15% chance of developing a second lesion in the same arch, and if a second arch lesion does develop, there is about a 25% chance that he will develop a third primary. Cryosurgery can be utilized repeatedly for these recurrent lesions. It is especially helpful in elderly patients in the treatment of primary lesions or with lesions that have not been eliminated by radiation therapy or composite resection. More extensive surgical procedures can be avoided after local application of this modality. Several patients with verrucous carcinoma of the palate have been

treated with partial excision followed by cryosurgery to the periphery, the architecture of the bone of the palate being thus maintained for an eventual prosthesis. Similar verrucous lesions of the tongue and lingual tonsillar region have been treated with cryosurgery to avoid composite resection in elderly people or in people who have had a previous failure with radiation therapy.

Because cryosurgery freeze-depth is not precise and because one may not know the

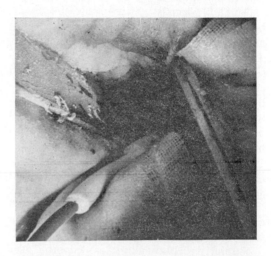

FIG. 38B–6. Protective packing and thermocouple in place. Retromolar carcinoma.

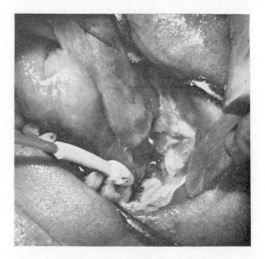

FIG. 38B–7. Thermocouple in place in frozen retromolar carcinoma.

exact depth of a carcinoma of the tongue and its frequent tumor pseudopods, the technique has only been helpful as a palliative measure in large carcinomas of the tongue. If the lesion is small, such as a T_1 lesion of the tongue, it can be treated primarily by cryosurgery, by local excision, or by radiation therapy. Also, small recurrent multicentric carcinomas of the tongue and the floor of the mouth can be treated successfully using cryosurgery after radiation and surgical failures; the technique can also be used as a palliative measure.

Ameloblastomas which invade the alveolar ridge, producing large cavities, often necessitate resection of the mandible and reconstruction. Several patients with this lesion have been successfully treated with cryosurgery only, liquid nitrogen being delivered through a 1-mm spray tip. The cavity becomes replaced with new bone and fibrous tissue and eventually is covered with mucous membrane.

Adamantinomas, which tend to grow up into the maxillary sinus, may require several surgical procedures to eradicate them. They have also been successfully treated with cryosurgery without necessitating another resection.

Similarly leukoplakia, as reported by Goode and others, has responded to superficial application of cryosurgery, using either the closed (preferable) or open probe. The mucous membrane readily regrows.

Gage has reported a high rate of cure using cryosurgery for the treatment of carcinoma of the oral cavity, but until more experience is gained, it is best to rely on the more certain modality of surgery, radiation or a combination of both. However, in those patients with medical or logistic problems, cryosurgery can certainly be used as a primary modality in the treatment of early carcinoma of the oral cavity.

Of particular interest is the use of cryosurgery in the treatment of lymphangiomas and cavernous hemangiomas. If located in the tongue, a large tumor could require a total glossectomy. This same tumor might be successfully managed by using a closed cryoprobe, two or three treatments being administered at intervals separated by many months. Treatment near the cheek runs the

risk of causing a fistula unless the freeze is carefully controlled by a thermocouple. Depigmentation of the skin may occur.

Recurrent carcinomas of the floor of the mouth, extending to the alveolar ridge, that are radiation failures can be treated by cryosurgery with one or two courses. The sequestrated bone can be removed as an office procedure many months later. Five-year "cure" rates have been established in many such patients.

NASOPHARYNX

The management of nasopharyngeal angiofibroma can be complicated by excessive bleeding. Cryosurgery has been very effective in the care of such tumors, mainly because of two factors: (1) its adherent qualities as the freeze develops on the angiofibroma; and (2) the many small vessels, arteries, and veins that are thrombosed or undergo complete vascular stasis during the period of the freeze. The cryoprobe can then be used as a handle on the tumor, which is usually quite rubbery. This enables the surgeon to deliver the tumor with its many lobulations via a transpalatal or transantral approach or a combination of both, using finger dissection, electrocautery, or scissors dissection. Should several pseudopods of tumor remain, the cryoprobe can be reapplied to those areas. It is rare for an angiofibroma to be destroyed by cryosurgery

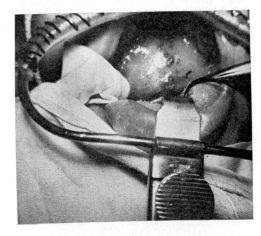

Fig. 38B–8. Huge cavernous hemangioma of the nasopharynx and palate.

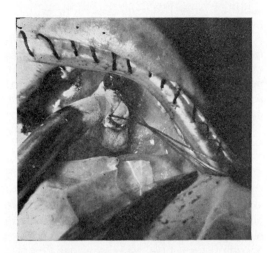

FIG. 38B–9. Closed probe attached to frozen hemangioma of the nasopharynx and palate. Patient is free of gross tumor 7 years after surgery.

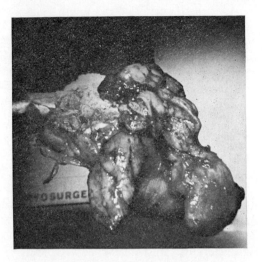

FIG. 38B–11. The probe is still attached to the fibroma after removal.

The use of cryosurgery in nasopharyngeal cancer is limited. The recurrent primary tumor, which has already undergone a full course of radiation therapy, can be treated palliatively to rid the patient of gross tumor, bleeding, slough, odor, and frequently pain. It can also be used in successive intervals as indicated.

EAR

Cryosurgery has been effective in the treatment of tumors of the ear. Most patients with ear cancer referred for cryotherapy have already had surgery and/or radia-

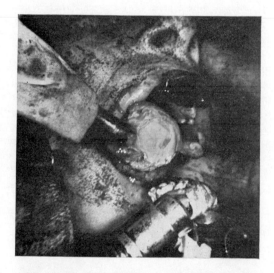

FIG. 38B–10. Closed cryoprobe used as handle to remove a juvenile angiofibroma.

alone unless it has a very small pedicle, and this is quite rare. The resultant reduction of loss of blood has been striking, however, in most patients so treated. Embolization of Gelfoam through the angiographic catheter 2 days prior to surgery and subsequent utilization of the cryosurgical technique after sufficient exposure of the tumor surgically have reduced the number of transfusions necessary for patients with these tumors.

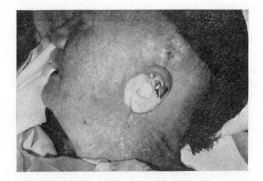

FIG. 38B–12. Persistent carcinoma of the middle ear and external auditory canal after radiation and surgical failure. The figure shows the frozen tumor.

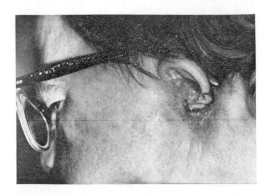

FIG. 38B–13.   Patient shown 4 years after cryosurgery.

tion therapy, with facial nerve paralysis, invasion of bone, and often intracranial involvement through the jugular foramen and hypoglossal foramen. Patients are treated by a liquid nitrogen spray at $-196°C$. Four of 6 patients so treated are now free of disease, one for over 5 years. One must of necessity produce a facial nerve paralysis and destruction of the inner ear with loss of vestibular function if this has not already occurred. As much surgery as possible should be done to expose the area to be frozen. The tegmen should be preserved whenever possible, and if not, care must be taken not to apply the open spray to the region of the dura. A flat disc closed cryoprobe can be applied to that area to obtain minimal destruction. Recurrent carcinoma about the ear can be treated palliatively as well, and cryosurgery may be used in repeated courses determined by the size and rate of regrowth of the carcinoma.

Chemodectoma of the middle ear can be kept under control and often completely destroyed by using cryosurgery. A closed probe is preferred in this area in an attempt to prevent facial nerve paralysis or labyrinthitis. Several patients have been maintained with cryosurgery given at intervals of 3 to 5 years, which kept an extensive tumor under control with a minimum of symptoms.

It is possible to utilize a catheter embolization of the vessels feeding a glomus jugulare tumor, followed within a few days by cryosurgery to the region of the glomus tumor. Use of the closed probe should not be attempted without good surgical exposure of the tumor. The alternative may require

subtotal temporal bone resection, with its high morbidity rate.

Tumors of the auricle which have extended to the scalp and invaded the cortex of the parietal and temporal bones have been eradicated completely by cryosurgery. Regrowth of epithelium covering the denuded bone occurs over a period of many months.

NOSE AND SINUSES

The use of cryosurgery in the nose or sinuses requires exteriorization of the target area. If a lesion of the nasal vestibule is to be treated, a partial lateral rhinotomy with elevation of the alar region must first be accomplished. One must consider the fact that cartilage is easily destroyed when this modality is used. Should maxillectomy be required for a carcinoma of the antrum with residual or recurrent disease, cryosurgery is not easily employed because of the proximity and vulnerability of the eye and optic nerve. It is easier to successfully utilize cryosurgery for residual disease in the greater wings of the sphenoid or the ethmoidal region if the patient has had an orbital exenteration along with maxillectomy. The sequestrated residual ethmoid bone and cribriform plate area eventually are easily removed and the dura covered by epithelium and fibrous tissue. The longest tumor-free period in a patient so treated is now 9 years. Thus, cryosurgery can be delivered at the time of the primary orbital exenteration and maxillectomy if residual tumor remains, or later if it is recurrent. However, if the tumor has invaded the skull by passing through the foramina, cryosurgery is of little help.

CARCINOMA OF THE SKIN

Basal and squamous cell carcinoma of the skin have been treated repeatedly by cryosurgery with a 98% cure rate. Use of the cryospray unit or the closed copper disc cryoprobe has been very effective in the treatment of these lesions; it can be performed as an outpatient procedure, usually with local anesthesia. This is a particularly useful modality in patients with lesions on the cheek near the alar region, inner canthus, lower eyelid, or external auricle, or in areas that normally require a pedicle flap to

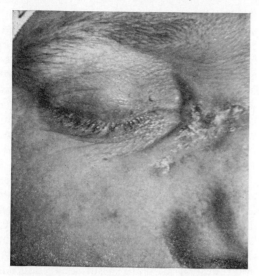

FIG. 38B–14. Recurrent basal cell carcinoma of the nose and inner canthus of the eye —a radiation failure.

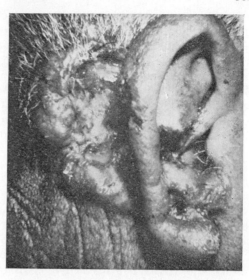

FIG. 38B–16. Basal cell carcinoma of the auricle and scalp with evidence of temporal bone involvement.

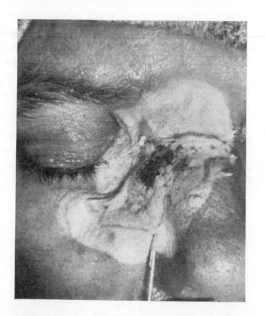

FIG. 38B–15. Frozen basal cell carcinoma with thermocouple in position.

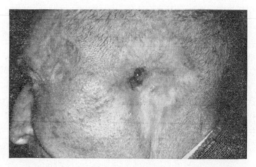

FIG. 38B–17. Appearance 2½ years after cryosurgery. Pale area shows previously exposed bone with regrowth of skin over defect.

of a local protein toxicity or lymphatic obstruction in the region of the freeze. It begins a few hours after the treatment and may last for 1 to 2 days.

close a surgical defect. It lessens the need for radiation therapy in this area. One should be aware of the fact that edema of the eyelids takes place easily in facial lesions treated with cryosurgery. Freezing a lesion within 6 cm of the eye may result in moderate eye edema. This may be the result

LARYNX

Dating back historically to Billroth's first total laryngectomy, the aim of the laryngologist in the treatment of carcinoma of the larynx has been to eliminate the cancer and preserve the life of the patient if possible— usually, however, at the expense of the larynx. Attempts to preserve voice production while eliminating the cancer soon led to partial operations on the vocal cords. In the 1930's the value of good radiation therapy in the cure of cancer, with preservation of the voice, began to obtain a foothold. As radiotherapeutic techniques, with supervoltage cobalt therapy, and knowledge increased in this field, more larynges were saved, and the cancer was eradicated in a high percentage of cases. The search for a method of eradication of this disease and preservation of some or all of the function of voice production continues. Radiation has its possible complications; conservation surgery has its problems and limitations. Cryosurgery to eliminate the disease while preserving the larynx has reached a point of clinical application which indicates increased use in the future.

When radiation of T_1N_0 lesions of the larynx is used, the 5-year "cure" rate is 89%. Of the 11% failures, an additional 6% can be salvaged, usually by total laryngectomy. Cryosurgery can be used in the 11% not controlled by irradiation, and if successful, it preserves the voice, of course. Our first clinical report revealed that 13 out of 17 patients so treated were free of disease for 1 to 5 years, with subsequent recurrence in 2 patients necessitating total laryngectomy. The technique was performed through the laryngoscope with Lewy suspension using the small 3.2-mm Brymill cryoprobe. Erroneous preclassification was made in four patients in whom the treatment subsequently failed. It was noted technically that one could not produce the necessary freeze-depth in T_2 lesions. It is likely that larger lesions might respond to the freezing techniques if the correct application of a larger cryoprobe could be made under proper visualization.

In January of 1974, Mulvaney and Miller embarked on a study to overcome some of the problems inherent in treating carcinoma of the larynx transorally with cryosurgery. Use of the more penetrating open spray in the larynx with liquid nitrogen from above often destroyed more tissue than desired. Good vision was disturbed by the "smoke" of the vapor produced. Use of petrolatum-impregnated gauze to protect nontarget tissues was not entirely satisfactory. As a result, a two-phase project with an assessment of time, temperature, and freeze-depth relationships with different-sized closed cryoprobes via a larynx-splitting operation on large dogs was inaugurated. The authors were able to determine by thermocouple studies what would occur with various closed cryoprobes in terms of tissue destruction. They were also able to determine the probability of the nondestructive effect on the lamina of the thyroid cartilage. Double-freeze applications provided the most efficient destruction.

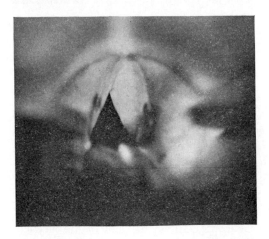

FIG. 38B–18. Cryosurgery has just been applied to the right vocal cord for recurrent carcinoma (T_1N_0) after a full course of cobalt 60 radiation therapy.

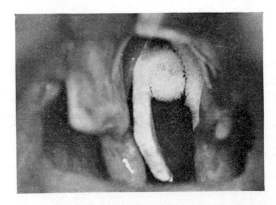

FIG. 38B–19. Dog. Frozen vocal cord and cryoprobe adjacent. Styrofoam paddle protects left vocal cord.

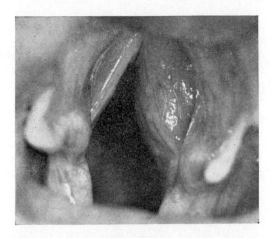

FIG. 38B–20. Dog. Forty-five minutes after cryosurgery.

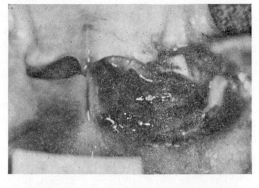

FIG. 38B–22. Dog. Seven days after cryo-surgery.

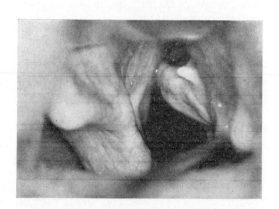

FIG. 38B–21. Dog. Five days after cryosur-gery.

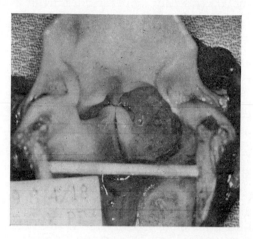

FIG. 38B–23. Dog. Nine weeks after cryo-surgery.

From this study it became apparent that the 3.2-mm probe with a surface of 8 sq mm produced nothing more than a superficial freeze below −20°C. A slight increase in the diameter of the tip from 3.2 to 5 mm, making it 20 sq mm, permitted greater freeze delivery to deeper tissue levels. Subsequently, a rectangular closed cryolaryngeal probe with a surface of 45 sq mm was developed, which has further extended the perimeter of the tissue destroyed.

The second phase of the project entailed determining the practical considerations involved in creating a cryolesion via a tracheostomy, but visually controlled by direct suspension laryngoscopy. A Styrofoam paddle was fashioned and inserted from above to protect the opposite vocal cord. This procedure, using a 45 sq mm cryoprobe, has been proved successful in destroying an entire vocal cord with preservation of the cartilage of the lamina. There is no interference with swallowing. The larnyx heals in 4 weeks, and the tracheostomy is usually closed within 4 to 5 days. The liquid nitrogen is passed through the closed cryoprobe (SP5 Brymill unit). The technique appears to have great promise. One minute of cryosurgery is used, beginning the count only when the liquid nitrogen has vented from the delivery arm. A double-freeze cycle is performed. Time and experience will determine the size of the tumor of the larynx that can be so treated.

Table 38B–1.   Papillomas of the Larynx

Number of patients treated with cryosurgery (1968-1973)	21
Adults treated	15
Children treated	6
Number of direct laryngoscopies and cryosurgery	55
Number free of disease up to 5 years	16

Papillomas of the larynx respond better to a combination of excision, cryosurgery, and microcautery, through direct laryngoscopy. It has taken one to five such courses, and occasionally more, at intervals of 3 to 11 months to eradicate most papillomas. If a child's larynx is treated, tracheostomy should be performed because of edema. If an adult's larynx is treated, tracheostomy is rarely, if ever, necessary.

COMPLICATIONS OF CRYOSURGERY

Protection of the nontarget tissue involves use of 8-ply petrolatum gauze to wall off the areas away from the tumor. Cryosurgery using the open spray is not as precise as that using the closed probe, and when anatomically irregular areas involving various ridges are treated, undesired destruction of tissue may result. The choice of the aperture size for delivery of the liquid nitrogen is important. This ranges from 0.25 to 1 cm. The 1-mm spray aperture is probably the most commonly used and can reach the depth desired for thin but wide tumors. Using a thermocouple inserted into the periphery of the target area, one can decide on the duration of treatment. Usually about 2 to 3 minutes of freezing, repeated in a second course of freezing after the first ice ball has thawed, is desired. For buccal mucosa lesions, the thermocouple should be placed as close to the skin as possible within the oral cavity. Occasionally liquid nitrogen may seep through improperly packed petrolatum gauze, and the nitrogen may slip into the oropharynx or over the lip and cause destruction of tissue which may interfere with function later. Liquid nitrogen may leak through the protective packs onto the lip around the intratracheal tube and produce destruction of the skin and contracture of the lip. It is most important to pack carefully about the intratracheal anesthesia tube at the angle of the lip. Cryosurgery applied to lesions of the retromolar triangle, in which the tumor extends up into the pterygoid palatine region, may eventually cause trismus. It is important to spend as much or more time on protecting the nontarget area as on applying sufficient freeze to destroy the target areas.

When cryosurgery is to be used for tumors in the oral cavity involving periosteum, the patient and his family should be told of the probability of exposure of and destruction of some of the mandible. If one applies cryosurgery to the base of the tongue, one must be concerned with secondary infection, aspiration, and pulmonary complications, even if a tracheostomy is performed prior to the delivery of the freeze. Even with a tracheostomy and intermittent cuff protection, gram-negative organisms may invade the cold-produced gangrenous lesion in the base of the tongue and produce secondary pulmonary problems of infection.

REFERENCES

Amoils, S. P., and Walker, A. J.: The Thermal and Mechanical Factors Involved in Ocular Cryosurgery. Proc. R. Soc. Med., *59*:1056, 1966.

Cooper, I. S.: A Cryogenic Method for Physiology Inhibition and Production of Lesions in the Brain. J. Neurosurg., *19*:853, 1962.

Cooper, I. S.: Cryogenic Surgery: A New Method of Destruction or Extirpation of Benign or Malignant Tissues. New Engl. J. Med., *268*:743, 1963.

Cooper, I. S.: Cryobiology as Viewed by the Surgeons. Cryobiology, *1*:44, 1964.

Gage, A., et al.: Cryotherapy for Cancer of the Lip and Oral Cavity. Cancer, *18*:1646, 1965.

Goldstein, J. C.: Cryotherapy in Head and Neck Cancer. Laryngoscope, *80*:1046, 1970.

Goode, R. L., and Spooner, T. R.: Office Cryosurgery for Oral Leukoplakia. Tr. Am. Acad. Ophthal. Otolaryngol., *75*:968, 1971.

Miller, D.: Cryosurgery for the Treatment of Neoplasms of the Oral Cavity. Otolaryng. Clin. North Am., *5*:377, 1972.

Miller, D.: Does Cryosurgery Have a Place in the Treatment of Papillomata or Carcinoma of the Larynx? Ann. Otol. Rhinol. Laryngol., 82:656, 1973.

Miller, D., and Metzner, D.: Cryosurgery for Tumors of the Head and Neck. Trans. Am. Acad. Ophthal. Otolaryng., 73:300, 1969.

Miller, D., and Mulvaney, T.: Cryosurgery as a Modality in the Treatment of Carcinoma of the Larynx. Laryngoscope, 85:1281, 1975.

Miller, D., et al.: Cryosurgical Treatment of Carcinoma of the Ear. Trans. Am. Acad. Ophthal. Otolaryng., 76:1363, 1972.

Neel, H. B., III, and DeSanto, L. W.: Cryosurgical Control of Cancer: Effects of Freeze Rates, Tumor Temperatures, and Ischemia. Ann. Otol. Rhinol. Laryngol., 82:716, 1973.

Rowbotham, G. F., et al.: Cooling Cannula for Use in the Treatment of Cerebral Neoplasms. Lancet, 1:12, 1959.

Sherman, J. K., and Kim, K. S.: Correlation of Ultrastructure Before Freezing, While Frozen, and After Thawing in Assessing Freeze-thaw Induced Injury. Cryobiology, 4:16, 1967.

Smith, M. F. W., and Lipson, L.: Angiofibroma: Role of Cryosurgery. J. Cryosurg., 2:12, 1969.

Smith, M. F. W., et al.: Cryosurgery Techniques in Removal of Angiofibromas. Laryngoscope, 74:1071, 1964.

Wang, C. C.: Treatment of Glottic Carcinoma by Megavoltage Radiation Therapy and Results. Am. J. Roentgen. Radium Ther. Nucl. Med. 120:157, 1974.

Wilson, W., et al.: Juvenile Nasopharyngeal Angiofibroma. Laryngoscope, 82:985, 1972.

Zacarian, S. A.: Cryosurgery in Dermatologic Disorders and in the Treatment of Skin Cancer. J. Cryosurg., 1:70, 1968.

Zacarian, S. A., and Adham, M. I.: Cryotherapy of Cutaneous Malignancy. Cryobiology, 2:212, 1966.

Chapter 39
Defects of Speech

G. Paul Moore and Thomas B. Abbott

Laymen casually accept the ability to communicate and associate that process generally with the mouth, ears, nose, and throat. These persons, along with the more sophisticated and the professional users of voice, often turn to physicians, particularly otolarygologists, for help when either **speech, language, or voice is impaired or** fails to develop normally. The health of the organs of communication is the special province of the otolaryngologist, while training or rehabilitation of speech problems is usually managed by speech pathologists. However, since adequate functioning of the vocal organs is intimately linked to their health and structure, the medical specialist is often challenged by his patients to provide guidance that extends well beyond his customary training. Many otolaryngologists are properly reluctant to offer rehabilitation in areas other than the treatment of disease because they do not feel qualified; yet patients inevitably seek answers to questions about communication disorders. The physician becomes, in fact, a mixture of speech pathologist, audiologist, and counselor. Persons with speech disorders are often intensely concerned about their handicaps and thereby force the conscientious otolaryngologist who is unable to refer his patients to assume an additional role.

A second and extremely important relationship between communication and the medical specialist rests in the surgery or other treatment which he elects. The conscientious physician naturally must consider the significance and consequences of his therapy in order to select, insofar as possible, that procedure which is least detrimental to the patient's capacity to speak or hear. A basic understanding of the communication process is essential to fulfill such a responsibility.

This chapter does not, and in fact could not, present sufficient information for the conduct of a speech rehabilitation program. Its purpose, instead, is to provide some insight into the common communicative disorders and the intimate relationships that exist between the physiologic and communicative functions of the nose, mouth, ears, and throat. The ultimate reason for having such information is the more complete guidance of patients and parents who request help for defective speech, language, or voice.

The Communication Process

Oral communication ordinarily involves two or more persons and is a process that can be represented as a chain of functions containing such links as thinking, symbolizing (usually in verbal language), speaking, transmission of the sound, hearing, listening, and perceiving. The first three links are associated primarily with the speaker, who encodes and utters the message; the last three refer essentially to the listener, who hears and decodes the message. The transmission of the sound is the acoustic link in the chain that connects the speaker and listener. Impairment of any of the mechanisms used in this sequence—that is, the nervous system, the organs of speech, the mechanism of hearing, or the complex combinations of psychological factors called learning—may cause a communicative disorder and consequently present a problem of concern to speech pathologist and audiologist. It is the breadth of the problems and the involvement of structures in the domain of otolaryngology that creates an interdependent relationship between otolaryngology, speech pathology, and audiology. The contribution of audiology cannot be overestimated, but since its role is discussed in other chapters, this presentation will emphasize the speaking rather than the listening aspects of communication.

Defects of Speech

A recent report from the National Advisory Neurological and Communicative Disorders and Stroke Council estimated that there are approximately 17 million persons in the United States (roughly 7%) with speech disorders. Within this total there are approximately 8 million with articulatory problems, 6 million with faulty language formulation, and 3 million divided equally between stuttering and voice disorders. A review of many surveys in schools covering various populations suggests that about 7% of students have speech disorders and that about three fourths of these have articulatory problems. However, most of the disorders are age-related, with larger numbers occurring among the younger children. A survey of 32,500 children in a large school population revealed approximately 6% with voice disorders deviant enough to justify special attention, including 1.5% with problems sufficiently serious to interfere with intelligibility or progress in school. No broad survey of speech or voice defects among adults has been conducted; consequently, definitive numbers are not available. How-

ever, many voice problems, unlike stuttering and articulatory disorders, develop in adulthood. Speech pathologists recognize that a substantial segment of the adult population as well as the younger groups have serious voice defects, the problems which involve otolaryngologists most directly.

Individuals who speak abnormally often have a combination of two or more types of speech problems, but for systematic study and convenience in discussion, the disorders can be divided into four major categories. First and most common are the articulatory defects (dyslalias). These problems include defective language sounds and sound combinations which may be distorted, omitted, substituted, or added as accessory sounds. Sometimes articulatory disorders cause unintelligible speech, but more commonly these problems encompass a relatively small number of sounds and are popularly, but often incorrectly, called lisping, baby talk, lalling, or tongue-tie. A second type of disorder is the impairment of the rhythmic flow of speech, which is called stuttering or stammering. Stuttering is characterized by repetition of sounds or words, by prolongations, by atypical pauses, or by word substitution, all of which produce linguistically meaningless interruptions in the expected continuity of the utterance. A third category is variously labeled language impairment, linguistic disability, or faulty symbolization, which refers to disorders in the expression of thought in language. The category includes a variety of problems from delayed speech to aphasia. The fourth type of disorder encompasses deviations in vocal pitch, loudness, or quality, which are classified as voice defects. A vocal problem is present when either pitch, loudness, or quality is atypical compared with the voices of most other persons of the same age, sex, and cultural group.

Some concept of the complexity of communicative disorders is revealed in this classification. That therapy is equally complex is emphasized by the fact that both organic and functional causes are present in all of the problems, with the possible exception of stuttering. Those communicative problems that can be diagnosed as functional result from the faulty behavior of normal organs of speech and are causally related to either psychological or environmental factors. The organic defects result from malfunction of one or more parts of an impaired speech-producing mechanism, which encompasses the nervous, muscular, skeletal, glandular, and circulatory systems.

SPEECH DEVELOPMENT IN THE CHILD

The normal acquisition of speech may be expected to follow much the same pattern as the motor, adaptive, and personal-social behavior of the child. As in all other types of learned behavior, speaking depends upon the process of maturation. There appears to be a "speech readiness period" between the ninth and twenty-fourth months of life, when the child acquires the ability to develop speech as a method of communication. However, this capacity represents the cumulative learning of many bits and pieces of language that begin within the first few weeks of life.

The infant is not born with the desire or the need to use oral language, except as crying may be considered a form of oral language. The child learns to talk only because those in his immediate environment speak to each other and to him. Before he can learn to use an arbitrary array of oral symbols as a form of social behavior, he normally lives through a series of prelingual overlapping stages of sound production. The child's physical, emotional, and intellectual needs are served and expressed in each stage. Furthermore, the emergence of speech in the "normal" child serves as an excellent index of his physical, intellectual, and emotional status.

The Cry. The development of speech is usually classified into a sequence of five stages, each of which has distinctive characteristics that blend cumulatively. The first stage is crying, which includes both the undifferentiated and the differentiated cry. The former is part of a total body reflex response to the environment; it is nonspecific during the first month or two and does not identify sensations of hunger or pain, heat, cold, or other kinds of discomfort. However, regardless of the lack of differentiation in the early

crying of the infant, this vocal response, like speaking, is produced primarily on exhalation.

Differentiated crying appears within the first few months, and although it continues to be part of a total body response, it begins to be associated with the situation, and the mother soon learns to interpret variations in the cry as signals of immediate needs or desires. Lewis states that "a child's progress in speech will to some extent depend on the way in which others respond to his cries and gurglings. If he is frequently allowed to cry for long periods without anyone coming to him, then his cries will not easily be connected by him with the satisfaction of his needs, and his crying will tend to remain aimless." On the other hand, the same author points out that some persons may anticipate every need of the infant and thereby weaken his incentive to gurgle and cry for attention.

Babbling. The second stage in the development of speech is called babbling. The infant does not abandon differentiated crying, but usually by the third or fourth month he produces a variety of sounds at random, and he may appear to be "listening" as well as responding to sounds in his environment.

The speech development of the congenitally deaf child will differ from that of the child with normal hearing beyond the babbling stage. The deaf child does not continue babbling for as long as the hearing child, and his speech does not progress to the next stage, the self-imitative repetition called lallation.

Lallation. This third stage, lallation, begins during the second 6 months. At first, the sounds produced are carried over from babbling, but later the infant appears to be responding more selectively to the sounds of others.

Echolalia. Echolalia, the name given to the fourth stage, begins somewhere around the ninth to tenth month, when the baby repeats sounds which he hears in his environment. It is unlikely that he comprehends the meaning of such sounds, but as in lallation, he seems to produce sounds that are pleasurable to him and that another individual is initiating for him. It is during babbling and lallation that the baby acquires an inventory of sound complexes which he later will use in learning to speak and in developing a vocabulary.

Intentional Speech. The fifth stage is the acquisition of speech as a practical tool for communication. Before the child enters this final but ever-expanding stage, he must have established a functional understanding of conventionalized speech patterns.

It is difficult to provide meaningful time sequences for the mastery of speech sounds because there are many factors that influence and regulate their acquisition. Girls generally surpass boys in learning speech sounds and tend to be accelerated in articulation skill from about 4½ years on. Girls normally approximate mature articulation by the age of 7, whereas boys usually take an additional year to reach the same degree of proficiency. Children living in orphanages and similar institutions do not develop speech as rapidly and clearly as do children in the conventional home environment.

Poole studied the genetic development of consonant sounds in children and formulated the following norms:

Age in Years	Sounds Developed
3½	p, b, m, w, h
4½	d, t, n, g, k, ng, j
5½	f
6½	v, zh, sh, l
7½	z, s, r, th, wh

These norms should be used for recording the use of consonant sounds at the listed ages and not for determining the exact onset of the sound. In general, research indicates that the average child of 36 months should have acquired a vocabulary of approximately 1000 words and should be using short meaningful sentences. In all probability there will be errors in his articulation; nevertheless, 80 to 90% of his conversational speech should be intelligible to an interested listener. If a child is not speaking acceptably by the age of 7 years, it may be due to any one or a combination of the following: (1) defective hearing; (2) poor motor coordination; (3) physical defects; (4) poor speech models in the family environment; (5) insufficient language stimu-lation; (6) mental retardation; or (7) emotional disturbance.

DEFECTS OF ARTICULATION (DYSLALIA)

Dyslalia may be described as faulty or atypical production of sounds in the spoken language. It encompasses many kinds of articulatory defects and constitutes the most frequent type of speech disorder. Articulatory defects are usually subclassified into four types as follows:

1. *Substitution.* One sound is substituted for another in the initial, medial, or final position within the word. For example, the sound *w* is frequently substituted for *r*, producing *wed* for *red; t* or *d* may replace *th,* and *mother* becomes *mudder* and *something* changes to *someting; th* may substitute for *s,* and *miss* becomes *mith.* The most frequently misarticulated sounds are those which are mastered last in the course of speech development (*s, z, r, l, th*).

2. *Omission.* Sounds are omitted in a word and are not replaced by a substitute. The child may produce *tep* for *step, air* for *where,* or *daw* for *dog.*

3. *Distortions.* The sound is produced, but it is modified so that the acoustic result is inaccurate. The *s* and *z* are among the most misarticulated speech sounds because adjustments of the tongue, teeth, and bite relationships are so exacting that minor deviations easily occur. The distortion of one or more of the sibilant consonants (*s, z, sh, zh*) is called lisping or sigmatism.

4. *Additions.* Extra sounds are added which are not part of the word; examples are *warsh* for *wash* or *plass* for *pass.* Additions are not as common as substitutions, omissions, and distortions.

Functional Dyslalia

When a defect or disorder is designated *functional,* it is frequently assumed to be more elementary or simple than when it is called *organic.* That this assumption is not entirely true may be demonstrated by the resistance to therapy that some individuals show when no organic etiology is present. Conversely, the speech pathologist fre-

phonetic analysis of the articulatory errors. Other phases of this motor disorder must not be neglected. . . . Psychological factors (emotional, intellectual, etc.) may reflect in the speech problem. . . ."

Treatment of Dysarthria. Eisenson suggests that "if the involvements are peripheral the patient is likely to distort or slur sounds, or to speak slowly and laboriously because his articulatory mechanism has become cumbersome. Improvement is likely to take place spontaneously as innervation improves. If there is residual paresis, the patient, through a basic phonetic approach, may be taught compensations for some of the speech sounds which continue to be difficult to produce. Articulatory drill may be of some help, as will any drill which improves the tonus and control of the articulatory muscles. . . . If the dysarthria is of central origin, it may be of help in later stages of training to make the patient aware of his errors and to use a phonetic approach in training." The person with neural impairment may not be able to achieve perfect or even good speech, but a treatment program can aim for serviceable communication and adaptation to the circumstances.

When dysarthria is associated with cerebrovascular trauma, Buck states that "the major consideration in personal and language adjustment of the stricken patient involves far more than language drills in isolation. . . . As far as any language retraining is concerned, some repetitive drill will be of little value until the overlying psychological disruptions are well controlled. Undue pressures in solving unrealistic language drills may markedly interfere with both psychological and physical adjustments." Wepman states that he "has never insisted upon correctness in articulation as an early goal for the patient. Rather it is felt that the ability to express one's self in free and easy speech and the use of all of the communicating forms of language are the important areas for the therapist to consider. Accuracy of enunciation is a comparatively easy, although specialized, area which can be treated separately if necessary after the patient has learned to function on an adult level in terms of ability to use speech and language."

Wood cautions that dysarthria in children should not be confused with dyspraxia, although the symptoms are similar in both problems. Dyspraxia involves the child's inability to perform a specific motor function voluntarily. Although the organs of speech are intact, the child has little or no control of them. Dysarthria is frequently observed in children with cerebral palsy; however, it may present itself also in children who do not demonstrate involvement of the extremities.

Wood further states that "children with dysarthria are unable to control the fine jaw or tongue movements necessary for speech, which when dysarthria is present, is slurred and frequently unintelligible. These children talk as if the entire length of their tongue were rooted to the floor of their mouth. Not only is the child with dysarthria unable to move his lower jaw and tongue independently when he wants to or when requested to do so, but he is unable to use his tongue and jaws adequately for chewing or eating. Swallowing is difficult for him also." These children frequently require therapy which extends over a long period of time. It is necessary for them to learn to control the movements of the tongue and jaw in order to acquire acceptable speech, provided no other serious involvements are present.

DEFECTS OF RHYTHM (STUTTERING)*

Stuttering is one of the most enigmatic of speech defects encountered by the speech pathologist. It is a difficult phenomenon to define because "no two stutterers are alike" and no one stutterer is the same from one time until the next. A workable definition of stuttering that has been acceptable to all speech pathologists has not yet been formulated. However, there appears to be a general agreement among professional personnel in the following description:

The dictionary and the general public may define stuttering as "hesitating or stumbling in uttering words" but to the speech pathologist

*The terms *stuttering* and *stammering* are synonymous, the former being preferred in the United States.

this definition is not complete unless it is qualified by at least three statements: (1) the speaker has no discernible physical or mental abnormality that is functionally related to the disfluent speech, (2) he regards his way of talking as unusual and considers it a problem or a difficulty, and (3) he seeks to contend with this difficulty by means of avoidance reactions that interfere with his speech, including the attempt to force trouble-free speech.

The committee on the Midcentury White House Conference of the American Speech and Hearing Association (1952) estimated the incidence of stuttering among school-age children to be 7 per 1000, or 0.7%. Robinson reports that stutterers constitute approximately 1% of each generation's population. More recent estimates from a report presented in 1969 by the National Institute of Neurological and Communicative Disorders and Stroke, National Institutes of Health, indicate that the percentage of stutterers in the population remains constant. Research has confirmed the clinical observation that stuttering is more common among boys than girls, the former exceeding the latter in a ratio of approximately 4:1. Furthermore, the stuttering phenomenon usually begins before puberty and persists longer in the male.

The literature presents a variety of theories regarding the origin of stuttering. However, there again appears to be general agreement that the child's environmental conditions are speech-centered and that the origin or onset of stuttering usually occurs during the speech development period of the child's life. Yet, it is also apparent that a large majority of children experience a period of "normal nonfluency" during their early years. Metraux reports that at the age of 18 months, children repeat syllables or words and that these repetitions are easy and unforced and can be terminated by the child or by the response of others. The 24-month-old child may exhibit a kind of compulsive repetition of a phrase or word. There may be a variation in the phrase, but it seems necessary to the child to repeat it. Metraux further states that the 30-month-old child "will repeat a phrase or word occasionally, but some of them will continue interminably with more force, higher pitch

and volume each time . . . it often seems to be the external stimuli which increase repetition since the child is attempting more and more to use speech as a tool to command others to his needs." However, the same author reports that at 36 months "most children are again on an easy repetitive basis with none of the compulsion noted earlier . . . occasional repetition of the beginning syllable and (Λ) (uh-uh)* or (ΛM) (uhm-uhm)* is often used as a starter for speech." At 42 months repetitions are frequent and seem "to be related to another person, in demand for attention, information, or encouragement." Luper and Mulder have suggested that when a child begins to "stutter" or show signs of beginning to stutter, the prognosis for improvement is as good as it will ever be. At this point, the speech of the child is a "problem" because someone in his environment views it as such. When the young child becomes overly aware of his own speech and builds up anxiety-tensions that cause him to fear and avoid speaking situations, then his speech presents a problem. When stuttering can be restricted to the "normal" hesitations and repetitions that frequently characterize the early stages of speech development, they often disappear spontaneously, and "direct" clinical assistance is rarely required. However, when these patterns advance into a more severe stage, accompanied by anxiety-tension, overt word substitutions, facial or body grimaces, and the desire to avoid speaking situations, followed by feelings of frustration and guilt, then the problem is of clinical concern. It has been observed that the stutterer frequently comes from a home environment in which demands for adult speech and social behavior have been excessive or in which there may have been a physical separation between the child and parent resulting in verbal and emotional disruption. The family may have criticized the child's speech productions or commented unfavorably with such remarks as "he stutters," "stop and start again," or "you don't have to talk like that," thereby creating a false self-image within the child regarding his ability to speak. It is also pos-

*Present authors' addition.

sible that criticism of the child's general behavior may have been superabundant and praise for his accomplishments meager.

Almost all stutterers have periods of relative freedom from hesitancies, repetitions, blocks, or prolongations. The stutterer can usually sing or speak in unison without disruption in his flow of speech, and he usually has no difficulty when he speaks aloud to himself or to his animal pets. The degree of communicative stress in a speaking situation appears to govern the degree of stuttering severity. Van Riper suggests that "the more one stutters, the more he fears certain words and situations. The more he fears, the more he stutters. The more he stutters, the harder he struggles. The more he struggles, the more penalties he receives, and the greater become his fears." Johnson believes that the average stutterer is not basically different from the nonstutterer, except in his usage of speech and his reactions to his own speech.

Common Questions about Stuttering

What is *primary* stuttering? This term is sometimes used to describe a child's speech when it is marked by effortless repetitions or prolongations of words, phrases, or syllables without an awareness on the child's part that these mannerisms are different or abnormal. Johnson states that "practically all stutterers are originally diagnosed (regarded as 'stutterers' or as 'not talking right' or as 'having difficulty saying words,' and so forth) by laymen, not speech specialists. They are usually diagnosed by their parents, more often than not the mother being the first to become concerned.

What is *secondary* stuttering? The term is used to describe the speech of an individual who exhibits mannerisms of hesitating or stumbling in speaking and who has an awareness that his speech is different. He may attempt to avoid difficulty by developing a complex pattern of verbal avoidances, grimaces, and gestures in order to release his tension or conceal his anxiety. Secondary or advanced stuttering tends to increase when the act of oral communication becomes more meaningful to the speaker and the listener. Stuttering behavior then becomes a self-perpetuating problem, and the stutterer may easily develop other problems because the stuttering behavior appears to superimpose itself upon his total existence.

Is stuttering hereditary? There is no clear evidence to support the view that stuttering is a characteristic which can be transmitted, in a biological sense, from one generation to another.

Does stuttering run in families? The research studies pertaining to the families of stutterers and nonstutterers indicate that to a limited extent stuttering does tend to run in families. The reason appears to be more a matter of tradition than heredity. When parents have had a background of experience with stuttering, they appear to react to the speech imperfections of their children differently from parents who are unfamiliar with the condition. The parent with stuttering in his background may be so conditioned in attitude, policies, and concern that he views his child's normal speech imperfections as stuttering.

Does confused laterality (handedness) cause stuttering? The basic concept of this theory gained popular acceptance in the 1920's and 1930's. It was the belief that stutterers were individuals who lacked adequate margins of unilateral dominance for the purpose of speech. However, research and clinical observation have pointed out that changing a child's handedness per se does not cause him to stutter but rather that the environmental influences, such as the emotional tone involved in the change, might do so.

Is stuttering caused by imitation? Parents frequently are concerned about the possibility of a child becoming a stutterer if he associates with a stuttering child. Imitation in and of itself does not cause stuttering. If this were true, the incidence of stuttering would be considerably higher than that currently reported. Children have been exposed to stuttering for years in public and private schools, and no "epidemic" has ever been recorded.

Do inflexible parent-child relationships tend to increase stuttering? As previously discussed, the child who stutters may come from a home which is not conducive to the natural growth and development of speech.

Moncur studied the environmental factors of stuttering and nonstuttering children and concluded that "it may be that the parents of the stuttering children are (as a group) dominant parents." Johnson and co-authors have suggested that the child with a speech defect may become less self-reliant because the parents may tend to be oversolicitous and sympathetic. They further state that the parents may "in subtle indirect and even seemingly kindly ways, reject him in refusing psychologically to accept the speech defect. . . ." Abbott found that mothers exhibited strong and consistent tendencies to overprotect their stuttering children. Any impaired relationship between parent and child makes for more dysfluent speech, and the child's speech production is closely tied to parental ego.

Why do more boys than girls stutter? Studies have shown that male stutterers outnumber female stutterers by about 4 to 1. Although there appears to be a great need for more research in this area of stuttering, Schuell has suggested that "a tenable hypothesis would seem to be that the male child, whose physical, social, and language development proceeds at a slower rate than that of the female, encounters more unequal competitions, and consequently more frustrations, particularly in relation to language situations, than the female child, and that as a result he exhibits more insecurity, more hesitancy, and more inhibitions in speech. If the frustrating situations are too many, if his speech behavior is compared unfavorably with that of other children, or if he becomes aware of unfavorable reactions toward it on the part of other people, it is conceivable that anxieties and tensions and the overt behavior regarded as stuttering might develop."

Treatment of Stuttering

It is essential that parents of a young child who demonstrates minor hesitations and repetitions in his speech remain unemotional about these speech patterns in order to prevent the development of undue awareness and concern on the part of the child. The young child with incipient stuttering should not be subjected to direct speech therapy or any type of therapy that he can relate to his speech production. All treatment should be directed through parent education and environmental reorganization.

The advanced or secondary stutterer should seek the assistance of a qualified speech pathologist. The stutterer or his family should be warned against treatment employing unethical procedures, such as gimmicks, devices, pills, or the guarantee of a "cure for stuttering." The treatment should always be conducted by individuals who have had academic training and experience in the areas of speech pathology, clinical psychology, or psychiatry. Psychotherapy, as well as speech therapy, may be recommended. Therapeutic objectives may include a modification of the stutterer's attitudes regarding himself, his speech, and his social environment. It is important that the advanced or secondary stutterer see himself as a person who stutters and is in need of therapy. Frequently the family of the secondary stutterer is also in need of appropriate treatment. Johnson has said, "You cannot give an adequate account of a speech defect except by describing the person who has it and the people who react to it."

DEFECTS OF SYMBOLIZATION (LANGUAGE)

Language may be defined as an organized symbolic representation of thought and action used as a means of communication on an abstract level by human beings. Therefore, preceding the act of speaking is the process of symbolization, which involves the comprehension and formulation of language. When this process is disturbed, the resultant may be classified as a communication disorder which is manifested in the inability or limited ability to use linguistic symbols as a means of oral communication. The general term *aphasia* (dysphasia) refers to the difficulty experienced in the comprehension (receptive-sensory) and use of linguistic symbols (expressive-motor) in verbal communication.

Congenital Aphasia

There has been considerable controversy about the existence of aphasia as a type of language disorder in children. Myklebust has stated that "there has been rather wide confusion relative to the area of aphasia in children. Much of this is due to semantic difficulties. For example, some adhere to a literal definition of the term aphasia, which is 'the loss of speech.' This literal definition of the word aphasia perhaps is inaccurate and inappropriate as far as any language or symbolic disorder is concerned, whether it be in children or adults. . . . Aphasia is not a speech disorder as such. Rather it is an impairment or inability to relate a language symbol to experience. . . . Some authorities continue to think of aphasia as a 'loss of speech' and imply that, if an individual has not acquired speech, he has no speech that he can lose and thus cannot be correctly or appropriately referred to as an aphasic. . . . We speak of 'congenital deafness' to differentiate it from deafness which has been sustained after birth. Likewise, in aphasia the causal concept, that is, a symbolic disorder due to neurological involvements, should not be confused with the time concept of when such a difficulty was sustained. The term congenital appropriately used is simply a time-of-onset concept. Therefore, congenital aphasia simply means that neurological involvements which have caused the verbal language disorder have been present from the time of birth."

Another point of view has been expressed by Sugar, who states that "bilateral brain damage does occur in so-called 'cerebral palsy,' but such children are not properly considered to have 'congenital aphasia' any more than a mentally retarded child has aphasia. Delayed or deficient development of speech function does occur; it is often associated with uncertainty in selection of a dominant hand. A child of 1 would not be properly termed a 'congenital aphasic,' for he has not yet developed speech, although the apparatus of speech is present. . . . 'Congenital aphasia' should refer to disability in speech in children who are intellectually and physically capable of speaking. In the sense of aphasia as it occurs in adults, this type of aphasia does not occur permanently in children, and certainly could not be said to occur as a congenital phenomenon. Rather one should use the phrase 'de-layed or failure of development of speech,' clumsy though it may be, for it gives a more accurate description of the disability. It implies brain damage or maldevelopment, and should lead to the consideration that such children are not intellectually normal (as an aphasic adult may be considered)." Gens and Bibey have attempted to resolve these differences when they state that "the term 'aphasic-like' is used instead of 'aphasic' because it is difficult to make a diagnosis of aphasia in a child who does not present definite neurological symptoms. A significant number of exogenous children present no accompanying motor or paralyzing involvements. In many cases, neurological examinations do not produce supportive evidence for neuropathologies. Without these positive findings there are those who would be reluctant to make a definite diagnosis of aphasia. Clinically, however, these children present aphasic-like symptomatology. Where these children respond to specialized aphasic training after having failed to respond to normal school teaching methods, more support is gained for the tentative diagnosis of congenital aphasia."

Parents frequently seek professional assistance after their child has been "diagnosed" erroneously as mentally retarded, deaf, or emotionally disturbed. The child may appear mentally retarded because he does not perform satisfactorily on standardized intelligence tests; the label *deaf* may be applied because he is unable to use verbal symbols which require hearing for response. The emotionally disturbed classification may seem appropriate because he exhibits behavioral problems, yet more inclusive evaluation of all the data usually will differentiate the several problems and identify the aphasic child.

Diagnosing aphasia in children is a complex process requiring the united efforts of many specialists, including the neurologist, pediatrician, psychologist, otologist, audiologist, speech pathologist, language pathologist, and educational consultant. Each of these specialists must seek to uncover the vestigial factors and look beyond the overt symptoms. It is only through the combined efforts of these specialists using a systematic, diagnostic approach that the child will be led to a more directive type of educational training.

Treatment of Aphasia in Children

Wood has suggested that "the approach to the child with aphasia has three basic objectives: First, the child with aphasia requires a special approach to his speech, language and educational problem which is designed to provide meaningful experience so that the child has an opportunity to associate verbal symbols (that is, words) with appropriate objects, people, places, and things. Second, education of these children must be aimed at helping them organize incoming stimuli so that they can understand and comprehend incoming information for use in communication with others. Third, these children must be introduced to a system whereby speech is no longer a rote articulation of sounds but, rather, a method of expressing ideas which are organized and meaningful."

The diagnosis and prescribed training program for the aphasic child would be woefully incomplete if the emotional factors of the family constellation were not considered. The family may protect or shield the child excessively, or it may coerce him or reject him. The presence of an aphasic child in the family unit may be deeply disturbing; the situation calls for a thorough appraisal of both the family structure and the need for therapeutic counseling.

The prognosis for most aphasic children is considered to be good; consequently, an educational program appears to be justified. However, the availability of appropriate educational facilities in the United States is limited.

Aphasia (Dysphasia) in Adults

Aphasia is associated with cortical disturbances or lesions resulting from vascular impairment (thrombosis, embolism, hemorrhage), tumors, degenerating and infectious disease, and trauma. Wepman has stated that "aphasia is any language problem resulting from organic disturbance of cortical tissue in which the defect is not due to faulty innervation of the musculature of speech, dysfunction of the peripheral sense organs, or general mental deficiency. The language problem manifests itself in the areas of symbolization, comprehension, and reproduction of concepts while the individual is using or attempting to use conventional spoken or written symbols. The brain defect which produces the aphasia is seen to produce also many other far-reaching symptoms beyond the realm of language."

The linguistic disturbances of the aphasic have been classified in numerous ways that reflect the clinical experience of the classifier and his concepts of cortical function related to language. These classifications have attempted also to recognize the major types and specific forms of language disturbance. One classification that has influenced the field for many years, particularly in the development of inventories for aphasia assessment is that designed by Weisenberg and McBride, and summarized by Eisenson as follows: (1) *predominately receptive*—a term designating a disturbance of the individual's ability to comprehend spoken or written symbols; (2) *predominately expressive*—a name indicating that the primary fault is a reduced ability to express ideas in speech and writing; (3) *amnesic*—a term suggesting that the patient's chief difficulty is in recall of appropriate names for persons, objects, conditions, relationships, and qualities; amnesic impairment is, in effect, a subtype of expressive disturbance; (4) *expressive-receptive*—a designation referring to disturbances in both receptive and expressive language functions, a condition that is likely to be present in a great many patients in the early stages of aphasic involvement. However, only a comparatively few patients continue to manifest equally severe disturbances of both reception and expression. Usually, receptive functions improve spontaneously to a greater degree than do expressive functions.

Wepman and coworkers have recognized three types of aphasic persons: "(1) those who cannot relate in language to a stimulus, internal or external (pragmatic aphasia), (2) those whose problem lies in the semantic act of symbol formation (semantic aphasia), and (3) those whose grammar and syntax are faulty or absent (syntactic aphasia). . . ."

In pragmatic aphasia the patient may experience extreme difficulty in using words and may be almost speechless. He may lack the ability to comprehend words, especially names, numbers, etc. Semantic aphasia involves the inability to recognize the true or associated meaning of language, i.e., a word or expression may be understood but the individual is unable to reproduce or clearly comprehend the actual meaning. Syntactic aphasia indicates the inability of the individual to place words or symbols in an intelligible sequence, resulting in a type of "jargon."

The emotional language of the adult aphasic is usually better than his propositional language. He may find it easier to swear, count, or to use other forms of automatic speech or nonpropositional forms of speech. However, he is at a loss when requested to develop this emotional language into abstract or propositional language situations. He experiences difficulty in combining simple linguistic symbols into more complex linguistic units. His ability to use language propositionally has been impaired. It is not that he is without words but rather that he cannot quickly command the response which is appropriate to the situation.

Prognosis for the recovery of the aphasic patient must be based on many factors, including his general health, attitude toward self and environment, age and educational attainment, vocation and avocations, and family attitude and degree of cooperation. Assuming that these and other factors are relatively positive, considerable recovery may be expected from the overall linguistic impairments as well as physical impairments. Spontaneous improvement may be noted during the first few months after the onset without structured training. This may give false hope to the patient and his family for additional recovery without seeking professional assistance. Depending on the degree of involvement, the family, with the physician's guidance, should enlist the services of a physical therapist, occupational therapist, speech pathologist, psychologist, and vocational counselor in formulating a personalized rehabilitation program. Ideally, the adult aphasic should be started on a program of rehabilitation as soon after the traumatic episode as possible.

DIFFERENTIATION BETWEEN SPEECH AND VOICE

The earlier sections of this chapter dealt primarily with the defects of speech and language—problems related to phonetic, linguistic, and symbolic factors in oral communication. In that presentation allusions were made to phonation and vocal sound, but these aspects of speaking and the disorders of voice have been reserved for separate attention in the remaining part of the chapter.

The contribution of phonation to the normal communication process is demonstrated succinctly by its absence; speech without phonation is whispering. In whispered speech the vocal cords do not vibrate; there is no phonation; the voice is aphonic. When this condition is present, the speaker uses language but he has no vocal pitch in the musical sense, and the sound is a relatively weak noise composed of breath sounds produced when the air becomes turbulent as it rushes past the irregularities that jut from the walls of the respiratory tract. In contrast, when the vocal cords vibrate, there is vocal sound that has pitch, loudness, and many of the distinguishing vocal qualities that identify individual voices.

NORMAL AND ABNORMAL VOCAL CORD VIBRATION

Normal vibration of the vocal folds consists of relatively regular, repetitive, simultaneous, synchronous lateral and medial movements, followed in each sequence by a period in which the cords contact each other to close the glottis and momentarily interrupt the air flow. Vibration begins when the breath pressure against the undersurfaces of the approximated folds is sufficient to force them apart, thereby allowing the pressure to drop until the elasticity of the folds and the flow of air through the glottis (the Bernoulli effect) close them. When the air pressure below the glottis again becomes great enough to overcome the resistance of the vocal folds, they are forced open as before, and the cycle repeats itself. The repetitive interruption and release of the breath stream create trains of pressure pulses that are modified by resonance in the upper respiratory tract and are transmitted as sound waves to the ear of the listener.

The pitch of the sound produced is directly related to the frequency at which the pulses are released, a rate that is determined primarily by the mass and elasticity of the vocal folds in relation to their length. When the folds in any normal larynx are shortened, their cross section becomes more massive and their elasticity is reduced. Conversely, when the vocal cords are elongated, they become thinner and their elasticity is increased; as a result, when the air stream pushes them apart, they return to their approximated positions more quickly. This reaction results in increased frequency and higher pitch. Frequency of vibration may also be altered by isotonic tension in the muscles of the vocal folds. This type of contraction increases the stiffness of the folds and consequently causes them to vibrate more rapidly. Another factor influencing pitch is the overall size of the vocal folds. Large folds produce a lower pitch than smaller folds because the larger ones vibrate more slowly.

Loudness of the voice is related to the sound pressure created by the released pulsations, i.e., sound pressure is directly proportional to the volume-velocity of the air flow in the glottis. Greater volume-velocity increases the amplitude of the sound waves, causing greater excursions of the ear mechanism and a sensation of louder sound. Increased air pulse pressure is acquired through a delicate balance between greater resistance at the vocal cords and stronger subglottal breath pressure.

The quality of voice is determined by both vocal fold vibration and resonance. The phonatory aspect includes the manner of air pulse release related to the vibratory pattern of the vocal cords. The opening, closing, and closed phases of the glottal cycle can vary in relation to each other, and the shape of vocal fold movement is more or less unique to each larynx. Each of these factors can influence the number and relative intensity of the partials composing the complex vocal sound and, consequently, the quality of the voice. Modification of the sound as it travels through the pharynx, mouth, and nose results from selective emphasis and deemphasis of the overtones and other partials in the complex sound generated in the larynx.

Abnormal vocal fold vibration takes many forms, most of which are not visible to the unaided eye. Ultraslow-motion films and, to a limited degree, stroboscopy have revealed that one vocal cord may move faster than the other; one may have a greater lateral excursion; vibration may be limited to one vocal fold; there may be no glottal closure; closure may occur at a paramedian position; vibratory patterns may be dissimilar at different regions along one or both folds; and the vibratory periods and amplitudes may be randomly variable in consecutive glottal openings. It is readily apparent that the potential complexity of vibratory patterns resulting from combinations of these cyclic abnormalities and sequential irregularities is almost endless. Accordingly, if hoarseness in its various forms can be presumed to result from abnormal vocal cord vibration, its origin should be found in one or more of the deviations which have been mentioned.

CLASSIFICATION OF VOICE DISORDERS

Voice disorders involve the components of speech to which reference has been made: pitch, loudness, and quality. When one or more of these factors in an individual's voice differs noticeably from that which is heard in the voices of the majority of persons of the same sex, age, and cultural group, his voice is considered to be defective.

Pitch disorders are present when the voice is consistently higher or lower (in relation to the musical scale) than would be expected for a particular individual, or when the sound is tremulous, monotonous, or bizarre, i.e., when the pitch patterns do not convey the ideas being expressed.

Disorders of loudness may also be classified into three categories that parallel those used with pitch deviations. The voice may be too loud or not loud enough in relation to the place and circumstances, or there may be variations that are not appropriate to the meaning of the utterance.

Voice quality disorders are the most common and the most complex of the vocal problems. They encompass both resonance and phonatory components, which may be mixed in a variety of ways and which are complicated further by changes in the degree of severity from moment to moment. The several phonatory deviations can be placed along an auditory continuum extending from aphonia to hoarseness, with such intervening and intermixing qualities as breathiness and harshness. The resonance disorders are also complex but are composed primarily of hyper- and hyponasality. These problems often affect intelligibility of speech more than do the phonatory disorders, and they constitute speech disturbances that carry potentially significant diagnostic clues that are often ignored.

Causes of Abnormal Vocal Pitch

An involuntary high-pitched voice in the adult male is one of the most distressing of voice defects. It resembles the female voice and consequently suggests a lack of masculinity, with all the associated social implications. The vocal pitch itself does not interfere with communication; and if it were produced by a female, it would probably not be considered unpleasant. The defectiveness, therefore, is not the sound itself; it is the inappropriateness of the sound to the circumstances.

High-pitched male voices frequently have functional origins, but this does not mean that the individual who has this voice defect is capable of lowering his habitual pitch voluntarily. Some persons, for various reasons, do not learn to use an adult vocal pitch, or, more accurately, some boys at the normal period of voice change maintain the juvenile voice and carry it into adulthood as the only method of voice production which they know. To tell a person with this type of voice that he has nothing wrong with his larynx and that he should go home and speak normally may reassure him, but it does not help him, and usually it serves

only to increase his frustration. He is already speaking "normally" and needs to be taught how to phonate in a way that is "abnormal" for him. Most of these patients respond readily to voice therapy and adopt the new voice after a brief period of self-consciousness. Those with normal structure who wish to maintain the high pitch rarely seek assistance; if they do ask for help, they deserve the attention of a psychiatrist.

Although the majority of abnormally high-pitched voices are probably caused by functional problems, cases with organic etiology are not uncommon and may be classified into four categories. One is the underdeveloped larynx which has small vocal cords that vibrate more rapidly than larger cords and consequently create a higher pitch. The small larynx may accompany a general structural retardation or be part of a hereditary familial body size. The larynx may also fail to develop as a result of hormonal imbalance, which is usually revealed simultaneously in the retardation of other secondary sex characteristics.

Another organic cause of the high-pitched voice is laryngeal web, which may be congenital or cicatricial. When this structure is small enough not to interfere with breathing or does not contribute to a stridor, it may go undetected until the voice is observed as being abnormal. A web need not extend far along the borders of the vocal folds to create a voice problem. Its effect is to shorten the free portions of the folds and thereby produce faster vibration and a resulting higher pitch. The vocal tone in children with webs resembles falsetto and tends to be weak. Hoarseness may be present also, accompanied by the audible evidence of vocal strain, particularly with adult males who have attempted to force a lower pitch.

A third organic cause for chronic high pitch is abnormal approximation of the vocal cords. In this condition a structural asymmetry may cause the vocal process of one arytenoid cartilage to slide on top of or below its opposite member in such a manner that posterior parts of the membranous vocal cords are pressed together, thereby effectively shortening their vibrating portions. The adjustment approximates that which is often observed in the male larynx when a high-pitched, falsetto voice is produced.

A fourth condition and one which may be overlooked or ignored as the cause of excessively high pitch is enlargement of the glottal margin of one or both vocal cords adjacent to the anterior commissure. A localized protrusion no more than 1 mm high and 2 mm long on the glottal margin is sufficient to shorten the vibrating length of the folds and to produce a higher than normal pitch. This lesion can be seen only when the anterior commissure is visualized, while the folds are widely abducted. During adduction the protruding areas are compressed into the underlying tissue and create the illusion of a prominent commissural attachment without significance. The location of the offending lesion at the anterior attachment where the folds converge enables it to modify the vibratory pattern more extensively than it would if it were located more posteriorly. That is, when a protruding mass is located where it is not pinched between the vocal folds, it usually does not shorten the vibrators and consequently does not raise vocal pitch; instead, it often causes a lower pitch accompanied by hoarseness or breathiness.

Defects of vocal pitch encompass the abnormally low voice as well as the deviations of high pitch which have been discussed in the preceding paragraphs. Excessively low pitch in both the male and female is usually associated with organic change; however, there are many persons who attempt to speak at a pitch below that which is optimum for the structures involved.

An abnormally low pitch or masculine-type voice in a female is as distressing to the woman possessing it as is the high-pitched voice in the male and for the same kinds of psychosocial reasons. Virilization of the female voice following hormone therapy in young women has been reported with increasing frequency. Recovery of normal pitch in these patients does not occur with interruption of medication, and at the present time there seems to be no specific counter-agent. The larynges of women with virilized voices appear to be normal in all aspects except perhaps for some general enlargement of the vocal folds toward their glottal margins. However, this observation must be considered as tentative at this time because the involved larynges have been seen only after the condition has developed; consequently the premorbid appearance cannot be described. Furthermore, the effects of compensatory vocal adjustments upon the size and condition of the structures is not known.

A form of excessively low pitch that is used by adolescent boys and young men in an effort to "sound more masculine" is often called "vocal fry" or glottalization. The voice is characterized by a low-frequency popping or ticking sound that is produced normally when only very little breath pressure is exerted against the vocal folds. The problem is almost always functional and usually disappears with mature emotional development, but occasionally it persists into adulthood and may be the cause of more serious voice problems. Furthermore, this type of voice can also have organic causes; it has been heard in relation to postirradiation conditions and with edematous vocal folds.

Vocal pitch deviations such as persistent tremulousness and extreme monotony are rare in young persons and are usually considered to be psychogenic. However, in older individuals these vocal characteristics may be symptomatic of deterioration or injury to the nervous system. In instances of brain stem involvement, the vocal changes may appear among the early symptoms and consequently deserve careful consideration in the diagnosis. On the other hand, when either tremulousness or monotony develops as a secondary symptom, other impairments are usually so prominent that the voice, as an entity, is relatively unimportant.

Causes of Loudness Deviations

Disorders in which the voice is too loud or not loud enough in relation to the environmental circumstances are usually functional in origin. These vocal differences often reflect the behavior of such personality types as the overly aggressive, the shy, and the socially insecure. There are also two organic conditions of importance that may influence vocal loudness: hearing impairment and paresis or paralysis. When a loss of hearing is sufficient to cause the individual to speak louder than circumstances warrant, the hearing problem is usually evident, and the offending vocal symptom is approached through treatment of the hearing loss. When a paresis or paralysis is present in the laryngeal muscles, the vocal folds cannot close the glottis firmly, and a relatively weak, breathy sound is produced.

A tangential aspect of loudness is the need of some persons to speak loudly in their occupations. This vocal requirement often creates laryngeal trauma, subsequent changes in the vocal organs, and consequent voice disorders. Excessively loud speaking is recognized as one of the principal types of vocal abuse and a difficult problem to manage when the basic occupational conditions persist. However, voices can be trained to meet most requirements if the patient is willing to learn how to use his voice. Before public address systems were available, preachers, politicians, and public lecturers devoted considerable attention to the development of loud voices; opera and concert singers still must do so. It would be beneficial to the modern professional speaker, as well as to workmen in noisy environments, to acquire "big voices."

The focal problem with the occupational voice disorder, when work requires daily vocal abuse, is the lack of opportunity to recover from traumatic effects and to institute a period of training to prepare the voice for unusual demands.

Causes of Voice Quality Disorders

Defects of voice quality arise from two sources, the larynx and the spaces of the respiratory tract. The problems associated with the larynx are known as phonatory defects, and those that are related to the respiratory spaces are called resonance disorders. The phonatory defects have been classified under many terms, but for this presentation they are reviewed under four headings: aphonia, breathiness, harshness, and hoarseness. The resonance disorders are described as, and are limited to, hypernasality, hyponasality, and muffled quality.

Phonatory Problems. There is a tendency for authors reporting in the medical literature to classify all voice disorders under the headings *aphonia* and *hoarseness*. These terms are useful but not adequate for a discussion of the variety of existing phonatory defects. Since many of the physiologic factors related to phonatory problems are known, it is possible to enlarge the classifications somewhat and to differentiate among the disorders on a physiologic basis. That is, certain voice defects can be associated with specific, atypical vocal cord movement, which can, in turn, be related to types of laryngeal disorder. The basic science is still incomplete, but certain principles can be used as the foundation for the immediate discussion of voice quality disorders.

Aphonia, the absence of phonated sound, is revealed as whispered voice and indicates that the vocal cords are not vibrating. This condition exists when the vocal folds do not approximate sufficiently to be activated by the air stream or when the folds themselves are not capable of vibrating even when approximated. The underlying causal factors include lateral fixation of the arytenoid cartilages, massive intrusion of some neoplasm, absence of vocal cord tissue, or excessively stiff, nonmotile vocal cords. The associated diseases range from psychogenic problems through neural impairment to various tumors and other localized laryngeal lesions.

There are persons who are intermittently aphonic: some whisper most of the time, others are aphonic only occasionally. The underlying conditions in these patients are similar in type to those in persons with chronic aphonia, but there is usually less impairment in those factors influencing vocal cord vibration.

Breath pressure can also be an important factor in intermittent aphonia, since relatively inactive vocal cords may be vibrated when the flow of air is sharply increased during exhalation. The additional air activates slightly abducted folds by alternately pushing them laterally and drawing them medially by the negative pressure of the Bernoulli effect. It should also be observed that any generalized swelling of the glottal margins that improves approximation without stiffening the folds contributes to vibration and sound generation. This fact is illustrated by those patients whose voices become louder when they have laryngitis or mild edema.

Chronic breathiness is quite common and can be heard in many varieties. It is generally characterized by the presence of excessively audible breath-flow noise which is accompanied by a relatively low overall loudness level. The vocal cords vibrate in the production of a breathy voice, but they are unable to hold back the air stream long enough for much increase in infraglottal pressure. The cords may either stand too far apart to permit them to meet during the medial excursion of their vibratory movement, or they may form a partial closure while a limited opening remains. This latter situation occurs when the arytenoid cartilages do not approximate or when some protrusion occurs on the glottal margin that prevents a complete closure. The air flows more or less continuously, thereby producing audible turbulence with weak phonated component.

One of the authors (G.P.M.) stated in a previous publication (1957): "The etiologic factors related to breathy voice are similar to those associated with aphonia and thereby serve to stress the fact that the laryngeal condition is rarely specific to the type and extent of vocal involvement. The degree of approximation permitted by an obstruction or paralysis, the amount of relaxation, and the urgency of the vocal effort, as reflected in both the flow of air and the muscle tension in the larynx, can determine whether the voice is aphonic, breathy, or hoarse at any particular moment.

"Discussions of the breathy voice traditionally suggest that this quality is associated with the adequacy of breath supply. Adequacy may be expressed in two ways: the amount of air available; and the force with which it is expelled. Clinical evidence indicates that a reduced air supply, such as that resulting from the collapse or removal of one lung, is not, in itself, a cause of breathiness. The condition may result in shorter phrases and in 'shortness of breath,' particularly under stress, but this is not a true breathiness. There are many persons with a low vital capacity who have normal voices. There is also substantial clinical evidence that reduced breath pressure alone is not a cause of breathiness. If low pressure produced the defect, a person with a normal voice would necessarily have a breathy voice whenever he uttered a tone of low intensity. It is obvious that trained singers can intone a clear nonbreathy voice which is scarcely audible. The critical element is the adjustment of the vocal cords in relation to the breath pressure.

"In view of the foregoing observations, recognition should be made of the fact that persons who are fatigued or ill or who have a paralysis involving the muscles of breathing often have a breathy voice. Under most circumstances, the breath factor is only part of the involvement. In these cases, the basic condition is usually not limited to the muscles of respiration, but includes also the muscles of the larynx. The laryngeal component is responsible for the voice defect, but the combination of reduced breath pressure and weakened vibratory control in the larynx tends to exaggerate the vocal defect which would have resulted from the laryngeal weakness alone. The heightened effect comes, at least in part, from the person's lessened ability to compensate in some measure for the reduced muscular control. That is, patients with only the laryngeal involvement probably learn to regulate the breath stream for maximum possible efficiency of voice production. Those with paralysis limited to the breathing musculature probably learn compensatory laryngeal adjustments."

The basic physiologic cause of the breathy voice has been described as the failure of the vocal cords to close the glottis completely during the vibratory sequence. When the opposite condition pertains, i.e., when the vocal cords remain in contact a disproportionately long time in the vibratory cycle as the result of reduced subglottal air pressure or excessive sphincteric squeezing of the intrinsic laryngeal musculature, a voice quality known as harshness results. This vocal problem is usually functional, is quite common in its milder aspects, and is usually interpreted as a symptom of a stressful situation. It suggests boredom in its milder manifestations; it frequently reflects attempts of boys and young men to lower vocal pitch to "sound more masculine"; and it is often prominent in the voices of hyperactive, aggressive individuals. Organic causes for this type of voice include edematous vocal cords, neoplasms, and any other structural alteration that tends to prolong the glottal closure in the vibratory cycle.

Harshness in its more prominent forms is often called hoarseness, and indeed these two qualities may be heard in the same voice within the same sentence. Auxiliary adjustments of the larynx for changes of pitch and loudness and variation in breath pressure are probably responsible for such differences.

Hoarseness varies from mild to severe and is so common in the population that it evokes little concern unless it is marked or chronic. The differentiating, audible feature of hoarseness is a roughness that results from random variations in the periodicity and/or the intensity of consecutive sound waves. Normal musical sound, whether produced by an instrument or the larynx, results from repetitive vibrations that are similar to each other in time and intensity or that vary progressively as the pitch shifts upward or downward. When the regularity of vibratory patterning is lost, the resulting vocal sound is heard as hoarseness.

The conditions that cause the random aperiodicity are not completely understood at this time, but they are recognized as being extremely complex. It is probable that the vibratory phenomena result from a combination of transient and interference factors. Any disease or condition in the larynx that changes the size or stiffness or surface characteristic of one or both vocal cords, or that causes excessive squeezing of one cord against the other, may create the condition for hoarseness. Enlargements due to tumor or edema, reductions resulting from surgery or atrophy, flaccidity subsequent to neural involvement, or functional hypercontraction of the adductory muscles represent the kinds of changes to which reference has been made. It is also possible under certain circumstances for tissue and structures above the vocal cords, such as the ventricular folds or epiglottis, to be set into more or less in-

dependent vibration and thereby create hoarse or rough sounds. The concept being stressed is that vocal sound is generated by the motions of the vocal cords in conjunction with the breath stream that activates them, and that any condition that alters their regular, repetitive, synchronous vibration may create the sounds that are called hoarseness. The descriptions of the many laryngeal diseases and anomalies that are potentially related to hoarseness occupy much of this volume. The possible effects of some of these conditions are summarized in the subsequent section on voice therapy.

Resonance Problems. The two most common resonance defects are too much nasal resonance and insufficient nasal resonance. The first is caused by inadequate closure of the nasopharyngeal valve, the second by blockage of the nasal passageway. The incomplete velopharyngeal closure results from one or more of five possible causes: (1) congenital deformity, such as cleft palate, submucous cleft, excessively deep pharynx, or short palate; (2) paralysis of pharyngeal or palatal muscles; (3) destructive disease; (4) surgical procedure in which adenoidal tissue vital to velopharyngeal closure has been removed; and (5) imitation of hypernasal speech.

The second general condition, blockage of the nasal passageway, causes denasality (cold in the head speech), which also results from one or more of five causes: (1) growths such as adenoid tissue, papillomas, polyps, and nasal spurs; (2) hypertrophy resulting from chronic disease; (3) swollen mucosa associated with allergies; (4) trauma to the nose; and (5) imitation. It should be noted that a blockage situated anteriorly in the nasal passageway may contribute to hypernasality instead of hyponasality, since the posterior nasal areas will act as resonators if an opening is present at the velopharyngeal valve.

A resonance disorder identified as muffled quality or "hot potato speech" is often difficult to identify since it is similar to some rural dialects. It results from space-occupying lesions in the vallecula between the epiglottis and the base of the tongue. Confusion with dialects occurs because some speakers habitually retract the base of the tongue into the pharynx on sounds that customarily do not employ that adjustment. The detrimental lesions are masses of lymph tissue or tumors.

The two separate sources of voice quality disorders, the larynx and resonance cavities, are capable of functioning independently; consequently, quality deviations can be generated in both concurrently. This condition provides the means by which many combinations of phonatory and resonance disorders may be produced simultaneously and presents a basis for the great variety of voice quality disorders which exist. The potential complaint is compounded additionally by the fact that both organic and functional deviations may be present at the same time. It is apparent that vocal disorders deserve careful evaluation and diagnosis; it is equally clear that vocal rehabilitation may require more than one form of therapy.

THERAPY FOR VOICE DISORDERS

The long history of medicine has demonstrated that medical and surgical treatment may eliminate voice disorders, but it is also evident that such treatment cannot always restore normal function. Nonmedical, rehabilitative measures may be necessary to help compensate for altered anatomic and physiologic conditions, and re-educative procedures almost always are indicated in the treatment of habitual or functional disorders.

The rehabilitative steps that are used in the management of voice problems are adapted to the patient and his problem, as such measures are in most therapeutic procedures. The preceding presentation has suggested the potential complexity of the disorders; since this discussion must play a relatively minor role in a volume on otorhinolaryngology, the suggestions for therapy have been limited to basic or universal recommendations that can be used by the physician who cannot devote much time to vocal rehabilitation. When greater depth is needed, there are detailed books and extensive reports in the periodical literature to which reference should be made to support systematic therapy. The purposes of this volume are best served by directing the physician's attention to the following four aspects of voice therapy: (1) the patient's general health and conditions affecting his larynx, (2) his environment, (3) his psychological adjustment, and (4) his voice.

Conditions Affecting the Larynx

It is probably redundant to stress the need for careful and complete medical evaluation and treatment of the individual who presents a voice disorder. Laryngologists particularly are aware that voice problems are among man's most subtle disorders; they reflect certain aspects of his thinking, his behavior, his health, and his diseases. They require definitive evaluation and they deserve careful treatment. The range of causal organic factors suggested in the preceding section indicates the array of etiologies that may be found in the medical literature. These causes of voice disorders may be arbitrarily grouped into the following six categories:

1. Structural modifications that result from misuse of the voice, such as thickened vocal cord tissue, myasthenia laryngis, vocal nodules, and contact ulcer. Furthermore, vocal abuse combined with infection may cause such chronic conditions as laryngitis, corditis with hypertrophic and hyperplastic laryngitis, and atrophic laryngitis.

2. Diseases and growths, including infections not related to vocal abuse; paralyses of central, peripheral, and myopathic origin; cysts; and both benign and malignant tumors.

3. Mechanical and chemical irritants affecting the mucosa; fumes, irritating vapors and gases, dry air, dusts, allergens, and silver nitrate.

4. Substances causing noninflammatory edema, such as internal medicaments, mechanical compression of venous blood flow, glandular imbalance, and allergy.

5. Congenital anomalies.

6. Destruction of laryngeal tissue by surgery, trauma, or disease.

Conditions leading to chronic fatigue, such as anemia, malnutrition, and inadequate rest, can also affect the voice adversely, but vocal symptoms are rarely linked with such factors in the literature on voice disorders. This is unfortunate, since on the one hand, the vocal sound may be a revealing diagnostic clue to a specific disease or to a generalized condition, and on the other hand, the treatment of the fundamental problem is basic to any direct voice therapy.

Environmental Factors

A program of voice therapy that does not recognize the demands of the environment upon the communication needs of the patient is incomplete and may be doomed to failure. The person who must talk more or less continuously in a noisy environment may develop detrimental vocal habits, and he may also abuse the larynx and create tissue changes. Parallel situations exist in some families and in recreational activities, in which the individual competes or fights vocally and yelling is the method of disciplining or direction. In some families the excessive and harmful use of the voice is so common or so subtle that the persons involved are not aware of the excess and do not associate the behavior with the voice.

Therapy for a voice disorder that is generated and nourished within an environment often presents great problems. Frequently, the patient cannot move to another job or otherwise modify his living situation; when such changes can be made, however, the restoration of the voice is simplified. When the environmental conditions cannot be altered, the voice therapy must include a review of the situation with the patient, or with the parents if children are involved, in order to provide insight and a rationale for adjustment to the environment. The physician, as well as the speech clinician, recognizes the incredible difficulty that may be present in these suggestions concerning environmental adjustment, yet to ignore the patient's setting is as hazardous as it would be to disregard a site of known infection in the treatment of a related disease.

A certified speech pathologist is qualified to handle the environmental aspects of voice therapy, but the physician may find it necessary to use a family counselor, a social worker, or a clinical psychologist. When such professional substitution is made, it may be desirable for the referring physician to outline in some detail the environment-voice relationship with the professional associate and to specify the reasons for his request.

Psychological Factors

An individual's attitude toward himself and his environment is reflected in such vocal elements as the rate at which he speaks, his choice of words, his vocal pitch, the loudness of his voice, and his vocal quality. These factors often indicate his degree of poise, his anxieties, his emotional states, his feelings of friendship or hostility, and his belief about his acceptance or rejection. When these concepts cause the individual to use an unpleasant, inadequate, or defective voice, it is apparent that any successful modification of the problem must include a consideration of the person's concepts about himself, his environment, and his speech.

Often the factors influencing vocal behavior are not deep-seated or abnormal. The boy who attempts to emulate a movie hero or the adolescent who forces his pitch to an abnormally low level to "sound more masculine" will usually change quickly when the situation is discussed with him and his behavior is described. In our Western culture the low-pitched male voice seems to be identified strongly with concepts of masculinity, and unless the young man realizes that a tenor voice is just as masculine as a bass one, he is apt to develop firm habits that are carried into adulthood. This voice characteristic is heard often in mature men who develop voice disorders and who report that they tried to affect low-pitched voices when they were young.

Children as well as adults sometimes use loud voices or rough-sounding, hoarse voices to dominate, to control, or to compete in their family or social groups. The chronic laryngeal changes that may result have been mentioned earlier; the focus of attention here is on the fact that the attitudes and needs of the individual that led to vocal nodules or thickened vocal cord tissue must be considered in any program of vocal rehabilitation.

Individuals occasionally demonstrate overwhelming anxieties in such vocal disorders as hysterical aphonia, intermittent dysphonia, and tremulousness. In these conditions it is usually desirable to seek psychiatric assistance, and if any work on the voice is recommended, it is carried on as a supporting activity in close cooperation with the psychiatrist.

The preceding paragraphs have suggested that psychological factors of many degrees of severity may cause voice disorders. It follows that successful vocal rehabilitation must include appropriate psychotherapeutic procedures when indicated.

Direct Voice Therapy

There are two general types of instruction that relate specifically to direct voice therapy: the first can be classified as "recovery," the second as "training." Recovery procedures presume a need for healing, for a return of the structures to normal; they are based on the premise that the vocal organs will restore themselves if abusive behavior is discontinued. Recommendations commonly given to achieve these goals include complete vocal silence for a week or two (or sometimes longer) with no whispering; limited vocal use in which speaking is allowed only when absolutely necessary; reduced vocal intensity; elimination of all singing; limitation of physical exercise and activity that cause the breath to be impounded by the closure of the glottis; and avoidance of coughing and clearing of the throat whenever possible.

These recommendations are essentially passive, and although they may be desirable early in therapy, they have little or no effect on improvement of voice production. For example, if a phonatory voice disorder has been caused by habitual vocal abuse and if recovery procedures have allowed the larynx to become more normal, the resumption of phonation will ordinarily result in a relapse because the old habits will be reestablished since they are the only ones the individual knows. Therefore, to be successful, voice therapy must include a period of training which modifies previous habit patterns and replaces them with more efficient phonatory behavior.

Direct training procedures for vocal rehabilitation can be grouped under six general headings. Methods vary widely, and this underscores the fact that there is more art than science in voice therapy. However, there appears to be considerable agreement about the general objectives of the methods employed. The following suggestions are intended to be used as general guides by the otolaryngologist or other physician when he is unable to refer his patient to a speech pathologist or vocal specialist. There is no presumption that these recommendations provide a program of voice therapy.

Description of the Voice Problem. Defective voices usually are not consistently abnormal in the same degree under all circumstances. A voice that is hoarse at a low pitch may be completely clear in falsetto; vocal sound may be more normal during the production of certain vowels than with others; and the characteristics of vocal defects often change with loudness or vocal effort. It is essential that the individual who provides voice therapy know the capacities and limitations of the patient's voice, since this information not only provides diagnostic data but also determines the pattern of rehabilitation. Therapy begins with what the patient can do; he cannot practice something he cannot do.

To determine the dimensions of a voice disorder, the clinician should evaluate systematically and individually the pitch, loudness, and quality characteristics of the voice. The patient should be asked to sing a vowel, such as *ah,* up and down a musical scale to the limits of his range. It may be necessary to provide a tone for him to imitate, because many patients with voice disorders have poor pitch discrimination. The adequacy of the pitch range should be noted, as well as any changes in vocal quality that occur at different positions on the scale. This procedure should be repeated at various vocal loudness levels with at least two other vowel sounds, *ee* and *oo.* The patient should also be required to read a few paragraphs of simple material to reveal his typical vocal habits.

Generous samples of the patient's vocal production should be recorded during the evaluation process. Recordings are essential for objective listening to the voice, and they serve as a basis for determining improvement or regression during the course of therapy.

The vocal evaluation should answer the following questions: Is the pitch of the voice which the patient uses in conversation and while reading aloud normal for a person of his age, sex, and size? Are there any unusual inflections or atypical pitch variations? Is there a satisfactory pitch range, e.g., a minimum of five to six tones? Can the patient match the pitch of a given tone, and can he voluntarily go up and down a scale? Is the loudness of the voice appropriate to the circumstances? Is there any evidence of a hearing loss? Is the quality of the voice predominately normal? Is it aphonic? Or breathy? Or harsh? Or mildly hoarse? Is it severely hoarse? Does the voice quality change when the pitch is high or low? Does the speaker appear to be using too much or too little effort in his speaking? Does too much sound seem to come out through the nose? Does too little sound pass through the nose on the *m, n,* and *ng* sounds? Is there any tremulousness? Is the general precision of speech commensurate with the socioeconomic background of the patient? Under what conditions of pitch, vowel sounds, and loudness levels does the subject produce his best vocal sound?

Patient's Evaluation of His Voice Problem. Two basic premises support the concept that a person must evaluate his own voice problem if he wishes to modify it. First, an individual does not hear his own voice as others hear it; second, the clearer and more specific a goal or task can be made, the faster it will be reached. The corollary of these concepts is that unless an individual can recognize his voice problem and can form a clear concept of the improved vocal sound that he wishes to produce, his remedial efforts will be relatively ineffective.

The process by which a person evaluates his own voice is systematic listening, sometimes called "ear training." The most effi-

cient approach is through tape recording. Samples of the patient's voice should be recorded at appropriate intervals during therapy, and these should be studied carefully with frequent comparison of the vocal features in the several recordings. The clinician should choose one vocal element at a time for special attention, and he must avoid both discouraging the patient and overwhelming him with the reeducative task. This purposive listening requires great clinical skill to make it meaningful and to keep the patient motivated. Inexperienced listeners do not hear many of the elements of vocal sound, particularly their own, until they are instructed; this is the function of the clinician. The temptation to send the patient home to listen to his own recording as a therapeutic measure should be resisted until there is assurance that he can identify specific faults.

Another aspect of evaluative listening is detailed analytic study of the vocal characteristics of other persons with both good and poor voices. This type of exercise improves the patient's ability to identify specific vocal features and augments his efforts to modify his own production through imitation and experimental variations.

Imitation and Experimentation. Soon after the patient learns to hear specific flaws in his own voice, he should be encouraged to experiment with voice production in an effort to modify his specific faults and also to develop greater control over his voice. It is often helpful to use two recorders, one of which plays a voice sample and the other records the patient's efforts to imitate. If the second machine is recording when the sample is played as well as when the patient speaks, the second tape will contain both items and they can be compared readily when it is replayed. It is a procedure which is often difficult but highly rewarding because it is frequently the principal pathway to vocal recovery.

Relaxation. In those voice disorders in which vocal abuse is present, the patient usually has excessive tension in the muscles of the larynx as well as elsewhere throughout the body. Unless this tension can be controlled, vocal therapy cannot progress.

The patient needs to relax. This is a truism that is easier to advise than to accomplish because the faulty vocal habits are usually firmly established.

The term *relaxation* commonly has two meanings: it may refer to the absence of muscle contraction; or it may signify coordination in which the opposing sets of muscles exert just enough reciprocal tension upon each other to accomplish a desired movement with perfect control. Both types of relaxation can be learned and sometimes must be learned for the successful alleviation of a voice disorder. Learning to relax involves both muscle training, which can be approached directly through exercise, and emotional control, which is managed through modification of attitudes, anxiety, worry, and comparable problems. It is difficult to achieve relaxed control of phonation if the patient is in a chronic mental turmoil. The efficient, coordinated type of movement so desirable in phonation is based on the ability to relax voluntarily and incorporates the capacity to produce the optimum voice as determined through evaluative listening.

Pitch Adjustment. Many persons, particularly men, attempt to use a vocal pitch that is lower than that which is normal for their laryngeal structures. This behavior not only produces an unpleasant voice but also traumatizes the laryngeal structures. If this vocal tendency is observed, its inadequacy should be explained and assurance provided that a more normal pitch will supply a satisfactory masculine image. Subsequently, direct instruction can be given to establish a habitual pitch that averages four or five musical notes above the lowest tone that the patient can produce. It is an interesting clinical observation that an average shift of as little as one tone will "feel" much higher to the speaker and will make him reluctant to accept the change. Furthermore, he is usually surprised to discover that he cannot hear much change in his recording, and he is startled when the average listener does not recognize a change of as much as several tones in his speaking pitch.

Vocal Practice. If the physician finds it necessary or desirable to direct the vocal practice of a patient, the focus of the suggestions should be on the use of a quiet voice. More specifically, practice sessions of 5 to 10 minutes should be advised in which vowel sounds are prolonged gently at various pitches, and short selections from magazine stories and other sources are read aloud. If the subject has experimented successfully with various voice qualities and is able to relax adequately, such practice will prove to be beneficial. However, if the patient uses detrimental vocal behavior when he reads aloud, this practice should be postponed.

Vocal practice requires patience and constancy. Patients are often disturbed when they are told that they may not detect much improvement in 3 months or more and that 6 months may be required to achieve some skill in the use of new vocal habits. One of the most difficult and important aspects of voice therapy is motivation of the patient.

LARYNGEAL CANCER AND VOCAL REHABILITATION

Cancer in the larynx sometimes has no influence on the voice, but in more than half of the patients, hoarseness is present and is frequently accompanied by pitch change and reduction in loudness. A recent report by Lowry and others of a retrospective study of 260 laryngeal carcinomas stated: "Hoarseness was the predominant symptom in all four stages of glottic and supraglottic lesions. In the supraglottic lesions hemoptysis, dysphagia and weight loss combined to give a nearly equal number with hoarseness." However, clinical experience has demonstrated that any disease, trauma, or systemic disorder that can alter the size, contour, mass, or elasticity of even one vocal fold usually produces vocal symptoms of hoarseness associated with pitch change and vocal weakness. This observation emphasizes three factors: (1) vocal (phonatory) abnormalities signal the presence of modifications in the function or physical features of the vocal folds, not a specific disease; (2) the sound of the voice is often the first evidence of disease; and (3) increased sensitivity of the laryngologist to the quality, pitch, and loudness of the voices of all his patients is the most direct route to early detection of laryngeal cancer.

Impact of Medical Management Upon Vocal Rehabilitation

When the laryngologist finds cancer in a larynx and decides upon therapy by either irradiation, partial laryngectomy, total laryngectomy, or a combination of irradiation and surgery, he sets the course not only for the treatment of the disease but also for the pre- and postmedical stages of rehabilitation. Each medical procedure influences the patient in a distinctive way, and each affects vocal re-education uniquely.

According to the 1974 report of the American Cancer Society, approximately 9500 new cases of laryngeal cancer were anticipated in the United States in that year; 8300 of this expected total were men, 1200 women. A tentative estimate indicates that about one fourth of these patients can anticipate irradiation as primary therapy, a similar number will undergo partial laryngectomy, and the remaining half will be treated by total laryngectomy. Only a relatively small number of those receiving the conservative therapies will require vocal rehabilitation, and these patients can be managed by standard vocal therapy techniques similar to those used with unilateral paralysis, weak voices, and hoarseness. The remaining 4000 or 5000 receiving total laryngectomy will need a special form of speech rehabilitation. It is these patients who are the focus of the comments in the remainder of this chapter.

Presurgical Therapy

Most of the presurgical management of the person who must have his larynx removed is composed of advice and guidance by the surgeon and allied personnel in preparation for the medical and other types of rehabilitation. The preparatory phase is extremely important in the total therapy and should be handled with great care. Most laryngeal surgeons have developed effective procedures for informing and advising their patients about the surgery and its sequelae. However, a recent study by Snidecor of approximately 150 laryngectomies indicated that some aspects of the presurgical management could be improved. Of those patients studied, 85% believed they had been counseled well and at the right time, but the majority of these patients also stated that they would have benefitted from more specific counseling for themselves and their spouses about the operation, the postsurgical physical conditions, and the speech. Only 53% learned about the kinds of available replacement speech from their surgeons. The remainder got their information from other laryngectomees, speech pathologists, and the American Cancer Society. At the time the diagnosis of laryngeal cancer was reported to the patients, about three fourths of them were accompanied by their spouses, which was considered helpful and desirable, but more than half of the spouses were "shocked, anxious, and deeply concerned."

The same study confirmed what most laryngologists know, that patients who have been told they have cancer and need surgery are filled with anxiety and many fears. They fear the cancer and the possibility of death, they fear the surgery, they fear the loss of voice and its consequences, and they are distressed about the potential effects of vocal impairment upon their work, family life, and social relationships. Such fears and anxieties are probably to be expected, but the sensitive counselor who acknowledges such feelings and whose experience allows him to anticipate the postsurgical conditions can often reduce the apprehensive attitudes.

Advisability of Presurgical Speech Training

Some laryngeal surgeons regularly introduce a good esophageal speaker to the patient prior to surgery. Others believe that this practice is unwise. Clinical experience suggests that the introduction of a well-adjusted, fluent laryngectomized person is beneficial when a male patient has accepted the need for surgery and wants to move forward without delay. However, women are almost always depressed by esophageal speech, whether it is produced by a woman or a man; consequently, women usually should not be introduced to this form of speech prior to surgery. Similarly, men who are greatly disturbed by the diagnosis and those who are naive about the nature of postsurgical speech tend to reject esophageal speech and also the voice produced by artificial devices. These men are negative because they are unable to adjust emotionally to the concept of alaryngeal speech and because they cannot comprehend a condition of voicelessness and the great advantage of esophageal speech over voicelessness. It follows that men of this type and all laryngectomized women should not be introduced to even a good laryngectomized speaker before surgery.

The laryngeal surgeon often needs to consider the advisability of speech therapy in the period between diagnosis and surgery. Some surgeons and speech pathologists recommend it, while others are opposed. The former believe that the initiation of procedures for developing an esophageal air supply and an eructation noise is easier while the larynx is present than after the laryngectomy, and the postsurgical therapy is shortened. Those who hold an opposing position point out that the period of time between diagnosis and surgery is usually too brief for the successful development of esophageal sound, and when failure occurs, the consequent apparent lack of success may result in further depression. Furthermore, esophageal speech learned when a diseased larynx is present may not be transferable to a mechanism that has been extensively altered by surgery. An additional objection to presurgical speech training primarily applies to those overly eager patients who attempt to practice esophageal speech before healing is complete and thereby create fistulas or other surgical problems. Reliable estimates on the prevalence of presurgical speech training are not available, but it seems that relatively few speech pathologists currently advise this practice.

Perhaps the most satisfactory way to plan for postsurgical speech in the presurgical period and to handle the many questions about work, family, and social relationships is to introduce a mature speech pathologist who has had extensive experience with laryngectomized persons. Of course, such an individual will not attempt to answer the medical, financial, and other questions which may be asked. His function is to encourage and motivate the patient and to make plans for the postsurgical period. He does not promise fluent speech or that the learning will be easy, since according to Gardner, approximately 30% of laryngectomized patients do not learn to speak well with esophageal speech. However, he can express confidently that verbal communication is almost always possible with either esophageal speech or with an artificial larynx.

Early Postsurgical Period

Within a few days following surgery, the patient begins to assess his new condition. He is relieved that the operation is successfully past and that he is alive, but he discovers new problems and fears to add to those that linger. He is bothered somewhat by breathing and coughing through his stoma. He is dismayed by the reality of voicelessness; his attempts to whisper are frustrating. During convalescence at home, anxieties often grow about employment, personal appearance, family relationships, and association with friends. The inability to talk leads to depression and withdrawal from social situations, a condition that becomes progressively more difficult to reverse. If the person who loses his larynx could resume talking immediately after the laryngectomy, his concern would be no greater than that associated with any other major surgery. Unfortunately, when his means of communication is disrupted, he feels isolated and at a great disadvantage. It is apparent that the early restoration of the ability to talk is a major consideration in successful rehabilitation.

Methods of Restoring Speech Communication

The normal larynx generates undifferentiated sound without phonetic value. This sound is transformed into specific vowels and consonants in the upper respiratory tract by relatively consistent adjustments of the pharynx, velum, tongue, mandible, and lips. Since structural adjustments above the larynx create the spoken language, any complex sound that can be put into the upper airway can be substituted for the laryngeal sound and be molded into speech. This basic phonologic concept combined with the need to restore speech to the laryngectomized has enabled engineers, surgeons, speech pathologists, and others to devise various means for producing sound that can substitute for the larynx.

The engineering approach involves the development of artificial sound generators. These can be separated into two general types according to the driving force used in the production of sound. One kind is powered by the breath stream, the other by electricity from batteries. There are several forms of breath activated instruments, but they have three elements in common: (1) a flexible tube that conveys the breath from the tracheal stoma to a small capsule held in one hand; (2) the capsule which contains a reed or membrane that is vibrated by the breath, thereby generating the sound; and (3) a second, smaller tube that carries the sound from the capsule into the mouth, where it is articulated into speech.

The electrical instruments employ either of two basic concepts. In one the sound is generated by a small buzzer about the size of a hearing aid phone that is held in the hand and from which the sound travels by way of a tube into the mouth. Some manufacturers put the sound generator into the bowl of a tobacco pipe and conduct the sound to the mouth through the pipe stem. The second type of electrical instrument is a hand-held unit which transmits a buzzer type sound through the tissues of the neck into the pharynx, mouth, and nose, where the sound is articulated into speech in the customary manner. The vibrating element of these units is a disc which is placed against the skin of the neck and is activated by an electrical power source controlled by a switch similar to that on a flashlight.

The surgical efforts to provide a sound-producing mechanism have also followed two basic concepts. The more common entails the construction of a shunt connecting the tracheal stoma area with the pharynx or esophagus in such a way that the inner end of the shunt will vibrate to generate a

sound when the breath passes through it. Ordinarily the shunt lies collapsed until the patient blocks the stoma with his finger or other cover, thereby diverting the breath through the shunt and causing it to flutter at its inner end, which produces sound that is readily articulated into speech. The second concept employed in the surgical construction of sound-producing mechanisms is either the implantation or the external attachment of an artificial breath-activated sound generator that discharges its sound into the pharynx. The sound is developed by a vibrating reed or membrane located in an enclosure that can be implanted in a shuntlike arrangement so that diversion of the breath through it by closure of the stoma will create a sound; alternatively, the enclosure with the vibrator may be kept outside of the patient, where it is attached by two tubes, somewhat like the breath-activated, hand-held instruments mentioned previously. However, in the external unit, instead of the sound being led from the sound-generating unit into the mouth, it is introduced into the pharynx through a tube inserted into a surgically produced fistula which passes through the skin and tissue of the neck into the pharynx.

The third approach to speech recovery for laryngectomees is the development of esophageal speech. This procedure enables the patient to control and refine the natural eructation sound as the basis for speech. The techniques associated with this approach are presented in some detail in a subsequent section and consequently will not be elaborated here.

Positive and Negative Features of the Methods of Speech Restoration. *Breath-powered Artificial Larynges.* Breath-powered, hand-held, artificial larynges have several attractive features. They are inexpensive and offer the patient an early means of talking with little or no special instruction. The speech sound can be relatively loud, phrasing and sentence length are normal, and speech is intelligible, even though it has a monotonous pitch.

Unfortunately, the disadvantages attending the use of these simple instruments are substantial; consequently, few of them are currently in use. The problems can be listed as follows: moisture from the exhaled breath condenses relatively quickly at the vibrator, causing malfunction and the necessity of draining or drying it; the tube conveying air from the stoma to the vibrator becomes congested with mucus from the trachea, causing both esthetic and hygienic problems; saliva seeps into the sound-conducting tube, contributing to vibrator problems and necessitating frequent change and washing of the tube to keep it clean. Since the unit is held by one hand, it interferes with two-handed activities; furthermore, since it must be transported by the user and kept readily available for speaking, it becomes a nuisance.

Electrical Artificial Larynges. Battery-powered artificial larynges share with the breath-activated units such advantages as low cost, early and easy restoration of speech, and good intelligibility. The electrical tissue-vibrating units have the additional positive features of freedom from hygienic problems, moisture condensation, and instrument care which accompany the breath-powered instruments.

On the negative side, electrical artificial larynges continuously require one hand for operation and must be carried most of the time. An additional disadvantage of the electrical vibrating disc models is the field noise which they generate. That is, some noise from the unit is transmitted directly to the surrounding air, which competes with the sound that enters the subject and is transformed into speech. The ambient noise and the continuous sound generation also contribute to an artificiality of the speech. Breathing and phrasing are interrelated in normal speech. When the basic sound is produced more or less continuously, as with the electrical instruments, utterance tends to become more "mechanical." However, experienced users of these units learn to start and stop the sound to approximate the needs of the sentences.

Surgical Shunts. There are at least four advantageous features associated with the surgical creation of a shunt for the production of voice. It provides an almost normal manner of speaking, and utterance is produced on exhalation; consequently, phrases and pauses are typical, occasionally slight

pitch variations are achieved, and little or no training in the use of the method is needed.

The major disadvantages from a speech standpoint are (1) one hand must be used to close the tracheal stoma whenever sound is produced; (2) the quality of the voice is abnormal, being similar to that of esophageal speech; and (3) vocal intensity is often reduced. While these disadvantages are important, they are relatively minor when compared to the attendant medical and health problems. Shunts frequently do not remain closed sufficiently to prevent the leaking of fluids from the pharynx into the trachea or to the outside of the neck, depending upon the location of the orifice. Inflammation and infection may occur in the shunt or trachea, requiring additional surgery to close or remove the shunt.

External Artificial Larynx With Fistula. The surgical creation of a fistula through the neck tissues into the pharynx, permitting the connection of an external artificial sound source, appeals to many laryngectomized persons, particularly those who have been unable to learn esophageal speech and who do not want to use one of the hand-held artificial larynges. Advantageous features of the surgical fistula and attached mechanical device include the capacity to produce fluent speech with customary phrasing and the utterance of sentences of normal length. The speech is highly intelligible, being equivalent in quality and intelligibility to good esophageal speech. This use of an artificial sound source which contains an automatic air valve enables the speaker to control the flow of air with breath pressure, thereby freeing both hands.

The disadvantages of this system are (1) the obvious esthetic, hygienic, and clothing annoyances caused by a device attached at both the tracheal stoma and the fistula; (2) the special surgical procedure that is necessary to create the fistula; (3) the hygienic care of the fistula and instrument; and (4) the fact that when the tube which passes through the fistula is removed for sleeping or other reasons, a stopper must be inserted into the fistula to prevent leakage.

Esophageal Speech. The advantages of esophageal speech are (1) natural physiologic structures and functions are used, thereby obviating the need for an artificial device; (2) both hands are free for normal activities during speech; and (3) the good esophageal speaker presents a relatively normal appearance and speaking manner.

The disadvantages of esophageal speech are (1) it is often difficult to learn and frequently requires 3 months or more to achieve fluency; (2) phrasing is usually changed, so that fewer words than normal are uttered in a sequence without pause for phonatory air; and (3) the voice lacks sufficient loudness to be heard easily over common environmental noise.

All of the substitute methods of creating voice except the battery-powered, disc-type artificial larynges encounter maximal problems when the patient eats. Swallowing food and the stimulation of salivary secretion complicate speaking and frequently embarrass the patient in social situations. Esophageal voice production and the artificial larynges with oral tubes are probably more adversely affected while eating than the other methods discussed.

Selecting a Method of Speech Rehabilitation

If some presurgical training was given the patient, it should be resumed as soon as the postsurgical condition warrants. On the other hand, if no previous instruction was provided, the rehabilitative program should begin with an assessment of the individual's needs by both the laryngologist and the speech pathologist to determine the advisability of using an artificial larynx. If immediate communication is necessary in the employment situation, if the patient lives where he cannot receive adequate training, if he cannot write, if he has a serious hearing loss, or if some other condition is detrimental to the learning of esophageal speech, an instrument may be advisable. However, when esophageal speech can be developed, which means the majority of cases, including even those who have undergone radical procedures, it is the preferred method.

If the decision is made to use an artificial larynx, either temporarily or permanently, the patient should be taught how to apply it most effectively and how to care for it. Manufacturers customarily include printed instructions, but usually these need to be supplemented by demonstration and personal experimentation. The best location on the neck for electrical vibrator-type instruments needs to be determined with each patient, and instruction about more careful articulation of the speech sounds is helpful. Persons with reed and electrical instruments that lead the sound into the mouth through a tube must experiment with the placement of the tube and the regulation of the reed or the switch on the vibrator. The patient also needs to learn to coordinate his speaking with the operation of the instrument. The basic sound is no longer automatic; consequently, considerable practice is necessary to acquire satisfactory timing in the use of the artificial sound source. Frequently, persons who initially accept an instrument learn esophageal speech and discard the artificial device.

Procedures for Developing Esophageal Speech

It was asserted earlier that any sound put into the mouth can be articulated into speech. When the normal sound generator, the larynx, is not present, it is logical to substitute the most available vicarious sound source, which is the eructation mechanism. Its location in the hypopharynx is ideal from a language-producing standpoint because it permits normal articulation of almost all speech sounds. It is also desirable because it is universal; almost everyone has produced a burp sound at some time, and most people learn at an early age to regulate it to some degree.

It is recognized that the air used in ordinary eructation comes from the stomach and that the sound usually does not result from voluntary acquisition and expulsion of air. However, there are many persons who learn to take air into the esophagus and expel it without allowing it to reach the stomach. The air in the esophagus is put under some pressure by respiratory movements and escapes in vibratory pulses through the sphincter mechanism at the upper end of the esophagus. This organ does not produce sound as effectively as the larynx, but its phonation function is similar, and it is subject to considerable regulation. The ability to control the air and consequently the moment of sound production is the primary problem in learning esophageal speech.

Before air can be expelled from the esophagus, it must be taken in. If it is allowed to enter the stomach, it cannot be returned readily for voice; consequently, it must not be swallowed in the sense that water is swallowed. Instead, it must either be "inhaled" or "injected" into the esophagus. Experience proves that either of these procedures is serviceable, for each has been employed by good esophageal speakers. Indeed many of these speakers use both methods interchangeably.

If the esophagus were held open as the trachea is, the ordinary respiratory expansion of the thorax would draw air into the esophagus as readily as into the lungs. Many laryngectomized persons can learn to relax the upper esophageal sphincter at the moment of inhalation and thereby allow air to be pulled into the esophagus. However, in the initial stages of learning this procedure, before the laryngectomee is able to relax the esophageal valve readily, he can facilitate the intake of air by momentarily covering his stoma with a finger. This action suddenly decreases the pressure in the thorax, causing the air in the pharynx to be drawn into the esophagus. As soon as the air has been taken in, it can be expelled by increasing the thoracic pressure, as in exhalation. This return flow is interrupted intermittently by the vibration of the tissues of the pseudoglottis, thereby producing sound.

The "injection" method of putting air into the esophagus employs a different principle from that used in the inhalation procedure just described. In "injection" the air is forced, pumped, or squeezed from the mouth and pharynx into the esophagus. Injection is accomplished by closing the lips and the velopharyngeal valve to provide an air-tight oropharyngeal area simultaneously thrusting the back of the tongue upward from the *d* position. This movement pumps the air out of the mouth into the pharynx, and since it is not permitted to escape through the nose and no longer has access

to the larynx and trachea, it passes into the esophagus. Squeezing the air from the mouth into the esophagus can also be achieved by compressing the lips and buccal spaces as in a *b* sound and simultaneously lifting the mandible. A further application of this injection principle employs syllables, words, and sentences that are loaded with plosive sounds, *p, b, t, d, k, g*. The normal production of each of these sounds requires intraoral breath pressure, which causes some of the impounded air to be pushed into the esophagus, where it adds to the supply for phonation.

Understanding these various techniques provides insight and a basis for instruction, but experience indicates that verbal description is less effective than demonstration and imitation. Consequently, the instructor of the laryngectomized person should learn to burp and to speak a few words of esophageal speech at will. It is also advantageous to have one or more good laryngectomized esophageal speakers on the instructional team. It is not unusual for beginning laryngectomees to observe the production of esophageal sounds and to develop their own skills without hearing any discussion of the theory or anatomic structures involved. In fact, some of the most effective instruction in this field is being done by laryngectomized persons who have learned how to teach. Unfortunately, there are some laryngectomees who have presumed that they were automatically qualified as instructors simply because they learned to speak.

An important adjunct to the development of esophageal speech is relaxation. The laryngectomee should be told that he will learn to use his new voice more rapidly if he remains relaxed. Tensions created by anxiety, fears, and even the eagerness to talk make speaking more difficult. Experienced esophageal speakers universally report that talking is more difficult when they become tense or excited.

After the laryngectomee has learned to produce sound, he advances quickly to words of one syllable, then two, three, four, and more, with concurrent introduction of phrases and short sentences. He should be urged to practice frequently for short periods during his early training and advised to avoid fatigue. At this stage of rapid development, the patient sometimes becomes so eager to rejoin the conversing world that he slights his practice, tries short cuts, and develops various detrimental habits such as whispering, expelling air noisily from the stoma, phrasing sentences carelessly, and articulating speech sounds poorly. As a consequence, many listeners will not exert the extra effort necessary to follow the comments of the speaker; the latter senses the withdrawal, struggles harder in his ineffective way with increasingly poor results, and finally gives up completely and stops speaking. The physician or speech clinician can anticipate this behavior and help the patient avoid it in the systematic instructional sessions. There is much helpful and interesting practice material available to keep him working and improving. Some of this appears in the bibliography. There are also a number of manuals and instructional booklets that are available through local cancer societies.

It is often necessary for the person working with a laryngectomee to help with suggestions about everyday hygiene and appearance. The instructor should be able to advise on such items as care of the tracheal tube, cleanliness, coverings for the stoma, suitable neckwear for men and women, precautions related to bathing, difficulties of speaking while eating, and similar personal problems. The clinician should also be able to help the laryngectomee join a Lost Cord club for instruction, practice, and recreation. Addresses of these groups can be obtained from the International Association of Laryngectomees listed at the end of the references or from the local Cancer Society.

REFERENCES

Abbott, T. B.: A Study of Observable Mother-Child Relationship in Stuttering and Non-Stuttering Groups. Unpublished Ph.D. Dissertation, University of Florida, 1957.

Anonymous: Need for Speech Pathologists and Audiologists. American Speech and Hearing Association Committee on Legislation, ASHA, 1:138, 1959.

Anonymous: Speech Correction. American Speech and Hearing Association Committee on the Midcentury White House Conference. J. Speech Hearing Disorders, 17:202, 1952.

Anonymous: Stuttering Words. No. 2. Memphis, Speech Foundation of America, Dec. 1960.

Brodnitz, F. S.: Vocal Rehabilitation. Minneapolis, Whiting Press, 1959.

Brodnitz, F. S.: Goals, Results and Limitations of Vocal Rehabilitation. Arch. Otolaryng., 77:148, 1963.

Buck, M. W.: The Language Disorder. J. Rehabilitation, 29:37, 1963.

Damsté, P. H.: Virilization of the Voice due to Anabolic Steroids. Folia Phonat. (Basel), 16:10, 1964.

Denes, P. B., and Pinson, E. N.: The Speech Chain: The Physics and Biology of Spoken Language. Garden City, N.Y., Anchor Press/Doubleday, 1973.

Eisenson, J.: Aphasia in Adults. In Travis, L. E. (Ed.): Handbook of Speech Pathology. New York, Appleton-Century-Crofts, 1957.

Eisenson, J.: Aphasia in Adults: Basic Considerations. In Travis, L. E. (Ed.): Handbook of Speech Pathology and Audiology. New York, Appleton-Century-Crofts, 1971.

Eisenson, J.: Therapeutic Problems and Approaches with Aphasic Adults. In Travis, L. E. (Ed.): Handbook of Speech Pathology and Audiology. New York, Appleton-Century-Crofts, 1971.

Eisenson, J., and Ogilvie, M.: Speech Correction in the Schools. 2nd ed. New York, Macmillan Co., 1963.

Eisenson, J., et al.: An Investigation into the Ability of Voice Defectives to Discriminate among Difference in Pitch and Loudness. J. Speech Hearing Disorders, 23:577, 1958.

Fairbanks, G., and Lintner, M. V. H.: A Study of Minor Organic Deviations in Functional Disorders of Articulation: 4. The Teeth and Hard Palate. J. Speech Hearing Disorders, 16:273, 1951.

Fairbanks, G., and Spriestersbach, D. C.: A Study of Minor Organic Deviations in Functional Disorders of Articulation: 1. Rate of Movement of Oral Structures. J. Speech Hearing Disorders, 15:60, 1950.

Flanagan, J. L.: Some Properties of the Glottal Sound Source. J. Speech Hearing Research, 1:99, 1958.

Fletcher, S. G., et al.: Tongue-Thrust Swallow, Speech Articulation, and Age. J. Speech Hearing Disorders, 26:135, 1961.

Gardner, W. H.: Laryngectomee Speech and Rehabilitation. Springfield, Ill., Charles C Thomas, Publisher, 1971.

Gens, G., and Bibey, M. L.: Congenital Aphasia: A Case Report. J. Speech Hearing Disorders, *17*:32, 1952.

Jackson, C., and Jackson, C. L.: *Diseases of the Nose, Throat and Ear.* Philadelphia, W. B. Saunders Co., 1959.

Johnson, W.: *People in Quandaries.* New York, Harper & Brothers, 1946.

Johnson, W., et al.: *Speech Handicapped School Children.* 3rd ed. New York, Harper & Brothers, 1956.

LaBarge VoiceBak Prosthesis. LaBarge, Inc., St. Louis, Missouri.

Lewis, M. M.: *How Children Learn to Speak.* New York, Basic Books, Inc., 1957.

Lowry, L. D., Marks, J. E., and Powell, W. J.: 260 Laryngeal Carcinomas. Arch. Otolaryngol. *98*:147–151, 1973.

Luper, H. L., and Mulder, R. L.: *Stuttering Therapy for Children.* Englewood Cliffs, N. J., Prentice-Hall, Inc., 1964.

McEvery, E. T., and Gaines, F. P.: Tonguetie in Infants and Children. J. Pediatr., *18*: 252, 1941.

Mase, D. J.: *Etiology of Articulatory Speech Defects.* Contributions to Education, No. 921. New York, Teachers College, Columbia University, 1946.

Mason, R. M., and Proffit, W. R.: The Tongue Thrust Controversy: Background and Recommendations. J. Speech Hearing Disorders, *39*:115, 1974.

Metraux, R. W.: Speech Profiles of the Preschool Child 18 to 54 Months. J. Speech Hearing Disorders, *15*:37, 1950.

Milisen, R.: The Incidence of Speech Disorders. *In* Travis, L. E. (Ed.): *Handbook of Speech Pathology and Audiology.* New York, Appleton-Century-Crofts, 1971.

Moncur, J. P.: Parental Domination in Stuttering. J. Speech Hearing Disorders, *17*: 155, 1952.

Moolenaar-Bijl, A. J.: Consonant Articulation and the Intake of Air in Oesophageal Speech. Folia Phonat., *58*:212, 1953.

Moore, G. P.: Voice Disorders Associated with Organic Abnormalities. *In* Travis, L. E. (Ed.): *Handbook of Speech Pathology.* New York, Appleton-Century-Crofts, 1957, pp. 653–703.

Moore, G. P.: *Organic Voice Disorders.* Englewood Cliffs, N.J., Prentice-Hall, Inc., 1971.

Moore, G. P.: Voice Disorders Organically Based. *In* Travis, L. E. (Ed.): *Handbook of Speech Pathology and Audiology.* N.Y., Appleton-Century-Crofts, 1971.

Moore, G. P.: Voice Problems Following Limited Surgical Excision. The Laryngoscope, *85*:619, 1975.

Moore, G. P.: Observations on Laryngeal Disease, Laryngeal Behavior and Voice. Ann. Otol. Rhinol. and Laryngol. *85*:553, 1976.

Murphy, A. T.: *Functional Voice Disorders.* Englewood Cliffs, N. J., Prentice-Hall, Inc., 1965.

Myerson, M. C.: *The Human Larynx.* Springfield, Ill., Charles C Thomas, Publisher, 1964.

Myklebust, H.: Aphasia in Children. *In* Travis, L. E. (Ed.). *Handbook of Speech Pathology.* New York, Appleton-Century-Crofts, 1957.

National Advisory Neurological Diseases and Stroke Council: *Human Communications and and its Disorders—an Overview.* Bethesda, Maryland, NINDS, 1969.

Patton, F. E.: A Comparison of the Kinaesthetic Sensibility of Speech Defective and Normal-speaking Children. J. Speech Hearing Disorders, *7*:305, 1942.

Peacher, W. G.: Dysarthria. *In* Levin, N. M. (Ed.): *Voice and Speech Disorders: Medical Aspects.* Springfield, Ill., Charles C Thomas, Publisher, 1962.

Peacher, W. G.: The Etiology and Differential Diagnosis of Dysarthria. J. Speech Hearing Disorders, *15*:252, 1950.

Poole, I.: Genetic Development of Articulation of Consonant Sounds in Speech. Elementary English Review, *11*:159, 1934.

Rieber, R. W., and Brubaker, H. S. (Eds.): *Speech Pathology.* Amsterdam, North-Holland Publishing Co., 1966.

Robinson, F. B.: *Introduction to Stuttering.* Englewood Cliffs, N. J., Prentice-Hall, Inc., 1964.

Schuell, H.: Sex Differences in Relation to Stuttering: Part I. J. Speech Hearing Disorders, *11*:277, 1946.

Senturia, B. M., and Wilson, F. B.: Otorhinolaryngic Findings in Children with Voice Deviations. Ann. Otol. Rhinol. Laryngol., *77*: 1027, 1963.

Sisson, G. A., McConnell, F. M. S., Logemann, J. A., and Yeh, S.: Voice Rehabilitation after Laryngectomy. Arch. Otolaryngol. *101*:178–181, 1975.

Snidecor, J. C.: *Speech Rehabilitation of the Laryngectomized.* Springfield, Ill., Charles C Thomas, Publisher, 1962.

Snidecor, J. C.: The Family of the Laryngectomee. *In The Family as Supportive Personnel in Speech and Hearing Remediation.* Proceedings of a Post-graduate Short Course, University of California, Santa Barbara.

U. S. Dept. of Health, Education and Welfare, 1971, pp. 12–24.

Snow, K.: Articulation Proficiency in Relation to Certain Dental Abnormalities. J. Speech Hearing Disorders, 26:209, 1961.

Sugar, O.: Congenital Aphasia: An Anatomical and Physiological Approach. J. Speech Hearing Disorders, 17:301, 1952.

Van Riper, C.: Stuttering. Chicago, National Society for Crippled Children and Adults, Inc., 1948.

Van Riper, C.: Speech Correction: Principles and Methods. 4th ed. Englewood Cliffs. N. J., Prentice-Hall, Inc., 1963.

Van Riper, C., and Irwin, J. V.: Voice and Articulation. Englewood Cliffs, N. J., Prentice-Hall, Inc., 1958.

Weinberg, B., and Riekena, A.: Speech Produced with the Tokyo Artificial Larynx. J. Speech Hearing Disorders, 38:383, 1973.

Weisenburg, T., and McBride, K.: Aphasia, A Clinical and Psychological Study. London, Commonwealth Fund, Oxford University Press, 1935.

Wepman, J. M.: Recovery from Aphasia. New York, Ronald Press Co., 1951.

Wepman, J., et al.: Studies in Aphasia: Background and Theoretical Formulations. J. Speech Hearing Disorders, 25:323, 332, 1960.

Wood, N. E.: Delayed Speech and Language Development. Englewood Cliffs, N. J., Prentice-Hall, Inc., 1964.

Zwitman, D. H., and Calcaterra, T. C.: Phonation Using the Trachea-esophageal Shunt After Total Laryngectomy. J. Speech Hearing Disorders, 38:369, 1973.

Pertinent Organizations

American Speech and Hearing Association
9030 Old Georgetown Road
Washington, D.C. 20014
International Association of Laryngectomees
c/o American Cancer Society, Inc.
219 E. 42nd Street
New York, New York 10017

PART 4
THE EAR

David F. Austin

Chapter 40
Anatomy and Embryology

THE TEMPORAL BONE

The temporal bone not only contains the sense organs of hearing and balance, together with the sound conduction apparatus, but also contributes to the cranial vault and zygoma. The temporal bones are situated at the sides and base of the skull and consist of five parts: the squama, mastoid, petrous, tympanic, and styloid process (Figs. 40–1 to 40–3).

The *squamous portion* of the temporal bone is largely thin and convex outward. Its external surface affords attachment to the temporalis muscle, which is bounded inferiorly by the temporal line, an important surgical landmark. The suprameatal triangle, another landmark, is a fossa situated just superior and posterior to the external meatus. The triangle is bounded at the meatus by the suprameatal spine (spine of Henle). This triangle approximates, on the external surface of the temporal bone, the position of the mastoid antrum. The zygomatic process projects forward from the lower part of the squama and with the squama and tympanic bone serves to bound the mandibular fossa. A suture line runs through the fossa, the petrotympanic fissure (glaserian fissure), which leads to the middle ear and transmits the tympanic branch of the internal maxillary artery. A canal separated slightly from the fissure, the canal of Huguier, transmits the chorda tympani nerve.

The *tympanic portion* is an incomplete cylinder which, together with the squama superiorly, forms the bony external auditory meatus, a canal roughly 2 cm in length by 1 cm in diameter. Anteriorly it also serves to bound the mandibular fossa. The medial end of the tympanic bone contains a sulcus which holds the fibrous annulus of the tympanic membrane. A thin plate extending posteriorly contains a socket in which the styloid process is held. The posterior margin of the tympanic bone articulates with the mastoid portion to form the tympanomastoid fissure, which transmits the auricular branch of the vagus nerve.

The greatest volume of the temporal bone is formed by the *mastoid portion* posteriorly and inferiorly. Since it is extensively pneumatized, however, it has no greater mass than the other portions. The mastoid process projects inferiorly behind the external meatus. This serves as the attachment for the sternocleidomastoid, splenius capitis, and longissimus capitis muscles. From the inferior aspect there is a deep groove, the mastoid notch (digastric fossa), which holds the digastric muscle. In the interior of the mastoid process when a mastoidectomy is being performed, this groove presents as the digastric ridge and is an important landmark, since the stylomastoid foramen which transmits the facial nerve is located at the anterior extremity of this ridge. The superior surface of the mastoid is a thin plate of

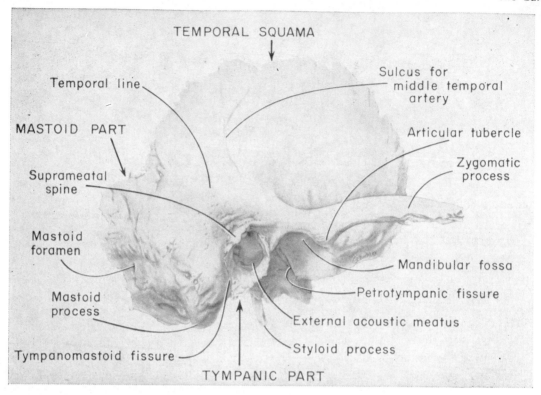

TEMPORAL SQUAMA

Temporal line

Sulcus for
middle temporal
artery

MASTOID PART

Articular tubercle

Suprameatal
spine

Zygomatic
process

Mastoid
foramen

Mandibular fossa

Petrotympanic fissure

External acoustic meatus

Mastoid
process

Tympanomastoid fissure

Styloid process

TYMPANIC PART

FIG. 40–1. Right temporal bone, lateral view. (Anson, B. J., and Donaldson, J. A.: *Surgical Anatomy of the Temporal Bone and Ear.* Philadelphia, W. B. Saunders Co., 1967.)

bone overlying the tympanic antrum, known as the tegmen mastoideum. Posteriorly, together with the posterior surface of the petrous portion, it forms the anterior border of the posterior cranial fossa. Here it has a deep groove formed by the lateral or sigmoid sinus. Two smaller channels directed medially contain the superior and inferior petrosal sinuses.

The *petrous portion* is usually called the petrous pyramid and contains the otic labyrinth. Superiorly it forms the inferior surface of the middle cranial fossa and posteriorly, bounded by the attachment of the tentorium cerebelli, helps to form, together with the mastoid portion, the anterior face of the posterior cranial fossa. The superior face of the petrous is marked by the arcuate eminence, which is the protrusion formed by the superior semicircular canal. Anterior to this is the fossa containing the geniculate ganglion, occasionally covered by a thin plate of bone, and a groove extending for-

ward from this fossa, which contains the greater superficial petrosal nerve and a branch of the middle meningeal artery. Medially there is a depression in which lies the semilunar ganglion. The posterior face of the bone presents several landmarks, the most obvious being the porus acusticus, or mouth of the internal auditory canal, which transmits the seventh and eighth cranial nerves as well as the internal auditory artery. The lateral end of the internal auditory meatus is divided horizontally by the crista falciformis. The superior compartment contains the facial nerve anteriorly and the superior branch of the vestibular nerve posteriorly. The inferior compartment transmits the cochlear division anteriorly and the inferior branch of the vestibular nerve posteriorly. A shallow depression in the middle of the posterior face ends in a duct running posteriorly under a thin ledge of bone and marks the external position of the endolymphatic sac. The cochlear aqueduct opens

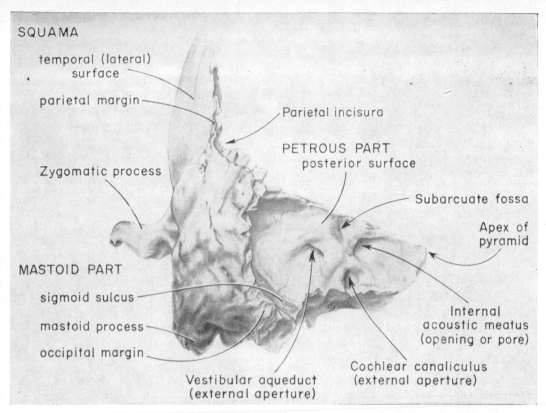

SQUAMA
  temporal (lateral) surface
  parietal margin
  Parietal incisura
  PETROUS PART
  posterior surface
  Zygomatic process
  Subarcuate fossa
  Apex of pyramid
MASTOID PART
  sigmoid sulcus
  mastoid process
  occipital margin
  Internal acoustic meatus (opening or pore)
  Vestibular aqueduct (external aperture)
  Cochlear canaliculus (external aperture)

FIG. 40–2. Left temporal bone, posterolateral view. (Anson, B. J., and Donaldson, J. A.: *Surgical Anatomy of the Temporal Bone and Ear*. Philadelphia, W. B. Saunders Co., 1967.)

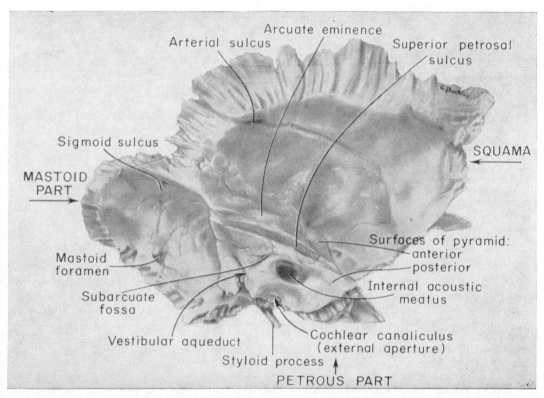

  Arcuate eminence
  Arterial sulcus
  Superior petrosal sulcus
  Sigmoid sulcus
  SQUAMA
MASTOID PART
  Mastoid foramen
  Surfaces of pyramid: anterior posterior
  Subarcuate fossa
  Internal acoustic meatus
  Vestibular aqueduct
  Cochlear canaliculus (external aperture)
  Styloid process
  PETROUS PART

FIG. 40–3. Left temporal bone, medial view. (Anson, B. J., and Donaldson, J. A.: *Surgical Anatomy of the Temporal Bone and Ear*. Philadelphia, W. B. Saunders Co., 1967.)

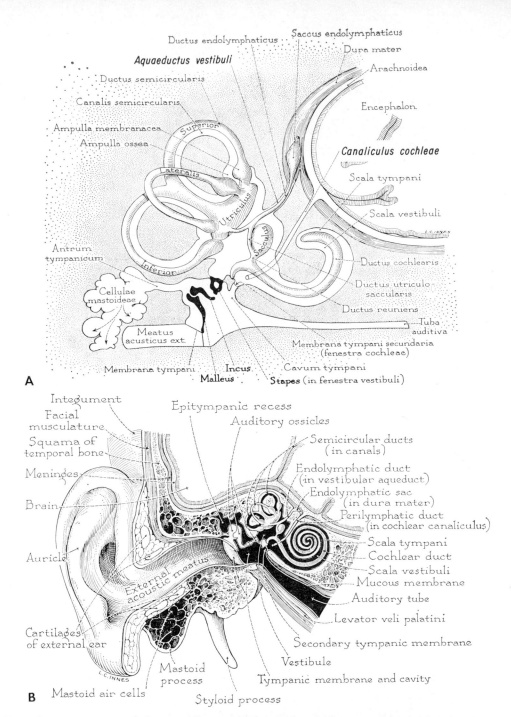

FIG. 40–4.   A, Parts of the ear (diagrammatic): the membranous duct system for the endolymph; the surrounding osseous labyrinth containing the perilymph; the tympanic cavity; the
auditory tube and pneumatic spaces (with which the cavity is continuous); and the contained
auditory ossicles. The tympanic cavity (of the middle ear) is separated from the external acoustic
meatus (of the outer ear) by the tympanic membrane and from the vestibule (of the inner ear)
by the base, or footplate, of the stapes, anchored in the vestibular (oval) window by the annular
ligament. The labyrinths are not wholly sequestered systems. The perilymphatic spaces of the
osseous labyrinth communicate with those of the cranial arachnoid through the cochlear canaliculus (or aqueduct); the endolymphatic sac of the membranous labyrinthine system is lodged
in the dura mater, which it reaches through the vestibular aqueduct. (Courtesy **Dr. Barry J.
Anson.**) B, General relationships of parts of the ear (semidiagrammatic). (From Anson, B. J.,
and McVay, C. B.: *Surgical Anatomy.* 5th ed. Philadelphia, W. B. Saunders Company, 1971.)

just below the internal auditory canal at the base of the petrous bone. The lateral aspect of the petrous bone constitutes the medial wall of the middle ear and will be described under that section. At the petrous apex a hiatus is present between the tentorium and the petrous, which forms a canal for the passage of the fifth cranial nerve (Meckel's cave). The sixth cranial nerve runs through a notch just below the posterior clinoid process (the medial attachment of the tentorium) and above the articulation of the petrous and sphenoid (Dorello's canal). Disease in the petrous apex will thus produce irritation and dysfunction of the fifth and sixth cranial nerves—Gradenigo's syndrome.

THE EAR

Both anatomically and functionally the ear is divided into three parts: the external ear, the middle ear, and the inner ear (Fig. 40-4, A, B).

The External Ear

The external ear is that portion of the ear external to the tympanic membrane. It consists of the auricle and the passage leading to the tympanic membrane, the external auditory canal.

The auricle is a convoluted plate of elastic cartilage covered with skin and fixed in position by both muscles and ligaments. The major convolutions of the auricle are the helix and antihelix, the tragus and antitragus, and the concha, which is a funnel-like

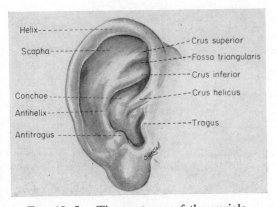

Helix
Scapha
Conchae
Antihelix
Antitragus

Crus superior
Fossa triangularis
Crus inferior
Crus helicus
Tragus

FIG. 40–5.   The anatomy of the auricle.

depression leading into the meatus (Fig. 40-5). The lobule is the only portion of the auricle which contains no cartilage. The cartilage of the auricle is continuous with that of the external meatus.

The external auditory canal is formed in its outer one third by an extension of the cartilage of the auricle and in its inner two thirds by the tympanic and squamous portion of the temporal bone. It is bounded medially by the tympanic membrane. The cartilaginous portion of the canal differs markedly in structure from the bony portion. The cartilage is firmly attached to the temporal bone but maintains some mobility due to fibrous channels in the cartilage, the fissures of Santorini, which may also transmit infection or tumor between the canal and the parotid gland. The skin covering the cartilaginous portion of the canal is loosely applied and contains numerous hair follicles and ceruminous and sebaceous glands.

The bony external canal is curved anteriorly and inferiorly and narrows in its midportion to form an isthmus. It constitutes two thirds of the total length of the meatus, which averages 3½ cm. The diameter of the canal varies but averages 7 by 9 mm, the vertical dimension being the greater. The skin of the bony canal is closely applied to bone, the subcutaneous layers condensing to form the periosteum. Fibrous tissue enters the two suture lines in the canal, making elevation of the canal skin particularly difficult over these sutures. As the tympanic membrane is approached, the skin gradually thins, forming a layer 5 to 7 cells thick over the meatal surface of the tympanic membrane. The drum and bony canal skin have a self-cleaning property owing to migration of the keratin layer of epithelium from the drum outward to the cartilaginous portion. This migration is rather rapid near the attachment of the malleus handle, decelerates circumferentially from the umbo, and becomes quite slow as the canal is reached.

The tympanic membrane is composed of three layers, the squamous layer bounding the external ear medially, the mucosal layer bounding the middle ear laterally, and the fibrous layer lying between. The fibrous layer is composed of both circumferential and radial fibers and gives the tympanic membrane its shape and consistency. The radial fibers insert into the perichondrium of the malleus handle and into the fibrous annulus, creating the functionally significant conical shape. The circumferential fibers give strength without interfering with free vibration, while some tangential fibers reinforce the architecture. These architectural characteristics of the tympanic membrane allow it to approach the ideal in radiation of vibratory energy.

The most prominent landmark in the tympanic membrane is the manubrium (handle) of the malleus whose superior limit is marked by the lateral or short process, a short thumblike projection directed laterally. The manubrium is flat and rounded inferiorly, ending at the apex or umbo of the tympanic membrane. Because of the conical shape of the drum, a typical light reflex projects anterior-inferiorly from the umbo. At the periphery of the tympanic membrane the fibrous layer thickens and coalesces to form the tympanic annulus which is inserted into the sulcus of the tympanic bone. Superiorly, the tympanic ring is incomplete so that the fibrous layer is bounded by the anterior and posterior mal-

lear folds. The superior arch of the margin of the tympanic membrane formed by the squamous portion of the temporal bone is termed the incisura tympanica or notch of Rivinus. The segment of tympanic membrane superior to the mallear folds and bounded by the rivinian notch is completely lacking a fibrous layer and is thus called the pars flaccida (Shrapnell's membrane). The larger, inferior portion is called the pars tensa of the tympanic membrane.

The Middle Ear

The middle ear consists of the space between the tympanic membrane and the capsule of the inner ear, the ossicular and muscular contents of this space, and the appendages; the auditory (eustachian) tube; and the mastoid air cell system (Fig. 40-6). The superior and inferior limits of the tympanic membrane serve to divide the tympanic cavity into the epitympanum or attic, the mesotympanum, and the hypotympanum.

The *hypotympanum* is a shallow space lying inferior to the tympanic membrane. Its bony surface presents a scalloped appearance because of the presence of cuplike

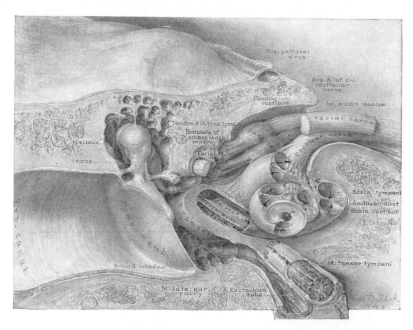

Fig. 40-6. Section through the middle ear and labyrinth. (From *Three Unpublished Drawings of the Human Ear*. Max Brodel, W. B. Saunders Co., 1946.)

air cells. This wall covers the jugular bulb. Occasionally a dehiscence permits the jugular to present in the lower tympanic cavity.

The *mesotympanum* is bounded medially by the otic capsule, inferior to the level of the tympanic portion of the facial nerve. The curved eminence covering the basal turn of the cochlea lies immediately medial to the drumhead and is termed the promontory. Several shallow channels in the promontory contain the nerves making up the tympanic plexus. Posterior to the promontory, located superiorly and inferiorly, respectively, are the oval (vestibular) and round (cochlear) windows, each placed at the bottom of a niche. These two depressions communicate at the posterior limit of the mesotympanum by a deep curved fossa, the tympanic sinus. The oval window contains the stapedial footplate, which is placed in the sagittal plane. The round window is protected from view because it is placed in a mostly transverse plane anterior to a lip extending from the promontory. The round window is closed by a thin membrane, the secondary tympanic membrane. The posterior wall of the mesotympanum is formed by the bone covering the descending portion of the facial nerve. This bone is usually pneumatized with the cells, often communicating with the mastoid air cell system. Superiorly on this wall a conical projection, the pyramidal eminence, encloses the stapedius muscle and transmits its tendon. A branch of the seventh nerve runs to the muscle. Lateral to the pyramidal eminence is the foramen for the chorda tympani nerve which runs inferiorly through a curved canal to join the facial canal near or at the stylomastoid foramen.

A clinically important space, the posterior sinus or facial recess, occurs immediately lateral to the facial canal and pyramidal process, being bounded laterally by the posterosuperior tympanic annulus and superiorly by the short process of the incus inserting into the incudal fossa (Fig. 40–7). The space leads from the posterosuperior middle ear cavity to the aditus ad antrum and frequently hides disease. Approaching this space from the mastoid antrum allows exposure of the structures of the posterior tympanum and the facial nerve.

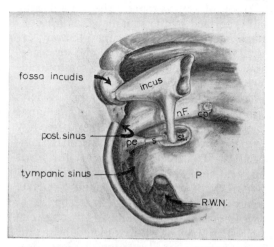

FIG. 40–7. Recesses of the posterior tympanum. *RWN,* Round window niche; *P,* promontory; *pe,* pyramidal eminence; *s,* stapedius tendon; *st,* stapes; *nF,* facial nerve; *cp,* cochleariform process.

The anterior extremity of the tympanic portion of the facial canal is marked by a hooklike projection of the posterior end of the canal of the tensor tympani muscle, the cochleariform process, which serves to turn the tendon of the tensor laterally into the middle ear. The canal of the tensor tympani runs forward into the superior surface of the eustachian tube and marks the anterosuperior limit of the mesotympanum.

The anterior wall of the mesotympanum contains the tympanic orifice of the eustachian tube superiorly and forms the bony covering of the ascending carotid canal inferiorly. This wall is usually well pneumatized and may have bony dehiscences.

The *epitympanum* contains the bulk of the incus and malleus. Superiorly it is bounded by a thin projection of the petrous, the tegmen tympani, which is continuous with the posterior tegmen mastoideum. The otic capsule forms the medial attic wall, which is marked by the bulge of the lateral semicircular canal. Anteriorly the ampullary region of the superior canal may be approached, and anteriorly yet is the region of the geniculate ganglion, marking the anterior extremity of the attic space. The anterior wall is separated by a narrow space from the malleus head and may contain entrances of some of the air cells pneumatizing

form the short neck. The crura are bowed, the posterior more than the anterior, and terminate by fusing with the flat oval base. The obturator aspect of the neck and crura is extensively excavated, leaving a hollow shell of periosteal bone. The stapedius tendon inserts on a small prominence on the posterior surface of the neck of the stapes.

Tympanic Muscles. Two muscles are contained within the middle ear; the tensor tympani and the stapedius (Fig. 40–9).

The tensor tympani muscle arises from the walls of the semicanal of the tensor tympani. This canal lies just superior to the bony auditory canal and is open toward the auditory canal, thus the term "semicanal." The muscle fibers collect and become tendinous at the tympanic end of the semicanal, which is marked by the cochleariform process. This process serves to turn the tendon lateralward into the middle ear. The tendon inserts on the upper portion of the neck of the malleus. The tensor tympani is innervated by a branch of the fifth cranial nerve. Its action causes the drumhead to be pulled inward, thus tensing it and raising the resonant frequency of the sound conduction system as well as attenuating low frequency sound.

The stapedius muscle arises within its canal in the pyramidal eminence, the fibers being attached to the periosteum of this canal. The fibers collect and form the stapedius tendon, which inserts on the posterior aspect of the neck of the stapes. The stapedius is innervated by a branch of the seventh cranial nerve given off as it passes the stapedius during its second turn. The action of the stapedius pulls the stapes posteriorly around a pivot at the posterior lip of the stapes base. This stiffens the stapes, attenuating sound transmission and raising the resonant frequency of the ossicular chain.

These actions can be controlled voluntarily by some individuals but are usually a part of reflex activity of the ear. Although the purpose of this activity was thought to be to protect the inner ear from the trauma of loud sounds, animal investigation has indicated the possibility of vegetative and species survival function (Simmons).

Tympanic Folds. As the mucosa invests the tympanic space during fetal development, various folds arise in relationship to the ligaments, tendons, and blood vessels to form mesentery-like membranes which serve to delineate various clinically important compartments within the middle ear. Except for two openings, one between the stapes and tensor tendon and one between the short process of incus and pyramidal process, the attic space is completely isolated from the mesotympanum by these folds (Figs. 40–10 to 40–13). Anteriorly, the tensor fold runs forward from the tensor tympani along the anterior mallear ligament and semicanal of the tensor tympani to separate completely the anterior attic from the anterior mesotympanum. This fold usually prevents attic cholesteatoma from entering the anterior mesotympanum. Running transversely through the superior ligament of the malleus is the superior mallear fold, dividing the attic into anterior and posterior spaces. Lateral to the neck of the malleus between the lateral mallear ligament and Shrapnell's membrane lies Prussak's space, which is the first space to be occupied by a young cholesteatoma. The lateral incudal fold extends between the inferior border of the incus to the lateral attic wall. This fold may prevent the extension of posterosuperior marginal squamous ingrowth into the attic with consequent formation of secondary acquired cholesteatoma. Primary acquired cholesteatoma may, however, leave Prussak's space posteriorly and extend under the lateral fold to involve the posterior mesotympanum. A full description and discussion of these spaces has been given by Proctor.

Auditory (Eustachian) Tube. The auditory tube extends from the anterior superior wall of the mesotympanum to the nasopharynx. The anatomy of the tube varies considerably, ranging from its pharyngeal cartilaginous portion to the tympanic bony portion. The pharyngeal orifice is surrounded by a hook-shaped cartilage within the torus tubarius. Contraction of the anteriorly attached tensor veli palatini muscle causes the cartilaginous tube to assume a more cylindrical shape and become patent. The mucosal lining of the cartilaginous por-

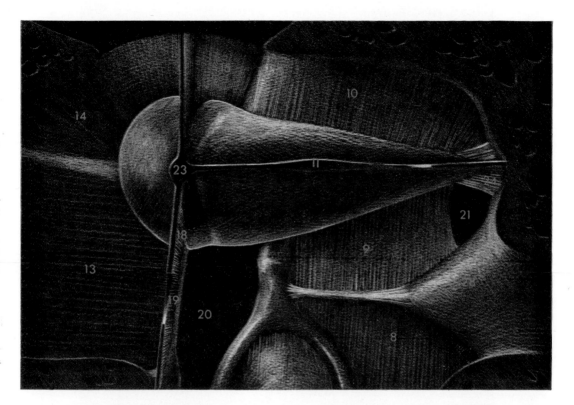

FIG. 40–10.   Floor of attic viewed from above. The mesotympanum is almost completely separated from the attic by the ossicular chain folds. The only constant communication is supplied by the isthmus tympani anticus and the isthmus tympani posticus. *5*, Obturatoria stapedis fold; *8*, plica stapedis fold; *9*, medial incudal fold; *10*, lateral incudal fold; *11*, superior incudal fold; *13*, tensor tympani fold; *14*, anterior mallear fold; *18*, superior mallear fold; *19*, incisura tensoris; *20*, isthmus tympani anticus; *21*, isthmus tympani posticus; *23*, superior mallear ligament; *24*, posterior incudal ligament. (Proctor, B.: J. Laryngol., *78*:631, 1964.)

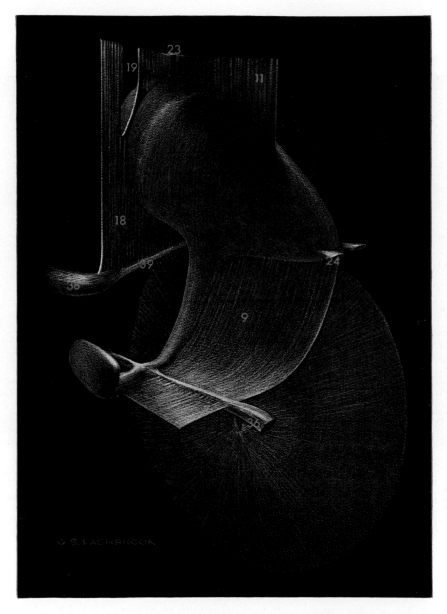

FIG. 40–11.   Posterior, superior, and medial views of the ossicles. The medial incudal fold extends medially and posteroinferiorly from the incus crura to the stapedial tendon. *8,* Plica stapedis; *9,* medial incudal fold; *11,* superior incudal fold; *18,* superior mallear fold; *19,* incisura tensoris; *23,* superior mallear ligament. (Proctor, B.: J. Laryngol., *78*:631, 1964.)

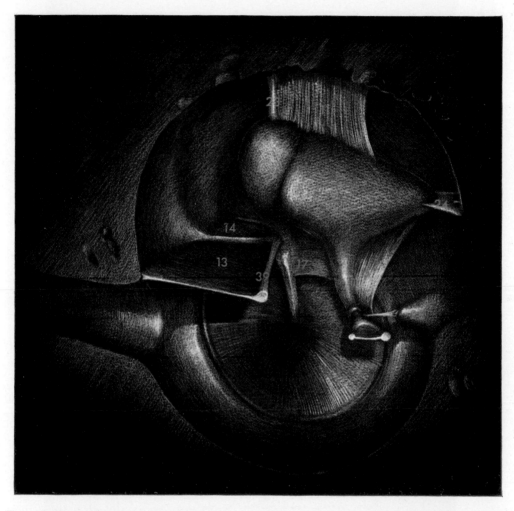

FIG. 40–12. Note the anterior compartment of the attic with the tensor fold as the floor, the interossicular fold between the malleus and incus, and the medial incudal fold with the isthmus tympani posticus behind. *9,* Medial incudal fold; *11,* superior incudal fold; *13,* tensor tympani fold; *14,* anterior mallear fold; *17,* interossicular fold; *23,* superior mallear ligament. (Proctor, B.: J. Laryngol., *78*:631, 1964.)

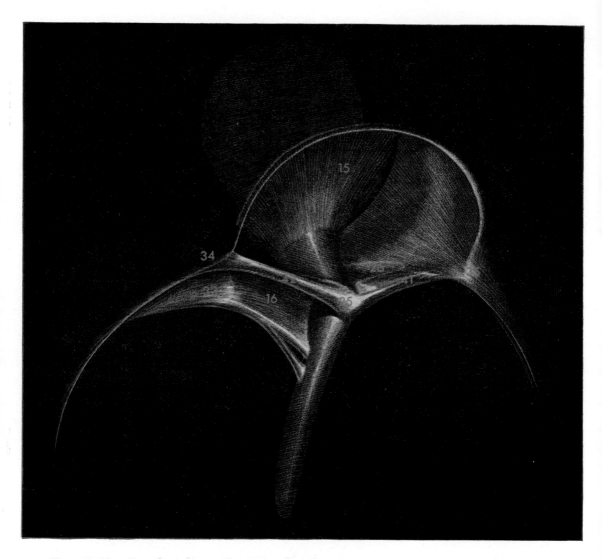

FIG. 40–13. Terminal fibers of annulus fibrosis spread out to help form the boundaries of Prussak's space. The roof is formed by the lateral mallear fold which fans out to attach along the rim of the notch of Rivinus. *15,* Lateral mallear fold. (Proctor, B.: J. Laryngol., *78*:631, 1964.)

tion is similar to that of the pharynx, having many mucous glands. The submucosa contains numerous lymphoid aggregates. The cartilaginous portion runs posteriorly, superiorly, and medially for two thirds of the total length of the auditory tube (4 cm), where it joins the bony or tympanic portion of the tube. The point of union is the narrowest part of the tube, the isthmus, and there is a gradual widening to the largest diameter at the tympanic orifice. During this course the mucosa gradually thins to become similar to the cuboidal or low columnar tympanic mucosa. A few mucous glands continue through the tympanic portion. The inferior wall of the bony auditory tube overlies the carotid canal. The superior wall contains the semicanal of the tensor tympani muscle.

Nerve Supply of External and Middle Ear. The auricle and external meatus receive sensory branches from the auriculotemporal branch of the fifth nerve anteriorly, from the greater and lesser auricular nerve posteriorly, and by branches arising from the glossopharyngeal and vagus nerves.

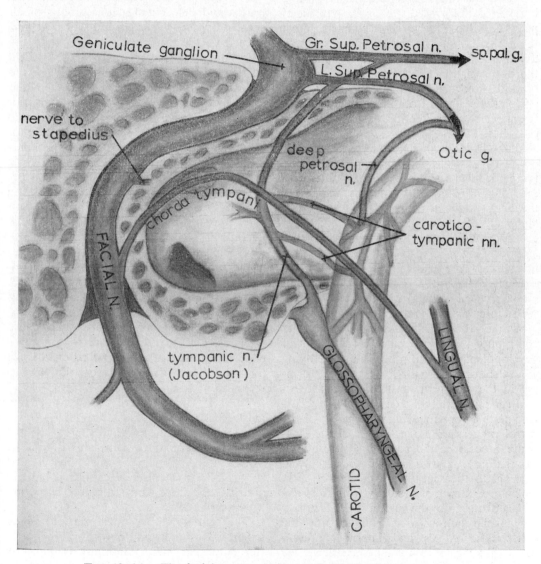

FIG. 40–14.   The facial nerve and its relationships (diagrammatic). *sp.pal.g.,* Sphenopalatine ganglion.

The branch from the vagus is known as Arnold's nerve, the stimulation of which may cause a cough reflex when the external ear is being cleaned. The posterior superior portion of the bony canal may be supplied by sensory branches of the facial nerve (Fig. 40-14).

The promontory of the middle ear contains the tympanic plexus (Jacobson's plexus). This receives Jacobson's nerve, a branch of the glossopharyngeal arising from the petrosal ganglion below the ear. After entering the tympanic plexus, the fibers run forward, leaving the middle ear with a branch of the facial, the lesser superficial petrosal nerve. After a short course through the cranial cavity on the anterior aspect of the temporal bone, the fibers terminate in the otic ganglion to innervate primarily the parotid gland. The tympanic plexus receives sympathetic fibers from the carotid plexus by superior and inferior caroticotympanic branches.

The chorda tympani enters the middle ear just below the posterosuperior lip of the tympanic sulcus and runs forward lateral to the long process of the incus, then under the neck of the malleus just above the attachment of the tensor tympani tendon. It exits through the petrotympanic fissure after running medial to the anterior mallear ligament.

Mastoid Anatomy. *Pneumatic.* The pneumatic air cell system arises in conjunction with the enlarging temporal bone as an outgrowth of the middle ear and antrum. Air cell groups may be classified by the point of developmental origin. The cells developing from the antrum are the largest group, forming in the enlarging mastoid process. *Mastoid cells* are external to a commonly occurring plate of bone marking the fusion of the antral process of the petrous and the tympanic process of the squama (petrosquamous suture), known as Körner's septum. Internal to the septum are the *antral cells,* which are extensions medially from the original antrum into the petrous. These may invade the petrous deeply to outline the semicircular canals and internal auditory canal. The sigmoid sinus may be surrounded with a *sinus group,* and the squama may be invaded. An anterior and lateral extension of these cells may invade the zygoma (*zygomal cells*) and communicate with the attic. The *mastoid tip cells* occasionally form a large coalescent area in the extremity of the mastoid process.

The middle ear tympanic cells form several divergent groups which pneumatize the petrous. The largest of these is made up of the *carotid air cells* which surround the carotid canal and merge with the *subtubal group* of air cells arising from the auditory tube. The *apical cells* of the petrous arise mainly from this group, as do the *precochlear cells.* Also differentiated are *precarotid, postcarotid,* and *supracarotid* groups of air cells. A *supracochlear* group of air cells may arise from the medial attic wall and extend above the cochlea and around the geniculate ganglion, sometimes merging with antral cells around the superior semicircular canal. Cells arising from the posterior middle ear may communicate anterior to the facial nerve with the mastoid cells or even serve as a point of origin for the mastoid cells. The *retrofacial cells* arise from the tympanic sinus and pneumatize the petrous medial to the facial nerve. Eradication of disease from these last two groups of air cells presents a surgical risk to the facial nerve.

The extent of pneumatization of the temporal bone varies greatly between individuals. This is apparently determined by both hereditary and environmental factors. Otitis in infancy and childhood can definitely inhibit further pneumatization as well as cause sclerosis. On the other hand, there is evidence that limited pneumatization of the temporal bone may predispose the ear to infection.

Surgical. The surgical anatomy of the mastoid deserves special study since it involves picturing the internal margins of the mastoid after removal of the air cell system. This anatomic configuration is thus created surgically and consists of exposing, but not injuring, the important structures bordering the *mastoid cavity.*

The posterior limit of the mastoid cavity is formed by the bone overlying the posterior dura. The major landmark is the large convex channel running from the superolateral corner to the posteromedial corner formed by the lateral sinus. The superior limit of this wall forms an acute angle with the mastoid tegmen, the sinodural angle. The tegmen forms the upper wall of the cavity. Inferiorly the mastoid tip forms the wall superficially, with the concave digastric ridge projecting into the space medial to the tip. The cavity is limited anteriorly by the posterior wall of the external auditory canal and the vertical segment of the facial nerve lying at the base of this wall (Fig. 40–15). This portion of the facial nerve extends roughly from the fossa incudis to the anterior end of the digastric ridge.

The medial wall of the mastoid cavity presents several landmarks. The lateral and posterior semicircular canals occupy the major portion of this wall. The triangle between the external prominence of these canals and the posterosuperior corner of the mastoid is known as Trautmann's triangle, from which a group of antral cells invade the petrous deeply to the region of the internal auditory canal. Visualization

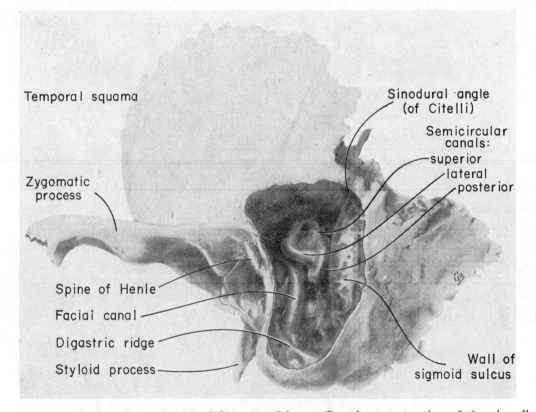

Fig. 40–15. Mastoid cavity in a left temporal bone. Complete exenteration of the air cells. Demonstrating the relation of the facial (Fallopian) canal to the semicircular canals and to the sulcus for the sigmoid part of the transverse (venous) sinus of the dura mater. The facial canal, in passing lateralward and downward, lies close to the mastoid wall of the tympanic cavity. Surgically, the tip cells are removed with the facial canal as the anterior limiting boundary and the wall of the sigmoid sulcus serving as the posterior boundary. The sulcus, on the medial wall of the mastoid part of the temporal bone, curves from above and behind in a direction downward and forward. The floor of the space is elevated by the so-called digastric ridge. On the external surface of the mastoid process a corresponding depression occurs; this is the mastoid incisure (or digastric fossa of the older terminology). The sigmoid sulcus meets the "roof" of the cavity at an acute angle; externally the angle thus formed is represented by the junction of the middle with the posterior cranial fossa. The roof is the bone of the anterior surface of the petrous pyramid; it is covered by the meningeal layers of the cerebrum. (From Anson, B. J., and Donaldson, J. A.: *Surgical Anatomy of the Temporal Bone and Ear*. Philadelphia, W. B. Saunders Company, 1967.)

of the medial wall may be confused by the presence of Körner's septum, which divides the cells into superficial and deep regions. The antrum is not reached until this septum is removed and the previously mentioned landmarks identified.

The Inner Ear

Contained within the petrous portion of the temporal bone is the otic capsule, in turn containing the periotic labyrinth which surrounds the essential structure of the inner ear, the otic labyrinth (Fig. 40–16). The otic labyrinth is that continuous series of epithelial lined tubes and spaces of the inner ear which contains the otic fluid or endo-lymph. The otic labyrinth is divided into three interconnected parts with separate functions; the pars superior or vestibular labyrinth, the pars inferior or cochlea, and the endolymphatic duct and sac.

The *vestibular otic labyrinth* consists of the saccule, the utricle, and the semicircular ducts. The semicircular ducts arise and end at the utricle, each being directed in a plane perpendicular to the other in the axis of the petrous pyramid. These are the superior, posterior, and lateral or external ducts. The posterior limb of the superior duct joins into

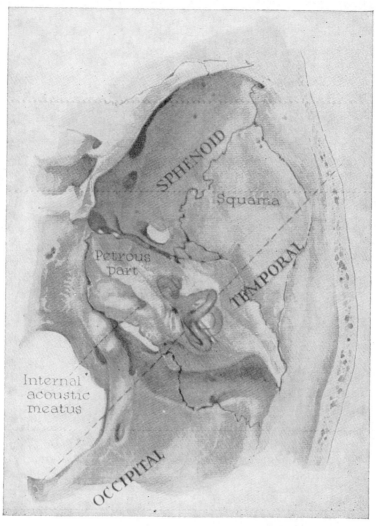

FIG. 40–16.   Position of the right osseous (perilymphatic) labyrinth in the skull. (Anson, B. J. [Ed.]: *Morris' Human Anatomy.* 12th ed. New York, McGraw-Hill Book Company, 1966.)

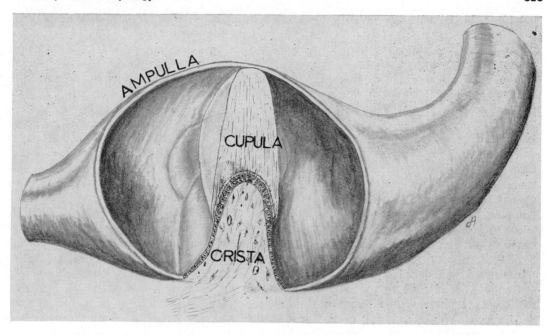

FIG. 40–17.   Section (diagrammatic) through the ampulla of a semicircular duct.

a common crus with the superior limb of the posterior duct to enter the utricle, while each of the remaining limbs are separate. Near the origin of each semicircular duct is a cystic dilatation termed the ampulla, which contains the endorgan of balance, the crista.

The sensory organs within the inner ear are constructed of essentially the same elements, but each is organized in a specialized manner to respond to a particular type of mechanical stimulus. These elements include supporting cells; sensory cells containing nonmotile cilia on their free surface, the hair cells; and a gelatinous, cushionlike structure lying on the hair cells principally composed of mucopolysaccharides which are secreted by the supporting cells.

The crista ampullaris forms a ridge across the ampulla perpendicular to the direction of fluid motion. This ridge is capped by a layer of hair cells supported between flask-shaped cells. A semilunar cap of gelatinous material, the cupula, extends from the hair cells to the opposite wall of the ampulla to form a valve which is deflected by the smallest fluid motion in either direction (Figs. 40–17 and 40–18). Two types of cuboidal cells, light and dark, run along the base of

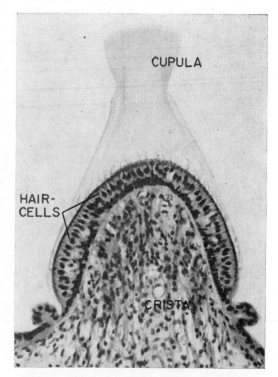

FIG. 40–18.   Photomicrograph of crista ampullaris. (Unpublished photomicrograph provided by Dr. M. Igarashi.)

the ridge, then up on the walls of the ampulla at each end of the crista to form the planum semilunatum, which seems to have both a secretory and an absorptive function. The cupula has a definite structure, with channels running through it which contain for at least part of their length the cilia of the hair cells. There is a thin, clear zone between the hair cells and the cupula.

The otic semicircular ducts are eccentrically located within the surrounding periotic space (semicircular canals), being attached along their greater curvature to the endosteum of the otic capsule. The remaining space within the semicircular canals is crossed with sparsely distributed arachnoid-like trabeculae through which circulates the periotic fluid (perilymph). The periotic spaces join anteriorly into a single large cistern, the vestibule, containing the utricle and saccule. The lateral wall of this space contains the oval window, closed by the stapes footplate (Fig. 40–19). Connective tissue outpouchings anterior and posterior to the oval window, the fissula ante fenestram and fossula post fenestram, will be described in the embryology section.

In addition to serving as a reservoir for the semicircular duct fluid flow, the utricle has an otolithic endorgan or macula lying on its floor in the horizontal plane and occasionally extending slightly up the anterior wall. The maculae are flat structures composed of hair cells between supporting cells (Fig. 40–20). The gelatinous cushion (otolithic membrane) overlying the hair cells is flat and firmly attached to the cilia. There is a free space between the undersurface of the otolithic membrane and the free surface of the hair cells through which the cilia project. Embedded on the surface of the otolithic membrane are numerous small calcareous deposits adding additional mass.

The utricular duct leaves the anterior face of the utricle and curves posteriorly around the anterior wall, creating a deep, valvelike fold over the orifice of the duct first described by Bast and termed the utriculo-endolymphatic valve. The valve is structured to permit inflow of endolymph but not outflow. An actual valvular function has yet to be demonstrated. The utricular duct joins with a similar channel from the saccule, the saccular duct, to form the endolymphatic duct (Figs. 40–21 to 40–23). After an initial dilatation, the sinus of the endolymphatic duct, it narrows to enter a bony channel through the otic capsule, the vestibular

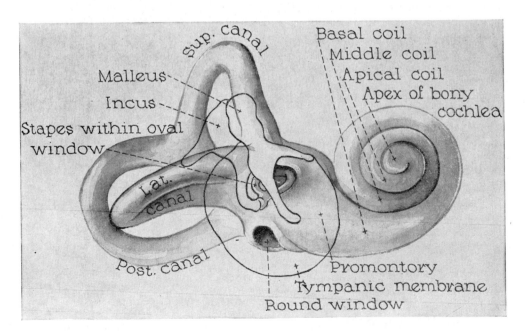

FIG. 40–19.   Relationship of the tympanic membrane and ossicles to the bony labyrinth.

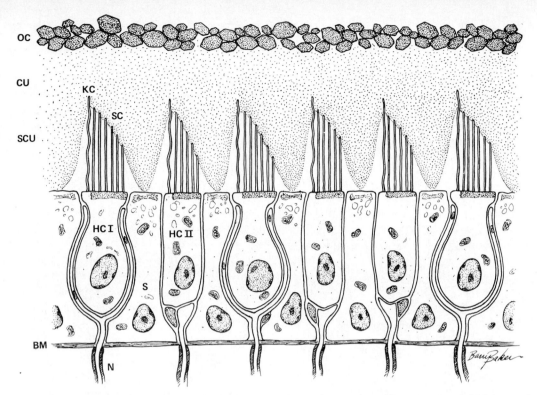

FIG. 40–20. Schematic drawing of a cross section of a macula. The gelatinous substance is divided into cupular (*CU*) and subcupular (*SCU*) layers. There are two types of hairs: kinocilia, labeled *KC* (one per hair cell), and stereocilia, labeled *SC* (many per hair cell). *OC*, Otoconia; *HC I*, type I hair cell; *HC II*, type II hair cell; *N*, nerve fiber; *BM*, basement membrane; *S*, supporting cell.

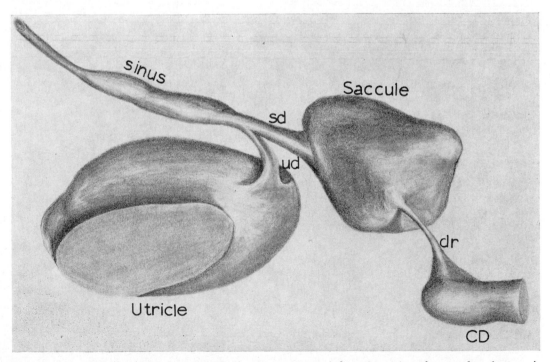

FIG. 40–21. Detail of the endolymphatic duct system (after Anson). *sd*, saccular duct; *ud*, utricular duct; *dr*, ductus reuniens; *CD*, cochlear duct.

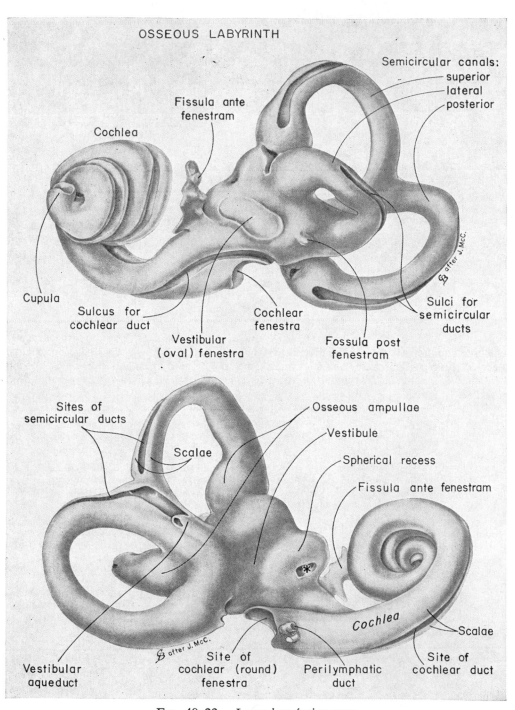

FIG. 40–22.   *Legend on facing page.*

aqueduct. The aqueduct parallels the common crus of the posterior and superior semicircular canals, then swings in a lateral and posterior direction to emerge on the posterior face of the petrous bone, usually just medial to the lateral extremity of the posterior semicircular canal. The vestibular aqueduct gradually enlarges and contains abundantly vascular connective tissue around the endolymphatic duct. Within the terminal portion of the aqueduct, the duct enlarges and the lining membrane becomes rugose to form the proximal portion of the endolymphatic sac, which is contained within the bony aqueduct. The distal external portion gradually becomes relatively smooth and is contained within the dural covering of the posterior face of the petrous pyramid. The end of the sac terminates in close relationship to the sigmoid sinus. Numerous active granular cells similar to others with secretory activity are found in the lining membrane of the endolymphatic sac.

The saccule is much smaller than the utricle but similar in structure. The saccule supports a macular structure on its medial wall in the vertical plane extending slightly onto the anterior wall. Both the utricle and saccule are entirely surrounded by perilymph except where the nerves enter at the macular region. A small duct leaves the wall of the saccule to run along the floor of the vestibule and enter the cochlear duct. This is termed the ductus reuniens and is the sole endolymphatic communication of the cochlea with the remainder of the labyrinth.

Cochlea. The pars inferior of the labyrinth is formed in a spiral of 2½ to 2¾ turns, with a total length of approximately 35 cm. Both the cochlear duct and the periotic space are complexly structured, forming a system of three tubular chambers, the

---

Fig. 40–22. Membranous labyrinth. Adult anatomy, demonstrated by a reconstruction (6-month-old infant) and by a semidiagram.

a, The utricle communicates broadly with the common arm of the superior and posterior semicircular ducts; together they assume the form of an open V. The tube-shaped utricle, lying in the elliptical recess of the vestibule, is continuous with the three semicircular ducts. On its anterolateral surface is situated the acoustic macula. The saccule has the form of an elongate oval. It occupies the spherical recess. Whereas the utricle opens widely into its canalicular ducts, the saccule is connected with the cochlear part of the system by narrow intermediary conduits; namely, the saccular and reuniting ducts. These enter and leave the saccule on the latter's inferior surface; as a result, the saccule is set off from its dependent communications. The acoustic macula is situated on the anteromedial surface. The saccule is connected with the utricle indirectly, through the saccular and the utricular (or utriculoendolymphatic) ducts; in the opposite direction (toward the cochlea) the connections are the reuniting duct (*ductus reuniens*) and the vestibular cecum, a cul-de-sac of the cochlear duct proper.

b, The endolymphatic duct, far from being a quill-like tube with a mushroom-shaped terminal expansion, is regionally modified in a constant fashion. The opening into the utricle, for example, is slitlike in form, the orifice being bounded by a folding of the apposed walls of the utricle and the endolymphatic duct. The proximal part of the latter duct is expanded into a sinuslike enlargement that occupies the internal aperture of the vestibular aqueduct. Continuing toward the external aperture, the duct narrows into an isthmus. While still intraosseous, the duct becomes a flattened cecal dilatation, the endolymphatic sac. The *saccus* is prolonged beyond the aperture, to rest in a shallow impression on the posterior surface of the petrous pyramid.

The cochlear part of the membranous labyrinth is formed by the cochlear duct. It begins in a recess of the vestibule, extends within the osseous spiral canal, through basal, middle, and apical coils, where it ends blindly in the cupular cecum. The cochlear duct is in large part triangular in cross section. Its outer wall is held by periosteal connective tissue to the osseous cochlea. It contains the spiral organ (Corti), a highly differentiated structure that contains the termination of the cochlear nerve. (From Anson, B. J., and Donaldson, J. A.: *Surgical Anatomy of the Temporal Bone and Ear.* Philadelphia, W. B. Saunders Company, 1967.)

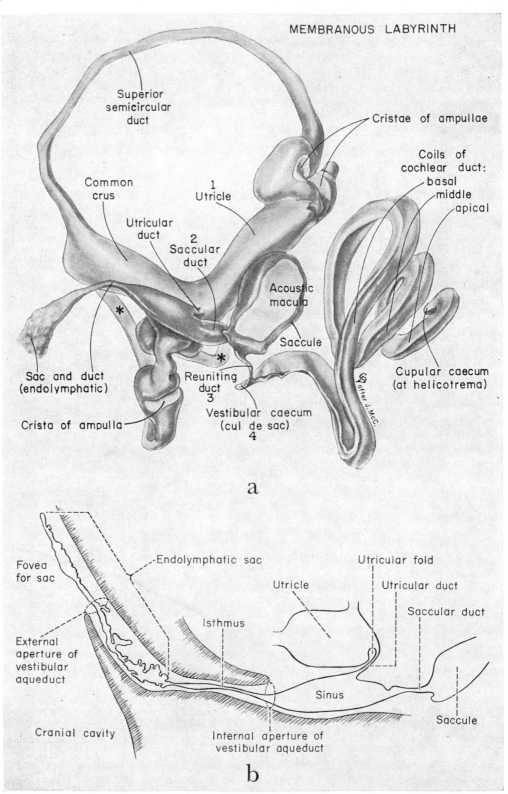

MEMBRANOUS LABYRINTH

Superior semicircular duct

Cristae of ampullae

Coils of cochlear duct:
basal
middle
apical

Common crus

1
Utricle

Utricular duct

2
Saccular duct

Acoustic macula

Saccule

Sac and duct (endolymphatic)

Reuniting duct
3

Cupular caecum (at helicotrema)

Crista of ampulla

Vestibular caecum (cul de sac)
4

a

Fovea for sac

Endolymphatic sac

Utricular fold

Utricle

Utricular duct

Saccular duct

External aperture of vestibular aqueduct

Isthmus

Sinus

Saccule

Cranial cavity

Internal aperture of vestibular aqueduct

b

FIG. 40–23. *Legend on facing page.*

scala vestibuli, the scala media or cochlear duct, and the scala tympani (Fig. 40–24).

The cochlea is supported by the modiolus, a central spiral of membrane bone anchored to the otic capsule by septa which serve to separate and delineate the turns of the cochlea. The fibers of the auditory portion of the eighth nerve ascend within the modiolus, reaching their termination at the hair cells through small channels in the osseous spiral lamina, a projection outward from the modiolus which anchors the cochlear duct centrally. The cell bodies of these neurons are grouped along the modiolus at the base of the spiral lamina to form the spiral ganglion.

The cochlear duct (scala media) is triangular in shape, expanding from a narrow attachment at the bony spiral lamina to a broad attachment external to the otic capsule by means of a band of fibrous tissue, the spiral ligament. The boundary adjacent to the scala tympani forms the principal attachment, being a strong, radially fibrous extension of the bony spiral lamina called the basilar membrane, which supports the endorgan of hearing, the organ of Corti, on its surface. The border between the scala vestibuli and the cochlear duct is formed by a delicate two-cell layer membrane, Reissner's membrane. Externally, a vascular strip extends along the cochlear duct, containing a surface of granular secretory type cells, the stria vascularis.

The periotic spaces, scala vestibuli and scala tympani, around the cochlear duct are joined only at the termination of the cochlear spiral. Here the bony spiral lamina ends in a hooklike projection, the hamulus, which forms a round opening with the top of the

---

FIG. 40–23.   Osseous labyrinth, shown by a reconstruction of the contained perilymphatic system of spaces.   Lateral and medial aspects.

The bony labyrinth, here represented as the contained perilymphatic space, consists of three parts: a middle, the vestibule; the cochlea, situated anteromedially; the three semicircular canals, placed posterolaterally in the petrous part of the temporal bone.

The vestibule is roughly oval-shaped. The medial wall (see lower figure) forms part of the fundus of the internal meatus. Two deepened areas of unequal size are present on this wall; the posterior one, the elliptical recess, serves for reception of the utriculus; the anterior small rounded area, the spherical recess, receives the saccule. In the latter the perforated area (medial cribrose macula, at *) transmits the saccular branch of the vestibular nerve.

The bony semicircular canals are three curved tubes, each of which is continuous at two points with the space of the vestibule. The lateral, or "horizontal," canal produces the *prominentia* in the wall of the epitympanic recess. Its plane is not exactly horizontal. The other two canals run in approximately vertical planes. The superior canal stands at a right angle to the axis of the petrous pyramid; it gives rise to the *eminentia arcuata* on the anterior surface of the pyramid. The posterior canal lies almost parallel to the posterior surface of the pyramid. One of the two ends of each semicircular canal presents a flask-shaped enlargement, the osseous ampulla (entrance for an ampullary nerve at * in lower figure). The nonampullated ends of the superior and posterior canals unite to form a *crus commune*. The corresponding semicircular duct occupies the periphery of the canal (represented here by sulci between scalae).

The cochlea, or "snail," is cone-shaped with the axis placed horizontally. The base, with the modiolus, is directed toward the fundus of the internal acoustic meatus. It curls upon itself into about two and three-quarter turns. The basal turn projects into the tympanic cavity as the *promontorium*. The cochlear duct, like each of the semicircular ducts, occupies the outer aspect of a coil (here shown as a continuous sulcus). In the macerated bone (that is, in a skeletal preparation) the perilymphatic space is carried into three offsets, which cross the bone to the opposite surface of the pyramid. These appendages are the following: vestibular aqueduct, cochlear canaliculus (or aqueduct), fissula ante fenestram (and, inconstantly, a fossula post fenestram). The so-called perilymphatic "duct" is the network of interstices among the fibrils of periotic connective tissue in the canaliculus. (From Anson, B. J., and Donaldson, J. A.: *Surgical Anatomy of the Temporal Bone and Ear.* Philadelphia, W. B. Saunders Company, 1967.)

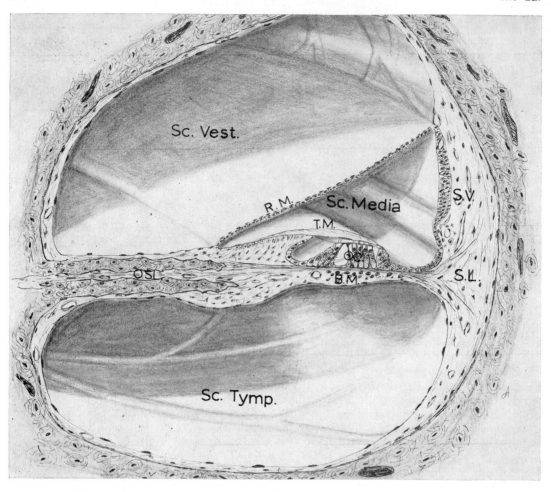

F<small>IG</small>. 40–24.   Section (diagrammatic) through the cochlea. *Sc. Vest.*, Scala vestibuli; *R.M.*, Reissner's membrane; *Sc. Media*, scala media; *T.M.*, tectorial membrane; *O.C.*, organ of Corti; *B.M.*, basilar membrane; *S.V.*, stria vascularis; *S.L.*, spiral ligament; *O.S.L.*, osseous spiral lamina; *Sc. Tymp.*, scala tympani.

modiolus, the helicotrema. Through the helicotrema the two periotic scalae communicate. The scala tympani ends proximally in a blind pouch into which the fenestra rotunda (round window) opens. The scala vestibuli opens directly into the vestibule. A bony passage communicates between the termination of the scala tympani and the subarachnoid space, the cochlear aqueduct. This contains a trabecular network of connective tissue, the so-called periotic duct, which may allow exchange of spinal fluid and perilymph. Paralleling the cochlear aqueduct is a separate channel containing the cochlear vein.

The *organ of Corti* is a complex structure consisting of the three basic parts: supporting cells, hair cells, and a gelatinous contacting membrane—the tectorial membrane (Fig. 40–25). Together with its supporting structure, the basilar membrane, it varies continuously throughout its length. At the basal end, the basilar membrane is narrow and stiff, becoming broad and more flaccid in the apical portion. The tectorial membrane and organ of Corti follow a similar variation in structural characteristics along their length, resulting in a "tuning" of the cochlear duct. As a result of these characteristics, high-frequency sound energy is

Chemically the fluid resembles extracellular fluid, being high in sodium content and low in potassium (140 mEq/L versus 5.5 to 6.25 mEq/L). The protein content averages 200 mg per 100 ml, which is considerably greater than that of the CSF. Other chemical differences outlined in Table 40–1 indicate the probability that perilymph is largely formed as an ultrafiltrate of plasma from the vessels in the walls of the periotic spaces. Perilymphatic fluid balance would thus be largely under the control of the balance of hydrostatic and osmotic pressure, as is most extracellular fluid. An important but yet unmeasured factor in this balance is the amount and state of polymerization of mucopolysaccharides present in this fluid.

Endolymph. Although it has long been thought that the stria vascularis is responsible for the formation of endolymph, it is now evident that many other areas play a role. It has also been found that certain spaces within the otic ducts contain substances dissimilar to endolymph.

Endolymph, as shown in Table 40–1, is high in potassium content (140 to 160 mEq/L) and low in sodium (12 to 16 mEq/L), as is intracellular fluid. The protein content is slightly lower than that of perilymph. Radioactive labeling experiments have shown the basilar membrane to be impermeable to these ions, while Reissner's membrane is actively engaged in transporting K^+ into the scala media against this concentration gradient. The transport activity is shown by rapid appearance of the labeled K^+ from the scala media into the capillaries of the stria vascularis. Cells of the stria are actively engaged in both absorption and secretion of endolymph. In a similar fashion cells of the planum semilunatum of the ampullae and on the slopes of the cristae are also active in the formation and absorption of endolymph.

Studies have long shown that there is a longitudinal flow of endolymph to the endolymphatic sac. Small particulate matter and radioactive sulfur have been seen to gravitate to this structure. Fluid found in the sac is dissimilar to endolymph elsewhere in that it has a high concentration of protein (5 g per 100 ml), with a concentration of so-dium and potassium similar to that of serum. These findings would tend to indicate a high absorption of fluid in this region. Absorptive type cells contained in the rugose walls of the sac give an anatomic basis for this assumption.

Fluid within the tunnel of Corti ("cortilymph") is found to be different from endolymph, and one investigator (Rauch) has suggested that it is formed from CSF passing along the fibers of the auditory nerve through the canaliculi of the bony spiral lamina. Neurophysiologic knowledge supports this view, since neural transmission should be impossible in the high potassium concentration of endolymph and the fibers terminating on the outer hair cells pass through the tunnel of Corti.

The space between the hair cells and the overlying membranes (cupula, otolithic, and tectorial) contains a substance different from endolymph. Only little is known of this material, but it has a high viscosity, is structureless, and resembles in other characteristics a concentrated mucopolysaccharide. This is apparently secreted by the supporting cells of the sensory organs.

Fluid Pressure Dynamics. It has become apparent that another function of the intracranial extension of both the otic and periotic spaces is the maintenance of equilibrium between perilymphatic and endolymphatic fluid pressure. Normal vestibular and cochlear function depends upon stability of fluid pressures. Not only are variations in hydrostatic pressure constantly present, as with change in body position, coughing, or straining, but also the inner ear is exposed to changes in the atmospheric pressure in the middle ear through the round and oval windows. The endolymphatic sac can compensate for changes in perilymphatic pressure, since similar CSF pressure changes will be transmitted to both fluid systems simultaneously, maintaining equilibrium. Air pressure variations directed into the perilymphatic space may be compensated for by a reservoir action of the endolymphatic sac and slight release of perilymph through the cochlear aqueduct.

Although the details of this mechanism remain largely conjectural, it is obviously

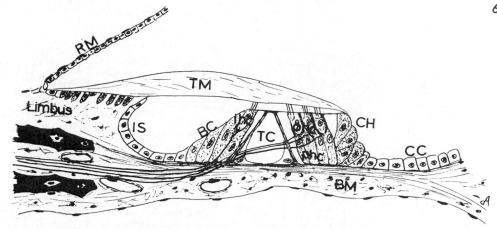

FIG. 40–25. Detail of organ of Corti. *RM,* Reissner's membrane; *IS,* inner sulcus; *BC,* border cells; *ihc,* inner hair cells; *TM,* tectorial membrane; *phc,* phalangeal cells; *CH,* cells of Hansen; *TC,* tunnel of Corti; *ohc,* outer hair cells; *CC,* cells of Claudius; *BM,* basilar membrane.

concentrated at the basal end of the cochlea, while lower frequencies spread progressively along the length of the organ of Corti.

The hair cells are arranged in a single row of inner hair cells and three to five rows of outer hair cells. These are separated by an inverted V formed by the tonofibrils of the inner and outer pillar cells, resulting in a strong central supporting structure. The space between the pillars is called the tunnel of Corti, which seems to contain a fluid other than endolymph, termed "cortilymph."

The hair cells are supported by elongated phalangeal cells. The free ends bear nonmotile cilia which rest against the inferior surface of the tectorial membrane. The remainder of the supporting cells have a changing shape, being tall near the hair cells and becoming shorter away from them to give the organ of Corti a sloping shape. These cells are named the cells of Hansen, the cells of Claudius, and the border cells. The tectorial membrane is supported centrally by the limbus, a thick plate of cells resting on the bony spiral lamina. The limbus also serves as the attachment for Reissner's membrane. The tectorial membrane is attached firmly at its free edge to the cells of Hansen, creating a space between the hair cells and the tectorial membrane containing the cilia of the hair cells. This space is continuous with a rather large space medially between the tectorial membrane and the medial edge of the basilar membrane, the internal spiral sulcus. The medial boundary of this space is lined by a distinct group of cuboidal cells, the inner sulcus cells.

The basilar membrane averages 32 cm in length. The width varies about sixfold, averaging 0.08 mm at the base to 0.498 mm at the apex. There are about 24,000 transverse fibers along the length of the membrane.

The organ of Corti contains about 15,500 hair cells. These are grouped in an inner row of 3500 and three to five outer rows containing 12,000. Near the base there are three rows of outer hair cells. Another row is added in the middle turns and occasionally a fifth row near the apex. The cross-sectional area varies about 4½ fold, ranging from 0.0053 mm at the base to 0.0223 at the apex.

The spiral ligament and tectorial membrane also vary in a similar fashion and degree along their lengths.

There are about 26,000 ganglion cells in the spiral ganglion of an adult with good hearing. There is a greater concentration of cells near the basal portion than in the upper turns.

The hair cells receive the termination of several neurons which form a basket around the base. Two types of nerve endings are found, one being efferent, the other afferent in function. Single neurons split to end on several hair cells. The neurons run through the canaliculi of the spiral ganglion at the base of the lamina. The axons then run through channels in the core of the modiolus, coiling to form the auditory portion of the eighth nerve. These fibers enter the pons in the region of the two cochlear nuclei, dorsal and ventral.

The nerve fibers of the vestibular labyrinth are slightly more complexly arranged, as they are separated into superior and inferior divisions. The superior division is made of fibers from the cristae of the lateral and superior semicircular canals and from the macula of the utricle. The inferior division receives fibers from the crista of the posterior canal and from the macula of the saccule. The ganglion containing the cell bodies of these fibers, Scarpa's ganglion, is contained within the internal acoustic meatus. The nerve trunk then runs medially to enter the pons near the auditory portion of the acoustic nerve, where the fibers are intricately divided among several vestibular nuclei (Chapter 42).

Fluids of the Inner Ear. It was formerly thought that there were two fluid systems of the inner ear, the endolymph and the perilymph (otic fluid and periotic fluid). The perilymph was thought to be derived from spinal fluid, entering through the periotic duct. The endolymph was thought to be formed by secretory cells of the stria vascularis and absorbed by the endolymphatic sac. Recent observations have thrown great doubt on these traditional concepts; not only have the sites of fluid formation and absorption been doubted, but also the possibility of two or three separate types of fluid being contained within the otic labyrinth has been added.

Perilymph. Much evidence has accumulated in recent years to indicate that little, if any, perilymph originates from cerebrospinal fluid. Anatomically the cochlear aqueduct is a narrow channel filled with loose areolar tissue without true ductal tissue. Fluid ingress through this channel should be slow at best. Clinically this is verified at stapes surgery, when only a slow renewal of perilymph is usually seen. Abnormally patent cochlear aqueducts have been seen in temporal bone specimens which are correlated with a massive flow of perilymph when the oval window is open. These patients usually demonstrate diminished cochlear function prior to surgery.

Table 40–1. Chemical Composition of Inner Ear Fluids

Mean Value	Perilymph	Endolymph	Cap. Serum	CSF
Na$^+$ (mEq/L)	143	12–16	141	141
K$^+$ (mEq/L)	5.5–6.25	144.3 (140–160)	5.9	2.9
Protein (mg%)	200 (89–326)	150?	7170	30
Glucose (mg%)	104		104	67
Free cholesterol (mg%)	1.5			0.035
Total cholesterol (mg%)	12		28	
MDH (IU)	95.6–136		63.5	18.3
LDH (IU)	127–155		151	1.9
PO$_3^-$(mM/L)	0.72		0.95	0.36
Ca^{++} (mM/L)	1.16	1.07	2.44	1.12
Lactate (mM/L)	6.78		4.63	3.94

MDH = Malate dehydrogenase
LDH = Lactate dehydrogenase

effective as demonstrated by the ability of man to function both in the depths of the sea and in the reaches of outer space.

BLOOD SUPPLY TO THE EAR

The blood supply to the ear is formed in two completely independent circulations—one that supplies the external and middle ear, and one that supplies the inner ear—with a complete lack of anastomosis between the two.

The external ear is supplied mainly by the auriculotemporal branch of the superficial temporal anteriorly and by branches of the posterior auricular division of the external carotid artery posteriorly.

The middle ear and mastoid are supplied by an abundant anastomosing arterial circulation. The anterior tympanic branch of the external maxillary artery enters through the petrotympanic fissure. The anterior wall of the mesotympanum also transmits small branches from the carotid artery to the tympanum, the caroticotympanic arteries. Superiorly, the middle meningeal gives off the superior tympanic branch, which enters the middle ear through the petrosquamous fissure. The middle meningeal also gives off the superficial petrosal artery, which runs with the greater superficial petrosal nerve to enter the facial canal at the hiatus containing the geniculate ganglion. This vessel anastomoses with a branch of the posterior auricular artery, the stylomastoid artery, which enters the facial canal inferiorly through the stylomastoid foramen. A branch of this last artery, the posterior tympanic artery, runs through the canaliculus of the chorda tympani to enter the middle ear with this nerve. An important artery enters from the inferior aspect of the middle ear, the inferior tympanic branch of the ascending pharyngeal artery. This is the major supplier of glomus jugulare tumors of the middle ear.

The ossicles receive an anastomosing blood supply from the anterior tympanic artery, the posterior tympanic artery, a vessel running with the stapedius tendon, and branches from the plexus of vessels on the promontory. The vessels run in the mucosal covering of the ossicles, sending nutrient vessels into the bone. The long process of the incus seems to have the most tenuous blood supply, commonly suffering necrosis when there is inflammatory or mechanical interference with its circulation.

The inner ear receives its blood supply from the internal auditory artery, usually arising from the anterior inferior cerebellar artery but occasionally arising directly from the basilar artery (Fig. 40–26). This is an end artery receiving no known anastomosing vessels.

Soon after entering the internal auditory meatus, the artery divides into three branches. One branch accompanies the vestibular nerve and supplies that nerve, the semicircular ducts, utricle, and saccule. The second branch, the vestibulocochlear artery, supplies the saccule, utricle, posterior semicircular canal, and basilar turn of the cochlea. The terminal branch is the cochlear artery. This enters the modiolus, where it gives rise to the spiral vessels running through the base of the bony spiral lamina. Twigs leaving the spiral arteries run through the canaliculi to the base of the organ of Corti. Other twigs leaving the spiral arteries supply the walls of the scala vestibuli and scala tympani, both terminating at the stria vascularis.

Two other vessels enter the inner ear without anastomosis. One enters at the subarcuate eminence to supply the intercanalicular bone, while the other supplies the endolymphatic sac and duct.

The venous drainage of the external and middle ear is accomplished by vessels accompanying the arterial supply. A mastoid emissary vein communicates between the external mastoid cortex and the lateral sinus.

The venous drainage of the inner ear is accomplished by three routes. The cochlear return is by the internal auditory vein draining the middle and apical turns. The cochlear vein drains the basilar turn of the cochlea and the anterior vestibule, leaving through a channel paralleling the cochlear aqueduct to empty into the inferior petrosal sinus. A third venous channel follows the endolymphatic duct to drain into the sigmoid sinus. This plexus drains the posterior labyrinth.

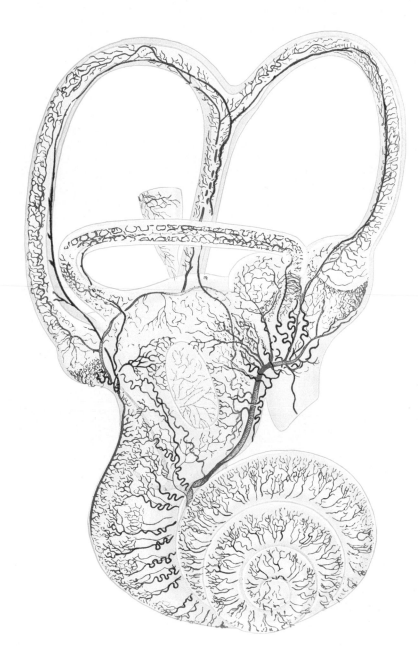

Fig. 40–26.   The circulation of the labyrinth (Shambaugh).

FACIAL NERVE

The facial nerve (see Fig. 40–14) leaves the pons in two functional divisions, the motor division and the nervus intermedius, the latter containing the special sensory fibers of taste and parasympathetic fibers. The nerve enters the temporal bone through the internal acoustic meatus, running along the anterosuperior portion. The nerve then enters a bony channel, the facial canal (fallopian canal), which runs through the temporal bone from the anterosuperior fundus of the internal auditory canal to the stylomastoid foramen. Initially the nerve runs a lateral and superior course between the cochlea and superior semicircular canal to approach the junction of the petrous with the middle ear. Here in a shallow fossa just under the dura covering the superior face of the petrous is the geniculate ganglion. A branch, the greater superficial petrosal nerve, runs forward through a channel in the petrous to innervate the lacrimal gland. A smaller branch runs into the middle ear, the lesser superficial petrosal nerve, to join the tympanic plexus.

The trunk of the facial nerves makes a right angle turn to enter the middle ear just above the cochleariform process and runs posteriorly just inferior to the lateral semicircular canal. During this course it forms a portion of the superior wall of the oval window niche. This part of the facial canal is often dehiscent, allowing the nerve trunk to bulge into the oval window niche, partially occluding it.

In the region above the pyramidal eminence and medial to the fossa incudis, the facial makes a second downward turn to begin its vertical portion. At this turn the nerve gives off a twig to the stapedial muscle. As the facial canal nears its inferior limit, a tributary channel, the canaliculus of the chorda tympani, is given off at an acute angle to return to the posterosuperior middle ear. This canaliculus contains the fibers of the chorda tympani nerve. The facial nerve then leaves the temporal bone through the stylomastoid foramen, after which the main trunk turns forward to run between the superficial and deep lobes of the parotid gland to be distributed to the muscles of the facial expression.

EMBRYOLOGY*

The ear, more than any other structure, demonstrates the phylogeny of the human. Consisting of a primitive endorgan of balance, a more recently developed auditory sensor, and a sound conduction mechanism derived only after the aquatic environment was left, the human ear repeats these stages in an orderly sequence of development. The inner ear is the first organ in the body to be developed; it reaches adult size and configuration by midterm. The middle and external ear, on the other hand, have not completely formed at birth, and the temporal bone continues to grow and change in form into puberty.

Otic Labyrinth (Membranous Labyrinth)

The otic labyrinth begins to differentiate at the end of 3 weeks with the appearance

*When I refer to the inner ear, I will use the terminology outlined by Anson, which is in conflict with the current BNA terminology. This terminology has been completely outlined in *Temporal Bone and the Ear* (see References). The reasons for this usage were best outlined by Anson in *Morris' Human Anatomy* in a footnote on pages 1214 and 1215 and are directly quoted: "The terminology employed in describing the internal ear is both inadequate and misleading. The term 'osseous labyrinth' is inappropriate, since its use is based on the fallacious notion that a bony wall may be shelled away, as an independent investment for the system of continuous labyrinthic spaces which contain the perilymph. This is not possible in the temporal bone after it has assumed adult consistency—which it actually does in the fetus. Thereupon the bone of the primordial bony capsule fuses with the compact periosteal bone surrounding it.

Now, were the term otic labyrinth used for the ectodermal epithelial tube system (as a substitute for membranous), the space between the otic labyrinth and the capsule would become 'periotic labyrinth.'

The name 'otic labyrinth' would have logical appeal, on the basis of its derivation from the otic vesicle, the latter in turn differentiated from the otocyst. The names 'otic fluid, periotic fluid, and periotic tissue' would be equally logical, as would 'otic duct' and 'otic sac' (replacing endolymphatic duct and endolymphatic sac, respectively). The term 'endolymphatic' would then become an inclusive name, applied to the whole system of epithelium-lined labyrinthic channels."

of the auditory placodes. These ectodermal thickenings lie on either side of the midportion of the hindbrain. Before a week has passed, the placode has invaginated to form the auditory pit, which in turn dilates to form a patent sac which then becomes sealed by growth at the mouth to form the auditory vesicle. A process of migration, growth, and elongation of the vesicle then ensues, and soon enfoldings of the wall of the sac clearly delineate three major divisions of the auditory vesicle—the endolymphatic duct and sac, the utricle with its semicircular ducts, and the saccule with its

outgrowth, the cochlear duct (Fig. 40–27). This differentiation progresses from the sixth week through the tenth week of fetal life, at which time the definitive relationships obtaining in the adult ear have been established (Fig. 40–28).

The initial fold in the wall of the otic vesicle deepens finally to contact the opposite wall of the labyrinth and in doing so delineates the endolymphatic duct and sac. The free edge of this fold persists to form the utriculoendolymphatic valve of Bast. As this process is completed (ninth week), the semicircular ducts and the cochlear duct are

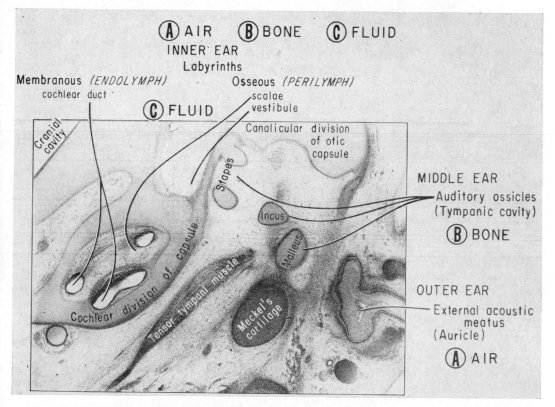

Fig. 40–27. Anatomic development of the auditory mechanism—its branchial and labyrinthine sources in the human ear—shown in a transverse section in the series from a fetus of 3 months (62 mm CR length). (Wisconsin Collection. Courtesy of Dr. Barry J. Anson.)

The primary element is the membranous labyrinth, derived from the otocyst (ectoderm of the embryo), around which develop the perilymphatic spaces and the osseous otic capsule.

The secondary elements, which constitute the links in the acoustic "chain" from environmental air to perilymph in the osseous labyrinth, are modifications of the branchial apparatus of lower vertebrates (entoderm and mesoderm of the embryo). The external acoustic meatus, auricle, and outer layer (cutaneous stratum) of the tympanic membrane come from the first visceral groove; the auditory ossicles arise chiefly from the first and second visceral arches; the auditory (eustachian) tube, tympanic cavity (with the associated air spaces), and inner layer (mucosal stratum) of the tympanic membrane originate from the first pharyngeal pouch.

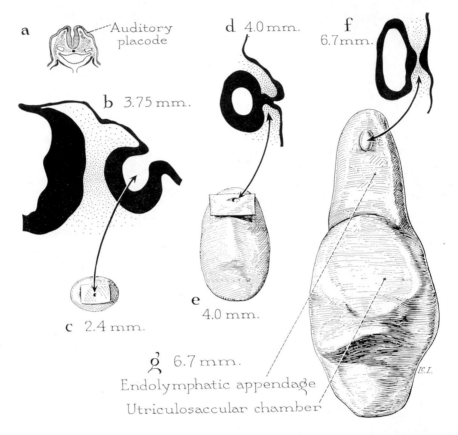

a — Auditory placode

b 3.75 mm.

d 4.0 mm.

f 6.7 mm.

c 2.4 mm.

e 4.0 mm.

g 6.7 mm.
Endolymphatic appendage
Utriculosaccular chamber

FIG. 40–28. Development of the otocyst and otic vesicle. Progress in approximately a two-week period. Demonstrated by drawing of sections (*a, b, d,* and *f*) and of reconstructions (*c, e,* and *g*).

a. The primordium of the paired membranous labyrinth is a platelike thickening of the ectoderm opposite the developing hind brain of the embryo.

b and *c,* The thickened placode is invaginated into the mesenchymal tissue (*b*). It appears on the surface as the otic pit, still continuous with the surface ectoderm from which it was derived (*c,* where, as in *e,* the ectoderm is retained in the model as a rectangular piece).

d and *e,* The vesicle enlarges rapidly, growth being chiefly downward(*e*). The aperture of the pit narrows, then becomes a stalk by meeting of its wall (*d*).

f and *g,* When the original continuity of the vesicle with parental ectoderm is lost, the area of connection remains for a short time in the form of apposed thickenings; one on the surface layer of the embryo (*f*), the other on the lateral aspect of the developing endolymphatic duct, near the latter's apex (*g*). The other adult subdivisions are also forecast at this stage in the presence of a utriculo-saccular chamber and a cochlear part (downward directed).

(From Anson, B. J. [Ed.]: *Morris' Human Anatomy.* 12th ed. Section X. New York, McGraw-Hill Book Company, 1966.)

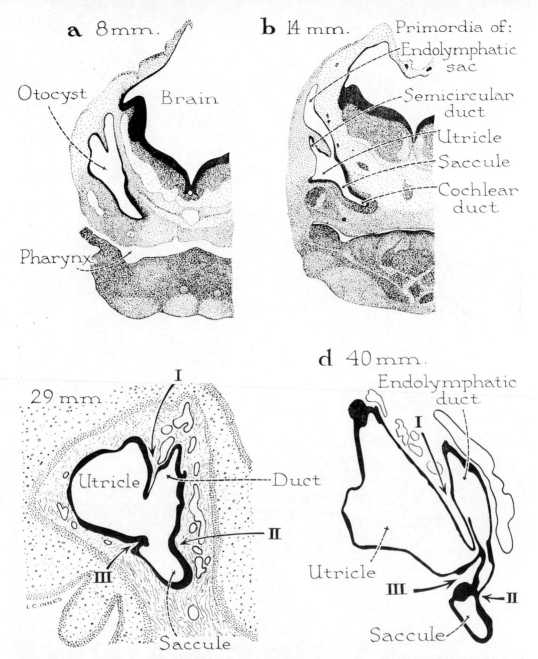

a 8 mm.

Otocyst

Brain

Pharynx

b 14 mm.

Primordia of:
Endolymphatic sac
Semicircular duct
Utricle
Saccule
Cochlear duct

29 mm

I

Utricle

III

II

Duct

Saccule

L.C.INNES

d 40 mm.

Endolymphatic duct

I

Utricle

III

II

Saccule

FIG. 40–29. Otocyst and its derivatives in man: progress in the formation of the major chambers and the intercommunicating channels of the membranous duct system in approximately a 5-week period (5th to 9th week). Drawings from tracings of sections. *a,* Embryo of 8 mm., crown-rump length (5 weeks). *b,* Embryo of 14 mm. (6 weeks). *c,* Fetus of 29 mm. (8½ weeks). *d,* Fetus of 40 mm. (10 weeks).

a, In the 8-mm. specimen the future divisions of the membranous labyrinth are already indicated in the presence of an upward-directed offset (future endolymphatic duct and sac), a downward-directed prolongation (future cochlear duct) and an intermediate chamber (future utricle and saccule).

b, At the 14-mm. stage the utricle is identifiable through the presence of outpocketings which will become the semicircular ducts.

c and *d,* Infoldings of the epithelial wall, present as ledges (when seen in sections), subdivide the main chamber into parts. The perilymphatic space is predicted (*c*) in the presence of a reticulum around the membranous labyrinth.

Transverse sections. Harvard Collection of Comparative Embryology. (From Anson, B. J.: In *Otolaryngology.* Edited by Walter H. Maloney, Hagerstown, Harper & Row, 1973, Chapter 1.)

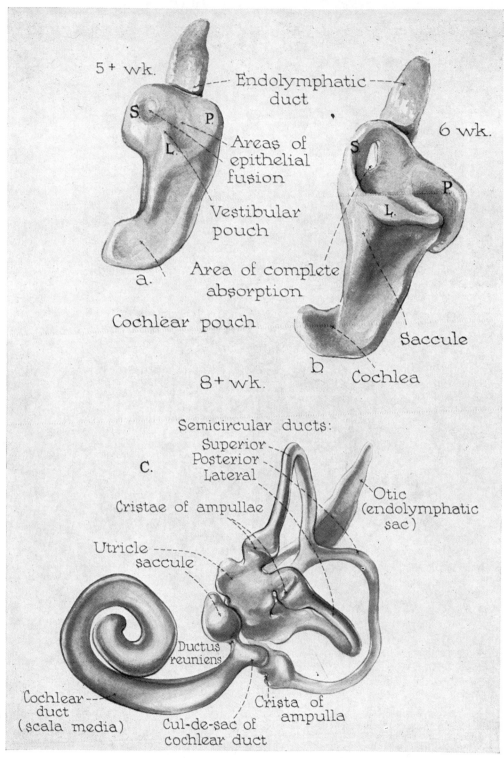

FIG. 40–30. *Legend on facing page.*

also nearing adult form. The semicircular ducts have formed through disclike outpouchings of the utricle beginning in the fourth week. The centers of the discs gradually compress until at the sixth week the walls fuse and then disintegrate, leaving a semicircular duct opening at each end into the utricle, with the exception of the posterior and superior duct, which share a common opening posteriorly (Figs. 40–29 and 40–30). The cochlear duct has formed as an outpouching of the saccule at the sixth week. By the seventh week it has formed one turn, and by the tenth week it has completed a full 2½ to 2¾ turns. The cochlear duct remains joined to the saccule by the relatively slender ductus reuniens. The cochlear duct continues to grow in size until midterm but does not increase in the number of turns.

At the beginning of this period of differentiation of the auditory vesicle (sixth week), the mesenchyme surrounding it changes into precartilage and by the ninth week has matured into true cartilage. The growth of the now differentiated labyrinth takes place within this wall of cartilage through two processes. There is an extensive regression of cartilage around the semicircular ducts, which is accompanied by connective tissue ingrowth. At the same time the cartilage at the advancing arcs of the semicircular canals is becoming undifferentiated, while the cartilage at the receding margin is being rebuilt. The superior canal reaches adult size first (twentieth week), followed shortly by the posterior canal and lastly, by the lateral semicircular canal. Ossification of the surrounding cartilage has started about the sixteenth week and is completed by the twenty-fourth week shortly after the membranous labyrinth has reached full size.

The neuroepithelial structures of the otic labyrinth are basically similar in cell type but are modified in form, depending upon the particular stimulus to which each must respond. Each of these sensory endorgans has formed from the simple squamous epithelium of the otic labyrinth and consists of sensory hair cells, supporting cells, and an overlying gelatinous structure in which the cilia of the hair cells are embedded. These structures are the cristae ampullares of the semicircular canals, the maculae of the utri-

---

Fig. 40–30. Membranous labyrinth. Developmental anatomy demonstrated by reconstructions. *a,* Embryo of 8 mm. (5 weeks). *b,* Embryo of 13 mm. (6 weeks). *c,* Fetus of 30 mm. (8 weeks).

a, In the 5-week embryo the otic vesicle undergoes elongation in the dorsoventral direction. The slender, ventral part will become the cochlear duct. In the dorsal part the formation of the semicircular ducts is indicated; the intermediate region will soon subdivide into utricle and saccule.

b, At the 6-week stage the semicircular ducts appear as two flattened pouches—the superior and posterior ducts arising from a single pouch (see S and P), the lateral duct (L) from a separate horizontal outpocketing of the vesicle. Conversion of the secondary pouches into ducts begins with the superior outpocketing. In each case, the walls flatten and fuse centrally to form an epithelial plate; thereby a canal is left at the periphery that retains communication with the remainder of the otic vesicle. The central part of the plate breaks down, setting the duct free except at its ends.

c, By the eighth week the semicircular canals and the endolymphatic duct are well formed; the main chamber has become divided into utricle and saccule. The cochlear duct has coiled into one and a half turns. Superior and posterior ducts have a common limb which communicates with the utricle; their opposite ends and the rostral end of the lateral duct are dilated to form the *ampullae.*

In the twelfth week the adult configuration of the labyrinth has been attained. At that stage the utriculosaccular communication is narrower, the semicircular ducts are longer, the ampullae more prominent, and the cochlear duct has become coiled into its two and one-half turns.

Transverse sections, Wisconsin Collection, series 178, 180, and 92. (From Anson, B. J., and McVay, C. B.: *Surgical Anatomy.* 5th ed. Philadelphia, W. B. Saunders Co., 1971.)

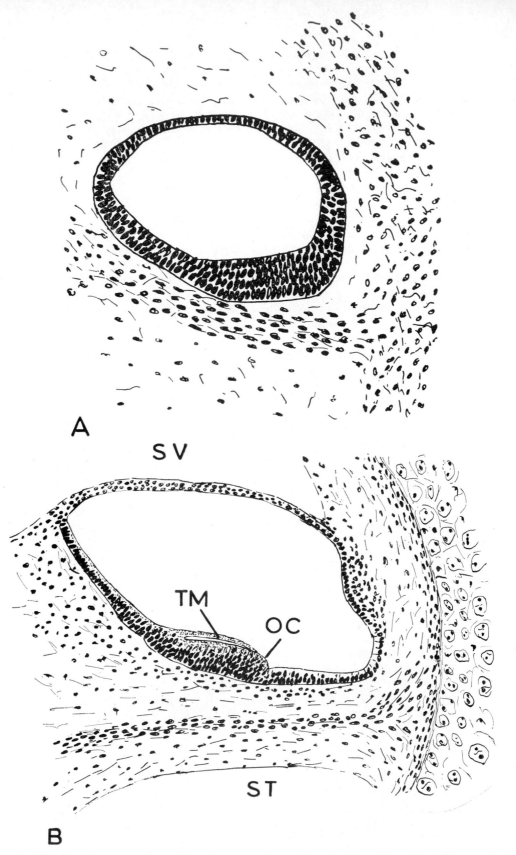

FIG. 40–31.   Development of cochlear duct: *A*, 11 weeks; *B*, 16 weeks. *SV*, Scala vestibuli;
TM, tectorial membrane; *OC*, organ of Corti; *ST*, scala tympani.

cle and saccule, and the organ of Corti of the cochlear duct.

The maculae develop from the epithelium of the utricle and saccule at the point where the nerves enter their walls. This process begins in the seventh week, at which time there is a heaping up of cells to form a complex pseudostratified layer. By the twelfth week two cell types are apparent: the supporting cells, which also secrete the gelatinous mucopolysaccharide layer, and the hair cells, which bear a row of bristlelike hairs at their free end. By the fourteenth to sixteenth week, calcareous deposits (otoconia) have formed in the gelatinous layer, the otolithic membrane, and the structure has an adult form.

The cristae ampullares form within the ampullae, again at the point where the nerve fibers enter. The ampullae are located on the anterior limb of the superior and lateral semicircular canals and on the inferior limb of the posterior semicircular canal near their origin from the utricle. The cristae begin their development at the same time as the maculae, but instead of remaining a flat pad, they become elevated into a ridge with the gelatinous layer, the cupula, forming a valvular cap extending across the ampulla so that every movement of otic fluid causes a deflection of the cupula. The cristae and cupulae are always formed so that their ridge is at right angles to the direction of flow of the endolymph.

The development of the organ of Corti within the cochlear duct, being a much more complicated structure than the cristae or maculae, is a much more complex process (Fig. 40–31) involving, however, only morphologic changes in the same three basic elements: hair cells, supporting cells, and gelatinous membrane. The cells of the wall of the cochlea are in a stratified form when the duct is first differentiated. The walls then begin to thin, leaving only the inferior wall stratified. This process, like the development of the cochlear duct as a whole, proceeds in time from the basal end to the apical portion. By the twelfth week, both cell types may be distinguished and a layer of gelatinous material, the tectorial membrane, lies on the free surface of these cells. In the 15-week-old fetus, a separate type of cell may be seen in the lateral wall of the cochlear duct resting on a vascular connective tissue which forms the stria vascularis with its glandular type of epithelium. The cells of the inferior wall fold inward slightly to form the internal sulcus, while at the same time the tunnel of Corti is forming through a process of cell migration.

The periotic spaces have formed by the eighth week; they then begin to fuse with the walls of the cochlear duct to form Reissner's membrane by the union of the scala vestibuli with the scala media and the basilar membrane and by the fusion of the scala tympani with the inferior wall of the scala media. Because these periotic scalae are wider medially than the cochlear duct, the osseous spiral lamina forms within the connective tissue between the two scalae, extending to the modiolus which has formed separately as the only membrane bone within the otic capsule. The adult configuration has been obtained by the twenty-fifth week of development.

Periotic Labyrinth (Osseous Labyrinth)

The precartilage immediately surrounding the otic labyrinth forms the periotic space through a process of dedifferentiation. This process is occurring as the outer zone of precartilage is becoming true cartilage. As described previously, growth of the otic labyrinth is accommodated by regression of the already formed cartilage into precartilage. These two zones are apparent by the eighth week, and as growth of the otic labyrinth ensues, the inner zone of precartilage gradually modifies to form three zones; an inner layer of condensed areolar tissue surrounding the otic labyrinth, a middle layer of loose arachnoid-like tissue filled with fluid (perilymph or periotic fluid), and an outer condensation which becomes the endosteum of the otic capsule. These changes begin with the formation of a reticulum, which is first evident in the region between the stapes and saccule. The meshes of the reticulum of the middle layer enlarge and coalesce to form the periotic space proper, which is first evident at 9 to 10 weeks. The vestibule forms soon after the scala vestibuli and scala tympani are evident, and shortly thereafter spaces develop around the otic semicircular ducts. The periotic spaces gradually enlarge and fuse until a continuous periotic labyrinth has formed. The scala tympani communicates with the scala vestibuli only at the distal end of the cochlear duct through an opening called the helicotrema. The periotic spaces do not completely surround the otic system, since the semicircular ducts are attached to the cartilaginous wall of the otic capsule along their greater curvature, the cochlear duct is attached at the strial wall, and the saccule and utricle are attached at the point of entrance of their nerve supply. The periotic spaces have completely formed by the fifth month of fetal life.

Three important appendages of the periotic space are formed in this same period; the so-called periotic duct within the cochlear aqueduct, the fissula ante fenestram (Figs. 40–32 to 40–35), and the fossula post fenestram. The so-called periotic duct

forms in the region of the cochlear vein as a rarefication of the precartilage, which forms a syncytial tissue mass leading from the region of the glossopharyngeal nerve to the scala tympani. This syncytial tissue gradually loosens to form a trabeculated passage from the subarachnoid space. The cochlear vein runs in a separate passage through the capsule.

The fissula ante fenestram and fossula post fenestram form as outpouchings of the vestibule anterior and posterior to the oval window. This can be seen as early as the eighth week when the vestibule is first beginning to form. The course of the fissula can be seen as a stripe of altered precartilage which gradually undergoes necrosis and is replaced by connective tissue. By the fourteenth week this process has approached the stapedial area, with enlargement and extension of the fissula. As this process is extending from the vestibule, a vascular bud is

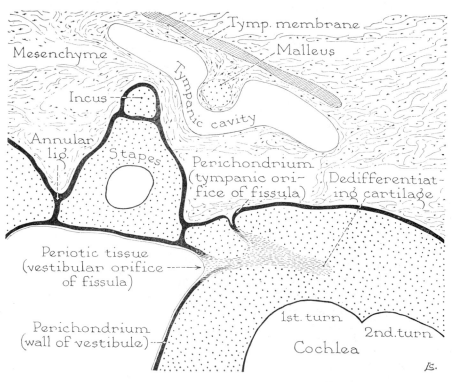

Fig. 40–32. Fissular and related areas of the cartilaginous otic capsule in a human fetus (semidiagrammatic), showing the way in which the periotic tissue invades the antefenestral portion of the capsule and its relation to the perichondrium. (Bast, T. H., and Anson, B. J.: *The Temporal Bone and the Ear.* Springfield, Ill., Charles C Thomas, Publisher, 1949.)

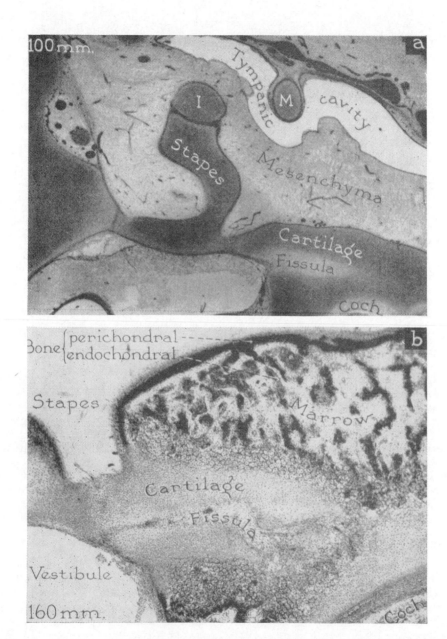

FIG. 40–33.   Development of fissula ante fenestram; *a*, 14 weeks; *b*, 19 weeks. (Bast, T. H., and Anson, B. J.: *The Temporal Bone and the Ear.* Springfield, Ill., Charles C Thomas, Publisher, 1949.)

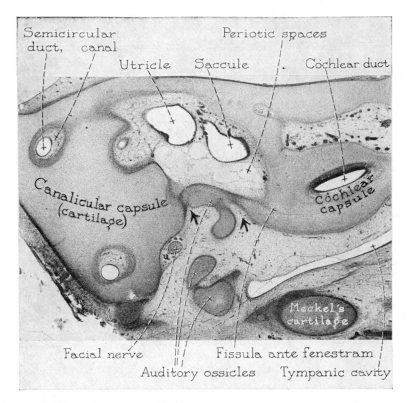

Fig. 40–34. Middle and inner ear. Preosseous stage in development of the otic capsule and the auditory ossicles. Fetus of 10 weeks (48 mm.). The parts of the membranous labyrinth have attained definitive form. The perilymphatic system of spaces of the future osseous labyrinth are predicted in the presence of a periotic reticulum around the semicircular ducts, utricle and saccule, and cochlear duct. The position of the vestibular (oval) window is indicated (at arrows) by a retrogressive change in the cartilage of the capsule circumferential to the differentiating tissue of the base (footplate) of the stapes. The branchial arch origin of the ossicles is suggested by the presence of Meckel's cartilage (first, or mandibular, arch). The pharyngeal diverticulum (from the first branchial pouch) is nearing the malleus, which like the incus and stapes, will be enveloped by its further advance and concurrent expansion. The future facial canal is represented by a sulcus on the wall of the canalicular division of the otic capsule.

Transverse section. Wisconsin Collection, series 202. (Courtesy of Dr. Otto A. Mortensen and Dr. Barry J. Anson.)

growing into the developing capsular cartilage anterior to the stapes, causing erosion of the cartilage and fusing with the vestibular extension of the fissula. The growth of the fissula occurs concurrently with growth of the cartilaginous otic capsule and has reached a maximum by the time ossification starts. During ossification the layer of perichondral tissue at the edges of the fissula forms an irregular layer of cartilage, which cause reduction in the size of the fibrous core of the fissula. Variations in the size, shape, and amount of cartilage around the

fissula are common, giving a great inconsistency in the adult.

The fossula post fenestram develops in a similar way posterior to the stapes but is more of a saccular extension of the vestibule, communicating with the middle ear in only 25% of cases. Its presence is common but not invariable, being seen in about 67% of cases. Cartilaginous and bony changes in the fossula post fenestram are much less common than in the fissula ante fenestram, being present in about 5% of specimens.

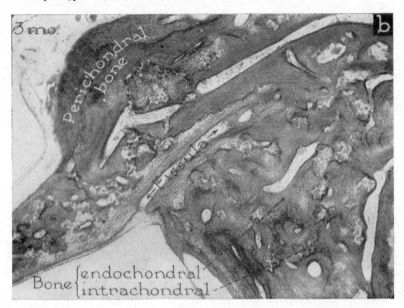

FIG. 40–35. Fissula ante fenestram in 3-month-old infant. (Bast, T. H., and Anson, B. J.: *The Temporal Bone and the Ear*. Springfield, Ill., Charles C Thomas, Publisher, 1949.)

Otic Capsule

The major developmental changes in the otic capsule have already been described: the change from precartilage into cartilage, the method of growth to encompass the expanding otic labyrinth, and the conclusion of the growth process by the fifth fetal month. Ossification of the otic capsule then proceeds from midterm to completion shortly before birth. With the exception of the modiolus, the otic capsule develops from a preexisting cartilage model and thus is cartilage bone but has some distinct characteristics. Unlike other cartilage bones, it is neither long nor flat but rather a boxlike structure enclosing the inner ear. Since it is full-sized before ossification occurs, replacement of the endochondral bone does not occur, this middle layer persisting throughout life. Intrachondral bone (persistent islands of calcified cartilage whose lacunae have been invaded by osteocytes) may be seen in many areas where the primary cartilage has not been replaced with enchondral bone.

Ossification of the capsule proceeds from 14 centers which appear at succeeding intervals, enlarge, and fuse with preexistent centers. The first center appears on the outer part of the capsule on the beginning of the basal turn of the cochlear with others appearing in turn: near the ampulla of the posterior canal (#2), near the ampullae of the superior and lateral semicircular canals (#3), above the round window (#4) on the lateral surface of the internal auditory canal (#5), inside the cochlear capsule at the entrance of the fibers of the cochlear nerve (#6), in the upper medial wall of the internal meatus (#7), over the course of the cochlear duct (#8), at the inferior medial margin of the internal canal (#9), at the posterior arch of the superior semicircular canal (#10), at the superolateral aspect of the cochlea (#11), between the cochlea and entrance of the superior branch of the vestibular nerve (#12), immediately below this last center (#13), and the last center in the lateral arch of the posterior semicircular canal (#14).

The modiolus develops as a membrane bone beginning at the twentieth to twenty-first week and becomes well ossified by the twenty-fifth week. It is anchored to the cochlea by bony partitions extending between the turns of the cochlear duct.

The process of ossification takes place in several ways. The internal and external peri-

chondral layers become modified into periosteum with the appearance of osteoblasts
and vascular bonds and the laying down of
calcareous deposits within the perichondral
layers. These layers, termed the endosteal
and periosteal, continue development exactly
as in the long bones with the appearance
of haversian systems. Osteogenic buds which
are highly cellular invade the cartilage capsule with resultant necrosis of the now calcified cartilage. Osteoblasts form in these
centers of necrosis and deposit bone in these
hollow nests. Vascular buds appear, and ex-
cavation of the calcified cartilage ensues,

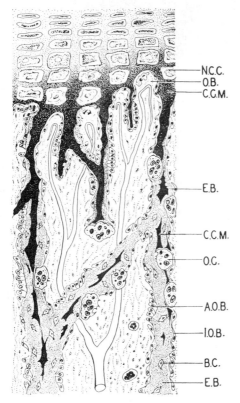

Fig. 40–36. Development of endochondral
bone (diagrammatic). The successive stages in
the transformation of cartilage into endochondral bone are reported in order from top to
bottom of the diagram. *A.O.B.,* Active osteoblasts; *B.C.,* bone cell; *C.C.M.,* calcified cartilage matrix; *E.B.,* endochondral bone; *I.O.B.,*
inactive osteoblast; *N.C.C.,* necrotic cartilage
cell; *O.B.,* osteogenic bud; *O.C.,* osteoclasts.
(Bast, T. H., and Anson, B. J.: *The Temporal
Bone and the Ear.* Springfield, Ill., Charles C
Thomas, Publisher, 1949.)

with laying down of bone in the resultant
spaces (Fig. 40–36). Many islands of calcified cartilage remain whose cells are replaced by osteoblasts to become intrachondral bone. The replacement of the cartilage
is slower than the formation of the periosteal bone. Shortly before birth, however,
this process becomes rapid with the filling
of the excavated spaces with bone to form
the enchondral layer, which then remains
constant throughout life without further remodeling.

External and Middle Ear

The structures of the middle and external
ear are derived from the endodermal first
pharyngeal pouch, the ectodermal first and
second branchial arches with their contained
branchial groove, and the intervening mesodermal mesenchyme. The space contained
within the first pharyngeal pouch will form
the eustachian tube and middle ear, while
the branchial groove forms the primitive
external meatus (Figs. 40–37 and 40–38).
The auricle, tympanic ring, and ossicles form
from the contained mesenchyme of the
branchial arches.

The pharyngeal pouch is evident by the
third week of development and by the sixth
week has elongated and flattened at its distal
end to lay against the first branchial groove.
Connective tissue soon grows between these
approximated surfaces which will form the
tunica propria of the tympanic membrane
and the manubrium of the malleus. By 8
weeks the flattened fundus of the pharyngeal
pouch has expanded to form the early middle ear space. This space is present only in
the lower half of the middle ear, the remainder containing connective tissue. The proximal portion of the pouch has constricted
and elongated owing to growth of the head
to form the definitive eustachian (auditory)
tube.

The first branchial groove, which for a
short time during the fourth week had been
in approximation with the distal end of the
pharyngeal pouch, soon becomes separated
by growth of the head. A rather thick layer
of connective tissue separates these structures, and the groove becomes funnel-
shaped. A core of epithelial cells grows to-

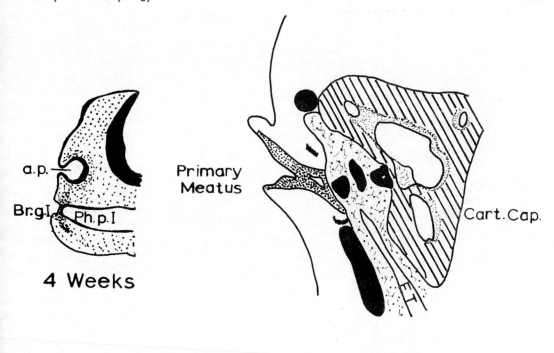

a.p.

Br.g.I Ph.p.I

Primary
Meatus

4 Weeks

Cart.Cap.

8 Weeks

FIG. 40–37. Development of the external and middle ear in relationship to the labyrinth (diagrammatic). *a.p.,* Auditory pit; *Br.g.I,* branchial groove I; *Ph.p.I,* pharyngeal pouch I; *Cart. Cap.,* cartilaginous capsule; *E.T.,* eustacian tube.

ward the middle ear in the sixth week to again approach the pharyngeal endoderm. The layer of connective tissue intervening will differentiate into the fibrous layer of the drum. The malleus handle has already appeared as an area of condensed mesenchyme. The solid external meatus expands with cranial growth until the bony tympanic ring has formed at the periphery of the tympanic membrane in the third fetal month. At this stage the epithelial core splits to form the epithelial lining of the bony external canal which, as the tympanic ring grows outward, forms the inner two thirds of the external meatus.

During this same period a series of six hillocks have appeared on the surface of the first and second branchial arches. These fuse to form the human contours of the auricle.

The mesenchyme of the superior portion of the middle ear begins to show areas of condensation. One area is situated at the cranial end of the second visceral bar (hyoid

or Reichert's cartilage), which is the stapedial primordia. Within a week the incus and malleus are evident as a single unit at the upper end of the first visceral bar (Meckel's cartilage). The stapes is in the form of a ring pierced by the stapedial artery, which is relatively large at this stage. The connection to Reichert's cartilage becomes quite tenuous, with only a thin strand of cells which will differentiate into the head of the stapes and the stapedius tendon and muscle. By the seventh week the stapes has enlarged to approach closely the otic capsule. The tissue is becoming cartilaginous, the incus and malleus have become separated, and the long process of the incus is approximated to the head of the stapes. The malleus and incus differentiate quickly into cartilage while this process in the stapes seems to be timed to that of the otic capsule.

In the eighth week the stapes is pressed firmly into the otic capsule, which is slightly concave in this region. Change into cartilage

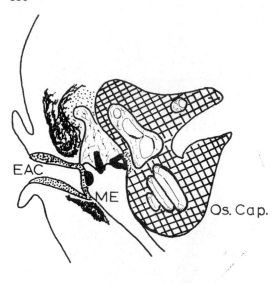

EAC

ME

Os. Cap.

20 Weeks

FIG. 40–38. Development of the external and middle ear in relationship to the labyrinth (diagrammatic). EAC., External auditory canal; *ME,* middle ear; *Os.Cap.,* osseous capsule.

is occurring in the stapes and the otic capsule with the exception of the base of the stapes and fenestral region. Here the tissues are changing in character so that the outer layer of the lamina stapedialis of the otic capsule changes to a dense fibrous layer which will become the perichondrium of the vestibular surface of the stapes footplate. The outer surface of the footplate becomes the external perichondrium. With further development, the capsular tissue at the border of the stapes footplate differentiates and then condenses to form the annular ligament. The appearance of the annular ligament is delayed, however, until the footplate of the stapes has reached its final size, since growth of the footplate is obtained by progressive change in the bordering otic capsule.

Ossification of the ossicles begins in the incus with the formation of a shell of periosteal bone around the long process in the fifteenth week. This extends up to the body of the incus and is also apparent on the head of the malleus in another 2 weeks.

Ossification begins on the obturator surface of the stapes in another week and then spreads up each crura. The ossicles, with the exception of the malleus handle, ossify initially with a shell of periosteal bone. Later, replacement bone with marrow spaces forms within the ossicles. This process on the inner surfaces of the stapedial crura and head results in their erosion and dissolution, leaving only the outer shell of perichondral bone remaining in a U-section as seen in the adult. The handle of the malleus develops endochondral replacement bone only, leaving a shell of cartilage which remains throughout adult life.

In the fifth month of development the ossicles have assumed adult configuration. Meckel's cartilage is undergoing regression in the region of the malleus with the anterior spine, which has formed separately on Meckel's cartilage and migrated to attach to the neck of the malleus, now present. The remainder of Meckel's cartilage has disappeared to form the fibrous anterior suspensory ligament of the malleus. Both the stapedius muscle and the tensor tympani muscle are differentiated. Meckel's cartilage will finally disappear, leaving, in addition to the malleus and incus, the anterior mallear ligament, the sphenomandibular ligament, and the mandible. Reichert's cartilage also disappears after forming the stapes, stapedius tendon and muscle, styloid process, stylohyoid ligament, and lesser horn of the hyoid bone.

By the fourth month the bony confines of the middle ear have been defined by growth of the tympanic process of the temporal squama, the osseous tympanic ring, and the tympanic membrane. The contained connective tissue is beginning to loosen, and the tympanic cavity begins to expand through growth of the mucosa. This growth gradually extends into the middle ear, where the ossicles are invested with mucosa in a manner similar to the formation of the visceral peritoneum. The antrum is formed by the growth of this space into the region between the tympanic process of the squama and the newly formed periosteal-antral bone from the posterior otic capsule. These two bones meet and fuse lateral to the antrum to give rise to the mastoid process. By the seventh month the antrum is well defined and pneumatized.

Pneumatization of the temporal bone seems to occur concurrently with its growth. As new marrow spaces form within the enlarging bone, the older spaces are undergoing coalescence and dissolution, with subsequent ingrowth from the mucosal lining of the antrum and middle ear. In this way the mastoid bone does not have time to form bone marrow unless the process of pneumatization is arrested by some unknown factor. The process of pneumatization is thus present before birth and continues long after birth.

Postnatal Change

Although the inner and middle ear have reached full size by the sixth month of development, growth of the head and temporal bone continues until puberty. Involved in this growth are the external auditory meatus, the squama, and the mastoid process.

At birth the canal is quite short due to the lack of much outward growth of the tympanic ring. The tympanic membrane is positioned nearly horizontally, closing the canal with a marked, upwardly directed bevel. The mastoid process has not developed below the level of the tympanic ring.

The tympanic ring grows rapidly outward, so that by the first year the normal relationship of one-third cartilaginous canal to two-thirds bony canal prevails and the drum has assumed a more erect position. The remainder of development occurs with enlargement and pneumatization of the mastoid process and growth of the temporal squama.

REFERENCES

Anson, B. J. (Ed.): *Morris' Human Anatomy*. 12th ed. New York, McGraw-Hill Book Co., 1966, Chapter X, Part II.

Anson, B. J., and Bast, T. H.: *In* Schenck, H. P. (Ed.): *The Ear and Temporal Bone in Otolaryngology*. Vol. I. Hagerstown, Prior, 1955, Chapter I.

Bast, T. H., and Anson, B. J.: *The Temporal Bone and the Ear*. Springfield, Ill., Charles C Thomas, Publisher, 1949.

Dohlman, G. F.: Secretion and Absorption of Endolymph. Ann. Otol., *73*:708, 1964.

Ormerod, F. C.: Research in Otology. J. Laryngol., *79*:845, 1965.

Proctor, B.: Development of Middle Ear Spaces. J. Laryngol., *78*:631, 1964.

Rauch, S.: Membrane Problems of the Inner Ear and Their Significance. J. Laryngol., *80*:1144, 1966.

Simmons, F. B.: Perceptual Theories of Middle Ear Muscle Function. Ann. Otol., *73*:724, 1964.

Chapter 41
Radiology of the Temporal Bone

Galdino E. Valvassori

The temporal bone is unique in the human body since it contains in the small volume of a cubic inch a concentration of vital osseous and membranous structures surrounded by a more or less extensive system of pneumatic cells. Because of the different densities of its bony components and the air- and fluid-filled spaces around and within them, the temporal bone lends itself to accurate radiographic visualization. This may be achieved either by conventional radiography or by special tomographic techniques. Conventional radiography should be used first as a screening procedure for those cases which may need a more sophisticated tomographic study.

CONVENTIONAL RADIOGRAPHY

Technique

In order to obtain a consistently satisfactory examination, a head unit should be used because of the flexibility present in this equipment. The table top should be small so that the patient's shoulder can fit under it during the upright examination, resulting in closer approximation of the head to the film. A transparent table top facilitates the proper centering on the area of interest, allowing a visualization of both the entrance and exit points of the central x-ray beam. The unit should be equipped with a tube with a small focal spot (0.3 mm) in order to increase the definition. For the same purpose a slow to average speed screen-film combination should be employed.

The port size should be as small as possible for the area under investigation. This reduces scattered radiation which tends to fog the film, resulting in a loss of sharpness. No grid is necessary for small ports; however, a fixed or moved grid must be used to control scatter whenever the port exceeds 3 inches in diameter. The use of a small port requires proper positioning of the patient's head and an accurate centering. This may only be obtained if the radiologic technologist has a knowledge of the basic anatomy of the area to be investigated.

Projections

Special projections are indispensable for the study of the temporal bone. Each projection may be particularly useful for the demonstration of one or more structures which are seen in the proper axis and become free of confusing superimpositions. By summation of the findings obtained in the various projections it is possible to obtain a satisfactory visualization of the entire area under examination and therefore to reach a more meaningful interpretation. The use of stereoscopic views is helpful, since they add dimension to the images due to a combination of superimposed structures.

Different projections are obtained by rotation of the patient's head and/or by direction of the central x-ray beam. The selection of the projections is based upon two basic radiographic principles.

1. The structures closest to the film appear sharper and less magnified than those farther from the film. Therefore the side to be examined should always be positioned closer to the x-ray film.

2. By creating an angulation of either the x-ray beam or the head, the superimposition of structures otherwise located in the same plane is avoided. The structures close to the table top are projected on the adjacent portion of the x-ray film, while the structures farther from the film are moved away from the point of interest according to the direction of the x-ray beam. The angle necessary to avoid superimposition depends upon the proximity of the two structures; structures in close proximity require a greater angle than those farther apart. For example, to separate the two mastoids in the lateral view, an angle of 15 degrees is sufficient, but to avoid superimposition of the middle ear upon the labyrinthine block of the same side, an angle of at least 35 degrees is required.

The projections discussed here include those used for a conventional radiographic study of the mastoids and petrous pyramids. General views of the skull, including the Towne's projection, may offer value in particular situations, but they will not be included here since they are not of specific diagnostic value.

THE RADIOGRAPHIC STUDY OF THE MASTOID AND MIDDLE EAR

This examination consists of three basic views: Schuller's, Owen's, and third projection of Chausse.

Schuller's or Rungstrom's Projection

This is the simplest and most easily reproducible of the views. It allows an almost undistorted view of the mastoid and of the position of the lateral sinus (Fig. 41–1).

Technique. The Schuller's projection is a lateral view of the mastoid obtained with a cephalocaudad angulation of the x-ray beam of 25 to 30 degrees. The patient's head is turned so that the sagittal plane of the skull becomes parallel to the table top and the side under examination is closer to the film. Proper centering is obtained by placing the external auditory meatus of the side to be examined 1 cm above the center of the film or of the table top.

Interpretation. The extent of the pneumatization of the mastoid, the distribution of the air cells, the degree of aeration, and the status of the trabecular pattern are the main features of this projection. The anterior wall of the vertical portion of the sigmoid sinus (corresponding to the most lateral part of the posterior aspect of the petrous pyramid) casts an almost vertical line, slightly concave posteriorly in its upper portion, superimposed upon the air cells. At its upper extremity this line joins another line which slopes gently forward and downward, forming the most lateral portion of the petrous angle, the sinodural angle of Citelli. The latter line is formed by the superior aspect of the lateral portion of the petrous pyramid. The more medial portion of the superior petrous ridge, from the arcuate eminence to the apex, has been displaced downward by the angulation of the x-ray beam and casts a line which extends forward and downward, crossing the epitympanic area and more anteriorly the neck of the mandibular condyle. Above this line the upper portion of the attic with the head of the malleus is usually visible. Finally, the temporomandibular joint is clearly outlined.

Owen's Projection

The purpose of this view is the study of the attic and of the upper portion of the tympanic cavity including the ossicular chain. This view resembles the Mayer's projection but offers the advantage of less distortion (Fig. 41–2).

Technique. The patient's head is first positioned as for a Schuller's projection in a lateral view, and it is then rotated with the face away from the table top for an angle of 30 degrees. During this rotation it is important to maintain the contact of the mastoid with the table top. The x-ray beam

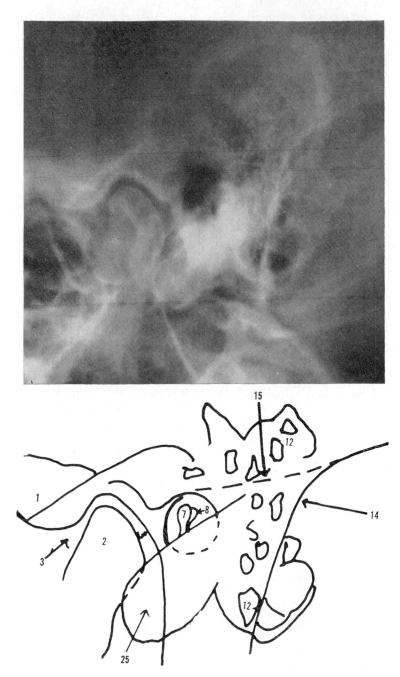

Fig. 41–1. Schuller's projection: *1*, root of the zygoma; *2*, condyle of the mandible; *3*, temporomandibular joint; *7*, malleus; *8*, incus; *12*, air cells; *14*, anterior plate of the sigmoid sinus; *15*, dural plate; *25*, petrous apex.

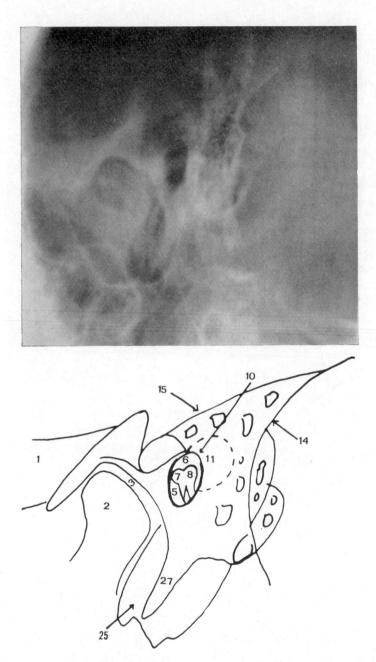

FIG. 41–2.   Owen's projection: *1*, root of the zygoma; *2*, condyle of the mandible; *3*, temporo-mandibular joint; *5*, tympanic cavity; *6*, attic; *7*, malleus; *8*, incus; *10*, region of the aditus; *11*, mastoid antrum; *14*, anterior plate of the sigmoid sinus; *15*, dural plate; *25*, petrous apex; *27*, styloid process.

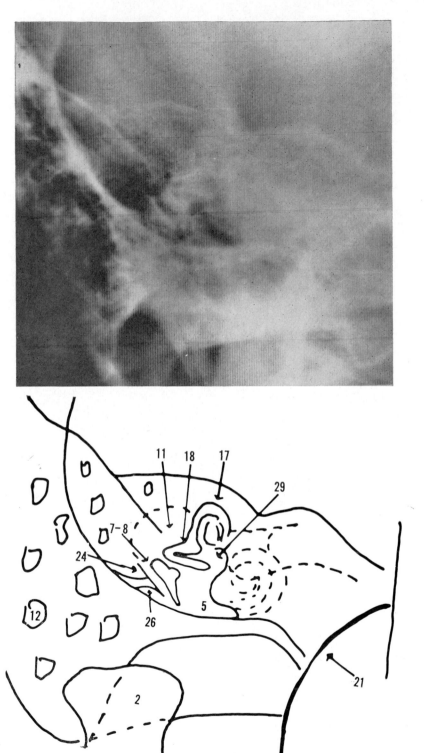

FIG. 41–3.   Third projection of Chausse: *2*, condyle of the mandible; *5*, tympanic cavity; *7–8*, malleus and incus; *11*, mastoid antrum; *12*, air cells; *17*, superior semicircular canal; *18*, horizontal semicircular canal; *21*, orbital rim; *24*, lateral wall of the attic; *26*, superior wall of the external auditory canal; *29*, vestibule.

is directed cephalocaudad with an angle of 35 degrees.

Interpretation. By the rotation of the patient's head, the petrous pyramid, which in the Schuller's view was obscuring most of the attic and the middle ear cavity, is displaced downward and posteriorly. An oval radiolucency is now well outlined due to the superimposition of the attic and upper portion of the tympanic cavity upon the external auditory canal. Within the radiolucency the entire malleus and a variable portion of the incus are clearly detectable. In pathologic cases the decrease or absence of the normal air-borne interface between the ossicles and the surrounding air makes the recognition of the ossicular structures more difficult. The dense bony ring surrounding the middle ear cavity appears thin or almost open superoposteriorly. This area represents the region of the aditus into the mastoid antrum. The pneumatic system of the mastoid, the anterior wall of the vertical portion of the sigmoid sinus, and the temporal mandibular joints are again visible, although they are more distorted than in the Schuller's view.

Third Projection of Chausse

The purpose of this projection is the study of the attic, aditus, and mastoid antrum, especially of the anterior portion of the lateral wall of the attic (Fig. 41–3). This wall from front to back runs first slightly inward, forming an average angle of 10 degrees with the sagittal plane of the skull, then turns outward to form the lateral margin of the aditus (Fig. 41–4). The Chausse view is therefore complementary of the Owen's projection since it shows the anterior portion of the lateral wall of the attic, seen in profile, whereas the Owen's shows the posterior or aditus portion of it.

Technique. The patient is positioned with the occiput on the film, the head rotated approximately 10 degrees toward the opposite side to the one under examination and the chin flexed on the chest. The central x-ray beam should be directed just above and lateral to the orbital process of the frontal bone of the side under examination and run in a plane crossing the external auditory canal.

Interpretation. The lateral wall of the attic, seen on end, casts a well-defined linear density which meets inferiorly the superior wall of the external auditory canal. Medial to the lateral wall of the attic, the ossicles are recognized as a triangular density with the base upward. The lateral portion of the triangular mass is formed by the body of the incus, the medial portion by the head of the malleus, and the apex by the handle of the malleus. The prominence of the horizontal semicircular canal is well outlined, and above it can be seen the radiolucency of the antrum with the tegmen antri.

THE RADIOGRAPHIC STUDY OF THE PETROUS PYRAMID AND INNER EAR

The petrous pyramids lie in the base of the skull at an angle of approximately 45 degrees to the sagittal plane. The internal auditory canal enters the petrous pyramid from its posteromedial surface at the junction of the anterior two fifths with the posterior three fifths. The long axis of the canal forms a right angle with the sagittal plane of the skull and an angle of about 45 degrees with the long axis of the petrous pyramid. The porus of the canal, on the other hand, has a shape much like the bevel of a needle, with its maximum diameter in the same axis of the petrous pyramid (Fig. 41–4). The posterior, superior, and inferior lips of the porus are prominent and made up of dense bone, while the anterior lip is usually poorly demarcated so that the anterior wall of the canal blends in smoothly with the posteromedial wall of the petrous apex. The internal auditory canal in cross section usually has an oval shape, with its vertical diameter being slightly larger than its horizontal diameter. The shape of the canal may change at the porus owing to the presence of bony projections.

The lateral end of the canal is closed by a vertical plate, the lamina cribrosa. Arising from the lamina cribrosa is a horizontal crest, the crista falciformis, which divides the lateral end of the internal auditory canal into two unequal portions, with the larger

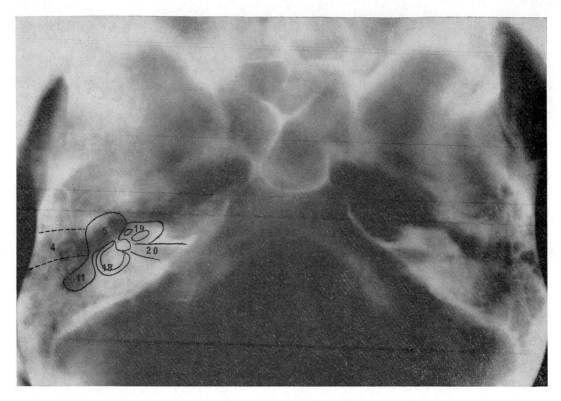

FIG. 41–4. Horizontal tomographic section of a dry skull: *4*, external auditory canal; *5*, tympanic cavity; *11*, mastoid antrum; *18*, horizontal semicircular canal; *19*, cochlea; *20*, internal auditory canal.

portion being the inferior one. Beneath the crista falciformis are three sets of foramina: the anterior set for the cochlear nerve, and the two posterior sets for the two branches of the inferior vestibular nerve. Above the crista falciformis are two sets of foramina: the anterior set for the facial nerve and the nervus intermedius, and the posterior set for the superior vestibular nerve.

From the above anatomic description of the internal auditory canal one can deduce that the best projections for its study are the frontal and axial views for a demonstration of the canal in its full length and the lateral for the visualization of the canal on end. The Stenvers' view is unsatisfactory for the visualization of the internal auditory canal, which is markedly foreshortened due to its obliquity to the plane of the film, but is useful for the demonstration of the porus of the canal which is seen on face.

Transorbital Projection

The purpose of this projection is the visualization of the petrous pyramid and internal auditory canal through the radiolucency of the orbit (Fig. 41–5).

Technique. This view can be obtained with the patient either facing the film or with his back to the film. In view of the fact that the petrous pyramids are located in the middle of the skull, the use of an anteroposterior view which produces a considerable magnification of the orbit and therefore an easier centering may be preferable. The patient's head is flexed on the chin until the orbitomeatal line is perpendicular to the table top. For better details each side should be obtained separately and the central x-ray beam directed at the center of the orbit of the side under examination and perpendicular to the film.

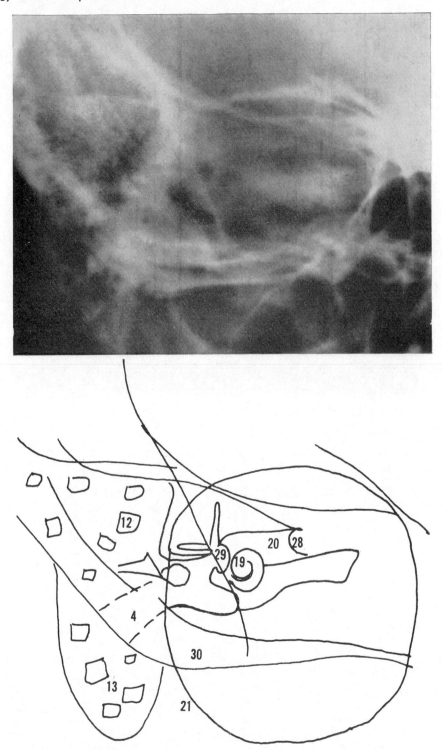

FIG. 41–5. Transorbital projection: *4*, external auditory canal; *12*, air cells; *13*, mastoid process; *19*, cochlea; *20*, internal auditory canal; *21*, orbital rim; *28*, medial lip of the posterior wall of the internal auditory canal; *29*, vestibule; *30*, base of the skull.

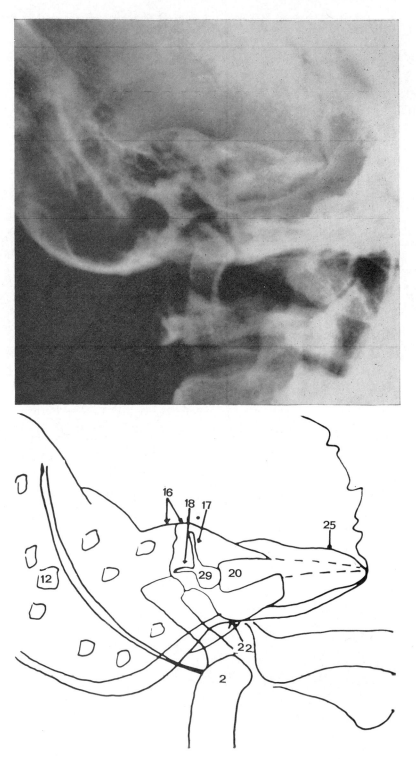

F<small>IG</small>. 41–6. Stenvers' projection: *2*, condyle of the mandible; *12*, air cells; *16*, arcuate eminence; *17*, superior semicircular canal; *18*, horizontal semicircular canal; *20*, internal auditory canal; *22*, basilar turn of the cochlea; *25*, petrous apex; *29*, vestibule.

Interpretation. The petrous apex is clearly outlined but foreshortened because of its obliquity to the plane of the film. The internal auditory canal is visualized in its full length as a horizontal band of radiolucency extending through the petrous pyramid. At the medial end of the canal the free margin of the posterior wall casts a well-defined and smooth margin, concave medially. Quite often the radiolucent band of the internal auditory canal seems to extend medially to the lip of the posterior wall into the petrous apex. This image is not due to the internal auditory canal but is merely produced by the prominence of the upper and lower lips of the porus and of the interposed groove. Lateral to the internal auditory canal, the radiolucency of the vestibule and of the superior and horizontal semicircular canals is usually detectable. The apical and middle coils of the cochlea are superimposed upon the lateral portion of the internal auditory canal, whereas the basilar turn is visible underneath it and the vestibule.

Stenvers' Projection

The purpose of the view is the visualization of the petrous pyramid in its full length (Fig. 41–6).

Technique. The patient is positioned facing the film, with the head slightly flexed and rotated 45 degrees toward the side opposite to the one under examination. By doing so, the lateral rim of the orbit of the side under investigation should lie in close contact with the table top. The x-ray beam is angulated 14 degrees caudad.

Interpretation. The entire petrous apex is visualized in its full length lateral to the orbital rim. The porus of the internal auditory canal seen on the face appears as an oval-shaped radiolucency open medially and limited laterally by the free margin of the posterior canal wall. Lateral to the porus the internal auditory canal appears quite foreshortened. The vestibule and semicircular canals, especially the posterior which lies in this projection in a plane parallel to the film, are usually recognizable. On the outside, the entire mastoid is outlined, with the mastoid process free from superimpositions.

Submental Vertex or Axial Projection

Without entering into details about this routine view of the skull, I would only like to stress the importance of this projection for the study of the following structures:

1. The anterior aspect of the petrous pyramid and of the adjacent floor of the middle cranial fossa.

2. The posterior aspect of the petrous pyramid, especially of the region of the jugular fossa. In order to obtain a better visualization of this area, the extension of the patient's head should, however, be slightly decreased so that the base line of the skull, rather than being parallel to the table top, forms with it an angle of 20 degrees open anteriorly.

3. The middle ear cavity in cases of atresia or stenosis of the external auditory canal, since the lack of the normal radiolucency of the external auditory canal bars the use of the Owen's projection.

TOMOGRAPHY

Technique

When compared with tomography, conventional radiography has the advantage of being a simpler, less time-consuming study which can be accomplished with standard radiographic equipment available in most departments. It has the intrinsic defect, however, of producing a picture which is the summation on a single plane of structures located at different depths in the three-dimensional body. Each point on the x-ray film represents the summation of multiple points crossed by each x-ray beam as it travels through the body under investigation. It is clear that in such a system small structures are lost in the confusing superimposition and that dense structures obscure others of lesser density.

The introduction of body section radiography or tomography in the early 1930's seemed to overcome the limitation of conventional radiography. However, it was only 30 years later, following modification of the equipment, that tomography became sufficiently refined to open to roentgenology a new and challenging field of investigation.

Tomography is the method of examining tissue structures by blurring out objects above and below the desired plane. Although this effect can be obtained by different techniques, the principle of body section radiography remains constant. In summary, it is a system in which focus and film move in opposite directions, with a constant ratio between their velocities. The film describes a translational motion in relation to the object. In such a system, the rays incident on a fixed point of the film will have a point of intersection that is stationary in relation to the object during the exposure. As each point of the film has a point of intersection, all points of intersection will form a plane, the focal plane. The thickness of the plane in focus decreases with the widening of the angular opening of the scanning movement for a given focal film distance. The blurring of the structures outside the focal plane increases with the length of the scanning movement.

Unidirectional or linear body section radiography, initially used when this technique was first being explored, proved unsatisfactory for the study of small structures of the temporal bone. With linear tomography, the coefficient of cancellation of the structures outside the focal plane is quite limited and uneven because of the short scanning movement and because those structures whose long axis is parallel to the longitudinal axis of the trajectory are not effaced but merely elongated.

Multidirectional tomographic equipment is now available. In our study we used the polytome made by Philips, which has a hypocycloidal or cloverleaf trajectory. The Polytome allows a thickness as small as 1 mm of the plane in focus and a blurring effect about five times as great as the one obtained with a linear trajectory of the same angle.

Our tomographic examination of the temporal bone consists of multiple sections obtained 1 or 2 mm apart in different planes. A small field is used, approximately 1.5 to 2 inches in diameter, at the plane in focus. A movable cassette tray allows multiple exposures on a 10×12 film.

An important consideration is the total x-ray exposure of the patient involved in this technique. Careful computation shows that, owing to the small size of the port, the patient's gonads and bone marrow receive no measurable x-ray exposure. The lens of the eye is protected by a lead shield 2 mm thick, which cuts the dose for a tomographic study involving 36 exposures of an average adult from 15 to 2 rads.

Tomographic Projections of the Temporal Bone

Five different radiographic projections and planes of section are commonly used by this author (G.E.V.) in the study of the temporal bone: (1) coronal or frontal, (2) sagittal or lateral, (3) semiaxial of the petrous pyramid or 20-degree coronal oblique of the skull, (4) horizontal or basal, and (5) axial of the petrous pyramid or Poschle.

The selection of the projections to be used in each particular case depends upon the anatomic structure or structures under investigation and the type of pathologic process or processes under consideration.

Coronal or Frontal Projection. This projection is quite satisfactory for the study of all three portions of the ear, is comfortable for the patient, and is easy to obtain and reproduce. We consider it a basic projection and use it in all instances except for the study of the vestibular aqueduct. It is obtained with the patient lying on the table either prone or supine with the line running from the tragus to the external canthus perpendicular to the table top. Figures 41–7 and 41–8 are two representative frontal sections of a normal ear, one obtained at the level of the anterior portion of the attic and cochlea and the second at the level of the oval window, vestibule, and internal auditory canal.

Sagittal or Lateral Projection. This projection is complementary to the coronal projection, since it shows the anterior to posterior aspects of the structures seen in their lateral to medial relationships in the coronal projection. It is particularly satisfactory for studying the mastoid, external auditory canal, ossicles, vertical portion of the facial nerve canal, semicircular canals, internal auditory canal, and vestibular aqueduct. The patient lies prone on the table with the sag-

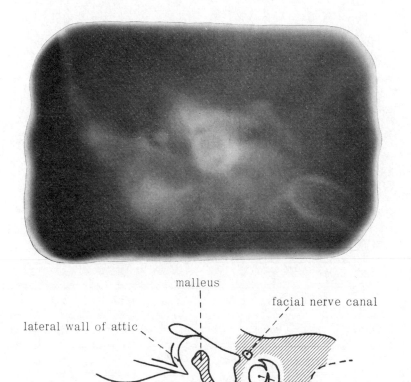

FIG. 41–7. Frontal section of normal ear at the level of the anterior portion
of the attic and cochlea.

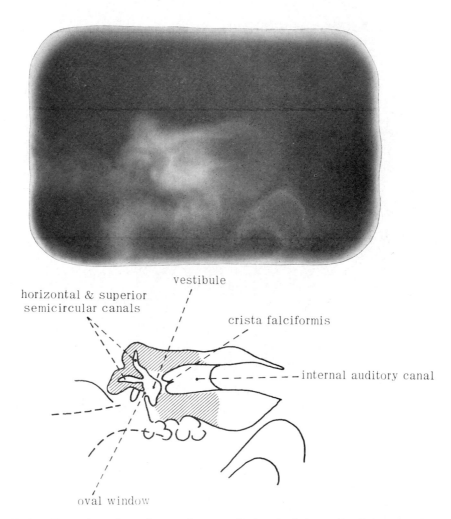

FIG. 41–8.   Frontal section of normal ear at the level of the oval window, vestibule, and internal auditory canal.

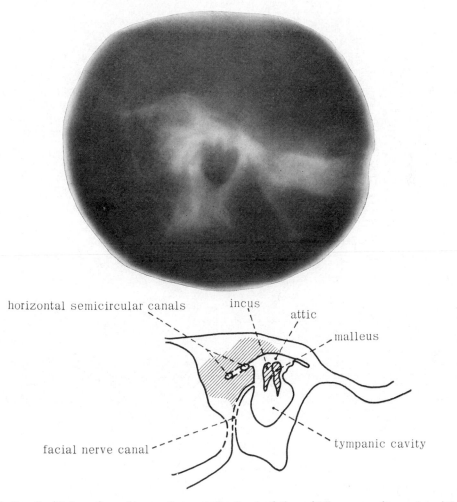

Fig. 41–9.   Sagittal section of normal ear at the level of the middle ear cavity and ossicles.

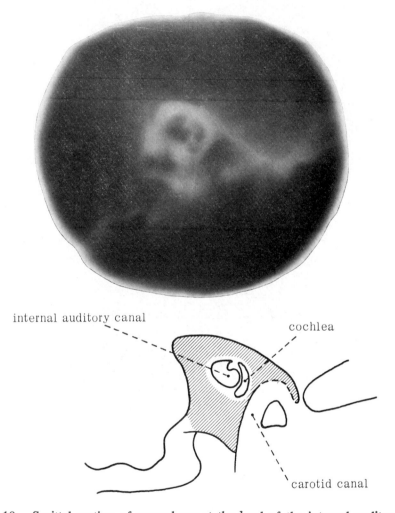

FIG. 41–10.   Sagittal section of normal ear at the level of the internal auditory canal.

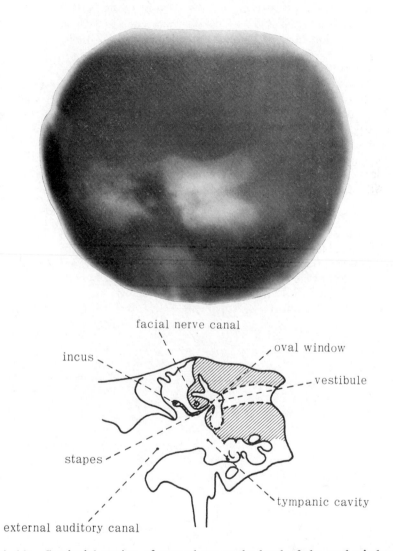

FIG. 41–11. Semiaxial section of normal ear at the level of the oval window.

ittal plane of the skull parallel to the table top. The side away from the table is examined in order to facilitate the centering, particularly when the skull is asymmetric. Figures 41–9 and 41–10 are two representative sections of a normal ear, one at the level of the middle ear cavity and ossicles and the second through the internal auditory canal.

Semiaxial Projection of the Petrous Pyramid or 20-degree Coronal Oblique of the Skull. This projection is particularly useful for the study of the medial or labyrinthine wall of the middle ear cavity. It is mandatory for the evaluation of the oval window, the promontory, the horizontal semicircular canal, and the horizontal segment of the facial nerve canal. The patient lies supine on the table with the head rotated 20 degrees toward the side under examination. By this rotation, the medial or labyrinthine wall of the middle ear cavity, which forms an angle, open posteriorly, of 15 to 25 degrees with the sagittal plane of the skull, becomes perpendicular to the plane of film and therefore to the plane of section. Figure 41–11 is a representative section of a normal ear obtained at the level of the oval window.

Horizontal or Basal Projection. This projection is quite satisfactory for the study of the temporal bone, especially in patients with congenital malformations and tumors. Its use is limited by the fact that it is very uncomfortable for the patient and that it requires a higher radiation exposure than the other projections. The patient lies on the table with his head overextended until the plane running from the tragus to the external canthus is parallel to the table top.

A 15-degree flexion of the head is advisable, however, whenever the jugular fossa and the adjacent posteromedial aspect of the petrous pyramid are under investigation.

Axial Projection of the Petrous Pyramid or Poschle. This projection is useful for the study of the vestibular aqueduct and cochlear capsule. The section or sections through the long axis of the modiolus allow good visualization on end of several segments of the cochlear coil. It is obtained with the patient lying on the table either supine or prone with his head rotated 45 degrees so that the long axis of the petrous pyramid becomes perpendicular to the plane of the film and therefore to the plane of section.

REFERENCES

Compere, W.: *Radiographic Atlas of the Temporal Bone.* Book I. Am. Acad. Ophthal. Otol., 1964.

Mundnich, K., and Frey, K.: *Das Rontgenschichtbild des Orhes.* Stuttgart, Georg Thieme, 1959.

Valvassori, G.: Laminagraphy of the Ear: Normal Roentgenographic Anatomy. Am. J. Roentgen., 89:1155, 1963.

Valvassori, G.: *Radiographic Atlas of the Temporal Bone.* Book II. Am. Acad. Ophthal. Otol., 1964.

Valvassori, G.: Radiologic Diagnosis of Cochlear Otosclerosis. Laryngoscope, 75:1563, 1965.

Valvassori, G., and Buckingham, R.: *Tomography and Cross Sections of the Ear.* Stuttgart, Georg Thieme, 1975.

Valvassori, G., and Pierce, R.: The Normal Internal Auditory Canal. Am. J. Roentgen., 92:449, 1969.

Chapter 42

The Physiology of the Auditory and Vestibular Systems*

Alfred C. Coats and Bob R. Alford

EXTERNAL EAR

Traditionally, the external ear has been regarded as a sort of funnel to collect sound and thereby increase overall auditory sensitivity. Since man is endowed with a much less impressive pinna than many lower vertebrates, this traditional view forces the pinna into a rudimentary role in human hearing. Relatively recently, however, evidence has been found that the pinna's primary function is sound localization. Batteau described a simple experiment, demonstrating this function, as follows: "W. McLean jingled keys in front of me with my eyes closed and I pointed accurately to them. Then he had me bend the tops of my pinnae down and jingled the keys again; I missed by 90°. Since anyone can perform this experiment, I recommend it to you."[11]

Additional evidence involved the demonstration of accurate sound localization in subjects with monaural hearing and loss of this localization when the pinna of the hearing ear was strapped to the head. Also, abnormally poor sound localization around an "imperfectly" remodeled pinna has been reported.[10,11]

Studies of models of the human pinna suggest that the pinna extracts information about sound location by changing the transmission characteristics of different frequencies according to the sound source's location relative to the pinna.[10,11,146,183]

To the surgeon remodeling the pinna, the possibility that it may have a sound-localizing function is important because it suggests that the surgery may have more than a cosmetic effect. Additional investigation is needed to isolate the anatomic aspects of the pinna that are particularly important in sound localization.

MIDDLE EAR

Figure 42–1 diagrams the anatomy of the middle and inner ears. The middle ear ossicles form a lever system to transmit sound energy from the tympanic membrane to the oval window. We shall divide our discussion of the middle ear into two categories: (1) "impedance matching" between air (the external environment) and fluid (perilymph and endolymph), and (2) middle ear muscle reflex.

The widespread use of surgical modification of middle ear structures to improve hearing and the recent rapid growth of impedance audiometry make the concept of

* The authors gratefully acknowledge the advice of Dr. James Jerger in their discussion of the middle ear, and Dr. Makoto Igarashi in their discussion of the vestibular apparatus.

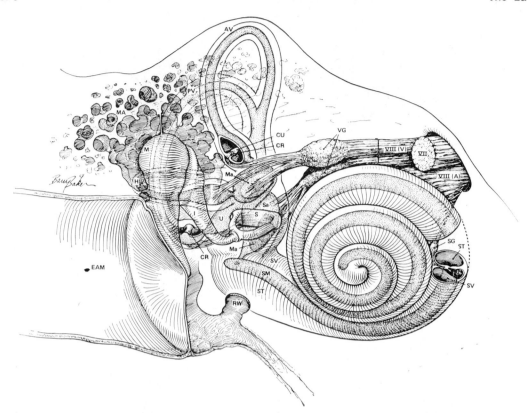

FIG. 42–1. Schematic drawing of the inner ear (labyrinth), which consists of a series of tunnels hollowed out of the petrous portion of the temporal bone. The osseous labyrinth (outer tunnel) is clear, and the membranous labyrinth (inner tunnel) is stippled. SV, Scala vestibuli; ST, scala tympani; SM, scala media; SG, spiral ganglion, containing the cell bodies of the auditory nerve; VG, vestibular ganglion, containing the cell bodies of the vestibular nerve; VIII (A), auditory part of the eighth cranial nerve; VIII (V), vestibular part of the eighth cranial nerve; VII, facial nerve; Ma, macula; CU, cupula; CR, crista; Sa, sacculus; U, utriculus. Semicircular canals are labeled AV (anterior vertical), PV (posterior vertical), and H (horizontal). EAM, external auditory meatus; RW, round window; M, malleus; I, incus; S, stapes; MA, mastoid air cells in temporal bone.

acoustic impedance and its relationship to middle ear function very important to the otologist. Accordingly, our discussion will include some basic principles of acoustic impedance.

Transmission of Acoustic Energy through the Middle Ear

Figure 42–2 diagrams the transmission of sound energy through the middle ear into the inner ear. The tympanic membrane moves the handle of the malleus. The long process of the incus and the handle of the malleus move together because the malleo-

incudal joint is fixed.* In contrast, the joint between the incus and the stapes is flexible. Therefore, since the stapes is fixed at its posteroinferior border, tympanic membrane movement causes it to rock in and out of the oval window. The pressure changes caused by the stapes moving in and out of the oval window are transmitted via perilymph through the cochlear partition, then out the round window. Pressure transmission through the cochlear partition causes the partition to bulge either upward or downward, depending on the direction of the

* In man, it is probably capable of limited motion.

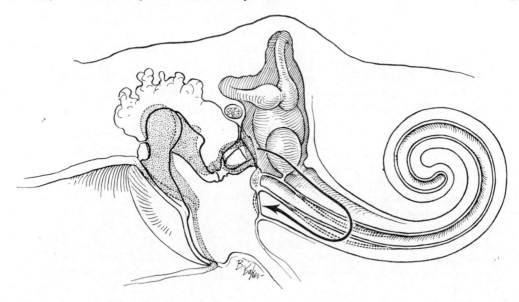

FIG. 42–2.   Transmission of tympanic membrane movement into the cochlea via the ossicles. The system at rest is unstippled. The stippled ossicles and dashed cochlear partition illustrate the system when the tympanic membrane is pushed inward by a sound wave.

pressure change. As will be discussed, this bulging causes the hair cells in the organ of Corti to stimulate the auditory nerve endings.

At very high sound intensities (around 100–110 dB SPL), the mode of vibration of the ossicular chain changes; instead of rotating about its short axis, as shown in Figure 42–2, the stapes footplate rotates about its long axis.[14, p. 113] This change results in less efficient sound transmission through the middle ear but is probably less effective in protecting the inner ear from loud, steady sounds than the stapedius reflex, since the stapedius reflex has a much lower threshold (70–80 dB sensation level). It is of interest, however, that the change in vibration mode occurs at the threshold of feeling. This suggests that the somatic sensation caused by very loud sounds is due to perception of altered ossicular vibration by middle ear bone and tendon receptors.

Impedance Matching by the Middle Ear

Auditory function in land-dwelling animals requires transmission of sound from air to fluid. As swimming underwater and attempting to listen to sounds generated even a few inches above the surface demonstrates, direct transmission across an air/water boundary is extremely inefficient. The inefficiency occurs because the specific acoustic impedances of air and water differ greatly, and whenever energy is transmitted between media with different specific impedances, much of the energy is reflected back at the boundary between the two media. The middle ear matches impedances of air and cochlea (415 and 56,000 rayles, respectively[232, p. 40]) and thereby greatly increases the efficiency of energy transmission into the cochlea.

Impedance means, essentially, *the opposition of a system to movement.* Thus, the more force required to move a mechanical system at a given speed, the greater its impedance. Figure 42–3 illustrates the principles of mechanical impedance. If the force applied to a system and the speed that it moves in response are known, the impedance of the system may be calculated as follows:

$$\text{Mechanical impedance} = \frac{\text{force}}{\text{velocity}}$$

As Figure 42–3 illustrates, the physical parameters which determine mechanical impedance are *mass, stiffness,* and *frictional resistance.* Friction is the *resistive component* of impedance. It consumes energy and is independent of driving frequency. Stiffness and mass comprise the *reactive component of impedance.* They store energy (e.g., once the weight in Figure 42–3 is set in motion, it will tend to continue because of inertia, and if the spring is compressed, it will tend to push backward). As shown by the formula at lower right in Figure 42–3, *stiffness reactance* decreases with frequency (f), and *mass reactance* increases with frequency. This formula also demonstrates that stiffness and mass reactance are of opposite sign. Therefore, there will be a particular "resonant" frequency when stiffness reactance equals mass reactance; hence total reactance will be zero. At this resonant frequency, impedance will be minimal.

Acoustic impedance is a special type of mechanical impedance in which force is replaced by pressure (force per unit area), and the system is driven by sound. Figure 42–3 could be converted into a diagram of an acoustic system by interposing a piston, or membrane, between the force and the mass.

When air transmits sound, the stiffness component of its acoustic impedance is determined by elastic coupling between air molecules; the mass component is determined by the molecules' mass; and the frictional component is determined by frictional resistance between air molecules. Since water is much denser and less compressible than air, it might seem at first that mass and stiffness create the main difference between the cochlea's acoustic impedance and that of air. However, reference to Figure 42–2 shows that transmission of energy into the cochlea does not involve compression of the cochlear fluid itself. Also, the elastic restorative forces of the cochlear partition and round window tend to cancel out the effect of the fluid's mass. Thus, the effective acoustic impedance of the cochlea is primarily resistive.[150,223, p. 72]

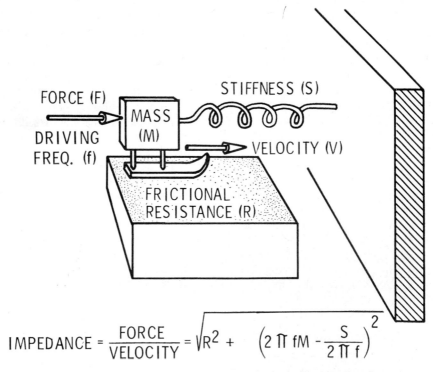

$$\text{IMPEDANCE} = \frac{\text{FORCE}}{\text{VELOCITY}} = \sqrt{R^2 + \left(2\pi fM - \frac{S}{2\pi f}\right)^2}$$

FIG. 42–3.   Principles of mechanical impedance. The diagram could be converted to a representation of acoustic impedance by interposing a cylinder, or diaphragm, between the driving force and the driven mass and expressing the displacing input as pressure (force per unit area).

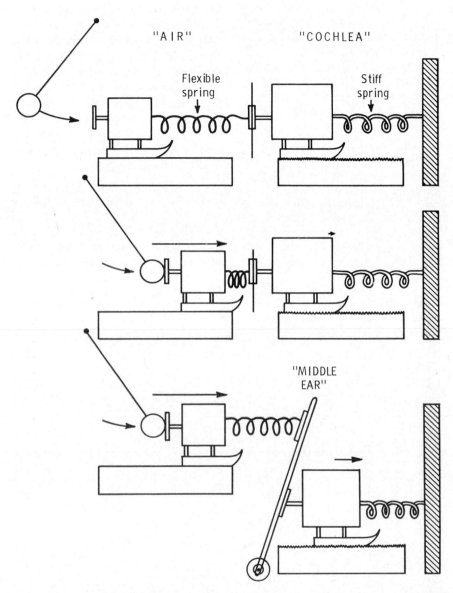

FIG. 42–4. Principle of mechanical impedance matching by "levering down" the driving force. The upper two drawings depict transmission directly across the air/cochlea boundary. With impedances unmatched, energy will be reflected off the air/cochlea boundary, and transmission into the cochlea will be inefficient. The reflection may be visualized by looking at the middle drawing and imagining the next event, which would be expansion of the "flexible spring" to push the pendulum backward. As shown in the bottom drawing, adding a lever to increase driving force and thereby "match" impedances improves transmission into the cochlea. In actual middle ears, driving force is concentrated both by a lever action and by a difference in membrane areas (tympanic membrane versus oval widow).

The middle ear "matches" the low impedance of air with the high cochlear impedance by concentrating the incident sound pressure from the large area of the tympanic membrane onto the small area of the oval window. The ossicular chain also contributes to the middle ear's "transformer action" by levering down the vibration amplitude. In the human, the area ratio of the tympanic membrane and the oval window is about 20:1, but the tympanic membrane does not vibrate as a whole;[14, p. 101,113,209] hence, the effective area ratio is only about 14:1.[223, p. 111] The ossicular chain/lever ratio is around 1.3:1.[71]

Figure 42–4 shows why the middle ear's transformer action improves energy transmission. The top two pictures depict attempted direct transmission into the "cochlear fluid." Very little movement in the "cochlea" occurs, and much of the energy will be reflected back into the "air" (i.e., the next thing that will happen is that the flexible spring will expand, pushing the pendulum backward). The bottom picture shows how increasing the effective force applied by the incident energy improves transmission into the high-impedance medium. It is possible to "overmatch" impedances; i.e., if the lever ratio in Figure 42–4 were made too large, energy transmission into the high-impedance medium would again become inefficient.

In actuality, the middle ear somewhat undermatches the acoustic impedances of air and cochlea.[34, p. 113,232, p. 40] Tonndorf and Khanna[208] pointed out that this undermatching has the teleological advantage of broadening the ear's frequency response.

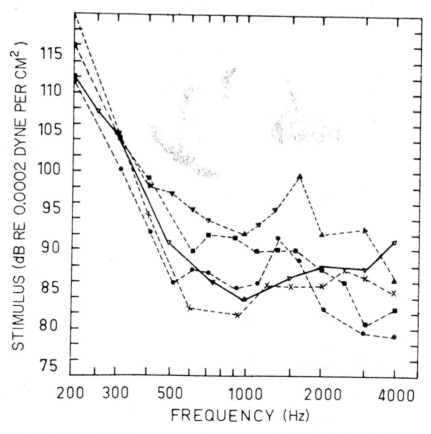

FIG. 42–5. Sensitivity of the human acoustic reflex. Dashed lines from four subjects plot intensities required to elicit an acoustic reflex with 10% of the maximum obtainable amplitude (measured with an impedance technique). The solid line is the threshold of audibility raised 80 dB. (Møller, A. R.: Ann. Otol. Rhinol. Laryngol., *71*:86, 1962.)

Middle Ear Muscles

Causes of Middle Ear Muscle Contraction. In primates, the stapedius contracts reflexly in response to sound stimuli, but the tensor tympani probably does not.[66,180] The efferent limb of the stapedius reflex is the facial nerve, and the reflex pathway probably goes no higher than the superior olive.[17]

Figure 42–5 plots stapedius reflex threshold versus sound frequency. The pure tone reflex threshold curve parallels the audibility threshold curve but is 80 dB above it.[100,148] White noise stimuli elicit the reflex more effectively than do pure tones.[73,148,149] The stapedius reflex threshold decreases with increasing stimulus duration with a time constant of about 200 msec.[57,232] This approximates the time constant of temporal summation of loudness and sensitivity. These observations, coupled with the clinical observation that the stapedius reflex demonstrates "recruitment" in cochlear hearing losses,[102,143] suggest that the acoustic reflex threshold correlates with subjective loudness rather than with absolute sound intensity.

A number of nonauditory causes of middle ear muscle contraction have been reported, including (1) spontaneous contractions, (2) body movements,[180] (3) vocalization[56,180] (contractions start *before* vocalization begins), (4) movement of facial muscles[180] (tensor tympani only), (5) stimulation of the ear canal,[114,115] and (6) voluntary contractions.[168,188]

Effect of Middle Ear Muscle Contractions. As Figure 42–6 illustrates, the stapedius pulls the stapes footplate backward and into the oval window, and the tensor tympani pulls the handle of the malleus inward. Figure 42–7 illustrates the effect of these contractions on sound transmission through the middle ear.[168,188] Transmission of low-frequency sounds is attenuated by contraction of either muscle,[151] but the stapedius is probably a somewhat better attenuator than the tensor tympani.

Time Course of the Acoustic Reflex. The human acoustic reflex has been studied by recording (1) the middle ear muscle electromyogram,[180] (2) pressure change in the external canal,[96] and (3) impedance

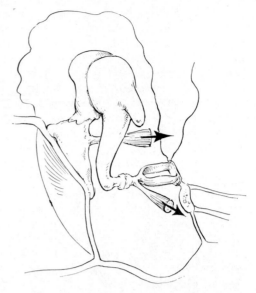

Fig. 42–6. Action of the middle ear muscles. The view is from behind the head. The muscles are not drawn to scale. The tensor tympani muscle (above) attaches to the handle of the malleus and pulls it backward, tensing the tympanic membrane. The stapedius muscle (below) attaches to the neck of the stapes and pulls the posterior-inferior border of the stapes down and into the oval window.

change.[102,149] Figure 42–8 shows a stapedius reflex recorded by the impedance change method. The latency (time to first detectable change) generally varies from 10 to 50 msec. The reflex decays over about 500 msec after the sound has been turned on. The initial reduction in impedance is a recently discovered phenomenon and is frequency-dependent.[101]

Function of the Middle Ear Muscles. The middle ear muscles support and stiffen the ossicular chain[223, p. 189] and are generally thought to protect the inner ear against overstimulation by loud sounds. Since the acoustic reflex attenuates transmission of loud, low-frequency sounds, and since these are the most damaging acoustic stimuli, assigning the acoustic reflex a protective function seems reasonable. However, recently Simmons[185] cast doubt on this protective function by pointing out that the loud, low-frequency sounds against which the reflex is supposed to afford protection do not exist in nature.

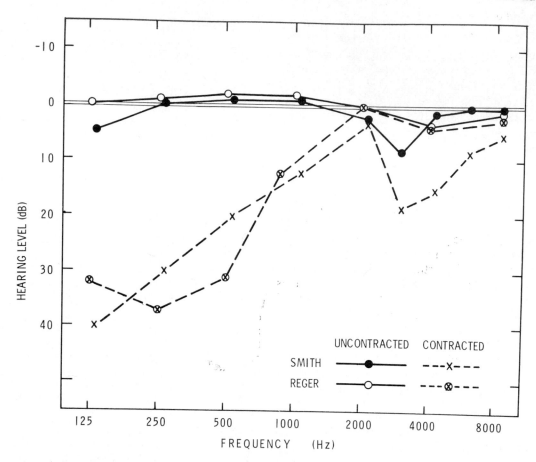

FIG. 42–7. Effect of middle ear muscle contractions on pure tone thresholds. The curves were obtained from normal subjects with the ability to voluntarily contract their middle ear muscles.[168,188] Although the effect of voluntary contraction may differ from the effect of normal involuntary contraction, the general observation that middle ear muscle contractions preferentially attenuate low frequencies is probably valid.

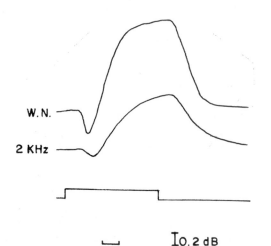

FIG. 42–8. Time course of human stapedius contractions in response to white noise (W.N.) and 2KHz pure-tone stimuli. Bottom trace shows stimulum time course. The stimuli were 90 dB above normal threshold and were delivered to the right ear. The muscle contractions were recorded from the left ear by the acoustic impedance change method. (Records courtesy of Dr. James Jerger.)

An alternative middle ear muscle function could be to attenuate low-frequency masking sounds which might otherwise interfere with auditory function. Contractions during chewing and other face and body movements could attenuate the resultant internal body sounds (which are largely low-frequency) while preserving sensitivity to high-frequency external sounds.

The low-frequency attenuation produced by contractions prior to vocalization may also be functionally important. The following observations support a middle ear muscle role in vocalization: (1) patients with otosclerosis demonstrate significant deficits when administered the delayed feedback test for malingering;[94] (2) stutterers have a deficit in the prevocalization middle ear muscle contraction.

COCHLEA

The cochlea has two basic functions: (1) it *transduces* the sound energy into a form suitable for stimulating the auditory nerve endings, and (2) it *codes* acoustical parameters so that the brain can process the information contained in the sound stimulus. We shall consider each of these functions in turn.

Transducer Function

Anatomy. As Figure 42–1 shows, the cochlea is divided into three tunnels (*scalae*). The middle tunnel (*scala media*) is the cochlear extension of the membranous labyrinth and is filled with a potassium-rich, sodium-poor electrolyte fluid (*endolymph*). The outer two tunnels (*scala vestibuli* and *scala tympani*) constitute the osseus labyrinth (which the scala media divides in two) and are filled with a sodium-rich, potassium-poor electrolyte fluid (*perilymph*). When the cochlea is activated by sound, the scala media and its contents tend to move as a unit. The space enclosed by Reissner's and basilar membranes have therefore been termed the "cochlear partition."[14, p. 11]

Figure 42–9 diagrams the scala media's contents. The auditory nerve fibers synapse at the hair cell bases in the *organ of Corti.*

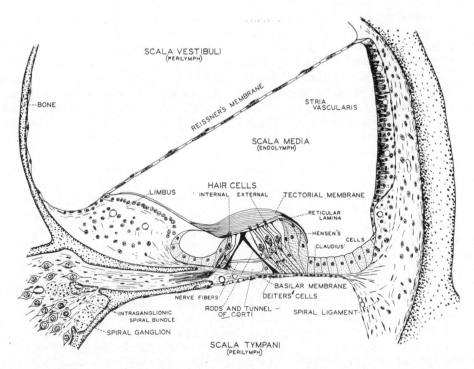

FIG. 42–9. Semidiagrammatic representation of a cross section of the guinea pig cochlear duct. (Davis, H., *et al.*: J. Acoust. Soc. Am., *25*:1180, 1953.)

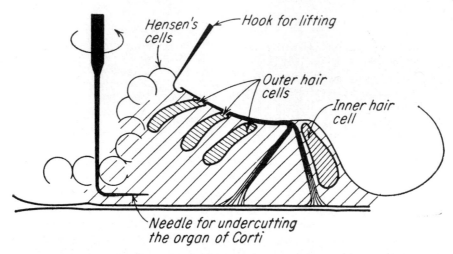

Hensen's cells

Hook for lifting

Outer hair cells

Inner hair cell

Needle for undercutting the organ of Corti

FIG. 42–10. Effect of undercutting the reticular lamina with a bent needle and lifting its outer edge. Von Bekesy made this observation on the living guinea pig cochlea, using a slit-lamp microscope. (Von Bekesy, G.: *Experiments in Hearing.* New York, McGraw-Hill, 1960.)

They enter the scala media through the *habenula perforata,* where they lose their myelin sheaths.

The *reticular lamina* and the *tectorial membrane* are two membranes in the organ of Corti which are particularly important in cochlear transduction. The reticular lamina resembles a very stiff net whose webbing enmeshes the tops of the hair cells. The rods of Corti are attached to, and support, the reticular lamina. Thus, the *rods of Corti* and the reticular lamina provide the skeletal support of the organ of Corti. Figure 42–10 diagrams von Bekesy's experiment which elucidated these mechanical properties.[14]

It is particularly noteworthy that the boundary between high-potassium and high-sodium electrolytes is not the basilar membrane but the reticular lamina. However, the fluid between basilar membrane and reticular lamina probably differs from both perilymph and endolymph in chemical content[7,64] (although its electrolyte content is the same as that of perilymph). The term *cortilymph* has been coined for this fluid.[64]

The tectorial membrane resembles a rather stiff, oval, gelatinous tube. It is attached to the limbus by a flexible, membranous band that allows it to move up and down like the cover of a book.[14, p. 489]

The cilia on the outer hair cells are of varying lengths. The longer cilia attach to the tectorial membrane's undersurface. It is unclear whether the shorter outer hair cell cilia attach to the tectorial membrane. The inner hair cell cilia are shorter than the outer hair cell cilia and probably do not attach to the tectorial membrane.[111,123,124,190]

Mechanical Transduction. The final mechanical event in the cochlear transduction process is bending of the hair cell cilia. Figure 42–11 illustrates the mechanism. Basilar membrane deformation causes a shearing action between the reticular and tectorial membranes. The long outer hair cell cilia are attached to both membranes and thus are bent. Since the inner hair cell cilia, and possibly also the shorter outer hair cell cilia (not shown in Figure 42–11), are not attached to the tectorial membrane, some mechanism other than displacement shear must bend them. The mechanism may involve fluid streaming between the sliding parallel plates formed by the two membranes.[34, p. 202,194] Such fluid streaming would be generated by the relative velocities of the membranes rather than by their relative displacement. Dallos and coworkers[36] selectively damaged outer hair cells with kanamycin and found changes in cochlear potentials that convincingly demonstrated that the inner hair cells are velocity sensors, in contrast to the outer hair cells which are displacement sensors.[14, p. 684]

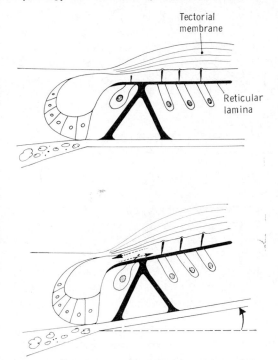

Tectorial
membrane

Reticular
lamina

FIG. 42–11. Translation of basilar membrane displacement (as shown in Fig. 42–2) into bending of the hair cell cilia. Shearing action between the tectorial membrane and the reticular lamina bends the outer cilia, which are attached to both structures. Streaming movement, imparted to the fluid between the reticular lamina and the tectorial membrane, may bend the inner cilia, which are not attached to the tectorial membrane. Inner cilia deflection may be longitudinal (i.e., perpendicular to the page) rather than radial, as depicted.

Von Bekesy pointed out that the shearing action between reticular and tectorial membranes has the effect of reducing the displacement amplitude of the stimulating energy while increasing its force.[13,14, p. 703] Therefore, this shearing action may serve to match impedances of fluid and solid transmission media as the middle ear matches air and fluid impedances.

Cochlear Electrical Potentials. Three cochlear bioelectric events have been identified: the *endocochlear potential,* the *cochlear microphonic*, and the *summating potential*. The endocochlear potential is present at rest; the other two potentials appear only when sound stimulates the ear.

Endocochlear Potential. The endocochlear potential is a constant (DC), 90–115 mV potential,[159] which may be recorded with an electrode in the scala media.[12,202] The stria vascularis generates the endocochlear potential.[41,205] Since the endocochlear potential is very sensitive to anoxia and chemical agents interfering with oxidative metabolism,[44,117,118,147,181] its existence probably depends on active metabolic processes in the stria vascularis.

Figure 42–12 shows the endocochlear potential's distribution in the scala media. The endocochlear potential is probably bounded by the reticular lamina and not by the basilar membrane,[159,202] thus providing further evidence for a significant boundary at the hair-bearing ends of the hair cells.

The voltage drop across the hair-bearing ends of the hair cells is probably important in both vestibular and cochlear transduction.[204] The hair cell's negative intracellular potential creates a voltage drop, but the endocochlear potential approximately doubles this voltage drop and thereby presumably improves transduction.

Cochlear Microphonics and Summating Potentials. When the appropriate stimulus

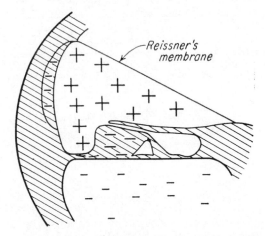

Reissner's
membrane

Fig. 42–12. Distribution of steady (DC) voltages inside the cochlear partition. Plus signs and minus signs indicate electrical polarity, and the signs' sizes indicate approximate voltage magnitude. The large positive voltage in scala media is the endocochlear potential. Voltages are referred to perilymph above Reissner's membrane. (Von Bekesy, G.: *Experiments in Hearing.* New York, McGraw-Hill, 1960.)

is applied, most sensory end organs generate bioelectric events called *sensory end organ potentials*. These potentials differ from action potentials in that they are graded rather than being all-or-none, have no latency, are not propagated, and have no apparent postresponse refractoriness.[42] Summating potentials and cochlear microphonics are the sensory end organ potentials of the cochlea.

The cochlear microphonic reproduces the waveform of the stimulating sound (hence the name "microphonic").[42,203,222] The summating potential is a DC shift that follows the "envelope" of the stimulating sound.[40] Figure 42–13 illustrates this waveform. An electrode in the cochlea records a composite potential, consisting of cochlear microphonics, summating potentials, and action potentials; therefore, to visualize the summating potential, one must mentally separate its waveform from the recorded composite waveform.

A much longer portion of the cochlear partition generates cochlear microphonics than generates the summating potential (see Fig. 42–19). Because of its more restricted

source, recording the summating potential requires an electrode located relatively close to the organ of Corti. In animal experimentation, summating potentials are usually recorded with an electrode inside the cochlea, whereas cochlear microphonics can be recorded with a round window electrode. In keeping with its more diffuse origin, averaged cochlear microphonics can be recorded from the external ear canal in man[30,63,230] (see Fig. 42–29), whereas a promontory electrode is required to record human summating potentials.[60,61]

Both cochlear microphonics and summating potentials are generated across the hair cells' hair-bearing ends.[119,202] The cochlear microphonic probably comes from the outer hair cells.[41] At low stimulus intensities, the summating potential also comes from the outer hair cells, but as intensity is increased, the inner hair cells contribute a progressively larger proportion of the recorded summating potential until, at high intensities (above around 60 dB re 0.0002 dynes/cm^2), the inner hair cell contribution predominates.[35]

Cochlear microphonics and summating

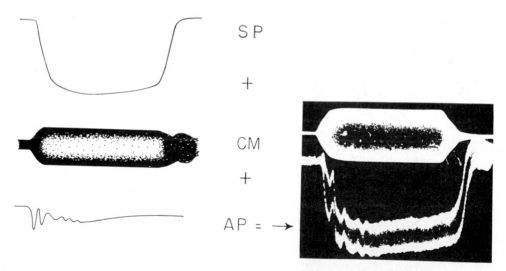

SP

+

CM

+

AP = →

Fig. 42–13.   Waveform of the summating potential response to a tone burst (upper oscilloscope trace at lower right of figure). The recorded response (electrodes in basal turn) is a composite of summating potential (SP), cochlear microphonic (CM), and auditory nerve action potential (AP). The recorded response is the lower oscilloscope trace at lower right of figure. The frequency of the tone burst is too high to allow resolution of the individual cycles, which appear as a "snowy" area in the sound stimulus and cochlear microphonic records. The line drawings at the left show how the separate bioelectric events combine to give the composite potential actually recorded. (Davis, H., *et al.*: Am. J. Physiol., *195*:251, 1958.)

potentials differ not only in their origin and waveform but also in their response to varying sound intensity. As Figure 42–14 demonstrates, summating potentials predominate at high intensities, whereas cochlear microphonics predominate at low intensities.[40]

Role of Cochlear Potentials in Transduction. Wever and Bray's discovery of the cochlear microphonic[222] led to the hypothesis that the auditory nerve endings are stimulated electrically.[43] However, relatively recent electron microscope observations of humoral synapselike structures at the hair cell/auditory nerve junction (see Fig. 42–24)

have led to the current view that a humoral mediator stimulates the auditory nerve endings.[38,70,218] This leaves the role of the cochlear sensory end organ potentials uncertain. However, these potentials are probably either directly involved in the cause and effect chain leading to auditory nerve stimulation or intimately related to a process which is directly involved.[34, p. 378, 35,38]

Coding in the Cochlea

The cochlea must "code" acoustic parameters into parameters of nervous activity.

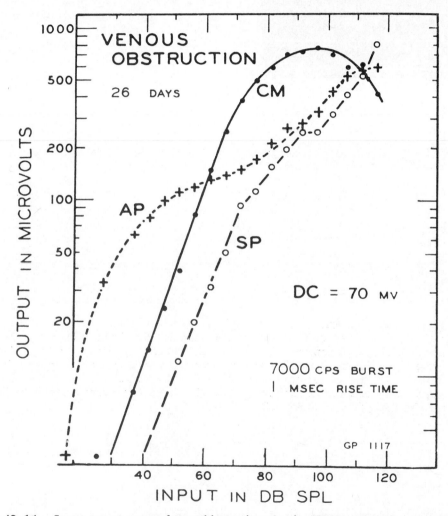

FIG. 42–14. Input-output curves for cochlear microphonic (CM), summating potential (SP), and action potential (AP) recorded from a guinea pig cochlea. Although the venous outflow of the stria vascularis was obstructed, the curves were essentially normal. (Davis, H., *et al.*: Am. J. Physiol., *195*:251, 1958.)

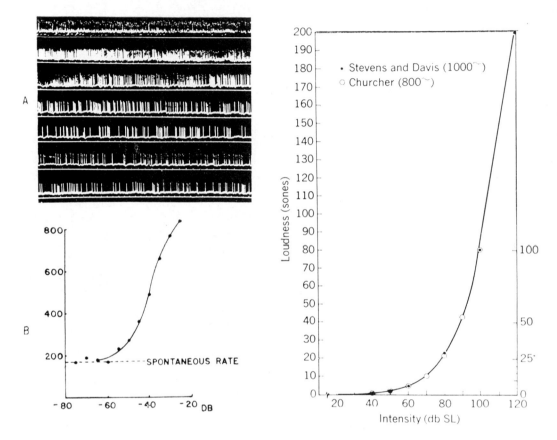

FIG. 42–15.   Effects of sound intensity on subjective loudness (right) and auditory nerve fiber firing rate (left). The shapes of the curves are similar, but the dynamic range of the single auditory nerve fiber is much narrower than that of the auditory system as a whole. Above the auditory nerve firing rate curve are shown single-fiber responses to sounds of progressively increasing intensity. (Subjective loudness curve from Gulick, W. L.: *Hearing, Physiology and Psychophysics.* New York, Oxford University Press, 1971; auditory nerve curve from Katsuki, Y., *et al.*: J. Neurophysiol., *21*:569, 1958.)

The basic acoustic parameters to be coded are *intensity, frequency,* and *temporal pattern.* The basic parameters available for neural coding are *place, amount* of neural firing, and *temporal pattern* of firing. In this section we shall discuss cochlear coding of intensity and frequency.

Intensity Coding. "Loudness" is the approximate subjective correlate of sound intensity. It is generally assumed that the neural correlate of loudness is "amount" of nervous activity; amount means the total number of action potentials delivered by a population of nerve fibers. Thus, loudness is coded as a combination of the number of fibers firing and the rate at which they are firing.

Figure 42–15 compares plots of sound intensity versus single auditory nerve fiber firing rate, and sound intensity versus subjective loudness. The agreement in the general shapes of the curves supports the view that amount of auditory nerve firing codes loudness. However, on closer scrutiny, we note that firing rate changes only over a 20-dB sound intensity range, whereas loudness varies over a 100-dB range.[109, p. 79] This does not disprove the amount of firing code for loudness, since increasing sound intensity causes more auditory units to fire. However, it does require that the neural code emphasize the number of units firing.

Frequency Coding. *Classic Theories.* Two opposing theories of frequency coding in the auditory periphery were proposed in the late nineteenth century. These theories have had a fundamental influence on subsequent thinking about cochlear frequency coding. *Helmholtz's place theory*[95] held that the basilar membrane acts as if it were a series of tuned resonators, analogous to a set of piano strings. Each tuned resonator vibrates sympathetically to a different frequency and thus selectively stimulates a particular nerve fiber. *Rutherford's frequency theory,* later termed *telephone theory,*[179] proposed that all frequencies activate the entire length of the basilar membrane, which transmits, essentially unchanged, the temporal pattern of the auditory stimulus. It then remains for more central neural structures to "decode" the acoustic parameters.

Evidence for Place Coding. Von Bekesy used optical methods to make the first direct observations of *mechanical place analysis* of frequency in the cochlea.[14, p. 19] Recent observations with more sensitive techniques (Mosbauer, capacitive-probe, and fuzziness detection under laser illumination) have confirmed the general nature of von Bekesy's results (although probably differing in several as yet unresolved details) and extended his observations to lower sound intensities.[116,169,225]

Figure 42–16 illustrates the mechanical response which von Bekesy observed. Each pure tone cycle elicits a traveling wave that moves along the cochlear partition from base to apex.[14, pp. 448,461,462] As it travels, the wave's amplitude increases slowly, passes through a maximum, then declines rapidly (Fig. 42–16, *A*). Tones of progressively higher frequencies elicit traveling waves with maximum amplitude points located progressively closer to the oval window. The inset at the bottom of Figure 42–16, *B* shows how this traveling wave pattern causes each cochlear partition point to respond maximally to a different stimulus frequency. Fall-off of vibration amplitude is gradual when frequency is reduced below the maximum and abrupt when frequency is increased above it.

Although von Bekesy supported the general concept of frequency place coding envisaged by Helmholtz, he disproved Helmholtz's tuned resonator concept of the place coding mechanism with the following observations:

1. A singe, sharp, cochlear partition displacement causes only a brief, highly damped oscillation.[14, pp. 460,643] A series of tuned resonators would be expected to continue ringing for an appreciably longer time.

2. The basilar membrane is not under transverse tension, as would be expected if it functioned as a series of tuned resonators.[14, pp. 465,472,643]

3. The asymmetrical traveling wave pattern is completely unlike the pattern that a series of tuned resonators would produce.[14, p. 494]

The mechanism by which cochlear mechanical place coding is achieved is imperfectly understood. However, the basilar membrane's physical properties play a crucial role; it is nearly a hundred times stiffer at the base than at the apex, and its width increases systematically from base to apex.[14, pp. 467,468,476]

Microelectrode recordings of single-fiber action potentials provide evidence that further supports the frequency place coding theory. As shown in Figure 42–17, plots of single auditory nerve fiber thresholds against sound frequency yield *neural frequency response areas* that resemble inverted cochlear mechanical tuning curves.[106,109,201] Such curves would be expected if the cochlear partition place code were transferred intact into the central nervous system.

Sharpening of the Mechanical Place Code. One difficulty with a strict place code theory is that tuning of the cochlear partition points is not nearly sharp enough to account for our subjective ability to discriminate sound frequencies. Below 2k Hz, the subjective frequency difference limen is about 3 Hz; above 2k Hz, it is about 2 to 3% of the base frequency.[184] The mechanical tuning shown in Figure 42–16 is obviously not this sharp. Thus, a place code theory must postulate "sharpening" of cochlear mechanical tuning curves. There is good evidence that

such sharpening does occur, both in the cochlea itself and in the central nervous system.

Figure 42–17 compares mechanical and neural tuning curves. Neural and mechanical curves show the same general shape (gradual low-frequency cutoff and sharp high-frequency cutoff), but the neural curves tend to be more sharply tuned than the mechanical curves.[65,194] The mechanism of this cochlear sharpening is not known. However, at least in part, it may be a mechanical process. To understand this process, we must look at the cochlear partition vibration pattern in more detail.

For clarity, we have discussed shearing between the tectorial membrane and the reticular lamina as if it occurred only in the radial direction (across the organ of Corti). In actuality, however, both longitudinal and radial shearing occur. Figure 42–18, *A* diagrams the three-dimensional displacement pattern of the uncoiled cochlear partition at one instant during traveling wave propagation.[207] At the amplitude maximum, the curvature is primarily across the cochlea (arrows labeled *Ra*); hence, at this point, most of the shearing action is radial, as illustrated in Figure 42–11. However, apicalward from the amplitude maximum,

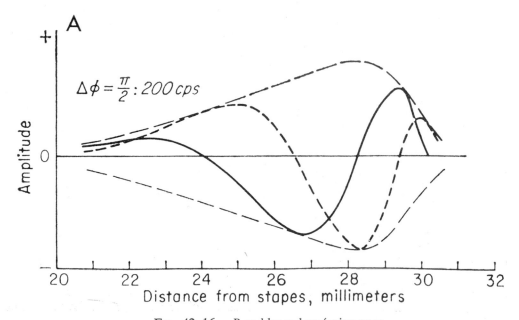

FIG. 42–16.   *B and legend on facing page.*

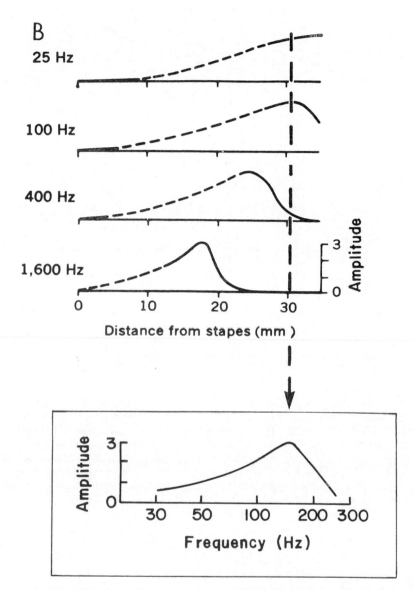

FIG. 42–16.   Mechanical place coding in the cochlea. *A,* The traveling wave response of the cochlear partition to a pure tone stimulus. The solid and dashed lines show the cochlear partition's displacement patterns at two successive instants within one cycle. The lines with the longer dashes are drawn through displacement maxima and therefore show the traveling wave's envelope. *B,* The top four curves are envelopes of traveling wave responses to pure tone stimuli of varying frequencies. Each envelope depicts only the upper half of the envelope traced in *A.* At bottom, the response of a single cochlear partition point approximately 30 mm from the stapes (indicated by the vertical dashed line) is plotted against frequency. This is the mechanical tuning curve of this point. (Von Bekesy, G.: *Experiments in Hearing.* New York, McGraw-Hill, 1960.)

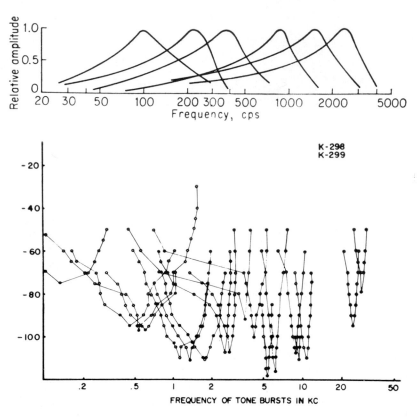

Fig. 42–17. Mechanical and neural tuning curves. The mechanical tuning curves (above) were obtained from fresh human temporal bone preparations at various cochlear partition positions, as shown in Figure 42–16 *A*. The neural tuning curves (below) were obtained from single auditory nerve fibers of cats. "Thresholds" are the sound intensities at which spike discharge rate noticeably increased above the spontaneous firing rate. Even allowing for horizontal scale differences, the neural tuning curves at high frequencies are noticeably sharper than the mechanical tuning curves. (Mechanical curves from Von Bekesy, G.: *Experiments in Hearing*. New York, McGraw-Hill, 1960; neural curves from Kiang, N. Y. S.: *Discharge Patterns of Single Fibers in the Cat's Auditory Nerve*. Cambridge, Mass., M.I.T. Press, 1965.)

the curvature, hence most of the shearing, is longitudinal (arrows labeled *Lo*). Figure 42–18, *B* shows cochlear shear movements during traveling wave propagation, actually observed by von Bekesy.[14, p. 497] The longitudinal shear is apicalward from the radial shear, as expected from the pattern shown in Figure 42–18, *A*.

At the tectorial membrane's inner border, longitudinal shear is more effective in producing an electrical hair cell response, whereas radial shear is more effective at the tectorial membrane's outer border.[14, p. 707] Therefore, the inner hair cells are probably sensitive to longitudinal rather than radial

shear. As discussed above, inner hair cells also respond to cochlear partition velocity rather than displacement. Mathematical treatments of cochlear partition traveling wave patterns suggest that both longitudinal[108] and velocity displacement[194] patterns are more narrowly tuned than the transverse displacement tuning curves illustrated in Figures 42–16 and 42–17. Therefore, if the neural tuning curves shown in Figure 42–17 come from inner hair cell units, we would expect them to be sharper than the mechanical tuning curves. Since the large majority of auditory nerve fibers come from inner hair cells, it is not unreasonable to assume

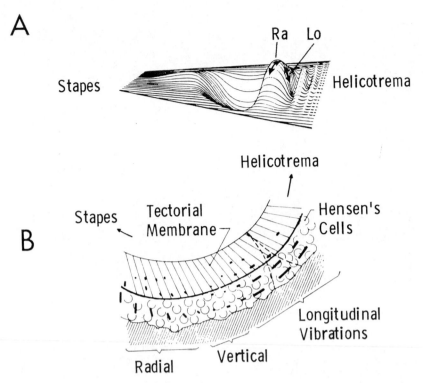

FIG. 42–18.   Longitudinal and radial shearing movements in the cochlear partition. *A*, Three-dimensional displacement pattern of the cochlear partition at one instant during traveling wave propagation. The cochlear partition is uncoiled. The area of maximal radial (across the cochlea) shearing is shown by the arrows labeled *Ra*. The area of maximal longitudinal shearing is shown by the arrows labeled *Lo*. Maximal longitudinal shearing is toward the helicotrema from maximal radial shearing. *B*, Radial and longitudinal shearing movements in guinea pig organ of Corti. View is through Reissner's membrane. Solid lines on tectorial membrane and Hensen's cells show vibrations of these structures relative to the basilar membrane. As expected, longitudinal shearing is apicalward from radial shearing. (*A* from Tonndorf, J.: *In* Rasmussen, G. L., and Windle, W. F. (Eds.): *Neural Mechanisms of the Auditory and Vestibular Systems.* Springfield, Ill., Charles C Thomas Publisher, 1960, pp. 91–104; *B* from Von Bekesy, G.: *Experiments in Hearing.* New York, McGraw-Hill, 1960.)

that most published neural tuning curves come from inner hair cell units.

The effect of varying stimulus frequency on cochlear microphonic and summating potential amplitude, shown in Figure 42–19, supports the above-outlined mechanical explanation of cochlear sharpening.[35] The cochlear potentials were recorded from the basilar turn. The changes in cochlear microphonic voltage parallel fairly closely the cochlear partition's displacement response in the basilar turn (Fig. 42–16). The narrowed, apically displaced, summating potential frequency response area is predictable if (1)

inner hair cells generate the summating potential (at this sound intensity, they probably generate most of it[35]), and (2) the inner hair cells respond to longitudinal velocity shearing rather than radial displacement shearing.

The auditory place code is probably sharpened not only mechanically but also neurally by a mechanism known as "lateral inhibition." Figure 42–20 illustrates the principle of response area sharpening by lateral inhibition. Each neuron inhibits neurons coming from adjacent areas of the basilar membrane ("receptor surface").

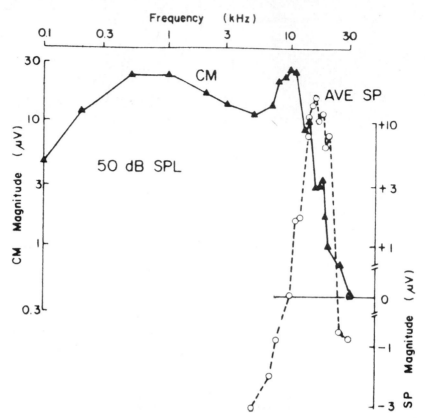

FIG. 42–19. Effect of stimulus frequency on cochlear microphonic (CM) and summating potential (SP) amplitude, recorded with basilar turn electrodes across the cochlear partition (guinea pig). (Dallos, P.: *In* Møller, A. R. (Ed.): *Basic Mechanisms in Hearing.* New York, Academic Press, 1973, pp. 335–372.)

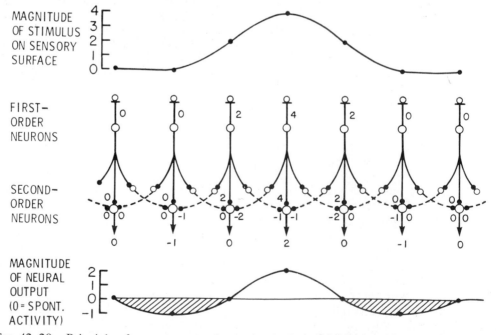

FIG. 42–20. Principle of response area sharpening by lateral inhibition. Numbers by the neural units indicate magnitude of neural activity. Dashed lines indicate inhibitory neurons. It is assumed that the response of inhibitory neurons is 50% of the response of excitatory neurons.

Neurons from the maximally stimulated area inhibit their neighbors more strongly than their neighbors inhibit them. Hence, neurons at the periphery of the stimulated area are inhibited, and the output tends to localize to the center of the stimulated area.

Figure 42–21 demonstrates sharpening of an auditory frequency response area by lateral inhibition.[92] The shaded frequency-intensity areas define the sound stimuli that reduced the unit's spontaneous activity. These inhibitory areas surround the excited area, as would be expected if lateral neural inhibition were occurring.

Sharpening of the frequency place code in the auditory system is an example of neural contrast enhancement by lateral in-

hibition, which appears to be a general operating principle of sensory systems.

Psychophysical Estimates of the Place Code. Figure 42–22 compares cochlear partition displacement maxima[14, p. 442,232] (Fig. 42–16) with three psychophysical estimates of the frequency place code. The psychophysical estimates are based on (1) quantitative pitch measurements[196] (assuming that subjective difference in pitch is related to distance along basilar membrane), (2) integration of frequency difference limina[195] (assuming that a frequency difference limen represents a constant distance along the basilar membrane), and (3) critical bandwidth of masking noise[72] (assuming that a critical band constitutes a constant basilar mem-

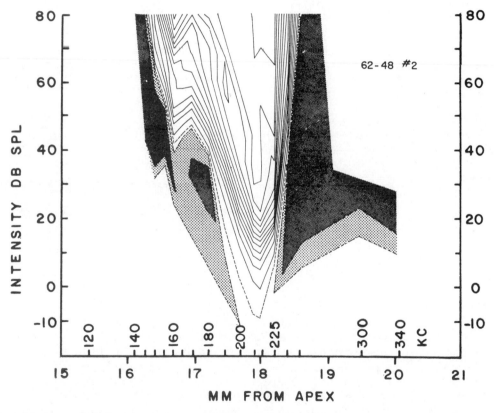

FIG. 42–21.   Inhibitory regions surrounding the excitatory frequency response area of a single unit in the cat cochlear nuclear complex. The crosshatched areas show regions in which spontaneous activity was suppressed by three standard deviations. The dotted areas show regions in which activity was suppressed by one to three standard deviations. The dashed line shows threshold and is comparable to the neural tuning curves shown in Figure 42–17. The solid lines inside the neural tuning curve trace frequency-intensity combinations that evoked the same number of spikes. (Greenwood, D. D., and Maruyama, N.: J. Neurophysiol., *24*:863, 1965.)

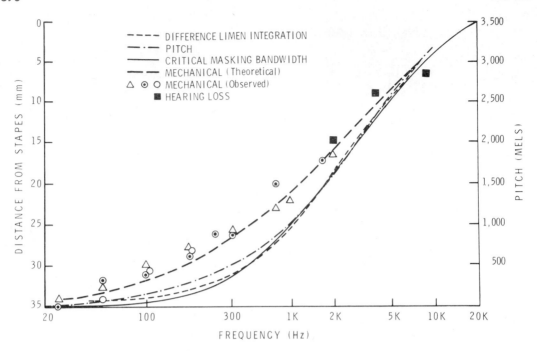

FIG. 42–22. Psychophysical estimates and mechanical observations of the cochlear frequency place code in man. Particularly for low frequencies, the psychophysical estimates (difference limen integration,[195] pitch,[196] and critical masking bandwidth[72]) tend to be displaced away from the stapes (toward the helicotrema) from points of maximum mechanical movement. The mechanical maxima refer to transverse displacement, as plotted in Figure 42–16, *A*. The mechanical place code plot includes three different observations of mechanical maxima and a theoretical treatment based on known mechanical properties of the cochlear partition.[232] Also plotted are three points obtained by correlating hearing losses with histologic cochlear damage.[33]

brane distance). The similarity in general shape of the psychophysical and mechanical curves provides some evidence in favor of a frequency place code. However, the psychophysically estimated places are displaced toward the helicotrema from the vibration maxima. This apical displacement would be partly explained if velocity and longitudinal shear maxima rather than amplitude maxima constituted the frequency place code. However, an alternative explanation (discussed below) is that the psychophysical estimates' underlying assumption (i.e., that all audio frequencies are place-coded) is incorrect.

Evidence for Telephone Coding. The above-cited evidence for place coding has not invalidated Rutherford's telephone theory,[179] because there is also considerable evidence for a telephone code, particularly at low frequencies. For example, critical

inspection of the mechanical and neural tuning curves in Figure 42–17 discloses that both neural and mechanical tuning become progressively poorer as frequency is lowered, and below about 100 Hz, there are no cochlear partition amplitude maxima and no tuned auditory units. Thus, the physiologically observed frequency place code becomes progressively worse as frequency is lowered.

A neural telephone code has been demonstrated which, in contrast to the place code, becomes progressively better as frequency is lowered. Figure 42–23, *A* shows a recording of single auditory nerve fiber spike discharges, demonstrating "phase-locking" to the individual cycles of the stimulating tone and thus preserving the temporal pattern.[80] Compiling large numbers of single-unit spikes into histograms,

A

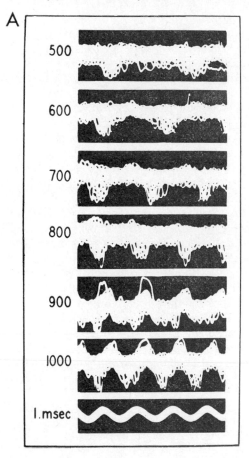

FIG. 42–23. Neurophysiologic demonstrations of telephone coding in the auditory pathway. *A*, Single auditory unit spike responses (cochlear nucleus), superimposed on cochlear microphonic response to pure tones from 500 Hz to 1k Hz. Each record is the photograph of many oscilloscope sweeps. The single unit spikes are sharp, downward deflections; the cochlear microphonics are sinusoidal curves following the lightest areas of the photographed traces. *B*, Period histograms (dotted bar graphs), showing the probability of auditory nerve fiber firing at a particular time, correlated with the waveform of a complex stimulating sound (solid line). (*A* from Galambos, R., and Davis, H.: J. Neurophysiol., *6*:39, 1943; *B* from Brugge, J. F., *et al.*: J. Neurophysiol., *32*:386, 1969.)

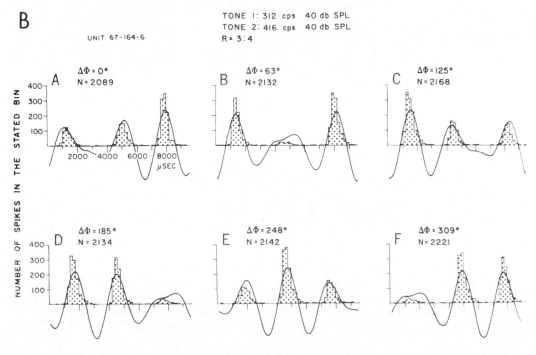

as shown in Figure 42–23, *B,* has demonstrated an impressive ability of single auditory unit discharges to reproduce the stimulating sound's waveform. Analogous waveform-reproducing whole nerve responses have been recorded.[19,130,220, p. 157] The ability to reproduce sound waveforms becomes progressively poorer as frequency is increased. The upper limit is generally estimated at about 4k Hz, but critical inspection of quantitative single-unit data suggests that phase locking becomes quite poor at around 2.5k Hz.[24,121,171]

A bit of psychophysical evidence against place coding is the fact that amplitude modulating a sound at a regular rate creates the sensation of a pitch at the frequency of amplitude modulation. Frequency analysis of the amplitude-modulated sound shows little energy at the perceived *periodicity pitch,* making its existence difficult to explain on the basis of a mechanical frequency place coder.[186] Periodicity pitch occurs only at frequencies below 1k Hz.

Another psychophysical observation arguing against place coding is that below 4k Hz, changes in phase relationship can be subjectively appreciated as changes in the quality of a complex sound and as changes in sound localization.[93, p. 195, 156,210,220, p. 404] A mechanical frequency place coder would not detect phase differences.

Figure 42–24 illustrates a recent observation that supports the existence of a telephone code for low frequencies.[142] This figure plots frequency discrimination achieved by deaf patients fitted with electrically stimulating cochlear implants. The electrical waveform follows the stimulating sound, and the stimulus is applied over most of the patient's basilar turn. Thus, the implant preserves the temporal pattern of the acoustic stimulus but does no place coding. It is therefore a "pure" telephone coder. Below 200 Hz, the patient's nervous system is able to utilize the telephone code to achieve essentially normal frequency discrimination (indicated by the horizontal solid line at 2.5

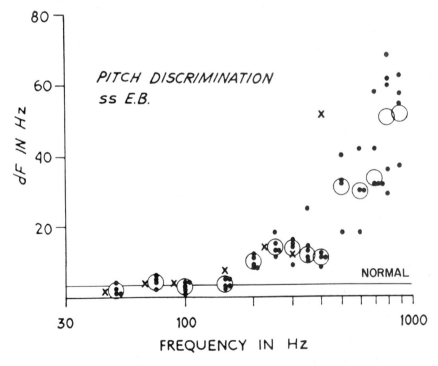

Fig. 42–24. Frequency discrimination, achieved with mass electrical stimulation of the cochleas of deaf patients. The solid horizontal line shows the approximate normal frequency difference limen (about 3 Hz). (Merzenich, M. M., *et al.*: Ann. Otol. Rhinol. Laryngol., *82:* 486, 1973.)

Hz). Between 0.2 and 1k Hz, the ability to discriminate frequency rapidly deteriorates, suggesting that a telephone code operates in the 0.2 to 1k Hz range but becomes progressively less dominant as frequency is increased.

Telephone Place Theory of Frequency Coding. In 1949, Wever published an auditory frequency coding theory which he termed the *volley* theory but which has since become known as the *telephone place* or *frequency place* theory. Currently, this is probably the most influential of the viable theories of hearing. It states that low frequencies (below 400 Hz) are telephone-coded and that high frequencies (above 4000 Hz) are place-coded; in the middle-frequency range (400–4000 Hz), the auditory system utilizes place and telephone information to discriminate frequencies.[220,221]

Since the maximum "driven" firing rate of a single auditory unit is only 150 to 250 action potentials per second,[109, p. 83, 175] the telephone place theory must account for the ability of the system to telephone-code 4000-Hz tones. To do so, it invokes the "volley" principle, which states that individual auditory units always fire at the same point in the stimulus cycle but skip several cycles. Thus, the entire responding fiber population produces a burst ("volley") of action potentials at each stimulus cycle, but different fibers contribute to different volleys.[220, p. 166] Above 4000 Hz, the volley mechanism fails, and the peripheral auditory system can no longer generate synchronized neural responses.[19]

The telephone coding hypothesis encounters some difficulty in accounting for intensity coding at low frequencies. The telephone code assumes more rapid firing as frequency is increased, but according to the generally accepted view of intensity coding, such increased firing rate ought to be perceived as increased loudness. Wever circumvented this difficulty by assuming that the intensity code is the number of impulses per individual volley.[220, p. 172]

Wever advanced an interesting evolutionary argument in support of the telephone place code theory. Primitive ears (as found in fish, amphibians, and lower reptiles) are telephone coders that cannot analyze high audio frequencies because of the inherent limitation on the rate at which nerve fibers can respond. Therefore, as evolution progressed, place coding had to be added to allow analysis of high frequencies. In Wever's words:

The evolutionary significance of the extension of range to the high tones is clear. These tones are much more serviceable than the low tones in indicating the direction as well as the character of sounds, and they provide useful information about the shape and texture of objects from which they are reflected. Therefore, they aid in the identification of enemies and possible prey, and they assist in orientation to objects in the vicinity.

Our own use of sounds in communication is greatly aided by our keen sensitivity in the region of 1000 to 4000 cycles, and though our sensitivity falls off beyond 4000 cycles, we still depend on the higher frequencies for many of our discriminations of speech and sharp transients. . . . The appearance and elaboration of the place principle for frequency representation therefore was a major event in the evolution of the ear.[221]

Inner versus Outer Hair Cell Function. It is thought that the inner and outer hair cells represent separate receptor systems. The outer hair cell system is a sensitive, low-level detecting system which has poor place coding ability (possibly the outer hair cell system also codes loudness). The inner hair cell system carries place code but is relatively insensitive. The rod (night vision) and cone (day vision) systems are possibly analogous to the outer and inner cochlear hair cell systems.

The following observations support the dual cochlear receptor system concept.

Anatomy. Figure 42–25 illustrates inner and outer hair cell anatomy. There are many consistent differences between the cell types, including (1) overall cell shape ("bottle" shape for inner hair cells, "cylindrical" shape for outer hair cells), (2) nerve endings ("chalice" shape for inner cells versus basal "bouton" shape for outer cells), and (3) arrangement of cilia. The anatomic differences support differing functions for the two cell types.[7]

The anatomic location of the inner and outer hair cells also supports the dual re-

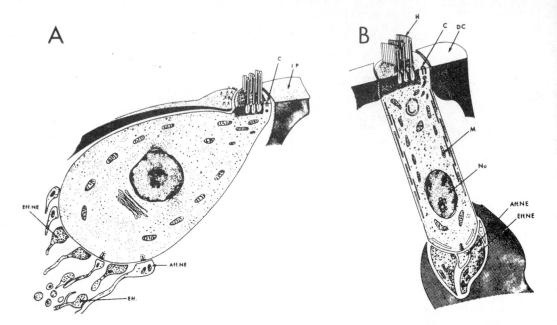

FIG. 42–25. Schematic drawing of an inner hair cell (*A*) and an outer hair cell (*B*). *C*, centriole; H, hair cell cilia; Aff. NE, afferent nerve ending; Eff. NE, efferent nerve ending; IP, inner pillar; DC, Deiters' cell; M, mitochondrion; Nu, nucleus. (Wersäll, J., *et al.*: Cold Spring Harbor Symp. Quant. Biol., *30*:115, 1965.)

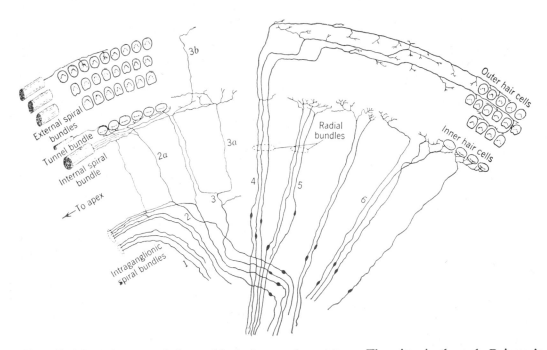

FIG. 42–26. Diagram of the cochlea's innervation pattern. The view is through Reissner's membrane, looking "down" on the organ of Corti. Principal fiber bundles are: *1* and *2*, intraganglionic spiral bundles (fibers labeled 1 are efferent olivocochlear fibers); *2a* and *3a*, internal spiral fibers; *4*, external spiral fibers, traveling in radial bundle to innervate outer hair cells; *5* and *6*, radial fibers, innervating inner hair cells. The "V" shape of the cilia pattern on the outer hair cells and the shallower "U" pattern on the inner hair cells are shown in the upper corners of the diagram. (Wever, E. G.: *Theory of Hearing.* New York, John Wiley & Sons, 1949.)

ceptor system concept. The outer hair cells are located in the center of the basilar membrane, where maximum deflections occur, while the inner hair cells are located at the edge of the basilar membrane, where they are partly protected by the osseous spiral lamina. That outer hair cells are more "exposed" to acoustic activation of the cochlea is supported by the fact that they are more susceptible to acoustic trauma.[39]

Innervation Pattern. Figure 42–26 diagrams the innervation pattern of the inner and outer hair cells.[67,126] Inner hair cell innervation via radial fibers is point-to-point, i.e., each radial fiber innervates inner hair cells covering only a small basilar membrane area. In contrast, outer hair cell innervation is diffuse, i.e., each outer spiral fiber turns basalward and travels as far as one third of a cochlear turn, giving off collaterals to outer hair cells along its entire length. Since their diffuse innervation pattern allows many hair cells to stimulate a single nerve fiber, this pattern is suited to a sensitive sensory system but cannot transmit a place code.

Transducer Mechanism. As previously discussed, the velocity-sensitive inner hair cell transducer action is better localized than the displacement-sensitive outer hair cell transducer action and hence is more likely to generate a usable place code.

EFFERENT AUDITORY SYSTEM

Anatomy

Rasmussen established the existence of a chain of descending auditory neurons which links auditory cortex to hair cells and which parallels the classic afferent projection pathway[167] (discussed in the next section). The *olivocochlear bundle,* the final link in the descending chain,[166] has two components. The "crossed bundle," comprising three fourths of the fibers, originates in the medial superior olivary nucleus, crosses the midline just beneath the floor of the fourth ventricle, and enters the vestibular nerve root. At this point, it is joined by the "uncrossed bundle," which originates in the lateral superior olive. The combined olivocochlear fibers travel in the vestibular nerve until, at the saccular portion, they cross to the auditory nerve via the *vestibulocochlear anastomosis.*[77]

At the spiral ganglion, the efferent fibers turn apicalward and form the *intraganglionic spiral bundle* (see Fig. 42–26). Efferent fibers are distributed to the cochlea from this bundle.

In the organ of Corti, the efferent endings can be distinguished from the afferent endings because they contain vesicles. The vesiculated endings synapse directly with the outer hair cells but terminate on the afferent fiber endings of the inner hair cells.[77,112, 187,192] The outer hair cell vesiculated endings are concentrated mostly in the basilar turn and thin out toward the apex. At the apex they are found only on the inner row of hair cells.[77] There are a great many efferent endings in the cochlea; hence, the olivocochlear fibers must undergo extensive terminal branching.[37]

Function

Electrical stimulation of either the crossed or the uncrossed olivocochlear bundle causes inhibition of the auditory nerve response to sound stimuli.[49,68,79] Stimulation of higher portions of the descending pathway may also inhibit transmission across higher-level afferent synapses[48,161] (see, however, Comis and Whitfield[32]). Thus, the efferent system is probably inhibitory. The fact that the efferent fiber hair cell endings are vesiculated suggests that the olivocochlear inhibitory effect is humoral. Several neuropharmacologic observations support a humoral mechanism and suggest that the mediator is acetylcholine (ACh).[51,69,167]

The role of the auditory efferent system in hearing is unknown. The small number of efferent fibers and their widespread cochlear ramifications make any sort of "place" analyzer unlikely. Since auditory stimulation activates olivocochlear fibers,[68] the system may have some sort of recurrent or "feedback" inhibitory function. The system inhibits responses to low-intensity, low-frequency acoustic signals.[49,189,224] Dewson[52] suggested that this characteristic ideally suits the efferent system to screen out low-level masking noise and thus improve perception of acoustic signals in a noisy environment. Supporting this hypothesis is the observation that the monkey's perception of masked speech sounds deteriorates after section of the olivocochlear bundle. It has also been suggested that the system may be part of the central attention mechanism, suppressing auditory input when it is desired to attend to some other sensory modality (e.g., vision).[48]

CENTRAL AUDITORY PATHWAY

Each of the five primary senses sends transduced and coded information into the brain via two separate pathways: a direct or *specific pathway* and a *nonspecific pathway*. The nonspecific pathway involves structures in the core of the neuraxis, collectively known as the *reticular system*. In the reticular system, all sensory modalities share the same gross neural structures (hence the name "nonspecific"). Ascent via the nonspecific structures is multisynaptic and hence is characterized by long delay times.

The direct pathways for each sensory modality are separate and involve long axonal processes, with a minimal number of synapses; hence, compared to the indirect pathway, transmission along the direct pathways involves minimal delay times. The synapses of the direct pathways tend to congregate in well-defined neural structures called *nuclei*.

Clinically, lesions of the central auditory system are localized according to their level in the direct projection pathway. Therefore, our discussion will emphasize this pathway.

Anatomy

Figure 42–27 diagrams the direct auditory projection pathway. The numbers in each nucleus indicate neuronal "order" (determined by the number of synapses). The auditory projection pathway is more complex than the pathways of other sensory systems, possibly because it developed relatively late on the phylogenetic scale and had to incorporate bits and pieces of other already-developed neuronal systems. However, the following general principles should

clarify the pathway's more important characteristics.[77]

1. All cochlear nucleus input is ipsilateral; at all higher levels, representation is bilateral.

2. The cochlear nucleus (except possibly dorsal cochlear nucleus) contains second-order neurons; brain stem nuclei contain third- and fourth-order neurons, and thalamocortical neurons are fourth- and fifth-order.

3. No axons bypass the cochlear nucleus, medial geniculate, and (possibly) inferior colliculus.

4. The contralateral pathway tends to contain lower order neurons than the ipsilateral pathway because many contralateral second-order neurons bypass the superior olive, whereas no ipsilateral neurons do so.[88,158,215]

Internal Organization of the Direct Projection Pathway

Neuronal Population. Table 42–1 lists the number of neurons at different levels of the projection pathway (estimated by a sampling method).[26] Neuronal populations in the projection pathway increase dramatically as the pathway is ascended.[4,5,84,170,172,213,227]

Tonotopic Organization. Both neurophysiologic and anatomic observations show that cochlear place is represented in an orderly way throughout the projection pathway. Figure 42–28 shows neurophysiologic demonstrations of tonotopic organization in the cochlear nucleus[172] and inferior colliculus.[173] As the electrodes penetrate the nuclei, they encounter neural units with restricted frequency response areas, whose

Table 42–1. Estimates of Neuronal Populations at Various Levels of the Auditory Projection Pathway

Auditory nerve	31,000
Cochlear nuclei	88,000
Inferior colliculus	392,000
Medial geniculate	422,000
Auditory cortex	10,200,000

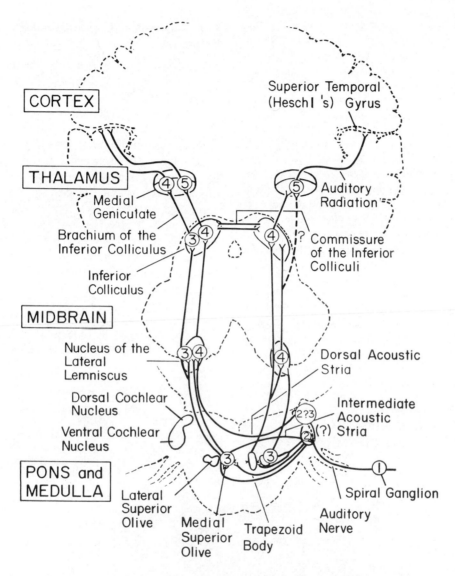

CORTEX

Superior Temporal
(Heschl 's) Gyrus

THALAMUS
Medial
Genicuate

Auditory
Radiation

Brachium of the
Inferior Colliculus

Commissure
of the Inferior
Colliculi

Inferior
Colliculus

MIDBRAIN

Nucleus of the
Lateral
Lemniscus

Dorsal Acoustic
Stria

Dorsal Cochlear
Nucleus

Intermediate
Acoustic
(?) Stria

Ventral Cochlear
Nucleus

PONS and
MEDULLA

Spiral Ganglion

Lateral
Superior
Olive

Auditory
Nerve

Medial
Superior
Olive

Trapezoid
Body

Fig. 42–27. Diagram of the direct auditory projection pathway. Numbers indicate approximate neuron "order," as determined by the number of synapses traversed. Dashed lines labeled with question marks indicate two areas of uncertainty: (1) whether the dorsal cochlear nucleus primarily contains second- or third-order neurons; and (2) whether any nerve fibers bypass the inferior colliculus.

best frequencies progress in an orderly fashion from low to high or from high to low.

Multiple Representation of the Receptor Surface. Figure 42–28 demonstrates not only tonotopic organization but also "multiple representation." Note, for example, that in the cochlear nucleus (Fig. 42–28, *A*) there are two breaks in the orderly progression of best frequencies (indicated by heavy lines between best frequency numbers). In the inferior colliculus (Fig. 42–28, *B*), a similar break occurs at the boundary between the external (*ex*) and central (*C*) nuclei. Electrical stimulation of discrete cochlear locations evokes responses at several discrete primary auditory cortex locations, thus providing further evidence for multiple tonotopic representation of the cochlea in the projection pathway.

Multiple representation of the receptor surface in the direct projection pathway occurs in all sensory systems. Nerve fiber branching is probably the anatomic basis of this multiple representation.[125] The number of receptor surfaces represented probably increases as the pathway is ascended. At least three cochleas are represented in the cochlear nucleus,[170] while at least six cochleas are represented in the auditory cortex.[227]

Auditory-Evoked Electrophysiologic Responses

In most neurophysiology laboratories, microelectrode recording of action potentials generated by one or a few neurons has, in recent years, supplanted the classic technique of recording from many synchronously responding neurons with a gross electrode. Recently, however, averaging techniques have made it possible to record from humans, with surface electrodes, gross, synchronized, electrical responses reflecting the entire auditory pathway, from cochlea to cortex.[29,104,122,131,163] The potential clinical applications of this technique have revived the importance of the classic gross electrode observations. Since recording techniques and general clinical significance are the same for all human auditory electrophysiologic responses, we shall include in this discussion responses occurring before (cochlea and au-

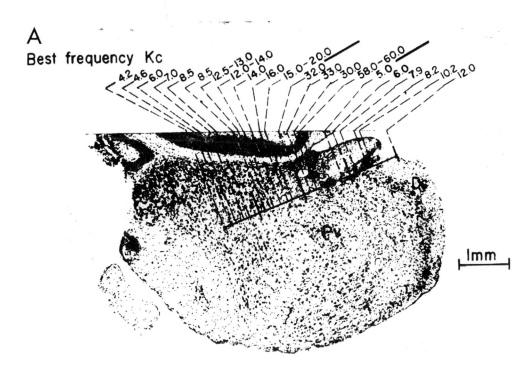

FIG. 42–28. *B and legend on facing page.*

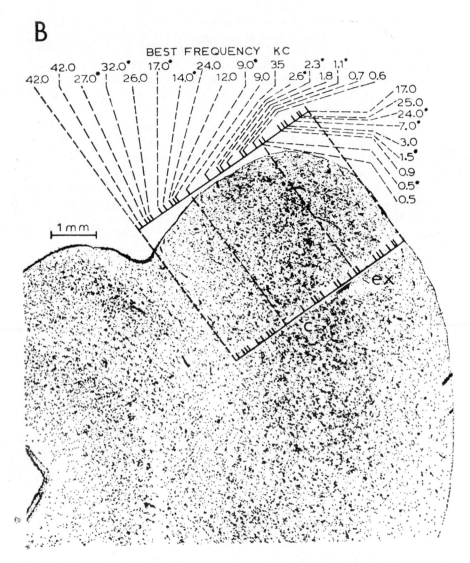

Fig. 42–28. Neurophysiologic demonstrations of tonotopic organization in the cochlear nucleus (*A*) and inferior colliculus (*B*) of the cat. In each photomicrograph, a solid line through the nucleus indicates the pathway of a microelectrode. Dashed lines intersect each electrode tract, indicating where single units were encountered. The dashed lines point to numbers, indicating the unit's best frequency. In both nuclei, best frequencies change in an orderly fashion, except for "breaks," indicated by heavy lines between best-frequency numbers in the cochlear nucleus and between the external (ex) and central (C) nuclei of the inferior colliculus. (*A* from Rose, J. E., *et al.*: Bull. Johns Hopkins Hosp., *104*:211, 1959; *B* from Rose, J. E., *et al.*: J. Neurophysiol., *26*:294, 1963.)

ditory nerve) and after (myogenic and vertex) direct projection pathway responses.

Auditory Nerve Action Potentials. In animals, a synchronized auditory nerve action potential, elicited with an impulsive acoustic stimulus (either a broad-band "click" or a narrower-band "tone pip"), can be recorded with an electrode anywhere on the temporal bone.[30,177] However, the preferred electrode location is either directly on the auditory nerve or on the round window. Human auditory nerve action potentials, cochlear microphonics, and summating potentials are recorded clinically, either with an electrode on the external auditory canal wall[30,62,229] or with a transtympanic needle,[8,61] with the tip resting on the promontory. In clinical application, this technique is known as *electrocochleography* (ECochG).

Figure 42–29 shows human and cat auditory nerve action potential and cochlear microphonic responses to a click stimulus.[30] The auditory nerve action potential has two negative peaks (N_1 and N_2). Each peak is about 1 msec in duration. The amplitude of N_2 is always less than that of N_1. Increasing stimulus intensity reduces action potential latency and increases amplitude. The action potential can be distinguished from the cochlear microphonic because it is "masked" (i.e., its amplitude is reduced) by the simultaneous presentation of a continuous sound (white noise is the most efficient masker). Increasing stimulus rate to above about 10/sec also reduces action potential amplitude but leaves microphonic amplitude unaffected.[30,47]

Central Auditory-Evoked Responses. Figures 42–30 and 42–31 show click- or tone pip-evoked potentials from more cen-

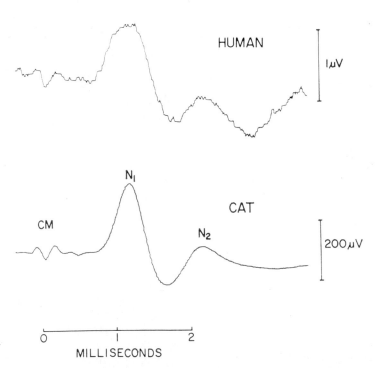

FIG. 42–29.   Averaged click-evoked auditory nerve action potentials, recorded from human (needle electrode in external canal) and cat (silver ball electrode on round window). Plotter gain was adjusted to produce equal N_1 amplitudes. CM is cochlear microphonic response to the click. N_1 and N_2 are the two negative peaks of the action potential. Click intensity was 55 dB re normal threshold. The record from the human was obtained by averaging 1024 responses and that from the cat by averaging 20 responses. (Coats, A. C., and Dickey, J. R.: Ann. Otol. Rhinol. Laryngol., *79*:844, 1970.)

tral locations in the human auditory system. All of these responses can be recorded with a vertex electrode, referred to an electrode located anywhere on the lower half of the head (the earlobe is a common location).

Figure 42–30 compares latencies of the very early series of peaks (labeled II through VI) with peak latencies of evoked responses recorded directly from animals' auditory projections pathways.[1,48,50,105,152,176,193,228] This comparison suggests that this very early wave complex comes from the lower auditory projection pathway (cochlear nucleus

to inferior colliculus). Clinical application of the very early response has been termed *brain stem audiometry*.

The middle-latency response, labeled N_0, P_0, etc. (Fig. 42–31), occurs between 8 and 40 msec after the stimulus and probably is a combination of auditory-cortex and scalp-muscle responses.[16,134,163]

The relatively high-amplitude, late response, labeled P_1, N_1, etc. (commonly called the *vertex potential*), occurs between 50 and 250 msec after the stimulus. It is a cortical response, but its latency is much too

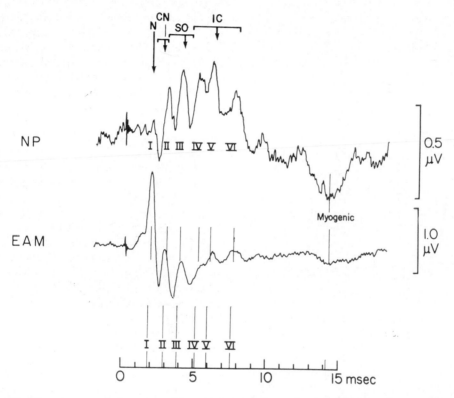

FIG. 42–30. Averaged human click-evoked auditory nerve action potential (EAM) and brain stem response (NP). The auditory nerve action potential was recorded with a needle electrode in the external auditory meatus, and the brain stem response was recorded with a nasopharyngeal electrode. Roman numerals identify the auditory nerve peak (I) and the generally recognized brain stem peaks (II-VI). Upward deflection represents negativity at the active electrode. Click intensity was about 50 dB re normal threshold. The crossbars over the brain stem response compare peak latencies of published cat brain stem auditory-evoked responses with the waveform of the human evoked response. Peak latency values were adjusted to a "normalized" N_1 latency of 1.7 msec (N) where auditory nerve action potentials were included. CN, SO, and IC are evoked responses from cochlear nucleus, superior olive, and inferior colliculus, respectively. Crossbars show peak latency ranges, and arrows show means. (Martin, J. L., and Coats, A. C.: Brain Res., *60*:496, 1973.)

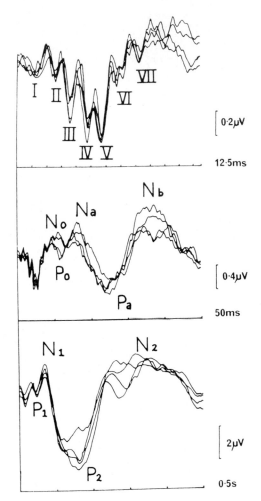

FIG. 42–31. Averaged human click-evoked potentials, recorded with vertex-mastoid electrodes. Upward deflection represents negativity at the vertex. From top to bottom, the time base is slowed to demonstrate progressively later responses. At top is the brain stem response (polarity is opposite the response recorded with a nasopharyngeal electrode); in the center is the middle latency response; and at bottom is the late "vertex" response. Each tracing represents the average of 1024 single responses. Several tracings are superimposed in each record to give an idea of variability. Roman numerals and letters identify individual peaks of the various responses according to accepted convention. (Picton, T. W., et al.: Electroencephalogr. Clin. Neurophysiol., *36*:179, 1974.)

long to come from primary auditory cortex; it comes from "associative" (probably frontal) cortex.[45,163,165]

Activity of Central Auditory Units. Although microelectrode studies of single-unit auditory activity have proliferated in the past decade, they have thus far yielded no unifying principles about the brain's data processing mechanisms. We can, however, make the following general comparisons of auditory unit function at different projection pathway levels.

Spontaneous Activity. Most single units at all projection pathway levels fire spontaneously. Units may respond to stimulation by either increasing (a *facilitory* response) or decreasing (an *inhibitory* response) their firing rates. These appear to be general operating principles of all sensory systems.

Temporal Patterns of Responses to Acoustic Stimuli. Single-unit responses become increasingly complex as the projection pathway is ascended. All primary neurons respond with an increased firing rate at the stimulus onset, followed by a gradual decline as the stimulus progresses. In contrast, central units respond with a variety of patterns—for example, a brief burst only at stimulus onset ("on-responder"), a brief burst followed by a period of inhibition followed by a sustained response ("pauser"), or a series of alternate inhibitory-facilitory responses ("chopper").[110,162] At the geniculate and cortical levels of the pathway, most units respond with an "on-responder" pattern.[24,25,59]

Response to Varying Stimulus Intensity. All peripheral units increase their firing rates when stimulus intensity is increased.[107] However, many central units demonstrate a "rollover" in their intensity versus firing rate plots. Firing rate increases with increasing intensity until a "critical" intensity is reached, after which the firing rate declines with further intensity increase.[87,173]

Localization of Sound in Space. Localization of sound in the horizontal plane provides the most straightforward relationship that has been observed between central auditory single-unit behavior and psychophysical function. Slight binaural differences in intensity and/or arrival time provide the auditory cues for localization of sound in the horizontal plane (sound lateralization). The acoustic image seems to be located on the side of the louder or earlier sound. At all levels in the auditory projection pathway above the trapezoid body, there are units that are very sensitive to binaural time and intensity differences.[20,23,24,85,174] The medial superior olive is the lowest level at which these units have been found. Since this is the first nucleus to receive converging input from both ears, it is ideally situated to make binaural comparisons.

The medial superior olivary nucleus contains transversely oriented neurons that receive exclusively ipsilateral cochlear input on one terminal dendrite and exclusively contralateral input on the opposite terminal dendrite.[197] As sound to one ear is made progressively louder or earlier than sound to the opposite ear, these units change abruptly from an inhibitory to a facilitory response.[81,85] By assuming a facilitory contralateral input and an inhibitory ipsilateral input (or vice versa), these units' neurophysiologic behavior can be explained in a straightforward way. An orderly variation in amount of ipsilateral versus contralateral inhibition from neuron to neuron would place-code binaural time-intensity differences.

Functional Deficits after Projection Pathway Lesions. *Experimental Procedures.* A typical animal experiment designed to elucidate the auditory function of a neural structure consists of (1) teaching a conditioned response that requires an auditory discrimination, (2) making the desired brain lesion, and (3) retesting to determine if the conditioned response is retained or can be relearned. Usually, the surgery abolishes the conditioned response, and the animal's ability to make the auditory discrimination is judged by its ability to relearn the response.

Pure Tone Thresholds. In both cats and monkeys, pure tone thresholds remain essentially normal after removal of virtually all auditory cortex.[157] Early work by Ades and coworkers[2] demonstrated that, in cats, localized medial geniculate lesions produced hearing losses at localized frequencies. However, the maximum losses were only about 25 dB, and in most cases were less than 15 dB. Furthermore, this study did not investigate the possibility of relearning the conditioned response. Unfortunately, there is apparently no data on pure tone threshold changes following lower brain stem lesions. However, severe auditory nerve damage produces surprisingly little change in pure tone thresholds,[153,182] so it seems likely that brain stem lesions would also produce relatively little threshold change.

Intensity Discrimination. Extensive lesions of auditory cortex leave intensity difference limina essentially normal. Bilateral ablation of the inferior colliculus or its brachium causes a slight intensity discrimination deficit.[157] Lesions at lower midbrain and pontine levels probably cause more severe intensity discrimination deficits.[120,164,178]

Frequency Discrimination. In cats, complete bilateral removal of auditory cortex produces no deficit in a simple frequency discrimination task.[55,90] In monkeys, a similar ablation reduces frequency discrimination ability, but the deficit is much more severe for high frequencies (above 4k Hz)[132] than for low frequencies (below 1k Hz).[133] In cats, section of the brachium of the inferior colliculus produces a severe, permanent frequency discrimination deficit.[89]

Temporal Pattern Discrimination. As the above discussion indicates, extensive auditory cortex ablations create very little deficit in simple auditory tasks, i.e., sound detection, and in discriminating frequency and intensity. However, in both cats and monkeys, auditory cortex ablations impair the ability to discriminate temporal patterns (e.g., a high-low-high versus a low-high-low tone burst pattern).[53,55] Possibly related to the temporal pattern deficits are observations that decorticated monkeys lose the ability to discriminate speech sounds.[54] This deficit is increased if the association cortex surrounding primary auditory cortex is also ablated.

Short-Term Auditory Memory. The early frequency discrimination experiments yielded contradictory results, and the resolution of the contradictions uncovered evidence that the auditory cortex is essential for short-term auditory memory. If several seconds elapse between different frequency stimuli, the animal is unable to relearn a frequency discrimination. If, however, the two frequencies are presented in immediate succession, the discrimination can be relearned.[90,206]

Localization of Sound in Space. Lesions at all levels of the cat's auditory projection pathway (except lesions confined to the inferior colliculus[137]) create deficits in the ability to localize sound in space. However, the nature of the deficit differs according to the level of the lesion.

If the trapezoid body is transected, the ability to discriminate interaural time differences is completely lost,[136] but only a mild deficit in sound-localizing ability is created.[154] In contrast, auditory cortex ablations create very severe deficits in sound-localizing ability[154,155,198] but do not abolish the ability to discriminate interaural time difference (although they diminish it).[135] The effects of lesions at intermediate levels of the projection pathway (lateral lemniscus[136] and brachium of the inferior colliculus[137,199]) are similar to those of cortical lesions.

These observations suggest that the superior olive encodes binaural time differences, and the higher centers integrate the encoded information with information from other sources to create a subjective "auditory space." Thus, we would expect that interrupting the major contralateral superior olive input (the trapezoid body) would abolish the animal's ability to perceive binaural time differences. However, since other cues (e.g., those provided by rotating the head and pinna) are still available, the final sound-localizing deficit is slight. In contrast, with higher lesions the animal loses its perception of auditory space and hence has a severe sound-localizing deficit. However, the low-level "binaural comparator" is still intact; hence, the animal retains a rudimentary ability to discriminate binaural time differences.

Correlation with Central Auditory Deficits in Humans. *Lateralization of Hearing Deficits.* It is a well-known clinical maxim that a central lesion involving one side of the projection pathway causes a hearing deficit in the contralateral ear. This does not correlate with the pathway's gross anatomy, since from the superior olive upward, both ears are represented on each side. However,

studies of animal auditory projection pathways provide two more subtle correlates: (1) as previously described, the contralateral path to the temporal cortex has fewer synapses, and (2) evoked responses from the contralateral pathway are consistently of higher amplitude and shorter latency than evoked responses from the ipsilateral pathway.[1,129]

Localization of Function at Different Projection Pathway Levels. The preceding discussion of the animal auditory projection pathway demonstrates that the pathway's anatomic organization, single-unit responses, and deficits produced by lesioning all become more complex as the pathway is ascended. These characteristics suggest a hierarchy of data processing tasks, with processing complexity increasing as the pathway is ascended. Audiometric deficits in humans correlate in a general way with this concept. Thus, pure tones can be used to detect a cochlear lesion, whereas simple speech materials (e.g., single words) are necessary to detect an auditory nerve or pontomedullary lesion, and considerably more complex speech materials (e.g., sentences, interfered with by a contralateral competing message) are required to detect a cerebral hemisphere lesion.[103]

VESTIBULAR APPARATUS

General Principles

The nonauditory part of the inner ear (termed the "vestibular apparatus") consists of two functional subdivisions: the *semicircular canals* (two *vertical* and one *horizontal*) and the *otolith organs* (the *saccule* and the *utricle*). The semicircular canals sense head rotation (more accurately, angular acceleration), and the otolith organs (primarily the utricle) sense head position (more accurately, linear acceleration). The function of the saccule is unknown; in higher vertebrates, it probably has minimal balance and equilibrium function and may be a low-frequency auditory receptor.[9,98,99, 140, p. 37,141,216]

Conventionally, we regard the vestibular system as one of three sensory systems that function to maintain body balance and equilibrium. The other two are the somatosensory (chiefly proprioceptive) and visual systems. Loss of proprioception (e.g., as in tabes dorsalis) or vision causes more significant balance and equilibrium difficulty than does loss of vestibular function. With bilateral vestibular function loss, difficulties occur only when one of the other systems is disrupted (e.g., as when walking in the dark or on a soft surface). Thus, in man, under physiologic conditions, the vestibular system is probably the least important of the three balance and equilibrium sensory systems. The most significant functional deficits occur when the vestibular system suffers acute, asymmetrical damage and generates "false" head position or head rotation signals.

Anatomy

Figure 42–1 illustrates the general anatomic plan of the vestibular apparatus.

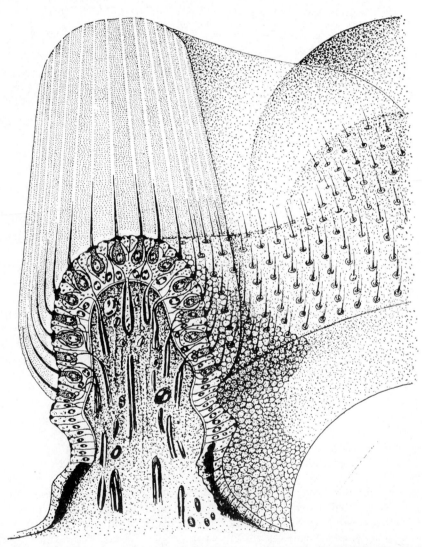

FIG. 42–32. Schematic drawing of one half of a crista and the gelatinous cupula atop it (stippled). The nerve fibers are shown ascending in the center of the crista and fanning outward to terminate at the bases of the hair cells. The sensory hairs pass from the surfaces of the hair cells into fine channels in the cupula. (Wersäll, J.: Acta Otolaryngol. (Stockh.) [Suppl.], *126*: 1, 1956.)

23

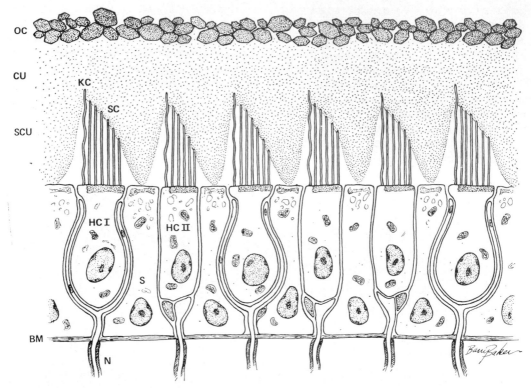

OC
CU
KC
SC
SCU
HC I
HC II
S
BM
N

Fig. 42–33. Schematic drawing of a cross section of a macula. The gelatinous substance is divided into cupular (CU) and subcupular (SCU) layers. There are two types of hairs: kinocilia, labeled KC (one per hair cell), and stereocilia, labeled SC (many per hair cell). OC, Otoconia; HC I, type I hair cell; HC II, type II hair cell; N, nerve fiber; BM, basement membrane; S, supporting cell.

There are many similarities with cochlear anatomy. For example, both end organs are located in a tunnel, hollowed out of the petrous portion of the temporal bone (embryologically, both organs come from the same tunnel), which is divided into an outer, perilymph-filled, *osseus labyrinth* and an inner, endolymph-filled, *membranous labyrinth*. Also, as in the cochlea, the receptor cells of the vestibular apparatus are ciliated, and the cilia extend into a gelatinous matrix.

The three semicircular canals are at right angles to each other. They can be thought of as lying in the lower corner of a room: the *horizontal* (or *lateral*) canal is in the plane of the floor, and the *anterior-vertical* (or *superior*) and *posterior-vertical* (or *posterior*) canals are in the planes of the two walls. In man, the entire canal complex is tilted upward about 30 degrees. In the physiologic position, the head is bent forward about 30 degrees; therefore, the 30-degree upward tilt puts the horizontal canal in the horizontal position under everyday conditions.

The semicircular canals' sensory organs (*cristae*) are located in enlarged areas at one end of each canal (*ampullae*). Figure 42–32 shows the anatomy of the crista. It is a saddle-shaped mound of tissue, attached to the ampulla's wall. The hair cells are on the mound's surface. The ampullar nerve fibers travel through the center of the crista to synapse at the hair cell bases. The hair cell cilia protrude from the crista's surface into a gelatinous mass called the *cupula*. The cupula covers the top of the crista and extends to the opposite ampullar wall.

The *sacculus* and *utriculus* are two sacs in the membranous labyrinth, located in the *vestibule* (entrance) portion of the inner

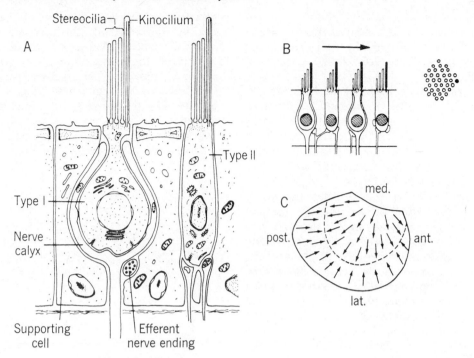

FIG. 42–34.　Microanatomy of the vestibular hair cells. *A*, Schematic drawing of two hair cell types. *B*, Diagram showing morphologic polarization of the hair cells. Arrow shows direction of cilia bending that produces excitation. At right is a cross section through the hair-bearing end of the hair cell, showing many stereocilia (open circles) and one kinocilium (filled circle). *C*, A diagrammatic surface view of the human utricular macula. Arrows indicate direction of polarization. Dashed line is the linea alba. (*A* from Brodal, A.: *Neurological Anatomy in Relation to Clinical Medicine.* New York, Oxford University Press, 1969; *B* and *C* from Lindeman, H. H. and also from Wersäll, J., *et al.*: *In* de Reuck, A. V. S., and Knight, J. (Eds.): *Myotatic, Kinesthetic and Vestibular Mechanisms.* Boston, Little, Brown and Co., 1967, pp.105–120.)

ear. Their receptor organs, called *maculae,* can be seen in Figure 42–1 as patches of epithelium on the membranous labyrinth wall. Figure 42–33 shows the macula's structure. It consists of hair cells, surrounded by supporting cells. The hair cell cilia are attached to a gelatinous membrane. On the top of the gelatinous membrane is a layer of calcium carbonate concretions called otoliths.* The otoliths are the densest structures in the inner ear.

Figure 42–34 summarizes two important facts about hair cell morphology which electron microscope observations have provided. First, as shown by Figure 42–34, *A,* there are two types of hair cells in both the macula and the crista.[218,219] *Type I hair cells*

* *Nomina Anatomica* lists "statoconia" as standard nomenclature, but "otoliths" is the most widely used term among clinicians.

are bottle-shaped and have "chalice"-type nerve endings that surround all but the hair-bearing end. *Type II hair cells* have a cylindrical shape and have several small nerve endings only at the cell's base. Type I hair cells are concentrated in the apex of the crista and the central part of the macula; type II hair cells are concentrated in the remaining end organ areas.[191,217]

The electron microscope has also demonstrated two types of cilia: *kinocilia* and *stereocilia*[191] (Fig. 42–34, *B*). Each hair cell has only one kinocilium and a bundle of 60 to 100 stereocilia. Stereocilia are homogeneous, clublike rods, with dense roots extending deep into the cuticular plate. Kinocilia are relatively flexible and end in a well-defined *basal body,* located just beneath the hair cell membrane. Within each kinocilium, there are nine peripheral filaments, arranged regularly around two central filaments. This nine-plus-two pattern is found in many motile cilia (e.g., respiration epithelia, oviduct epithelium, unicellular flagellates).[191]

On each hair cell, the single kinocilium is located to one side of the bundle of stereocilia. In both maculae and cristae, hair cells in the same area tend to have kinocilia on the same side of the stereocilia bundle. Thus, the vestibular sensory epithelium has a morphologic "directional polarization."[218, 219] Figure 42–34, C illustrates the directional polarization of the utricular macula. The kinocilia all tend to point toward a line running across the macula's approximate center, called the *linea alba*. In the saccule, the kinocilia point away from the linea alba. In the horizontal canal crista, kinocilia point toward the utricle, while in the vertical crista, they point away from the utricle. Thus, vertical and horizontal cristae are morphologically polarized in opposite directions.[191]

Transduction and Coding

Mechanical Events. As in the cochlea, the final mechanical event in vestibular ap-

paratus transduction is **bending of the hair cell cilia.** Figure 42–35 illustrates transduction by the macula. When the macular surface is tilted, the heavy otoliths tend to slide downward, carrying the gelatinous membrane and attached hairs with them.

Figure 42–36 illustrates transduction by the cupula. When the head rotates, the endolymph's inertia causes movement relative to the canal walls and cupula. The endolymph

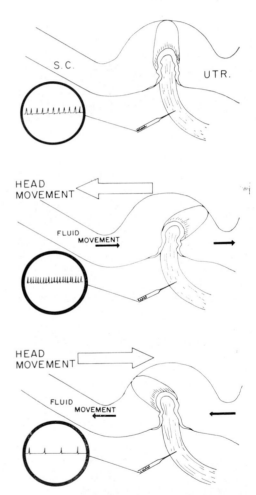

FIG. 42–36. Conversion of head rotation to bending of hair cell cilia by the crista and cupula. Arrows show direction of endolymph movement. Also shown is the effect of this bending on horizontal ampullar nerve firing rate. A microelectrode is inserted into a representative nerve fiber, and the oscilloscope record of the fiber's action potentials is shown to the left. S.C., semicircular canal; UTR, opening into utriculus.

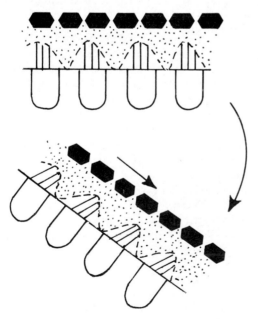

FIG. 42–35. Conversion of head tilt to bending of hair cell cilia by the macula (diagrammatic representation).

Physiolog

The c
of the v
However
ferior nu
significar
bellum.
ceives ir
but this
sparse. '
fore app
lar func

Cortical

Whet
a direct
controv
lary to
can co
to vest
has ge
subject
stimula
motor
is diff
mary
power

Ex
tion
strate
tical
monk
adjac
sory
fore
cated
area
Deel
the
the
proj
the
the
the

Ve

vess
aff
at
co
dis

pushes the cupula, which swings like a trap-door, carrying the embedded cilia with it.[58] There may be a space between the crista surface and the cupula, suggesting that the cupula also slides along the crista surface, thus adding a shearing action.

Bioelectric Events. Several observations suggest that vestibular electrophysiologic events, analogous to cochlear electrophysiologic events, accompany vestibular transduction.[181,211,212] In both the semicircular canals and the otolith organs, there is a constant potential of about 8 to 20 μV across the hair-bearing ends of the hair cells, with the endolymph side positive and the perilymph side negative. This is exactly analogous to the endocochlear potential's polarity and distribution. Thus, although the vestibular resting potential is much smaller than the endocochlear potential, it may well have an analogous function.

Cupular deviation modulates the ampullar resting potential in much the same way as bending of cochlear hair cell cilia modulates the endocochlear potential to produce cochlear microphonics and summating potentials. The effect of direction of cupular deflection on this modulation differs in the vertical and horizontal canals. In the horizontal canal, bending the cupula toward the utricle (utriculopetal) decreases the resting potential, and bending it away from the utricle (utriculofugal) increases the resting potential. In the vertical canal, this directional effect is exactly opposite. Thus, we observe a bioelectric analog of the crista's morphologic polarization.

Stimulating the macula by tilting the head modifies the macular DC potential in a way exactly analogous to crista stimulation.[212] Flöck's[74] extensive studies of hair cell receptor potentials in fish lateral line organs argue strongly that bending of hair cell cilia, with resultant generation of a graded receptor potential, is a general operating principle of hair cell mechanoreceptors of all types.

Neural Output. Figure 42–36 illustrates the neural output of the semicircular canals. Most ampullar nerve fibers fire continuously when the head is at rest (the *resting discharge*). The resting discharge is increased by bending the hair cell cilia in one direction and decreased by bending them in the opposite direction. Thus, rate of discharge of ampullar nerve fibers reflects amount and direction of hair cell cilia bending, which in turn (under normal conditions) reflects amount and direction of head rotation.[3,86,128,191] By a similar process, the utricular macula "codes" head tilt as rate of neural firing.[3,127]

The directionality of the horizontal and vertical canals' neural output is opposite. In the horizontal canal, utriculopetal cupular movement increases neural resting discharge, while utriculofugal movement decreases resting discharge. The directional effects in the vertical canal are opposite.

We have said that the morphologic polarization and the effect of cupular deviation on the sensory end organ potential are oppositely directed in the vertical and horizontal canals. We may, therefore, make the following statement about the directionality of the crista's hair cell function: bending the stereocilia toward the kinocilium depresses the crista's DC resting potential and increases ampullar nerve firing rate; bending the stereocilia away from the kinocilium has exactly opposite effects.[74]

CENTRAL VESTIBULAR PATHWAY

Motor Reflex Connections

The vestibular system functions primarily as an afferent reflex input to the motor system. In general, vestibular pathway–mediated reflexes involve three muscular systems: *extrinsic oculomotor, cervical* and *antigravity*.

As might be expected, the major central connections of the semicircular canals (rotation sensors) are to the extrinsic oculomotor and cervical muscles (i.e., to the muscles that compensate for head rotation), whereas the major central connections of the otolith organs (position sensors) are to the antigravity muscles. Also, as might be expected of a motor reflex system, there is heavy reciprocal innervation between the vestibular pathway and the cerebellum. Figure 42–37 outlines these three major central vestibular connections.[21,22, p. 382] It is to be emphasized that the figure diagrams *major* connections only. A multitude of lesser con-

responses are toward the stimulated ear; if the current is negative, these responses are away from the stimulated ear.

Because the galvanic stimulus probably acts at a retrolabyrinthine location (either vestibular nerve, Scarpa's ganglion, or more central locations), it has been suggested as a means of differentiating vestibular end organ from vestibular nerve lesions. However, this procedure has not found widespread clinical acceptance, possibly because of uncertainty over the exact locus of action. For example, patients with their vestibular nerves sectioned intracranially still have a recognizable body-sway galvanic response,[15,27,91] suggesting that at least part of the galvanic stimulus's action is central to the vestibular nerve (brain stem or possibly cerebellum).

When a fistula communicates between the vestibular apparatus and the middle ear, pressure change applied to the oval window induces an abnormal vestibular reaction called the *fistula response*. When the pressure change is acoustic, the fistula response is called the *Tullio phenomenon*.[212] Sound stimulation elicits a *vestibular microphonic*

(analogous to the cochlear microphonic) from animals with artificial inner ear fistulas but not from animals with normal inner ears.[97,211] This is the electrophysiologic analog of the Tullio phenomenon.

The *fistula test* is a clinical procedure for demonstrating the presence of a labyrinthine fistula. It is positive when pressure applied to the tympanic membrane (hence, via the ossicular chain, to the oval window) elicits vertigo and nystagmus. Pressure may be applied by closing the patient's external ear canal with his tragus and pushing on the tragus, or with a Politzer's bag or an otoscope with bulb attachment.[140]

Figure 42–38 illustrates the mechanism of the fistula response. Normally, the membranous vestibular apparatus is located in a blind, rigid-walled cavity, which prevents applied pressure from deforming the vestibular structures; instead, the pressure is equalized through the round window, deforming the cochlear partition in the process (see Fig. 42–2). When, however, a fistula opens the blind cavity, as shown in Figure 42–38, pressure is equalized through this

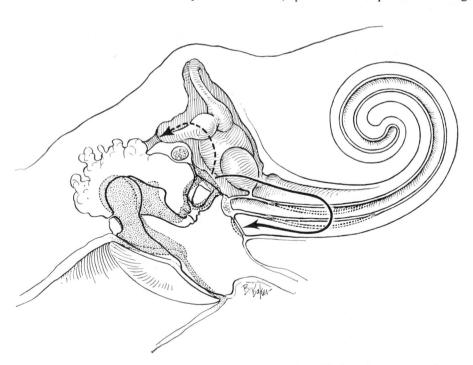

FIG. 42–38.   Mechanism of the fistula response. Pressure applied at the oval window is equalized through the fistula (dashed line with arrow) as well as through the round window. Equalization of pressure through the fistula deforms and thereby stimulates vestibular structures.

opening as well as through the round window and therefore deforms (hence, stimulates) vestibular as well as cochlear structures.

It will be noted that at least some peripheral vestibular function must be present to elicit a fistula response. A fistula response cannot be elicited from a "dead" labyrinth.

Vestibular Nystagmus

Compensatory Eye Movements and Rotational Nystagmus. One of the most important functions of the semicircular canals is to elicit eye movements that keep the eyes steady during head movement and thereby facilitate visual fixation. When the head rotates, the endolymph, because of its inertia, lags behind; hence, relative to the skull, it moves opposite the direction of head rotation and thus causes cupular deflection and end organ stimulation, as shown in Figure 42–36. A compensatory eye movement is illustrated in Figure 42–39. A basic rule is that the eyes rotate in the direction of endolymph movement.

Vestibular nystagmus occurs when the semicircular canal system is overstimulated. Thus, if the head is continuously rotated in one direction at an ever-increasing speed, the semicircular canal–initiated compensatory eye movement becomes repeatedly interrupted by rapid, snap-back movements and hence becomes a *rotational nystagmus*. Since the relatively slow compensatory eye movement phase of the nystagmus comes from the semicircular canal system, it is called the *vestibular* or *slow phase* of the nystagmus. Since the fast, snap-back eye movement comes from the brain, it is called the *central* or *fast phase* of the nystagmus.

Caloric Nystagmus. *Caloric nystagmus* is produced by a temperature change in the region of the vestibular apparatus. In the clinical laboratory, this temperature change is usually produced by running cold or warm water into the external auditory canal. The temperature change is conducted through bone to the semicircular canals. Since the horizontal semicircular canal is closest to the irrigating water, it is the most affected; hence, caloric nystagmus is almost entirely in the horizontal plane.

Figure 42–40 illustrates the mechanism of caloric nystagmus. The subject is in the supine position, with his head elevated 30 degrees to bring the horizontal canal into the vertical position. The caloric irrigation cools the endolymph in part of the horizon-

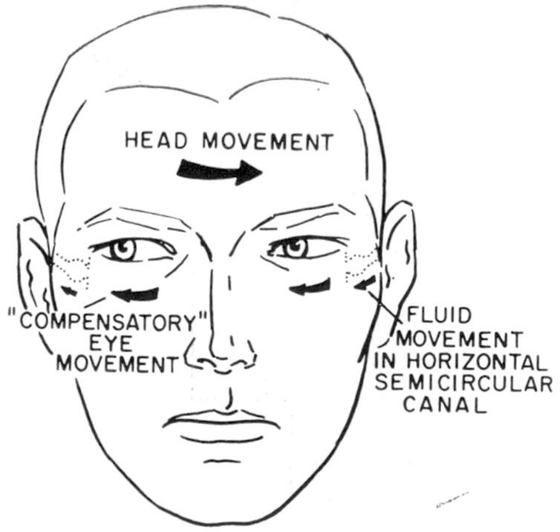

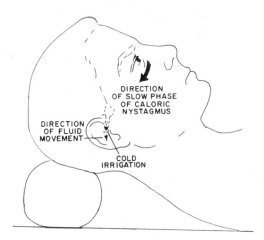

FIG. 42–39. A compensatory eye movement, initiated by the horizontal semicircular canals. The eyes move in the direction of endolymph flow. If rotation of the head is continued at an ever-increasing speed, the compensatory eye movement becomes the slow phase of a rotational nystagmus.

FIG. 42–40. The mechanism of cold caloric nystagmus. The density of the cooled portion of the endolymph (darkened) is increased, causing it to fall, thereby producing endolymph movement. The slow phase of the caloric nystagmus is in the direction of endolymph movement.

115. Klockhoff, I. H., and Anderson, H.: Recording of the Stapedius Reflex Elicited by Cutaneous Stimulation. Acta Otolaryng. (Stockh.), *50*:451, 1959.

116. Kohllöffel, L. U. E.: Observations of the Mechanical Disturbances Along the Basilar Membrane with Laser Illumination. *In* Møller, A. R. (Ed.): *Basic Mechanisms in Hearing.* Royal Swedish Academy of Sciences Symposium Series 1. New York, Academic Press, 1973, pp. 49–67.

117. Konishi, T., *et al.*: Effect of Anoxia on Cochlear Potentials. J. Acoust. Soc. Am., *33*:349, 1961.

118. Konishi, T., and Kelsey, E.: Effect of Cyanide on Cochlear Potentials. Acta Otolaryng. (Stockh.), *65*:381, 1968.

119. Konishi, T., and Yasuno, T.: Summating Potential of the Cochlea in the Guinea Pig. J. Acoust. Soc. Am., *35*: 1448, 1963.

120. Kryter, K. D., and Ades, H. W.: Studies of the Function of the Higher Acoustic Nervous Centers in the Cat. Am. J. Psychiatry, *56*:501, 1943.

121. Lavine, R. A.: Phase-Locking in Response of Single Neurons in Cochlear Nuclear Complex of the Cat to Low-Frequency Tonal Stimuli. J. Neurophysiol., *34*:467, 1971.

122. Lev, A., and Sohmer, H.: Sources of Averaged Neural Responses Recorded in Animal and Human Subjects during Cochlear Audiometry (Electro-Cochleogram). Arch. Klin. Exp. Ohren. Nasen. Kehikopfheilkd., *201*:79, 1972.

123. Lim, D.: Morphological Relationship between the Tectorial Membrane and the Organ of Corti—Scanning and Transmission Electron Microscopy. J. Acoust. Soc. Am., *50*:92, 1971.

124. Lindeman, H. H., *et al.*: The Sensory Hairs and the Tectorial Membrane in the Development of the Cat's Organ of Corti. Acta Otolaryng. (Stockh.), *72*: 229, 1971.

125. Lorente de Nó, R.: Anatomy of the Eighth Nerve: The Central Projection of the Nerve Endings of the Internal Ear. Laryngoscope, *43*:1, 1933.

126. Lorente de Nó, R.: The Sensory Endings in the Cochlea. Laryngoscope, *47*:373, 1937.

127. Löwenstein, O., and Roberts, T. D. M.: The Equilibrium Function of the Otolith Organs of the Thornback Ray. J. Physiol. (Lond.), *110*:392, 1949.

128. Löwenstein, O., and Sand, A.: The Mechanism of the Semicircular Canal. A Study of the Responses of Single-Fibre Preparations to Angular Accelerations and to Rotation at Constant Speed. Proc. R. Soc. Lond. [Biol.], *129*:256, 1940.

129. Marsh, J. T., *et al.*: Differential Brainstem Pathways for the Conduction of Auditory Frequency-Following Responses. Electroencephalogr. Clin. Neurophysiol., *36*:415, 1974.

130. Marsh, J. T., *et al.*: Auditory Frequency-Following Response: Neural or Artifact? Science, *169*:1222, 1970.

131. Martin, J. L., and Coats, A. C.: Short-Latency Auditory Evoked Responses Recorded from Human Nasopharynx. Brain Res., *60*:496, 1973.

132. Massopust, L. C., Jr., *et al.*: Increases in Auditory Middle Frequency Discrimination Thresholds after Cortical Ablations. Exp. Neurol., *28*:299, 1970.

133. Massopust, L. C., Jr., *et al.*: Changes in Auditory Frequency Discrimination Thresholds after Temporal Cortex Ablations. Exp. Neurol., *19*:245, 1967.

134. Mast, T. E.: Short-Latency Human Evoked Responses to Clicks. J. Appl. Physiol., *20*:725, 1965.

135. Masterton, R. B., and Diamond, I. T.: Effects of Auditory Cortex Ablation on Discrimination of Small Binaural Time Differences. J. Neurophysiol., *27*:15, 1964.

136. Masterton, R. B., *et al.*: Role of Brainstem Auditory Structures in Sound Localization. I. Trapezoid Body, Superior Olive, and Lateral Lemniscus. J. Neurophysiol., *30*:341, 1967.

137. Masterton, R. B., *et al.*: Role of Brainstem Auditory Structures in Sound Localization. II. Inferior Colliculus and its Brachium. J. Neurophysiol., *31*:96, 1968.

138. McCabe, B. F., *et al.*: Medial Vestibular Nucleus: Nuclear and Internuclear Activity. Laryngoscope, *74*:806, 1969.

139. McCabe, B. F., *et al.*: Further Experiments on Vestibular Compensation. Laryngoscope, *82*:381, 1972.

140. McNally, W. J., and Stuart, W. A.: *Physiology of the Labyrinth.* Chicago, American Academy of Ophthalmology and Otolaryngology, 1967.

141. McNally, W. J., and Tait, J.: Ablation Experiments on the Labyrinth of the Frog. Am. J. Physiol., *75*:155, 1925.

142. Merzenich, M. M., *et al.*: Neural Encoding of Sound Sensation Evoked by

Electrical Stimulation of the Acoustic Nerve. Ann. Otol. Rhinol. Laryngol., 82:486, 1973.

143. Metz, O.: Threshold of Reflex Contractions of Muscles of Middle Ear and Recruitment of Loudness. Arch. Otolaryng., 55:536, 1952.

144. Miller, E. F., II: Counterrolling of the Human Eyes Produced by Head Tilt with Respect to Gravity. Acta Otolaryng. (Stockh.), 54:479, 1962.

145. Miller, E. F., and Graybiel, A.: A Comparison of Ocular Counterrolling Movements between Normal Persons and Deaf Subjects with Bilateral Labyrinthine Defects. Ann. Otol. Rhinol. Laryngol., 72: 885, 1963.

146. Mills, A. W.: Auditory Localization. In Tobias, J. V. (Ed.): Foundations of Modern Auditory Theory. Vol. 2. New York, Academic Press, 1972, pp. 301-348.

147. Mishray, G. A., et al.: Effects of Localized Hypoxia on the Electrophysiological Activity of Cochlea of the Guinea Pig. J. Acoust. Soc. Am., 30:705, 1958.

148. Møller, A. R.: The Sensitivity of Contraction of the Tympanic Muscles in Man. Ann. Otol. Rhinol. Laryngol., 71:86, 1962.

149. Møller, A.: Acoustic Reflex in Man. J. Acoust. Soc. Am., 34:1524, 1962.

150. Møller, A. R.: An Experimental Study of the Acoustic Impedance of the Middle Ear and its Transmission Properties. Acta Otolaryng. (Stockh.), 60:129, 1965.

151. Møller, A. R.: The Middle Ear. In Tobias, J. V. (Ed.): Foundations of Modern Auditory Theory. Vol. 2. New York, Academic Press, 1972, pp. 135-194.

152. Moushegian, G., and Rupert, A.: Medial Superior-Olivary-Unit Response Patterns to Monaural and Binaural Clicks. J. Acoust. Soc. Am., 36:196, 1964.

153. Neff, W. D.: The Effects of Partial Section of the Auditory Nerve. J. Comp. Physiol. Psychol., 40:203, 1947.

154. Neff, W. D.: Neural Structures Concerned in Localization of Sound in Space. Psychol. Beitrage, 6:492, 1962.

155. Neff, W. D., et al.: Role of Auditory Cortex in Discrimination Requiring Localization of Sound in Space. J. Neurophysiol., 19:500, 1956.

156. Nordmark, J. O.: Time and Frequency Analysis. In Tobias, J. V. (Ed.): Foundations of Modern Auditory Theory. Vol. 1. New York, Academic Press, 1970, pp. 55-83.

157. Oesterreich, R. E., et al.: Neural Structures Mediating Differential Sound Intensity Discrimination in the Cat. Brain Res., 27:251, 1971.

158. Osen, K. K.: Projections of the Cochlear Nuclei on the Inferior Colliculus in the Cat. J. Comp. Neurol., 144:355, 1972.

159. Peake, W. T., et al.: Microelectrode Recordings of Intracochlear Potentials. In Quarterly Progress Report No. 94. Cambridge, Mass., M.I.T. Research Laboratory of Electronics, 1969, pp. 293-304.

160. Pfaltz, C. R. P., and Koike, Y.: Galvanic Test in Central Vestibular Lesions. Acta Otolaryng. (Stockh.), 65:161, 1968.

161. Pfalz, R.: Efferent Crossed Inhibition in the Ventral Cochlear Nuclei. In Møller, A. R. (Ed.): Basic Mechanisms in Hearing. Royal Swedish Academy of Sciences Symposium Series 1. New York, Academic Press, 1973, pp. 773-781.

162. Pfeiffer, R. R.: Classification of Response Patterns of Spike Discharges for Units in the Cochlear Nucleus: Tone Burst Stimulation. Exp. Brain Res., 1:220, 1966.

163. Picton, T. W., et al.: Human Auditory Evoked Potentials. I. Evaluation of Components. Electroencephalogr. Clin. Neurophysiol., 36:179, 1974.

164. Raab, D. H., and Ades, H. W.: Cortical and Midbrain Mediation of a Conditioned Discrimination of Acoustic Intensities. Am. J. Psychol., 59:59, 1946.

165. Rapin, I., et al.: Evoked Responses to Clicks and Tones of Varying Intensity in Waking Adults. Electroencephalogr. Clin. Neurophysiol., 21:335, 1966.

166. Rasmussen, G. L.: Further Observations of the Efferent Cochlear Bundle. J. Comp. Neurol., 99:61, 1953.

167. Rasmussen, G. L.: Anatomic Relationships of the Ascending and Descending Auditory Systems. In Fields, W. S., and Alford, B. R. (Eds.): Neurological Aspects of Auditory and Vestibular Disorders. Springfield, Ill., Charles C Thomas, Publisher, 1964, pp. 5-23.

168. Reger, S. N.: Effect of Middle Ear Muscle Action on Certain Psychophysical Measurements. Ann. Otol. Rhinol. Laryngol., 69:1179, 1960.

169. Rhode, W. S.: An Investigation of Post-Mortem Cochlear Mechanics Using the Mössbauer Effect. In Møller, A. R. (Ed.):

and below center. Gaze is maintained for 30 seconds in each of the eight eye positions.

Gaze nystagmus may be present but not recorded, either because its amplitude is too low or because it is rotary. Also, paretic eye movements may be easier to observe visually than to record. Therefore, during the gaze test it is very important to observe the patient's eyes visually as well as to record their movements.

Diagnostic Significance

Gaze nystagmus and gaze paresis usually indicate the presence of central nervous system pathology. Particularly if persistent for a month or more, these findings further suggest brain stem involvement.[30,33,96, p. 271] Figure 43–5 shows a recording of gaze nystagmus in a patient with a brain stem glioma.

The major exceptions to the above statements of the significance of gaze nystagmus are (1) intense spontaneous nystagmus (visible only behind closed eyelids), causing a unilateral horizontal gaze nystagmus;[25] and (2) diphenylhydantoin (Dilantin)[61] or barbiturates,[13] causing bilateral equal horizontal gaze nystagmus.

SINUSOIDAL TRACKING TEST

Technique

The sinusoidal tracking test is done by having the patient fixate on a spot that is moving in a sinusoidal pattern.[12,57,72] We test with frequencies of 0.3 and 0.6 Hz, and the pattern subtends an angle of ± 30 degrees from center gaze. We obtain tracking movements in both the vertical and horizontal directions.

Diagnostic Significance

A normal individual should be able to track the pattern smoothly, although brief fixations on other objects may occasionally interrupt the smooth sinusoidal pattern. In the abnormal sinusoidal tracking patterns, saccadic eye jerks in the direction of spot movement repeatedly "break up" the smooth sinusoidal pattern. Figure 43–6 illustrates these normal and abnormal patterns.

I have encountered an additional, helpful, abnormal sinusoidal tracking pattern—a tendency for gaze nystagmus to appear in an enhanced form at the extremes of the sinusoidal pattern. Figure 43–7 shows this pattern in a patient with an up-beating vertical

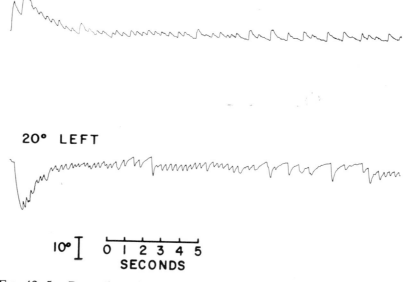

FIG. 43–5. Recording of a bilateral, unequal, horizontal gaze nystagmus from a patient with an intrinsic pontine glioma.

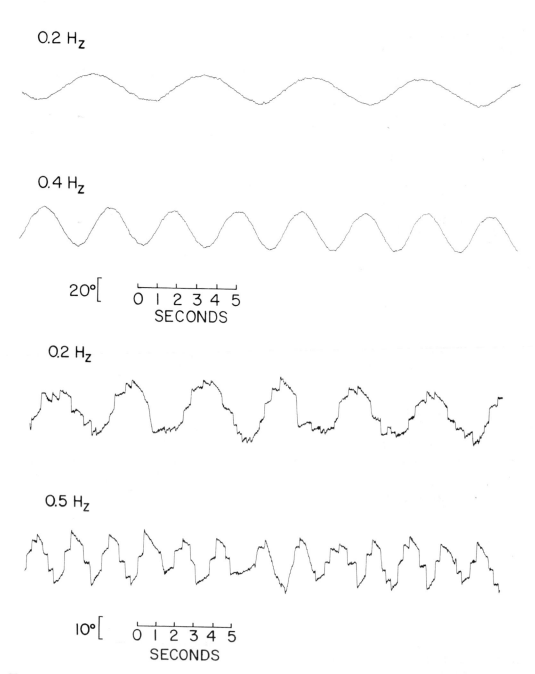

0.2 Hz

0.4 Hz

20°[0 1 2 3 4 5
SECONDS

0.2 Hz

0.5 Hz

10°[0 1 2 3 4 5
SECONDS

FIG. 43–6. Sinusoidal tracking test, demonstrating normal smooth-pursuit movements (above) and abnormal "break" of smooth-pursuit movements in a patient with amyotrophic lateral sclerosis (below).

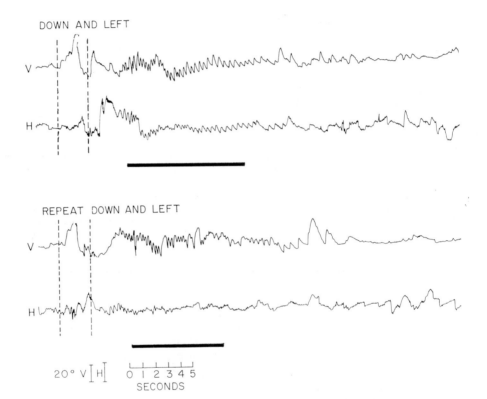

FIG. 43–11. Hallpike test. Example of "nonclassic" type of paroxysmal nystagmus. Vertical eye movements (*V*); horizontal eye movements (*H*). Most of the recordable response is in the vertical direction. The response is nonclassic because it does not fatigue.

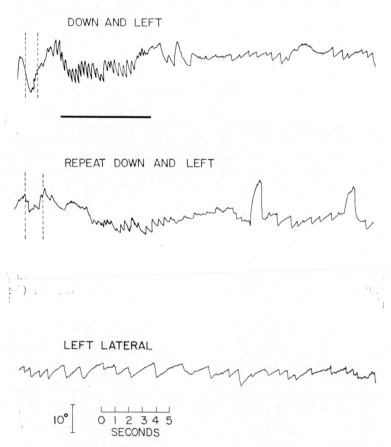

DOWN AND LEFT

REPEAT DOWN AND LEFT

LEFT LATERAL

10° 0 1 2 3 4 5
SECONDS

FIG. 43–12.   Paroxysmal nystagmus and position tests. "Classic" paroxysmal nystagmus, with oppositely directed positional nystagmus. When the patient was brought rapidly from the sitting to the head-hanging-and-left position, a burst of intense right-beating nystagmus appeared (above). However, when the patient was moved slowly into the left lateral position, a persistent, moderate, left-beating nystagmus was present (lowermost tracing). After the transient paroxysmal nystagmus disappears, the patient's left-beating positional nystagmus can be seen in the records of the paroxysmal nystagmus test (top two tracings). The solid black bar below the top record indicates approximate duration of dizziness. The dashed lines show the period during which the patient was being moved.

example of this. It therefore seems evident that "positional nystagmus of the benign paroxysmal type" is dependent not upon the final head position but upon the violent maneuver preceding it. Hence, I prefer not to use the word "positional" in describing a positive response to the Dix-Hallpike maneuver.

Diagnostic Significance

I have found it helpful to distinguish between *classic* and *nonclassic* paroxysmal nystagmus. Classic paroxysmal nystagmus is what Dix and Hallpike originally described; Figure 43–12 shows an example. The essential criteria of classic paroxysmal nystagmus are (1) *dizziness,* accompanying the nystagmus, (2) a *latent period* of 0.5 to 8.0 seconds between the arrival at the test position and the beginning of the nystagmus, (3) *transient* nystagmic response, and (4) *fatigability* of the response from one maneuver to a second maneuver.

Classic paroxysmal nystagmus suggests peripheral vestibular pathology. Usually the pathologic ear is the ear that is down when the nystagmus is elicited. My experience parallels Schuknecht's,[82] that patients with classic paroxysmal nystagmus tend to cluster into the following clinical types: (1) *elderly* (over 65), (2) *post-traumatic dizziness,* (3) *middle ear pathology,* and (4) *surgical manipulation of the stapes or round window.*

Nonclassic paroxysmal nystagmus is a positive response to the Dix-Hallpike maneuver which fails to meet one or more of the criteria of a classic response (e.g., it does not fatigue when the maneuver is repeated). Cawthorne[19] and Harrison[45] suggested that

nonclassic paroxysmal nystagmus indicates central nervous system pathology. However, in my experience, this finding, although more likely due to central pathology than a classic response, nevertheless is frequently of peripheral origin. I therefore regard a nonclassic positive Dix-Hallpike test as a nonlocalizing sign.

POSITION TEST

Technique

The position test explores a series of standard head positions to determine if the patient has positional nystagmus. Unlike the paroxysmal nystagmus test, movement into each position is as slow as possible to exclude the effects of movement. In our laboratory, eyes-closed records of at least 30 seconds are obtained with the patient in the sitting (head upright), supine, right lateral, left lateral, and head-hanging positions. In addition, records are obtained with the patient supine and neck twisted to the right (head right) and to the left (head left).

Classification of Positional Nystagmus

Most authorities use Aschan and coworkers'[4] modification of Nylén's classification, as outlined in Table 43–2.[9,36,53,64]

Figures 43–13 and 43–14 show examples of the persistent forms of positional nystagmus (types I and II). Type III includes all varieties of pathologic transitory positional nystagmus. A transitory positional nystagmus is usually a partially elicited paroxysmal nystagmus, and some authors regard type III positional nystagmus and paroxysmal nystagmus as synonymous.[3] However,

Table 43–2. Classification of Positional Nystagmus

I. Persistent—continues for at least 1 minute after assuming the test position.
   A. Type I (direction changing)—beats in one direction in one (or more) position(s). Figure 42–13 shows an example.
   B. Type II (direction fixed)—beats in the same direction whenever present. Figure 42–14 shows an example.

II. Transitory—goes away within 1 minute after assuming the test position; called "type III positional nystagmus"; also called "positioning nystagmus."

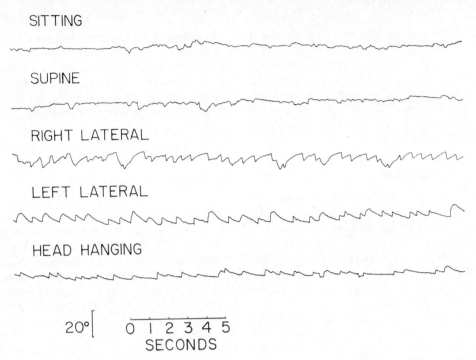

SITTING

SUPINE

RIGHT LATERAL

LEFT LATERAL

HEAD HANGING

$20°\lceil$ 0 1 2 3 4 5
SECONDS

FIG. 43–13. Position test. Example of a moderate-to-intense, direction-changing positional nystagmus (left-beating in right lateral position, and right-beating in left lateral and head-hanging positions). The patient was a 65-year-old man with "senility" and a presumptive diagnosis of "abnormal cerebral blood flow."

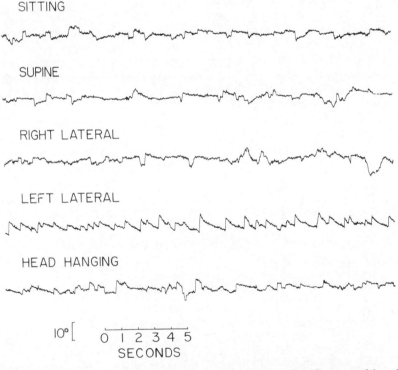

SITTING

SUPINE

RIGHT LATERAL

LEFT LATERAL

HEAD HANGING

$10°\lceil$ 0 1 2 3 4 5
SECONDS

FIG. 43–14. Position test. Example of a moderate, direction-fixed positional nystagmus (right-beating in left lateral position). The patient was a 21-year-old man with sudden left hearing loss 3 weeks before testing. Caloric test showed borderline left unilateral weakness.

739

a small minority of the transient positional responses either do not have a typical "paroxysmal" time course or are accompanied by a negative Dix-Hallpike test. Therefore, in agreement with Henriksson and coworkers[48] and Stenger,[88] I prefer to replace the term "type III positional nystagmus" with "positioning nystagmus."

Diagnostic Significance

Low-Intensity Positional Nystagmus. As with spontaneous nystagmus (see Table 43–1), a positional nystagmus with a slow-phase speed of less than 7°/sec is encountered in about 20% of apparently normal subjects.[11,15,24,29,40,62] Low-intensity positional nystagmus is therefore of questionable pathologic significance.

Drugs Causing Positional Nystagmus. Alcohol,[5,50] sedatives (particularly barbiturates), and salicylates (quinine and aspirin) may cause direction-changing positional nystagmus.[70] Therefore, when a direction-changing positional nystagmus is encountered as an isolated finding, the possibility of drug ingestion must be ruled out.

Moderate- and High-Intensity Positional Nystagmus. Although some authors report a statistical tendency for direction-changing positional nystagmus to occur in central lesions and direction-fixed positional nystagmus to occur in peripheral lesions,[48,70] it is generally agreed that this tendency is not sufficiently strong to be useful clinically.[6,53,56,81] Therefore, positional nystagmus with a slow-phase speed of more than 7°/sec, whether type I or type II, is a nonlocalizing abnormality.

Positioning Nystagmus. Because it is very uncommon, there has been little or no systematic study of the diagnostic significance of positioning nystagmus. Therefore, until better information is available, this finding must be considered nonlocalizing.

BITHERMAL CALORIC TEST

Technique

The bithermal caloric test consists essentially of obtaining cold and warm caloric responses from each ear, with the temperatures equally above and below body temperature.[39] Figure 43–15 illustrates a caloric irrigation. The patient is supine, with head inclined 30 degrees, to bring the horizontal canal into the vertical position. In our laboratory, each ear is irrigated for 40 seconds at temperatures of 31°C and 43°C. A rest period of at least 5 minutes is allowed between the disappearance of one caloric response and the beginning of the next irrigation. Because of the possibility of large fluctuations in corneoretinal potential amplitude,[1] we repeat the amplitude calibration before each irrigation.

In order to minimize central suppression of the caloric responses,[10,22] the patient is instructed to perform aloud a "concentration task" (e.g., subtracting serial seven's) during each response. The task's difficulty is adjusted to match the patient's ability.

Quantification Methods

Table 43–3 lists various caloric response measurements proposed by different writers.

Table 43–3. Alternative Measurements of Caloric Response Magnitude

I.	Response duration—time elapsed from first beat to last beat
II.	Total response magnitude
	A. Total number of beats during response
	B. Total amplitude (sum of the amplitudes of all beats occurring during the response)
III.	Maximum response magnitude
	A. Maximum amplitude
	B. Maximum frequency
	C. Maximum slow-component speed

A

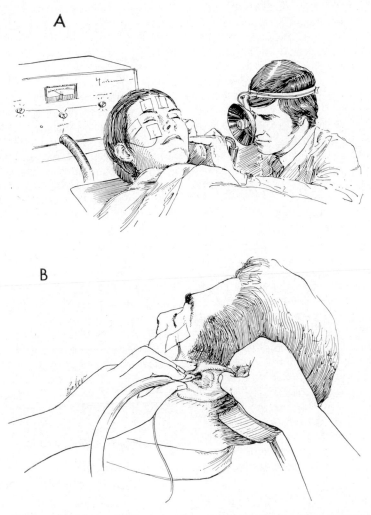

B

FIG. 43–15.   Performing the caloric irrigation (*A*). Dual, constant-temperature reservoirs can be seen behind the patient. The outlet is controlled by a footswitch-operated timer. The tube leading to the subject's ear is insulated with foam rubber. A head lamp is used to visualize the position of the irrigating tube in the ear canal. Insert (*B*) shows technician's view of inserted tube. A catch-basin, normally placed under the patient's ear, is not shown.

It is generally agreed that maximum speed of slow component (SSC) is a better measure of caloric response magnitude than is duration because (1) maximum SSC correlates better with stimulus intensity,[2,47] and (2) in patients with unilateral sensorineural hearing loss, maximum SSC demonstrates vestibular pathology much more often than does caloric response duration.[41,47,56,59,86]

The other caloric response measurements are not as unequivocally inferior to SSC as is duration.[42,85,92] However, the other measurements have not been studied as extensively as the SSC.

The most direct way of determining SSC is to measure its amplitude and duration and divide duration into amplitude. In terms of the record's appearance, this determines slow-phase *steepness* or *slope*. Figure 43–16

illustrates "exact" and approximate (shortcut) methods of determining SSC. The effect of random slow-phase speed fluctuations is minimized by averaging SSC's across several (at least ten in our laboratory) beats. The approximate measurements may occasionally yield false-negative results.[47] Therefore, a borderline significant difference in caloric responses obtained by an approximate measurement may prove significant if the responses are remeasured the "exact" way.

Maximum SSC's cannot be used directly to evaluate the vestibular system because absolute values in normals vary widely.[6,52,57,85] Therefore, comparative measurements are used.[52] Two comparisons are made: (1) a comparison of the responses from the right versus the left ear (*unilateral weakness*

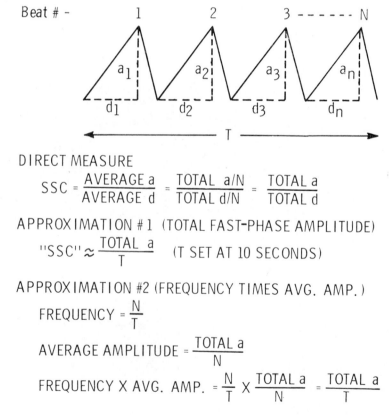

DIRECT MEASURE

$$SSC = \frac{AVERAGE\ a}{AVERAGE\ d} = \frac{TOTAL\ a/N}{TOTAL\ d/N} = \frac{TOTAL\ a}{TOTAL\ d}$$

APPROXIMATION #1 (TOTAL FAST-PHASE AMPLITUDE)

$$"SSC" \approx \frac{TOTAL\ a}{T} \quad (T\ SET\ AT\ 10\ SECONDS)$$

APPROXIMATION #2 (FREQUENCY TIMES AVG. AMP.)

$$FREQUENCY = \frac{N}{T}$$

$$AVERAGE\ AMPLITUDE = \frac{TOTAL\ a}{N}$$

$$FREQUENCY\ X\ AVG.\ AMP. = \frac{N}{T} \times \frac{TOTAL\ a}{N} = \frac{TOTAL\ a}{T}$$

FIG. 43–16.   Exact and approximate methods of determining slow-phase speed. N beats occur during the period over which the average is obtained. a = Slow-phase amplitudes; d = slow-phase durations; T = total duration of nystagmus record measured. The two approximate methods yield essentially the same results.

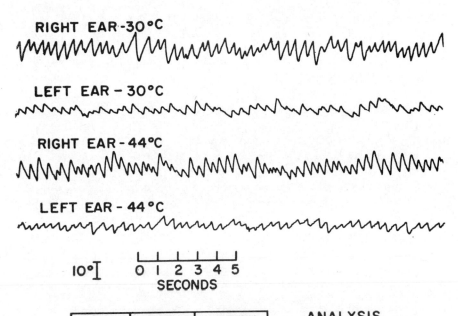

	LATENCY OF NYS (SEC)	DURATION OF NYS (SEC)	MAXIMUM SPEED SLOW COMP.
R 30°C	15	224	27.1°/SEC
L 30°C	27	248	13.3°/SEC
R 44°C	23	188	28.4°/SEC
L 44°C	32	209	12.6°/SEC

ANALYSIS OF MAX. EYE SPEED

% TOTAL EYE SPEED

UNIL. WEAKNESS
RT. EAR (RW+RC) 68.2%
LT. EAR (LW+LC) 31.8%

DIRECTIONAL PREP.
RT. BT. (LC+RW) 51.2%
LT. BT. (RC+LW) 48.8%

TOTAL EYE SPEED 81.4°/SEC

FIG. 43–17. Caloric nystagmus. Caloric test, showing a unilateral weakness on the left. The large difference between ears shown by the maximum slow-phase speeds (right-hand column in box at bottom) was not demonstrated by caloric-response duration (time from first to last beat). The patient was a 59-year-old man with intermittent dizziness and severe sensorineural hearing loss on the left.

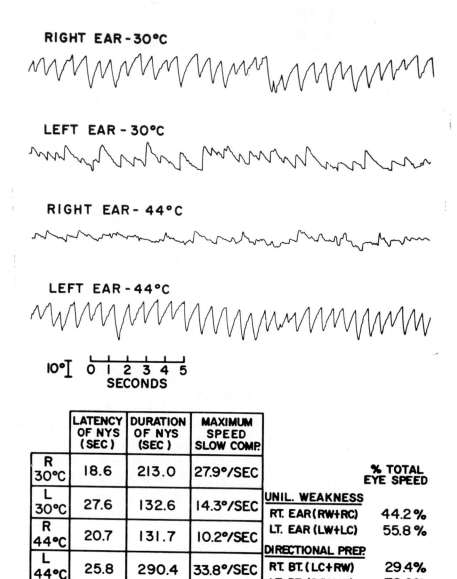

FIG. 43–18. Caloric nystagmus. Caloric test, showing a relatively large directional preponderance to the left. The patient was a 75-year-old woman with moderate left sensorineural hearing loss, tinnitus, and occasional episodes of dizziness.

or *canal paresis*); and (2) a comparison of right-beating versus left-beating nystagmus (*directional preponderance*). Figure 43–17 shows a left unilateral weakness, and Figure 43–18 shows a directional preponderance to the left.

Absolute differences between ears and between right-beating and left-beating responses become more variable as the responses become more intense.[56] Therefore, we express unilateral weakness and directional preponderance in relative terms, i.e., as a percentage of the total of all four response intensities.

Normal Limits

Unilateral Weakness (UW) and Directional Preponderance (DP). Table 43–4 summarizes the results of six independent normal bithermal caloric test series. UW standard deviations vary from 5.3 to 11.5%. It is standard practice to set the normal limit of a quantitative clinical test at twice the standard deviation. In our laboratory, the normal limit of UW is set at 20%, thus assuming a "true" standard deviation of 10%.

In all but one of the normal series,[47] DP was more variable than UW. DP's greater variability makes its normal limit less well-defined than that of UW. Further complicating the determination of DP's normal limit is the possible existence of a "physiologic" DP in some normals.[22,43,55] In our laboratory, a DP of 20 to 30% is regarded as "questionably pathologic"; a DP greater than 30% is considered pathologic.

Bilateral Weakness (BW). Although absolute maximum SSC's vary widely in normals, it is a general clinical impression that a very weak (or absent) caloric response from both labyrinths is abnormal. Presently available normative data on absolute maximum SSC's suggest that average maximum SSC's of less than 7.5°/sec from each ear indicate abnormal bilateral weakness.[47,76] Figure 43–19 shows a caloric test that demonstrates BW.

Failure of Fixation Suppression (FFS). In normal individuals, visual fixation either suppresses or abolishes caloric nystagmus. Several reports suggest that failure to suppress caloric nystagmus with visual fixation is a pathologic sign, indicating central nervous system pathology.[46,66,69,78] I termed this sign "failure of fixation suppression" and defined it as "SSC with eyes open and fixed as great or greater than with eyes closed."[25] Figure 43–20 contrasts FFS with the normal effect of visual suppression on caloric nystagmus.

Table 43–4. Standard Deviations of Normal Caloric Unilateral Weakness
and Directional Preponderance
(Measured by Maximum Slow-Component Speeds)

Reference and Methods	UW	DP
Aschan *et al.*[6] 30-sec irrigations at 30°C and 44°C, eyes closed. 25 subjects, 25–50 years old.	8.6%	8.8%
Henriksson.[47] 40-sec irrigations at 30°C and 43.6°C, in dark. 25 subjects, 19–45 years old.	9.5%	8.5%
Jongkees *et al.*[55] 30-sec irrigations at 30°C and 44°C, eyes closed. 47 subjects.	7.5%	8.7%
Preber.[76] 40-sec irrigations at 30°C and 44°C, eyes closed. 50 subjects.	5.3%	5.8%
Coats.[21] 40-sec irrigations at 30°C and 44°C, eyes closed. 30 subjects.	9.5%	13.2%
Brookler and Pulec.[18] 30-sec irrigations at 30° and 44°C, eyes closed. 839 "patients without neurootologic disease."	11.5%*	13.5%*

*Measured by the author from frequency distribution curves.

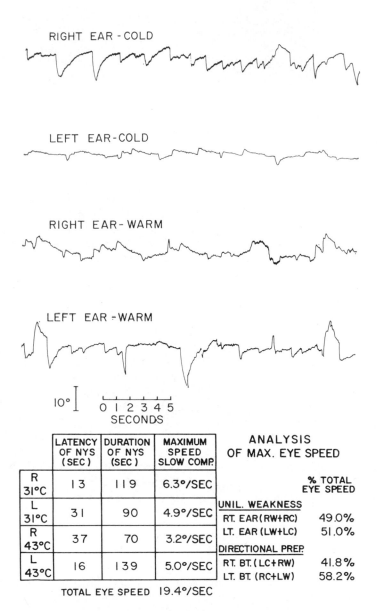

RIGHT EAR - COLD

LEFT EAR - COLD

RIGHT EAR - WARM

LEFT EAR - WARM

10° | 0 1 2 3 4 5
        SECONDS

	LATENCY OF NYS (SEC)	DURATION OF NYS (SEC)	MAXIMUM SPEED SLOW COMP.
R 31°C	13	119	6.3°/SEC
L 31°C	31	90	4.9°/SEC
R 43°C	37	70	3.2°/SEC
L 43°C	16	139	5.0°/SEC

TOTAL EYE SPEED 19.4°/SEC

ANALYSIS OF MAX. EYE SPEED

% TOTAL EYE SPEED

UNIL. WEAKNESS
RT. EAR (RW+RC)   49.0%
LT. EAR (LW+LC)   51.0%
DIRECTIONAL PREP.
RT. BT. (LC+RW)   41.8%
LT. BT. (RC+LW)   58.2%

FIG. 43–19. Caloric nystagmus. Caloric test, showing bilateral weakness in a patient with possible streptomycin toxicity. The average response from each ear is less than 7.5°/sec. For example, the average response from the right ear is: $\dfrac{RC + RW}{2} = \dfrac{6.3 + 3.2}{2} = 4.8°/\text{sec}$ (where RC = right 31° SSC and RW = right 43° SSC).

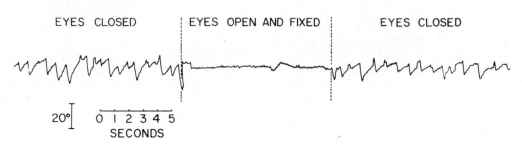

LEFT EAR WARM

EYES CLOSED | EYES OPEN AND FIXED | EYES CLOSED

20° | 0 1 2 3 4 5
SECONDS

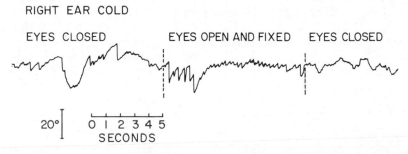

RIGHT EAR COLD

EYES CLOSED   EYES OPEN AND FIXED   EYES CLOSED

20° | 0 1 2 3 4 5
SECONDS

FIG. 43–20. Demonstration of "failure of fixation suppression" (FFS) of caloric nystagmus. The record above demonstrates normal suppression of caloric nystagmus by visual fixation. It was obtained from a patient with a small right acoustic neurinoma. The record below demonstrates FFS. It was obtained from a patient with multiple sclerosis.

Diagnostic Significance

Unilateral Weakness. A caloric UW can only be caused by a lesion of the vestibular end organ or the primary vestibular nerve fibers. It is therefore a peripheral finding.[2,6,52,57,85]

Directional Preponderance. A caloric DP can be due to either peripheral or central pathology.[17,20,39,59] It is therefore a non-localizing abnormality.

Bilateral Weakness. Caloric BW may be due either to bilateral peripheral vestibular pathology, such as that which streptomycin toxicity might produce, or to central pathology that interferes with the vestibulo-ocular reflex arc. However, most BW's are due to bilateral peripheral pathology. Furthermore, the occasional patient with BW due to central pathology almost always has associated central oculomotor signs. In particular, the OKN test is usually abnormal. Thus, I consider BW a peripheral sign, with,

however, the proviso that brain stem oculomotor pathology has been ruled out.

Failure of Fixation Suppression. FFS is a central sign. However, two benign causes of FFS have been demonstrated and must be ruled out: (1) sedation, particularly by barbiturates;[25,79] and (2) contact lenses, particularly if they are new or uncomfortable. In addition, as with all central ENG abnormalities, peripheral ocular pathology must be ruled out in the patient demonstrating FFS.

ROTATION TEST

Advantages and Disadvantages

Rotational nystagmus has been used as long as caloric nystagmus for clinical vestibular system evaluation, but, compared to the caloric test, the rotation test's disadvantages are generally thought to outweigh its advantages. Therefore, in recent years the clinical rotation test has been seldom used. However, the recent development of the torsion swing chair has caused a partial resurgence of the rotation test as a clinical tool.

The major *advantages* of the rotation test over the caloric test are:

1. It creates less patient discomfort. This makes the rotation test particularly suitable for pediatric patients.

2. The rotational stimulus can be quantified with greater precision than the thermal stimulus. This makes the rotation test particularly suitable for pharmacologic studies.

3. It is much easier to test the vertical semicircular canals with the rotational stimulus.

The major *disadvantages* of the rotation test are:

1. It stimulates both labyrinths simultaneously; hence, it cannot assess the function of individual labyrinths.

2. Until the introduction of the torsion swing chair, rotation testing equipment was expensive and occupied an inordinate amount of laboratory space.

One of the most important clinical applications of the rotation test is the assessment of congenital otologic abnormalities in pediatric patients.[35,90] Since congenital abnormalities are usually bilateral, the inability of the rotation test to assess individual labyrinths is not a serious problem in this group of patients. On the other hand, the rapidity of the test procedure and the absence of patient discomfort are particular advantages in these patients.

Test Technique

Basically, the clinical rotation test consists of eliciting oppositely directed rotational responses at equal accelerations. Usually, rotation is applied in one of the following three patterns: the *Barany test, cupulometry,* or the *torsion chair test.* Each of these acceleration patterns will be discussed separately.

Barany Test. The patient sits in a rotating chair (the *Barany chair*), which may be either manually rotated or motor-driven. The chair is accelerated at a constant rate until a predetermined velocity is reached.

The patient is then rotated at this constant velocity for several seconds, then decelerated at the same constant rate until the chair stops.[48,85,90] Figure 43–21, *A* plots the chair's velocity against time and shows recommended "standard" parameters for clinical testing. During chair rotation, the patient's head may be positioned to place any pair of semicircular canals in the horizontal plane so that that pair will be selectively stimulated.

The nystagmic responses to the Barany rotation test consist of the following:

1. During acceleration, there is a "perrotatory" nystagmus, beating in the direction of rotation.

2. During constant velocity, a "postrotatory" nystagmus, beating opposite the direction of rotation, appears. This nystagmus dies out during the period of constant velocity.

3. During the deceleration period, there is a second "perrotatory" nystagmus, beating opposite the direction of rotation.

4. After the chair stops, a final "postrotatory" nystagmus appears, which normally dies out after a few seconds.

Cupulometry. Figure 43–21, *B* illustrates the "cupulometry" rotation pattern.[48] The Barany chair is also used for this test. The chair is accelerated at a constant rate for 1 to 4 seconds, then is decelerated rapidly. A perrotatory nystagmus appears during the initial constant acceleration. The abrupt deceleration generates a postrotatory nystagmus in the opposite direction. Usually, a series of "post-post" responses follow the first burst of postrotatory nystagmus. By repeating the rotation pattern at progressively lower initial acceleration rates, the vestibular threshold can be determined.[51,68,94]

Torsion Chair Test. The torsion chair utilizes the principle of a torsion pendulum to apply a damped sinusoidal rotation, as shown in Figure 43–21, *C*.[35,56,73] The chair is turned 90 degrees to a preset "stop," then released. The torsion pendulum causes the chair to rotate back and forth sinusoidally, at a progressively decreasing amplitude. Figure 43–22 shows the normal nystagmic response to this rotation pattern. A series of rotational nystagmus bursts appear. Each burst is opposite the direction of the pre-

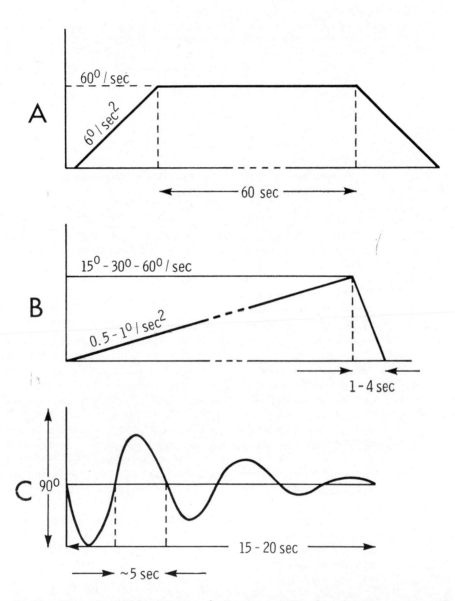

FIG. 43–21. Recommended patterns of angular acceleration for three types of rotation testing: the Barany test (A), cupulometry (B), and the torsion chair test (C). (Henriksson, N. G., et al.: A Synopsis of the Vestibular System. Basel, Gasser & Cie, 1972.)

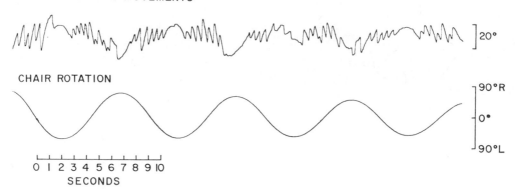

HORIZONTAL EYE MOVEMENTS

CHAIR ROTATION

0 1 2 3 4 5 6 7 8 9 10
SECONDS

FIG. 43–22. Normal nystagmic response to the back-and-forth sinusoidal rotation of the torsion chair.

ceding burst. The bursts are superimposed on a sinusoidal eye rotation. As the chair's rotation rate declines, the nystagmic bursts decline in intensity.

The torsion chair has the following advantages over the conventional Barany chair: (1) since it does not rotate all the way around, slip-rings are not required to record the nystagmic signal; (2) the torsion pendulum is a more economical and reliable method of controlling rotation than is the Barany chair's gear-motor mechanism; (3) the torsion chair applies a wide range of acceleration rates in a short period of time, thus permitting a much shorter clinical test procedure.

The disadvantages of the torsion chair, compared to the Barany chair, are that: (1) it does not quantify rotation rates as accurately; (2) it is not as flexible, since the Barany chair can be programmed to deliver a wide range of acceleration rates and patterns; (3) it is more difficult to measure the slow-phase velocity of the nystagmic response to torsion chair rotation, because the nystagmus is superimposed on a sinusoidal eye movement.

Clinical Significance

All of the above-described rotation tests may detect one of three abnormalities: "areflexia," "hyporeflexia," or "directional preponderance." *Areflexia* is an absence of rotational nystagmus in both directions.

Hyporeflexia is an abnormally depressed rotational nystagmus in both directions. Both of these findings suggest bilateral peripheral vestibular pathology (e.g., as in ototoxicity or congenital deafness). However, as with caloric BW, occasionally a central abnormality that interferes with the vestibulo-ocular reflex arc causes areflexia or hyporeflexia.

As with caloric DP, either central or peripheral vestibular pathology can cause *rotational DP*. Rotational DP is therefore a nonlocalizing sign.

Occasionally, the caloric and rotational test results do not agree. For example, there may be a rotational DP but no caloric DP; or there may be caloric BW but normally intense rotational nystagmus. Animal experiments suggest that such *caloric-rotational dissociation* may be a central sign.[89] However, this possibility has not been studied systematically in humans.

CERVICAL VERTIGO AND NYSTAGMUS

Definition and Pathophysiology

Cervical (also termed "neck-torsion") vertigo and nystagmus are abnormal responses to neck-twisting. Factors predisposing to cervical vertigo include (1) arteriosclerosis, (2) abnormalities of the cervical spine (e.g., osteoarthritis, disc herniation), and (3) whiplash injury.[14,37,75]

Table 43–5. Diagnostic Significance of ENG Abnormalities

Test	Nonlocalizing	Peripheral	Central (R/O Ocular for All Signs)
Calibration			Ocular dysmetria ("calibration overshoot") (R/O eye blinks)
Gaze test			Gaze nystagmus: Vertical Unilateral (R/O intense spontaneous NYS) Bilateral, equal (R/O sedation) Bilateral, unequal
Optokinetic test			Asymmetry (R/O intense spontaneous NYS) Bilateral diminution (R/O lack of voluntary visual fixation and sedatives)
Sinusoidal tracking test			"Breakup" of smooth pursuit (R/O sedation)
Position test	Vestibular spontaneous NYS and positional NYS greater than 7.5°/sec behind closed-eyelids		Central spontaneous NYS
Paroxysmal nystagmus test	Nonclassic	Classic	
Bithermal caloric test	DP greater than 30%	UW BW (R/O central V-O reflex interruption)	FFS (R/O sedation)
Rotation test	DP greater than 30%	BW (R/O central V-O reflex interruption)	Caloric rotational dissociation

Abbreviations: R/O, rule out; NYS, nystagmus; V-O, vestibulo-ocular; DP, directional preponderance; UW, unilateral weakness; FFS, failure of fixation suppression; BW, bilateral weakness.

Two basic pathophysiologic mechanisms of cervical vertigo have been postulated: "vascular" and "neurosensory." The *vascular* theory holds that cervical vertigo occurs because of vascular occlusion due to neck-twisting.[7] Since there is a rich collateral blood supply to the brain, the vascular hypothesis requires the presence of an already compromised cerebral circulation. This could occur because of mechanical compression of the vertebral arteries, as, for example, in the scalenus anticus syndrome or with osteoarthritic spurring or disc herniation. A compromised cervical circulation could also be due to internal occlusion (e.g., as in atherosclerosis) or to congenital absence or atresia of strategic vessels (e.g., the circle of Willis). Arteriographic studies have convincingly demonstrated a vascular etiology in some cases of cervical vertigo.[37]

The *neurosensory* theory of cervical vertigo postulates that, since both the semicircular canal system and the cervical proprioceptive system sense head rotation, derangement of the cervical proprioceptive system ought to produce pathologic nystagmus, just as does derangement of the semicircular canal system. In support of the neurosensory theory of cervical vertigo, it has been observed that after unilateral sectioning of the cervical nerve roots in the rabbit, twisting of the animal's neck generates a pathologic nystagmus.[14,75] It has also been observed that injecting procaine into the neck muscles of humans can produce cervical vertigo-like attacks.[54]

Test Technique

To test for cervical vertigo, the effects of vestibular stimulation must be separated from the effects of neck-twisting. Bos and Philipszoon[16] proposed a variation of the torsion swing test, in which the patient's head is fixed while the body is rotated back and forth. In the office, a simple desk swivel chair can be used for this test. Normally, this maneuver generates sinusoidal eye movements at the same rate as the neck-twist, with a few nystagmus-like beats superimposed on the sinusoidal movements. Cervical vertigo can be diagnosed if the neck-twisting generates intense nystagmus, vertigo, or asymmetrical eye movements.[54]

Another test for cervical vertigo consists of placing the patient's entire body in a particular position (e.g., right lateral), then placing only his head in the same position by twisting his neck (e.g., patient supine, head turned right). A nystagmus appearing with the neck twisted but not with the neck straight is considered cervical in origin. In my experience and that of others,[9] this latter "static" test for cervical vertigo rarely yields positive results. Bos and Philipszoon's "dynamic" test apparently yields positive results more frequently.[54] Therefore, the dynamic test is probably the procedure of choice for detecting cervical vertigo.

SUMMARY

In the introduction to this chapter, I noted that the vestibulometric examination may help localize an abnormality to the peripheral vestibular system or may yield only "nonlocalizing" signs (signs that indicate the presence of an abnormality but, by themselves, give no localizing information). Table 43–5 classifies the abnormal findings of the vestibulometric examination as central, peripheral, or nonlocalizing. Because of the special nature of its localizing significance, the test for cervical vertigo does not fit readily into this classification and therefore has been omitted.

REFERENCES

1. Aantaa, E.: Light-induced and Spontaneous Variations in the Amplitude of the Electro-oculogram. Acta Otolaryng. (Stockh.) [Suppl.], *267*:1, 1970.
2. Aschan, G.: The Caloric Test: A Nystagmographical Study. Acta Soc. Med. Upsal., *60*:99, 1955.
3. Aschan, G.: The Pathogenesis of Positional Nystagmus. Acta Otolaryng. (Stockh.) [Suppl.], *159*:90, 1961.
4. Aschan, G., et al.: The Effect of Head Movement on Positional Nystagmus—Electro-nystagmography with an Electric-driven Posture Table. Laryngoscope, *67*:884, 1957.
5. Aschan, G., et al.: Positional Nystagmus in Man During and After Alcohol Intoxi-

cation. Quart. J. Stud. Alcohol, *17*:381, 1956.

6. Aschan, G., *et al.*: Nystagmography. Recording of Nystagmus in Clinical Neuro-otological Examinations. Acta Otolaryng. (Stockh.) [Suppl.], *129*:1, 1956.

7. Aschan, G., and Hugosson, R. B.: Vestibular Symptoms Provoked by Head and Neck Rotation after Bilateral Carotid Ligation. Acta Otolaryng. (Stockh.), *61*:49, 1966.

8. Barany, R.: Diagnosis of Disease of the Otolith Apparatus. J. Laryngol. Otol., *36*: 229, 1921.

9. Barber, H. O.: Positional Nystagmus: Testing and Interpretation. Ann. Otol. Rhinol. Laryngol., *73*:838, 1964.

10. Barber, H. O., and Wright, G.: Release of Nystagmus Suppression in Clinical Electronystagmography. Laryngoscope, *77*, 1016, 1967.

11. Barber, H. O., and Wright, G.: Positional Nystagmus in Normals. Adv. Otorhinolaryngol., *19*, 276, 1973.

12. Benitez, J. T.: Eye-tracking and Optokinetic Tests. Diagnostic Significance in Peripheral and Central Vestibular Disorders. Laryngoscope, *80*:834, 1970.

13. Bergman, P. S., *et al.*: The Effects of Drugs on Normal and Abnormal Electrically Recorded Eye Movements. Trans. Am. Neurol. Assoc., *76*:232, 1951.

14. Biemond, A., and De Jong, J. M. B. V.: On Cervical Nystagmus and Related Disorders. Brain, *92*:437, 1969.

15. Bos, J. H., *et al.*: On Pathological Spontaneous and Positional Nystagmus. Pract. Otorhinolaryngol. (Basel), *25*:282, 1963.

16. Bos, J. H., and Philipszoon, A. J.: Neck Torsion Nystagmus. Pract. Otorhinolaryngol. (Basel), *25*:339, 1963.

17. Brookler, K. H.: Directional Preponderance in Clinical Electronystagmography. Laryngoscope, *80*:747, 1970.

18. Brookler, K. H., and Pulec, J. L.: Computer Analysis of Electronystagmography Records. Trans. Am. Acad. Ophthal. Otolaryng., *74*:563, 1970.

19. Cawthorne, T.: Positional Nystagmus. Trans. Am. Otol. Soc., *42*:265, 1954.

20. Cawthorne, T. E., *et al.*: Studies in Human Vestibular Function. III. Observations on the Clinical Features of Meniere's Disease, with Especial Reference to the Results of the Caloric Tests. Brain, *65*: 161, 1942.

21. Coats, A. C.: Electronystagmographic Examination: History, Technique and Interpretation. Med. Rec. Ann. (Houston), *58*:48, 1965.

22. Coats, A. C.: Directional Preponderance and Spontaneous Nystagmus as Observed in the Electronystagmographic Examination. Ann. Otol. Rhinol. Laryngol., *75*: 1135, 1966.

23. Coats, A. C.: Central and Peripheral Optokinetic Asymmetry. Ann. Otol. Rhinol. Laryngol., *77*:938, 1968.

24. Coats, A. C.: The Diagnostic Significance of Spontaneous Nystagmus as Observed in the Electronystagmographic Examination. Acta Otolaryng. (Stockh.), *67*:33, 1969.

25. Coats, A. C.: Central Electronystagmographic Abnormalities. Arch. Otolaryng., *92*:43, 1970.

26. Cogan, D. G.: Ocular Dysmetria: Flutter-like Oscillations of the Eyes and Opsoclonus. Acta Ophthalmol. (Kbh.), *51*: 318, 1954.

27. Cogan, D. G.: *Neurology of the Ocular Muscles.* 2nd ed. Springfield, Ill., Charles C Thomas, Publishers, 1956.

28. Cogan, D. G., and Loeb, D. R.: Optokinetic Response and Intracranial Lesions. Arch. Neurol. Psychiatr., *61*:183, 1949.

29. Collins, W. E., *et al.*: Some Effects of Alcohol on Vestibular Responses. Adv. Otorhinolaryngol., *19*:295, 1973.

30. Daroff, R. B., and Hoyt, W. F.: Supranuclear Disorders of Ocular Control Systems in Man. Clinical, Anatomical and Physiologic Correlations—1969. *In* Bach-y-Rita, P., Collins, C. C., and Hyde, J. E. (Eds.): *The Control of Eye Movements.* New York, Academic Press, 1971, pp. 175–235.

31. Davidoff, R. A., *et al.*: Optokinetic Nystagmus and Cerebral Disease. Arch. Neurol., *14*:73, 1966.

32. Dix, M. R., and Hallpike, C. S.: Pathology, Symptomatology and Diagnosis of Certain Common Disorders of the Vestibular System. Proc. R. Soc. Med., *45*:341, 1952.

33. Dow, R. S., and Manni, E.: The Relationship of the Cerebellum to Extraocular Movements. *In* Bender M. B. (Ed.): *The Oculomotor System.* New York, Harper & Row, 1964, pp. 280–292.

34. Ellenberger, C., Jr., *et al.*: Ocular Dyskinesia in Cerebellar Disease. Evidence for the Similarity of Opsoclonus, Ocular Dysmetria and Flutter-like Oscillations. Brain, *95*:685, 1972.

35. Eviatar, A.: The Torsion Swing as a Vestibular Test. Arch. Otolaryng., *92*:437, 1970.

36. Fernandez, C., and Lindsay, J. R.: Positional Nystagmus in Man and Animals. J. Nerve. Ment. Dis., *130*:488, 1960.

37. Fields, W. S.: Vertigo Related to Alteration in Arterial Blood Flow. *In* Wolfson, R. J. (Ed.): *The Vestibular System and Its Diseases*. Philadelphia, University of Pennsylvania Press, 1966, pp. 472–483.

38. Fields, W. S., and Alford, B. R. (Eds.): *Neurological Aspects of Auditory and Vestibular Disorders*. Springfield, Ill., Charles C Thomas, Publisher, 1964.

39. Fitzgerald, G., and Hallpike, C. S.: Studies in Human Vestibular Function. I. Observations on the Directional Preponderance (Nystagmusbereitschaft) of Caloric Nystagmus Resulting from Cerebral Lesions. Brain, *65*:115, 1942.

40. Fluur, E., and Eriksson, L.: Nystagmographic Recording of Vertical Eye Movements. Acta Otolaryng. (Stockh.), *53*:486, 1961.

41. Fodor, F.: Electronystagmography: Its Perspective, Advantages, and Limitations in Routine Vestibular Testing. *In* Wolfson, R. J. (Ed.): *The Vestibular System and Its Diseases*. Philadelphia, University of Pennsylvania Press, 1966, pp. 309–321.

42. Gulick, R. D., and Pfaltz, C. R.: The Diagnostic Value of Caloric Tests in Otoneurology. Ann. Otol. Rhinol. Laryngol., *73*:893, 1964.

43. Hallpike, C. S., et al.: Abnormalities of the Caloric Test Results in Certain Varieties of Mental Disorder. Acta Otolaryng., *39*:151, 1951.

44. Haring, R. D., and Simmons, F. B.: Cerebellar Defects Are Detectable by ENG Calibration Overshoots. Arch. Otolaryng., *98*:14, 1973.

45. Harrison, M. S.: Benign Positional Vertigo. *In* Wolfson, R. J. (Ed.): *The Vestibular System and Its Diseases*. Philadelphia, University of Pennsylvania Press, 1966, pp. 404–427.

46. Hart, C. W.: Ocular Fixation and the Caloric Test. Laryngoscope, *77*:2103, 1967.

47. Henriksson, N. G.: Speed of Slow Component and Duration in Caloric Nystagmus. Acta Otolaryng. (Stockh.) [Suppl.], *125*:1, 1956.

48. Henriksson, N. G., et al.: *A Synopsis of the Vestibular System*. Basel, Gasser & Cie, 1972.

49. Higgins, D. C., and Daroff, R. B.: Overshoot and Oscillation in Ocular Dysmetria. Arch. Ophthalmol., *75*:742, 1966.

50. Hill, R. J., et al.: Influence of Alcohol on Positional Nystagmus over 32-Hour Periods. Ann. Otol. Rhinol. Laryngol., *82*:103, 1973.

51. Hulk, J., and Jongkees, L. B. W.: The Turning Test with Small Regulable Stimuli. II. The Normal Cupulogram. J. Laryngol. Otol., *62*:70, 1948.

52. Jongkees, L. B. W.: Value of the Caloric Test of the Labyrinth. Arch. Otolaryng., *48*:402, 1948.

53. Jongkees, L. B. W.: On Positional Nystagmus. Acta Otolaryng. (Stockh.) [Suppl.], *159*:78, 1961.

54. Jongkees, L. B. W.: Cervical Vertigo. Laryngoscope, *79*:1473, 1969.

55. Jongkees, L. B. W., et al.: Clinical Nystagmography. A Detailed Study of Electronystagmography in 341 Patients with Vertigo. Pract. Otorhinolaryngol. (Basel) *24*:65, 1962.

56. Jongkees, L. B. W., and Philipszoon, A. J.: Electronystagmography. Acta Otolaryng. (Stockh.) [Suppl.], *189*:1 1964.

57. Jung, R., and Kornhuber, H. H.: Results of Electronystagmography in Man. The Value of Optokinetic, Vestibular and Spontaneous Nystagmus for Neurologic Diagnosis and Research. *In* Bender, M. B. (Ed.): *The Oculomotor System*. New York, Harper & Row, 1964, pp. 428–482.

58. Kestenbaum, A.: *Clinical Methods of Neuro-ophthalmologic Examination*. 2nd ed. New York, Grune & Stratton, 1961.

59. Koch, H., et al.: Directional Preponderance and Spontaneous Nystagmus in Eyespeed Recording. Acta Otolaryng. (Stockh.), *50*:517, 1959.

60. Kris, C.: Vision: Electro-oculography. *In* Glasser, O. (Ed.): *Medical Physics*. Vol. 3. Chicago, Year Book Medical Publishers, 1960, pp. 692–700.

61. Kutt, H., et al.: Diphenylhydantoin and Phenobarbital Toxicity. Arch. Neurol., *11*:649, 1964.

62. Lansberg, M. P.: Latente Idiopathische Nystagmus. Ned. Tijdschr. Geneeskd., *106*:398, 1962.

63. Lindsay, J. R.: Postural Vertigo and Positional Nystagmus. Ann. Otol. Rhinol. Laryngol., *60*:1134, 1951.

64. Lindsay, J. R.: Paroxysmal Postural Vertigo and Vestibular Neuronitis. Arch. Otolaryng., *85*:544, 1967.

65. Lipman, I. J.: "Voluntary Nystagmus"— Ocular Shuddering. Dis. Nerv. Syst., *33*: 200, 1972.

66. Maccario, M., et al.: Paradoxical Caloric Response in Altered States of Consciousness. Neurology (Minneap.), *22*:781, 1972.

67. Marg, E.: Development of Electro-oculography: Standing Potential of the Eye in Registration of Eye Movement. Arch. Ophthalmol., *45*:169, 1951.

68. Montandon, A., et al.: A New Technique of Vestibular Rotatory Stimulation and of Electrical Recording of Nystagmus in Man. Ann. Otol. Rhinol. Laryngol., *64*: 701, 1955.

69. Naito, T., et al.: The Effect of Eye-closure upon Nystagmus. Acta Otolaryng. (Stockh.) [Suppl.], *179*:72, 1963.

70. Nylén, C. O.: Positional Nystagmus (A Review and Future Prospects). J. Laryngol. Otol., *64*:295, 1950.

71. Nylén, C. O.: The Posture Test. Acta Otolaryng. (Stockh.) [Suppl.], *109*:125, 1953.

72. Ohm, J.: Auslösung des Optokinetischen Pendelnystagmus und des Willkürlich-Optokinetischen Rucknystagmus. Graefe's Arch. Ophthalmol., *142*:482, 1940.

73. Oosterveld, W. J.: The Torsion Swing Test. Pract. Otorhinolaryngol. (Basel), *27*:309, 1965.

74. Orzechowski, C.: De l'Ataxie Dysmetrique des Yeux. J. Psychol. Neurol. (Lpz.), *35*: 1, 1927.

75. Philipszoon, A. J.: Compensatory Eye Movements and Nystagmus Provoked by Stimulation of the Vestibular Organ and the Cervical Nerve Roots: Pract. Otorhinolaryngol. (Basel), *24*:193, 1962.

76. Preber, L.: Vegetative Reactions in Caloric and Rotatory Tests. A Clinical Study with Special Reference to Motion Sickness. Acta Otolaryng. (Stockh.) [Suppl.], *144*: 1, 1958.

77. Preber, L., and Silfverskiöld, B. P.: Paroxysmal Positional Vertigo following Head Injury (Studied by Electronystagmography and Skin Resistance Measurements). Acta Otolaryng. (Stockh.), *48*: 255, 265, 1957.

78. Preber, L., and Silfverskiöld, B. P.: Vascular Paramedian Pontine Lesion Associated with Vestibulo-ocular Disturbances. Acta Otolaryng. (Stockh.), *51*:153, 1960.

79. Rashbass, C., and Russell, G. F. M.: Action of a Barbiturate Drug (Amylobar-bitone Sodium) on the Vestibulo-ocular Reflex. Brain, *84*:329, 1961.

80. Rosborg, J., et al.: Vertical Optokinetic Nystagmus. Acta Neurol. Scand., *48*:621, 1972.

81. Schiller, F., and Hedberg, W. C.: An Appraisal of Positional Nystagmus. Arch. Neurol., *2*:309, 1960.

82. Schuknecht, H. F.: Cupulolithiasis. Arch. Otolaryng., *90*:113, 1969.

83. Smith, J. L.: Vertical Optokinetic Nystagmus. Neurology (Minneap.), *12*:48, 1962.

84. Smith, J. L.: *Optokinetic Nystagmus.* Springfield, Ill., Charles C Thomas Publisher, 1963.

85. Stahle, J.: Electro-nystagmography in the Caloric and Rotatory Tests. Acta Otolaryng. (Stockh.) [Suppl.], *137*:1, 1958.

86. Stahle, J., and Bergman, B.: The Caloric Response in Meniere's Disease: An Electronystagmographical Study in 300 Patients. Laryngoscope, *77*:1629, 1967.

87. Stahle, J., and Terins, J.: Paroxysmal Positional Nystagmus—An Electronystagmographic and Clinical Study. Ann. Otol. Rhinol. Laryngol., *74*:69, 1965.

88. Stenger, H. H.: Über Lagerungsnystagmus unter besonderer Berücksichtigung des gegenläufigen transitorischen Provokations-nystagmus bei Lagewechsel in der Saggitalebene. Arch. F. Ohren. Nasen U. Kehlkopfheilkunde, *168*:220, 1955.

89. Stroud, M. H., et al.: Vestibular Dysfunctions after Midline Lesions in the Brain Stem of the Cat. Ann. Otol. Rhinol. Laryngol., *80*:750, 1971.

90. Tibbling, L.: The Rotatory Nystagmus Response in Children. Acta Otolaryng. (Stockh.), *68*:459, 1969.

91. Toglia, J. U., and Moreno, S.: Labyrinthine versus Central Nystagmus: Electronystagmographic Observation. Dis. Nerv. Syst., *32*:623, 1971.

92. Torok, N.: Differential Caloric Stimulations in Vestibular Diagnosis. Arch. Otolaryng., *90*:78, 1969.

93. Tos, M., et al.: Horizontal Optokinetic Nystagmus in Cerebral Diseases. Acta Neurol. Scand., *48*:607, 1972.

94. van Egmond, A. A., et al.: The Turning Test with Small Regulable Stimuli. I. The Method of Examination: Cupulometria. J. Laryngol. Otol., *62*:63, 1948.

95. von Noorden, G. K., and Preziosi, T. J.: Eye Movement Recordings in Neurological Disorders. Arch. Ophthalmol., *76*:162, 1966.

96. Walsh, F. B., and Hoyt, W. F.: *Clinical Neuro-ophthalmology*. 3rd ed. Baltimore, Williams & Wilkins, 1969.

97. Williams, H. L.: The Present Status of the Diagnosis and Treatment of Endolymphatic Hydrops. Ann. Otol. Rhinol. Laryngol., 56:614, 646, 1947.

98. Wolfson, R. J. (Ed.): *The Vestibular System and Its Diseases*. Philadelphia, University of Pennsylvania Press, 1966.

Chapter 44

Audiology

James Jerger and Robert Frisina

The accurate measurement of hearing and hearing loss is vital to the assessment of communication handicaps and to otologic diagnosis. To understand how modern hearing tests can contribute to the total evaluation of the hearing-impaired patient, it is necessary to consider the nature of sound, the measurement of sound intensity, and the limits of human hearing. This initial material is followed by sections on pure tone audiometry, speech audiometry, special diagnostic audiometry in adults, testing of children, and the nature of and indications for aural rehabilitation.

Nature of Sound

Sound in air results from the alternate compression and rarefaction of air particles. The rate at which this compression and rarefaction takes place is the *frequency* of the sound. A single compression and rarefaction is called a *cycle*. Frequency is the number of such cycles occurring in each second of time. The unit of frequency, formerly the number of *cycles per second,* has recently been changed to *hertz* and is abbreviated *Hz.* Thus a 1000-Hz sound is one in which there are 1000 complete cycles of compression and rarefaction each second.

The magnitude or *intensity* of a sound is most conveniently described by the alternating *pressure* it exerts. The unit of sound pressure is the *dyne per square centimeter,* commonly abbreviated dyne/cm².

The Decibel Scale of Sound Intensity

The range of sound pressures to which the normal ear responds is so great that the numbers involved are difficult to handle. Near the threshold of hearing, sound exerts a pressure of about $\frac{1}{10,000}$ of a dyne/cm². This pressure must be increased 10 million fold, however, before that same sound becomes painfully loud. The *decibel* (dB) scale is employed in order to keep within tractable limits the numbers involved in such a range. This is done by selecting some arbitrary point on the pressure scale as a base, expressing all other points on the scale as ratios of this base, taking the common logarithm of the ratio, and finally multiplying this logarithm by 20.

For example, an arbitrary base that might be selected is 12 dyne/cm². Now consider another point on the pressure scale, 1200 dyne/cm². This is a pressure 100 times greater than the base. In order to express this second pressure of 1200 dyne/cm² on a decibel scale in which 12 dyne/cm² is zero, we first form the ratio 1200/12. This ratio is 100. Now we take the common logarithm of 100. The common logarithm of a number is the number of times that 10 must be multiplied by itself (the exponent of 10) in order to produce the original number. For example, if $10^x = y$, then X is the logarithm of y. In our example above, 2 is the logarithm of 100, since $10^2 = 100$. Two, therefore, is the logarithm of the pressure ratio. In order to put this number into decibel units we must multiply it by 20. Since $20 \times 2 = 40$, 40 is the number of decibels that 1200 dyne/cm² is above 12 dyne/cm².

Note that it is meaningless to talk about decibels unless the starting point is specified. A sound at any given pressure can have several different decibel values, depending on what pressure is chosen as the zero or starting point on the scale. In actual practice there are three commonly used starting points for decibel scales. One is 0.0002 dyne/cm², which was chosen because at one time it was considered to be the sound pressure corresponding to best human hearing. Another base is the average normal hearing threshold itself. Finally, 1 dyne/cm² (1 microbar) is frequently used as a reference pressure, particularly in the calibration of microphones.

The scale based on 0.0002 dyne/cm² is called the *Sound Pressure Level* (SPL) scale. Thus 60 dB SPL means a pressure 60 decibels above 0.0002 dyne/cm². The scale based on average normal hearing is called the *Hearing Threshold Level* or *Hearing Level* (HL) *Scale*. Thus 60 dB HL means a pressure of 60 decibels above the standard threshold reference pressure corresponding to average normal hearing at that frequency.

One essential difference between these two scales is that the SPL scale is based on a physical starting point (0.0002 dyne/cm²), whereas the HL scale is based on a psychological or behavioral measurement starting point, average normal hearing.

The decibel markings on the hearing loss dial of an audiometer represent a Hearing Level (HL) scale. The zero point on the dial at any frequency is, in fact, the sound pressure level that corresponds to the average normal threshold of hearing at that frequency, as defined by the International Standards Organization (ISO–64) or the American National Standards Institute (ANSI–69).

Limits of Human Hearing

Roughly, humans can hear frequencies in the range of 20 to 20,000 Hz. This is only a coarse generalization, however, because the ability to hear very high frequencies de-

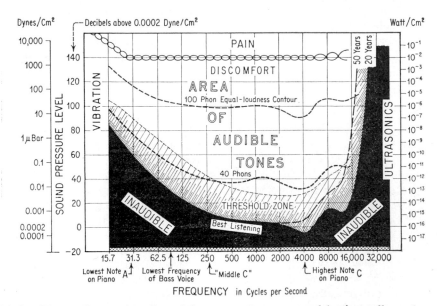

FIG. 44–1. The auditory area. Sound frequency is represented horizontally and sound intensity vertically. The upper frequency boundary is the most difficult to define because of its marked decline with age. (Davis, H., and Silverman, S. R.: *Hearing and Deafness*. New York, Holt, Rinehart and Winston, 1960.)

clines gradually with age. We know that this decline begins as early as the third decade of life and may reduce the upper limit to as little as 10,000 Hz or even less by the sixth decade of life. Furthermore, it is becoming clear that young children may hear higher frequencies than we had previously suspected. Ultimately the upper limit may have to be set as high as 30,000 Hz.

The intensity boundaries of human hearing can be identified with greater precision. The sound pressure level of just audible tones varies somewhat with frequency. In the region of best sensitivity (1000 to 4000 Hz), it is close to 0.0002 dyne/cm². The upper intensity boundary is about 140 dB above 0.0002 dyne/cm². At this level, sounds of any frequency become painful and cannot be long endured.

The *auditory area* defined by those boundaries is graphically illustrated in Figure 44–1.

The Audiogram

The most common form in which the results of hearing tests are displayed is called an *audiogram*. The purpose of the audiogram is to provide a graphic plot of the patient's loss in threshold sensitivity at each test frequency. The audiogram is, in fact, nothing more than the central part of the auditory area defined in Figure 44–1, but with two important changes. First, it is turned upside down so that intensity increases downward rather than upward as in Figure 44–1. Second, the zero line is not 0.0002 dyne/cm². Instead, it is the sound pressure level corresponding to average normal hearing at each frequency. Thus the decibel scale on the audiogram means decibels above average normal hearing, and any departure from zero indicates departure from "normal." For many years this scale was actually called "hearing loss." More recently, however, it has been relabeled "hearing threshold level" or simply "hearing level" (HL). The term *hearing level* is meant to imply status relative to some average norm, whereas the term *hearing loss* is meant to imply deviation from a given individual's previous state.

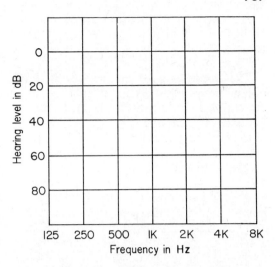

FIG. 44–2. The audiogram. Frequency is represented horizontally in octave intervals. Hearing level is represented vertically in decibels and increases downward. Each octave covers the same distance as 20 dB.

Figure 44–2 shows an example of a typical audiogram form. It covers the frequency range from 125 Hz to 8000 Hz, and the intensity range from −10 to + 100 dB hearing level.

AUDIOMETRY

There are three necessary conditions for audiometry: an audiometer, a suitable testing environment, and a competent audiometrist.

The Audiometer

Commercially available audiometers consist of six essential parts: (1) an *oscillator*, which generates the various pure tones; (2) an *amplifier*, which increases the intensity of the pure tone to a useful level; (3) an *interruptor* circuit, which permits the tester to turn the pure tone on and off smoothly and without audible clicks; (4) an *attenuator*, which allows the tester to increase or decrease the intensity by known amounts; (5) an *earphone*, which converts the electrical signal generated by the audiometer into actual sound; (6) a *masking noise generator*, which is often needed to exclude the ear not under test.

Audiometers produce pure tones at octave or half-octave intervals from 125 to 8000 Hz and permit variation of the intensity over a range of 110 dB.

The importance of an adequately functioning interruptor circuit cannot be overemphasized. Unless the tone can be turned on and off smoothly and quickly without overshoot and other types of distortion, audiometric results may be equivocal.

The amplifier and attenuator are important to the accuracy of the intensity calibration of the audiometer. The attenuator is more familiarly known as the hearing-level dial of the audiometer. It is ordinarily marked off in 5-dB steps. At the higher frequencies it is not uncommon for attenuators to "leak" (i.e., fail to attenuate properly) at the very low hearing levels (0 to −10 dB hearing level). When this happens, the responses of people with normal hearing all tend to cluster around the lowest level on the hearing loss dial (usually −10 dB). In this event nonlinearity or "leaking" of the attenuator must be suspected.

Although the proper care of an audiometer requires attention to all of these parts, the place where trouble is most likely to occur is the earphone or the earphone cord. Earphones should always be treated gently and the cords replaced at regular intervals. This will go a long way toward reducing the amount of service that an audiometer will need.

In diagnostic audiometry it is essential to have available a source of noise with which to "mask out" the ear not under test when the need arises. A good masking noise is "white noise," a type of noise that sounds much like escaping steam or rushing wind. White noise has many desirable properties that recommend it over other types of noise such as "sawtooth," "complex," or 60-cycle hum. Narrow-band masking noise is simply white noise that has been filtered to remove energy that is not useful in masking the particular tone under consideration.

Suitable Testing Environment

Precise audiometry cannot be carried out unless the background noise level is low enough so that the sensitivity of normal hearing listeners will not be masked by the background noise. The problem is greatest for low frequencies, especially 125, 250, and 500 Hz. Generally speaking, the lower the test frequency, the more likely it is to be affected by environmental noise.

The best method of coping with background noise is to situate the patient in a specially constructed sound booth that has been designed to minimize the transmission of sound through its walls. Although rooms of this type can be constructed from raw materials, it may be just as desirable to obtain prefabricated rooms that have been especially designed for audiometric use.

Although certain earphone headsets produce considerable attenuation of background noise, they are ordinarily not sufficient as replacements for actual sound booths. The problem with headsets is that they do not produce much attenuation in the low-frequency range from 100 to 500 Hz, the range most important for audiometry. In this low range, only a thick wall accomplishes much sound attenuation.

Competent Audiometrist

Adequate audiometry cannot be carried out by personnel who have not received suitable training and experience. In order to obtain accurate and useful clinical information, the audiometrist must have a satisfactory grasp of the basic principles underlying behavioral measurement. He must, in addition, be familiar with the audiologic patterns associated with the various types of hearing disorders. Finally, he must understand the limitations of electroacoustic instruments.

PURE TONE AUDIOMETRY

Air Conduction Audiogram

The purpose of air conduction audiometry is to measure the sensitivity of the entire hearing mechanism—the outer and middle ear and the sensorineural mechanism of the cochlea and auditory nerve.

The air conduction audiogram is obtained by presenting short pulses of tone to the test ear via the audiometer earphone. At each test frequency the audiometrist varies the intensity systematically in order to find the patient's "threshold" hearing level for the test tone. *Threshold* is usually understood to mean that level at which the patient responds to the tone just 50% of the time. In practice this is a difficult level to pinpoint exactly, since the intensity is ordinarily changed in relatively large steps (5 dB). In seeking the threshold level it is important that the test tone be presented only in short spurts by means of the interruptor switch of the audiometer. The tester initially presents the tone at a level well above threshold, decreases the intensity of successive tone bursts until the patient ceases to respond, then increases the intensity until a response reappears. The tester then continues this crisscrossing until he has identified that level at which a response occurs about half of the time. For a detailed description of the preferred method for threshold audiometry, consult Carhart and Jerger.

The patient may signal his response in a number of ways, but most audiometrists prefer to have him raise his finger each time a tone is heard. The advantage of this method of signaling is that it provides a direct visual contact between patient and tester at all times.

Most audiometrists begin the audiometric exploration at 1000 Hz because of a prevalent feeling that threshold is somewhat more stable at this frequency than at any other. There is no good evidence that the order in which the various frequencies are tested has any marked effect on the results obtained. It is important, however, that the first frequency tested be at least as high as 500 Hz, since patients have ordinarily had no previous experience in listening to low-pitched tones. Practice at 500 Hz and above greatly facilitates the subsequent test at 250 and 125 Hz.

As each threshold hearing level is identified, it is entered directly on the audiogram form. Red O's denote the right ear. Blue X's denote the left ear. The various symbols are then joined by short lines. Figure 44–3 shows an example of a complete air conduction audiogram for right and left ears.

It sometimes happens that there is a substantial difference between threshold hearing levels in the two ears. Whenever this differ-

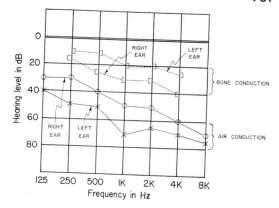

FIG. 44–3. Method for recording audiometric findings. Air conduction is represented by red O's for the right ear and blue X's for the left ear. Bone conduction is represented by red ['s for the right ear and blue]'s for the left ear. The direction in which the latter symbols face is based on visualization of the patient's head as seen from the front by the examiner.

ence exceeds the interaural attenuation factor for air-conducted sounds, it is necessary to put a suitable masking noise into the better ear when testing the poorer ear. Unless this is done, one runs the risk that the sound presented to the poorer ear will cross around the head and be heard in the good ear. The problem of cross-hearing of the test signal from the test ear to the nontest ear arises in *air conduction* whenever there is a sensitivity difference of 30 to 50 dB between ears. In this circumstance a tone presented to the poorer ear at or near "threshold" could travel around and/or through the head, by both air conduction and bone conduction routes, and be heard in the better ear. Unless this better ear is "masked" out by noise, one cannot be sure in which ear the patient is actually hearing the tone. In fact, experimental evidence shows that patients with total unilateral losses will show audiometric curves at about a 50-dB hearing level on the poorer ear when the opposite normal ear is not masked. Such false results are called "shadow curves" because they follow or "shadow" the contour of the audiometric curve on the normal ear but are displaced downward by the amount that the sound is attenuated (i.e., decreased in intensity) in its trip around

Figure 44–6 illustrates the audiometric contour typical of unilateral Meniere's disease. Hearing is normal in the left ear, but the right ear shows a flat loss of moderate degree, with interweaving air and bone indicating that the loss is sensorineural rather than conductive.

Figure 44–7 illustrates the audiometric contour typical of bilateral presbycusis, the decline in hearing associated with aging. Air and bone curves interweave, indicating a sensorineural loss. The curves show a mild loss that increases gradually with frequency.

Within any given category of hearing loss one must expect considerable variation in both degree of loss and exact conformity to these illustrative examples. Nevertheless, the recognition of these characteristic audiometric contours has proved to be of immense value in the refinement of otologic diagnosis.

SPEECH AUDIOMETRY

The introduction of the concept of speech audiometry is probably the most important single contribution of audiology to the evaluation of hearing impairment. Broadly speaking, there are two kinds of speech audiometric measures, those concerned with *sensitivity* and those concerned with *understanding*.

Measures of Sensitivity

Measures of sensitivity are designed to answer the question, "What is the faintest level at which speech can be understood by the patient?" The problem has been approached in the same fashion as pure tone sensitivity testing, by presenting individual words at different hearing levels and seeking the level at which the patient correctly repeats just 50% of the test words—in other words, his *threshold* for speech.

Spondaic words (i.e., two syllables, equally stressed) have been traditionally used as the test stimuli. Recorded versions of spondaic threshold tests are available as Central Institute for the Deaf (CID) Auditory Tests W–1 and W–2.

The relation between the threshold for speech and the threshold for pure tones forms the basis for the clinical application of speech sensitivity measures. Ordinarily the threshold HL for spondaic words should agree closely with the average threshold HL for pure tones at 500, 1000, and 2000 Hz. The only serious qualification to this rule occurs in the case of patients with sharply falling audiometric contours in the mid-frequency region. In such patients the threshold HL for speech will agree more nearly with the average threshold HL of the two lowest frequencies, 500 and 1000 Hz.

Measures of Understanding

Measures of understanding ask the question, "How adequately can the patient understand speech that is well above his threshold?" If speech is made loud enough to overcome the patient's sensitivity loss but he still cannot understand all of it clearly, then he is said to have a *discrimination loss* for speech.

In the past, tests for discrimination loss have employed, almost exclusively, the phonetically balanced (*PB*) *word* lists originally developed to test the adequacy of speech transmission systems.

Typically, each of the 50 words in a PB list is delivered to the patient's ear at a level 20 to 40 dB above his spondaic threshold, and he is asked to repeat each word. The tester then scores his responses as either correct or incorrect. The percentage of the 50 words correctly repeated is the patient's *discrimination score*. The percentage of incorrect responses is the *discrimination loss*. Recorded versions of PB word tests are available as CID Auditory Test W–22.

Patients with purely conductive hearing problems ordinarily show little or no discrimination loss, but patients with sensorineural loss may show any degree of discrimination loss from very slight to very severe. The most marked discrimination losses seem to occur in patients with active eighth nerve lesions, such as acoustic neurinoma. However, the variability among patients and the degree of overlap between clinical categories are so great that discrimination loss per se is not a precise tool for differential diagnosis.

Measures of understanding for speech do,

however, have two important clinical applications. First, they give us indispensable information about the extent of the patient's communication handicap. They form the basis for predicting the problems which the patient will face in day-to-day living. Second, they tell us a good deal about the prognosis for the successful use of a hearing aid.

Unfortunately the conventional tests for speech discrimination loss, the PB word lists, are not entirely satisfactory as predictors of the patient's ability to understand actual running speech. We need, for this purpose, test materials that more closely simulate the "everyday speech," and, more importantly, the "everyday hearing," typical of the normal communication process. Workers in many laboratories and clinics are currently attacking this problem.

DIAGNOSTIC AUDIOMETRY

Impedance Audiometry

Impedance audiometry is one of the most important new developments in audiology during the past decade. The advent of the inexpensive, simple to operate, and clinically feasible electroacoustic impedance bridge has wrought a minor revolution in audiologic evaluation.

Impedance audiometry consists of three components. The first, tympanometry, measures how the impedance characteristics of the middle ear mechanism change as air pressure is varied in the external auditory meatus. The change in impedance as a function of changing air pressure is called a tympanogram, and the resulting measure is called tympanometry.

The diagnostic value of tympanometry lies primarily in the fact that different types of middle ear disorder modify the shape of the tympanogram in characteristic ways. The normal, or type A, tympanogram, for example, is attenuated or made shallow (type A_S) by ossicular chain fixation but is deepened (type A_D) by ossicular chain discontinuity. Negative pressure in the middle ear space shifts the peak of the tympanogram in the negative direction (type C), while fluid or other mass effects in the middle ear flatten out the ordinarily sharp peak (type B).

Thus the shape of the tympanogram, considered in relation to the nature of the audiogram and the acoustic reflexes, can have considerable diagnostic significance.

The second component of impedance audiometry is the absolute impedance or static compliance. This refers to the ease with which the middle ear system can be set into vibration in comparison with the normal middle ear. Again the diagnostic value of the static compliance measure lies in the fact that the absolute value is modified in characteristic fashion by middle ear disorder. Unfortunately, however, the wide range of variability of this measure in the normal population makes it the least useful member of the impedance battery.

The third component of impedance audiometry is the stapedius or acoustic reflex. The stapedius muscle is connected from the head of the stapes to the posterior wall of the middle ear cavity. When it contracts, it draws the stapes inward and backward, tensing the chain and producing a characteristic impedance change. The acoustic reflex can be elicited by an acoustic signal in either ear. The measurement is carried out by varying the intensity of the acoustic signal until the muscle contraction occurs. Contraction of the muscle is detected by the impedance bridge.

The nature of the acoustic reflex in patients with hearing disorders is, paradoxically enough, at once the most ambiguous and the most useful member of the impedance team. While the absence of the reflex per se can be attributed to a variety of diverse problems, the complex interaction of the audiogram, the tympanogram, and both crossed and uncrossed reflex data provides an unusually incisive diagnostic description of the hearing disorder.

The modern electroacoustic impedance bridge contains all of the necessary components for carrying out the three components of impedance audiometry: tympanometry, static compliance, and the stapedius reflex. The probe tip of the impedance bridge is sealed in the external canal by a small rubber tip, and an earphone is placed over the opposite ear. The probe tip contains the tube which permits variation of air pressure in the external canal and the necessary instrumentation for monitoring the impedance characteristics of the middle ear system. Sounds of various frequencies can be delivered to an earphone, by an audiometer which is an integral part of the impedance bridge, for measurement of the acoustic reflex.

Impedance measures permit four broad categories of prediction: (1) the differentiation of conductive loss and sensorineural loss, (2) the nature of the conductive loss, (3) the nature of the sensorineural loss, and (4) the quantification of degree and slope of sensorineural hearing loss.

The actual clinical application of impedance audiometry, however, involves extremely complex interpretations. For a more detailed treatment of this important subject, consult the *Handbook of Clinical Impedance Audiometry* (Jerger, 1975).

Although impedance audiometry has been found to be extremely useful in the evaluation of virtually all patients with hearing problems, its diagnostic value is most dramatically illustrated in the evaluation of young children. In these patients, conventional behavioral techniques and/or physiologic recording techniques are often incomplete or ambiguous. The additional data afforded by the impedance battery can therefore provide extremely valuable confirmatory evidence. Table 44–1 illustrates how the overall pattern of impedance results can be helpful in confirming or denying clinical impressions based on behavioral audiometric tests. For example, the following impedance results would confirm an impression of unilateral conductive loss: (1) type B or C tympanogram on the bad ear, type A tympanogram on the good ear; (2) static compliance measures lower than normal on the bad ear and within the normal range on the good ear; and (3) acoustic reflexes absent in both ears. In contrast, the following impedance pattern would confirm an impression of unilateral cochlear loss with loudness recruitment: (1) type A tympanogram on both ears; (2) static compliance measures within normal limits on both ears; and (3) acoustic reflexes elicited at normal hearing levels on both ears.

The impedance patterns in Table 44–1 can be particularly helpful in the evaluation of very young children with either no audiometric data or sound-field behavioral results only. For example, if a child seems to be responding behaviorally in the sound field at moderate sound levels yet acoustic reflexes are bilaterally absent in spite of normal static compliance and normal type A tympanograms, then the validity of the behavioral responses is questionable. Similarly, if

Table 44–1. Ways in Which Results of Impedance Audiometery Help to Confirm Audiometric Impression in the Evaluation of Young Children

Tympanometry	Static Compliance	Acoustic Reflex	Confirm Behavioral Audiometric Impression of
A in both ears	Normal in both ears	Normal bilaterally	Bilateral normal hearing or bilateral mild-moderate sensorineural loss or unilateral mild-moderate sensorineural loss
A in both ears	Normal in both ears	Absent bilaterally	Severe bilateral sensorineural loss
A in one ear; B or C in other ear	Normal in A ear; low in B or C ear	Absent bilaterally	Unilateral conductive loss
B or C in both ears	Low in both ears	Absent bilaterally	Bilateral conductive loss

there is no observable response to sound at any level yet acoustic reflexes occur at normal levels bilaterally, then the behavioral impression of profound deafness is not supported. Other possible reasons for the child's failure to respond behaviorally must be entertained. Impedance results can also be helpful in identifying middle ear disorders in children whose bone conduction levels cannot be validly measured either because of age or because the sensorineural loss is too severe.

These examples illustrate just some of the many ways in which impedance audiometry can supplement conventional behavioral techniques. The combination of impedance results and conventional audiometric findings offers valuable information that cannot be obtained from either test procedure alone.

OTHER DIAGNOSTIC TESTS

A number of special audiometric test procedures have been developed to assist in otologic diagnosis. Properly used, they can contribute valuable information on the probable locus of the hearing disorder. In general, they are all based on observations that lesions at different points along the auditory system alter the patient's response to certain sound stimuli in different ways. This kind of specialized audiometry requires, however, rather sophisticated electronic instrumentation and considerable training in auditory test administration and interpretation.

The following diagnostic audiometric procedures are helpful in the differentiation of cochlear and eighth nerve disorders:

1. Alternate binaural loudness balance (ABLB) (Jerger, 1962)

2. Bekesy audiometry (Jerger, 1962) and its modifications (Jerger, 1973): the forward versus backward continuous sweep frequency tracings (Jerger and Jerger, 1974) and the Bekesy comfortable loudness (BCL) tracings (Jerger and Jerger, 1974)

3. The threshold tone decay test (TDT) (Carhart) and the suprathreshold adaptation test (STAT) (Jerger and Jerger, 1976)

4. The acoustic reflex decay test (Jerger et al.)

5. The rollover effect (Jerger and Jerger, 1974) on the performance versus intensity function for speech materials

In addition to some of the above procedures, several other techniques are helpful in the evaluation of central auditory disorders:

1. The synthetic sentence identification (SSI) test (Jerger, 1973) contrasting performance in the presence of ipsilateral competing messages (ICM) and contralateral competing messages (CCM)

2. The staggered spondaic word (SSW) test (Jerger, 1973)

For a more complete discussion of these techniques and their interpretation, consult Chapter Three, Diagnostic Audiometry, in *Modern Developments in Audiology* (Jerger, 1973).

Some of the many tests especially useful in the detection and evaluation of functional hearing disorders are the following:

1. Electrodermal audiometry
2. Stenger test
3. Bekesy audiometry
4. Acoustic reflex test
5. Lombard test
6. SRT versus PTA discrepancy

For a more complete discussion of these techniques and their interpretation, see Chapter 6, Functional Hearing Loss, in *Modern Developments in Audiology* (Hopkinson).

AUDITORY TESTING OF CHILDREN

Children, in contrast to adults, have little if any reason for wanting to be tested. They frequently show a natural reluctance to become involved with strangers in an unnatural setting. Special effort is required to persuade children to listen attentively for sounds which, for the most part, are unrelated to their everyday interests. Also, the reliability of the child's response is often questionable. It is common, therefore, to modify adult procedures when using them with young clinical patients.

Neonatal Period (Birth to 2 Months)

The principal observable responses to sound which occur during the first 2 months of life are essentially gross all-or-none behavioral responses. These include the so-called Moro reflex, the auriculopalpebral reflex (APR), and the crying responses generated by percussive instruments emitting sharp, loud sounds of short duration. Pure tones ranging from 500 to 4000 Hz delivered through loudspeakers at intensity levels of 85 to 95 dB above normal threshold can elicit the APR during the first 2 weeks of life. However, pure tones or other controlled stimuli presented at or near normal threshold levels do not elicit behavioral responses.

The surge in infant screening programs has subsided. The accepted position at this time is that infant screening might best be limited to high-risk cases, as opposed to its general application to all newborns.

Infancy (2 to 24 months)

Near the end of the neonatal period, apparent neurologic maturation is reflected by changes in behavioral responses. The high-intensity sounds which heretofore evoked the Moro reflex and the APR seem to do so less regularly, although both responses are still present. An important change in auditory behavior occurs at about the eighth week. The infant begins to attend to sounds and is disrupted by them. At 16 weeks the high-intensity sounds elicit an auditory oculogyric (AOR) response (eye movement in the horizontal plane) rather regularly. Response to lower intensity levels in the form of localization of sound sources becomes apparent after approximately 24 weeks in the normal infant. The localization response has become an important diagnostic clue in infants. Speech stimuli, white noise, and familiar environmental sounds presented through loudspeakers at intensity levels within 20 dB of normal can be responded to consistently if the youngster is not too engrossed in other activities. Failure to localize mild and moderate intensity stimuli accurately by the age of 8 months is of diagnostic significance. However, failure to do so sometimes may be related to factors other than deafness. For example, children with developmental retardation associated with central nervous system involvement frequently do not localize the source of the sound accurately at 8 months.

The average 1-year-old infant comprehends auditory symbols. He can identify his parents, and, as he approaches the fifteenth month, he begins to identify parts of the body by name at normal intensity levels. He begins to produce two-word sentences at approximately 18 months. In the absence of these abilities in comprehension and expression, his auditory status should be questioned. Unfortunately, monaural threshold measurement utilizing behavioral responses has not been routinely successful below 2 years of age. At best, a good deal of clinical skill is involved in making judgments concerning auditory thresholds of children below 2 years of age. Moreover, in such instances the decisions must be based on factors other than purely auditory measurement.

Beyond Infancy

Pure tone audiometric thresholds can be obtained in clinical patients as young as approximately 22 months. Apparently the ability to associate an auditory stimulus with a specific volitional behavioral response requires nearly 2 years of neurologic maturation. Additional factors requiring consideration in the measurement of hearing with behavioral response techniques are: (1) the child must be assisted in overcoming the natural resistance to strangers and to an unfamiliar setting; (2) the child must accept earphones so that the ears can be measured separately; (3) a conditioning procedure must be used which allows the child to associate a stimulus with a specific response; and (4) the child must be assisted in maintaining the attention to the stimulus-response (S-R) task.

Standard or conventional audiometry (adult procedure) is applicable in normal children as young as 3 years of age. Normative data on such children indicate that auditory sensitivity in children is equal to that of young adults.

Several electrophysiologic responses have been used for research purposes in the human and in lower animals. Although declining in its usefulness, the most common clinical auditory test procedure utilizing an electrophysiologic response has been the *electrodermal response* (EDR, GSR, PGSR). When response criteria are defined precisely, the thresholds resulting from standard audiometry and EDR audiometry in adults are equivalent. This similarity in thresholds holds for groups of children with normal hearing and those with deafness as well. In the case of the latter, play audiometry is used to derive thresholds for comparison with those obtained from EDR audiometry. Electrocardiographic response audiometry has been attempted in neonates, but at present this approach is used neither clinically nor, to any great extent, experimentally in children.

Recently Hecox and Galambos demonstrated brain stem responses, presumably from the inferior colliculi, by averaging techniques following the input of clicks at the rate of 20 per second. This response seems to hold considerable promise in the evaluation of young children.

Pediatric patients generally referred for audiometric tests are those with acute middle ear involvement, those who have not learned to talk normally, and those with developmental deviations related either to central nervous system disorders or to emotional adjustment difficulties.

Testing for Middle Ear Loss

The extent and duration of a hearing loss due to middle ear infection usually do not influence greatly the child's ability to communicate. Thus the procedures used to obtain the pure tone air conduction audiogram in such children over 3 years of age are similar to those described by Carhart and Jerger.

Bone conduction audiograms are plotted according to the procedure used in determining air conduction thresholds. Masking is necessary in most young children because of low reliability in reporting lateralization. A simple explanation to the child indicating that he should ignore the noise and continue responding to the pure tones and a brief practice period are sufficient for successful bone conduction testing in most children 36

months of age and older who have middle ear disorders.

It is desirable to establish speech sensitivity thresholds because this provides an outside criterion with which to compare reliability and validity of the pure tone air conduction responses. This is accomplished by using selected spondaic words in a manner similar to that used with adult patients.

Testing for Sensorineural Loss

Varying degrees of discrimination loss occur when the site of the hearing disorder exists beyond the middle ear. The resultant inability to understand clearly the speech of others causes a delay in the development of the child's own speech production. Thus one finds that most pediatric sensorineural cases of hearing loss are brought to the attention of the otolaryngologist because of some manifest delay in speech development. Because of the communication problem which frequently exists in such children, standard pure tone and speech audiometric procedures cannot always be followed precisely.

Play audiometry is the modified procedure of choice at present in children 22 to 24 months of age and older who have retarded speech development which is presumed to be a result of hearing loss (Fig. 44–8). The child must first be led to accept earphones, so that the two ears can be

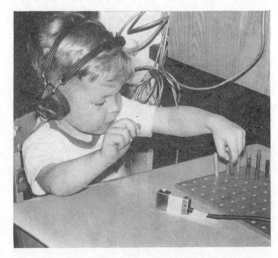

Fig. 44–8. A 3-year-old child participating in play audiometry.

measured separately. The air conduction pure tone audiogram is then completed in the following manner. Testing is begun at 500 Hz, because if any hearing remains, it is most likely to be present at 500 Hz, and if the loss is complete, a tactile response can often be elicited at this frequency. Attentiveness on the part of the patient can be maintained if the examiner conveys a demonstrable interest in the proceedings. Reward in the form of applause, a smile, a nod, activation of a toy, and so forth should be provided only when a correct response has been made. The child's response should be as simple as possible—for example, placing a ring on a peg, placing a block in a box, or executing any simple play activity. It is imperative that the child know when his response is correct. It is critical, too, that he not be rewarded for making false responses. Finally, the response must be in keeping with his mental age. In defining threshold the procedure should first determine the intensity that consistently elicits the play response. It is recommended that 10- to 15-dB intervals be used in the bracketing-of-threshold procedure and that positive stimuli (intensity level where consistent responses occur) be interspersed frequently so as to reduce the number of false responses, which a child often makes in attempting to please the examiner. It is common to find that the threshold (50% response point) is 5 dB above the zero response point and 5 dB less intense than the 100% response point. In other words, the dB range between consistent responses and no responses rarely exceeds 10 dB when the factors discussed are incorporated into the air conduction procedure.

Bone conduction testing in cases with sensorineural hearing loss follows the procedure used in plotting the air conduction audiogram. Forehead placement of the bone oscillator can be used to screen quickly the frequencies 250 through 4000 Hz at octave intervals. However, mastoid tip placement with masking of the opposite ear is used most commonly to determine threshold at each frequency.

Bekesy audiometry can be used with children as young as 6 or 7 years of age. The procedure must be modified for use below

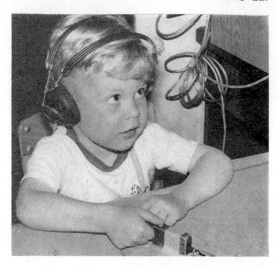

Fig. 44–9. A 3-year-old child participating in Bekesy audiometry.

these ages in order to provide information regarding different sites of lesion within the auditory system. Frisina and Johnson developed a modified approach to Bekesy audiometry for use with children who have communication disorders (Fig. 44–9). Deaf children as young as 3 years of age learned to perform this audiometric procedure following conditioning to a vibrotactile stimulus.

Speech audiometry is routinely applied to pediatric patients with sensorineural hearing loss. Since speech production in these children is likely to be limited, an alternate response is required. Instead of responding orally, the child must be taught to point to an appropriate picture representing the stimulus word. The procedure used for threshold determination in adults is followed. Only the response is altered. The threshold HL for spondaic words should agree closely with the average threshold HL for pure tones at 500, 1000, and 2000 Hz. In children who cannot satisfy the 50% correct response criterion, the *speech awareness threshold* (SAT) is determined. The child is conditioned to respond as in play audiometry. The SAT should agree with the 500-Hz threshold in cases with falling audiometric contours, or the frequency with the least hearing loss in cases with rising audiometric curves.

When age at onset is congenital or pre-lingual, children with sensorineural losses generally cannot participate validly in the measurement of discrimination loss. Their speech production anomalies make it impossible to score oral responses, and, as a rule, they are too young to write the response. Attempts can be made to have them select appropriate pictures, but the word lists available are of limited usefulness. Following professional assistance in the development of speech and general education training, many can speak or write the stimulus word heard, but for the most part the information is of little theoretical or practical value in those who cannot satisfy the 50% response criterion required for sensitivity threshold utilizing spondaic words.

MANAGEMENT OF DEAF CHILDREN

Each professional discipline applying its special talents to the management of deaf children has its unique definition of deafness. However, in the final analysis, the individual with deafness perhaps assesses the full impact of the hearing impairment on his overall functioning. If he depends principally upon vision for the intake of verbal and nonverbal information, he is likely to consider himself deaf. If he depends equally upon vision and hearing in adjusting to his verbal and nonverbal environment, he most likely considers himself hard-of-hearing. In either case, from an audiologic and communicative point of view, the effect of the hearing impairment on the understanding of speech is a most critical variable. The reduction in speech understanding is at the root of many of the developmental problems requiring special attention.

A Basic Problem of Deafness

The child who does not receive speech efficiently through the auditory channel prior to his development of speech and command of the English language is confronted with real obstacles. He must simultaneously learn to use a defective auditory system and learn the structure of the English language. The average 2½-year-old-child with normal hearing has learned to receive and produce spoken sentences of five to six words. This verbal ability has been developed primarily through the auditory system. His speech and language are elaborated upon for an additional 4 to 4½ years (principally through hearing), for it is not until he reaches 5 or 6 years of age that a nonauditory symbol system is introduced. This, of course, involves the use of reading.

The heavy reliance upon the auditory system during the so-called formative pre-school years places the child with deafness at a severe disadvantage. He is forced to transpose spoken words (he sees them essentially as lip or labial movements) from the auditory to the visual form. However, acoustic signals are coded for the ear, not the eye. This imposes restrictions upon the efficiency with which he receives the speech of those around him. He does not receive appropriate models of speech and thus does not comprehend spoken language. Moreover, his inability to decode the speech of others results in the reception of inadequate models which he might imitate. The auditory deficit he possesses precludes the monitoring of his own voice even if he were to receive the message of others through means other than speech. Thus deafness brings problems of inefficiency in receiving communication, inability to develop the structure of the English language, and the resultant inability to develop speech spontaneously. Unless special procedures are instituted, these deficiencies further complicate education and socialization of the individual.

Sensorineural hearing losses, which routinely result in some discrimination loss, have the unfortunate potential of influencing development in these critical areas. It is important, then, that such pediatric cases of deafness be discovered early and managed properly.

Development of Communication Skills

Certain approximate guidelines exist relative to the effect of hearing loss on the development of speech and language. If the HL is less than 35 to 40 dB, speech is expected to emerge in essentially a normal manner. Speech distortions and omissions occur when the HL approaches 45 to 50 dB. Hearing levels of 55 to 65 dB influence the quality and quantity of speech production. In such cases speech is likely to develop spontaneously without professional assistance but will consist of simple phrases and short sentences which are malarticulated. As the HL approaches 70 to 75 dB, speech will no longer emerge in a spontaneous fashion. Special teaching techniques are required in order to develop speech in such children.

Hearing Aid Use. An important early step in the educational treatment of deaf children is the selection of an appropriate hearing aid. Hearing aids serve to make sounds louder but cannot reverse the discrimination loss resulting from the defective auditory system. Therefore, use of a hearing aid with most hard of hearing and deaf children should be considered a supplement to, rather than a replacement for, special assistance in communication and education. As the discrimination loss and the hearing level become more severe, the individual relies increasingly on vision for the intake of verbal information. In such cases the hearing aid is used as a supplement to lipreading. Most hard of hearing and deaf children are more proficient lipreaders when they supplement visual with auditory cues than when they are forced to lipread only. In these cases speech production often improves as a result of hearing aid use.

Hearing aids are especially helpful in children whose HL ranges from 45 to approximately 75 dB. Beyond a hearing level of 75 to 80 dB, a quantitative improvement in the understanding of the speech of others or in one's own speech proficiency as a result of hearing aid use is difficult to demonstrate. In short, a hearing aid is used in an attempt to reduce the ambiguity inherent in the visual process called lipreading and to facilitate the monitoring of one's own voice production.

Speech Training. The term *deaf and dumb* is no longer used by those working with the deaf in the United States. The term *deaf* is used in reference to those with severe auditory impairment. The term *dumb*

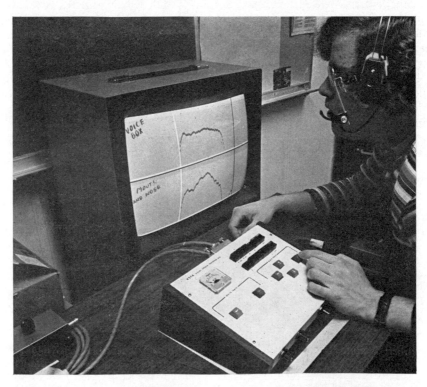

FIG. 44–10.   Electroacoustic visual display unit. (Courtesy National Technical Institute for the Deaf, Rochester, N.Y.)

has been eliminated because of its often incorrect connotation of an intellectual deficit. Educators of the deaf stress the fact that all deaf children, if provided appropriate training, are capable of learning to speak to some extent. Speech is taught in a variety of ways at this time in the many special schools and classes available for hard of hearing and deaf children in the United States. Much emphasis is placed on speech training in the preschool and primary school levels. The advent of wearable hearing aids and high-fidelity auditory training units has had a positive influence on the speech proficiency of those with deafness. Systematic research and development efforts regarding the use of electroacoustic visual display units in speech therapy with deaf students are presently under way at the National Technical Institute for the Deaf (Fig. 44–10).

Lipreading (Speech Reading). Prior to the availability of electronic hearing aids, the deaf and hard of hearing were chiefly dependent upon the visual skill of lipreading for the reception of speech. As a result, several methods of lipreading were devised. Formal training in this skill has receded sharply with the introduction of wearable hearing aids. However, those with a HL of 75 dB and greater are still dependent upon lipreading as a basic means of receptive communication. Deaf persons vary markedly in their lipreading performances as well as in their ability to improve in this specialized skill. The acquisition of lipreading skill and the process of lipreading have been the subject of many scientific investigations. Multifaceted and single correlational studies have shed very little light on how to teach lipreading or how to learn to lipread *well*. To assume that a course in lipreading will change the long-term needs of a deaf child is a gross oversimplification of the problem.

Reading. Learning to read well is not readily achieved in deaf children. The marked inefficiency in the reception and production of speech during the early years of a deaf child's life results in a paucity of information regarding the English language. His vocabulary is limited, and his knowledge of the structure of his native tongue is absent. When the hearing child learns to read, he is merely acquiring another vehicle

for representing the language he already has accumulated through acoustic symbols. It is a laborious task for the deaf child to learn the multiple meanings of words and to learn the meanings of larger units, such as idiomatic expressions and sentences, which have been readily assimilated by the child with normal hearing.

Manual Communication. Manual communication consists of fingerspelling and signing. The single-hand alphabet is used by many deaf persons in the United States. The letters of the alphabet are formed by positioning the fingers and thumb in 26 unique ways. This is the means by which Helen Keller communicated with her companion except that the positions were felt rather than seen by Miss Keller. The so-called "sign language" consists of a formal set of gestures which represent whole words. When one uses the sign language today, it is generally a combination of fingerspelled and signed words. Manual communication is used among many deaf persons because for them it is less ambiguous than acoustic symbols conveyed to them through hearing or via lipreading. The most vulnerable aspect of communication among even the highly educated deaf is the reception of speech. It is for receptive purposes that manual communication has sustained itself among the deaf and by many who must deal with the deaf on a daily basis educationally, socially, or in the business world. It is not used as a replacement for speech in those educational programs using manual communication. Rather, it is used as a supplement in the reception of speech which is perceived through the combination of hearing, lipreading, and signing.

Total Communication. The term total communication (TC) is in prevalent use today and refers to a philosophy of education of deaf children. Essentially, the advocates of TC promote the practices of speech training, hearing aid usage, lipreading training, reading instruction, and manual communication in the development of communication and linguistic skills in deaf children. In contrast to TC, the oral philosophy advocates recommend usage of all the above methodologies except manual communication.

BASIC TASKS IN PRESCHOOL TRAINING

Clarification of Problem and Interpretation to Parents

The diagnostic task requires the talents of several specialists, such as the pediatrician, otologist, psychologist, audiologist, and quite frequently the neurologist. With the cooperation of such specialists, the initial contact at the preschool level should be geared toward determination of biologic and psychological factors resulting in hearing, speech, and language deficiencies. In order to clarify the auditory status of the child, audiologic assessments should be repeated until reliable and valid test results are obtained. From these data the questions of amplification needs and type of amplification system are resolved. On-going psychological reappraisals should be conducted. From these reevaluations and other studies, special learning problems or idiosyncratic learning patterns can be determined and special programming can be devised.

Assistance to Parents

The program for parents should be organized around three areas. The first consists of information concerning general child development, the development of children with problems in audition, and the learning of language. Reading material and group discussions form an essential part of this first level of contact with parents.

The second area of attention provided parents should be the opportunity to participate in group discussions dealing with attitudes and feelings. The discussion need not be restricted to children with auditory and language disorders but should extend into parent-child and total family involvement. Ultimately, of course, references can be made to specific situations which can be handled according to accepted psychological principles.

The third area of interest deals with a limited number of parents who are in need of individual counseling. This is generally best accomplished through the cooperation of specialists in psychiatry and psychology.

A subtlety in working with parents of handicapped children is the danger that they will become too dependent upon the program and/or specific clinicians. A principal goal at the preschool level should be to make children and parents capable of accepting the fact that deafness requires more than routine attention as the child strives for adequate speech, language, and general educational development.

Preschool Experience

The basic purpose of this type of activity is to assist each child in his organization of behavior. More than lip service should be paid to individual differences. The history and determination of present status (through observation and utilization of objective tests) should be used as a point of departure with these children. Special attention should be given to auditory behavior, speech development, speechreading, reading, and writing.

Quantification of Techniques and Results

A final responsibility at the preschool level is the quantification of testing and treatment techniques. Cross-sectional research studies and a longitudinal study of each child are essential in dealing with such children. The application of quantifiable techniques will make it possible to determine the validity of existing audiologic and psychological tests. Hopefully, more reliable and hence more valid techniques will evolve as the result of such inquiries.

LONG-TERM ASPECTS OF DEAFNESS

Communication

In those children with hearing approximating HL 70 dB or greater in whom the age at onset of the deafness preceded the natural acquisition of speech, the reception of speech and the production of speech deviate in varying degrees from the normal. Although these children are aided materially by the availability of programs and early implementation of special training, the effects of deafness in the communication areas require many years of special attention. The development of speech appears to be most dependent upon and responsive to training and must be continued at least throughout the primary school years. Lipreading and auditory training (learning to use amplification devices) are less responsive to direct therapy but require practice and continued use over a period of years in order to contribute substantially to the overall communication proficiency of the individual.

Language

Acquisition of an understanding of the form and content of the English language is probably the most formidable obstacle confronting all deaf children. Idiomatic expressions, abstract concepts, and words with multiple meanings apparently are learned efficiently through hearing them repeatedly in meaningful contexts. The deaf child in comparison with his hearing counterpart perceives these unambiguously in markedly fewer instances. Perhaps it is not until the deaf child learns to read independently that the English language for the first time begins to gain some stability. A constant struggle for mastery of the English language remains with the congenitally deaf child throughout his lifetime, particularly in view of the new words and concepts introduced through the rapidly expanding technological and social changes taking place in our society.

Educational Requirements

Communication skills and language proficiency in large measure determine the efficiency with which a properly motivated child might learn the subject matter to which he is exposed. Regular classroom procedures are organized around acoustic signals (speech and hearing). The average deaf child is incapable of perceiving the speech of the teacher and the pupils efficiently. He is forced to make up for this inefficiency by working extra hours at home in an effort to keep pace with his classmates. This is in essence learning through a correspondence course rather than living the experience of spontaneous give-and-take in the classroom. The deaf student requires a classroom organized around visual stimuli augmented with auditory cues in order to make most effective use of classroom time. Even under these favorable conditions it is difficult for him to achieve in a manner similar to hearing students of comparable age.

TYPES OF EDUCATION PROGRAMS AVAILABLE

Schools for the Deaf

Day schools are those which children attend during the academic hours, after which they return home. *Residential schools* are those in which boarding facilities are provided following the academic hours. There are approximately 170 day and residential schools in the United States at this time (American Annals of the Deaf). Public day schools are generally part of the school systems of the cities in which they are located. Public residential schools are maintained as an attempt to ensure that every child in a given state is offered an appropriate educational program. If one is not available in his local community, he has recourse to private or public residential schools. Almost every residential school (public and private) encourages children to spend weekends at home whenever feasible. Also, all public and most private residential schools accept children on a day basis if they live within a reasonable commuting distance.

Classes for the Deaf

Frequently classrooms within a regular school are set aside for deaf children. Some 600 such classes are prevalent in metropolitan areas throughout the United States (Jerger, 1962). In areas of high population it is possible to provide adequate programs for deaf children. Sufficient space, modern electronic equipment, certified teachers, homogeneous grouping of children, limited teacher-pupil ratio, and a planned curriculum are among the important requisites for an adequate program for deaf children.

Classes for the Hard of Hearing

Special classes within local public school systems are available for children who need full-time special help. It is common to have rotating classes within which the hard-of-hearing student spends part of the day with other students with hearing problems and in addition attends classes with hearing students. Children with mild and moderate degrees of hearing impairment are frequently placed in regular classes. In many cities special communication and tutorial assistance is provided each day or at less frequent intervals.

Postsecondary Education

The postsecondary educational opportunities for deaf students have been expanding gradually. Two national programs sponsored by the Federal Government are now in existence. Gallaudet College (arts and sciences) in Washington, D.C., and the National Technical Institute for the Deaf (science and technology) in Rochester, New York, were founded through action of the Congress. In addition, some 25 conventional community colleges, technical-vocational institutes, and universities are providing special services which enable admission of deaf and hard-of-hearing students (Stuckless and Delgado).

REFERENCES

American Annals of the Deaf, *111*: 302, 1966.
Carhart, R.: Clinical Determination of Abnormal Auditory Adaptation. Arch. Otolaryng., *65*:32, 1957.
Carhart, R., and Jerger, J.: Preferred Method for Clinical Determination of Pure-tone Thresholds. J. Speech Hearing Disorders, *24*:330, 1959.
Frisina, D., and Johnson, D.: A Nonverbal Hearing Test for Children with Deafness. U. S. Office of Education Research Report No. 5–0962–4–11–3, 1966.
Hecox, K., and Galambos, R.: Brain Stem Auditory Evoked Responses in Human Infants and Adults. Arch. Otolaryng., *99*:30, 1974.
Hood, J. D.: The Principles and Practices of Bone Conduction Audiometry: A Review of the Present Position. Proc. R. Soc. Med., *50*:689, 1957.
Hopkinson, N.: Functional Hearing Loss. *In* Jerger, J. (Ed.): *Modern Developments in Audiology*. 2nd ed. New York, Academic Press, Inc., 1973, pp. 175–210.
Jerger, J.: Hearing Tests in Otologic Diagnosis. ASHA, *4*:139, 1962.
Jerger, J.: Diagnostic Audiometry. *In* Jerger, J. (Ed.): *Modern Developments in Audiology*. 2nd ed. New York, Academic Press, Inc., 1973, pp. 75–115.
Jerger, J. (Ed.): *Handbook of Clinical Impedance Audiometry*. Dobbs Ferry, N. Y., American Electromedics Corporation, 1975.
Jerger, J., and Jerger, S.: Audiological Comparison of Cochlear and Eighth Nerve Disorders. Ann. Otol. Rhinol. Laryng., *83*:275, 1974.
Jerger, J., and Jerger, S.: A Simplified Tone Decay Test. Arch. Otolaryng., *101*:403, 1975.
Jerger, J., *et al.*: The Acoustic Reflex in Eighth Nerve Disorders. Arch. Otolaryng., *99*:409, 1974.
Newby, H.: *Audiology*. New York, Appleton-Century-Crofts, 1958.
Stuckless, E., and Delgado, G.: *A Guide to College/Career Programs for Deaf Students*. Rochester, N. Y., National Technical Institute for the Deaf, 1973.

Chapter 45
Diseases of the External Ear

AURICLE

The skin on the external surface of the auricle is firmly attached to the underlying cartilage with the connective tissue of the dermis condensing to form perichondrium. The skin on the undersurface of the auricle, by contrast, has a true subcutaneous layer. This feature of the auricular integument combined with the exposed position of the auricle is responsible for the majority of clinical problems involving the auricle: trauma, exposure, and infection. Fluid accumulation consequent to these processes results in separation of the perichondrium from the cartilage. Unless this process is promptly relieved, necrosis of cartilage will result because of interference with its nutritional perfusion from the vessels of the perichondrium.

Trauma

Trauma to the auricle occurs frequently and may result in contusion, laceration, or, occasionally, loss of the entire auricle. In a number of instances, the auricle has been successfully resutured to the head with at least partial survival of the composite tissue. Repair of these injuries should follow ordinary principles of plastic surgery. Suturing of the anterior surface should be done with care and with complete control of hemorrhage because of the thin skin closely applied to the underlying cartilage. Extremely macerated areas may be removed by wedge excision with little resultant deformity com-

pared to the severe scarring which might otherwise occur.

Hematoma of the auricle is not confined to fighters but is also quite common in children. Trauma is the most common cause of this condition, although small hemorrhages secondary to blood dyscrasias have been described. The external surface of the auricle is usually affected due to its exposed position (Fig. 45–1).

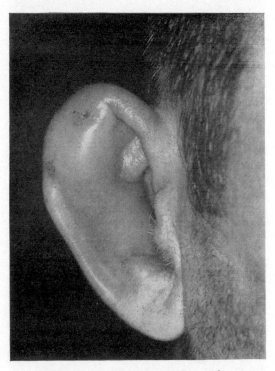

FIG. 45–1.   Hematoma of auricle.

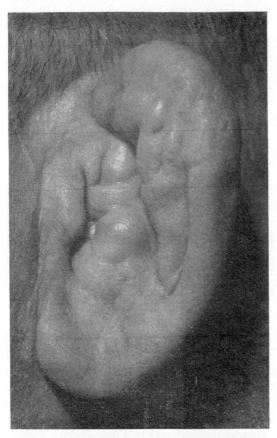

FIG. 45–2. Cauliflower ear. (Courtesy of Dr. Francis L. Lederer.)

The incision should be placed in the scapha, paralleling the helix. Sufficient exposure should be obtained to aspirate the entire hematoma. If delay has resulted in some organization, sharp ring curettes may be used to remove the clot. Small rubber drains may be used to prevent reaccumulation of blood or serum. If placed, they should not be left more than 48 hours because of the risk of infection.

A tight pressure dressing is placed for a minimum of 48 hours. If small residual blebs remain after this period, they may be aspirated with syringe and needle, again with aseptic technique. The antibiotic should be continued for a 5-day period, Frequent observation is necessary in order to detect perichondritis quickly if it should occur. The treatment of this complication is discussed later.

Frostbite

Frostbite is prevalent in the more northern climates, and the auricle is frequently involved because of its exposed position and the lack of subcutaneous or adipose tissue to insulate the blood vessels from the effects

Blood collects rapidly following the injury, dissecting between the perichondrium and cartilage. This creates a large bluish swelling usually involving the entire auricle, although it is sometimes confined to the upper half. If not treated early, the blood organizes into a fibrous mass causing necrosis of the cartilage due to interference with its nutrition. This mass of twisted scar, especially if formed from repeated trauma, creates the deformity known as "cauliflower ear" (Fig. 45–2).

Treatment is based on rapid evacuation of the collected blood. Because of the danger of perichondritis and its resultant severe scarring, aseptic surgical technique is required. Antibiotics whose spectrum includes *Pseudomonas aeruginosa (B. pyocyaneus)* should be used preoperatively and postoperatively, especially in those cases in which lacerations of the skin are also present.

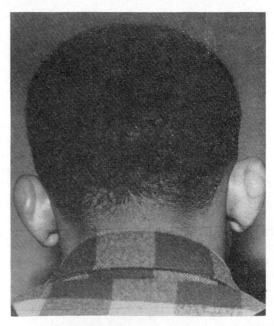

FIG. 45–3. Frostbite of auricle. Both auricles show massive vesiculation of the posterior surface.

of cold (Fig. 45–3). The severity of the trauma is dependent on the length and degree of exposure. The factors of wind and humidity, as well as temperature, are important determinants of the severity of exposure.

The pathogenesis of frostbite is primarily due to the effects of exposure on the blood vessels. Initially there is vasoconstriction, leaving the ear, especially the edges of the helix, blanched and cold to the touch. There follows a stage of hyperemia and edema due to a marked increase in capillary permeability. Ice crystallization of intracellular fluid may be primarily responsible for this, as well as cellular necrosis in the surrounding tissues. The ear now becomes swollen, red, and tender, and blebs of tissue fluid may appear under the skin. The final stage of frostbite is due to ischemia. The regional capillaries are filled with clumped red cells due to the slowed circulation through the distended capillaries and loss of serum through the capillary walls. If recovery of normal permeability does not occur within a few hours, intravascular clotting occurs, with permanent thrombosis and ischemic necrosis of the supplied tissue.

Treatment of frostbite is based on the above process and varies somewhat with its severity. The ear should be treated gently because of the risk of further damage to the already traumatized and devitalized tissue. Massaging with snow should thus be avoided, as should any other manipulation. Dressings should not be used, since they may further compromise the circulation.

The ear should be allowed to return slowly to body temperature. This may be done by placing the patient in a cool room or by directing a stream of cooled air over the affected area. With the onset of vasodilatation, burning and itching will be severe and should be controlled with analgesics. In children it may be necessary to restrain their hands to prevent them from rubbing their ears. In severe or prolonged exposure, the use of heparin to prevent blood sludging and intravascular clotting is recommended. This should be continued until the extent of final injury can be determined. In every case the parenteral use of conjugated estrogens (Premarin), bioflavonoids, and vitamin C is recommended to reduce the abnormal capillary permeability. Antibiotics may be necessary to prevent infection of the devitalized tissue.

If necrosis of portions of the auricle takes place, this should be allowed to delineate completely before any surgical excision is done. Spontaneous separation of the necrotic tissue will result in less loss of tissue and a better cosmetic result than if early surgery is undertaken. Infection of the gangrenous portion, however, indicates immediate surgical excision.

Perichondritis

Perichondritis of the auricle was once a complication of chronic otitis media or chronic external otitis. Since the popularization of endaural mastoid surgery, however, spread of infection through the incision has become the major etiologic factor. Trauma with laceration and hematoma is an occasional cause of perichondritis. The usual infecting organism is *Pseudomonas aeruginosa (B. pyocyaneus).*

The onset of perichondritis is marked by a diffuse red swelling of the auricle which becomes painful (Fig. 45-4). The auricle feels hot and is tender. The edema may

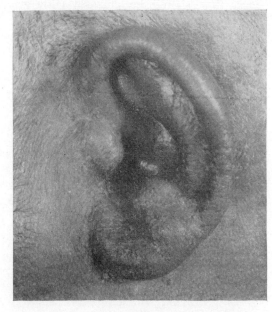

Fig. 45–4. Perichondritis of auricle.

spread to the postauricular region, causing the auricle to protrude. Elevation of temperature, regional adenopathy, and leukocytosis are common. Collections of serum in the subperichondral layer soon become purulent, giving rise to diffuse or localized fluctuation.

The *treatment* of perichondritis is difficult due to the antibiotic-resistant organism usually present. Prophylaxis, therefore, becomes paramount in dealing with perichondritis. Endaural incisions must avoid the auricular cartilage in any infected case. The most common errors involve making the meatal incision too far lateral, thus incising the concha or posterior cartilaginous wall of the canal, and making the superior incision too close to the helix, shaving its cartilage in so doing. An even more common error, and one more likely to cause perichondritis, is that of traumatizing the auricle with the shaft of the burr while drilling in the mastoid. This is often unnoticed since the operator's attention is directed to the point of the burr. Care must always be taken during mastoid surgery to avoid any trauma to the auricle. Early diagnosis aids treatment greatly, and to this end it is felt that pressure dressings over the ear should not be left for more than 48 hours. If circumstances dictate the need for prolonged dressings, they should be changed daily with aseptic technique.

If perichondritis should develop, rapid institution of treatment is needed. Heat should be applied to the auricle. Hot, moist packs are the most effective, but dry heat is required if the infection follows surgery. Cultures should be taken and antibiotic treatment which is directed toward a presumed infection with *Pseudomonas* started. If cultures reveal another organism to be causative, the antibiotic regimen may be changed at that time. The most effective systemic antibiotics are colistimethate (Coly-Mycin) and streptomycin. Neomycin and polymyxin B also are effective against *Pseudomonas* but have severe toxic potential when used systemically. Topical application is of little value in this problem other than its use in treating an otitis media or external otitis if present. The antibiotic should be continued for several days after apparent recovery because of the possibility of residual hidden areas of infection. The use of small doses of x-ray (300 to 600 R) has been of benefit in these cases. The appearance of fluctuation indicates the need for incision and drainage. This should be done as described under hematoma of the auricle. The drains should be left in place until the purulent discharge has ceased. Incision should not be done until localization has occurred.

Prognosis for a cosmetic result is poor in these infections because of the cartilage necrosis which occurs. Cosmetic reconstruction may be carried out, but this should be delayed for many months to ensure the complete elimination of residual infection.

EXTERNAL AUDITORY CANAL

The external auditory canal, being lined with squamous epithelium, is subject not only to all forms of dermatitis but also particularly to certain types of disease, many of which tend to become chronic. Many of these problems are self-inflicted because of the universal tendency to pick at the ears with the fingers or other suitably shaped objects. This introduces not only the danger of infection from trauma but also the risk of leaving a foreign body in the canal. Water, both clean and unclean, often enters the ear canal. Because of the gutter beyond the isthmus, it is difficult to dry the canal, which will then become macerated, creating a dank media ideal for the growth of bacteria and fungus. Often each of these problems interrelate: for example, the patient whose plug of cerumen traps water within the canal and whose efforts to remove the wax result in infection.

Cerumen

The ceruminous glands are contained in the superior canal wall and in the cartilaginous canal. Their secretion combines with the oily sebaceous secretion in the upper portion of the hair follicle to form a complex substance, cerumen. Cerumen forms a coating of the canal skin which mixes with the migrating keratin layer (see Chapter 40,

Anatomy and Embryology) to give a protective surface which seems to have antibacterial action. There is a great range in the amount and speed of migration of cerumen in that some individuals have a scanty amount, while others tend to form masses of cerumen which obstruct the canal periodically. It is these latter individuals who have the greatest problem, although the former may be subject to itching and maceration and thus induce infection.

Removal of cerumen may be done by irrigation or with instruments (Fig. 45–5). Irrigation is the most gentle means of cleaning the external canal but should be used only if the tympanic membrane has been previously examined. A perforation will allow contaminated solution to enter the middle ear and may cause otitis media. A too vigorous stream of water directed toward an atrophic drumhead may cause a perforation. The canal may be irrigated either with a syringe or more easily with a pressure-driven irrigating bottle. The canal is straightened by pulling the auricle up and back. Under direct visualization, the water stream is directed along the superior canal wall so that the returning stream may push the cerumen

from behind. The outflow is caught in a basin held tightly below the ear. An assistant is most helpful in this procedure.

The most useful instruments for cleaning the canal are wire loops, dull ring curettes, and delicate Hartmann forceps. The cerumen and desquamated layer of epithelium are first separated from the canal skin. A gentle touch is most important at this stage because the canal is extremely sensitive to instrumentation. The posterior and superior canal walls are less sensitive and the separation is best done on these surfaces. The loosened cerumen is then grasped with the forceps and teased out. Inspection of the drumhead may then show that further cleaning can be done with irrigation.

Suction is used to remove moist cerumen and to dry the canal. Cotton-tipped metal applicators may also be used for this purpose. Masses of impacted cerumen should be softened before removal to prevent trauma. A useful preparation for this is glycerite of peroxide used 2 or 3 days prior to cleaning. Cerumen-dissolving agents should be used cautiously, since their action depends on enzymes or chemicals which often irritate the canal and cause an external otitis.

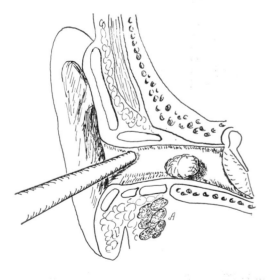 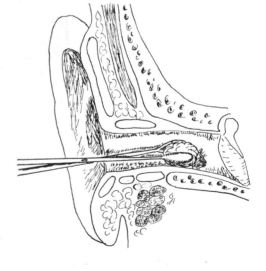

A   B

FIG. 45–5.   Methods of cleaning the external ear canal.   *A*, Irrigation—the stream of water is directed superiorly.   *B*, Instrumentation—a delicate Hartmann forceps is being used to grasp the object.

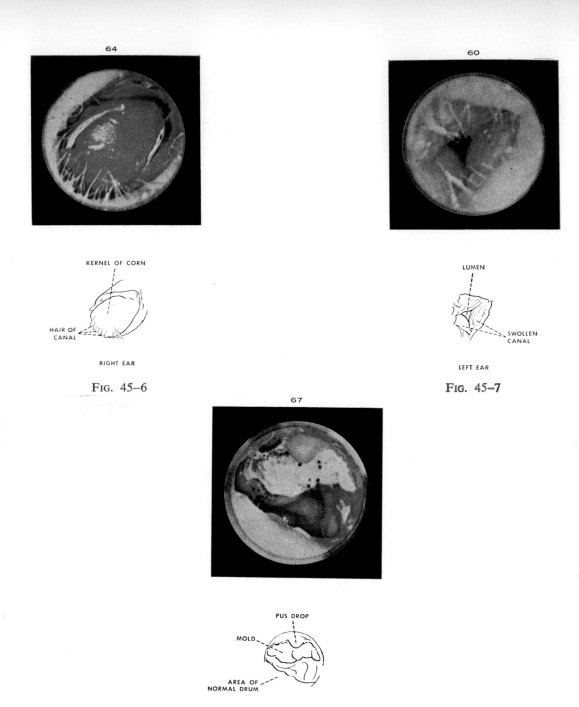

FIG. 45–6

FIG. 45–7

FIG. 45–8

FIG. 45–6. Foreign body. A kernel of corn is tightly impacted in external canal.

FIG. 45–7. Acute diffuse external otitis (swimmer's ear) with marked swelling of external canal.

FIG. 45–8. Chronic diffuse external otitis (otomycosis). The mold growth is confined chiefly to the upper half of the canal. A portion of normal membrane is seen inferiorly. A clog of purulent exudate is visible externally at the uppermost portion of the canal.

(Courtesy of Dr. Richard A. Buckingham. Abbott Laboratories, *What's New*, 196, 1956.)

Foreign Bodies

The list of objects which have been recovered from the ear canal is impressive for its variety (Figs. 45-6 to 45-8). These objects may be animate or inanimate, vegetable or mineral. Children are particularly prone to this affliction, with beans, beads, and pencil erasers being high on the frequency list. Among the poorer classes, maggots may follow a "night out," and campers return with a variety of insect life dwelling within the canal.

The major problem of foreign body removal is the isthmus of the canal. Attempts to remove the object occasionally result in pushing it beyond the isthmus. This trauma causes edema which can trap the object, thus making removal difficult. The foreign body, if smaller than the canal lumen, may be grasped with Hartmann forceps and removed. A larger object is removed by placing a hook or loop behind it and pulling it out. In some instances a stream of water may be directed superiorly to push the object out as described for cerumen removal.

Animate objects must be killed before removal. A cotton tampon well moistened with ether is effective. Its use for 5 minutes is sufficient to stupefy any insect, and then irrigation is used to flush the insect out.

Unless children are calm during foreign body removal, it is best to use general anesthesia. Many instances of traumatic injury to the tympanic membrane or the ossicles have been recorded because a child jumped during an attempt to remove a foreign body. In all patients in whom the object is lodged beyond the isthmus, removal should be done under anesthesia.

External Otitis

Under this general term are lumped all of the inflammatory processes involving the skin of the external auditory canal. Generalized skin disease may affect the ear, together with other parts of the body. The reader is referred to dermatologic texts for discussions of such disorders as psoriasis, pemphigus, and yaws. This discussion will cover those diseases peculiar to the ear or of sufficient frequency to constitute a significant problem.

For purposes of differentiation, these disorders may be classified as infectious, eczematoid, or seborrheic. They may also be acute, recurrent, or chronic. Although at least 58 forms of external otitis have been cataloged, the foregoing simple classification will include over 95% of patients with external otitis.

Symptoms. The symptoms of external otitis are common to the various forms, being dependent on the structure of the external canal rather than upon the etiology. The initial symptom is itching within the canal due to beginning inflammation. This symptom is often confused with a deep-seated tickle referred to the ear from the mouth of the eustachian tube and due to mild inflammation in this region. This referred sensation may be used as a guide to proper placement of a eustachian tube catheter. It is usually accompanied by a scratching sensation in the throat at the base of the tonsil. Movement of the palatal muscles will modify this tickle, while movement of the auricle has no effect. The reverse is true of the itching due to external otitis.

As the process becomes more severe, the itching progresses to a painful sensation which may become quite intense. This is due to the accompanying edema creating pressure against the confining auditory canal. Any movement of the auricle or cartilaginous canal, as in chewing, produces pain. Exudation and swelling now may cause hearing loss secondary to obstruction of the canal.

Discharge is initially watery but soon becomes purulent and thick when mixed with pus cells and desquamated epithelium. In chronic forms the discharge is scanty or absent, with a coagulum forming in the canal. This is usually musty- or foul-smelling due to the action of saprophytic bacteria or fungi in the canal.

Symptoms of toxicity with fever signify lymphatic spread. Adenopathy will become evident in the upper anterior cervical triangle, in the parotid region, or in the postauricular groups with this spread of infection.

Diagnosis A. *Inflammatory External Otitis.* Inflammatory external otitis may be divided both into localized and diffuse forms and into acute and chronic forms.

1. *Acute localized external* otitis is an infection of a hair follicle, beginning as a folliculitis but usually extending to form a furuncle. The infecting organism is usually *Staphylococcus.* The majority of these cases are brought on by the trauma of scratching the ear canal. An occasional case, usually involving a furuncle, is due to a blocked and infected sebaceous gland in the canal. Because heat and humidity seem to lower the canal skin's resistance to infection, these cases occur with slightly increased frequency during the summer months.

If the case is seen early, a diffuse red swelling can be visualized in one area of the cartilaginous canal, usually posteriorly or superiorly. The swelling may be sufficient to occlude the canal. As localization takes place, a pustule will be seen. Pain is severe in this condition, and examination is difficult for this reason. Discharge is not usually present until the abscess ruptures. Toxicity and adenopathy appear early because of the nature of the infecting organism.

2. *Acute diffuse external otitis (swimmer's ear)* is primarily a disease of the summer months and is the most common form of external otitis. The conditions of heat and humidity cause swelling of the stratum corneum of the skin, which blocks the follicular canals. Introduction of extraneous moisture from swimming or bathing increases the maceration of the canal skin and creates a condition favorable to bacterial growth. These changes may also cause itching of the canal, which adds the possibility of trauma from scratching. This may follow the actual onset of infection, however. Except in tropical climates where fungi are a significant infecting organism, *Pseudomonas aeruginosa* is the most common bacteria found.

As hyperemia and edema of the canal skin occur, there is intense itching which gradually becomes painful. The canal is diffusely inflamed and swollen, with tenderness on movement of the auricle. There is a copious serous discharge. As the disease progresses, the discharge becomes seropurulent and edema causes marked or complete closure of the canal, obscuring the drumhead. Although the process is usually limited to the canal, involvement of the intertragic notch and lobule may occur because of the irritation of the discharge. Small papules and vesicles are present on the surface of the skin, but these are not usually noticed because of the difficulty of examination.

Systemic manifestations may occur, but these symptoms are not as common as with gram-positive infections.

3. *Chronic diffuse external otitis,* being due to fungus infection, is relatively unusual in all but the most southern regions of the United States. It has become a common practice to diagnose all chronic itching or tickling of the ear as being due to "fungus," thus giving a false impression of the frequency of this type of external otitis.

Fungi, usually *Aspergillus niger, Actinomyces,* or yeasts, create a chronic superficial redness of the bony canal wall skin. A musty-smelling exudate forms which has a gray wrinkled appearance similar to wet blotting paper. On the surface of this rather thick membrane will be seen the filaments of the fungus. On removal of the membrane, the skin has a smooth red shine.

Itching is constant and intense in mycotic infection but seldom progresses to pain. Systemic manifestations are rare unless superimposed bacterial infection takes place, usually due to scratching of the ear.

B. *Eczematoid External Otitis.* This category includes all forms of hypersensitivity of the canal skin because of the common appearance of the lesion. The major causes of this type of external otitis are topical antibiotics or vehicles (dermatitis medicamentosa); allergy to various chemicals or metals used around the ear, such as hair sprays or ear rings (contact dermatitis or dermatitis venenata); atopic reaction due to ingested or inhaled antigen (atopic dermatitis); and infectious eczematoid dermatitis due to contact of the skin with middle ear discharge. Neurodermatitis and psoriasis might be included in this group of problems, but since they have multiple manifestations, they are best managed by dermatologists and will not be discussed.

Each of these types represents a distinct form of allergy. In contact dermatitis the local tissue contains the entire response, with no circulating antibodies present. Dermatitis medicamentosa is a particular variety of contact allergy. In atopy, circulating antibodies are present as well as a genetically determined defect of protein metabolism. In some instances examples of both the Shwartzman and the Arthus reactions may be present. Each of these forms of external otitis is characterized by histamine release in the tissues.

Eczematoid external otitis, because of its basic allergic nature, tends to be recurrent or chronic. Each episode of otitis serves to make the ear more susceptible to future attacks. In time, the ear usually loses this susceptibility, probably because of lessening of the allergic response.

The entire ear canal, concha, intertragic notch, and lobule are usually involved (Fig. 45-9), although in some cases of contact dermatitis the process is limited to the lobule. The appearance is that of a confluent mass of weeping, crusted lesions of the hyperemic and edematous skin. This is similar to any lesion of the same type anywhere on the body, such as poison ivy (which may be transmitted to the ear by the hands).

C. *Seborrheic External Otitis*. This form of external otitis is quite common and is as-

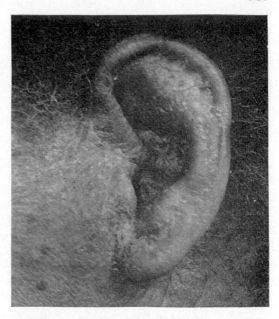

FIG. 45–10. Seborrheic external otitis. The typical greasy scaling is seen not only over the auricle but also anterior to the ear and in the scalp.

sociated with seborrheic dermatitis of other regions, particularly the scalp (dandruff). This condition is of unknown etiology but seems to have a hereditary factor.

The lesions are typified by a greasy scaling which has a yellowish appearance due to the abnormal sebum production (Fig. 45-10). Many patients are not aware of excess oilyness, feeling the scaling is due to a "dry skin." The external cartilaginous canal, concha, and postauricular regions are most often involved. The condition is usually recurrent rather than being continuously present.

Treatment of External Otitis. There are certain principles of management which must be observed in every case of external otitis. These are frequent inspection and cleansing of the canal; control of pain; use of specific medication appropriate to the type and severity of disease; acidification of the canal; and control of predisposing causes.

Frequent inspection, cleaning, and drying of the ear canal is undoubtedly the single most important factor in obtaining resolu-

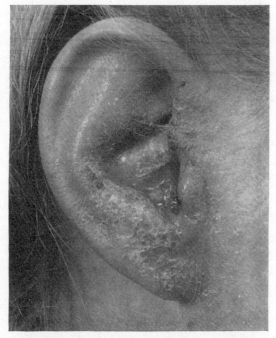

FIG. 45–9. Eczematoid external otitis. The external canal, concha, tragus, antitragus, and lobule are involved with confluent weeping, crusted lesions.

tion of all forms of external otitis. During the summer months with their high humidity, special efforts are needed to maintain dryness within the canal.

The most efficient method of cleaning the ear canal varies with the state of inflammation. In those with extremely edematous canals, cleaning must wait until the inflammation has subsided. If there is much soggy debris present, irrigation with 3% saline solution or dilute alcohol (10 to 20%) should be performed. This is followed by gentle suction drying. Blotting with cotton-tipped metal applicators is sometimes necessary (some children will not tolerate the noise of suctioning), but this is usually time-consuming and induces more trauma. Burow's solution is often used in acute moist ears to obtain rapid resolution of edema and crusting but, when used, requires special cleaning because of the abundant desquamative debris which forms. As soon as possible, these patients should be placed on a dilute alcoholic cleansing and drying solution (when its use will not cause burning). Seventy% alcohol acidified to a pH of 5 is efficient for this purpose.

Relief of pain is urgent in these cases and usually requires narcotics. Oral codeine or hydrocodone is effective. Since the pain is due to the edema and inflammation present, the use of heat and hydroscopic vehicles aids in the relief of pain.

Acute localized external otitis should be treated as is an abscess on any part of the body. If it is seen before suppuration has taken place, resolution may occur with the use of antibiotics only. These should be used both topically and systemically. Since this infection is usually staphylococcic, penicillin or tetracyclines in therapeutic dosage are administered for 5 days. Polymyxin B and/or neomycin in a liquid hydroscopic and acidified vehicle is used topically.

The patient should apply dry heat to the ear for at least 20 minutes three times a day. Bedrest is advisable in the more severe cases and is mandatory for those with toxic symptoms.

The ear should be inspected at least every 2 days until localization or resolution has occurred. With localization, incision of the abscess is necessary. This should result

in rapid resolution, during which time the above measures of heat and antibiotic administration are continued.

Acute diffuse external otitis should be treated during the early stages in such a way as to relieve rapidly the edema which blocks the lumen of the canal. To accomplish this it is usually necessary to insert cotton into the canal to carry the medication to the affected skin. A small tampon is best for this, since gauze wicks wad up and do not exert an even pressure. The cotton tampon is inserted gently with a fine Hartmann forceps after moistening with the medication. The patient is instructed to apply the liquid medication to the cotton once or twice daily. Within 48 hours the tampon should fall out of the canal owing to increase in the size of the lumen. After this time the medication may be applied directly into the canal.

Topical medication is usually effective in this form of otitis, although adenopathy and toxicity indicate the need for systemic antibiotics (see perichondritis). Polymyxin B and colistimethate are the most effective antibiotics against *Pseudomonas* and should be used in a hydroscopic vehicle, such as propylene glycol, which has been mildly acidified. Chemical agents such as gentian violet and dilute silver nitrate are bactericidal and may be applied directly to the canal skin. Two% aqueous gentian violet and 5% aqueous silver nitrate are the usual concentrations.

As the inflammatory response lessens, 70% alcohol may be added to keep the canal clean and dry. Patients should be advised to use this after any water enters the ear. The antibiotic drops should not be used longer than 2 to 3 weeks because of the risk of contact dermatitis from the medication itself.

The patient should be warned of the possibility of future episodes, especially after swimming. To avoid this, he should keep his ear dry by the routine use of dilute alcohol three times weekly and by drying his ear with alcohol whenever it comes in contact with water. He should also be warned against scratching the ear or using cotton applicators in his ear. Since infections are much easier to control at the onset, the patient should be told to return at any time the ear begins to itch rather than waiting until the infection has become more severe.

Chronic diffuse external otitis is usually of fungal origin and occurs in those whose canals are exposed to excessive moisture. In these patients, the preventive regimen outlined in the preceding paragraph is of special importance.

When initially seen, the moist membrane is removed by gentle irrigation and suction. The underlying skin is hyperemic and bleeds easily. The skin should be painted with metacresol acetate (Cresitin). If superimposed bacterial infection is present, the ear should be powdered with a mixture of polymyxin B and chloramphenicol. For this, 250 mg of polymyxin B powder is mixed with 3 g of chloramphenicol powder (usually removed from 12 oral capsules) and applied with a powder blower. When the hyperemia has begun to subside, dilute alcohol is added to the regimen and the powder and metacresol acetate gradually discontinued.

Although there is some evidence to indicate that *seborrheic external dermatitis* is linked to hormonal imbalance, treatment based on this etiology has been ineffectual. As will be pointed out in the discussion of eczematoid otitis, superimposed infection is often present in this condition and must be controlled before the basic seborrhea is treated. This is carried out as outlined under acute diffuse external otitis.

It has been found that control of seborrheic dermatitis of the scalp is necessary to control the external otitis. The best agent for this is selenium sulfide in a shampoo (Selsun) used once a month. At other times a detergent-type shampoo should be used and oily rinses avoided. The canal and concha are painted with 10% silver nitrate and dilute alcohol used daily to keep the canal clean and dry.

This condition is particularly bothersome in some individuals, being most common in the fourth and fifth decades. It seems to regress as middle age is reached, although recurrence is common. During the age of activity, these patients should be seen periodically and urgently should there be any symptom of exacerbation.

Eczematoid external otitis is perhaps the most difficult of all forms of external otitis to treat, since the provocative agents usually remain undiagnosed. It may follow infectious external otitis or otitis media as a reaction either to the infecting organisms or to the medication used to treat them. It may seem psychosomatic at times, since it may follow emotional trauma. Atopic individuals may exhibit external otitis after being sensitized to milk, peanuts, or other foods. Once the canal skin has become a target tissue, allergens other than the original sensitizing agent may provoke an episode of external otitis, thus producing an extremely chronic recurrent disease.

The prime agents for producing a rapid response are the corticosteroids. Since infection often accompanies the acute episode, topical antibiotics are usually combined with the steroid in the otic solution. Although this type of ear drop has become popular, steroids are not indicated for use in other types of external otitis. Another agent which has proved to be most efficient, particularly in the chronic forms of eczematoid otitis, is heparin. Heparin forms a chemical complex with histamine, preventing the local tissue reaction. In practice, heparin (1 ml containing 10,000 or 15,000 units) is added to a commercially prepared steroid-antibiotic otic solution to produce more rapid clearing of the otitis.

Contact dermatitis may call for skin testing to find the offending chemical. The more common causes, such as hair spray or nail polish, can usually be detected by history. Any ear preparation used for more than 10 days may produce an eczematoid reaction. Polymyxin B and penicillin are both prone to rapid sensitization. Atopy is detected by a family history of allergy plus such manifestations as asthma or hay fever in the past. Skin manifestations in other areas of the body may be of great help in diagnosis and in directing avoidance treatment.

The use of gentian violet is of help in drying and coating weeping areas. In chronic cases characterized by hypertrophy and fissuring of the skin, 10 and 25% silver nitrate painted on the canal is helpful. Dilute alcohol cleansing should be used between episodes to keep the canal clean and dry. Frequent inspection of the canal, even in quiescent periods, may help to treat subacute manifestations. In these cases, treatment must be individualized, and experience plus an open-minded acceptance of non-response to the first tried treatment so that another course may be adopted without undue delay is paramount to success.

Chronic Stenosing External Otitis

This disease is an extreme form of hypertrophic reaction to uncontrolled external otitis. In these cases, there is fibrous tissue proliferation in the subcutaneous layers combined with hyperkeratosis. Occasionally a foreign body hidden deep within the canal may be responsible for this reaction, and in rare instances neoplastic tissue has been found incident to treatment.

These changes in the skin of the canal are irreversible and may also be responsible for the chronic infection due to retention of moisture and debris in the narrow canal. Occasionally, fibrous hyperplasia of the pars media of the tympanic membrane may occur, resulting in a thick functionless tympanic membrane.

The best treatment in most of these cases is surgery. The operation consists of complete removal of the involved skin, enlargement of the bony canal, especially if it is smaller than normal, and grafting with split-thickness skin. In many instances, the operation may be done with a meatal incision. In those cases with involvement of the cartilaginous canal, an endaural incision provides improved exposure. When an endaural incision is made, Lempert's technique of excising a semilunar segment of conchal cartilage is recommended (see Chapter 50, Incisions, p. 838.) This enlargement of the canal orifice gives the advantage of improved access for postoperative care. The abnormal canal skin is entirely removed, using sharp dissection. If the drumhead is involved, the fibrous tissue is removed until a layer of normal thickness remains. The denuded canal is enlarged, using burrs, to an optimum size, increasing gradually in diameter toward the exterior. A 10-mil split-thickness graft is removed with a dermatome. This should be from an inconspicuous, hairless area such as the inguinal region ("bikini area") or the inner surface of the upper arm. The skin is placed into the canal to cover all exposed surfaces. If the tympanic membrane epithelium is removed, the skin is brought onto the drumhead. A firm, resilient packing is placed within a lining of surgical rayon or nylon. Some overlapping of the graft is unavoidable but will not cause difficulty because the superfluous skin will slough. In those cases in which skin removal is limited to the bony canal, it is not necessary to place a graft, as the epithelium will regenerate without stenosis.

The canal is left alone for 2 or 3 weeks, after which it is cleaned and any granulating areas touched with 25% silver nitrate. Inspection and cleaning are carried out at biweekly intervals until healing is complete.

Keratosis Obliterans

Keratosis obliterans is a relatively rare condition, but it has received much attention in the literature. Also referred to as destructive or invasive keratitis or canal cholesteatoma, it is characterized by the accumulation of large plugs of desquamated keratin in the bony portion of the external canal. Erosion of the bony canal occurs, usually of the inferior or posterior walls. These erosions may be so extensive as to undermine the tympanic annulus and expose the hypotympanum. Occasionally the descending portion of the facial nerve may be uncovered, calling for care in the removal of the keratin debris.

This condition is usually asymptomatic, being discovered incidental to examination for conductive hearing loss. Removal of the keratin plug will reveal the erosion of the canal. Occasionally the eroded area will become a source of irritation and infection, producing pain and discharge from the canal.

The etiology of this condition is unknown. It has been seen in association with chronic pulmonary disease and sinusitis. Bronchiectasis has been present in a high percentage of these cases, especially those with an onset under the age of 20.

The disease may be controlled in most cases by periodic cleaning. It may be necessary to remove the accumulated debris as often as every 3 months. The use of dilute alcohol irrigations or glycerite of peroxide drops three times weekly is of help. Those cases in which erosion and infection are marked or uncontrollable may benefit by surgery. In these cases a free tissue graft is placed under the skin in the affected region. In this procedure, a transmeatal skin flap is elevated to expose the eroded bone. This elevation sometimes will include the annulus. A free graft of temporalis fascia is removed through an incision above and behind the auricle. In cases with deep erosion, some muscle tissue may be left attached to the fascia to increase the thickness of the graft. The tissue is placed into the erosion and the skin flap replaced over the graft. A light packing of absorbable gelatin holds the flap in place. Healing is usually rapid and the chronic infection eliminated. Periodic cleaning may still be necessary after this surgery, however.

TRAUMATIC PERFORATION OF THE TYMPANIC MEMBRANE

The incidence of traumatic perforation has always been high. The causes are varied, with water sports (diving or water skiing) being a major source. Blows to the ear, usually with the cupped hand, and objects entering the ear with some force are fairly frequent causes of perforation of the drumhead. Occasionally, the patient will have been injured by an explosion or by too forceful irrigation of the ear canal.

Today a high percentage of these cases are the subject of litigation, so that complete and frequent examination of the ear and hearing is important. Since the energy of the traumatic force may be transmitted by the ossicular chain to the inner ear, an audiometric evaluation is important in every case. When severe force has caused the perforation, temporal bone and skull x-ray films should be made to determine if a fracture is also present.

The particular nature of the injury will cause the appearance of the tympanic membrane to vary. Usually there is a severe but rapidly abating pain at the time of the injury. The tympanic membrane on examination will be injected. The perforation is ragged and stellate in most instances. There will be a clot of blood around or over the site of tearing, and hemotympanum is not uncommon. Injuries caused by water may become rapidly infected, causing a seropurulent discharge. Without infection, there is usually a serous discharge for a few days after the injury. Welders are prone to perforation by hot chips of metal flying into the ear canal. These perforations will be round with cauterized edges. This cauterization prevents healing in most of these cases, resulting in a persistent perforation.

During the first 2 weeks following a perforation, inspection only should be done. Instrumentation and cleaning should be avoided. The patient should wear a cotton plug in the ear to prevent water or dirt from entering the canal. He should be advised against washing his hair or the skin around the ear. Most of these perforations heal rapidly, and after 2 weeks any crust remaining on the tympanic membrane may be removed under magnification to see if healing is complete.

Infection of the middle ear, if present, should be treated with antibiotics as described in Chapter 48 under acute otitis media, p. 823. A persistent perforation may follow infection, although in most cases closure of the perforation ensues as the infection subsides.

Persistent perforation calls for special measures. If the perforation has not healed within 1 month, an attempt may be made to close it in the office. The method developed by Derlacki is successful in closing a high percentage of these persistent perforations. The method consists of stimulating the margin of the perforation and then covering it with a moist cotton disc for a few weeks. The margin is stimulated with either trichloroacetic acid or by incision with a tiny right-angled pick. A cotton patch moistened with Euthymol (a proprietary mixture of eucalyptol, methyl salicylate, menthol, thymol, boric acid, and benzoic acid in 20% alcohol) is placed over the perforation and remoistened two times a day at home with one or two drops of the same solution.

Five% urea in normal saline solution may be used in those cases giving no response or reacting adversely to the Euthymol. This procedure is carried out at 10- to 14-day intervals until closure is accomplished. If there is no response after a 3-month period, or if there is intolerance of the treatment, as evidenced by repeated discharge after patching, surgical closure should be recommended (see Chapter 50, Myringoplasty, p. 840). Variations on this technique using dry patching with cigarette paper, gelatin, collagen film, or silastic film glued to the drumhead have been described. The moist technique seems to give the highest percentage of success—slightly over 70%.

REFERENCES

Derlacki, E. L.: Repair of Central Perforations of the Drum. Arch. Otolaryng., *58*: 405, 1953.

Jones, E. H.: *External Otitis; Diagnosis and Treatment*. Springfield, Ill., Charles C Thomas, Publisher, 1965.

McLaurin, J. W.: Persistent External Otitis. Laryngoscope, *75*:1699, 1965.

Paparella, M. M., and Kurkjian, J. M.: Surgical Treatment for Chronic Stenosing External Otitis. Laryngoscope, *76*:232, 1966.

Proud, G. O.: Surgery for Chronic, Refractory Otitis Externa. Arch. Otolaryng., *83*:436, 1966.

Senturia, B. H.: *Diseases of the External Ear*. Springfield, Ill., Charles C Thomas, Publisher, 1957.

Chapter 46
Tumors of the External and Middle Ear

Most tumors of the ear are similar to those occurring in other portions of the body. These tumors derive from skin or its appendages, from bone, from neural tissue, or from connective tissue. The major problem today, as in the past, is early diagnosis so that treatment may be carried out with a minimal loss of tissue, function, and life. Since the methods of removal of the neoplasms depend primarily on their location, the discussion will be subdivided by location and whether the tumor is benign or malignant.

BENIGN TUMORS OF THE AURICLE

Angioma

Angiomas are congenital tumors and are the most common tumors of childhood. They may involve the auricle together with other areas of the face and neck. These tumors occur in various forms. *Capillary hemangioma* consists of masses of capillary-sized vessels and may be in the form of a large flat mass, the "port-wine stain," or in the form of the spider nevus, which is a branching network of capillaries fed by a central larger vessel. The spider nevus is not a major problem, being small and fixed in size. Treatment, when deemed necessary, usually consists of needle coagulation of the central vessel. The port-wine stain is much more of a problem, increasing in size gradu-

ally until adolescence is reached and generally being quite disfiguring.

Cavernous hemangioma is the most alarming of these lesions, consisting of raised masses of blood-filled endothelial spaces. Often termed a "strawberry tumor," it in-

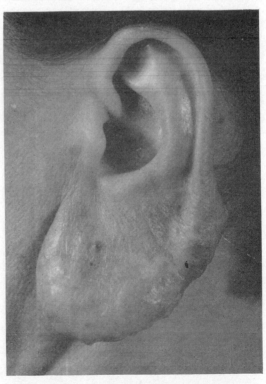

Fig. 46–1. Lymphangioma of auricle. (Courtesy of Dr. Francis L. Lederer.)

791

creases rapidly in size during the first year of life but usually regresses thereafter.

Much less common is the *lymphangioma*. This has the appearance of multiple pale circumscribed lesions, like a cluster of fish or frog roe (Fig. 46–1).

The major problem in these tumors is cosmetic. In general, the lesion should be allowed to regress maximally and the residual tumor treated. Various modalities have been recommended, including cryosurgery, surgical excision and skin grafting, radiation, electrolysis, and tattooing for port-wine stains. Most of these cases are handled by plastic surgeons, and consultation with those specializing in this field is recommended.

Cysts

Sebaceous cysts are common around the ear. They usually occur on the posterior surface of the lobule, in the skin over the mastoid process, and in the skin of the inferior or posterior cartilaginous canal (Fig. 46–2). These soft, nontender swellings are not difficult to diagnose. They may become infected and at these times may be confused with furuncle.

Treatment of sebaceous cyst is total excision. Incision and curettage, which has been recommended in the past, is followed by recurrence. Infection, if present, should be treated with heat and antibiotics before surgery is attempted so that the surgical field is free of inflammation. The cyst is removed by sharp dissection, care being taken to keep the walls intact to ensure complete removal. The ductal tissue leading to the cyst as well as its external opening should be removed by including this tissue with a small segment of the overlying skin outlined by the initial incision.

Preauricular cyst and/or fistula is of congenital origin, arising because of dysunion of the hillocks of the first and second branchial arches forming the auricle (see Chapter 40). It presents as a small opening in the skin anterior to the insertion of the helix (Fig. 46–3). From this opening a long branched tract may run under the skin between the helix and tragus and anterior to the tragus. The tract, which is lined with squamous epithelium, is often cystic, and the patient is frequently seen initially because of infection of the cyst.

Treatment of a preauricular fistula should be avoided unless recurrent infection is present because of the difficulty of complete re-

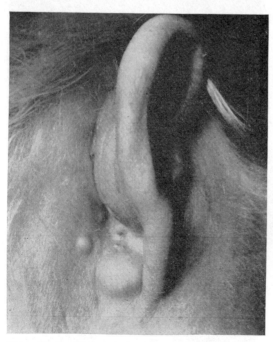

FIG. 46–2. Sebaceous cysts of retroauricular region.

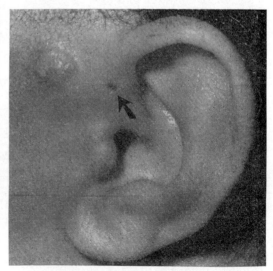

FIG. 46–3. Preauricular cyst and fistula. Arrow indicates the fistula opening. Anterior to this is an inflamed swelling due to an infected preauricular cyst.

moval. Incomplete removal is associated with the formation of draining sinuses, requiring even more difficult and radical surgery for their elimination. The difficulty of the surgery is due to the branching of the fistula, which makes it hard to define the complete extent of the tract. One suggestion to aid in removal is to inject the tract prior to surgery with methylene blue so that the stained tissue may be used as a guide to the extent of the fistula. It must be kept in mind that the dye may not enter all of the smaller ramifications, so that constant surveillance is needed during the dissection to detect small unstained channels. Some surgeons with experience in this disease feel that as experience is gained, the use of dye injection should be abandoned, since the dye spreads into the surrounding area, causing needless sacrifice of uninvolved tissue.

Fibroma

Fibromas occur only rarely about the external ear, most often in diffuse neurofibromatosis (von Recklinghausen's disease). They are firm, nontender, discrete swellings with slow growth (Fig. 46–4). Surgical excision is indicated when they occlude the canal or create a cosmetic problem.

Keloid tumors may represent a form of fibroma but more likely are pseudotumors due to genetic susceptibility (Fig. 46–5). The formation of a keloid is stimulated by trauma to the skin. The tumor is made up of massive collections of collagen interspersed with active fibroblasts and normal thin collagenous strands. Keloid formation is seen most frequently in the dark-skinned races, particularly in Negroes. Keloids around the ear are most frequently seen as pedunculated tumors on the lobule following ear lobe piercing. They may also occur in mastoidectomy scars, resulting in disfigurement or stenosis of the canal when the incision is placed endaurally.

Treatment is excision of the keloid followed immediately by a single dose of x-ray

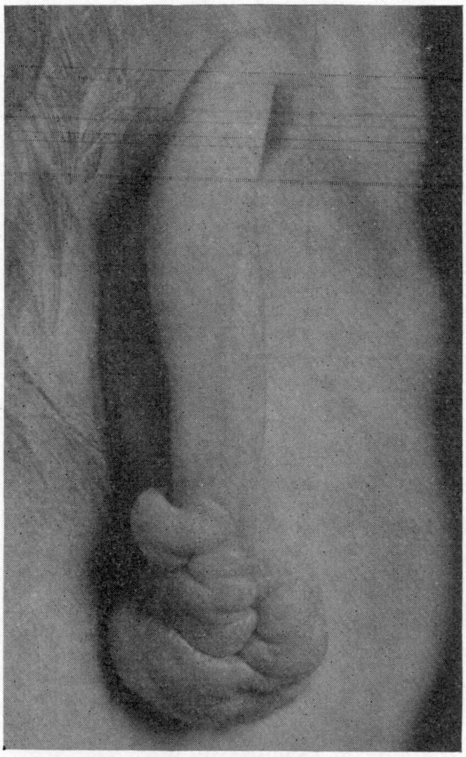

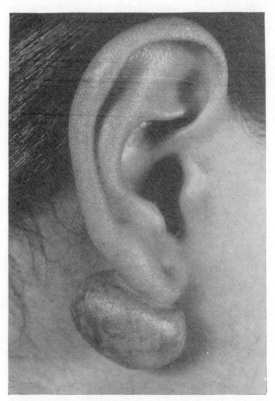

FIG. 46–4. Neurofibroma of auricle. (Courtesy of Dr. Francis L. Lederer.)

FIG. 46–5. Keloid of auricle that followed piercing of lobule.

radiation of 300 R to prevent recurrence. If the individual is known to form keloids, radiation should be used routinely after any surgical procedure. Another frequently used treatment to prevent keloid formation is the injection of a small amount (0.5 ml or less) of Kenalog into the surgical site.

Papilloma

Papillomas are seen in various forms both on the auricle and in the canal. These tumors arise in response to several sources of chronic irritation of the skin. The common wart is felt to have a viral etiology. The basic lesion consists of hyperplasia of both the basal and prickle cell layers of the skin. It is not rare for malignant changes to occur in these lesions, but benign papillomas will not have the pleomorphism, mitotic activity, or disruption of the basement membrane seen with malignancy.

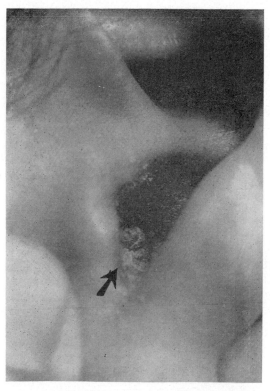

Fig. 46–6.   Papilloma of external auditory meatus. This is a common wart (verruca vulgaris) which, because of the marked keratinization, may be called a cutaneous horn.

A *cutaneous horn* is formed when there is a heaping up of keratin in a circumscribed papilloma, creating a rough, hard, brownish horn-shaped tumor (Fig. 46–6). This is seen most frequently on the rim of the helix in elderly individuals with long exposure to the elements. The curious appearance leads the individual to seek medical attention, which consists of surgical excision.

Keratoacanthoma is a rare lesion whose importance is due to its similarity to carcinoma and its premalignant nature. It occurs usually after the fifth decade in men who work outdoors. The lesion consists of a peripheral heaping up of prickle cells with a central crater filled with a mass of keratin. The lesion tends to grow rapidly after its initial appearance and then slowly regress, leaving a retracted scar. Although the disease is self-limited, excision biopsy is required to rule out the presence of a malignant tumor and is thus the most common treatment rendered.

Senile keratoses are raised, flat-surfaced lesions on exposed surfaces of the skin of elderly individuals. The lesion has a color distinct from the surrounding normal skin, usually yellow, brown, or black. The lesion consists of a marked increase in the outer layers of the epidermis with a dyskeratosis of the basal layers and underlying inflammation of the dermis. There is an increase in the number and depth of the rete pegs. Although these lesions are symptomless, they are the result of chronic exposure and atrophy of the skin and are in many instances premalignant lesions. The keratosis is usually untreated, but any change in its character dictates prompt excision, as outlined for carcinoma of the auricle.

Cylindroma

Cylindromas are tumors with cylindrical nests of epithelial cells surrounded by cords of hyaline material. They often involve the skin in areas other than the external ear, being common on the scalp, where they are called "turban tumors." These are multiple lobulated or mushroom-like masses which may occur in clumps resembling a cluster of grapes. The tumors are symptomless unless occlusion of the external auditory canal results in hearing loss.

The treatment is surgical excision, since rare instances of malignant degeneration have been reported. Radiation therapy has little or no effect.

Melanoma

Melanoma occurs fairly commonly on the auricle, usually being present since birth. In most cases these nevi are pigmented but may also be found without color. Malignant change is fortunately rare, but when it does occur, it is a serious problem. Excision is the best treatment because of the chance of malignant change. A rapid change in the size or color of a nevus is a definite indication for wide primary excision. If suspicion of malignancy exists, a biopsy should not be done because of the high incidence of spread from surgical trauma in this type of tumor.

Winkler's Disease

Painful nodular growth of the auricle is an interesting but rare tumor occurring on the top of the helix. It consists of tiny arteriovenous anastomoses with many nerve endings similar to a glomus body. It is seen mainly in men (90%) and is of unknown origin.

The main symptom and that causing the patient to seek medical attention is pain. The small nodule is tender, preventing some patients from sleeping on the ear. The lesion may be excised or injected with cortisone, which will relieve the pain in most instances.

BENIGN TUMORS OF THE EXTERNAL AUDITORY CANAL

Keloid, papilloma, sebaceous cyst, cylindroma, and melanoma, discussed above, may all involve the canal as well as the auricle.

Exostosis

Exostoses are the most common tumors of the external auditory canal. These benign outgrowths of bone are symptomless unless accompanied by the accumulation of debris against the tympanic membrane, resulting in infection or obstruction. Exostoses are usually seen as two or three smooth sessile protrusions on opposing surfaces of the bony canal near the annulus. In almost every case a history may be obtained of frequent swimming, often in cold water. This fact is probably of prime etiologic significance.

Osteoma occurs in the auditory canal as a single larger growth forming near the lateral end of the bony portion. These tumors are often pedunculated.

Each of these growths is benign and may be ignored unless of sufficient size to obstruct the canal or cause repeated infection from retention of debris. Surgical removal involves elevating the skin from the surface of the bony growth and then removing the growth with motor-driven burrs. When the normal canal lumen has been restored, the skin is replaced over the bone of the canal and held in place with a packing of absorbable gelatin sponge. In some instances, an exostosis will interfere with tympanic surgery, in which case the above described procedure becomes a part of the tympanoplasty with the skin flap becoming a tympanomeatal flap (see Chapter 50). A pedunculated growth may be removed by fracturing the base with a small chisel.

Adenoma

Adenomas of various sorts occur in the canal. These are derived from sweat glands (epithelioma adenoides cysticum or ceruminoma), sebaceous glands, or aberrant salivary gland tissue. Cylindroma as previously described may occur within the external auditory canal. Differentiation of these tumors depends on microscopic examination, since each appears as a smooth, skin-covered, polypoid mass arising from the canal wall. Symptoms are minimal unless the growth completely occludes the canal. Pain is a sign of malignancy and indicates the need for great suspicion if it occurs with a tumor within the canal.

The treatment is surgical excision. Some of these lesions occasionally become malignant, and pathologic examination is required in each case. Most of these adenomas may be removed through a transmeatal approach, although with larger growths an endaural incision may be needed (see Chapter 50).

Finally, any mass occurring within the external auditory canal, if persistent, should be removed for examination. Lesions thought to be polyps, granulomas, or other innocent forms have all on occasion proved to be malignant, usually squamous cell carcinoma. Since this disease is often associated with chronic discharge from the ear, patients with such discharge should be regarded with particular suspicion, especially if the discharge does not respond to adequate treatment.

BENIGN TUMORS OF THE MIDDLE EAR

Since cholesteatoma and middle ear polyps will be discussed in Chapter 49, Chronic Ear Disease, the principal lesion in this group is the glomus jugulare tumor (nonchromaffin paraganglioma).

Glomus Jugulare Tumor

Although vascular tumors of the middle ear have been described since the onset of the twentieth century, it was not until 1941 that the basic tissue of origin, the glomus jugulare, was discovered and described by Stacey Guild. In 1945, Rosenwasser reported the removal of a tumor of the middle ear whose microscopic appearance resembled that of a glomus jugulare. Since that year this tumor has proved to be the most common one arising in the middle ear.

The glomus jugulare is a tiny (0.5 × 0.5 × 0.25 mm) glandular structure similar to the carotid body. It consists of nests of nonchromaffin staining cells clustered among thin-walled vascular channels (Fig. 46–7). There are usually several of these in every temporal bone, being found on the top of the jugular bulb, along the course of Jacobson's nerve, the tympanic plexus, or Arnold's nerve. The function of these structures is unknown, the most probable being that they are chemoreceptors sensitive to CO_2 level or pH of the blood, as is the carotid body.

Histology. The glomus jugulare tumor is similar in cellular structure to the tissue of

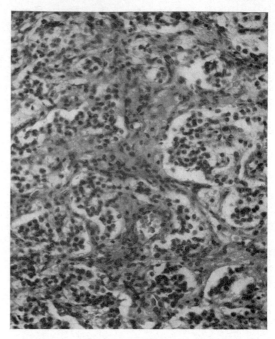

FIG. 46–7. Glomus jugulare tumor. Typical appearance of nests of large pale-staining cells surrounded by vascular channels.

origin. It usually arises in the hypotympanum at the site of entrance of Jacobson's nerve or in the adventitia of the jugular bulb. In many instances these tumors have been seen to arise on the promontory. They occur five times more often in women than in men. The tumors are extremely vascular, consisting of vascular sinuses supplied by the ascending pharyngeal artery which enters the tympanum along with Jacobson's nerve. Although the growth rate is variable, these tumors as a rule grow slowly, in some instances with 20 years elapsing between onset and diagnosis. These tumors only rarely metastasize, but they are destructive, growing by invasion into the surrounding structures. Instances of multicentric origin and association with carotid body tumors have been reported, indicating the need for a search for other similar tumors when a glomus tumor is found.

Symptoms. The earliest reported symptom is tinnitus, which is most often pulsatile. Hearing loss follows as the tumor enlarges; as it invades the tympanic membrane, bleeding and discharge due to secondary infection will occur. Isolated facial nerve paralysis is frequently present, and invasion along the course of the jugular will result in multiple involvement of the ninth, tenth, eleventh, and twelfth cranial nerves. Invasion of the cochlea and petrous tip is a late occurrence, resulting in sensorineural hearing loss and rarely paralysis of the fifth and sixth cranial nerves. Pain is not a common symptom, occurring more often with carcinoma.

Diagnosis. Examination in the early stages reveals a reddish swelling behind the tympanic membrane which, with magnification, may be seen to pulsate. If the drumhead is dull and the tumor is small, this appearance might be confused with the Schwartze sign in otosclerosis (see Chapter 52, Otosclerosis). As the tumor enlarges, it causes the inferior portion of the tympanic membrane to bulge (Fig. 46–8) and finally breaks through to form a smooth dark red polypoid mass which bleeds easily (and often massively) on manipulation. Application of pressure with a Siegle otoscope causes the tumor to increase in pulsation as the pressure is raised until sudden blanching occurs after the systolic pressure is exceeded (Brown's test). Radiographic examination is

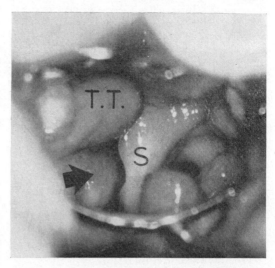

FIG. 46–9. Mirror view of nasopharynx showing extension of glomus jugulare down eustachian tube. At arrow the tumor is protruding through tubal orifice. T.T., Torus tubarius; S, the posterior end of the nasal septum.

of little value in early cases but as the tumor advances will reveal the extent of bony destruction. In advanced tumors, external carotid angiography is helpful in delineating the extent of involvement. Diagnosis is confirmed by biopsy, which must be done carefully in the hospital operating room because of the severe bleeding which may occur. With an intact tympanic membrane, the biopsy is best done through a tympanotomy approach and combined with total excision.

Alford and Guilford have introduced the concept of staging of glomus tumors, describing five clinical stages. The best treatment of the tumor will vary with the stage of the disease.

Stage 0. This stage is the earliest manifestation of a glomus tumor. The patient complains of hearing loss and/or pulsating tinnitus. There will be normal hearing or a conductive hearing loss. The drumhead is intact but discolored. Radiographs will be normal.

Stage I. Added to the above will be aural discharge due to involvement of the tympanic membrane by the tumor. Radiographs show clouding of the middle ear but no bone erosion. There is no nerve involvement.

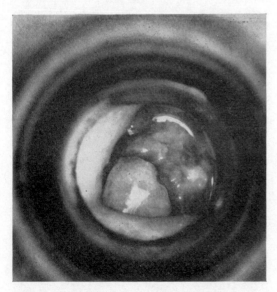

FIG. 46–8. Otoscopic appearance of glomus jugulare tumor. The tumor has eroded the tympanic membrane and is creating a serosanguineous otorrhea.

Stage II. Facial paralysis is now present, and there is sensorineural hearing loss. Radiographs show no bone erosion other than occasional enlargement of the jugular foramen.

Stage III. Involvement of the jugular foramen now adds paralysis of the cranial nerves IX, X, XI, and XII. There will be radiographic evidence of erosion of the petrous bone and enlargement of the jugular foramen.

Stage IV. Intracranial extension has taken place, and papilledema is present. Extensive involvement of the petrous bone has occurred, with paralysis of the third, fourth, fifth, and sixth cranial nerves.

Treatment. Treatment must be individualized, since many early cases may be cured through surgical excision, but slow growth of the tumor usually dictates palliation in the far-advanced cases. Tumors (Stage I) involving only the middle ear may be completely excised through a tympanotomy. The exposure should be primarily of the hypotympanum. This is done by extending the meatal flap to include the inferior canal wall and removing the inferior tympanic annulus with a diamond burr to expose the entire hypotympanic space. Extension into the attic or mastoid (Stage I or II) requires a radical mastoidectomy approach for adequate exposure. In extensive lesions hemorrhage may be life-threatening, so that ligation of the ascending pharyngeal artery should be done if surgery is contemplated. Cases involving the jugular foramen with cranial nerve paralysis (Stage III) have been successfully operated, but this is such a formidable procedure necessitating dissection and ligation of the lateral sinus and jugular vein in the neck that in most instances partial removal combined with radiation is employed. The easiest method of handling the tumor tissue is to expose the entire extent of the tumor and pack around it with small cotton or gauze packs while it is being removed to control the bleeding. A significant new modality now employed with these tumors is fractional destruction by cryosurgical freezing.

Radiation is often used in these cases, especially when complete removal is not possible. Although these tumors are somewhat radioresistant, x-ray has a definite effect on their course, causing a slow regression in the size of the tumor. Tumor doses of 2400 to 6000 R given over a period of 2 to 4 weeks have been employed. Long-term periodic examination must follow any type of treatment.

MALIGNANT TUMORS OF THE EAR

Carcinoma

The most common tumor of skin is squamous cell carcinoma; 90% of such cases occur on the face and neck and 6% on the auricle. Eighty-five% of cases of carcinoma of the ear present on the auricle, 10% on the external auditory canal, and 5% in the middle ear. Fortunately in clinical practice these percentages represent a small incidence, with large institutions seeing few cases. King's Hospital in London reported only 13 cases in the 10-year span between 1952 and 1961. This is an incidence of 4 or 5 carcinomas per 20,000 patients.

Etiology. Carcinoma of the auricle most often has its onset in the sixth or seventh decade, with about 80% of cases occurring in males. It is associated with chronic exposure of the skin, chronic eczema, or previous radiation of the ear. Carcinoma of the external auditory canal and middle ear is associated in over 75% of cases with chronic otorrhea.

Histology. These tumors may be present in three types; squamous cell carcinoma (75%), basal cell carcinoma (15%), and adenocarcinoma (10%). When these tumors are first seen, metastasis is present in about 20%, which may involve the postauricular, superior deep cervical, parotid, or submaxillary lymph node groups. Blood-borne metastasis is rare.

Squamous cell carcinoma (epidermoid carcinoma) consists of downgrowths and masses of enlarged epithelial cells which show marked variations and irregularity in their size. Many atypical mitoses will be seen. Typically there will be many concentric nests of keratinized cells forming keratin "pearls." These "pearls" and the presence of prickle cells are the main factors allowing differentiation from basal cell carcinoma. Basal cell carcinoma (rodent ulcer) is composed of cords and masses of cells with deeply basophilic nuclei. Mitotic figures are less frequent, and epithelial "pearls" are not as often present. Adenocarcinoma arises from the skin appendages or glandular elements of the middle ear. These form masses of cells arranged in alveoli and ducts interspersed with connective tissue.

These three types of carcinoma follow a somewhat different course. Basal cell carcinoma usually has an indolent course, existing for many months before a change in the lesion brings the patient to the doctor. At this time, the tumor usually will have modified into a squamous cell tumor, growing more rapidly and becoming ulcerated. Metastasis is more common with squamous cell carcinoma than with basal cell carcinoma, which is most often locally invasive. Adenocarcinoma follows the same type of course as squamous cell carcinoma, growing rapidly and producing frequent metastases.

Diagnosis. Diagnosis is not difficult with carcinoma arising on the auricle (Fig. 46–10). The lesion begins as a firm nodule which enlarges at a variable rate. Erosion of the surface occurs with the formation of a superficial crusted ulcer with hard, rolled edges. Occasionally there will be a pre-existing papilloma or keratotic lesion which will begin to enlarge and ulcerate. In some instances the tumor will be fungating. Auricular carcinoma is painless unless invasion and infection of the underlying cartilage occur.

Carcinoma of the canal or middle ear is much more difficult to diagnose early in its course. Usually associated with chronic infection, the tumor has a rough red surface which may be mistaken for a granuloma or polyp. For this reason any case of non-resolving ear infection should be regarded with great suspicion. All irregularities of the skin surface, granulomas, or polyps must be biopsied when present. The two most common symptoms associated with malignancy of the canal or middle ear are pain and bleeding. Since chronic infection usually causes neither of these symptoms, they constitute signs of malignancy. As the disease progresses, involvement of the facial nerve, progressing to paralysis, occurs regularly.

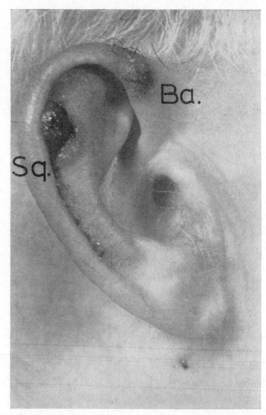

FIG. 46–10. Carcinoma of the auricle. The tumor on the anterior heli (Ba.) is a basal cell carcinoma, while the posterior mass (Sq.) is a squamous cell carcinoma.

Further spread may be to the regional lymph nodes or into the base of the skull with involvement of the lower cranial nerves.

Treatment. Treatment of carcinoma of the ear is dependent upon its position and size.

1. *Auricle.* Carcinoma of the auricle is usually discovered early and, if so, may be treated with minimal sacrifice of tissue. The cure rate is over 90% with lesions of the auricle. The tumor is excised with a wide margin of normal skin (at least 1 cm). The underlying cartilage is removed en bloc with the specimen. The methods employed most often are wedge resection with primary suture, which results in a smaller but normal-appearing ear (Fig. 46–11); resection with full-thickness skin grafting (Fig. 46–12); and resection with reconstruction and with postauricular staged pedicle flaps (Fig. 46–

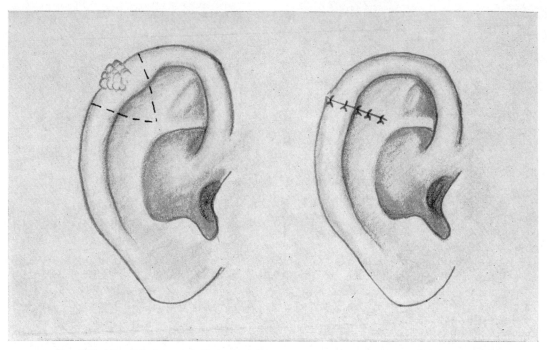

FIG. 46–11.   Wedge resection of auricle. The en bloc removal includes the full
thickness of the auricle.

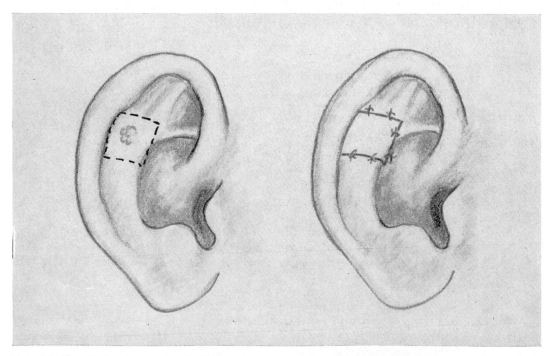

FIG. 46–12.   Resection with full-thickness skin grafting. The en bloc removal includes the skin
and underlying cartilage, but not the skin on the posterior surface of the auricle.

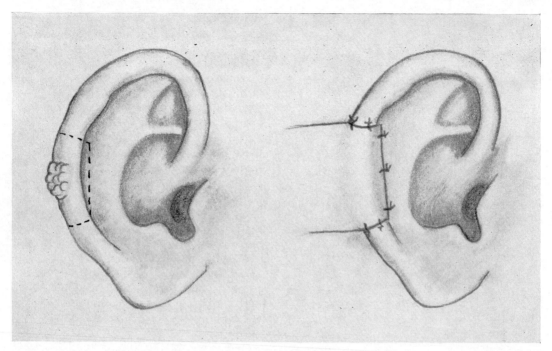

FIG. 46–13. Resection with pedicle flap repair. After healing has occurred following this procedure, a second procedure separates the pedicle, which is used to reconstruct the helix. The defect over the mastoid region is covered with a split-thickness graft.

13). Extensive tumors may require removal of the entire auricle with skin grafting of the surgical defect. When the tumor is associated with regional metastasis, resection of the ear is accompanied by radical neck dissection. In some cases partial or total parotidectomy must be included in this dissection, occasionally with sacrifice of the facial nerve. Preoperative or postoperative radiation is not usually indicated in these cases.

2. *External Auditory Canal.* The cure rate in carcinoma of the external auditory canal is poor, being less than 35%. Wide excision of the lesion dictates complete removal of the cartilaginous and bony auditory canal by means of a mastoid approach which removes the canal en bloc without disturbance of the involved tissue. The surgery is usually supplemented with a postoperative tumoricidal dose of radiation.

The surgical approach initially isolates the external meatus from the auricle by incisions made widely around the canal orifice through the tragus and concha (Fig. 46–14). A postauricular incision then gives access to

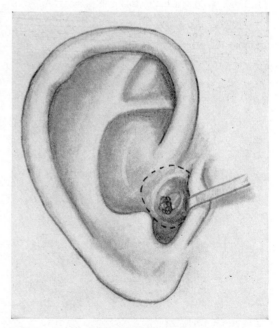

FIG. 46–14. Carcinoma of external auditory canal. The external meatus is isolated by the incision shown around the orifice of the canal (after Conley).

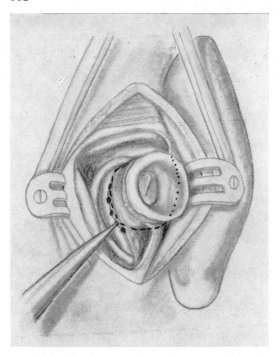

FIG. 46–15. Carcinoma of external auditory canal. The external auditory canal has been isolated by complete mastoidectomy and atticotomy. The facial nerve has been exposed and removed from the fallopian canal. A perforating burr is being used to outline a line which will be fractured through with chisel to free completely the entire auditory canal en bloc (after Conley).

the mastoid cortex to allow an atticomastoidectomy to outline completely the superior and posterior bony canal walls (Fig. 46–15). The intramastoid portion of the facial nerve is dissected to permit transection of the bony external canal at the level of the facial canal. A perforating burr is used to make multiple holes through the facial canal into the posterior sinus and tympanic sinus of the middle ear in order to make a controlled fracture at this level. The same technique is used to separate the anterior canal wall from the anterior extremity of the lateral attic wall. These fractures are made with a thin osteotome. With further separation of the surrounding soft tissues, an en bloc specimen is removed containing the entire cartilaginous and bony canal with the tympanic membrane and mal-

leus included. The resultant defect may be covered with a split-thickness skin graft.

3. *Middle Ear.* Carcinoma involving the middle ear and temporal bone has a poor prognosis, with a cure rate of less than 25%. Surgical excision of the temporal bone is a formidable procedure, with an operative mortality of about 30%. The complications of the surgery include meningitis, intracranial hemorrhage, cerebrospinal fluid leak, brain herniation, and wound infection. The surgical field is limited anteriorly by the carotid artery, posteriorly by the lateral sinus and posterior fossa dura, and superiorly by the middle fossa dura. Wide excision requires sacrifice of the facial nerve, parotid gland, and ramus of the mandible (Figs. 46–16 and 46–17). Blood loss can be considerable, and replacement of as much as 3 liters may be required. Surgery may be supplemented postoperatively by radiation therapy.

Extension of the tumor into the neck, base of the skull, tip of the petrous bone, or dura creates an incurable problem to date. Treatment in these far-advanced cases is limited to palliation, which may include limited surgery, radiation, or both.

Cystic Adenoid Epithelioma (Brooke's Tumor)

This tumor is a special form of carcinoma in which the cell type is thought to be derived from the germinal epithelium of the hair follicles and/or sweat glands. The lesion is exceedingly rare but may involve either the auricle or the external auditory canal.

Histologically there are immature epidermoid cells arranged in cords, clumps, and alveoli plus concentric rings of cornifying epithelium around a core of homogeneous material. These cells project from the basal layer of the skin or glandular ducts and commonly contain cystic areas filled with amorphous material.

Clinically these tumors appear after puberty and are more common in females. They present as small, painless, slowly enlarging nodules which do not ulcerate. Metastasis is rare, but the prognosis is poor be-

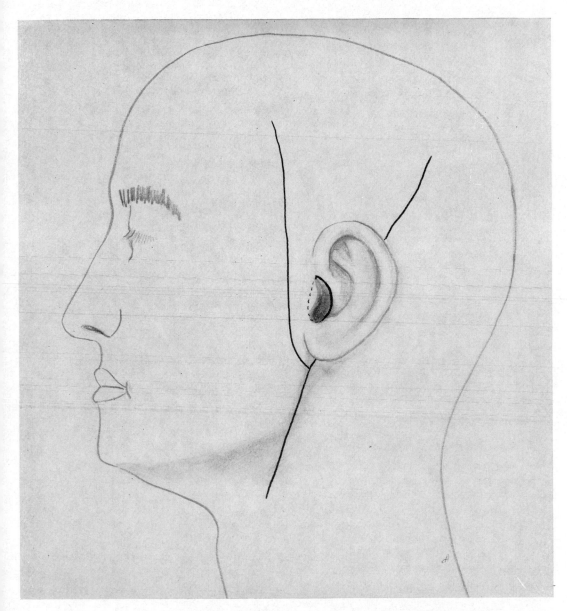

FIG. 46–16.   Carcinoma of middle ear and mastoid. The lines indicate the incisions used to develop the scalp flaps employed with total temporal bone resection (after Conley).

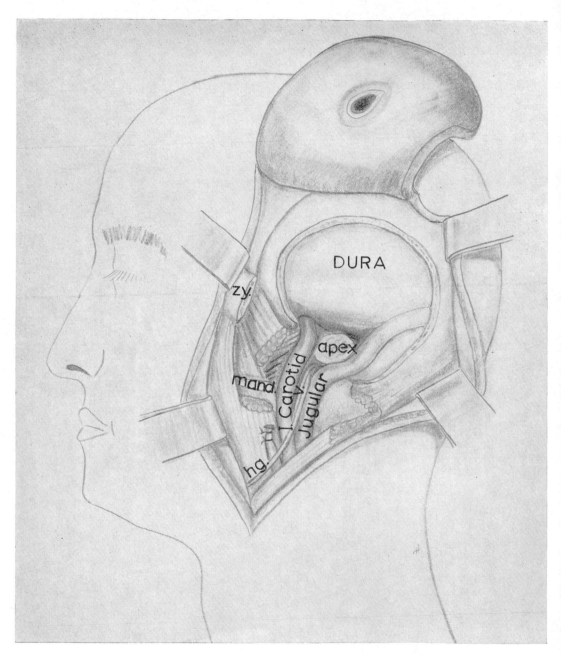

Fig. 46–17.   Carcinoma of middle ear and mastoid.   Residual defect after radical removal of temporal bone. hg., Hypoglossal nerve; mand., mandible; v., vagus nerve; zy., zygoma.

cause of insidious progress and recurrence despite seemingly adequate treatment.

Adequate surgical resection plus postoperative radiation is the preferred treatment to date. This follows the methods outlined under the discussion of carcinoma.

Sarcoma

Sarcoma occurs most often in much younger individuals than those with carcinoma, being the most common malignant ear tumor in childhood. The majority of these tumors are rhabdomyosarcomas with spindle cell sarcoma, fibrosarcoma, lymphosarcoma, and chondrosarcoma also being reported. In some instances the ear is invaded from the eustachian tube or from metastasis, but most often the tumor is primary in the middle ear or external auditory canal.

The prognosis is poor in these cases because of the rapid progress of the lesion. Often the tumor is beyond the bounds of surgical excision before the diagnosis is made. Radiation therapy is made difficult by the surrounding bone, which is often lost by radionecrosis after treatment. In those cases in which treatment is attempted, temporal bone resection followed by radiation therapy seems to offer the best prognosis.

Malignant Melanoma

Melanoma may occur either on the auricle or in the external canal, being more common in the former location. Diagnosis should be suspected with a pigmented lesion which begins to increase in size or changes in color. Since these lesions have a tendency to spread after surgical trauma, biopsy should be avoided. If the lesion is of short duration, an en bloc excision with wide margins of normal tissue should be done. Since lymphatic metastasis occurs unpredictably and often early, the prognosis should be guarded. Frequent follow-up examinations are needed to detect spread at the earliest possibility. If regional lymphatic spread is detected, radical neck dissection offers a chance of cure in some cases.

REFERENCES

Alford, B. R., and Guilford, F. R.: Tumors of the Glomus Jugulare. Laryngoscope, *72*: 765, 1962.

Ash, J. E.: Chapter 4, *In* Schenck, H. P. (Ed.): *Pathology of the Ear in Otolaryngology.* Vol I. Hagerstown, Prior, 1960.

Brown, J. S.: Glomus Jugulare Tumors. Laryngoscope, *77*:26, 1967.

Conley, J.: Cancer of the Middle Ear. Ann. Otol., *74*:555, 1965.

Conley, J. J., and Novack, A. J.: Surgical Treatment of Malignant Tumors of the Ear and Temporal Bone. Arch. Otol., *71*:635, 1960.

Eggston, A. A., and Wolff, D.: *Histopathology of the Ear, Nose and Throat.* Baltimore, The Williams & Wilkins Co., 1947.

Guild, S. R.: Glomus Jugulare in Man. Ann. Otol., *62*:1045, 1953.

Rosenwasser, H.: Carotid Body Tumor of Middle Ear and Mastoid. Arch. Otol., *41*: 64, 1945.

Rosenwasser, H.: Glomus Jugulare Tumor of the Middle Ear. Laryngoscope, *62*:623, 1952.

Shambaugh, G. E., Jr.: Surgical Approaches for Glomus Jugulare Tumors of the Middle Ear. Laryngoscope, *65*:185, 1955.

Tabb, H. G.: Cancer of the External Auditory Canal. Laryngoscope, *74*:634, 1964.

Chapter 47
Eustachian Tube Dysfunction

Diseases involving the eustachian tube are made manifest and cause their morbidity by interference with aeration and drainage of the middle ear. In some forms, this is associated with the accumulation of fluid in the middle ear which is either serous or mucoid, secretory otitis media. In all inflammatory disease of the middle ear, involvement of the eustachian tube plays a key role. When the cause of the disease is a chronic problem, the interference with hearing becomes a major symptom whose treatment can be difficult.

The causes of interference with eustachian tube function are numerous. Investigation of this problem must be thorough if an accurate etiologic diagnosis is to be made. Accurate diagnosis is essential in these diseases to achieve a satisfactory and lasting resolution.

Physiology

The essential features of eustachian tube anatomy contributing to disturbance in function are as follows: the medial two thirds of the eustachian tube run through a hook-shaped elastic cartilaginous framework whose open lateral aspect is closed by a membrane bounded by the tensor veli palatini muscle. The cartilaginous tube ends medially in the lateral nasopharyngeal wall, its cartilage projecting posteriorly beyond the meatus to form the torus tubarius. At rest, the cartilaginous tube is closed, with the lumen forming a vertical slit. The mu-

cosa is a thick, ciliated, columnar epithelium with numerous glandular elements and submucosal lymphoid aggregates. The cilia direct the flow of the mucous blanket toward the nasopharynx. The thickness of the mucosa lessens as the junction with the bony portion of the eustachian tube is reached. At this point, the isthmus, the tubal lumen reaches its smallest diameter, gradually re-expanding until the wide tympanic ostium opens into the anterosuperior mesotympanum. The mucosa of this portion is ciliated, but the cells are much shorter, usually cuboidal in form, with only rare glandular elements. Mucus is produced in the tympanum and bony eustachian tube mainly by scattered goblet cells.

The lumen of the cartilaginous tube is opened by action of the tensor veli palatini muscle pulling on the upper lateral projection of the tubal cartilage, thus giving a more circular form to the cartilage. This action is activated by the fifth cranial nerve and depends on synergistic action of the levator veli palatini muscle. The contraction of this latter muscle, mediated by the vagus nerve through the pharyngeal plexus, serves as a base against which the tensor may act to open the tube. The salpingopharyngeus and superior pharyngeal constrictor are also involved in this complex action. Under normal conditions, only the above muscular activity will open the tube for air exchange of the middle ear. Studies have shown that conscious and involuntary pharyngeal and palatal movement, as with swallowing, yawning, and speech, occurs several times a minute awake or sleeping. Normally no air exchange will take place without this muscular activity.

The basic information concerning the pressure differentials involved with air exchange of the middle ear was gathered by Hartmann in the last century but has been refined and added to by many workers since that time. The basic need for air exchange arises because of a constant gas flow across the capillary walls of the mucosa lining the middle ear and mastoid spaces, resulting in a mild but persistent relative negative pressure within these spaces (Fig. 47–1). This pressure differential, plus that created by barometric pressure variation, is equalized on contraction of the tubal musculature by an influx of nasopharyngeal air. In normal individuals, the pressure difference between the ear and nasopharynx needed to effect air flow is between 0.5 and 4 mm Hg.

Without muscular activity (as in the Valsalva maneuver), a much greater pressure differential of 20 to 40 mm Hg is required to force air into the middle ear. If the external air pressure is rapidly increased, as with caisson workers entering a pressure chamber or in rapid descent from high altitude, the eustachian tube cannot be opened after a differential of 80 to 130 mm Hg exists, even by swallowing. This last fact is due to the "flutter valve" action of the cartilaginous tube preventing influx of air when high atmospheric pressure causes collapse of the ostium. Escape of air from the middle ear through the closed tube will occur, however, with a pressure difference of as little as 12 mm Hg.

Measurement of Tubal Function

The evaluation of tubal function as an easily performed clinical procedure has not yet been accomplished. Since success in tympanoplastic surgery may be dependent on adequate tubal function, the importance of evaluation of tubal function is apparent.

The function of aeration is evaluated by determining the amount of pressure differential required to admit air to the middle ear. Early methods applied a positive pres-

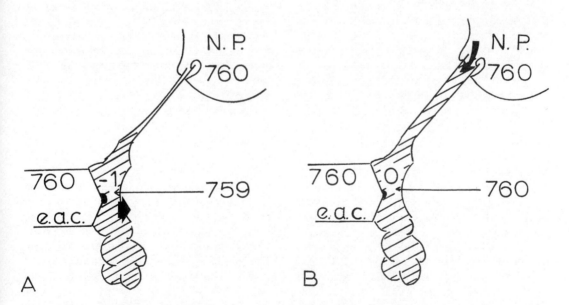

FIG. 47–1.   Aeration of middle ear. A, A constant transfer of gas into the capillaries of the middle ear (arrow) causes a relative negative pressure within the middle ear. The figures indicate an average value for this differential: 760 mm Hg atmospheric pressure in external auditory canal (e.a.c.) and nasopharynx (N.P.), 759 mm Hg pressure in middle ear, giving a relative negative pressure of 1 mm Hg. B, When the eustachian tube opens, the pressure differential causes the inflow of air to the middle ear (arrow), temporarily equalizing the pressures.

sure to the nasopharynx through an olive tip placed firmly in the nose while the palate is closed voluntarily. The difficulties of controlling and recording these measurements prevented this method from wide clinical application.

A recent method developed by Miller reverses the procedure by applying the pressure differential through a catheter sealed in the external auditory canal. The effect of swallowing on this pressure may be easily recorded on a paper writer, such as an ECG machine. The necessity of a perforate tympanic membrane has made the determination of normal values difficult, but this is not a problem in clinical practice, since most surgical patients have a preexisting perforation. The application of this method in patients with secretory otitis media requires placing a tube through the intact membrane. In practice the test is carried out by causing a negative pressure of 250 mm H_2O within the external auditory canal and observing the equalization of pressure as the patient swallows. With normal function, the pressure difference is eliminated after several swallows. Four gradations of abnormality have been described, the most severe being in those patients in whom no air flow occurs even with the application of a positive pressure of 250 mm H_2O, indicating complete functional obstruction of the tube.

Tympanometry (impedance audiometry) is an objective technique for evaluating tubal function which employs an acoustic bridge. This method uses an airtight ear plug containing tubes which vary sound pressure in the external auditory canal, measure the sound pressure, and vary the air pressure within the canal. One or more frequencies of sound may be used, the most common being 220 Hz. As the sound is applied, the air pressure within the canal is varied, and the probe measuring the sound level records the sound pressure within the canal. This sound pressure reaches a maximum when the air pressure in the canal balances that in the middle ear, thus indicating middle ear air pressure. Further, the recording provides a curve whose form may prove useful in differentiating various forms of middle ear pathology. (See Ch. 44 for a complete discussion.)

This technique is especially useful in children who are too young to test reliably with audiometry, principally because it is an objective procedure. It has been evaluated in several large school hearing screening programs and has been found to be the most reliable method of discovering middle ear problems in this age group.

Impedance (admittance) audiometry is at present in a period of development in terms of both instrumentation and potential applications. It is apparent now, however, that this tool is and will continue to be important in the evaluation of middle ear function and the differentiation of forms of pathologic processes within the middle ear.

Clinical estimation of tubal function without special equipment may be done, but reliable correlation with actual tubal adequacy is not always obtained. In this method the gradations are:

1. A patient who can inflate his ear easily by the Valsalva maneuver or who shows a positive reaction to the Toynbee maneuver. (The *Toynbee maneuver* is done by the patient swallowing while holding the nostrils closed. This causes a negative pressure in the nasopharynx, resulting in a flow of air from the middle ear. The tympanic membrane can be seen to be drawn inward during the swallow, returning to its normal position shortly after or on the next swallow, termed a "positive" reaction.)

2. A patient who can inflate his ear by the Valsalva maneuver only with much difficulty.

3. A patient who cannot inflate his ear by his own efforts but whose ear can be inflated using the Politzer technique.

4. A patient whose ear can be inflated only by tubal catheterization.

5. A patient whose ear cannot be inflated by any technique.

By adopting such a system of evaluation, there can be a more rational application of therapeutic methods for the individual patient.

Studies of the other tubal function, that of drainage of the middle ear, have been less adequately developed. These tests have been performed by placing a liquid substance into the middle ear and timing its appearance in the nasopharynx. The major problem is the determination of the end point or quantitation of these tests. Dyes such as fluorescein have been placed in the middle ear and the time of their appearance in the nasopharynx with swallowing used as an index of function. A method developed by Compere uses radiopaque material placed in the middle ear. The progress of the dye through the tube is then followed radiographically. This offers more information but at the expense of more time and difficulty. Fortunately drainage function usually correlates well with disturbance of aeration, so that the more simply applied tests of tubal function are adequate in most cases. The exception are the cases with "ball valve" pathology of the tympanic osteum preventing outflow from the middle ear while permitting inflation.

Pathologic Physiology

Obstruction of the eustachian tube may be partial or complete, functional or anatomic, and fast or slow in onset. This obstruction may also be accompanied by varying degrees of inflammation. It is these basic factors which determine the effect of the process on the middle ear.

When the function of aeration of the middle ear cleft through the eustachian tube is interfered with, the now static air within the middle ear and mastoid is absorbed by the blood vessels in the lining mucosa. This causes a negative pressure within these spaces. The reduced pressure results in a transudation of fluid from the mucosa as well as edema of the mucosa to compensate for the lack of air. If the blockage of ventilation is complete and long-standing, the air of the middle ear cleft will be completely replaced by fluid.

If inflammation or sudden pressure changes in the outside environment accompany this process, effusion as well as transudation occurs, and the process proceeds much more rapidly. On the other hand, chronic partial obstruction may result in no fluid accumulation at all, causing only an increased constant negative pressure within the middle ear. Cases described as "atelectasis of the middle ear" may result from this last mechanism.

Etiology

A wide variety of diseases causing eustachian tube obstruction have been cataloged:

Acute
  Upper respiratory infection
  Allergic rhinitis
  Adenoiditis or nasopharyngitis
  Sinusitis
Chronic or recurrent
  Chronic obstructive hyperplasia of adenoid
  Chronic nasopharyngeal lymphoid hyperplasia (other than adenoid)
  Chronic sinusitis
  Allergic rhinitis
  Adhesions or scarring in nasopharynx, especially in the fossa of Rosenmüller
  Scarring or hyperplasia of tubal mucosa
  Stenosis of bony portion of eustachian tube
  Malformation or cleft palate
  Paralysis of palatal muscles
Tumor of the nasopharynx

The reader is referred to the appropriate section for discussion of these problems.

Symptoms

The initial symptom is a sticking or cracking sound heard on yawning or swallowing as the opposing surfaces of the mouth of the eustachian tube tend to stick together. As progression occurs, a feeling of fullness develops in the ear, accompanied by a decrease in hearing. This is most often described as though something were occluding the ear canal. Pain is uncommon, although young children sometimes complain of mild "earache."

Tinnitus is commonly present. It is usually low-pitched and described as a "hum" or "sea shell" sound. It may be pulsating or continuous. Autophony is usually present, being described as hearing one's own voice loudly and with a hollow sound, like "having your head in a rain barrel."

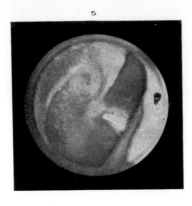

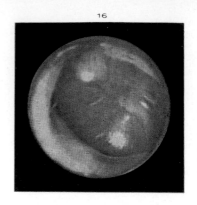

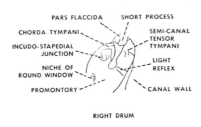

PARS FLACCIDA — SHORT PROCESS
CHORDA TYMPANI — SEMI-CANAL TENSOR TYMPANI
INCUDO-STAPEDIAL JUNCTION —
NICHE OF ROUND WINDOW — LIGHT REFLEX
PROMONTORY — CANAL WALL

RIGHT DRUM

FIG. 47–2

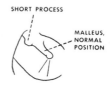

SHORT PROCESS

MALLEUS, NORMAL POSITION

LEFT DRUM

FIG. 47–3

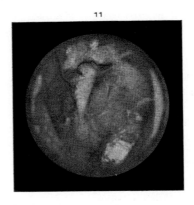

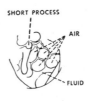

SHORT PROCESS

AIR

FLUID

RIGHT DRUM

FIG. 47–4

FIG. 47–2.   Otoscopic view of normal tympanic membrane.

FIG. 47–3.   Tympanic membrane in mild tubal dysfunction. The malleus handle is slightly fore-shortened and the short process prominent. The tympanic membrane is gray and lusterless.

FIG. 47–4.   After inflation, air bubbles in the thin secretion can be seen behind the tympanic membrane.

(Courtesy of Dr. Richard A. Buckingham. Abbott Laboratories, *What's New*, 196, 1956.)

Diagnosis

Otoscopy initially reveals retraction of the tympanic membrane. This is characterized by a foreshortening of the handle of the malleus owing to the fact that it is more parallel to the observer's line of sight (Fig. 47–3). At the same time, the short process of the malleus becomes more prominent, and the light reflex is distorted or lost.

As fluid accumulates in the middle ear, the drumhead becomes bluish, since more light is absorbed by the fluid. A yellowish cast is given to the drumhead if the fluid is serous. If air remains in the middle ear, a fluid level may be seen, appearing as a fine hairline on the drumhead. Bubbles of air may be seen occasionally, particularly following inflation of the middle ear (Fig. 47–4).

Hearing tests reveal an initial low-tone conductive loss as the reduced middle ear pressure causes increased stiffness of the tympanic membrane and ossicular chain. The accumulation of fluid results in increased mass and loss of high-tone conduction. The hearing loss may eventually reach a level of 30 to 40 decibels. Tympanometry reveals a reduced middle ear pressure (see Ch. 44).

The diagnosis may be confirmed by aspiration of the middle ear with a Gottschalk apparatus, which is a spinal needle attached to a small fluid trap. Aspiration not only will reveal the presence of fluid but also will provide a sample for analysis.

When the nature of the problem has been established by the above methods, a complete investigation must be undertaken to establish the underlying cause. This includes anterior and posterior rhinoscopy and sinus radiographs. Since eustachian tube obstruction is one of the earliest findings with nasopharyngeal tumors, this possibility must be kept in mind always.

Treatment

To be successful, treatment must be directed toward correcting the underlying cause as well as toward relieving the presenting symptoms. Removal of obstructing or chronically infected adenoids in children with a history of recurrent secretory otitis is particularly indicated. This is much more to the point than a procedure which removes fluid from the ear without resolving the reason for its being there.

Symptomatic treatment is directed toward relieving the obstruction to middle ear ventilation and replacing the fluid with air. To this end oral and topical decongestants are used, and various methods of inflating the middle ear are employed.

INFLATION OF THE EUSTACHIAN TUBE AND MIDDLE EAR

There are three common ways in which the ear may be inflated, the Valsalva maneuver, the Politzer method, and by catheterization. Each of these has specific indications and uses which should be familiar to the practitioner.

The purposes of inflation are to restore or equalize the air pressure on both sides of the tympanic membrane; to restore normal tension between drumhead, ossicles, and labyrinth; to restore normal circulation in the mucosal blood vessels and lymph spaces; to remove secretions from the eustachian tube and tympanic cavity; and to break down adhesions newly formed.

Valsalva Maneuver. This method of inflating the ear is of great usefulness, since it may be employed by the patient at all times with a frequency approaching that of normal tubal function. To be used successfully, the patient should be carefully instructed and told to inflate the ear every 15 to 20 minutes. More difficulty in getting air into the ear will be experienced on arising, since mucosal congestion is greatest at that time. This should be explained to the patient to prevent discouragement. The importance of inflating the ear should be emphasized to certain patients who have been told in the past that this is a dangerous procedure. Fear of inflation is perhaps the main source of difficulty with this method.

The method consists of forcing air into the ear by attempting to blow the nose with the nostrils held closed. This should be carried out without straining, because straining closes the glottis and prevents the rapid build-up of pressure necessary to open the eustachian tube. A more physiologic method but one more difficult to learn is to increase the nasopharyngeal pressure through contraction of the superior constrictor of the pharynx while the palate is closed, thus "squeezing" the air into the ears. This variation is termed the Frenzel maneuver for the German otologist first describing it.

Children can inflate their ears in this manner. They must first be taught to blow their nose effectively and forcefully while the mother holds the handkerchief. After this is learned, the child will be able to blow while the mother holds the nostrils partially or completely together. To be successful in most cases, the mother should learn to inflate her own ears by this method to understand what needs to be accomplished. Inflation may be continued as long as necessary to relieve the feeling of blockage.

Politzer Method. In 1863, Politzer introduced a method of inflating the middle ear cavities that is still of great use in otology. Inflation is accomplished by introducing air pressure through the nose while the patient closes his nasopharynx by swallowing or saying "K." For this purpose, either a rubber bulb fitted with an olive tip (Fig. 47–5) or a nasal tip on an atomizer powered by an air pressure supply may be used. The nasal tip is inserted into one nostril while the other is closed with the fingers (Fig. 47–6). As the patient swallows, pressure is applied by squeezing the bulb or triggering the air supply. Since the nose is closed anteriorly while the act of swallowing closes the nasopharynx, air is forced into the eustachian tube. The act of swallowing, if performed more than once or twice, may be-

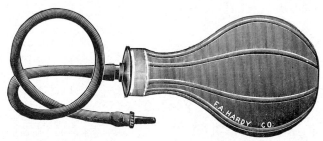

FIG. 47–5.   Politzer's bag and tube for use with a eustachian catheter or nasal tip.

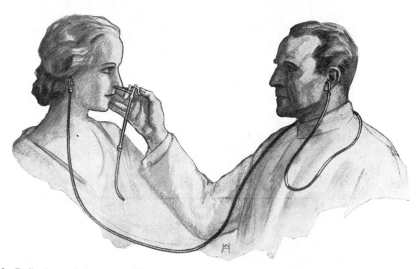

FIG. 47–6. Inflation of the eustachian tube by means of a catheter inserted beneath the inferior turbinate. The physician determines the accuracy of the inflation through the auscultation tube from the patient's ear to his own. The catheter is held in position with the left hand, although it is not thus shown in the illustration.

come difficult for the patient unless aided by a sip of water.

Auscultation during the use of the Politzer method shows two sets of sounds: one due to the entrance of air into the middle ear cavity; the other due to escape of air from the nasopharynx. The former is a soft, blowing murmur if the drumhead is intact, while the latter is rough, loud, and gurgling in character. If for any reason the tympanic murmur is not heard, the tympanic membrane should be observed while another inflates the ear to see if air enters the middle ear. In many instances, the patient is the best judge of whether air has entered the ear.

Politzerization with a regulated air supply may be used to determine the exact amount of pressure needed to inflate the ear at the time of primary examination. This method can be adopted for the office, but for bedside use, the Politzer bag still holds a distinct and useful place in otologic practice.

Catheterization. The usual method of catheterization consists of introducing the catheter through the inferior meatus of the nose into the nasopharynx, where it is turned outward and upward into the mouth of the eustachian tube. The curved tip of the catheter should be kept on the floor of the nose at the junction of the floor and the septum. When the tip touches the posterior wall of the pharynx, it is rotated outward into Rosenmüller's fossa, then drawn forward over the bulging posterior lip of the eustachian orifice into the mouth of the tube. The eyelet of the catheter indicates the direction of the curved tip which, when in the mouth of the tube, is generally turned outward and upward toward the outer canthus of the eye. In some cases the tip enters the tube when directed horizontally.

Another method of locating the tubal orifice is to rotate the tip of the catheter medially into the nasopharynx and then bring it forward to catch on the posterior end of the septum. This places the tip on line with the tubal mouth, which is entered by rotating the tip 180 degrees or more until the tip enters the tube. In instances of special need, it is sometimes possible to enter the eustachian tube with a catheter placed through the opposite nostril.

The catheter is anchored in place with the fingers, and air is forced through it as described for Politzerization. This method should not be used as a frequent routine because of the risk of further traumatizing the tubal mucosa.

FLUID REMOVAL FROM THE MIDDLE EAR

In cases of chronic fluid accumulation, it is often necessary to remove the fluid surgically. This will allow subsidence of mucosal edema and aeration by the normal route. Myringotomy and aspiration of the fluid is the simplest way of achieving this, but since the drum heals rapidly, the effects of the procedure are short-lived. Repeated myringotomy should be avoided, if possible, because of the possibility of associated scarring and permanent hearing impairment (see Bacterial Otitis Media for details of myringotomy, p. 820).

In order to achieve drainage and aeration of the middle ear over longer periods, it is

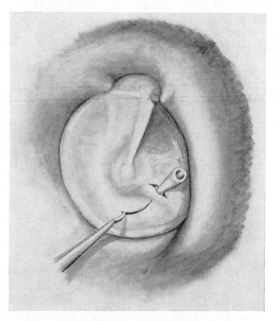

FIG. 47–7. Myringotomy and tympanic ventilation. The preferred position of a myringotomy incision is shown, being placed circumferentially in the inferior posterior portion of the drumhead. Long-term ventilation is done by placing a plastic tube through a radial incision in the anterior drumhead.

now the practice to insert plastic drains of polyethylene, Teflon, or Silastic through a large myringotomy incision (Fig. 47–7). These are allowed to remain in place until patency of the eustachian tube can be demonstrated. They may remain permanently but usually must be replaced every few months, since the migratory action of the drum epithelium carries them out into the canal.

The drains are usually flanged to prevent their rapid extrusion through the drum. Polyethylene is commonly used, since a flange may be formed by heating the end of the tubing. Another common shape is that of a "collar button" or "grommet" which has certain advantages over the longer single flanged tube. The tubes will remain in place longer when placed through a radial incision. The radial fibers will grasp the drain more firmly than do the circular fibers with a routine circumferential incision.

Drainage procedures should be carried out under the control of an operating microscope because of the increased visibility afforded and the ease of the procedure with magnification. In children, general anesthesia is usually necessary.

SPECIFIC DISEASES OF THE EUSTACHIAN TUBE

Acute Salpingitis (Acute Tubal Catarrh)

This is a disease secondary to inflammatory involvement of the nasopharyngeal mucosa by contiguity. It may occur during an acute nasopharyngitis, allergic rhinitis, acute sinusitis, etc. In children it is commonly associated with acute adenoiditis with inflammatory hyperplasia.

The pathologic condition consists of congestion, edema, and round cell infiltration. Severe or prolonged disease may produce damage to or loss of cilia. If the inflammation extends to the middle ear, the picture of acute secretory or bacterial otitis media is produced. Healing may produce fibrosis and scarring in severe cases.

The diagnosis is made by history and findings, as previously outlined. In most cases, there is retraction of the drum without fluid formation.

Treatment should be prompt and adequate, directed toward the primary disease. Since this is an early or developmental stage of acute otitis media, antibiotic therapy is indicated. Symptomatic relief is afforded by the use of decongestants and inflation.

Recurrent episodes are a definite indication for removal of adenoids when their presence is found.

Aerotitis Media (Acute Barotrauma)

Marked differences in barometric pressure from rapid altitudinal changes, as in flying, may affect the middle ear and mastoid, if the eustachian tube is obstructed from any cause. During ascent, the middle ear pressure is reduced with comparative ease, but as descent begins, the reverse action may not take place. Redundancy or edema around the pharyngeal orifice of the eustachian tube acts as a "flutter valve," covering over the orifice as higher atmospheric pressures are reached, preventing the normal passage of air to the middle ear. The reduced air pressure in the middle ear cavity produces a traumatic inflammation of the tympanic mucosa and indrawing of the eardrum.

If the relative vacuum is not relieved, serum will be produced and there may be small hemorrhages on the drum or on the mucosa of the middle ear.

Symptoms are discomfort, pain, tinnitus, and partial deafness. The pain frequently extends to the region of the parotid gland.

In mild cases, the tympanic membrane is injected, especially along the handle of the malleus and over Shrapnell's membrane. The drumhead is retracted unless the tympanic cavity is filled with blood or secretion, in which case the tympanic membrane may show bulging or marked inflammation. Repeated attacks may result in a chronic middle ear type of deafness.

Treatment. Altitude flying should not take place if an acute rhinitis is present or if the individual is unable to inflate the eustachian tubes at will. Periodic swallowing, chewing gum, or sipping fluids during the flight, especially during descent, may assist in keeping the eustachian tubes open. The ideal treatment, according to Hyde, is the reascent in a pressurized chamber or aircraft to the level at which successful middle ear ventilation is achieved, followed by a slow enough descent to allow the ears to be inflated periodically by the patient during the increase in atmospheric pressure.

Inflation of the eustachian tubes by catheter will restore the air equilibrium and ameliorate the symptoms and inflammation. Due to the severe edema produced in this problem, inflation is often impossible. If this is the case, myringotomy should be performed, which will result in rapid resolutions of the symptoms.

Analgesics and decongestants are indicated in the immediate post-trauma period.

Acute Secretory Otitis Media

This disease is most common in children and is usually associated with infectious or allergic hyperplasia of the adenoid. The fluid present in the ear may be either mucoid or serous. Mucoid fluid is thick and tenacious and has a high protein content. It is thought to be exudative. Serous fluid is a transudate, thin, light yellow, and low in protein content.

The exact cause of secretory otitis remains enigmatic. Adenoid hyperplasia or infection of the nasopharynx, even when occurring concurrently, does not always result in a fluid-filled ear. Likewise, removal of a large mass of adenoid does not always prevent recurrence of secretory otitis. There is a variation of incidence with racial types and with geographic location. A fair-skinned blonde or redhead living in a low northern area with high humidity and air pollution will have a high probability of being affected with secretory otitis. A significant fact is that the incidence of secretory otitis has risen markedly as the incidence of acute suppurative otitis media has fallen with the advent of the antibiotic era. Today over 10 per cent of school age children are afflicted at one time or another by the hearing loss attendant to loss of tubal function, as evidenced by the statistics of school hearing conservation programs. It may be that the majority of these cases would have proceeded to otitis media or to resolution had not the initial symptoms resulted in the "shot of penicillin" so often substituted for thoughtful evaluation and management of disease. The increasing awareness of atopy in children as a background for many symptoms may lead to the discovery of this as a significant factor in secretory otitis media.

Symptoms and findings have been previously outlined.

Treatment is directed toward relieving the immediate cause of obstruction, replacing the fluid in the ear with air, and preventing future occurrences of the disease through permanent control of the underlying pathologic condition. Frequent observation is necessary to guard against the occurrence of suppurative otitis media during the course of the disease.

The most common course of management of this problem is tonsillectomy and adenoidectomy coupled with myringotomy and aspiration of the fluid within the ear. Tubes may be placed at the time of this surgery. These procedures are not without complication, and a period of evaluation of the factors associated with the secretory otitis should precede surgery. Conservative management directed toward nasal hygiene, control of allergic factors, decongestion, and clearance of sinus infection is appropriate and may lead to resolution without surgery.

Adenoidectomy is definitely indicated in those children with long-standing or recurrent secretory otitis. Myringotomy is usually done as a part of the procedure, but some feel that resolution is not always hastened by aspiration of the fluid, even though hearing will be improved at least temporarily. In difficult cases of long-standing mucus accumulation, tympanotomy offers visualization of the middle ear and may reveal intratympanic pathology responsible for the fluid accumulation. The use of drains placed through the drumhead should be reserved for cases of chronic secretory otitis.

Chronic Secretory Otitis Media

This is a disease marked by a long-standing collection of fluid in the middle ear. The fluid in these cases is almost always thick and mucoid, creating the commonly used term of "glue ear." This group of patients is most often difficult to treat, since the basic cause is of a more severe and permanent form. In this category fall cases due to scar tissue formation, cleft palate, nasopharyngeal tumors, etc. It is usually necessary to provide aeration of the middle ear by the use of plastic drains while remedies are being sought for the underlying pathology. Even though a drain is inserted through the tympanic membrane, every effort should be made to have the patient inflate his ear by the Valsalva maneuver.

Treatment should be continued over a long period of time, since in some cases edema will subside slowly over 12 to 24 months, finally allowing inflation of the tube. Surgical procedures which destroy the tympanic plexus have been used with some success. This is proposed on the basis that in some cases there is excess mucus production due to hyperactivity of the parasympathetic fibers of the tympanic plexus. Surgical procedures directed toward restoring patency of the eustachian tube have proved largely unsuccessful. Efforts in this direction are still continuing.

This disease has a poor prognosis, particularly in regard to hearing improvement. It becomes important, therefore, to prevent the patient from becoming discouraged and to bend every effort toward solving this particular problem.

Abnormal Patency of the Eustachian Tube

An excessively open eustachian tube is frequently associated with atrophic changes in the mucosa of the nose, nasopharynx, and oropharynx. The process may not involve the entire eustachian tube but may be limited to the pharyngeal orifice. Some cases have been associated with certain debilitating diseases, with marked loss of weight, and with atrophy of fat about the cartilaginous portion of the tube. Perlman attributes many of the cases to lack of tonus of the tensor veli palatini muscles which are supplied by the fifth nerve. If the tube opens to pressures below 20 mm Hg, it may be considered pathologically patent.

The characteristic symptoms are the inward and outward movements of the drumhead synchronous with the respiratory movements and a soft, blowing murmur heard through the diagnostic tube, even without inflation. There may be autophony or the ringing of the patient's voice in his own ears. The voices of others sometimes give rise to the same disagreeable sensation. This symptom is somewhat different from hyperesthesia acoustica, in which there is a painful distinctness of hearing; in autophony, the patient's own voice seems to ring or roar in his head.

Treatment of this condition has been largely unsatisfactory in the past. It has consisted of various methods of inciting inflammation and scarring of the tubal mucosa. For this purpose, various cauterizing agents have been described, such as silver nitrate, trichloroacetic acid, salicyclic acid, and electrocautery.

Today an experimental method being employed for laryngeal disease holds promise. This is the submucosal injection of Teflon paste to secure lasting functional closure of the mouth of the tube.

REFERENCES

Armstrong, B. W.: New Treatment for Chronic Secretory Otitis Media. Arch. Otol., *59*: 653, 1954.

Armstrong, H. G., and Heim, J. W.: Effect of Flight on Middle Ear. J.A.M.A., *109*:417, 1937.

Bortnick, E., et al.: On the Egress of Fluid from the Middle Ear. Arch. Otol., *80*:297, 1964.

Davidson, R. A.: Ventilation of the Normal and Blocked Middle Ear. Ann. Otol., *74*: 162, 1964.

Ersner, M. S., and Alexander, M. H.: Chapter 10, *In* Schenck, H. P. (Ed.). *Otolaryngology.* Vol. I. Hagerstown, Prior, 1966.

Goodhill, V.: Hard of Hearing Child. Trans. Am. Otol. Soc., *61*:711, 1957.

Gottschalk, G. H.: Serous Otitis. Laryngoscope, *72*:1379, 1962.

Hartmann, A.: *Experimentalle Studien über die Function der Eustachischen Robre.* Leipsig, Veit. U. Comp., 1879.

House, W. F.: Function of Eustachian Tube. Arch. Otol., *71*:405, 1960.

McGovern, J. P., et al.: Allergy and Secretory Otitis Media. J.A.M.A., *200*:124, 1967.

Miller, G. F., Jr.: Eustachian Tube Function in Normal and Diseased Ears. Arch. Otol., *81*:41, 1965.

Perlman, H. B.: Chapter 3, *In* Schenck, H. P. (Ed.): *Otolaryngology*. Vol. I. Hagerstown, Prior, 1960.

Proud, G. O., *et al.*: Clearance Function of Eustachian Tube. Ann. Otol., *72*:563, 1963.

Sade, J.: Serous Otitis Media. Arch. Otol., *84*: 297, 1966.

Senturia, B. J., *et al.*: Middle Ear Effusions. Trans. Am. Otol. Soc., *64*:60, 1960.

Silverstein, H., *et al.*: Eustachian Tube Dysfunction. Laryngoscope, *76*:259, 1966.

Zalin, H.: Respiratory Catarrh in Children. Proc. R. Soc. Med., *52*:704, 1959.

Zollner, F.: Widerstandsmessungen an der Ohrtrompete zur Präfung ihrer Wegsamkeit. Arch. Ohren. Nasen. Kehlikopfheilkd., *140*: 137, 1935.

Chapter 48
Acute Inflammatory Diseases of the Middle Ear

Inflammatory disease of the middle ear has been greatly modified by the widespread use of antibiotics, so many forms of the disease as described in classic texts are no longer observed. The serious complications so dreaded in earlier years are also seldom seen. The most common forms of acute middle ear infection are:

1. Acute viral otitis media
2. Acute bacterial (suppurative) otitis media
3. Acute necrotizing otitis media

VIRAL OTITIS MEDIA

Viral otitis media accompanies the common cold and may best be described as an extension of the mucosal changes of the respiratory passages into the middle ear. The mucosa becomes thick and hyperemic, and a thin mucoid discharge is produced.

Symptoms usually consist of a sensation of "blockage" of the ears accompanying a cold. Pain, if present, is only slight.

Examination of the tympanic membrane reveals a slight thickening of the drum without marked hyperemia. There may be slight injection of the vessels along the malleus handle and posterior annulus.

The hearing may be slightly depressed for all frequencies but usually not more than 10 to 15 dB.

The treatment of viral otitis is directed toward the factors causing extension from the nasopharynx to the ear—namely, lessening the inflammatory edema obstructing the eustachian tube and maintaining ventilation of the middle ear. This is accomplished through use of mild shrinking nose drops and oral decongestants. The patient should also be instructed to maintain proper aeration of the middle ear by inflating with the Valsalva maneuver as frequently as necessary to avoid a blocked sensation. Antibiotics may be necessary to prevent secondary bacterial infection, although this can usually be avoided if treatment is instituted early. Because of this possibility, however, the patient should be carefully observed.

Frequent attacks of viral otitis media indicate the need for attention to the nose and throat to avoid this complication. This is particularly true in children in whom the presence of obstructive masses of adenoid tissue may indicate the need for adenoidectomy. Mild chronic sinusitis is also an occasional cause of increased susceptibility to upper respiratory infections.

Bullous myringitis is an unusual form of viral inflammation of the ear accompanying colds and influenza. This disease is initiated by the symptoms of blockage and fullness. Shortly after onset, severe ear pain occurs, which is particularly pronounced on movement of the eardrum or canal.

Examination will reveal formation of herpetic-like blebs on the lateral surface of the eardrum. The drum usually has a purplish hue.

Treatment is conservative and directed toward relieving pain. Puncture of the blebs may be of help, and the use of analgesic eardrops is indicated. The disease is self-limited, lasting from a few days to 2 weeks. Observation should be carried out during this time to watch for bacterial complications.

ACUTE BACTERIAL OTITIS MEDIA

Acute otitis media of bacterial origin is a common condition, especially in childhood. It may accompany the exanthems of children, particularly measles and scarlet fever, but is most often associated with infections of the nose and throat. It is a major public health problem, being most prevalent in infants and affecting those of lower socioeconomic status most severely.

The disease is most prevalent in the preschool years, peaking at age 2. This incidence falls rapidly after age 7. Race, nutrition, and economic conditions all influence the incidence of this disorder. At least 30% of Eskimo children are affected, and it is the leading reportable disease in the American Indian (8099 per 100,000 in 1967). In a study of poor, white Appalachians, 20% were found to be affected by acute otitis media by age 2. The incidence has also been found to vary directly with the amount paid for rent and with the gross national product on an international basis. The peak incidence occurs between December and March and is least during the summer.

Pathogenesis

Except in the relatively unusual case of traumatic introduction of bacteria into the middle ear through a ruptured tympanic membrane, most cases of otitis media arise from the nasopharynx and affect the middle ear secondarily. The stage for this complication is set by hyperemia and edema of the mucosa of the pharyngeal portion of the eustachian tube whose lumen is further encroached upon by lymphoid hyperplasia in the submucosa.

This impairment of middle ear ventilation is accompanied by exudative and transudative fluid collection in the middle ear. This results in extreme vulnerability of the middle ear to bacterial assault by direct extension from the infected tissues of the nasopharynx. The factors of host-resistance and bacterial virulence will then determine the progress of the disease from this point.

Bacteriology

Former texts indicate that beta-hemolytic streptococci were the causative agents in as many as 90% of the cases. Other common organisms were *Streptococcus viridans, Pneumococcus,* and *Staphylococcus.* In the past few years, widespread use of antibiotics has changed this picture radically. Hemolytic streptococci are now found in less than half the cases, and the presence of *Staphylococcus aureus* has increased markedly. Also assuming relatively more importance are the lower grade pathogens, *Streptococcus viridans* and *Staphylococcus albus.* In children under age 5, *Pneumococcus* and *Hemophilus influenzae* predominate as the infecting organisms.

An increasing problem is the increasing incidence of *Pseudomonas* and pyocyaneous infections, particularly in those individuals who have received prolonged antibiotic therapy. This is undoubtedly the result of overgrowth after the gram-positive organisms have been eliminated by the therapy. These infections can be most difficult to treat.

Stages

The course of otitis media follows a pattern in most cases, consisting of the following stages: (1) inflammation; (2) suppuration; (3) complication; (4) resolution.

Stage of Inflammation. The initial stages of acute otitis media are characterized by hyperemia and edema of the mucoperiosteum of the middle ear and mastoid. The eardrum is injected along the malleus handle and annulus. This is followed by exudation of serofibrinous fluid into the middle ear. The quantity of fluid increases until the middle ear cleft is filled and pressure is exerted against the drum.

Symptoms. A feeling of blockage is noted initially which increases to a deep-seated earache. This is accompanied by toxicity and fever. Hearing is only mildly affected at first, but more severe hearing loss develops as the ear fills with fluid.

Otoscopy. Examination of the drum at this stage reveals a dusky, bluish drum with injection along the handle of the malleus and annulus. As the course progresses, the drum becomes thick and angry red, with outward bulging of the pars tensa and loss of landmarks (Figs. 48–1 and 48–2). These later findings indicate that spontaneous perforation is imminent.

Treatment. In the early stages, prompt and adequate antibiotic administration is indicated (see discussion of bacterial infections of the respiratory tract, Chapters 8 and 9).

Because of the side effects of hypersensitivity, penicillin and sulfonamides are used more cautiously than formerly, although these drugs are effective in more than 90% of infections. Wide-spectrum agents, such as the tetracyclines, may be employed with less risk of complication. Chloramphenicol, streptomycin, and kanamycin should be used only in life-endangering situations because of the serious side effects of agranulocytosis in the case of chloramphenicol and the severe ototoxicity of the others. In children, ampicillin is the drug of choice because of the sensitivity of *Hemophilus influenzae* to this agent.

In addition to antibiotic treatment, decongestive therapy, using both oral and nasal agents, should be administered. This is necessary to relieve tubal obstruction and secure drainage through the eustachian tube. Inflation of the middle ear by means of the Valsalva maneuver promotes resolution by replacing the fluid content with air.

The patient should be advised to go to bed. Analgesics and local heat aid in obtaining necessary rest.

Myringotomy. If exudate accumulates under pressure, as indicated by a bulging tympanic membrane, myringotomy is indicated. This provides controlled drainage through an incision which heals with minimal scarring. Using a long narrow knife edge, a circumferential incision is made in the inferior portion of the drum below the malleus handle. Care must be taken to en-

sure against sudden head movement as the drum is incised, and general anesthesia is often necessary in young children. The point of the knife should just enter the middle ear and not touch the underlying mucosa which is sensitive. The incision should be long enough to accomplish good drainage, and the middle ear may be aspirated by gentle suction (see Fig. 47–7).

Cotton should be worn in the external canal and changed three or four times daily to absorb the drainage which will ensue.

Stage of Suppuration. If the disease progresses and myringotomy is not performed, the bulging drum will spontaneously rupture, usually in the anterior-inferior quadrant, but occasionally in the posterior half of the drum. The discharge is at first serosanguineous but soon becomes mucopurulent. The mucosa becomes markedly thickened and red, with the appearance of many new capillaries. This process is present throughout the entire middle ear and mastoid to the point of obliterating the smaller mastoid cells. The mucosal thickening may completely block the aditus ad antrum, preventing adequate drainage of the mastoid.

Symptoms. The onset of aural discharge relieves the pressure on the eardrum causing relief of the severe earache. The toxicity and fever also begin to lessen. The mucosal changes now produce more marked hearing loss. Tenderness and pain behind the ear may be felt if mucopus is trapped in the mastoid, warning of further difficulty.

Otoscopy. Otoscopy reveals a mucopurulent, often pulsating, discharge coming through a perforation of the pars tensa of the drum. The mucosa, if seen, is thick, red and velvety. A small perforation may have a protrusion of edematous mucosa with pus exuding from the center, a so-called nipple perforation.

Radiographs taken in the first two stages of acute suppurative otitis media will show "clouding" of the mastoid cell system due to the accumulation of fluid and mucosal edema. No destructive changes should be noted.

Treatment. At the onset of discharge, culture and sensitivity tests may be done to determine the most suitable antibiotic. Since these tests take a minimum of 24 to 48

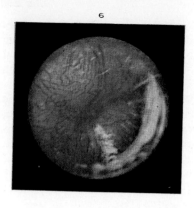

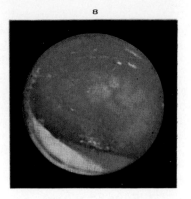

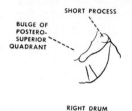

BULGE OF
POSTERO-
SUPERIOR
QUADRANT

SHORT PROCESS

RIGHT DRUM

FIG. 48–1

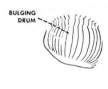

BULGING
DRUM

LEFT DRUM

FIG. 48–2

FIG. 48–1.   Early stage of acute otitis media. The tympanic membrane is moderately reddened; and there is definite bulging of the posterosuperior quadrant. The short process of the malleus can still be seen.

FIG. 48–2.   Severe acute otitis media is evident, with pronounced bulging and redness of the entire pars tensa. No landmarks can be identified. Myringotomy is urgently required to prevent complication and rupture of the tympanic membrane.

(Courtesy of Dr. Richard A. Buckingham. Abbott Laboratories, *What's New,* 196, 1956.)

hours, treatment is started promptly with a broad-spectrum antibiotic which can be changed if found to be an unsuitable agent.

With the advent of the discharge, topical antibiotics are suitable for use both to treat the mucosa of the middle ear and to guard the skin of the external canal against secondary external otitis.

The general measures of bedrest, decongestion, and inflation should be followed as previously outlined.

Stage of Complication. The major complication of mastoiditis, with its secondary extension to the venous sinuses, meninges, or labyrinth, is due to the prevention of adequate drainage through the aditus ad antrum because of mucosal thickening in the attic. As this occurs, the mastoid fills with edematous granular mucosa and mucopus under pressure. This process then causes adsorption of the thin osseous cell walls and, as it progresses to the periphery, extends along venous channels and dehiscences to the periosteum of the mastoid. The process in its earlier stages is reversible but later creates the need for surgical intervention to achieve adequate drainage and resolution before extension to the meninges or lateral sinus occurs.

Symptoms. After an initial period of relief from discomfort with the onset of aural discharge, milder symptoms recur. Low-grade fever and toxicity accompanied by pain over the mastoid region occur. This may occur in spite of a lessening of the amount of drainage, giving rise to the lay belief that the ear is now "draining inward," which is a grave danger signal. In this case the belief is well-founded.

If untreated, or with virulent infection, the disease may progress beyond the bounds of the mastoid, extending to the lateral sinus, the labyrinth, and the meninges or brain. These complications will be discussed in a later chapter (see Complications of Ear Disease, Ch. 51).

Findings. Tenderness and thickening of the periosteum over the mastoid cortex are present, progressing to the development of a fluctuant mass with the occurrence of subperiosteal abscess.

Otoscopy may reveal sagging of the posterosuperior canal wall. The eardrum will

not appear significantly different than before, and radiographs now show clouding of the mastoid cells and definite rarefaction and loss of distinctness of the mastoid cell walls.

Treatment. If previously untreated, it is possible to achieve resolution at this stage, in some cases, with the institution of antibiotic therapy. If this course is followed, however, the patient should be hospitalized and followed closely, since this is a late stage and surgical intervention may be urgently required.

Surgical evacuation of the mastoid to achieve drainage of abscessed areas is usually indicated at this stage of the disease. Simple mastoidectomy is performed and will be described in a later chapter (see Surgery in Chronic Ear Disease, Ch. 50). Fortunately, it is unusual for the disease to progress to this stage with early diagnosis and treatment, but in some regions and in neglected cases this procedure is still frequently necessary.

In determining the indication for surgical intervention, radiographs are useful. Care should be taken to differentiate simple clouding of the mastoid, which occurs with mucosal thickening, and fluid accumulation from the actual breakdown of cell septa and abscess formation. A febrile course and lack of response to treatment indicate the need for immediate surgical intervention.

Stage of Resolution. During this stage of acute inflammatory disease, the infection subsides and healing of the ear takes place. The discharge rapidly subsides. The mucosal thickening and edema resolve more slowly, but as return to normal occurs, hearing improves gradually to normal levels.

The small central perforation heals rapidly, usually leaving no residual scar, but sometimes causing a small atrophic scar. This is a weak point in the drum which will quickly break down if subsequent infection takes place, causing more rapid onset of discharge but accompanied by little otalgia.

Small collections of sterile fluid may persist for years in coalescent areas in the mastoid without causing symptoms. This is sometimes seen as isolated radiolucent areas on radiographic examination.

Treatment. Other than supportive measures and frequent observation to make certain of uneventful recovery, little is necessary at this stage. Failure of resolution within a 10- to 14-day period indicates the probability of persistent infection of the nose and throat.

Treatment should be directed toward prevention of future recurrence of acute otitis media. To this end, an effort should be made to acquaint the patient—child or adult—with the importance of maintaining middle ear aeration. Instruction in the Valsalva method of inflation should be given and the patient told to inflate his ear whenever it feels blocked or obstructed. This is particularly necessary with the occurrence of upper respiratory infections.

The nose and nasopharynx should be carefully evaluated for causative factors which should be eliminated to prevent future recurrence of otitis media. This includes radiographic survey of the paranasal sinuses and examination of the nasopharynx to evaluate the adenoid. Adenoidectomy should be performed if the presence of large or infected adenoid tissue is found.

In addition to these measures, the patient should be advised to seek medical help at the earliest sign of infection, since early institution of treatment will usually prevent a severe infection (see Treatment of Respiratory Infection, Chapters 8 and 9).

ACUTE NECROTIZING OTITIS MEDIA

This form of otitis media is characterized by a fulminating course accompanied by large areas of destruction of the tissues of the middle ear, drum, and ossicles. This form of otitis occurs in children and is a complication of measles, influenza, and, in former years, most commonly scarlet fever.

Fortunately in recent years, with increasingly prompt attention to the treatment of these diseases, this form of otitis media is becoming more unusual. Familiarity with its course is still necessary, for treatment must be efficient to prevent severe aftereffects.

Pathology. The essential pathology is a rapidly progressive, necrotizing infection of the mucosa of the middle ear and mastoid, usually due to beta-hemolytic streptococci. Rapid progress produces an early dissolution of the pars tensa of the drum. Necrosis of the mucoperiosteum often causes necrosis of portions of the ossicular chain, most often the long process of the incus. Thrombotic involvement may produce areas of sequestration in the mastoid. The tegmen and sinus plate as well as the septa of the mastoid cells may develop osteomyelitis.

The extent of the progress will depend upon the severity of the infection and the resistance of the host. Milder cases may be limited to destruction of the drum, while more severe infections will include all of the areas mentioned above.

Symptoms. This form of otitis media is similar in its symptoms to other types of otitis but is more severe and rapid.

Since early spontaneous rupture of the drum occurs, the first symptom may be the onset of a foul, thin, purulent discharge.

Findings. The most typical finding is a large central perforation of the drum which may continue to enlarge and become a nearly total loss of the tympanic membrane as the disease progresses. Bare bone may be seen through the perforation as the mucosa is lost, and friable granulation is commonly present. The aural discharge is thin, purulent, and foul.

Treatment. Antibiotic therapy should be instituted upon diagnosis and should be carried out with large parenteral doses to achieve a prompt high blood level.

Surgery is not indicated in the acute stage of the illness but may later become necessary to eliminate areas of bony necrosis causing persistence of infection and discharge.

Sequelae. Since destruction is so widespread in this disease, many end results are possible, most of which will require surgical reconstruction to restore function (see Surgery in Chronic Ear Disease, Ch. 50).

The picture seen after healing may vary from a large atrophic scar closing the tympanum with normal hearing to a total perforation and destruction of the ossicular chain with severe hearing loss.

Today, with tympanoplastic techniques, reconstruction is possible in a large percentage of these cases. This is sometimes indicated to relieve chronic infection but usually to restore hearing in these severely damaged ears.

REFERENCES

Glorig, A., and Gerwen, K. S.: *Otitis Media.* Springfield, Ill., Charles C Thomas, Publisher, 1972.

Lederer, F. L.: *Diseases of the Ear, Nose and Throat.* 6th ed. Philadelphia, F. A. Davis Co., 1955.

Mawson, S. R.: *Diseases of the Ear.* London, Arnold, 1963.

Shambaugh, G. E., Jr.: *Surgery of the Ear.* 2nd ed. Philadelphia, W. B. Saunders Co., 1967.

Wilson, T. G.: *Diseases of the Ear, Nose and Throat in Children.* 2nd ed. London, William Heinemann, Ltd., 1962.

Chapter 49
Chronic Ear Disease

Chronic diseases of the middle ear classically have been divided into benign and dangerous forms.

The danger of the bone-invading forms of chronic otitis media is due to the presence of squamous epithelium within the middle ear cleft and is better considered under the proper term *cholesteatoma*.

The benign forms of chronic ear disease are basically two in number: chronic suppurative otitis media and atelectatic ear disease. These benign forms have been seen, over time, to change their character with the development of secondary cholesteatoma, thus indicating the need for prompt surgical treatment in all patients with these problems. In the usual otologic practice, each of these problems — cholesteatoma, chronic suppurative otitis, and atelectatic ear disease — will share an equal incidence.

The onset of chronic ear disease is insidious, the patient usually presenting with fully developed symptomatic disease. Since the developmental stages of these diseases have not been observed or reported in the literature, the etiology and pathogenesis remain totally conjectural.

The morbidity of chronic disease of the middle ear is twofold. The primary disability is due to continuing or recurrent infection of the ear. The second area of disability is the attendant loss of function (hearing) due to damage to the sound conduction mechanism and to cochlear damage from toxicity or direct extension of the infectious process. Both these areas must be evaluated and treated in the patient with chronic ear disease in order to obtain complete resolution of the disease process.

CHRONIC SUPPURATIVE OTITIS MEDIA

Etiology and Pathogenesis. Since patients present with fully developed disease, the developmental period remains enigmatic. A theory as to pathogenesis appears in most modern texts and is commonly accepted as fact. This hypothesis states that a necrotizing otitis media occurs, mostly in childhood, resulting in a large drum perforation. Following the initial acute disease, the drumhead either remains perforate or heals with an atrophic membrane which then may collapse into the middle ear, creating the picture of atelectatic otitis.

This hypothesis ignores several factors which throw strong doubts on its plausibility:

1. Almost all cases of acute otitis media resolve with complete healing of the tympanic membrane. Scarring, rarely present, is usually characterized by thickening rather than atrophy.

2. Necrotizing otitis media is extremely rare since the use of antibiotics became established. This author (DFA) has seen fewer than a dozen instances in the past 15 years. The incidence of chronic ear disease, on the other hand, has not decreased over this period.

825

3. Patients with chronic ear disease do not give a history of such an acute episode of otitis as an initiating factor, but rather of a silent process gradually increasing in disability until help is sought some years after the patient became aware of the problem. Children are not brought to medical care until a hearing disability is found by testing at school or chronic discharge becomes an annoyance at home.

4. Pediatricians, observing children with acute otitis media, often recurrent, have not reported this development of chronic suppurative otitis, even with long-term follow-up.

At this time the pathogenesis of chronic suppurative otitis media remains unknown. It is most likely a primary process of the eustachian tube – middle ear – mastoid cell system. This process must have the characteristics of low-grade, insidious, and persistent activity, resulting in loss of portions of the tympanic membrane and establishment of factors conducive to further chronicity.

The factors responsible for chronicity in suppurative middle ear disease are varied. Among those factors are:

1. Chronic eustachian tube dysfunction due to:
   a. Chronic or recurrent nose and throat infection.
   b. Partial or complete anatomic obstruction of the eustachian tube.
2. Persistent perforation of the tympanic membrane.
3. Involvement of the middle ear with squamous metaplasia or other irreversible pathology.
4. Persistent obstruction to aeration of the middle ear or mastoid spaces. This may be caused by scarring, thickened mucosa, polyps, granulation tissue, or tympanosclerosis.
5. Areas of sequestration or persistent osteomyelitis in the mastoid.
6. Constitutional factors such as allergy, debility, or altered defense mechanisms of the host.

Pathology. Chronic suppurative otitis media is most often a recurrent rather than a constant disease. Chronicity is defined in time and stage rather than a uniform patho-

logic picture. Since the effects of tissue destruction, healing, and scarring are added to the overlying process of persistent or recurrent infection, the pathologic condition encountered is characterized by lack of uniformity. In general, the following patterns may be noted:

1. *The tympanic membrane* is perforated in its central portion. The size may vary from less than 20% of the drum area to the entire drum and portions of the annulus.

Healing efforts may result in ingrowth of squamous epithelium into the middle ear. This ingrowth may extend only through the perforation or may line the entire middle ear space. Occasionally, extension of this media layer into the attic region results in pocketing and secondary acquired cholesteatoma (see Atelectatic Otitis). The formation of an atrophic two-layer membrane lacking in fibrous elements may be seen. This membrane will be rapidly destroyed during active periods of infection.

2. *The mucosa* varies during stages of the disease. In quiescent periods, it will appear normal unless the effects of infection have produced thickening or metaplasia into transitional epithelium. Squamous metaplasia has been described.

During active infection, the mucosa becomes thickened and hyperemic, producing a mucoid or mucopurulent discharge. After treatment, the thickening and mucoid discharge may persist owing to chronic dysfunction of the eustachian tube. Allergic factors may also be responsible for this persistence of mucosal change. In some cases, this is a physical irritation due to exposure of the mucosa to the outside environment.

Mucosal thickening may completely seal the attic and mastoid spaces, resulting in filling of these spaces with mucus. With time, cholesterin crystals are deposited in these mucous pockets, resulting in cholesterol granuloma. This process is irritative, producing granulation of the mucous membrane and giant cell infiltration of the mucus-cholesterin fluid. This process may also be seen in the middle ear in chronic secretory otitis media.

During healing, the mucosa may exhibit the changes of tympanosclerosis. These consist of the formation of amorphous hyaline plaques in the submucosa, varying in size from thin layers to dense masses. In early stages, the mucosa assumes a thick, rubbery appearance. As healing progresses, the plaques become yellowish with a puttylike consistency. In time, calcium salts may be deposited, creating bony hard masses. The sites of predilection for this process are in the annular region of the tympanic membrane, particularly anterosuperiorly, and surrounding the ossicles. The process may result in fusion or complete fixation of the ossicular system, resulting in severe hearing loss.

The mucosa may also show the formation of granulation tissue and/or polyps. This process is associated with long-standing persistent discharge or active infection. Polyp formation is commonly associated with the presence of squamous epithelium in the middle ear. These masses may protrude through a small perforation, partially obstructing drainage and causing persistence of disease.

3. *The ossicles* may or may not be damaged, depending upon the severity of antecedent infections. Commonly, the long process of the incus has undergone necrosis due to thrombotic disease of the mucosal vessels supplying the incus. Necrosis less commonly involves the malleus and stapes unless secondary squamous ingrowth has occurred, in which case the arch of the stapes and the handle of the malleus may be destroyed. This process is not due to osteomyelitis but is said to be due to the formation of osteolytic enzymes or collagenase in the subepithelial connective tissue.

4. *Mastoid.* Chronic suppurative otitis media most often has its onset in childhood. Since *mastoid* pneumatization is most active between the ages of 5 and 10, this process of pneumatization is often halted or reversed by otitis media occurring at this age or earlier. As the chronic infection continues, the mastoid undergoes a process of sclerosis, resulting in a reduction of the size of the mastoid process. The antrum becomes smaller, and pneumatization is limited to a few air cell tracts in the immediate vicinity of the antrum.

This concept is contrasted with the fact that the degree of pneumatization of the mastoid varies between individuals. Those individuals with limited pneumatization (either from genetic cause or neonatal infection) are felt by some to have an increased susceptibility to chronic ear disease. Radiographs show these changes in the cellularity of the mastoid so commonly that a radiologic diagnosis of chronic mastoiditis is synonymous with the actual finding of a dense, small, sclerotic mastoid.

Severe forms of acute otitis media may also cause areas of osteitis or osteomyelitis of the walls or septa of the mastoid. This results, in time, in a continuous, foul, purulent discharge or sequestration of bone.

ATELECTATIC OTITIS MEDIA

Many terms are presently applied to this common chronic disease pattern of the middle ear. "Adhesive otitis media," "middle ear cholesteatoma," and "marginal or posterior-superior perforation" are used interchangeably in describing the process described here as "atelectatic otitis." Since "secondary acquired cholesteatoma" is a complication of this disease process, it will be discussed in this section rather than the section on cholesteatoma.

Etiology and Pathogenesis. In contrast to chronic suppurative otitis media, this type of chronic ear disorder develops over time. The typical patient has initially suffered from chronic secretory otitis, particularly in childhood but often extending into adulthood. Although many suffer from an unrelenting "blue drum" or "glue ear," recurrent acute secretory otitis may result in the same sequelae. Duration of the tubal ventilatory defect of the middle ear probably is a determining factor in these patients.

Over time, atrophy of the drumhead occurs, usually in the posterior-superior quadrant but also involving other portions, even including the entire tympanic membrane. Accompanying this atrophy is a collapse of the atrophic membrane into the middle ear —thus the term "atelectatic otitis." The degree of collapse is entirely dependent upon the extent of atrophy of the tympanic membrane. Loss of elasticity of the drumhead prevents normal ventilation of the middle ear and thus creates chronicity entirely subsequent to the nature of the pathology, even if the eustachian tube problem has cleared.

Progression of the retraction causes the atrophic membrane to drape over the incus and stapes, often resulting in necrosis of these structures. The aeration pathway to the attic is blocked, which, with time, results in the membrane retracting into these areas, causing secondary acquired cholesteatoma. This will have the same characteristics of all cholesteatoma: enlargement with keratin retention, bone destruction, and the onset of infection.

The above disease process seems clearcut, yet the pathogenesis of the tympanic membrane atrophy is still unknown. Perforation with healing by a two-layered membrane is often cited, but the atrophy has been seen to occur without perforation. It is most likely the result of activation of collagenase by the underlying disease, which causes breakdown of the fibrous layer of the tympanic membrane, leaving only the squamous and mucosal layers intact.

Pathology. The major pathologic features of "atelectatic otitis" have been described in the above section. The remaining pathologic feature is that of cholesterin granuloma. This process is the result of chronic blockage of the middle ear, attic, or mastoid ventilation pathways. These spaces fill with abnormal mucus ("glue"), and cholesterin crystals are deposited. The mucosa forms granulations, and breakdown of bony septa can occur. Apart from this sequela, infection of the middle ear is uncommon, occurring most often when contaminants are introduced through the canal, such as after swimming or showering. Extension of infection up the eustachian tube causes breakdown of the atrophic membrane and will convert the pathologic pattern to that described with chronic suppurative otitis media.

CHOLESTEATOMA

Cholesteatoma may be defined generally as the presence within the middle ear cleft of a squamous epithelial pocket or sac filled with keratin debris. Three types are recognized:

1. *Congenital cholesteatoma.* This is an epithelial cyst occurring within one of the

bones of the skull (usually the temporal bone) without contact with the external ear. It may occur deep in the temporal bone or in the squama. Increasing numbers are described occurring in the mastoid or attic space.

2. *Primary acquired cholesteatoma.* This type of cholesteatoma develops in continuity with a perforation of the pars flaccida of the tympanic membrane. It first fills Prussak's space and then may enlarge to occupy the attic, mastoid antrum, and portions of the middle ear.

3. *Secondary acquired cholesteatoma.* This type of cholesteatoma has been described under Atelectatic Otitis Media.

Etiology. The cause of primary acquired cholesteatoma has been the subject of debate since the latter half of the nineteenth century. There have been many theories proposed, but none as yet has been shown to be entirely causative in this disease. Among the postulates are:

1. Negative pressure in the attic, causing invagination of the pars flaccida and cyst

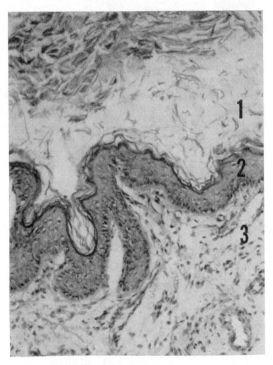

FIG. 49–1. Microscopic structure of cholesteatoma: *1,* keratin debris; *2,* epidermis (matrix); *3,* subepithelium.

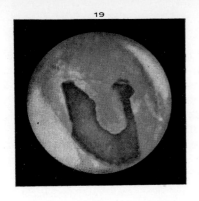

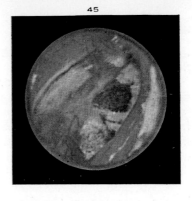

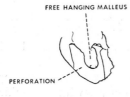

FREE HANGING MALLEUS

PERFORATION

LEFT DRUM

FIG. 49–2

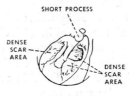

SHORT PROCESS

DENSE
SCAR
AREA

DENSE
SCAR
AREA

RIGHT DRUM

FIG. 49–3

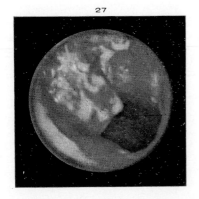

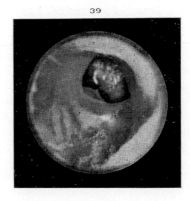

POLYP

CHOLESTEATOMA
BEHIND EAR DRUM

LEFT DRUM

FIG. 49–4.

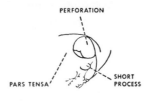

PERFORATION

PARS TENSA

SHORT
PROCESS

RIGHT DRUM

FIG. 49–5

FIG. 49–2.   Chronic otitis media.   Massive central perforation.   Recurrent discharge has been present for 30 years

FIG. 49–3.   Chronic otitis media.   Healing of previous infections has resulted in dense tympanosclerotic plaque of the submucosa of the tympanic membrane. Fixation of the ossicular chain by tympanosclerosis caused a 40-dB conductive hearing loss.

FIG. 49–4.   Cholesteatoma.   Polypoid granulation is forming at the mouth of an attic perforation. The posterior-superior tympanic membrane appears pearly white owing to downward growth of the cholesteatoma into this region of the middle ear.

FIG. 49–5.   Cholesteatoma. Large perforation of the pars flaccida leads into a cholesteatoma sac filled with hard black debris.

(Courtesy of Dr. Richard A. Buckingham. Abbott Laboratories, *What's New*, 196, 1956.)

formation (Habermann, Bezold, Tumarkin, Shambaugh, Jordan).

2. Metaplasia of middle ear and attic mucosa due to infection (Tumarkin).

3. Invasive hyperplasia followed by cyst formation of the basal layers of the epidermis of the pars flaccida due to the irritation of infection (Habermann, Nager, Hauze, Ruedi).

4. Congenital epidermal rests occurring in the attic region (McKenzie, Diamant, Teed, Cawthorn).

5. Invasive hyperkeratosis of the deep external meatal skin (McGuckin).

An important factor is the rapid proliferative ability of the drum epithelium, particularly in the pars flaccida and superior portion of the pars tensa.

Pathogenesis. Once a pocket or cyst of squamous epithelium has formed within the middle ear cleft, the progress of cholesteatoma is well-documented. Layers of desquamated epithelium interspersed with cholesterin crystals form and fill the sac. The surrounding epithelial matrix expands into the available spaces of attic, middle ear, and mastoid. Accompanying this process of expansion is bony destruction of the attic walls, the ossicles, and mastoid septa to accommodate the increasing size of the cholesteatoma.

It was formerly thought that pressure caused the bone destruction occurring with the expanding cholesteatoma. It has recently been shown that the bone erosion is caused by the secretion of osteolytic enzymes or collagenase by the subepithelial connective tissue.

The osteolytic process is accompanied by osteogenesis within the mastoid as sclerosis takes place, thus limiting free space available for expansion of the cholesteatoma. The process of sclerosis is accelerated by the superimposition of infection. Cholesteatoma which develops free of infection may allow normal pneumatization, creating the extremely difficult problem of a widely pneumatized mastoid filled with cholesteatoma. This is particularly true of congenital cholesteatoma.

Infection of the cholesteatoma not only causes rapid sclerosis of the mastoid but also increases the osteolytic process. This creates the danger of extension through the lateral semicircular canal, facial canal, attic and mastoid tegmen, and lateral sinus plate and rapid dissolution of the ossicular system. This creates the need for prompt diagnosis and surgical intervention in these cases.

If the disease is allowed to run its course, any of the above-mentioned complications may ensue (see Complications of Ear Disease, Ch. 51), or complete destruction of the mastoid, middle ear, and posterior canal wall, resulting in "nature's radical mastoidectomy," may occur. Other cases reach a stage of apparent equilibrium, remaining quiescent unless further stimulated by infection.

Diagnosis. Without question, otoscopic examination, particularly with magnification, is the most important facet of accurate diagnosis in chronic ear disease. By this means, appraisal of the extent of damage to the drum, ossicular system, and osseous walls of the middle ear may be made.

Complete examination should include critical scrutiny of the following areas:

1. The canal and drum must be carefully cleaned of wax and debris which may prevent a complete view of the drum.

2. The pars tensa is observed in all quadrants, and the size and location of any perforation are noted.

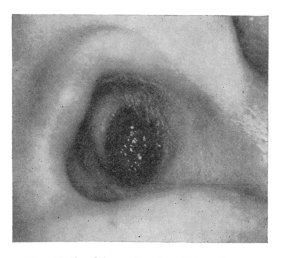

FIG. 49–6. Mucosal polyp filling the external ear canal in case of cholesteatoma. Surgical removal is necessary to secure drainage of middle ear and mastoid.

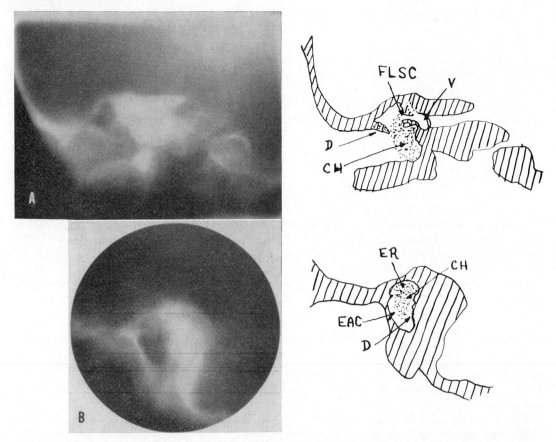

FIG. 49–7. Tomograms of middle ear in cholesteatoma. *A,* Front view indicates destruction of lateral attic wall (D) by cholesteatoma (CH). There is also erosion of the lateral semicircular canal causing a fistula (FLSC). *B,* Lateral view shows erosion of the attic (ER) with loss of ossicles. Destruction of the posterior annulus is indicated at D. EAC, External auditory canal; V, vestibule.

3. The presence of retraction or perforation of the pars flaccida is looked for.

4. The presence of squamous epithelium in the middle ear should be noted. The presence of debris behind the eardrum is a clue to this pathologic condition.

5. The condition of the mucosa seen through the perforation is noted. Any secretion present in the middle ear is removed by suction to allow complete visualization.

6. The nature of any secretion is noted.

7. The bony canal walls should be observed for evidence of destruction. Widening of the notch of Rivinus is a significant early finding of cholesteatoma.

8. The presence and location of granulation or polyps should be noted.

9. Finally, the area of the mouth of the eustachian tube should be inspected and evidence of patency noted. At this time, it is very useful to have the patient inflate the ear by the Valsalva maneuver while the ear is being inspected.

Audiometric Evaluation. Audiometric evaluation is necessary to determine the status of conductive and cochlear function. By the use of air and bone pure tone audiometry and speech discrimination scores, the amount of ossicular damage present may be estimated, and the hearing benefit to be gained by reconstructive middle ear surgery can be judged.

To aid in this evaluation, the following observations will be of help.

1. A simple perforation usually causes no more than a 15- to 20-dB conductive hearing loss.

2. Damage to the ossicular chain causes a 30- to 50-dB conductive hearing loss if a perforation is present.

3. Discontinuity of the hearing chain behind an intact drum causes a flat 55- to 65-dB conductive hearing loss.

4. Marked impairment of speech discrimination, regardless of the bone conduction, indicates severe cochlear damage.

Radiology. Radiographic examination of the mastoid in chronic ear disease is of limited diagnostic value compared to the benefits of otoscopy and audiometry. Carefully controlled radiographic examination may be of great value in diagnosing congenital cholesteatoma, osteitis, or osteomyelitis. The status of the ossicular system may also be demonstrated through careful technique. The views now generally used are:

1. *The Schuller view,* which shows the extent of pneumatization of the mastoid from laterally and above. This becomes of value in surgery by defining the position of the lateral sinus and tegmen. This is particularly helpful in a sclerotic mastoid to forewarn the surgeon and thus prevent entry into the dura or lateral sinus.

2. *The Mayer's or Owen's view* is taken from above and anterior to the middle ear. This throws the ossicles and attic into view and allows one to determine whether bone destruction has involved these structures.

3. *The Stenver's view* shows the length of the petrous pyramid and is more useful in showing the internal auditory canal, vestibule, and semicircular canals. It also throws the antrum in cross section and may give evidence of enlargement from cholesteatoma.

4. *The third projection of Chausse* gives a longitudinal view of the attic and shows early evidence of destruction of the lateral attic wall. In summary, to be differentiated are the following conditions:

Chronic Suppurative Otitis Media. This diagnosis is made in a patient with a history of repeated attacks of aural discharge and the finding of a central perforation without evidence of squamous epithelial ingrowth or bone necrosis. Granulation tissue or mucosal edema may be present, and the discharge is usually mucoid or mucopurulent. Hearing loss is usually present in varying degrees of severity.

Atelectatic Otitis. This diagnosis is made when otoscopy reveals atrophy of the tympanic membrane accompanied by collapse into part or all of the middle ear space. The usual history is one of insidious onset of progressive hearing loss, although today many patients mention that one or more myringotomies and/or ventilating tube insertions have been performed in the past. Infection is not a prominent feature of the history and, when present, creates difficulty in differentiation from chronic suppurative otitis.

Secondary acquired cholesteatoma. This is added to the above picture when retraction of the atrophic membrane has resulted in pocketing with retention of keratin debris and further bone destruction. The presence of granulation at the posterior-superior margin immediately lateral to the annulus is a common finding. Infection with continuous discharge is more common when the disease has reached this stage.

Congenital Cholesteatoma. This diagnosis is usually made in young individuals who have had careful medical observation. They have a history of slowly progressive hearing loss without antecedent infection. Examination shows the presence of a whitish bulge of the eardrum, usually in the posterosuperior quadrant. Until perforation of the drum takes place, hearing loss does not progress beyond 20 to 30 dB.

Primary Acquired Cholesteatoma. Infection in these cases often starts later in life, many times not until the second or third decade. Once aural discharge starts, it is persistent and usually constant. Examination reveals a perforation of the pars flaccida with destruction of the lateral attic wall. This area is often covered with a crust which must be removed to see the perforation. In advanced cases, there will be a perforation of the posterosuperior region of the pars tensa. Hearing loss is variable, depending upon the amount of ossicular destruction and whether the cholesteatoma sac is in a position to transmit sound.

Treatment. Effective treatment in chronic ear disease must be based on definition of the causative factors involved and upon the stage in which the disease is found. Thus the factors creating chronicity, the anatomic changes preventing good healing and proper function, and the infectious process involving the ear at the time of instituting treatment must all be evaluated. When cholesteatoma is diagnosed, surgery is absolutely indicated, but the following regimen may be used to control infection if it is present preoperatively.

Eustachian Tube. The most important function to be considered is aeration and drainage of the middle ear via the eustachian tube. The causes of interference with tubal physiology must be assessed and eliminated. Chronic infection or allergy affecting the nose and pharynx should be diagnosed and treated. Residual adenoids creating mechanical obstruction should be removed. Sinus radiographs are indicated to find hidden areas of low-grade infection.

The adequacy of the eustachian tube lumen is assessed by determining the ability of the tube to pass air (see Physiology of the Eustachian Tube, Ch. 47). This may be done by having the patient inflate the ear by the Valsalva method, by Politzerization, or by special manometric study of the tube. Obstruction of the tympanic end of the eustachian tube can often be determined by careful otoscopic inspection of this area while the patient is attempting to inflate the ear.

As a first step in treatment, the patient should be instructed in the Valsalva method of inflation and told to practice this many times each day.

Anatomic changes preventing proper aeration must be treated surgically if the portion of the eustachian tube involved is accessible.

Anatomic Factors. Permanent changes from normal anatomy commonly influence the response to medical treatment and cause chronicity of infection. Even as common a finding as a central perforation of the eardrum may be solely responsible for recurrent discharge from that ear. These alterations must be corrected surgically. Other types of purely surgical pathology are cholesteatoma, large polyps, masses of tympanosclerosis, and areas of bone necrosis from osteitis or osteomyelitis.

Alteration of hearing function by damage to the sound conduction system must be corrected surgically to obtain satisfactory restoration of hearing.

General Factors of Host Resistance. In dealing with chronic infection of any part of the body, special efforts should be made to investigate local and systemic factors affecting host resistance. Included in this group are dietary insufficiency, diabetes, debility, agammaglobulinemia, allergic disorder, adrenal cortical insufficiency, chronic leukemia, liver or kidney disease, etc. The presence of these conditions can be suspected by the general appearance of the patient plus a failure of response to treatment. Laboratory work-up should then reveal abnormalities leading to the proper diagnosis.

Treatment of Infectious Process. In chronic ear infection, saprophytic as well as pathogenic organisms may be involved. Not only will the bacterial flora vary from time to time, but also the effects of prior or present antibiotic treatment are extremely potent in effecting a change of organism. Prolonged antibiotic administration causes the emergence of resistant strains and will also cause the overgrowth of organisms such as *Pseudomonas* or *Pyocyaneous*. For this reason, culture and sensitivity tests assume an important role in planning therapy.

The presence of discharge implies a perforation of the eardrum, and for this reason, topical application of antibiotic therapy becomes practical and efficacious. Agents which are unsuitable for systemic administration because of toxicity are often applicable by this route. The most frequently used method of administration is by ear drops or insufflation of powder.

To be effective, a solution for use in the ear should be suspended in a hygroscopic vehicle. Propylene glycol is the best for this use. The antibiotics most frequently employed are polymyxin B sulfate and/or neomycin sulfate. The preparation is more effective when acidified to a pH of 5 to 5.5. Occasionally, corticosteroids may be added to control local allergic manifestations. Recently it has been shown that the addition of heparin is of value to control local histamine response in the tissues.

Powders should be chosen on the basis of bacterial sensitivity and solubility. An effective combination is 250 mg polymyxin B sulfate and 3 g of Chloromycetin. This is placed in a powder blower and insufflated two or three times a day.

The use of boric acid either in solution or as a powder is not indicated, since this forms an insoluble cake which is difficult to clean out of the ear and prevents antimicrobial agents from reaching the mucosa. Alcohol in strengths greater than 70% should be avoided, since it is both irritating and painful.

Before powder or drops are applied to the ear, discharge should be removed from the canal. Absorbent cotton wipes or suction is best for this. Cotton applicators are usually too bulky to be effective and sometimes cause external canal infection due to abrasion.

Systemic antibiotics are indicated in acute infections superimposed on the chronic infection. In this instance, a broad-spectrum antibiotic such as tetracycline is most commonly employed.

Infection of a cholesteatoma is difficult to treat because of the inability to obtain an antibiotic level within the sac where the infection exists. In these instances, removal of obstructing masses of debris or crusts from the mouth of the sac to obtain drainage is of great help. This is best done with gentle suction. Water in the ear must be avoided, since this causes the cholesteatoma to swell and may result in acute complication.

Granulations on the mucosa may be treated by applying mild (5 to 10%) solutions of silver nitrate. This can be followed by 2% gentian violet, which is drying and bactericidal. These agents are also useful in treating the external otitis which exists in most cases of chronic otorrhea.

Polyps or large masses of granulations are best removed with a biting forceps or snare and the raw surface touched with 25 to 50% silver nitrate. This may be necessary several times at intervals of 1 or 2 weeks to secure healing of the mucosa.

If the use of a thoughtfully applied regimen of therapy as outlined above does not succeed in controlling the disease, surgical intervention is indicated to control areas of inaccessible or irreversible pathology. These procedures will be outlined in the chapters on the surgery of chronic ear disease.

UNUSUAL FORMS OF CHRONIC EAR DISEASE

Tuberculous Otitis Media. Otitis media due to tuberculosis may arise from two sources: systemically through ingestion of nonpasteurized infected milk, and through direct contact with the bacillus from a patient with existent pulmonary tuberculosis. Both of these causes are becoming quite rare in this country as the incidence of contact is much less than in former times.

Middle ear involvement begins with a painless and insidious onset. The tympanic membrane becomes thickened and infiltrated. This is followed by spontaneous perforation, which either slowly enlarges or becomes multiple. This is associated with a thin, odorless discharge and an indolent, afebrile course.

Commonly there is a severe depression of hearing due to early labyrinthine involvement. This is much out of proportion to the other symptoms and findings and is a good clue to the diagnosis.

Treatment involves the use of modern antituberculous agents. Once the disease has been arrested, tympanoplastic surgery may be utilized to repair permanent damage to the middle ear if useful cochlear function remains.

Pneumococcus Type III Otitis Media (*Streptococcus mucosus*). This is a subacute, indolent form of otitis media which assumes importance because of the frequency of associated intracranial complication. Fortunately, widespread use of early antibiotic therapy has made this a rare entity.

After a short, mild acute phase, a latent period ensues with only mild symptoms of hearing loss. The drum is dull and thickened. The disease then proceeds to intracranial complication by causing bone destruction and direct invasion of the meninges, brain, or lateral sinus.

Treatment with antibiotics in the early

stages usually serves to prevent these complications (see Complications of Ear Disease, Ch. 51).

REFERENCES

Cawthorne, T.: Congenital Cholesteatoma. Arch. Otol., *78*:248, 1963.

Derlacki, E. L., and Clemis, J. D.: Congenital Cholesteatoma. Ann. Otol., *74*:706, 1965.

Diamant, M.: Chronic Middle Ear Discharge. Eye, Ear, Nose and Throat Monthly, *44*, 1965.

Diamant, M.: The "Pathologic Size" of the Mastoid Air Cell System. Acta Otol., *60*:1, 1965.

Hill, F. T.: Comprehensive Care in Chronic Otitis Media. Laryngoscope, *71*:587, 1961.

Jordan, R. E.: Secretory Otitis Media in Etiology of Cholesteatoma. Arch. Otol., *78*:261, 1963.

Juers, A. L.: Cholesteatoma Genesis. Arch. Otol., *81*:5, 1965.

McGuckin, F.: Chronic Otitis Media. Postgrad. Med. J., *36*:256, 1960.

McGuckin, F.: Concerning the Pathogenesis of Destructive Ear Disease. J. Laryngol., *75*:949, 1961.

Portmann, M.: Etiology of Chronic Suppurative Otitis Media. Arch. Otol., *78*:266, 1963.

Ruedi, L.: Acquired Cholesteatoma. Arch. Otol., *78*:252, 1963.

Tumarkin, A.: Attic Suppuration. J. Laryngol., *64*:611, 1950.

Tumarkin, A.: Pre-epidermosis. J. Laryngol., *75*:487, 1961.

Chapter 50
Surgery in Chronic Ear Disease

The recent past has brought great change in both the concepts and the techniques used in the surgery of chronic ear disease. The basic concepts of eradication of irreversible disease and adequate drainage, as pioneered by Schwartze, Stacke, Zaufel, and many others and refined by the father of modern otologic surgery, Julius Lempert, remain as the foundation of this surgical evolution. To this base has been added the present-day methods of reconstruction and surgical conservatism, resulting in the possibility of complete aural rehabilitation for the majority of individuals suffering from chronic ear diseases.

The indications for surgical intervention in chronic ear disease are basically twofold: the control of infection, and the restoration of function. Since hearing improvement is not usually possible unless disease is eliminated from the involved ear, this remains a primary consideration in surgery. The severe handicap of hearing loss, however, makes it mandatory to make every effort in order to improve hearing. With the potential of present-day techniques, this has become an equal consideration in the planning of surgical management.

The techniques most employed today in the management of these cases are:
1. Modified radical mastoidectomy
2. Tympanoplasty with or without mastoidectomy
3. Mastoid obliteration operation (musculoplasty)

Indications for Surgery. As mentioned above, the basic reasons for surgery in this group of diseases are control of infection and restoration of function. There may be defined, however, certain absolute indications for surgical intervention in the disease process. These indications are:

1. The presence of threatened or actual complication (see Complications of Chronic Otitis Media, Ch. 49, 51).
2. The presence of irreversible pathologic condition in the mastoid or middle ear, such as cholesteatoma, osteomyelitis, or sequestration.
3. The lack of response to an adequate medical regimen, indicating the presence of a surgical pathologic condition.

Relative indications usually consist of milder and recurrent infection or the presence of a conductive hearing loss due to past ear disease which may be surgically correctable. Absolute contraindications to surgery have not yet been defined, but it is agreed by most workers that severe eustachian tube dysfunction lessens the possibility of hearing restoration in most cases.

Preparation of the Ear for Surgical Procedure. Ear surgery is greatly facilitated when it is possible to work upon dry, healthy structures. Not only is vision enhanced because of the relative freedom from bleeding, but also the nature and extent of disease are more easily gauged when edema and granulation tissue are not present. To this end treatment, as outlined in the chapter on Chronic Ear Disease, should be rigorously administered. On the other hand, freedom from infection is not an absolute necessity prior to the surgical procedure, since a large percentage of these operations are performed in order to achieve a healthy ear. In any case, a needed surgical process should not be delayed because of poor response to an adequate period of medical treatment.

Approach to Surgical Management. There are two distinct philosophies current in the surgical management of chronic ear disease. One group maintains the classic and time honored idea that a fixed procedure is required to treat a certain ear disease and that deviation from this procedure will of necessity jeopardize the outcome. This is particularly applicable to the treatment of cholesteatoma in which modified radical mastoidectomy is done in a standardized manner in each case. In some instances this procedure, combined with forms of middle ear reconstruction, has been recommended as the operation of choice for all forms of chronic ear disease.

A more recent approach, fathered by the introduction of tympanoplasty by Zollner and Wullstein, takes a more conservative attitude. The followers of this approach believe that the nature and extent of the disease process should dictate the nature of the surgery required. By this approach the techniques of otosclerosis surgery, tympanoplasty, and traditional mastoid surgery may all be utilized as necessitated by the pathologic findings during surgery. Needless removal of healthy tissue is avoided, and if the disease is followed in a logical manner, eradication of infection is not compromised. This latter approach to chronic ear surgery will be outlined in this chapter, and in doing so the early techniques which have formed the foundation for this surgery must be considered last, since they are a final step in the eradication of severe or extensive disease.

Terminology. The following definitions of operations have been accepted by the Committee on Conservation of Hearing of the American Academy of Ophthalmology and Otolaryngology and include all the procedures to be discussed in this chapter.

1. *Myringoplasty.* An operation in which the reconstructive procedure is limited to repair of a tympanic membrane perforation.

2. *Tympanoplasty without Mastoidectomy.* An operation to eradicate disease in the middle ear and to reconstruct the hearing mechanism, without mastoid surgery, with or without tympanic grafting.

3. *Tympanoplasty with Mastoidectomy.* An operation to eradicate disease in both the mastoid process and middle ear cavity and to reconstruct the hearing mechanism with or without tympanic membrane grafting.

4. *Radical and Modified Radical Mastoidectomy.* An operation to eradicate disease of the middle ear and mastoid in which the mastoid and epitympanic spaces are converted into an easily accessible common cavity by removal of the posterior and superior external canal walls. Radical mastoidectomy also includes the mesotympanum in this cavity.

5. *Mastoid Obliteration Operation.* An operation to eradicate disease when present and to obliterate a mastoid or fenestration cavity.

Anesthesia. The level of anesthesia necessary in otologic surgery is related to the anxiety of the patient and to the amount of stimulation inherent in the procedure. The method of anesthesia most appropriate will vary with the individual situation of the surgeon and the degree of anesthetic skill available. All otologic procedures may be carried out with local anesthesia, but this may produce many difficulties due to apprehension of the patient. Adequate premedication is a partial help, but difficulties due to excessive bleeding and uncontrolled patient movement often arise.

In most instances the combination of local anesthesia with basal narcosis is satisfactory. The combination of narcotic agents, phenothiazine-type agents, and rapid-acting barbiturates, all given intravenously, has proved satisfactory for adults. Difficult anesthetic problems in adults and children may best be handled with general inhalation anesthesia through an endotracheal tube supplemented with local anesthesia, so that a lighter plane of anesthesia may be used.

Local anesthesia for transcanal operations is placed in four quadrants in the outer portion of the cartilaginous ear canal. In mastoid procedures the logical anesthetic agent is infiltrated anterior to the helix and over the mastoid cortex posterior to the pinna to block the temporal region completely.

Preparation of the Ear. At surgery, the ear canal should be cleansed of loose debris and accumulated cerumen, but without trauma which will lower local tissue resistance to infection. A detergent soap is used to irrigate the canal without wiping, and after suction drying, a protein-iodine complex is used to paint the area. The external ear is prepared in the same manner. In order to prevent painful stimulus of the middle ear, gelatin sponges moistened with a physiologic solution may be placed through the perforation to protect the mucosa while the canal is being prepared. It is not usually necessary to remove any hair, but it should be kept out of the field with adhesive spray and drapes.

Incisions. Three major approaches to the middle ear and mastoid are in use today: the transmeatal tympanoplasty incision, the endaural mastoid incision, and the postauricular incision. The transmeatal incision is used to approach the middle ear directly and is used in tympanoplasty. The latter two incisions provide access to the mastoid cortex for mastoidectomy. The endaural incision has the advantage of fewer complications due to complete closure of the mastoid defect with periosteum and a better cosmetic result. The postauricular incision provides a much better view of the mastoid and middle ear together, since the angle of view may be changed over a greater range, particularly from the posterior direction. This incision is preferred over the endaural for most operations involving preservation of the ear canal.

The *transmeatal* incision is carried out through an endaural speculum secured with a speculum holder. It is triangular, starting 3 to 4 mm above the anterior spine of the malleus and extending posteriorly to an apex 8 to 10 mm lateral to the annulus at the posterosuperior region of the canal (Fig. 50–1). The incision is then carried to the inferior canal region, again 3 to 4 mm from the annulus. Elevation of the canal skin and annulus provides exposure of the posterior two-thirds of the tympanum. Exposure ante-

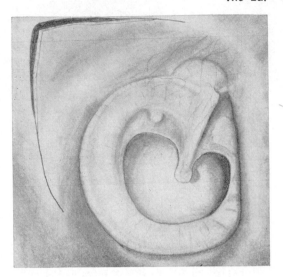

FIG. 50–1. The transmeatal incision.

rior to this, if necessary, is carried out by dissecting the drumhead from its attachment to the malleus.

The *endaural* incision is started inferiorly at the junction of the cartilaginous and bony portions of the canal (Fig. 50–2). It is carried upward through the posterior canal wall and then brought out between the tragus and helix for at least 2 cm. This portion of the incision is carried down to the temporalis

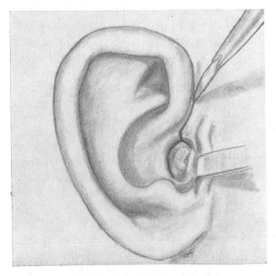

FIG. 50–2. The endaural incision.

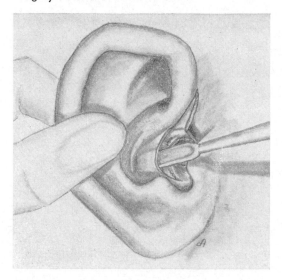

FIG. 50–3.   Elevation of the periosteum after endaural incision.

fascia. The periosteum is elevated from the mastoid cortex and a self-retaining retractor inserted (Fig. 50–3). Before the retractor is spread, a relaxing incision is made through the anterosuperior canal to prevent the retractor from tearing the skin away from the posterior bony canal. Separation of the retractor blades then provides a moveable window through which the entire mastoid cortex may be visualized (Fig. 50–4).

The *postauricular incision* is carried through the skin a few millimeters posterior to the retroauricular fold directly down to bone (Fig. 50–5). Its length should be sufficient to uncover the entire mastoid cortex. The periosteum is then elevated anteriorly and posteriorly, after which a self-retaining retractor is placed. Care should be taken to avoid the region anterior to the mastoid tip in order not to injure the facial nerve.

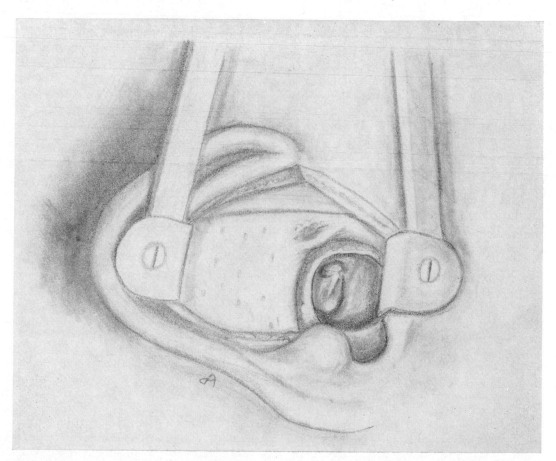

FIG. 50–4.   The endaural retractor is placed to create a mobile window over the mastoid cortex.

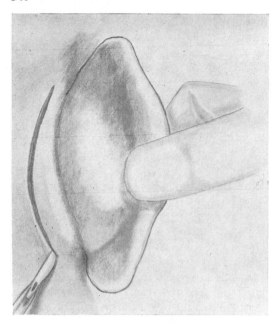

FIG. 50–5. The postauricular incision.

MYRINGOPLASTY

Since myringoplasty is a procedure which only corrects a defect in the eardrum when no other pathologic condition exists, this operation can properly be indicated only at the conclusion of the operation when it has been determined that these conditions, in fact, were present. Myringoplasty may be anticipated, however, in those cases in which chronic or recurrent infection has not been present or in perforations of traumatic origin accompanied by a hearing loss of less than 15 dB. In every instance, the middle ear should be inspected, since this adds little time to the procedure, does not increase the morbidity, and will occasionally reveal the presence of hidden or unsuspected pathology.

Graft Material. The first attempts to close drum perforations utilized split-thickness or full-thickness free skin grafts. Because of poor success rates, the predilection to infection, and the development of flap cholesteatoma (epithelial cysts originating from hair follicles and glands in the graft) with this material, its use has been largely abandoned. Today most grafts utilize connective tissue either alone or in combination with canal wall skin. For this purpose vein or tempo-

ralis fascia is frequently used. Other graft materials which have been used with satisfactory results are perichondrium, periosteum, and various preserved homograft materials, such as human tympanic membrane, dura, and heart valve. Preserved heterograft materials have also been used. The use of fresh autograft connective tissue such as vein or fascia avoids the complications of storage and offers the greatest degree of success.

The connective tissue graft is used to replace the missing fibrous elements of the drum, and the squamous layer and mucosa are allowed to regenerate over it. The rapidly proliferative squamous layer quickly carries blood to the graft, during which time it is able to survive by tissue perfusion. With the use of temporalis fascia, success rates as high as 98% have been reported.

Technique. Myringoplasty is usually performed by the transmeatal approach (see discussion of surgical incisions, pp. 838–839) or occasionally through a postauricular incision. The procedure consists of four steps: obtaining the graft, preparing the drum to receive the graft, inspection of the middle ear, and finally placement of the graft. Vein grafts are obtained from the larger arm veins, usually from the antecubital fossa. Since veins contain a high percentage of elastic tissue, a much longer segment of vein than the size of the perforation must be obtained. The vein is stretched, opened, and then put aside until used. Temporalis fascia is obtained through an incision above the hairline just superior to the auricle. Since fascia contains little elastic tissue, it does not tend to shrink before use and may be taken immediately prior to being placed.

The drum remnants are prepared by first splitting the edge of the perforation into two layers and then removing a 1- or 2-mm strip of mucosa from the undersurface of the drum (Figs. 50–6 and 50–7). This serves two purposes: to secure a raw edge of squamous epithelium around the entire periphery of the perforation from which regeneration will take place, and to ensure the removal of any ingrowth of squamous epithelium through the perforation into the middle ear. Failure to secure either of these objectives

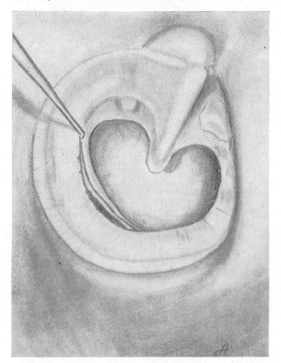

FIG. 50–6. Myringoplasty. The edge of the perforation is split into two layers.

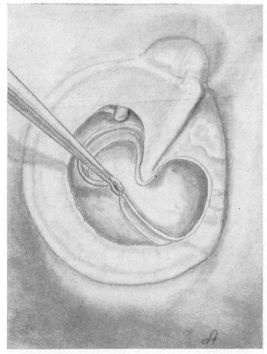

FIG. 50–7. Myringoplasty. The medial layer is stripped from the undersurface of the margin of the perforation.

may result in failure of the graft or in residual perforation.

An occasional difficulty encountered in this part of the operation is the inability to visualize the anterior margin of the perforation due to an extreme anterior curvature of the ear canal. This problem is usually over-

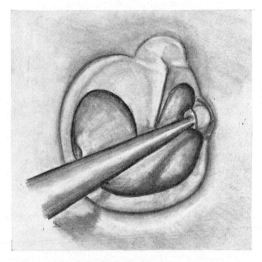

FIG. 50–8. The anterior margin of the perforation may be visualized by dissecting the annulus outward with a right-angled (reverse) elevator.

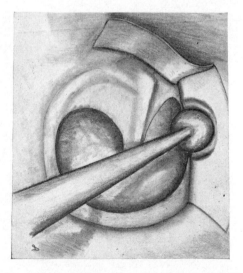

FIG. 50–9. When the anterior margin of the perforation is hidden behind a curved canal wall, it may be visualized by drilling or curetting away the bony canal after turning a skin flap.

27

come by either elevating the annulus outward into view (Fig. 50–8), or by removing this obstruction with a burr after first removing the skin from the area by turning a superiorly attached pedicle skin flap, which may be replaced at the end of the procedure (Fig. 50–9). Other surgeons elect the postauricular approach in these cases which allows a better angle of approach to this area.

Inspection of the Middle Ear. This is carried out by creating a tympanomeatal flap after making an endomeatal incision. A small amount of bone may be removed from the region of the posterosuperior annulus to visualize the lower portions of the posterior attic space, especially the long process of the incus and the incudostapedial joint (Fig. 50–10). Ossicular continuity and mobility should be checked at this time. Stapes fixation due to otosclerosis may occasionally be noted but should not be surgically corrected until a healed, closed middle ear space has been obtained by myringoplasty.

The creation of a skin flap is also of great value in the presence of posterior perforations, since a portion of the graft in this instance should be placed on the posterosuperior canal wall under the skin flap.

Placing the Graft. In order to exclude squamous epithelium from the middle ear, the tissue graft is placed on the inner surface of the drum remnant. If vein is used, the intima is placed toward the promontory; with fascia, there is no distinction as to surface.

In order to support the graft, the middle ear is filled with a nutrient, gelatinous substance. A good choice for this is a mixture of tiny pieces of gelatin sponge combined with blood (Figs. 50–11 and 50–12). The graft is then trimmed to fit the perforation,

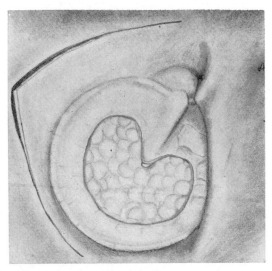

FIG. 50–11. Myringoplasty. To support the graft, the middle ear is filled with pledgets of gelatin sponge and blood clot.

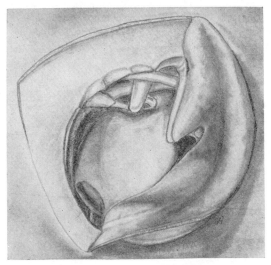

FIG. 50–10. Myringoplasty. The middle ear is inspected by elevation of a posterior tympanomeatal skin flap and, if necessary, by removal of a small amount of the posterosuperior lateral attic wall.

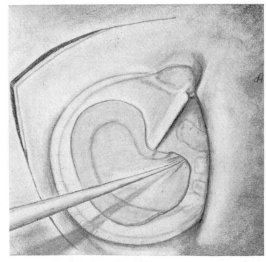

FIG. 50–12. Myringoplasty. The fascial graft is placed over the perforation. Then, starting anteriorly, the graft is tucked under the edges.

leaving enough excess to tuck under its edge and to bring onto the posterosuperior canal wall in the case of a large defect.

Another technique, evolved from the former method using skin grafts, is preferred by some surgeons. In this technique, the outer squamous layer of the drumhead is removed in continuity with the canal skin flaps. The connective tissue graft is placed over the denuded tympanic membrane remnant and the canal skin replaced over this. This author does not recommend this method because of a higher complication rate. Anterior blunting of the canal-drumhead junction, lateralization of the graft, and iatrogenic cholesteatoma secondary to entrapment of squamous epithelium beneath the graft have all been reported consequent to this procedure.

TYMPANOPLASTY

Tympanoplasty may be performed with or without mastoid surgery as dictated by the disease process or preferred by the surgeon. The tympanoplastic portion of the procedure is designed first to eliminate irreversible pathology and then to reconstruct the hearing mechanism by any of the several methods which is most appropriate to the pathology found. Since a perforation is usually present in these conditions, myringoplasty as just described becomes a part of the tympanoplasty.

TYMPANOPLASTY WITHOUT MASTOIDECTOMY

This is indicated in most cases of single chronic otitis media, chronic adhesive otitis, and the often present problem of tympanosclerosis. The procedure may be divided into several basic steps, including obtaining the graft (this has been described under Myringoplasty), and preparation of the drum remnant (this is carried out as in myringoplasty). Often in these cases an atrophic squamous epithelial layer has formed, and atrophic membrane may have retracted into the middle ear. This usually occurs in the posterosuperior portion of the middle ear (Fig. 50–13) but may involve the entire middle ear space. This presents a special problem, since the entire atrophic layer must be excised in order to prevent postoperative cholesteatoma formation and perforation of the drum. It has proved best to dissect this atrophic membrane from the middle ear spaces in continuity with the canal skin flap and then to excise it in its entirety in order to ensure the complete removal of this tissue (Fig. 50–14).

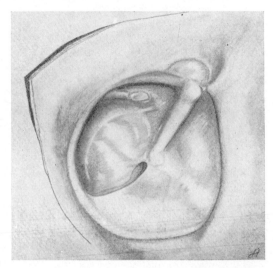

FIG. 50–13. Tympanoplasty. The presence of a retracted pocket of squamous epithelium in the posterior tympanum is a common surgical problem.

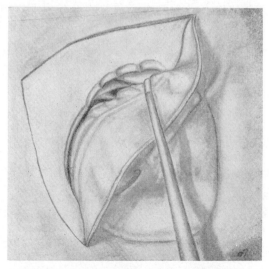

FIG. 50–14. Tympanoplasty. The atrophic epithelium is dissected free in continuity with the tympanomeatal flap, care being taken to maintain its integrity.

Exposure of the middle ear is accomplished by a tympanomeatal flap, as described previously. A small amount of the lateral attic wall may be removed to permit visualization of the attic and the contained ossicles. This exposure is necessary to determine the nature and extent of the pathologic condition so that the need for mastoid exposure can be carefully evaluated. If there is any question of irreversible disease extending into the mastoid cell system, mastoidectomy should always be performed as described in the next section (Tympanoplasty with Mastoidectomy).

Evaluation of the pathologic condition at surgery requires considerable experience to gauge its severity properly in all cases. It is always best to remove any questionable tissue rather than have it remain as a source of continuing infection. The main types of pathologic processes which may be encountered are squamous epithelium, mucosal infection, tympanosclerosis, osteitis, and osteomyelitis. Bone erosion may have caused dehiscence of normally protected areas, such as the facial canal, oval window, lateral semicircular canal, promontory, or jugular bulb. These areas must be dissected carefully when mucosal disease or granulation obscures the state of bony integrity. The surgeon must be rigorous in appraisal of difficult to expose areas, such as the sinus tympani and the tubal region, because retained irreversible disease will result in surgical failure.

Squamous epithelial ingrowth has been discussed under preparation of the drum and its removal in continuity with the skin flap described. Another source of squamous epithelium in the mesotympanum is the downward extension of attic cholesteatoma under the drum, which may perforate the drum, usually posterosuperiorly, prior to surgery. This type of squamous epithelium should not be removed in continuity but rather by carefully dissecting the drum or drum remnants from the lateral aspect of the cholesteatoma sac and then carefully removing the sac in toto from the mesotympanum. These techniques are necessary to ensure the complete removal of squamous epithelium. If the epithelium extends beyond visual control in the epitympanum, mastoid surgery with posterior tympanotomy should be carried out.

Mucosal disease may be encountered in every degree of severity from hyperemia and edema to thick fibrosis and tympanosclerosis. Polypoid degeneration is usually associated with the presence of squamous epithelium but may occur as an isolated finding. Granulation tissue is common and often covers osteitic bone. The milder forms of mucosal involvement are reversible and, unless associated with cholesteatoma or osteomyelitis, are usually avoidable by proper preoperative care (see Chronic Otitis Media, p. 825). Irreversible pathologic diseases, such as polyps, fibrosed mucous membrane, or masses of tympanosclerosis, should be removed. Retained islands of mucosa in the hypotympanum and eustachian tube will allow rapid regeneration of mucosa even with extensive removal. Small plaques of tympanosclerosis may be left if they do not interfere with free transmission of sound energy. The anterosuperior region of the mesotympanum should be carefully evaluated in this regard, since extension into the attic with fixation of the malleus is common with tympanosclerosis in this area. Dissection should be carried out carefully in the region of the footplate, facial nerve, and lateral semicircular canal, since extension of infection in these regions carries severe consequences.

Bone disease is difficult to differentiate at surgery and in general should be removed until healthy tissue is reached. Osteomyelitis is irreversible, extending to sequestration, and unless eliminated completely will result in continued infection. It should be remembered in dealing with ossicular bone that its blood supply is derived from mucosal vessels so that damage to this mucosa may result in necrosis.

OSSICULAR CHAIN RECONSTRUCTION

Ossicular chain reconstruction is based on certain definite principles, not only physiologic (see Ch. 42) but also empiric. These are: (1) The surgeon should use a technique which couples the vibrating elements of the sound conduction system in a way that maintains a lever advantage. (2) The surgeon should avoid the use of artificial prosthetic material, which has shown a high incidence of extrusion over time. The best prosthetic material has been ossicular bone, either autogenous or homogenous. (3) Less than adequate control of pathologic tissue results in residual infection, excessive scarring, and poor hearing.

Many techniques of ossicular reconstruction utilizing both artificial materials, such as polyethylene, Teflon, or stainless steel, and transposition of ossicular remnants have been described. These methods depend, of course, upon the particular ossicular pathologic condition involved and will be so outlined in this section. The most commonly encountered ossicular defects in order of their incidence are: long process of the incus (36.4%); arch of the stapes (18.0%); entire incus (17.0%); entire malleus (8.6%); head of the malleus (6.0%); handle of the malleus (4.3%). In addition to these naturally occurring types of pathologic processes, the problem of disease control may require surgical excision of portions of the ossicles. In the case of cholesteatoma, it is often necessary to remove the

head of the malleus and the body of the incus to ensure complete removal of matrix from the attic (Fig. 50–15). Severe tympanosclerosis with ossicular fixation often requires removal of the involved ossicles with subsequent replacement. It is especially true of this latter condition that compromise with the pathologic process frequently results in disappointing hearing results.

Use of Homograft Bone

Homograft ossicular bone provides the tympanoplastic surgeon with the most useful material for ossicular reconstruction. Although autograft bone is equally useful, in many instances it will not be available because of the extensive disease present. Bone surrounded by cholesteatoma matrix, when examined histologically, is usually extensively involved with osteomyelitic degeneration. Extension of squamous elements into the haversian system has also been found. Although some surgeons will autoclave the diseased bone, it seems preferable to use bone not involved with disease. Other patients will have extensive destruction through disease or past surgery and thus no ossicles present for prosthetic use. For these reasons, a homograft bone bank is needed.

Commercial bone banks have been established in several centers and can provide ossicles for prosthetic use. The surgeon may also establish a bank for his personal use. This author's practice is to have the pathologist remove ossicles through the tegmen during the course of head post-mortem examinations. These bones are then stored individually in 70% ethyl alcohol in the surgical refrigerator. They may then be employed for tympanoplasty after 2 weeks of storage. Cartilage and connective tissue may be preserved in a similar way and are useful for special applications to be described. At surgery, the needed bone or other tissue is removed from the alcohol and rinsed over a 1-hour period with several changes of physiologic irrigating solution.

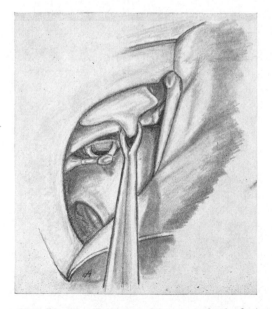

Fig. 50–15. Tympanoplasty—method of ossicular reconstruction. The incus is removed from the attic but is used for reconstruction only if healthy.

Systematic Reconstruction

A systematic approach to ossicular reconstruction is needed to avoid indecision or

	MALLEUS HANDLE	
	Present	Absent
STAPES ARCH — Present	A. Malleus-stapes assembly (59.2%)	C. Tympanic strut assembly (7.8%)
Absent	B. Malleus-footplate assembly (23.2%)	D. L shaped prosthesis (8.2%)

FIG. 50–16. Classification of the types of ossicular defects encountered during surgery. Within each block is the method of reconstruction used for that defect. The number within the block indicates the percentage occurrence of the defect in relation to all ossicular defects.

inappropriate application of technique. Since reconstruction is based on the remaining elements of the ossicular system rather than the missing portions, and since the critical portions are the malleus handle and stapes arch, a four-square diagram may be used to illustrate the choices available for reconstruction (Fig. 50–16).

The techniques to be described will follow this scheme:

A. Stapes Present, Malleus Present: Malleus-Stapes Assembly.

Falling within this category are two distinct types of ossicular problems. The first is ossicular fixation, either of the stapes or of the malleus head–incus body bloc located within the attic space. In both disorders the ossicular chain is intact but must be disrupted surgically to effect a hearing improvement.

Stapes fixation is often encountered in chronic ear surgery, being due either to otosclerosis or to tympanosclerosis. In either case, stapedectomy (as described in Otosclerosis, Ch. 52) is carried out as a staged procedure.

Fixation of the malleus head or body of the incus has a significant incidence as a cause of conductive hearing loss. When occurring together with other ossicular disease, it may be overlooked, resulting in postoperative hearing failure and necessitating revisional surgery. The cause of this fixation may be congenital, due to lack of differentiation of the suspensory ligaments of the

malleus and incus with consequent ossification. Acquired causes include hyperostotic healing of fracture of the tegmen, osteoma of the attic, and, particularly frequent in chronic ear disease, tympanosclerotic scarring of the attic. Tympanosclerosis has a predilection for the anterior attic space, often extending upward from the anterior-superior tympanic membrane and fixing the malleus due to involvement of the narrow premallear space. Effective treatment of all these conditions requires removal of the incus and malleus head, followed by reconstruction through malleus-stapes assembly described below.

The minimum defect of the incus is partial *erosion* of the tip of the long process or lenticular process. This erosion is often due to osteomyelitis and will progress to complete loss of the end of the long process even after healing of the tympanic membrane. To avoid this complication, the incudostapedial region should be carefully examined to determine the health of the mucosa and underlying bone. Tiny erosions may be ignored, while greater amounts of necrosis will necessitate sacrifice of normal ossicular continuity. A simple test of strength is to pull discreetly on the long process with a pick to see if it breaks easily. If the amount of disease falls between these two extremes, it is wise to proceed as though the long process were totally deficient. Erosion of the incus is uniformly associated with contact of retracted tympanic membrane and may be predicted when this is present. On the other hand, incus erosion is rare in simple central perforation without retraction and contact.

Reconstruction is carried out by fitting a bony prosthesis between the handle of the malleus and the stapes head: a *malleus-stapes assembly*. Either autograft or homograft bone is suitable, the guides previously stated being used to make a choice. The bony prosthesis may be constructed from either the malleus head or a portion of the incus body. Its length is sufficient to fit snugly between the malleus and stapes without either lengthy slack, which will result in displacement or poor hearing, or excessive pressure, which might result in stapes subluxation. A groove is formed in one end of

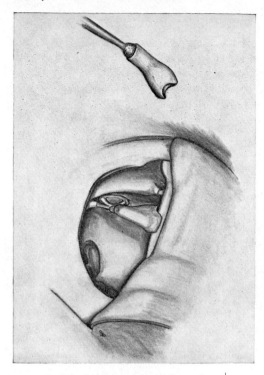

FIG. 50–17. Malleus-stapes assembly. A piece of ossicular bone, homograft or autograft, is drilled to fit between the malleus handle and stapes head (inset). It is then "snapped" into place as shown.

the prosthesis to fit against the malleus, and a socket is formed in the other end to fit over the stapes head (Fig. 50–17). A No. 4 diamond burr is the usual size used for this purpose. The socket of the prosthesis is placed over the stapes head. Then the malleus is gently pulled lateralward, using two instruments, while the prosthesis is "snapped" into position by a gentle push with the other instrument. Some practice is necessary to obtain proficiency in the techniques of drilling and positioning the prosthesis.

Compared to the former techniques of myringostapediopexy and incus repositioning, the results observed with this technique over a long period of time have been uniformly superior. Failures are usually technical, relating to an improper fit of the prosthesis. The good results reported are attributed to the excellent stability of the prosthesis, since neither the malleus nor the stapes will shift during the healing period.

This stability frees the ossicular graft from the shrinking process of the tympanic membrane graft during healing, which is responsible for many hearing failures occurring with former techniques.

B. **Malleus Present, Stapes Arch Destroyed: Malleus-Footplate Assembly.** The ossicular defect present in this category is found not only with destruction due to disease process but also postoperatively after the fenestration operation, and the reconstruction described below applies to both situations. The disease process associated with destruction of incus and stapes arch, sparing the malleus handle, is due to encroachment of squamous epithelium onto these ossicles, as seen in both primary acquired and secondary acquired cholesteatoma.

Malleus-footplate assembly (Fig. 50–18) is the reconstruction used for this type of defect. Again, the malleus handle serves as the lateral attachment for stability, the medial end resting on the footplate or oval

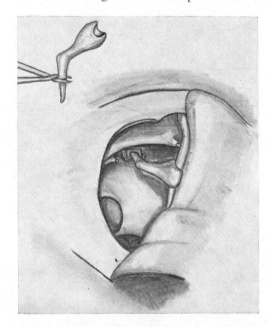

FIG. 50–18. Malleus-footplate assembly. A homograft malleus is carved as shown in the inset and fitted into place between the malleus handle and stapes footplate. It rests on a connective tissue pad over the footplate. This technique can also be used in revision of fenestration operations (see Otosclerosis, Ch. 52).

window membrane. The first such reconstructions used a straight prosthesis, usually an incus body, angled between the malleus and footplate. Slippage and bony contact with fixation were common complications with this method, however. Refinement of the technique involved the use of smaller and angled prostheses to avoid these poor results. The present method utilizes a homograft malleus for the prosthesis. The handle is shortened, the short process drilled away, and a groove drilled into the head to fit under the patient's malleus handle. In this way the narrow handle raises lateralward, avoiding contact with the oval window. The natural angle at the neck of the prosthesis allows the prosthesis to contact the undersurface of the malleus, always anterior to the midpoint of the oval window. Stability of the prosthesis may be further ensured by placing a piece of loose connective tissue as a "nonskid carpet" over the footplate. Again the prosthesis should fit snugly and be "snapped" into place. This can be accomplished only by accurately gauging the individual dimensions encountered. If a fixed footplate is found at the time of reconstruction, staging is necessary (p. 854), the prosthesis being placed and the tympanic membrane being grafted at the first operation. A second procedure follows complete healing, involving removal of the footplate and its replacement with a connective tissue graft upon which is placed the already incorporated prosthesis.

C. **Malleus Absent, Stapes Present or Malleus Absent, Stapes Absent: The Short or Long "L-shaped" Assembly.** Loss of the malleus handle occurs as a sequela of necrotizing otitis media. It may also be found as a postoperative result of radical mastoidectomy. As shown in Figure 50–16, presence or absence of the stapes arch is equally prevalent with loss of the malleus. The major goal in reconstruction with these findings is to incorporate a new strut or "malleus handle" within the tympanic membrane to collect sound energy and direct it to the oval window with a lever advantage. Although some surgeons prefer in these instances to use a tympanic membrane homograft with incorporated malleus handle to serve this function, this author has found to

date that optimum hearing results from a combination of connective tissue autografting of the tympanic membrane (see Myringoplasty) with the assembly described below.

"L-shaped" prosthesis assembly (Figs. 50–20 and 50–21) provides a lateral limb extending from the stapes head or footplate (as dictated by the defect present) and a tympanic limb extending across the tympanic membrane to replace the missing malleus handle as a collector of sound energy. For this purpose, the incus provides the best shape for the prosthesis. Either the long or short process may be chosen for the vertical limb, as dictated by the dimensions required. Usually the short process is fitted to the stapes head in a short "L-shaped" assembly, while the long process is needed in the long assembly. The bone is carved with diamond burrs, as indicated in Figure 50–19. The vertical limb is narrowed as necessary to avoid contact with the walls of the oval window niche. A socket is formed in the short assembly to fit over the stapes head. The assembly, which must extend to the level of the tympanic membrane graft, is stabilized by the middle ear packing (see Myringoplasty). The tympanic limb of the prosthesis should extend diagonally across the middle ear to be incorporated into the middle of the tympanic membrane. Again, as in malleus-footplate assembly, a "nonskid" layer of connective tissue over the footplate is of value in stabilizing the vertical limb of the long assembly.

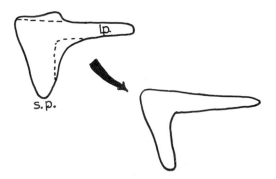

Fig. 50–19. A homograft incus is shaped as shown to provide an ossicular prosthesis when the malleus is not present. The vertical limb is short or long as dictated by the presence or absence of the stapes arch.

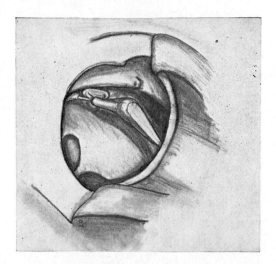

FIG. 50–20. The short "incus L" is placed on the stapes head with the horizontal limb extending across the middle ear under the defect to be grafted. It is supported by a bed of liquid Gelfoam and blood.

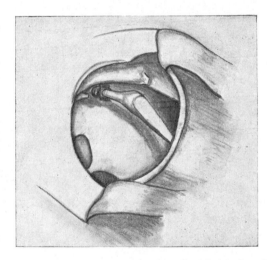

FIG. 50–21. The long "incus L" is placed on a connective tissue pad over the stapes footplate. Its horizontal limb is supported on a packing of Gelfoam and blood.

TYMPANOPLASTY WITH MASTOIDECTOMY

Extension of pathologic process into the mastoid air cell system requires exposure and removal. It has been demonstrated in recent years that this may be done without removing the bony canal walls, thus main-

taining normal tympanic anatomy. This gives a great advantage in the reconstruction of a functional sound conduction system. The decision to proceed to mastoid exploration is made during the exploration of the tympanum. The presence of cholesteatoma or mucosal polyposus or evidence of bone disease on radiographic examination dictates mastoid exposure. The procedure to be described is carried out after removal of tympanic pathologic condition and before ossicular reconstruction.

Posterior Tympanotomy

The incision for mastoid exposure is made postauricularly (see Incisions, p. 838). Extensive simple transcortical mastoidectomy is performed, the posterior and superior canal walls being maintained (Fig. 50–22). The dissection is carried anteriorly to the anterior attic wall. A most important part of this dissection is that of the "facial triangle." The bone lying between the second turn of the facial nerve and the chorda tympani nerve is removed in order to expose the posterior aspect of the middle ear. This enables the visualization of the stapes and the sinus tympani. The mastoid dissection should be sufficiently thorough to expose all diseased cell tracts but need not exenterate all cells, since the mastoid will be relined with normal mucosa.

The mastoid dissection is started in the region above the suprameatal triangle. The tegmen is found and followed medially toward the antrum, the cavity being enlarged externally as the bone removal is carried deeper, so that the surgical defect is either straight-sided or funnel-shaped. The antrum is identified by the curve of the lateral semicircular canal on its floor. The dissection is then carried forward through the aditus ad antrum until the fossa incudis is reached and the short process of the incus is identified. The lateral attic wall is removed, the superior canal wall being maintained until the space anterior to the malleus head can be completely visualized. The facial triangle is dissected by carefully removing the bone between the posterior annulus and facial nerve with diamond burrs to open the posterior sinus (Fig. 50–23). This allows a view

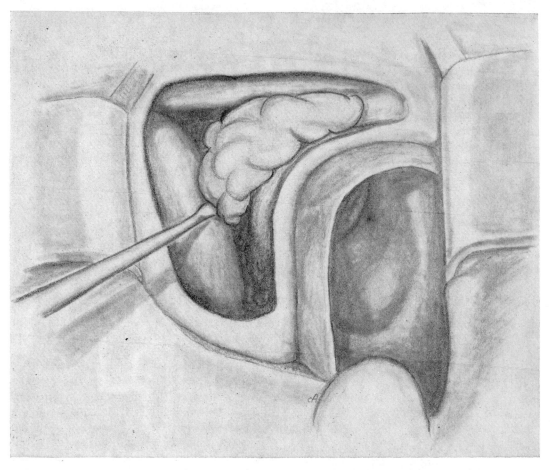

FIG. 50–22. Tympanoplasty with mastoidectomy. The mastoid cortex has been removed to expose a cholesteatoma which is removed intact if possible. The bony canal wall has been preserved at this stage.

of the posterior mesotympanum and sinus tympani from the mastoid aspect with much improved control of tympanic pathologic process. The mastoid dissection is completed by following the tegmen posteriorly to the lateral sinus, dissecting the sinodural angle in doing so, and then following the lateral sinus inferiorly toward the mastoid tip. When the pathologic condition has been encompassed, the dissection is completed. Since the second turn of the facial nerve has been well outlined by the initial dissection of the facial triangle, the position of the vertical segment of the nerve is defined, and injury should be no problem.

The mastoid cavity is allowed to fill with blood or may be filled with gelatin sponge unless there has been extensive destruction of the lateral attic wall. In this case, either the canal should be repaired or the mastoid segment should be obliterated as described under Mastoid Obliteration Operation. This procedure is used to reinforce the superior canal wall to prevent retraction of the graft into the attic and mastoid. Often small bony defects are created in the canal wall during dissection. In other patients, cholesteatomatous erosion occurs, creating canal defects. In each case repair must be carried out to prevent retraction through the defect and subsequent postoperative cholesteatoma formation. The most useful material for this purpose is homograft nasal cartilage. A thin slice of cartilage is cut with a surgical knife

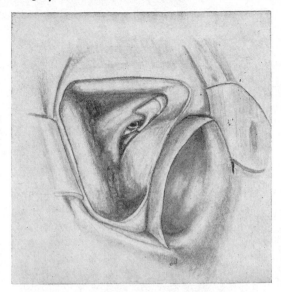

FIG. 50–23. Tympanoplasty with mastoidectomy. The entire attic and mastoid have been exposed and the diseased portion excised with the canal wall preserved. The facial recess (posterior sinus) has been opened to allow a posterior view of the oval window niche and sinus tympani. In most cases with cholesteatoma, the incus and head of the malleus would have been removed.

and inserted between the meatal skin or tympanic membrane graft and the bony defect, usually at the conclusion of the procedure. In most but not all instances, postoperative retraction will be prevented. Long-term observation is indicated to detect such occurrence, since early intervention will prevent the more severe complications of cholesteatoma. If retraction pockets become evident, mastoid obliteration seems to be the treatment of choice.

MODIFIED RADICAL MASTOIDECTOMY

Since the classic radical mastoidectomy removed all remnants of the middle ear, many attempts to modify the operation in order to preserve hearing have been described. One of the most successful of these was devised by Bondy. The pathologic indications for the operations were clearly delineated by Bondy but must be modified today owing to the refined surgical techniques now available. The object of radical mastoidectomy is to combine the middle ear, attic, and mastoid cavity into a single space draining through the external canal. The modified procedures preserved the middle ear space while draining the attic and mastoid. The element common to both these procedures is the removal of the posterior and superior canal walls.

During the course of the surgery as described under Tympanoplasty with Mastoidectomy, the extent and severity of the disease process are evaluated. A decision to proceed with modified radical mastoidectomy may then be made during the course of surgery based entirely on objective indications of the extent of the disease. The most important indication for this procedure is difficulty in obtaining needed visualization in canal preservation surgery, particularly in a small, nonpneumatized mastoid. These conditions will lead to unnecessary duration of surgery and increased risk of facial nerve injury or labyrinth exposure. Modified radical mastoidectomy should certainly be used by those surgeons untrained in posterior tympanotomy (see Ch. 51).

Technically the procedure entails removal of the superior canal wall, removal of the posterior canal wall to the level of the facial nerve, and creation of a canal skin flap which will be turned down to line the mastoid cavity and attic space (Figs. 50–24 and 50–25). This is most simply accomplished by thinning the bony canal walls from behind using drill and burrs. Initially, the dissection should be carried out lateral to the level of the facial nerve whose middle ear segment and second turn have already been visualized during the prior dissection of the facial triangle. The removal of the posterior canal wall is carried gradually outward to the level of the inferior wall. The final removal of bone is done with diamond burrs or rongeurs to avoid injuring the canal skin. The superior canal wall is removed anteriorly to the limit of the anterior attic space.

After removal of the bony canal walls, incisions are made in the remaining canal skin from the region of the tympanic annulus outward to the endaural incision, both anterosuperiorly and posteroinferiorly. This creates a tympanomeatal skin flap which, after the posterior annulus is dissected from the sulcus, is packed forward out of the way so that the remaining dissection of the facial ridge may be carried out. With diamond

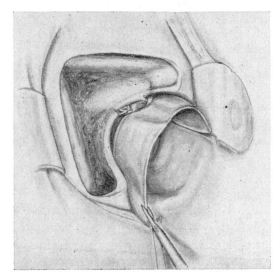

FIG. 50–24. Modified radical mastoidectomy. The superior and posterior canal walls have been removed, and the skin of the canal is being incised to fashion a pedicle flap attached near the annulus.

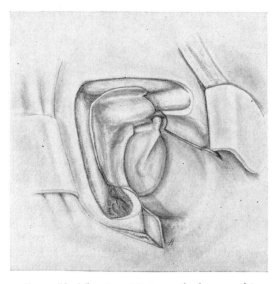

FIG. 50–25. Modified radical mastoidectomy. The skin flap is rotated over the facial ridge to line the mastoid cavity. If desired, a muscle flap may be placed behind the skin.

burrs, the remaining bone of the posterior canal wall is lowered to the inferior limit of the bony canal to create the facial ridge.

The severity of the pathologic conditions necessitating modified radical mastoidectomy has usually required the removal of the incus and the head of the malleus. If not, the tympanomeatal flap may be draped over the attic ossicular mass. Usually, the flap is brought down to lie on the bare bone of the medial attic wall and backward to partially line the mastoid cavity.

The modified radical procedure is concluded by repair of the tympanic membrane and ossicular chain, as described in the sections on myringoplasty and tympanoplasty. In many instances, staging is preferred, the tympanic membrane being grafted at the initial procedure and the ossicular repair being performed at a second stage (see Staging in Chronic Ear Surgery, p. 854).

As part of the closure, partial or complete mastoid obliteration may be carried out, if warranted by the pathologic condition present (see Mastoid Obliteration Operation, p. 853). The cavity is then packed with gelatin sponge and epithelization allowed to proceed from the skin edges. Postoperative dressings and manipulation should be delayed for a minimum of 2 weeks in order not to interfere with this process. Mastoid pressure dressings are applied and remain for 24 to 48 hours to control postoperative hemorrhage.

RADICAL MASTOIDECTOMY

Radical mastoidectomy is rarely indicated today, since it involves severe loss of function. Its application is reserved for tumors of the middle ear or external meatus, and in these procedures it may extend far beyond the operation formerly used for control of ear infection. This operation removed all middle ear structures including the tympanic membrane, ossicles (with the exception of the stapes), tensor tympani muscle, and mucosa. The orifice of the eustachian tube was occluded with bone chips or a cartilage plug. No grafting or skin flaps were used, the cavity being allowed to heal by secondary intention.

MASTOID OBLITERATION
OPERATION

The usefulness of mastoid obliteration procedures has been recognized for many decades. The incidence of chronic infection of mastoid cavities has not been reported, but it presents with persistent regularity in all otologic practices. Many procedures have been reported for this purpose. Most have used temporalis muscle for obliteration; others use fat or even space-occupying plastic materials, such as acrylic. Most of the early techniques have been abandoned because of failure to accomplish the primary purpose of obtaining a healthy ear by obliterating the mastoid cavity.

The advantage of these procedures seems to be the enrichment of blood supply to the skin lining the cavity and the provision of a soft tissue layer between this skin and the underlying bone. Obliteration provides a small or nonexistent mastoid cavity, making the problem of aftercare much easier. These procedures are thus indicated in the treatment of any chronically infected mastoid cavity and in the prevention of this complication after mastoid surgery by obliterating the mastoid primarily.

The contraindications to these procedures are extension of the disease process beyond the confines of the mastoid; threatened complication; or a disease process which may not have been controlled during the mastoidectomy, such as widespread cholesteatoma. The decision to do an obliterative procedure must be made at surgery and will vary with the experience and competency of the surgeon.

The technique to be described has been employed by this author and others for several years with uniform success in obtaining a good, long-lasting result. This technique employs a soft-tissue, anteriorly based pedicle flap from the mastoid surface, supplemented when necessary by autogenous bone paste and in rare instances by homogenous cancellous femoral head bone chips.

The incision for mastoid obliteration is, of necessity, postauricular. It is carried only through the skin, following which anterior and posterior undermining is done to expose a 4- to 5-cm area of subcutaneous fibrous

tissue lying on the mastoid cortex. A pedicle flap is then outlined, leaving it attached anteriorly at the level of the posterior meatus (Fig. 50–26). This is elevated from the underlying cortex with a periosteal elevator and kept free of the bony field by insertion under the anterior blade of the self-retaining retractor. At the completion of the mastoid dissection, this flap will be inserted into the cavity, terminating in the posterior attic and facial ridge to furnish a vascular connective tissue backing to the reformed canal wall. In small mastoid cavities, this flap is all that is necessary for obliteration.

The mastoid cortex is drilled away to expose widely the mastoid cavity. The bone dust is carried away through continuous suction irrigation, the aspirate being collected and saved in a 1-liter sterile trap bottle. Care is taken during this drilling not to dissect any diseased bone or squamous elements. The presence of infected bone contraindicates the use of bone in an obliteration procedure. When sufficient bone has been collected, the bone dust is strained through a fabric filter. The bony material then assumes the form of paste or mortar and as such is ideal for packing into the

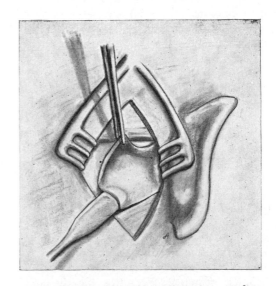

Fig. 50–26. Mastoid obliteration. Following the postauricular incision, the soft tissue over the mastoid cortex is exposed and elevated as an anteriorly based pedicle flap. It must be long enough to extend into the most medial depth of the mastoid cavity.

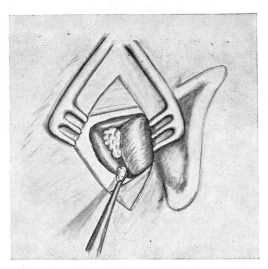

FIG. 50–27. Mastoid obliteration. The pedicle flap is fitted into the cavity, reforming the shape of the canal. Bone paste and bone chips (if needed) are packed in behind the soft tissue flap. The incision is closed without drainage.

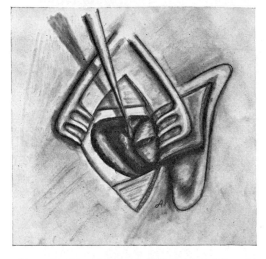

FIG. 50–28. Mastoid obliteration. The skin covering the mastoid bowl is elevated as a sheet to the level of the facial ridge. This will serve as the skin lining the obliterated cavity. The excess skin is excised.

space behind the pedicle flap. Osteogenic activity is rapid, causing a bony obliteration of the mastoid space (Fig. 50–27).

In the largest cavities, the space remaining is filled with small chips of cancellous bone obtained from homogeneous femoral heads. This bone material is widely available from our orthopedic colleagues. In actual use, the pedicle flap is first rotated inward and the remaining space gauged. If sufficient bone paste has not been collected, the homograft bone chips are placed posteriorly and the bone paste packed between the flap and bone chips to promote osteogenesis.

The steps of mastoid obliteration are then as follows:

1. The incision and development of the pedicle flap.

2. The removal of mastoid cortical bone to expose the mastoid cavity or, in primary operations, the underlying mastoid cell system.

3. In primary procedures the dissection is carried out as outlined under Modified Radical Mastoidectomy. In secondary procedures the skin lining the mastoid bowl is dissected free as a sheet from posterior to anterior, leaving this membrane attached along the medial attic wall and facial ridge. This membrane will serve as the new meatal wall skin and even if inflamed will rapidly heal. The excess mastoid skin is excised.

4. If tympanoplasty is required, it is performed as outlined earlier in this chapter.

5. The obliteration is performed as outlined in the paragraph above.

6. The incision is closed without drainage to avoid escape of the bone paste, and the canal is packed with moist Gelfoam pledgets as in other procedures.

Aftercare with this operation is minimal, since healing is usually complete within 4 weeks postoperatively.

STAGING IN CHRONIC EAR SURGERY

Hearing reconstruction may be carried out in either a one-stage or a two-stage procedure. This decision is based upon the severity of the disease and the type of reconstruction necessary. It is essential to a functional sound conduction system to have an air-filled middle ear space. All surgeons have experienced failure in reconstructive surgery due to collapse of the middle ear. This experience is more common in association with certain forms of pathology: total per-

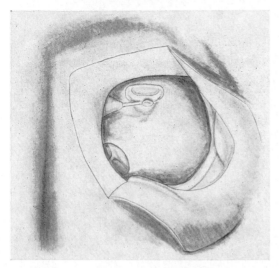

FIG. 50–29. Staged tympanoplasty may be needed for reconstruction of the middle ear, as in the case of a previously performed radical mastoidectomy, as illustrated.

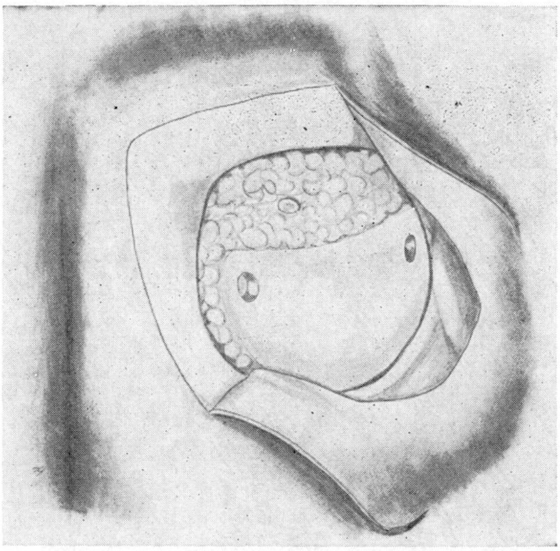

FIG. 50–30. Staged tympanoplasty. A plastic or paraffin mold is placed in the middle ear space and surrounded with gelatin sponge and blood clot.

foration, extensive and severe mucosal destruction, loss of the annulus through bone destruction, narrowing of the middle ear in modified radical mastoidectomy (Fig. 50–29), and total atelectasis of the middle ear. In these and other forms of pathologic process, based on the surgeon's experience, an improved success rate may be expected through staged tympanoplasty.

In staged tympanoplasty, to achieve better hearing results, the initial procedure consists of grafting the tympanic membrane perforation after first filling the middle ear space with a mold (Figs. 50–30 and 50–31). After the drumhead has healed and the mucosa has regenerated over the middle ear, a second procedure to repair the ossicular system is carried out, at which time the middle ear mold is removed. This method provides the obvious advantage of applying hearing reconstruction to a healed, air-filled middle ear.

Suitable for the purpose of filling the middle ear are three materials available today. Teflon molds and crescents, as well as Silastic films, are listed in surgical instrument catalogues and are commonly used. Gelfilm is an absorbable material which may be used for the same purpose, avoiding in many instances the need for a second operation.

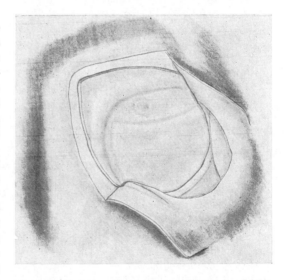

FIG. 50–31. Staged tympanoplasty. The graft is placed over the filled middle ear space. The mold is removed at a second operation after healing is complete.

When placed in the middle ear, it persists unchanged for 6 to 12 weeks, allowing sufficient time for regeneration of the mucosal elements with re-aeration of the middle ear.

The *second-look principle* is another important indication for staging in chronic ear surgery. Used with canal preservation surgery performed when cholesteatoma is present, the second look is carried out 6 to 12 months after the initial procedure to detect the presence of residual disease. After this period, any residual disease is easily detected in a healed mastoid or middle ear and may be removed without difficulty. These residua have the form of small pearls of cholesteatoma and thus can be completely eradicated without the need for radical surgery. This residual disease has been reported to occur in as many as 25% of cases, but a more common figure is 5% of cases. Cholesteatoma in a widely pneumatized mastoid is particularly prone to recurrence, and a second look is particularly essential in such patients. Another indication for reexploration is cholesteatoma matrix left over a fistula, in the oval or round window niches, or in inaccesible areas of the sinus tympani. At the conclusion of the primary surgery, the probability of residual disease is known to the surgeon, and reoperation should be indicated when this probability is present.

POSTOPERATIVE CARE

The use of *prophylactic antibiotics* has been the subject of much discussion in recent years. Opinion has varied between avoidance of antibiotics entirely; their use in selected cases; and routine use for several days in all cases. The most logical suggestion is to use antibiotics routinely, but only for the purpose of covering any possible contamination occurring at surgery (assuming no active infection is present). For this purpose 48-hour use of a broad-spectrum antibiotic is sufficient. The antibiotic should be started the night before the surgical procedure to achieve a blood level at the time of the operation. The antibiotic is discontinued 48 hours after the surgical procedure, usually at the time of discharge from the hospital.

Dressings for tympanoplasty may be limited to cotton tampons loosely applied in the concha and changed daily. When mastoid incisions are made, a pressure dressing should be applied to prevent hematoma formation. This dressing may be removed after 24 hours and a cotton tampon substituted.

The duration of hospitalization must be individualized. In general, a patient undergoing a simple tympanoplasty may be able to leave the hospital 1 day following surgery, while those with more extensive procedures may require 3 to 5 days' recovery. A 2-day stay postoperatively is average. The first dressing after surgery should be delayed for 2 to 3 weeks. This period allows adequate time for healing, so that cleaning the ear does not result in damage to the graft.

At the time of the first dressing, the state of healing of the ear canal and drum is assessed. Secondary infection of the canal is treated with topical antibiotics (see Chronic Otitis Media, Ch. 49). Excess granulation is painted with weak silver nitrate (5 or 10%), and 70% alcohol cleansing drops are prescribed to control the accumulation of serous discharge. Frequent inflation of the middle ear by the Valsalva technique (every 20 to 30 minutes) is reinstituted and continued for several weeks or months. Postoperative visits at bimonthly intervals should be made until healing is complete, after which examinations should be done at 6-month intervals. These examinations should be carried out periodically for several years, since a 10% regression rate is seen between the first and third years postoperatively, necessitating repeat surgery in these cases. A minimum of 5-years' observation should be advised in cases of cholesteatoma to guard against recurrence of the disease.

REFERENCES

Austin, D. F.: Vein Graft Tympanoplasty. Trans. Am. Acad. Ophthal. Otolaryng., 67: 198, 1963.

Austin, D. F.: Cholesteatoma. J. Laryngol., 78:384, 1964.

Austin, D. F.: Present Status of Vein Graft Tympanoplasty. Arch. Otolaryng., 81:20, 1965.

Austin, D. F. (Ed.): Chronic Ear Disease. Surg. Clin. North Am. Feb., 1972.

Brockman, S. J.: Cartilage Graft Tympanoplasty. Laryngoscope, 75:1452, 1965.

Committee on Conservation of Hearing: Standard Classification for Surgery of Chronic Ear Infection. Arch. Otolaryng., 81:204, 1965.

Corgill, D. A., and Starrs, L. A.: Intact Canal Wall Tympanoplasty. Trans. Am. Acad. Ophthal. Otolaryng., 71:53, 1967.

Farrior, J. B.: Ossicular Repositioning and Prosthesis. Arch. Otolaryng., 71:443, 1960.

Farrior, J. B.: Stapedectomy and Tympanoplasty. Arch. Otolaryng., 76:140, 1962.

Guilford, F. R.: Obliteration of the Cavity in Temporal Bone Surgery. Trans. Am. Acad. Ophthal. Otolaryng., 65:114, 1961.

Guilford, F. R.: Preoperative Evaluation in Chronic Ear Disease. Arch. Otolaryng., 78:271, 1963.

Jako, G. J.: Conservative Middle Ear Surgery. Laryngoscope, 76:1260, 1966.

Jako, G. J.: Posterior Tympanotomy. Laryngoscope, 77:306, 1967.

Jansen, C.: Cartilage Tympanoplasty. Laryngoscope, 73:1288, 1963.

Lempert, J.: Modern Temporal Bone Surgery. Laryngoscope, 60:740, 1950.

Proctor, B.: Chronic Middle Ear Disease. Arch. Otolaryng., 78:276, 1963.

Rambo, J. H. T.: Further Experiences with Musculoplasty. Arch. Otolaryng., 71:428, 1960.

Rambo, J. H. T.: Use of Paraffin. Laryngoscope, 71:612, 1961.

Rambo, J. H. T.: Musculoplasty. Ann. Otol., 74:535, 1965.

Shambaugh, G. E., Jr.: Surgery of the Ear. 2nd ed. Philadelphia, W. B. Saunders Co., 1967.

Sheehy, J. L.: Tympanic Membrane Grafting. Laryngoscope, 74:985, 1964.

Sheehy, J. L.: Surgery of Chronic Otitis Media in Otolaryngology. Vol. I, Chapter 10b. Hagerstown, W. F. Prior, 1965a.

Sheehy, J. L.: Ossicular Problems in Tympanoplasty. Arch. Otolaryng., 81:115, 1965b.

Smyth, G. D. L., and Kerr, A. G.: Homologous Grafts for Ossicular Reconstruction. Laryngoscope, 77:330, 1967.

Tabb, H. G.: The Surgical Management of Chronic Ear Disease. Laryngoscope, 73:363, 1963.

Thorburn, I. B.: Experiences with Pedicled Temporal Muscle Flaps. J. Laryngol., 75:885, 1961.

Wehrs, R. E.: Tympanoplasty with Aeration. Arch. Otolaryng., 82:18, 1965.

Wullstein, H.: Theory and Practise of Tympanoplasty. Laryngoscope, 66:1076, 1956.

Zollner, F., and Altmann, F.: Tympanoplasty in Otolaryngology. Vol. I, Chapter 10a. Hagerstown, W. F. Prior, 1960.

Chapter 51
Complications of Ear Disease

As modern chemotherapy has made otitic complications increasingly infrequent, it becomes more important to review the clinical patterns associated with these complications, since early diagnosis results in far more effective treatment. Formerly a high percentage of complications were associated with virulent acute otitis media (52%). Today most complications occur with chronic ear disease (76%) and are particularly frequent in conjunction with cholesteatoma. This has created a much more difficult therapeutic problem, since the underlying otitic disease must be effectively eliminated to prevent recurrence of the complication. These problems call for all the resources and skills available to the otolaryngologist.

The complications to be considered involve extension of disease process beyond the middle ear cleft to the meninges, lateral sinus, brain, or petrous portion of the temporal bone. The relatively common extension of mastoid infection through the cortex to form a subperiosteal abscess has been discussed under Acute Otitis Media, p. 819.

The intracranial complications in order of frequency are meningitis (34%); brain abscess (25%—temporal lobe, 15%, cerebellum, 10%); labyrinthitis (12%); otitic hydrocephalus (12%); thrombosis of dural sinuses (10%); extradural abscess (3%); petrostitis (3%); and subdural abscess (1%). Mortality and morbidity have been completely altered with the advent of antibiotic therapy. The overall fatality rate with intracranial complications has fallen from 35% in the preantibiotic era to 5% today, while the mortality rate for meningitis has been reduced from 80 to 22% and in brain abscess from 32 to 4%. These are remarkable advances indeed, but it must be remembered that the antibiotics have also made the diagnosis of these conditions more difficult due to the masking of the signs and symptoms of impending complication.

INTRACRANIAL COMPLICATION

Pathogenesis. In the progression of a middle ear infection to an intracranial complication there are three phases through which it must pass: (1) from the middle ear cleft to the meninges; (2) across the meninges; (3) into the brain tissue. Although hematogenous spread has been described on rare occasions, complication almost always occurs as a direct extension from the middle ear or mastoid. This results in involvement of either the middle or posterior cranial fossa with otogenic complication.

Spread to the meninges may result from several factors (Fig. 51–1). Preformed pathways, such as a temporal bone fracture line, a bony dehiscence, or a surgical defect, may promote easy egress of infection. The labyrinth may also be considered a preformed pathway once it has become infected, resulting in the possibility of spread to the posterior cranial fossa. Another route of extension is by thrombophlebitis of emissary

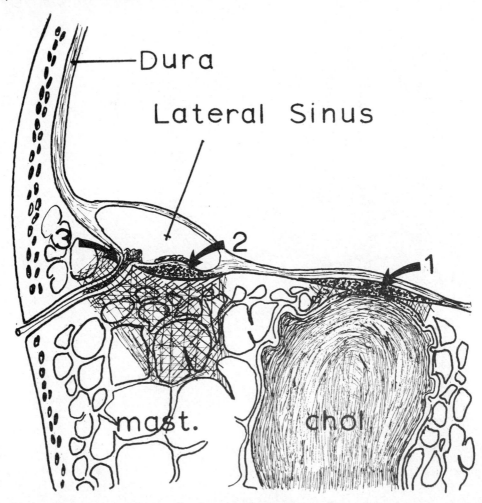

Dura

Lateral Sinus

2

1

mast.

chol.

FIG. 51–1. Pathogenesis of complications; methods of spread to the meninges: *1*, a cholesteatoma has caused erosion of the mastoid with the matrix lying against the dura; infection has resulted in an extradural abscess; *2*, osteitis of the mastoid has caused thrombophlebitis of the haversian system with resultant perisinus abscess; a mural thrombus is forming in the lateral sinus adjacent to the abscess; *3*, osteitis has involved a mastoid emissary vein; the infected thrombus is propagating into the lumen of the lateral sinus.

veins through the walls of the mastoid to the dura and dural sinuses.

Thrombophlebitis of the smaller haversian systems is a feature of osteomyelitis and osteitis and is the major factor in spread across the bony barrier of the mastoid and middle ear. This may result from a virulent otitis media and mastoiditis or a chronic otitis media. Complication in chronic ear disease usually follows an acute exacerbation of infection. This infection will then invade areas previously broken down or, in the case of cholesteatoma, will spread

through areas eroded by the cholesteatoma matrix which may be lying on bare dura.

The route of invasion of the infection is thus determined by many factors. The extent and course of mastoid pneumatization, the location and areas of erosion of cholesteatoma, the areas of involvement in previous mastoid infection, and sites of predilection created by prior surgery. As suppurative infection extends into the adjacent areas, local defense reactions are called into play, usually resulting in localized abscess formation. Extension through the mastoid cortex

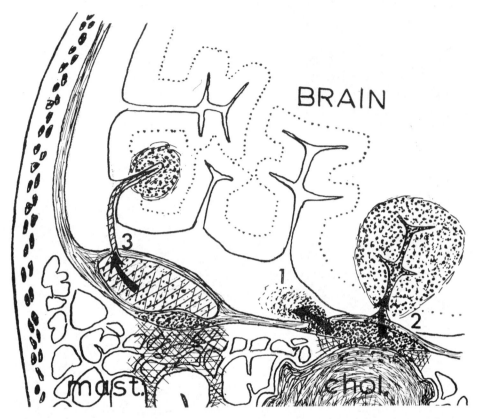

FIG. 51–2. Pathogenesis of complication; methods of spread across the meninges: *1,* an extradural abscess has broken through the dura, resulting in a subdural abscess or spread into the subarachnoid space and diffuse meningitis; *2,* the subarachnoid space has been obliterated through inflammatory reaction, resulting in direct invasion of the brain as the dura breaks down; this results in the "brain abscess with a stalk." *3,* the infected thrombus in the lateral sinus has extended along a communicating vessel, resulting in a cerebellar abscess.

has been described previously. Extension across the tegmen will result in extradural abscess of the middle fossa, while extension across the posterior wall of the temporal bone will result in either extradural abscess or perisinus abscess. An osteitis without bone necrosis may result in a localized extradural abscess without an obvious communication with the middle ear cleft.

Spread across the meninges is initiated as the disease reaches the dura, with a resultant pachymeningitis (Fig. 51–2). The dura is extremely resistant to the spread of infection, becoming thickened, hyperemic, and more adherent to the adjacent bone. Granulation tissue forms on the exposed dura, and the adjacent subdural space may be obliterated. If an extradural abscess forms across

the tegmen, it may become large because of the loose attachment of the dura to the temporal squama. In the posterior fossa the dura is much more tightly attached, and an abscess in this location will be much smaller. This is also true of the superior surface of the petrous bone medial to the arcuate eminence. If the primary area of involvement is adjacent to the sigmoid sinus, abscess formation is termed "perisinus abscess." In this region, thrombophlebitis of the dural vessels may propagate, or local sinus wall irritation may lead to mural thrombus formation. Both of these processes may lead to sinus thrombosis, which may be either aseptic or suppurative.

If these first local measures to limit the spread of infection fail because of necrosis of the dura, invasion of the subdural space takes place. Although this space has usually been obliterated by the preceding inflammatory response, empyema may occasionally take place with widespread diffusion through the entire plane even to the opposite hemisphere. Subdural infection is most often localized but may increase in size to involve underlying cortical tissue by thrombophlebitis with the formation of multiple small brain abscesses. In direct extension of the infection to the brain, the subdural and subarachnoid spaces have been obliterated, usually resulting in a direct tract to the brain substance forming an "abscess with a stalk."

Infection of the dura and subdural space promotes reaction of the pia-arachnoid with serous meningitis. Attempts at localization often produce an arachnoid cyst, particularly in the posterior cranial fossa. Enlargement of this cyst may produce symptoms because of encroachment on the cerebellum. Rupture of localized dural, subdural, or arachnoid abscesses results in sudden diffuse meningitis. Meningitis will often occur by direct extension through the dura without prior abscess formation. This is particularly true with virulent organisms or with markedly lowered resistance. Early in the development of meningitis a serous effusion occurs which proceeds to suppuration if the infection is not quickly controlled. Serous meningitis may occur as a reaction to dural irritation, in which case the spinal fluid is sterile and the symptoms of meningitis are milder (meningismus). As infection develops, bacteria and acute inflammatory cells appear in the spinal fluid, and severe symptoms and signs occur.

Spread into the brain tissue results in abscess formation usually in the region midway between the ventricle and surface of the cortex or in the center of a lobule of the cerebellum. This is a result of the method of progression of the infection into the brain tissue. This occurs by either thrombophlebitis or extension of the infection into the Virchow-Robin spaces terminating at the subcortical vascular area. Often sinus thrombosis results in thrombophlebitis of the communicating vessels with consequent cerebellar abscess explaining the frequent association of these complications.

Focal necrosis and liquefaction of the white matter is surrounded by an area of reaction. This edema and encephalitis may be extensive, causing more danger to life than the initiating abscess. Within several days the process of encapsulation takes place from the mobilization of microglia and fibrocytes. With capsule formation, the surrounding edema and encephalitis subside, resulting in a quiescent period.

Several courses may take place. The capsule of the abscess may calcify with subsequent complete healing. The abscess may rupture with the formation of one or more satellite abscesses. Rupture may take place into the ventricular system with subsequent meningitis. Enlargement of the abscess may result in external or internal hydrocephalus. Intermittent, inadequate drainage through the inflammatory tract into the subarachnoid space or mastoid cavity may cause intermittency in the symptomatology.

Reconsideration of these pathologic processes shows why multiple complications occur in at least one third of all cases. The disease may be arrested at any phase or may involve the total process. This requires not only knowledge of the symptoms of each specific complication but also the ability to recognize an impending or beginning intercranial extension of the disease. Great watchfulness is required during the treatment of the complication in order to recognize the progression of one complication to another, so that suitable adjustment of therapy can be made.

Diagnosis of Impending Complication. Thorough acquaintance with the normal progress of both acute and chronic ear disease is a prerequisite to diagnosis of a threatened complication. In general, if a total program of treatment as outlined in previous chapters (see Acute Otitis Media and Chronic Diseases of the Middle Ear) does not result in prompt remission of symptoms with cessation of discharge and otoscopic findings of resolution of the inflammation and fluid accumulation, the physician should become watchful. Except in the initial stages of acute disease, the patient is not ill, so that continued elevation of temperature, pain, or signs of toxicity may be danger signals. The development of headache, usually parietal or occipital, is a grave warning and may indicate that intracranial involvement has already taken place. Malaise, drowsiness or somnolence, nausea and vomiting, irritability all indicate extension of the disease. The signs of labyrinthine involvement will be discussed later. Children do not usually complain of headache and should be watched carefully. Their chief finding will be signs of toxicity and a continued febrile state.

Findings in these cases may be the recurrence of aural discharge after initial response to treatment. Usually the drumhead will remain inflamed, assuming at times a violaceous hue. In chronic ear disease, the signs of extension may occur after discharge has ceased, indicating the presence of purulent secretion under pressure. Frequent measurements of temperature should be made, since many of the complications are accompanied by a spiking temperature. Persistence of temperature elevation while the patient is on therapy or following completion of therapy is a definite sign.

X-ray examination at this time may be of help by showing evidence of breakdown of the walls of the mastoid. For these findings to be reliable, however, they must be of excellent quality and taken in several planes. Evidence of bony breakdown is an absolute sign of complication and indicates immediate surgical intervention.

Lumbar puncture should be performed in these cases when it has been determined that the danger of complication exists. The patient will have been hospitalized, and these findings are extremely helpful in arriving at an exact determination of the type of complication occurring. This examination should include determination of the pressure level, smear and culture for organisms, cell count, and chemical determination of protein, sugar, chloride content. Even if the findings are within normal limits, this information is of value as a base line if future spinal fluid examination should become necessary.

Specific Symptoms and Signs. Since the formation of an *extradural abscess* is the initiating process in the extension of disease, this complication was formerly common. Today most acute infections or exacerbations of chronic infection are quickly treated with antibiotics, which often limit or prevent this initial type of spread. If the antibiotics have not been effective, the initial symptoms will be little different from those of the ear infection itself. The first symptoms will be those described under Diagnosis of Impending Complication—namely, headache, toxicity, and a persistent mild febrile state. The most significant clue is the persistence of infection in spite of adequate treatment.

The most suspicious sign of extradural abscess is the gradual increase of the above symptoms, which are then suddenly relieved as the abscess spontaneously drains into the mastoid, causing an increase in aural discharge. This may occur several times, particularly if the abscess is not completely evacuated.

Extradural abscess may be localized at the petrous apex following petrositis, producing fifth and sixth nerve symptoms of facial pain and lateral rectus paralysis (Gradenigo's syndrome). In the middle fossa, lateral to the arcuate eminence, the dura is rather loosely attached to the calvarium. Extradural abscess in this region may become extensive, involving the entire temporal squama. Breakdown of the squama may occur with involvement of the periosteum above the external ear. Subperiosteal abscess may then form at a distance above the pinna, causing a fluctuant swelling (Pott's puffy tumor).

The advent of chemotherapy has reduced markedly the incidence of *sinus thrombosis* from 31% of complications in the preantibiotic era to 10% today. This complication, though occurring less frequently, is dangerous since the former mortality rate of 38% seems to have lowered only slightly. The reason for this is that sinus thrombosis is frequently (45%) associated with other complications, particularly meningitis, cerebellar abscess, and multiple sinus thrombosis occasionally extending to include the cavernous sinus.

Infection surrounding the lateral sinus causes the formation of a mural thrombus. This may progress to complete occlusion of the sinus lumen, with the possibility of growth in both directions and involvement of tributary vessels. Prompt treatment of the initiating infection may result in resolution, leaving a noninfected but thrombosed lateral sinus. This is usually asymptomatic, being discovered incidentally in later years at mastoid surgery. Invasion of the sinus by the infecting organism, usually hemolytic streptococci or type III pneumococci, results in purulent breakdown of the thrombus and resulting septicemia and bacteremia.

The onset of sinus thrombosis is marked by the appearance of a septic course typified by a high spiking temperature accompanied by marked toxicity, rapid pulse, chills, and sweating. During the frequent remissions, the patient looks and feels well, even euphoric. The fever quickly recurs, occasionally as often as every 4 hours. Nausea and vomiting may be present, and such severe symptoms as shock or convulsions occasionally occur. Headache, if present, is usually not severe and is not a prominent feature of this disease.

Involvement of the superior petrosal sinus may extend further into the cavernous sinus, causing the appearance of proptosis and chemosis, usually on the involved side. Pain in the lower jaw is frequently present in superior petrosal sinus thrombosis. Involvement of the jugular bulb may lead to paralysis of cranial nerves IX, X, and XI

The most typical and common finding in lateral sinus thrombosis is tenderness over the posterior mastoid at the exit of the mastoid emissary vein. Inflammatory response at this point may also cause redness and edema over the surface of the mastoid. Lumbar puncture shows normal spinal fluid, but the pressure may be increased, particularly with involvement of the larger sigmoid sinus or with spread to the confluence of sinuses. With increase of the cerebrospinal fluid pressure, papilledema is often present. The Tobey-Ayer test (comparing the rise in CSF pressure with alternate compression of each jugular vein) or the Queckenstedt test (bilateral simultaneous compression of the jugular veins) is helpful in determining the presence of lateral sinus thrombosis. The Lillie-Crow test gives the same indication by observing the retinal vein engorgement when the opposite jugular vein is compressed in the presence of lateral sinus thrombosis.

Blood cultures taken during the onset of a febrile period are positive in a high percentage of cases. This bacteremia may lead to the development of metastatic abscesses, particularly in the lung. The simultaneous occurrence of an ear infection with chest pain and productive cough should warn one of the possibility of pyogenic emboli from the lateral sinus.

Otitic hydrocephalus is most commonly a variant of sinus thrombosis. Typically this complication follows an acute ear infection about 10 to 20 days after resolution. The increase in spinal fluid pressure may be accompanied by headache, nausea and vomiting, vertigo, and occasionally lateral rectus paralysis causing diplopia. These symptoms are usually quite mild.

The marked increase in spinal fluid pressure (often above 300 mm H_2O) is accompanied by papilledema, while the spinal fluid chemistry remains normal.

The disease usually shows a slow resolution over a period of weeks to months without specific treatment. Persistence of papilledema may result in optic atrophy. To prevent this, frequent removal of cerebrospinal fluid by lumbar puncture may become necessary. In the case of bilateral sinus thrombosis with permanent increase of intracranial pressure, shunting procedures may be employed.

Subdural abscess, the purulent stage of pachymeningitis interna, is rare today. When it occurs, it must be regarded as a neurosurgical emergency, requiring immediate surgical intervention to prevent a fatal termination. Purulent effusion collects rapidly in the subdural space over the ipsilateral cerebral hemisphere extending to or into the falx cerebri. Reaction may produce loculation or obliteration by adhesion of the dura to the pia-arachnoid.

The clinical picture is characterized by a rapid onset of severe headache, toxicity, and somnolence proceeding to coma. Irritation of the cerebral cortex produces jacksonian seizures, whose pattern is a help in localizing the involved region. Paralysis of motor function consisting of contralateral hemiplegia or facial paralysis may occur. The cranial nerves may be affected by collections of purulent exudate causing, in many instances, oculomotor paralysis with ptosis and loss of conjugate deviation. Meningeal irritation is not predominant in this condition, and lumbar puncture helps to differentiate it from meningitis. The spinal fluid is usually clear without bacteria or change in chemistry. Spinal fluid pressure is usually moderately increased. Definite diagnosis is made by exploratory burr holes, which are also therapeutic with evacuation of the purulent exudate.

Otogenic meningitis may occur at any time during the course of complication of ear infection. Meningitis may cause labyrinthitis by extension through the internal auditory canal or may follow labyrinthitis by the reverse route. The usual method of spread is by direct extension, seldom with thrombophlebitis. The mortality rate with meningitis has been reduced in the antibiotic era, but it is still a serious problem, since death occurs in 25 to 35% of these patients. In cases of multiple complications, the fatality rate is greater than 50%.

The development of meningitis is usually divided into three stages: serous, cellular, and bacterial. As the infecting organism, usually streptococci, pneumococci, or staphylococci, less commonly *H. influenzae,* coliform, or pyococcus, invades the subarachnoid space, the pia-arachnoid reacts with the exudation of serous fluid which raises mildly the level of CSF pressure. Clinically this corresponds with mild symptoms of headache, slightly increased temperature, hyperirritability, and slightly positive signs of meningeal irritation. These signs are resistance to flexion of the neck (nuchal rigidity), which occurs in all degrees from slight resistance to a fixed hyperextension; Kernig's sign, which is the inability to extend the leg on a flexed thigh due to pain in the back; and Brudzinski's sign, which is flexion of the legs at the knee when flexion of the head is attempted.

Progression may be arrested at this stage, or the disease may progress to the cellular stage in which there is an effusion of leukocytes into the spinal fluid. In addition to the increase in cells (often to a concentration of 1000/ml or more), there will be an increase in the protein level and a mild decrease in chloride and sugar content. With the onset of the cellular stage there will be

an increase in the severity of the clinical picture as previously described: increase in the headache, now often described as "bursting pain," the appearance of vomiting and cerebral hyperirritability with periods of delirium, confusion, and drowsiness. Photophobia and withdrawal from tactile stimulation will now occur. During periods of irritation, the patient will lie on his side facing the wall in a fetal position to avoid all stimulation possible. The temperature will be continuously elevated from 101 to 102° F, usually with a lowered pulse rate.

The bacterial stage occurs with the appearance of frank pus in the spinal fluid. This is marked not only by the finding of bacteria on smear and culture of the fluid but also by the marked reduction (sometimes to zero) of spinal fluid sugar content because of bacterial utilization. If the disease is not arrested at this stage, the previous hyperirritability progresses to somnolence and coma with cranial nerve paralysis appearing, most often involving the extraocular muscles. Incontinence and death may rapidly follow. Opisthotonos often occurs in these late stages, particularly in children.

The diagnosis of meningitis is usually not difficult with the classic picture presented. Lumbar puncture usually results in prompt and accurate diagnosis. Sinus thrombosis or brain abscess coupled with meningitis may somewhat confuse the picture. In general, papilledema, epileptic seizures, or focal paralyses do not occur with uncomplicated meningitis and should point to other disease. A leaking brain abscess may produce recurrent signs of meningeal irritation. The possibility of concurrent disease must not be forgotten when dealing with otogenic meningitis, and appropriate diagnostic measures should be taken if the course does not seem typical.

Brain abscess is the ultimate complication both in severity and difficulty of management. Combining, as it does, the aspects of both a space-occupying and a space-consuming lesion, its presence implies deficits which are often significant to the patient even after a cure is effected.

Since this complication occurs almost always as a direct extension from mastoid disease (usually chronic), the temporal lobe or cerebellum is involved on the side of the disease. Brain abscess often occurs as one of many complications, which carries a much greater risk to life than when occurring alone (50% versus 5 to 10% mortality). Cerebellar abscess usually occurs with preceding sinus thrombosis and temporal lobe abscess with subdural or extradural abscess. A leaking brain abscess may cause recurrent episodes of meningitis.

The initial stages of brain abscess are accompanied by a wide surrounding zone of encephalitis, causing marked edema and resulting in an increase in cerebrospinal fluid pressure. Marked variation in symptomatology may occur, principally owing to variation in the degree of edema present. If virulence of infection does not result in rapid demise, encapsulation of the abscess proceeds, with a definite walling off occurring within 10 to 14 days. A fibrous capsule is formed within a 5- to 6-week period. Encapsulation of the abscess is accompanied by a marked reduction of symptoms due to regression of the surrounding encephalitis and edema. Exacerbation may take place, with rupture of the capsule and formation of satellite abscesses. Even after a firm fibrous capsule has formed this may occur. Eventually calcification of the abscess wall will take place.

The *general symptoms* of brain abscess are those of a space occupying lesion complicated by infection. There is an initial increase of intracranial pressure with the accompanying symptoms of headache, nausea, and vomiting. Somnolence and confusion sometimes combined with delusions or hallucinations are often present. These symptoms characteristically vary in degree, depending upon the state of edema, encapsulation, virulence, and response to treatment. Often these milder initial symptoms may be masked by the more striking features of other acute concomitant complications. With increasing severity, stupor and coma will ensue, accompanied by a slow pulse and subnormal temperature. Papilledema will not appear until 10 to 14 days after onset, but with a rapidly progressive case, tentorial herniation or herniation of the cerebellar tonsils will take place accompanied by fixation and dilatation of the pupils and finally respiratory paralysis. In cases of milder severity, the

varying general symptoms plus certain localizing symptoms and signs permit the diagnosis.

Localizing signs will vary depending on the site and degree of involvement. The signs of temporal lobe abscess depend upon whether the dominant side is involved. *Dominant temporal lobe* abscess commonly causes aphasia, which may be complete or partial. Abscess in either temporal lobe may cause homonymous hemianopsia due to interference with the optic radiations. Spread upward from the temporal lobe will cause initially a contralateral upper motor neuron facial paralysis with further progression resulting in upper limb and finally lower limb paralysis. Involvement of the minor temporal lobe, if small, is difficult to diagnose, causing vague symptoms of finger and body image agnosia. Often the general condition of these patients prevents the painstaking examination necessary to establish these findings.

The findings in *cerebellar abscess* may be few, even with one of massive size. The most typical findings are nystagmus, incoordination, and ipsilateral loss of muscle tone. Cerebellar nystagmus is spontaneous, slow, and coarse. It may be horizontal, usually with the quick component toward the involved side, rotatory, or vertical, which is an absolute sign of an intracranial involvement. Incoordination involves the side of the lesion primarily and is best tested by noting differences in fine motor coordination of the two sides. Such tests as grasping objects, finger to nose pointing, and one leg standing are most helpful in this regard. Dysdiadochokinesia is also present on the involved side. The patient falls to the side of the lesion, often telling of striking the door jamb when entering a room. Slurring of speech and difficulty in swallowing may also be present, representing another form of incoordination.

Diagnosis is based primarily on the clinical history, with confirmation helped by several forms of investigation. Lumbar puncture should be performed unless there is evidence of severely elevated intracranial pressure. This will usually reveal some elevation of pressure, protein, and cell count but may show no change from normal. Electroencephalography is of value and may show focal abnormality. A normal EEG does not rule out a brain abscess, however. Skull films may show shift of the pineal or even gas within the abscess. Electroencephalograms and arteriograms are of great value in localizing the site of the lesion. Brain imaging performed by computer-assisted axial tomography scanning has improved diagnostic efficiency. Ventriculograms may be necessary if the other methods have proved unsatisfactory but may be dangerous. Absolute diagnosis may be made by the finding of an abscess stalk or by needle aspiration at mastoid surgery.

Treatment. The treatment of the complications of ear disease must be twofold; not only must effective care of the complication be instituted, but also resolution of the primary disease must be accomplished. Often the severity of the complication requires delaying necessary mastoid surgery until the patient is well enough to tolerate the procedure. On the other hand, the complication, especially if impending or early in its course, may be treated with the same procedure which controls the primary disease. In brief, the essence of treatment consists of rapid institution of large doses of antibiotics, surgical management of the primary mastoid infection at the optimum time, and neurosurgical control of the intracranial lesion when required. Since neurosurgical and otologic cooperation has been utilized in the investigative phase, this team should continue in the combined management for the best outcome.

The antibiotic management of these problems is complicated by the blood-brain barrier, which prevents achieving a high concentration of many antibiotics in the cerebrospinal fluid. In the past, intrathecal administration was used to increase the concentration of penicillin, but this was quite irritating, and today the use of high parenteral doses of penicillin or tetracyclines is usually indicated. Treatment is initiated with 1 to 2 million units of penicillin given every 6 hours. Every effort should be made to obtain a positive culture for sensitivity, testing either from the primary mastoid infection or from the spinal fluid. If sensitivity tests or poor response to penicillin treatment indicate, another agent such as Chloromycetin

or streptomycin may be needed. The antibiotic should be continued until the febrile course has returned to a normal base line.

Surgical management ideally should be undertaken early in the course of the complication. In practice this is often a matter of determining the optimum time for intervention. The factors entering into this consideration are the diagnosis, the condition of the patient, and his response to antibiotic treatment. Continued spill or irritation from a cholesteatoma in the mastoid may cause a recurrent meningitis or progression in a brain abscess, so that control of the primary disease is essential for full recovery of the patient. In some instances drainage of a subdural empyema or drainage of an abscess must take precedence, but the mastoid surgery should be undertaken as soon thereafter as the patient's condition permits.

Surgical approach to the mastoidectomy in these cases should be such as to ensure complete removal of the inciting pathologic condition. In most instances this will require modified radical mastoidectomy, although extensive simple mastoidectomy may be performed if control can be obtained (see Surgery of Chronic Ear Disease). The essential part of this surgery is to expose and explore all possible routes of invasion of the infection. The bone overlying the sigmoid sinus should be thinned and removed. The posterior dural plate in Trautmann's triangle should be thinned, and the mastoid tegmen should be skeletonized in all cases.

Suspicion of underlying disease should be aroused by the presence of soft necrotic bone or violaceous granulation sometimes covered by purulent exudate. The dura is normally firm and pale blue, with the sinus a deeper blue. A freely bleeding inflamed surface on the dura indicates infection. Often the removal of necrotic bone releases the pus contained in a perisinus or extradural abscess.

Sinus thrombophlebitis is treated by opening the sinus after exposing it from the sinodural angle to the jugular bulb. All the necrotic or infected thrombus is aspirated and the sinus packed open (Fig. 51–3). Surgicel is a good material for this purpose, since it is slowly absorbed and obviates the necessity of delayed removal of gauze packing.

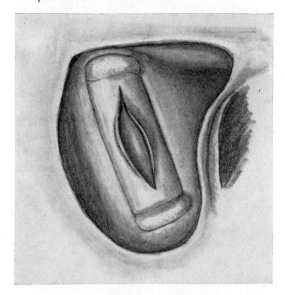

FIG. 51–3. Treatment of sinus thrombosis. After complete exposure of the mastoid extent of the lateral sinus, it is packed shut at each end and opened in its midportion. Infected or necrotic thrombus is removed, and firm thrombus is left in place to limit spread.

Firm fibrous clot need not be removed, since this helps prevent the extension of the infection.

The use of anticoagulants and jugular vein ligation have been advocated in the past to prevent the propagation of the thrombus. Neither of these measures has proved particularly effective in routine use, and they are not indicated in the average case. Anticoagulants may be used in those cases in which growth of the thrombus becomes widespread with involvement of the petrosal and cavernous sinuses or the confluence of sinuses. Jugular ligation is rarely needed today with the control of septic emboli by antibiotics. Rather, a continued septic course calls for reexploration of the sinus through the mastoid with further and complete removal of the infected thrombus. At this time the cerebellum should be needled for the presence of an abscess because of the common association of these two entities and the possibility of this causing the septic course.

Jugular ligation, if indicated, is performed through a 2- to 3-inch incision at the anterior margin of the sternocleidomastoid muscle just below the mastoid tip. The vein is doubly ligated and divided between the ligatures.

The presence of otitic hydrocephalus may require repeated spinal taps, especially if optic atrophy is threatened. Usually surgical treatment of the sinus thrombosis results in a gradual reduction of intracranial pressure.

Meningitis is treated primarily by antibiotic management. The possibility of an associated complication such as an abscess or thrombophlebitis should always be kept in mind and mastoid exploration undertaken if the expected response to treatment does not occur. Recurrence of otogenic meningitis is common, and it is felt that mastoid exploration should be performed in any case of recurrent meningitis regardless of the type of ear disease. In most of these an area of bone necrosis will be found occasionally associated with an extradural collection of pus. This unresolved disease is undoubtedly responsible for the reinfection in these cases.

Subdural abscess is a severe and life-endangering complication whose treatment is a neurosurgical emergency. Burr holes are made above and below the involved area, and the purulent collection is aspirated. Irrigation first with physiologic solution and then with an antibiotic containing solution is carried out, and the rubber drains are left in place so that frequent irrigation may be done. It is usually necessary to delay mastoid surgery until the empyema has resolved, but it should be done without more delay than is necessary for the neurosurgical treatment.

Brain abscess is again primarily a neurosurgical problem, although the initial diagnosis of a silent abscess may be made at mastoid surgery. Drainage of the abscess through the mastoid tegmen has been described in the past but is a risky procedure because of the possibility of herniation of the brain through the drainage site with the formation of a brain fungus. The best plan of management is to control the mastoid disease and associated extradural abscess through the mastoid and to treat the brain abscess from above through the cortex.

When the abscess has walled off and has been localized, it is treated either by tapping or by excision. Tapping is done through a burr hole. When the abscess has been reached, it is aspirated, and contrast material mixed with penicillin solution is instilled so that the progress of the abscess may be followed with radiographic examination. One aspiration may suffice, but usually several are required. A multilocular abscess presents a more difficult problem but is treated in essentially the same manner.

Excision of the abscess offers the opportunity to examine the dura and to control the route of invasion, as well as removing the diseased area.

It is a great help in these cases to correlate closely the mastoid and neurologic surgery. A continuous spill of infection into the brain tissue from the involved mastoid will result in poor response to treatment. Ideally both areas should be treated concurrently. Severely ill patients, of course, cannot be treated in this way, but as soon as control of infection has resulted in reduction of cerebral edema, the mastoid should be operated.

INFLAMMATORY DISEASES OF THE LABYRINTH

From a clinical viewpoint, diseases of the labyrinth based on some inflammatory process include the various circumscribed or diffuse forms of labyrinthitis due to most types of organisms capable of producing all inflammatory reactions. The most practical classification from a clinical and pathologic standpoint is:

1. Circumscribed
2. Diffuse serous
3. Diffuse suppurative
    a. Acute (manifest) stage
    b. Chronic (latent) stage

The acute (manifest) and chronic (latent) types of diffuse suppurative labyrinthitis are different stages of the same disease and are thus classified under the same subdivision.

Etiology. Infections of the labyrinth are usually the result of a direct invasion from the middle ear following an acute or chronic otitis. Labyrinthitis may also be secondary to a meningitis or a subdural abscess, or a necrotic process in the petrosa may erode

through the bony labyrinthine capsule, giving rise to a circumscribed or a diffuse form. It is possible for the infection to be transmitted through the fissula ante fenestrum. Transmission of the infection to the labyrinth by way of the vascular system also occurs.

Extension to the labyrinth from the middle ear is usually through the round window (most common) or the oval window. The round window is more deeply placed than the oval window, and this may promote stasis of the infected secretions in the round window niche beneath the rim of the promontorium and hence favor transmission of infection or toxins to the labyrinth. A fistula may or may not be present.

An erosion through the bony capsule of the labyrinth from a middle ear infection is usually secondary to a cholesteatoma producing erosion of the external portion of the lateral semicircular canal. A fistula with the characteristic signs and symptoms of a circumscribed labyrinthitis is the usual result. If the infection in any portion of the vestibular or acoustic labyrinth becomes walled off before a generalized labyrinthitis has developed, a circumscribed labyrinthitis, with or without a fistula, would occur.

If toxins penetrate the labyrinth (usually through the round or oval windows), a serous type of labyrinthitis may result. A fistula is usually not present in this form. If the serous labyrinthitis is secondary to a cholesteatoma with erosion into the lateral canal, the fistula test is usually positive.

Circumscribed Labyrinthitis

Definition. A circumscribed labyrinthitis is, as its name implies, an infection or inflammation of a portion of the labyrinth, usually the external limb of the lateral canal. Theoretically, any portion of the vestibular or cochlear labyrinth may be involved.

Etiology. The most common cause of circumscribed labyrinthitis is a cholesteatoma which has eroded into the lateral canal with the formation of a fistula. Occasionally, the oval window or the promontory is the pathway. At times, the superior or posterior canal is involved. The cochlea is less often affected, but when invasion does occur, the infection is more likely to result in a diffuse labyrinthitis.

A circumscribed labyrinthitis with a positive fistula sign may be observed at times in congenital syphilis, the various granulomas, or temporal bone tumors if a softened area is formed in the bony capsule over a semicircular canal which exposes the membranous structure of the canal.

Extension to the labyrinth is more likely to occur during an acute exacerbation of a chronic otitis media than during a quiescent period of the otitis.

Pneumococcal type III infection of the middle ear and mastoid cells tends to break through one or more of the semicircular canals by way of the perilabyrinthine cells, especially the retrolabyrinthine group. In type III pneumococcal infection of the labyrinth, an epidural abscess of the posterior fossa is almost invariably present, and purulent meningitis frequently follows.

Either circumscribed or diffuse labyrinthitis may follow a mastoidectomy in which the lateral canal or the stapes is disturbed or injured.

Pathology. A fistula, usually of the lateral semicircular canal, is present in probably more than half of the cases of circumscribed labyrinthitis. Fistulas may also form at the round (Figs. 51–4 and 51–5) and oval windows, at the promontorium, or at the tym-

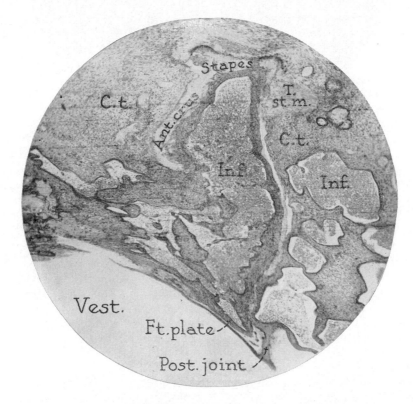

Fig. 51–4. Severe infection around the oval window. An acute suppurative process (*Inf.*) with some connective tissue in the region of the stapes and oval window. Mrs. T., aged 37, developed an otitis media (right), mastoiditis, and intracranial complications (*Streptococcus pyogenes.*) Autopsy, 16 days after the first symptoms revealed a subdural abscess, thrombosis of the sigmoid and inferior petrosal sinuses, and meningitis. In spite of the severe infection about the stapes, the internal ear was not involved in that region, but a circumscribed labyrinthitis with a fistula of the round window (Fig. 51–5) was found. The footplate and posterior joint of the stapes are shown. The anterior joint of the stapes and part of the crus do not show at this level of sectioning. The tendon of the stapedius muscle (*T.st.m.*) may be observed. × 36. (Courtesy of Dr. E. W. Hagens.)

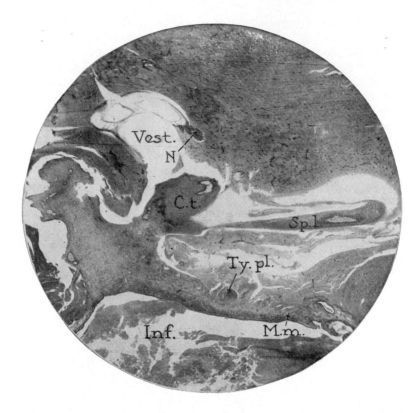

F<small>IG.</small> 51–5.   Circumscribed labyrinthitis with a fistula of the round window. Horizontal section at level of start of cochlea (Mrs. T., Fig. 51–4). Connective tissue (*C.t.*) formation has replaced the round window and grown into the vestibule (*Vest.*). The spiral ligament (*Sp.l.*) and the nerve (*N*) to the crista of the posterior semicircular canal are normal. Extensive infection (*Inf.*) in the tympanic cavity, with the thickened mucosa (*Mm.*) overlying the bony promontory, may be observed. The tympanic plexus (*Ty.pl.*) is normal. × 11. (Courtesy of Dr. E. W. Hagens.)

panic orifice of the eustachian tube. No portion of the labyrinth, vestibular or acoustic, would be exempt, however, from possible fistula formation.

The fistula usually erodes only the bony labyrinth but may extend into the membranous portion. In this latter event, the pathologic process is much more likely to become diffuse. Fistulas located in the round or oval windows, the promontory, or the tympanic mouth of the eustachian tube may involve the membranous cochlea and its nerves.

A fistula from any portion of the middle ear is formed by a primary breakdown of the middle ear mucosa, followed by resorption of a portion of the labyrinthine capsule to the endosteum. Bone resorption begins along the vascular canals. Erosion from a

cholesteatoma may occur without a primary bacterial invasion of the labyrinth.

Symptoms.   The acute stage of a circumscribed labyrinthitis lasts about a week. It begins with recurring attacks of dizziness and at times by nausea usually made worse by movements of the head and body. A spontaneous nystagmus toward the involved ear is present during the attacks. The temperature and hearing acuity are essentially normal. If there is any hearing loss, it is of the conductive type and of no greater degree than usually found in an otitis media. The temporary hearing loss in the diffuse serous forms of labyrinthitis is usually greater than in the circumscribed type.

In the chronic stage, intermittent attacks of vertigo, made worse or brought on by sudden movements of the head or at times by bending over, are usually noted. In some individuals, vertigo is absent. A low-grade spontaneous nystagmus may or may not be in evidence and, when present, may be in either direction.

The Fistula Sign. The presence of a fistula is determined by the fistula test in which either compression or aspiration of air in the external auditory canal is done. An airtight speculum of a Siegle's otoscope or a rubber bag with an olive tip is inserted into the external auditory meatus. Compression of the bag or relaxation of the compressed bag produces an increased or decreased air pressure within the canal, and if a patent fistula is present, a compression or expansion of the membranous labyrinth results. If a fistula is present (positive), vertigo and nystagmus are caused by either compression or a reduction of the air. The nystagmus will be to one side by compression and to the opposite by decreased pressure. The fistula sign may be absent (negative) if the fistula is blocked by granulations or other obstructions.

Diagnosis. The clinical diagnosis of a circumscribed labyrinthitis is based upon a history of recurrent attacks of vertigo and nystagmus in the presence of chronic ear disease and a positive fistula test. It is usually possible to demonstrate bony erosion of the labyrinth by polytomographic radiologic examination.

Treatment. The treatment of a circumscribed labyrinthitis is directed primarily toward the chronic otitis media and/or the cholesteatoma. (If the circumscribed labyrinthitis is in an acute stage, or before or after some surgical procedure, adequate treatment with antibiotics should be given.)

Surgical treatment should be directed toward, and be adequate for, control of the primary disease process. Cholesteatoma matrix is usually removed from the eroded labyrinth with deft and sharp technique, and the area is immediately covered with connective tissue (see Surgery in Chronic Ear Disease, Ch. 50).

Diffuse Serous Labyrinthitis

The acute form of diffuse serous labyrinthitis is frequently secondary to a pre-existing circumscribed labyrinthitis, or it may occur as a primary labyrinthitis following an acute middle ear infection in which toxins (and possibly bacteria) gain entrance to the labyrinth through the round or oval windows or through an erosion of the bony capsule. The erosion in this event reaches the endosteum by way of the vascular channels. The so-called diffuse serous induced labyrinthitis of Alexander and Ruttin frequently follows a mastoid operation, especially if the patient has had a previous circumscribed peri- or paralabyrinthitis. The symptoms in this event appear from the first to the fifth day after the operation. If serous labyrinthitis follows a direct injury to the labyrinth during the operation, the symptoms appear at once. This latter form may develop into a diffuse suppurative type within a few days. Edema of the middle ear may extend into the labyrinth producing serous labyrinthitis. Probably the most common cause of serous labyrinthitis is the absorption into the labyrinth of toxic products from bacterial activity in the middle ear and mastoid.

A mild form of serous labyrinthitis follows surgery on the inner ear. This is almost universal following the fenestration operation (see Otosclerosis, Ch. 52) and also occurs commonly after stapes surgery for otosclerosis. This form is short-lived and does not usually result in damage to hearing. The high tone hearing loss which occasionally follows this form of surgery is often ascribed to this cause.

Pathology. The essential pathology is that of a nonpurulent inflammation of the labyrinth. A section of the labyrinth examined histologically by Lindsay showed an early cellular infiltration with a serous or a serofibrinous exudate.

Symptoms. The symptoms and signs of an acute labyrinthine upset are spontaneous and rotational vertigo, nystagmus usually to the diseased side, nausea and vomiting at times, ataxia, and a beginning nerve type deafness. These symptoms and signs come on suddenly if the labyrinthitis is of the induced type, that is, not associated with a fistula or due to a circumscribed labyrinthitis. In the former event, prodromal labyrinthine symptoms are absent. The fistula sign would not be elicited. A history of an

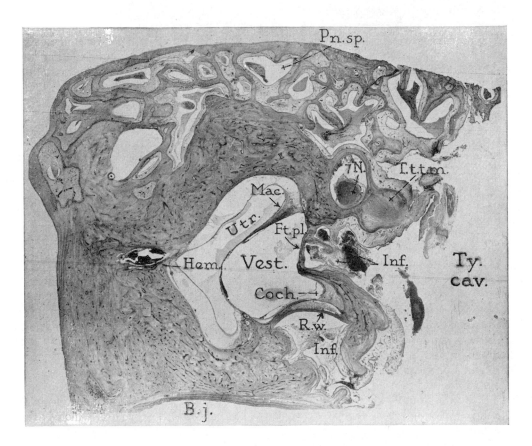

Fig. 51–6. Serous and suppurative labyrinthitis with extension of the infection to the laby-rinth through the round window. M.I., boy, 3 years of age, gave a history of a left otitis with fever and opisthotonus. Examination revealed a left otitis media, mastoiditis (mastoid operated), and meningitis (pneumococcal). At autopsy, a bilateral osteitis, otitis media, and labyrinthitis were found. The vertical coronal section shows the footplate of the stapes (*Ft.pl.*) resisting the extensive infection (*Inf.*), whereas the round window (*R.w.*) is infiltrated with cells. There is quite an accumulation of cells in the scala tympani at the start of the cochlea (*Coch.*). The utricle (*Utr.*) reveals a serous labyrinthitis. A hemorrhagic (*Hem.*) accumulation may be seen in the common crus of the semicircular canal. The facial nerve (*7 N.*), tendon of the tensor tympani muscle (*T.t.t.m.*), tympanic cavity (*Ty.cav.*), and jugular bulb (*B.j.*) may be seen. The extensive development of the infected pneumatic spaces (*Pn.sp.*) is unusual for a child 3 years of age. × 9. (Courtesy of Dr. E. W. Hagens.)

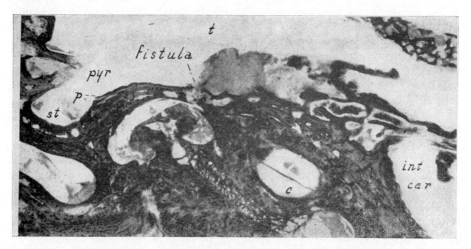

FIG. 51–7.   Fistula through the bony capsule into the promontory. The tympanic sinus (*st*) and the pyramid (*pyr*) housing the stapedius muscle are clearly seen. (Eggston A. A., and Wolff, D.: Histopathology of the Ear, Nose and Throat. Baltimore, Williams and Wilkins Co., 1947.)

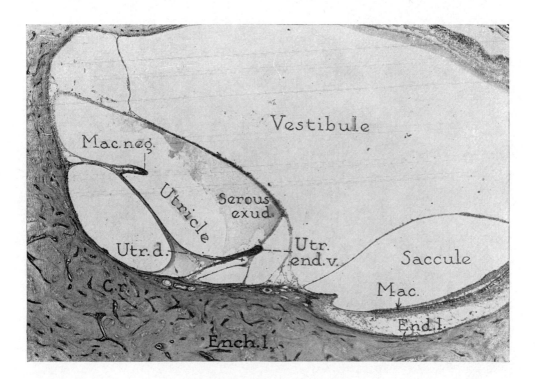

FIG. 51–8.   Acute circumscribed serous labyrinthitis. *CS.*, male, 10 years of age, gave a history of bilateral acute otitis media with headache and stiffness of the neck. The post-mortem examination revealed a streptococcal meningitis with a bilateral osteitis of the temporal bone and a circumscribed serous labyrinthitis of the utricle on the left side. Various structures may be seen, such as the utricular duct (*Utr.d.*); utriculoendolymphatic valve (*Utr.end.v.*); macula neglecta (*Mac.neg.*); macula (*Mac.*) of saccule; endosteal layer (*End.l.*) of the bony labyrinth; and endochondral (*Ench.l.*) wider layer with the cartilaginous rests (*Cr.*). × 32.5. (Courtesy of Dr. E. W. Hagens.)

acute otitis media or a preceding mastoid operation is usually obtained.

A serous labyrinthitis secondary to a circumscribed labyrinthitis would have similar but less severe symptoms due to some compensation that may have developed from the circumscribed labyrinthitis. The fistula test would be positive unless blocking of the fistula has occurred. A history of previous labyrinthine symptoms from the circumscribed labyrinthitis could be obtained. The temperature in serous labyrinthitis is normal or near normal.

Differential Diagnosis. The degree and permanence of the hearing loss are important in the differential diagnosis of the serous from the suppurative forms of labyrinthitis. In the serous type, the temporary hearing loss is usually not great, whereas in diffuse suppurative labyrinthitis, the hearing loss is total and permanent. If the hearing loss is great or complete in serous labyrinthitis, an early change into the diffuse suppurative type is possible.

If hearing loss is marked, masking of the good ear is necessary to prevent the transmission of sound to the better ear through bone conduction. If some hearing, however small, is present in the affected ear, a diffuse suppurative labyrinthitis has not occurred, and the vestibular tests are not necessary to demonstrate a partially functioning labyrinth.

Diffuse serous labyrinthitis should be differentiated from noninflammatory diseases of the labyrinth and eighth nerve.

Prognosis. The prognosis in serous labyrinthitis is good in terms of survival and usually complete restoration of labyrinthine function unless the serous form changes into the suppurative type. A severe temporary

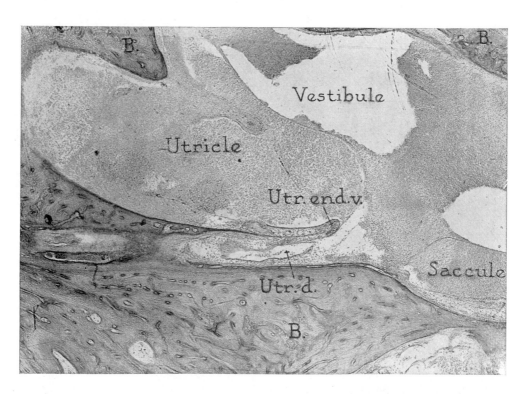

FIG. 51–9.   Acute suppurative labyrinthitis. E.M., female, 13 months of age, had a history of a bilateral otitis media with fever and convulsions. A mastoid operation done on the left ear was followed by death 2 weeks later. The post-mortem examination revealed a pneumococcal meningitis and a bilateral osteitis and labyrinthitis. This section shows extensive purulent exudate throughout the vestibule, saccule, utricle, and utricular duct (*Utr.d.*). The utriculoendolymphatic valve (*Utr.end.v.*) is shown very clearly. The bony labyrinth (*B*) is normal. × 32.5. (Courtesy of Dr. E. W. Hagens.)

type of deafness may result in some permanent hearing loss in serous labyrinthitis.

Treatment. Absolute bed rest is indicated during the acute stage. Mild sedation may be given. Antibiotics should be used in sufficient quantity and long enough to reach maximum efficiency.

Surgery is contraindicated. Adequate drainage of the middle ear should be maintained and in a later stage of an acute otitis media, simple mastoidectomy may be necessary. Tympanomastoidectomy may be advisable if a cholesteatoma with a fistula is present.

Acute Diffuse Suppurative Labyrinthitis

Acute diffuse suppurative labyrinthitis is characterized by complete deafness in the affected ear, associated with extreme vertigo (as a rule), nausea, vomiting, ataxia, and spontaneous nystagmus directed to the good ear.

Etiology. Suppurative labyrinthitis may follow a circumscribed type or it may develop from the induced serous form in which the infection enters through the round or oval windows. In many instances, the labyrinthitis is secondary to an acute or chronic otitis media or mastoiditis. In some cases, a subdural abscess or a meningitis extends into the interior of the bony labyrinth with or without a middle ear involvement.

Pathology. The pathology consists of an infiltration of the labyrinth with polymorphonuclear leukocytes, combined with destruction of the soft tissue structures (Figs. 51–10 to 51–13). The osseous labyrinth

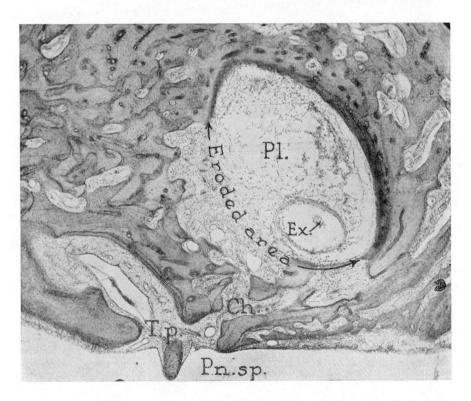

FIG. 51–10.   Acute diffuse suppurative labyrinthitis. R.B., male, 3 years of age, with a history of acute high fever and neck rigidity associated with a sudden onset of total bilateral deafness. The post-mortem examination revealed a meningococcic suppurative meningitis and a bilateral suppurative labyrinthitis. The section through the superior semicircular canal shows the perilymph space (*Pl.*) practically filled with cellular material, which as a result of the bone erosions is in continuity through channels (*Ch.*) with the tunica propria (*T.p.*) of a large pneumatic space (*Pn.sp.*). A cellular exudate (*Ex.*) can be seen in the endolymphatic canal. × 18. (Courtesy of Dr. E. W. Hagens.)

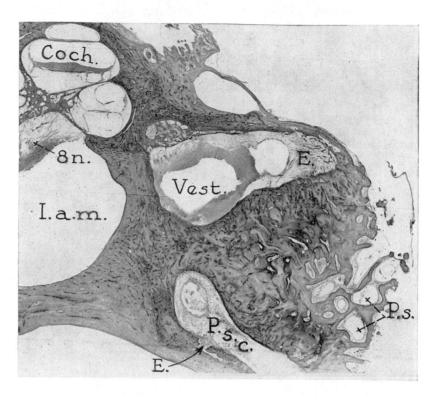

Fig. 51–11. R. B. Acute diffuse suppurative labyrinthitis with erosion through the posterior semicircular canal. Section through the right cochlea and vestibule shows extensive cellular exudate in the vestibule (*Vest.*). The utricle, saccule, and cristae are destroyed. Erosions (*E.*) are noted in the semicircular canal region. The cochlea in the left upper corner, the posterior semicircular canal, and the pneumatic space (*P.s.*) show cellular infiltration. *I.a.m.* is the internal auditory meatus. ×7.05. (Courtesy of Dr. E. W. Hagens.)

may become carious in part. Granulation tissue forms which may at times wall off a portion of the necrotic bone, forming one or more sequestra. Paralysis of the facial nerve may occur, or the infection may extend to the intracranial structures if it is virulent.

Symptoms. Nausea, vomiting, vertigo, and ataxia are severe if the onset of the suppurative labyrinthitis is rapid. In the slower-developing form, these symptoms may be somewhat moderated because of the compensating action of the opposite labyrinth.

The quick component of the horizontal rotary nystagmus is directed to the good ear. If the patient is observed in the first few hours of the disease before the function of the vestibular labyrinth has been destroyed, the nystagmus may be to the affected labyrinth.

Cochlear function is abolished, resulting in complete and permanent deafness in the affected ear. The temperature is normal or near normal, and if much elevation is present, it is probably due to other factors, such as the otitis media or mastoiditis. As a rule, there is an absence of pain, and if present, it is probably due to lesions other than the labyrinthitis.

During the acute stage the position of the patient is characteristic. The patient will lie on the sound ear and direct his eyes toward the affected side, i.e., in the direction of the slow component of the nystagmus. This position reduces the vertigo.

Reaction to caloric stimulus of the affected ear is absent. Neither caloric nor rotational tests should be done during the acute stage, as the vertigo would be greatly

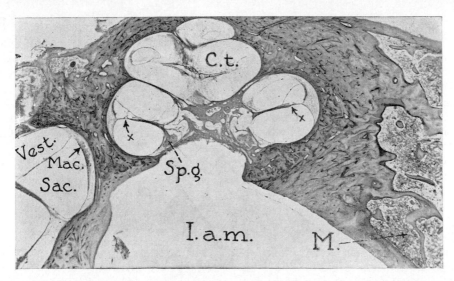

FIG. 51–12.   R. B. Acute diffuse suppurative labyrinthitis. The section through the left
ear shows the cochlea with only a rudimentary organ of Corti (x) in the basal coil. Considerable
connective tissue (*C.t.*) is seen throughout except in the scala tympani of the basal coil. The
spiral ganglion (*Sp.g.*) is present in the basal coil but is mostly absent elsewhere. In the vestibule
(*Vest.*), the saccule (*Sac.*) with its macula (*Mac.*) can be seen. At the level of sectioning the
eighth nerve does not appear in the internal auditory meatus (*I.a.m.*). Marrow spaces are seen,
as at M. ×8.9. (Courtesy of Dr. E. W. Hagens.)

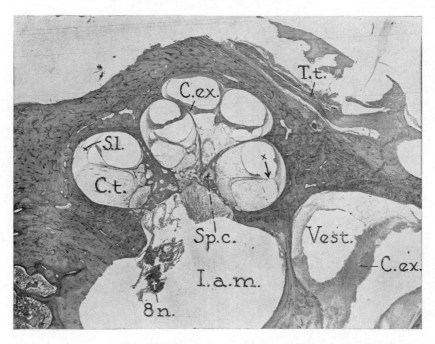

FIG. 51–13.   R. B. Acute diffuse suppurative labyrinthitis. The section through the right ear
shows connective tissue (*C.t.*) filling in the scala tympani of the cochlea and practically merging with the spiral ligament (*S.l.*). The organ of Corti has been destroyed, leaving only the basilar
membrane (x). Considerable cellular exudate (*C.ex.*) is noted in the middle and apical coils.
The spiral ganglion cells are practically absent from the spiral canal (*Sp.c.*). A part of the
eighth nerve (*8n.*) is in the internal auditory meatus (*I.a.m.*). An extensive cellular exudate (*C.ex.*)
in the vestibule (*Vest.*) and the tensor tympani muscle (*T.t.*) can be seen. × 8.9. (Courtesy of
Dr. E. W. Hagens.)

enhanced. If hearing in the involved ear is demonstrable, even though greatly reduced, it may be assumed that a diffuse suppurative labyrinthitis has not yet occurred. In other words, any hearing yet remaining indicates a partially functioning labyrinth, and the caloric and rotational tests are superfluous.

Diagnosis. The diagnosis is made from the history, signs, and symptoms of a labyrinthine upset in which a complete and permanent loss of function (acoustic and vestibular) of the affected labyrinth occurs. Roentgen-ray examinations of the middle ear, mastoid, and petrous pyramid may reveal some disease extraneous to the labyrinth. If meningeal irritation is suspected, spinal fluid examinations should be done.

Prognosis. An uncomplicated acute labyrinthitis has a favorable prognosis so far as

life is concerned. With modern antibiotic therapy, the prognosis of any complicating meningitis has been so successful that these agents rather than labyrinthine surgery should be given an adequate trial. If signs and symptoms of intracranial involvement persist despite adequate treatment with antibiotics, some form of labyrinthine drainage will give a better prognosis than if surgery is withheld.

Treatment. Absolute bedrest is essential during the acute phase, which may last for up to 6 weeks. Improvement usually occurs gradually, however, from the first day on. Mild sedation may be necessary in the early period. Phenobarbital, 32 mg (½ grain), given three or four times a day is satisfactory in most instances.

Adequate doses of antibiotics should be given for an extended period both to prevent

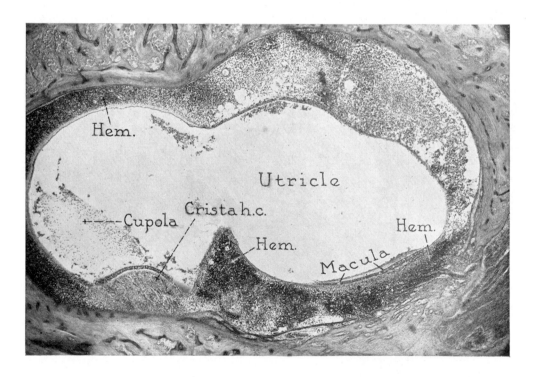

FIG. 51–14. Latent labyrinthitis. H.C., male, 5 years of age, had a history of acute drowsiness with stiffness of the neck. The necropsy revealed an influenza bacillus type of suppurative meningitis. The temporal bones showed a bilateral osteitis and labyrinthitis. The section through the vestibule demonstrates the characteristic findings of influenza in a hemorrhagic condition (*Hem.*) of the perilymph space. The macula of the utricle is seen, as well as the crista of the horizontal semicircular canal (*Crista h.c.*) with cells infiltrating the cupola. ×35. (Courtesy of Dr. E. W. Hagens.)

an intracranial extension and to cure the labyrinthitis. Cultures should be obtained to identify the organism and to demonstrate its antibiotic sensitivity. Prompt institution of treatment either with penicillin or with tetracyclines if the patient is penicillin-sensitive is indicated. Large doses administered parenterally are required. Clinical response supersedes sensitivity testing in determining continued administration or change in the antibiotic.

Drainage or removal of a portion of the destroyed labyrinth would be indicated if intracranial complication is present and is not responding to adequate antibiotic therapy. The presence of even a small amount of hearing in the affected side indicates a partially functioning labyrinth and contraindicates labyrinthine surgery.

Chronic (latent) Diffuse Labyrinthitis

The chronic or latent stage of diffuse suppurative labyrinthitis begins at or shortly after the acute vestibular symptoms have subsided. This may be from 2 to 6 weeks after the onset of the acute period.

Pathology. About the end of the tenth week after the beginning of the acute stage, the internal ear is almost filled with granulation tissue. Some infected areas may still be present, however. The granulations gradually change into fibrous tissue with a beginning calcification. New bone formation may partly or completely fill the labyrinthine spaces in from 6 months to several years in about 50% of the cases. Figures 51–14 to 51–16 show different stages of latent labyrinthitis.

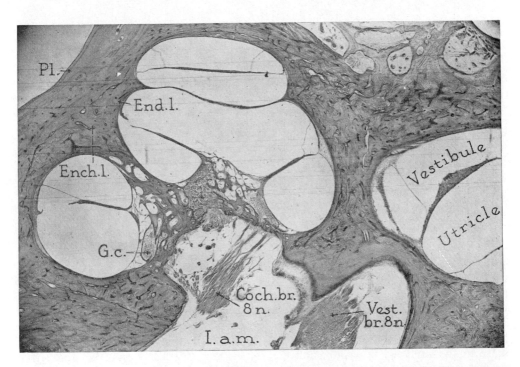

FIG. 51–15. Latent (atrophic) labyrinthitis. R. F., female, 14 years of age, gave a history of measles 1 year before, followed by a bilateral suppurative otitis media with severe bilateral deafness. There was an immediate history of headache, fever, and projectile vomiting accompanied by an acute right mastoiditis. The necropsy revealed an early meningitis and a mixed type infection pneumonia. The temporal bones showed an osteitis and an atrophic labyrinthitis, with a total absence of the organ of Corti. In the basal coil there are relatively few spiral ganglion cells (*G.c.*), and these are partly degenerated. In the internal auditory meatus (*I.a.m.*), the cochlear division of the eighth nerve, and also the vestibular branch, with Scarpa's ganglion cells, can be observed. The endosteal layer (*End.l.*) of the bony labyrinth, the wide endochondral layer (*Ench.l.*), and the periosteal layer (*P.l.*) are well demarcated. ×17. (Courtesy of Dr. E. W. Hagens.)

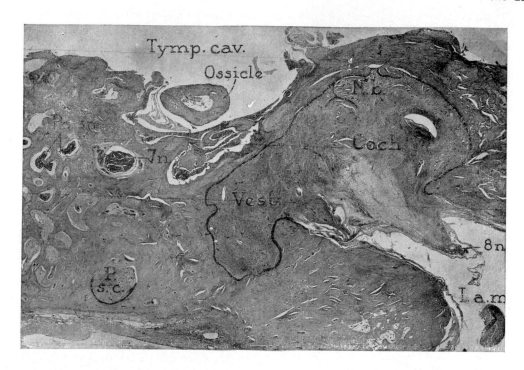

Fig. 51–16. Final stage of latent labyrinthitis. M.R., female, 35 years of age, had a history of unilateral otitis media and mastoiditis with late intracranial complications. The post-mortem examination revealed intracranial complications with a very latent stage of unilateral labyrinthitis. The section through the labyrinth shows an extensive fibrosis and new bone (*N.b.*) filling in the cochlea (*Coch.*) and vestibule (*Vest.*). All traces of the membranous labyrinth are gone. The eighth nerve, in the internal auditory meatus (*I.a.m.*), is partially destroyed; only a few Scarpa's ganglion cells are present. Pus has infiltrated the fibers. The incus (ossicle) can be seen in the tympanic cavity (*Tymp. cav.*). Infected pneumatic spaces (*Pn.sp.*) may be seen with the seventh nerve (*7n.*) close by. A cross section of the posterior semicircular canal (*P.s.c.*) is filled with fibrous tissue and bone. The border of the cochlea and vestibule and a portion of the posterior semicircular canal are outlined for better definition. ×8.5. (Courtesy of Dr. E. W. Hagens.)

Symptoms. Complete deafness in the affected ear is present. A slight vertigo and spontaneous nystagmus, usually toward the good ear, may persist for several months or until compensation by the remaining labyrinth has occurred. Caloric tests elicit no response in the involved labyrinth, and the fistula test is negative even though a fistula may be present. The discharge from the ear may be absent, or it may be present in a remaining focus in the labyrinth or other portions of the temporal bone.

Treatment. Local treatment should be directed toward any infection that may be present.

Surgical drainage or exenteration of the labyrinth is not indicated unless a focus of infection in the labyrinth or perilabyrinthine region has extended to, or is suspected of extending to, the intracranial structures and is not responding to antibiotic therapy.

A mastoidectomy may be done, if indicated. If a focus of infection in the labyrinth or the petrosa is suspected, the labyrinth may be drained by one of the labyrinthine operations. Any loose sequestra found should be removed, care being taken to avoid injuring the facial nerve. If the facial nerve is paralyzed, its canal should be decompressed as described in Chap. 57.

If temporal bone surgery is performed, adequate antibiotic therapy should be instituted both before and after the operation.

SEQUESTRUM OF THE LABYRINTH

Etiology. Various degrees of sequestration of the osseous labyrinth may be associated with or follow:

1. An acute or chronic suppurative labyrinthitis.

2. An injury to the osseous labyrinth, especially following an operative procedure on the temporal bone.

3. Any of the granulomatous diseases affecting the ear, such as tuberculosis, syphilis, etc.

4. A petrositis with necrosis extending to the bony labyrinth with sequestration of the labyrinth.

5. A dormant infection of the petrosal air cells flaring up and suddenly producing necrosis of the bony labyrinth.

Sequestration is more frequently observed in children but may be found at any age. Tuberculosis of the temporal bone in infants and children is especially prone to necrosis with sequestration of the labyrinth.

A circumscribed labyrinthitis with a fistula secondary to a cholesteatoma or a granuloma may produce localized sequestra of the labyrinth of varying sizes.

Pathology. The scanty blood supply of the middle or endochondral layer of the otic capsule results in a much reduced tendency to heal following an injury or an infection. This is not true of the thin, compact endosteal layer or of the outer or periosteal layer which contains haversian lamellae with many blood vessels. If an infection reaches the middle or endochondral layer by way of an erosion or injury through either the periosteal or the endosteal layers, the development of a labyrinthine fistula or the formation of an endochondral sequestrum is possible. Healing of defects of endosteal or enchondral layers is furnished from the periosteal layer by the formation of a compact lamellar bone.

The tendency toward a relatively greater pneumatization of the petrous pyramid superior and posterior to the labyrinth and medial to the arcuate eminence, combined with a constricted exit from these air cells, predisposes to necrosis with sequestration of a portion or all of the labyrinth. A tendency toward intracranial invasion is also enhanced thereby.

Diagnosis. A sequestrum of the labyrinth, while difficult to diagnose preoperatively, may be suspected if a persistent otalgia, profuse otorrhea, exuberant granulations, and a marked or complete loss of labyrinthine function in the affected ear are present following a labyrinthitis or a perilabyrinthitis.

Probing of the necrotic ear, while not always advisable, may detect the sequestrum.

Roentgen-ray studies may indicate an erosion or even suggest a sequestrum of the bony labyrinth.

Prognosis. The sequestrum in some instances may be absorbed, or it may be expelled spontaneously with or without alterations of the bony labyrinth. Drainage, surgical or otherwise, and removal of the sequestrum and all areas of infection in the temporal bone give a reasonably good prognosis. If drainage or removal of the infected and necrotic areas is not effected, extension to the intracranial structures or to the carotid artery may occur.

The facial nerve becomes involved in many instances, but complete recovery may take place after the subsidence of the infection, especially if the paralysis is only partial. If the nerve is partly destroyed, a nerve transplant may be necessary.

Treatment. If sequestration of the labyrinth is suspected, full and adequate doses of antibiotic should be given until there is evidence that further use of these agents is useless.

No hard and fast rule can be given as to the indications for surgical drainage and removal of the sequestrum. Each case should be judged by itself. In general, however, if a sequestrum can be diagnosed with reasonable certainty and total loss of labyrinthine function has occurred, some form of surgical drainage and removal of the necrotic areas should be done. If the sequestrum is firmly attached, removal may be deferred until the separation is more complete.

SURGERY OF SUPPURATIVE LABYRINTHITIS

The advent of effective antibiotic therapy, combined with early diagnosis and surgical correction of causative ear disease, has made labyrinthine drainage a rare procedure. However, suppurative labyrinthitis followed by signs of meningeal irritation requires prompt surgical drainage of the labyrinth. Many authors have described specific procedures for opening various segments of the labyrinth (Hinsberg, Jansen, Neumann, Bourget, Richards, etc.), but the variations in these operations are not truly significant.

Technique. Prior to opening of the labyrinth, a complete radical mastoidectomy should be performed, particular care being taken to remove all diseased mastoid cells which may otherwise be a source of infection. The details of this procedure are given under Surgery in Chronic Ear Disease, Ch. 50. As described in that chapter, the procedure is carried out with the operating microscope.

The drainage of the labyrinth is carried out by first opening the ampullae of the horizontal and vertical semicircular canals and joining these openings at their junction with the vestibule. The membranous contents are then removed with a pick and suction. The stapes is then removed and the oval and round windows joined in one opening by removing the bone of the promontory between the windows (Fig. 51–17). The drainage thus accomplished achieves effective control of the labyrinthine infection and removes the danger of its spread to the meninges and brain.

PETROSITIS

Petrositis is not really a complication of ear infection but rather an extension of the infection into the mastoid cells surrounding the labyrinthine capsule. Not only may infection follow this course, but cholesteatoma may invade these cells, creating an extremely difficult therapeutic problem. Fortunately, the mastoid sclerosis accompanying most

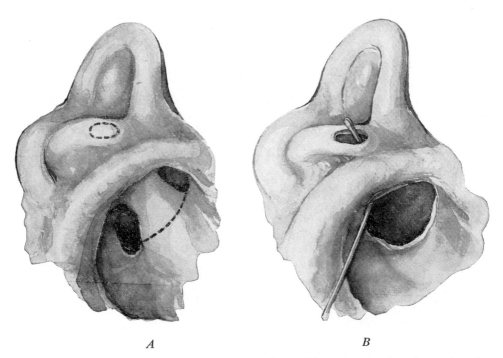

A   *B*

FIG. 51–17. The Hinsberg operation. *A,* The plate of bone, separating the oval and round windows, to be removed. *B,* A probe has been inserted through the newly created opening into the vestibule and out through the opening into the lateral canal. The facial ridge separates the two openings.

chronic ear disease blocks this avenue of spread, so that it is usually seen only in well-pneumatized temporal bones after acute otitis media.

Infection of the petrous cells occurs with most mastoid infections but does not constitute a separate problem, since it resolves as the total infection is treated. In the preantibiotic era, resolution of infection in these cells was usually delayed because of poor drainage. This caused an important problem not always solved by the simple mastoidectomy performed in treating the mastoiditis. These same factors are present today in resistant infections not treated with thorough mastoidectomy to open all diseased cell tracts. The retained infection has a tendency to break through the posterior or superior walls of the petrous bone, being a major source of otogenic meningitis.

Diagnosis. The diagnosis of petrositis is not made frequently today and, because of unfamiliarity, is sometimes missed. The diagnosis should be first suspected in any case with persistent infection and discharge after adequate treatment of otitis media and mastoiditis, or following mastoidectomy. Radiographs should be reexamined to detect clouding and rarefaction of the petrous cells. Deep-seated ear pain accompanying the persistent discharge is an even more definite clue to the presence of petrositis.

Gradenigo's syndrome involves otorrhea, pain around the eye, and diplopia due to abducens nerve paralysis. This is a definite indication of disease in the petrous apex. Also accompanying petrositis may be mild vertigo, transient facial nerve paralysis, and low-grade intermittent fever.

Treatment. The treatment of persistent petrous cell infection is to provide adequate drainage by opening the diseased cell tracts to the mastoid cavity (Fig. 51–18). This is best done by initial adequate mastoidectomy

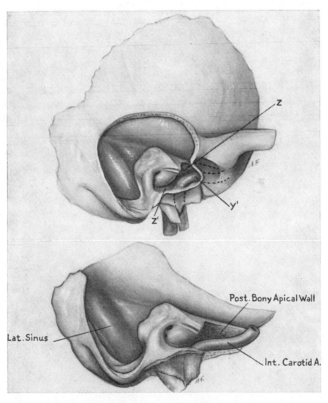

FIG. 51–18.   A dissection showing the areas of cellular spaces in the petrous portion of the temporal. It may be necessary to open any or all of these in petrositis. *y'*, Transverse apical portion of internal carotid artery; *z*, bony wall of posterior fossa at petrous apex approached anterior to cochlea and above carotid artery; *z'*, jugular bulb.

to visualize the involved groups of cells (see Surgery in Chronic Ear Disease, Ch. 50). The posterior cells proceed medially from Troutmann's triangle, outlining the labyrinthine capsule superiorly and posteriorly. Cells opening in the attic region may run through the arch of the superior semicircular canal or anterior to the canal over the cochlea. There may be a cell tract opening below the posterior semicircular canal running to the region below the internal auditory canal. The most difficult cell tracts to follow are those running anterior to the cochlea from the eustachian tube and carotid region. Opening these requires a preliminary radical mastoidectomy with sacrifice of the tympanic membrane and enlargement of the external auditory canal anteriorly. The cells are then followed by opening the medial wall of the eustachian tube just above the carotid artery.

Antibiotics selected by culture and sensitivity tests of the aural discharge are given for several days following surgery.

Fortunately, this disease is rarely seen today, so that the extensive surgery described above is not often needed. For this reason, it is recommended that the surgeon who undertakes this procedure have access to a temporal bone laboratory so that these dissections may be practiced periodically in order that familiarity with the highly complex, compact anatomy is not lost.

FACIAL NERVE PARALYSIS

Functional involvement of the facial nerve is not unusual in both acute and chronic disease of the middle ear and mastoid. This complication is discussed in Chapter 57.

REFERENCES

Dawes, J. D. K.: In Scott-Brown, Ballantyne, and Groves (Eds.): *Diseases of the Ear, Nose and Throat*. 2nd ed. London, Butterworths, 1965, p. 479.

Knauer, W. J.: Gradenigo's Syndrome. Arch. Otolaryng., 44:404, 1946.

Lederer, F. L., and Torok, N.: In Schenk, H. P. (Ed.): *Otolaryngology*. Vol. II, Chapter 16. Hagerstown, W. F. Prior Co., 1966.

Lempert, J.: In Schenk, H. P. (Ed.): *Otolaryngology*. Vol. II, Chapter 18. Hagerstown, W. F. Prior Co., 1960.

Lindsay, J. R.: Pathology of Vertigo Arising from the Peripheral Vestibular Apparatus. Ann. Otol. Rhinol. Laryngol., 56:541, 1947.

Proctor, B., *et al.*: Sequestration of the Osseous Labyrinth. Arch. Otolaryng., 37:819, 1943.

Proctor, C. A.: Intracranial Complications of Otogenic Origin. Laryngoscope, 76:288, 1966.

Shambaugh, G.: *Surgery of the Ear*. 2nd ed. Philadelphia, W. B. Saunders Co., 1967.

Chapter 52
Otosclerosis

Otosclerosis is a primary disease of the labyrinthine capsule characterized by foci of new bone formation. Clinically it is marked by conductive hearing loss due to stapedial fixation and in many instances by progressive sensorineural hearing loss.

Although the basic factors initiating the formation of otosclerotic bone are unknown, the tendency is known to be inherited. A great amount of the epidemiologic facts of otosclerosis were gathered by Stacy Guild, who studied a large number of temporal bones obtained at routine post-mortem examination. These and other statistics reveal that the disease is widespread, being noted in 9.3% of the specimens from a white population. Stapedial fixation was present in only 12% of the cases demonstrating otosclerosis, however. The disease is much less prevalent in Negroes, being noted in only 1% of these specimens. Otosclerosis is unequally distributed between the sexes, being present in 1 of every 8 females but in only 1 of every 15 males.

Pathology

The otosclerotic focus is similar in most respects to normal fibrous bone. The major difference lies in the microstructure of the bony matrix, which in normal capsular bone is lamellar or mosaic in appearance but in otosclerotic bone has a warp and woof pattern similar to that seen in healing bone or a callus.

Otosclerotic foci have been described in all portions of the labyrinthine capsule. Most often (80 to 90%) the focus occurs anterior to the stapes footplate in the region of the fissula ante fenestram—"the site of predilection." The border of the round window is the second most frequently involved site (30 to 50%). In about half the cases there is a single focus, and in the rest two or more foci. The endosteal layer of the capsule seems to limit the spread of the lesion, although an irritative hypertrophy of the endosteum has been described, and occasionally invasion of the vestibule or cochlea has been seen to occur.

In general, the otosclerotic focus consists of irregular areas of new bone formation with many vascular channels occurring on and within the dense bone of the labyrinthine capsule. The borders of the lesion are sharply defined but irregular, with projections along the vessels of the surrounding normal capsular bone. A border of blue-staining bone (with hematoxylin-eosin) is seen around a few of the vascular channels in the focus. These are called "blue mantles" and are typical of the otosclerotic lesion (Fig. 52–1).

The microscopic appearance has been divided into several forms, any or all of which may be present in a single otosclerotic lesion, consisting of a newly formed matrix with beginning mineralization, or in a mature inactive focus of compact bone. Wolff and Bellucci describe these forms as follows:

1. Classic type. This occurs in 31% of specimens. It is characterized by many vascular channels showing congestion and stasis accompanied by bony hypertrophy. Many osteoblasts and occasional osteoclasts are present.

2. Fibrotic type (17%). These lesions demonstrate bony hypertrophy, but with fibrous tissue replacement of former vascular spaces (Fig. 52–2). In these lesions osteoblasts and osteoclasts are not found, and areas of aseptic necrosis are present.

3. Osteoporotic type (11%). In this form the hypertrophic bone is also hypervascular, but the vascular spaces are devoid of content, giving the appearance of complete porosity (Fig. 52–3). Here, too, there is necrosis of the osteocytes.

4. Sclerotic type (rare). Few cases show this morphology singly, but the other forms commonly have areas of sclerosis. The bony tissue has been entirely replaced with calcium and contains no vascular channels or viable osteocytes (Fig. 52–4).

5. Hemangiomatous type (rare). This consists of a hypervascular overgrowth of

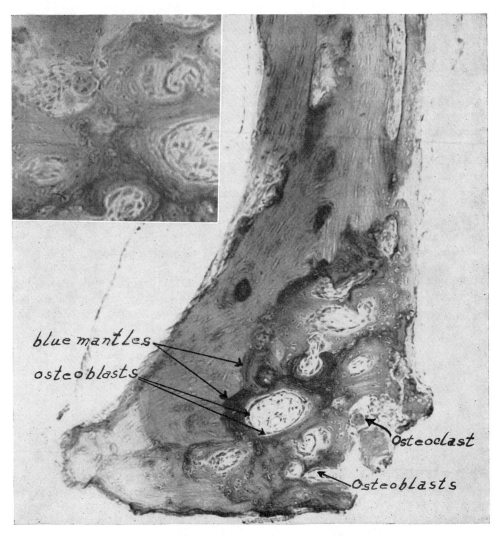

FIG. 52–1. Classic type of otosclerosis in localized area of anterior crus of stapes. Note hypervascularity, enlarged vascular channels bordered by osteoblasts, blue mantles, and viability of diseased bone. (Wolff, D., and Bellucci, R. J.: Arch. Otolaryng., 79:571, 1964.)

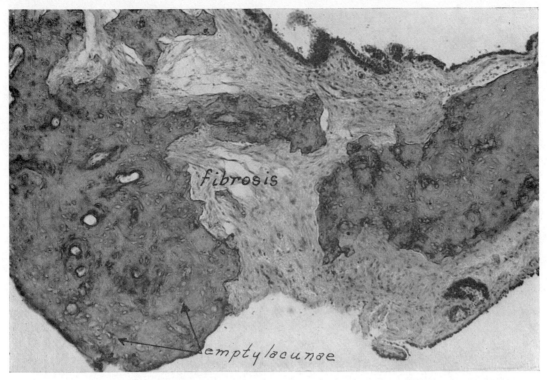

FIG. 52–2. Fibrotic type of otosclerosis. Note the irregularly gouged contour. The bone is partially necrotic with extensive fibrous replacement. (Wolff, D., and Bellucci, R. J.: Arch. Otolaryng., *79*:571, 1964.)

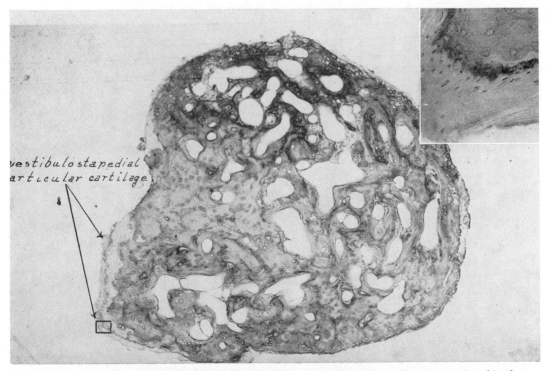

FIG. 52–3. Osteoporotic type of otosclerosis. Note the enlarged vascular spaces devoid of content. Inset shows ossified cartilage cells from anterior margin of footplate. (Wolff, D., and Bellucci, R. J.: Arch. Otolaryng., *79*:571, 1964.)

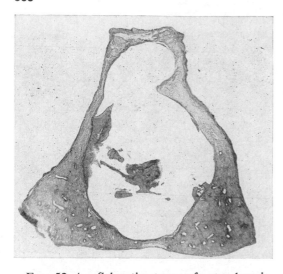

FIG. 52–4. Sclerotic type of otosclerosis. The bone is not viable in any region, and the vascular channels have no viable content. (Wolff, D., and Bellucci, R. J.: Arch. Otolaryng., *79*:571, 1964.)

mucosa, under which lies a large hypervascular bony tumor. This lesion often overgrows the oval window, with obliteration of the niche and invasion of the stapedial articulation.

6. Chelated type (13%). This picture consists of lytic dissolution of bone without osteoclasts but with an appearance of flowing or streaming of the cells of cartilage and bone. The lacunae shift and coalesce with each other (Fig. 52–5).

Wolff and Bellucci emphasize that these types should not be considered stages of the disease but rather variations in microscopic pathology. In most instances, the otosclerotic lesion will demonstrate many of the above types in different areas. This variation in the picture depends on the interaction of three important factors in bone physiology —the blood supply to the area, the state of acidity of the tissue fluids, and the enzymes and hormones contained in the tissue fluid.

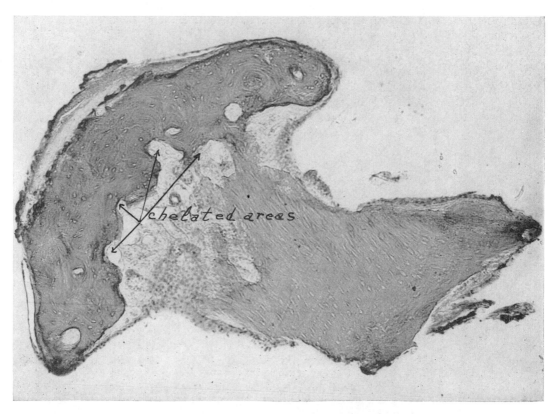

FIG. 52–5. Chelated type of otosclerosis. Chelated areas contain deposits of osteoid. (Wolff, D., and Bellucci, R. J.: Arch. Otolaryng., *79*:571, 1964.)

Pathogenesis and Etiology

The development of the above described lesions has long been shrouded in mystery, although investigations into this question have been undertaken since the lesion was first described (Politzer, 1893). The factors which influence the development of otosclerosis may be categorized as constitutional, local, and/or general activating factors.

The *constitutional* factors which have been best defined are heredity and race. A positive family history may be obtained in 50 to 60% of those suffering hearing loss from otosclerosis. This is indeed a high frequency, since histologic otosclerosis is much more common than clinical otosclerosis. Because of the difficulty of recognizing otosclerosis in the absence of hearing loss, the mendelian pattern has yet to be defined, since histologic study of temporal bones from complete families has not yet been done. The most thorough family studies indicate that otosclerosis is a monohybrid autosomal dominant inheritance with a penetrance of 40 to 50%.

Van der Hoeve's syndrome of osteogenesis imperfecta, blue sclera, and otosclerosis is rare but definitely hereditary, and both Fowler and Shambaugh have noted a correlation between blue sclera and otosclerosis in patients without frequent fractures.

Racial patterns have been noted in otosclerosis, with occurrence ten times more frequent in Caucasians than in Negroes. The disease is also more prevalent in India than in China or Japan.

Local Factors. Many local conditions have been cited as influencing the development of the otosclerotic focus. The most prominently mentioned is the presence of the fissula ante fenestram at the site of predilection of the lesion. This is a small channel filled with connective tissue in the adult, but in early stages of development it is surrounded by cartilage which may persist into adult life. It is felt that unstable cartilaginous elements may result in new bone formation or otosclerosis. Foci of otosclerosis posterior to the stapes may result from the presence of a similar structure—the fissula post fenestram—and foci at other areas result from cartilaginous rests which have been

seen to persist in many regions of the labyrinthine capsule long after ossification is otherwise complete.

This explanation has not satisfied many workers, and the theory of bony stress due to extrinsic forces or to intrinsic developmental torsion has been proposed by Mayer and by Sercer. These forces seem to develop the greatest strain at the site of predilection, and the tendency for new bone formation in this region is explained. Vascular and vasomotor influences upon the bone of the labyrinthine capsule have also been mentioned as possible local etiologic factors.

It has been pointed out by Frost that the basic cause of otosclerosis must lie in the formation of cementum by the osteoblasts, as controlled by their enzyme systems. Abnormal chemical constituents have been identified in the matrix of otosclerotic bone. At present, a great deal of research is concentrated in this area which will hopefully be able to define the genetically determined abnormal enzyme systems responsible for this disease.

General Activating Factors. Sex and age seem to be interrelated factors. The incidence in females is double that in males (65 versus 35%), and the period of activity of the disease correlates closely with the period of fertility. Only in rare instances has the disease been found before puberty or with an onset after 50. On the average, onset occurs between the ages of 20 and 25. In women with otosclerosis, more rapid progression of the hearing loss during or shortly after pregnancy is a common history in about 50%.

Diagnosis

Typically otosclerosis has its onset in early adult life, although the hearing loss may be ignored until middle age. After onset, the hearing deficit is slowly progressive. Female patients may tell of more rapid progression or onset during or shortly after pregnancy. Although a history of ear infection during childhood may be obtained occasionally, this is only a chance relationship and has no bearing on the hearing loss either historically or objectively. Only 1 to 2% of those with otitis media will suffer a concomitant otosclerosis. Although the hearing loss may be quite severe, speech discrimination is preserved except in the rare case of cochlear involvement. The patient may tell of being able to hear better in a noisy environment than in quiet, which is known as paracusia willisiana. Tinnitus is often present and is usually a low-frequency conductive type frequently accompanied by an audible pulse. Occasionally it is a high-pitched ringing, most often correlated with the presence of high-tone cochlear dysfunction. A positive family history of hearing loss occurring in early adult or middle age may be obtained in 50 to 60% of the cases.

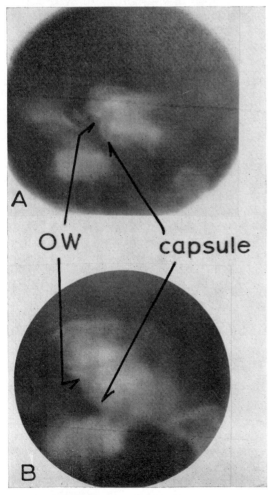

FIG. 52–6. Tomographic section of labyrinthine capsule demonstrating oval window and capsular involvement with otosclerosis. *A,* Normal; *B,* cochlear otosclerosis; *OW,* oval window. (Courtesy of Dr. Valvassori.)

Examination reveals a normal eardrum. Occasionally a pinkish blush may be seen on the promontory, especially with a translucent drumhead. This is the Schwartze sign and is indicative of a highly vascular otosclerotic focus. Pure tone hearing tests reveal a conductive loss of varying severity. Initially the major conductive component is in the lower frequencies due to stiffness of the annular ligament. As the mass of the lesion accumulates and with increasing friction, the conductive loss involves all frequencies. In addition, stapes fixation influences the measured bone conduction by increasing the impedance of the inner ear fluids, causing an apparent bone conduction loss which is maximum at 2000 cps—the "Carhart notch." This apparent loss of bone conduction averages 5 dB at 500 cps, 10 dB at 1000 cps, 15 dB at 2000 cps, and 5 dB at 4000 cps.

In recent times with the advent of tomographic techniques, it has been possible to visualize the otosclerotic focus by radiographic examination (Fig. 52–6). This technique is extremely useful in diagnosis of unusual symptomatology, such as vertigo coupled with mild hearing loss from otosclerosis, or in the severe cases in which bone conduction values cannot be obtained. Also of value in these latter cases is use of the speaking tube coupled with masking of the good ear with a Bárány noisemaker. In some of the patients with severe hearing loss, diagnosis is made by finding good discrimination with the speaking tube, a history of otosclerosis in the family, and a history of being able to use a hearing aid effectively in the past.

Otosclerosis must be differentiated from congenital conductive lesions and acquired ossicular defects due to infection but with an intact drum. Congenital hearing loss is, of course, present from birth and nonprogressive; however, in unilateral cases the date of onset may be equated with the date of discovery, and increasing severity may be mistaken for increasing notice of the defect. Acquired lesions are also nonprogressive but occur later in life, which may serve as a point of confusion. Aseptic necrosis of the incus is said to occur, but this is felt in most cases to be associated with mild ear infection not resulting in tympanic membrane perforation. Although accurate prediction of pathology is desirable, this differentiation is largely academic, since surgical exploration and restoration of hearing are indicated in all of these cases.

LABYRINTHINE OTOSCLEROSIS

It has long been felt by clinicians that there is a higher incidence of sensorineural hearing loss in patients with otosclerosis than in the general population. Statistical studies have not verified this, but temporal bone examination in otosclerosis has shown lesions which have definitely involved the cochlea. The major forms of pathology found in these cases are atrophy of the stria vascularis and degeneration of hair cells in the organ of Corti. In most cases the otosclerosis has been diffuse throughout the capsule, or there has been a large focus with involvement of the endosteum. In only rare cases has the otosclerotic focus itself been found to be sufficient in extent to explain the severity of the hearing loss. The two major theories explaining the presence of cochlear loss are that the otosclerosis releases toxic substances into the cochlea, or that the numerous arteriovenous shunts present in the otosclerotic focus impair the vascular supply of the stria vascularis. Since the degree of sensorineural hearing loss seems to correlate with the degree of involvement of the capsule adjacent to the stria, the latter idea seems to have much merit.

Large-scale studies of patients treated with sodium fluoride over periods of up to 10 years have shown the ability of this agent to prevent sensorineural hearing loss. Although these studies did not incorporate an adequate control group, less than 20% of those given sodium fluoride demonstrated progressive hearing loss, as compared to a much smaller group of untreated patients, 75% of whom had a progressive sensorineural loss. These studies, conducted both in the United States and in France, demonstrated that the optimum effect was obtained with administration of a 20-mg enteric-coated tablet of sodium fluoride twice daily. This dosage should be combined with additional calcium intake, through use of either calcium gluconate or supplementary milk to prevent calcium depletion.

Many instances of labyrinthine hydrops have been reported in association with otosclerosis, with the typical symptoms and findings of Meniere's disease. In some cases this seems to be related to irritative involvement of the vestibule by the otosclerotic focus. In at least one temporal bone a focus of otosclerosis was found obliterating the endolymphatic duct with associated cochlear hydrops. In most instances, stapedectomy will relieve the vertiginous symptoms.

TREATMENT OF OTOSCLEROSIS

Treatment of otosclerosis has been largely restricted to surgical efforts to circumvent the conductive hearing loss characteristic of the disease. The lack of any basic therapy for otosclerosis is related only to the lack of exact knowledge concerning the etiology and pathogenesis of the disease. Undoubtedly basic treatment will evolve as the nature of otosclerosis becomes clear, but until such time our efforts must be directed toward the improvement of hearing in these cases.

Surgery in otosclerosis has followed an interesting historical course. Initial efforts at correcting the stapedial fixation were directed toward breaking through the bony lesion by palpation of the incus and stapes through an incision in the drumhead. This was pioneered by Miot, who reported a series of 200 such procedures in 1890. In 1892, both Blake and Jack reported their experiences with extraction of the stapes for otosclerotic deafness. Although there were many good results reported, many prominent otologists expressed disapproval of these procedures in the early 1900's, and operative intervention was virtually abandoned. Holmgren, however, continued efforts to introduce sound into the cochlea by "decompressing the perilymph" through producing fistulas into the semicircular canals. Sourdille developed this work into a multi-stage fenestration of the lateral semicircular canal, which was later brought to perfection by Lempert with his one-stage fenestration operation. The reliability and predictability of this procedure (80% achievement of practical hearing in selected cases) made it the standard treatment for otosclerosis for 20 years.

In 1952, Rosen rediscovered stapes mobilization, and the obvious advantage of retaining the normal sound conduction mechanism made this a popular procedure. The process of bone healing with subsequent refixation of the stapes became rapidly noted, since less than 30% of these patients maintained hearing over a long term. The concept of bypassing the otosclerotic lesion at the oval window was introduced by E. P. Fowler, Jr., in 1956. He described the anterior crurotomy operation, in which the anterior crus was sectioned and an incision made through the footplate behind the focus of otosclerosis, thus freeing the posterior crus and attached segment of footplate. This procedure was much more successful in accomplishing permanent hearing improvement. A year later Shea again contributed the concept of eliminating disease from the oval window by removing the stapes. Stapedectomy as redefined by Shea with modern techniques and with application of auditory physiology has since become the universally applied operation for otosclerosis.

This is too short a period to be able to predict stabilization of surgical technique. With the passage of time and increasing permanency of results, it may be stated that stapedectomy is the standard procedure today for otosclerosis. The largely repressed thought that history repeats itself is still in the background, however, and the future may see a modified form of fenestration as the "standard" operation. This inconsistency of technique is due only to the nature of the surgical problem of restoring transmission of the maximum possible sound energy as complicated by the still active presence of the otosclerotic process.

SURGICAL LESION

The clinical lesion of otosclerosis at the oval window has several forms, each of which may present a distinct surgical problem. The Otosclerosis Study Group has defined these forms of otosclerosis as localized and diffuse otosclerosis.

The *localized* form may be further differentiated as predominantly an anterior focus, a posterior focus, or with extension around the margins of the oval window.

The *diffuse* forms involve the footplate. They may be *circumscribed*, in which the footplate has a distinct margin, and may be thin or thick (also called "biscuit" type). Diffuse *obliterative* otosclerosis is that in which the annular ligament is invaded and so the footplate has lost a distinct margin. In extreme cases of this type, the entire oval window may be filled with otosclerosis mounding between the promontory and facial nerve. The character of the otosclerosis bone may also vary from a soft hypervascular lesion to a focus of dense bone with little vascularity. The round window may be involved, in some instances to complete obliteration.

INDICATIONS FOR SURGERY

The prediction of hearing result in surgery for otosclerosis is of basic importance to both the surgeon and the patient. This prediction is based upon an accurate estimate of the cochlear reserve and upon an accurate knowledge of the surgeon's own success rate in accomplishing the theoretical ideal result with the particular type of operation performed. Cochlear reserve must be calculated for the individual patient, since pure tone bone conduction audiometry does not give an accurate measure of inner ear function. Fixation and increased mass of the stapes changes the mechanical impedance of the inner ear fluids and thus allows less energy transfer from the bone oscillator. Carhart has measured this loss in a large number of cases, as based on bone conduction threshold change with surgery. As mentioned under Diagnosis, this loss has been estimated at 5 dB at 500 cps, 10 dB at 1000 cps, 15 dB at 2000 cps, and 5 dB at 4000 cps. Correcting the bone conduction audiogram by these amounts will give a more accurate estimate of the functional capacity of the inner ear—the cochlear reserve. Comparing the speech discrimination ability with the pure tone audiogram will further define the rehabilitative capacity of the surgical venture.

The fenestration operation has been shown to have an average 25-dB conductive loss consequent to the loss of the normal middle ear mechanism secondary to this technique. Taking the average 10-dB Carhart notch into account, the successful fenestration will bring the air conduction to within 15 dB of the measured bone conduction for the three important speech frequencies (500, 1000, and 2000 cps). Since an average 30-dB threshold is considered necessary for practical hearing, patient selection is defined within rather narrow limits for the fenestration operation. Shambaugh has defined three categories of suitability for fenestration surgery. In group A is the ideal patient whose bone conductions for the three speech frequencies are within 5 dB of the 0 level after correction for the Carhart notch. Patients in group B are within 5 dB of the 0 level for two of the three speech frequencies, but one, usually 2000 cps, is worse than 5 dB. Patients in group C have two or three of the frequencies worse than 10 dB after correction. This last group is considered unsuitable for fenestration, since the resulting air conduction will average less than 40 dB even with a perfect result. Long-term results showed that 80% of ideal candidates will have a satisfactory hearing result after surgery. Four percent of these cases experienced loss of cochlear function.

Ideally, since stapedectomy completely eliminates the conductive hearing loss, estimate of the cochlear reserve should serve as the predictive level of postoperative hearing. The ideal result would then be an average 10 dB better than the preoperative bone conduction average (overclosure of the bone-air gap). Approximately 50% of patients will equal the predicted air conduction, and 90% will close the bone-air gap to within 10 dB. Loss of cochlear function occurs in less than 1% of stapedectomies. Because of this high probability of largely eliminating the conductive deficit in the otosclerotic patient, this procedure is not reserved for a particular category of patients but has been applied to patients with all degrees of hearing loss, including those with mild losses and those without measurable bone conduction. Stapedectomy may be employed in those patients with unilateral hearing loss, as well as in bilateral cases. It may be stated that stapedectomy may be applied to any patient with a conductive hearing loss whose correction will fill a definite need of the patient.

Surgery should be performed on the poorer hearing ear in all but the most exceptional cases. In the instances of the only hearing ear being considered for surgery, the extreme handicap of total deafness resulting from a bad result should indicate the recommendation of a hearing aid. Severe hearing loss cases may be operated with the understanding that a hearing aid will still be required after surgery. The great improvement in performance with a hearing aid is usually sufficient indication in these latter cases. Surgery may be performed on both ears, but only after a period of 6 to 12 months has passed since the initial surgery. This avoids the chance that a delayed complication might occur, resulting in a total hearing loss.

TECHNIQUE OF STAPEDECTOMY

Years have passed since the introduction of stapedectomy by Shea, but the technique has not yet stabilized to a point at which a "standard" operation exists. The basis of the procedure is to create a patent oval window, seal it with a membrane of either natural or artificial material, and provide a connection between the incus and the neomembrane cover of the oval window. In doing this either all or a part of the stapes footplate is removed; the oval window is covered with vein, mucous membrane, connective tissue, fat, Gelfoam, or collagen membrane; and sound transmission is reestablished with a stapes crus, polyethylene or Teflon tubing, a Teflon or stainless steel piston, stainless steel or tantalum wire, a platinum prosthesis, or a stapes carved from the patient's mastoid cortex. The above is *not* a comprehensive list of the variations of stapedectomy which have been described.

The technique of stapedectomy is further complicated by the variations in surgical pathology, as well as by variations in ossicular anatomy. Because of these factors it has become apparent that a single technique is not suitable for all cases of otosclerosis, and the surgeon must be able to vary his method according to the conditions found at surgery. The surgical approach followed by the author is to use partial stapedectomy with a tissue seal and repositioning of a crus (Hough) whenever possible (in about 90% of the cases). When anatomic or surgical difficulties preclude this, total stapedectomy with tissue seal and a preformed wire loop (House) is performed. In the case of obliterative otosclerosis, the piston technique (Shea) with either Teflon or stainless steel is used to reduce surgical trauma and prevent reclosure of the fistula. The various techniques will be outlined in this order.

The rationale for this series of procedures is based on the expected number of complications with each. Partial stapedectomy results in the most rapid closure of the oval window, because healing progresses both from the edge of the window and from the center where the transposed crus initiates mucous membrane growth. This method avoids the use of artificial prosthetic materials, thus provoking the least possible tissue reaction. A large series of cases in which this method was used resulted in the lowest incidence of cochlear damage reported to date (0.25%). The preformed wire loop and Gelfoam technique of House uses the least mass of foreign material and has the lowest incidence of cochlear damage of all methods using a prosthesis (0.6%). The piston technique of Shea has shown the highest percentage of maintained good hearing in obliterative otosclerosis with the lowest complication rate (80 to 85% success with 3 to 4% cochlear loss). The vein graft with polyethylene tube method first used resulted in a 70% success rate and a complication percentage of 10.

Preparation of the Ear. Stapedectomy is a transcanal operation, and since it is of great importance not to introduce pathogenic bacteria into the middle ear, care must be taken to evaluate the health of the external ear canal prior to surgery. All vestiges of external otitis must be eliminated, since this is felt to be one of the factors responsible for complication. Since many patients will be wearing a hearing aid in the ear to be operated, this should be removed at least 2 weeks prior to surgery. Patients with bilateral hearing loss should be advised to have an ear mold made for the other ear so

that communication will be possible during the immediate postoperative period.

At surgery, the ear canal should be cleansed of loose debris and accumulated cerumen but without trauma which will lower local tissue resistance to infection. Acetone mixed with alcohol in equal proportions is a good germicidal solvent for this purpose. A detergent soap is then used to irrigate the canal without wiping, and after suction drying a protein-iodine complex is used to paint the area. The external ear is prepared in the same manner. It is not usually necessary to remove any hair, but it should be kept out of the field with adhesive spray and drapes.

Anesthesia. Local anesthesia injected in the outer third of the cartilaginous canal and into the incision site is used in these procedures. Adequate patient relaxation is important to avoid positional discomfort and bleeding from increased arterial and venous pressure. For this purpose, heavy premedication is necessary using a combination of a narcotic, a barbiturate, and a tranquilizer. Often it is necessary to supplement this at surgery. At these times the use of a short-acting narcotic agent and a short-acting barbiturate given intravenously is helpful. The thiobarbiturates should be avoided because of their depressant effect, hangover, and risk of laryngospasm. Many new forms of chemical narcosis are being developed, so time will bring even more ideal methods of patient preparation in stapes surgery.

Exposure. Exposure of the oval window region is essential for meticulous operative technique. In this as in all temporal bone operations performed today, the operation microscope is an essential of technique. The use of a speculum holder is necessary to free both hands.

The incision is made in the posterior and superior canal wall (Fig. 52–7). This should be a sufficient distance from the annulus to provide an adequate skin flap to replace against bone regardless of the amount of bone removed from the canal wall for exposure. Bone is removed from the medial end of the posterosuperior canal wall until the entire oval window may be visualized. Curettes may be used for this purpose, but small

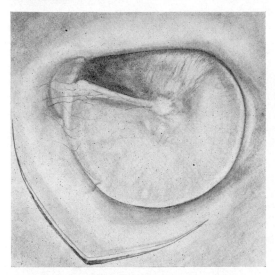

FIG. 52–7. Stapedectomy. The meatal incision is triangular, extending to an apex 7 to 10 mm from the annulus.

diamond burrs driven by a small electric-powered drill provide more speed and control of this dissection. Care should be taken to spare the chorda tympani nerve when possible. Needless sacrifice of the chorda results in a percentage of mild disability which may become more severe if surgery on the opposite ear results in loss of taste function. If the chorda tympani prevents good exposure of the oval window, however, it must be sectioned.

Evaluation of Pathologic Condition. Since selection of surgical technique is based on evaluation of the extent and type of otosclerosis, this should be evaluated at this point. The location and size of the otosclerotic foci, as well as the amount of footplate invasion, should be noted. Obliteration of the oval window with involvement of the crura dictates a piston technique. Total footplate invasion requires removal of the entire footplate, while if only a portion is involved, usually the anterior segment, the normal portion may be preserved. Anatomic factors will also enter into technique selection. A narrow, deep oval window niche may require a thin prosthesis, such as a wire, because use of even the patient's crus may result in scarring and restriction of mobility of the ossicular chain.

Partial Stapedectomy (Hough)

The initial step in every stapedectomy is to transect the footplate so that it may be removed in at least two pieces. This also prevents damage to the cochlea because of the transmission of large pressure waves to the vestibule through the intact footplate. The stapes crus which is involved in the otosclerotic focus, usually the anterior, is then sectioned as far laterally as possible. The most useful instrument for this purpose is a rotating crurotomy saw driven by the small drill. The stapedius tendon is then severed with a scissors and the posterior crus freed from any attachments to the posterior lip of the oval window. If the footplate is normal, a portion is left attached to the crus and freed from surrounding bone until complete mobility is obtained. If the entire footplate is involved with otosclerosis, as evidenced by thickening, the posterior crus is separated from its attachment to the footplate. The stapes is then elevated and placed out of the way on the promontory by upward traction with a right-angled pick placed under the arch of the stapes. The incudostapedial joint is loosened but can be kept intact during this maneuver. The remaining footplate is then removed, this having been made easier by the good visibility now present. In this as in other stapes procedures, dissection on the focus itself should be avoided, if possible, since it is felt that surgical trauma will stimulate bone growth in some cases. The remaining crus, with or without a segment of footplate, is replaced in the middle of the oval window, which is sealed with pieces of compressed Gelfoam placed anteriorly and posteriorly. The steps in partial stapedectomy are shown in Figures 52–8 to 52–10.

Bleeding is controlled throughout the operation with pledgets of Gelfoam moistened with epinephrine 1:1000. If at all possible, there should be no hemorrhage during the time the oval window is open. This is not because blood injures the cochlea but because it increases the risk of surgical trauma due to poor visibility and increased technical difficulty. Often a pause of a minute or two immediately before removal of the foot-

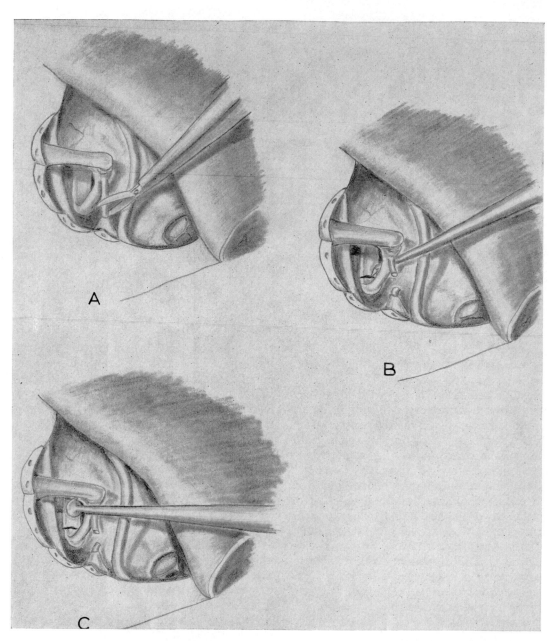

Fig. 52–8.   Partial stapedectomy. *A,* Sufficient bone has been removed from the postero-superior annulus to visualize the entire oval window, and the stapedius tendon is sectioned. *B,* The footplate is transected near the least involved crus. With footplate involvement, the crus is separated from its attachment to the footplate. *C,* The anterior crus is divided near the neck of the stapes.

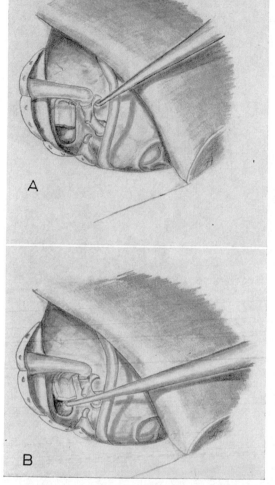

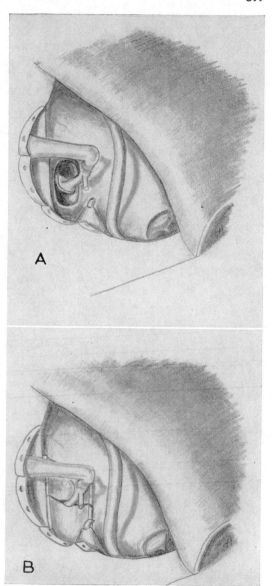

FIG. 52–9. Partial stapedectomy. *A*, The stapes arch is laid inferiorly by elevating the incus to allow this movement. *B*, The remaining footplate is removed from the oval window.

plate results in an entirely dry field and also will relax the surgeon before undertaking this crucial phase of stapedectomy.

The skin flap is carefully replaced and a small amount of packing placed over it to hold it in place. A piece or two of moistened Gelfoam is usually sufficient for this purpose. A small amount of antibiotic dusting powder is blown into the canal. A cotton tampon placed in the outer meatus is an adequate external dressing. Antibiotics are administered as outlined in Chapter 50, Surgery in Chronic Ear Disease.

FIG. 52–10. Partial stapedectomy. *A*, The stapes arch is replaced so that the footplate remnant or the end of the posterior crus lies in the middle of the oval window. A connective tissue membrane may be used to cover the oval window before the stapes is repositioned. *B*, Gelatin sponge is used to maintain the positioning of the stapes.

Total Stapedectomy (House)

Total stapedectomy may prove necessary due to a narrow oval window or accidental loss of the stapes crura. This latter is especially apt to occur if the crura are atrophic. In these cases the remainder of the stapes is removed by separating the incudostapedial joint. The entire footplate is removed, preferably in two pieces. The distance from the long process of the incus to the oval window is measured and the window immediately covered with a piece of compressed Gelfoam. A preformed wire loop as designed by House (or other suitable prosthesis of the surgeon's choice) of the proper length is selected. This should extend to the level of the oval window and not enter the vestibule by more than 0.25 mm. The hook is placed over the incus and the loop centered in the oval window. The hook is crimped so as to fit with some looseness around the incus. If the prosthesis fits too tightly, it may cause necrosis of the long

process due to interference with the blood supply. The prosthesis should be tight enough, however, to prevent its dislodgment during the immediate postoperative period, after which mucosal scarring will hold it securely. The skin flap is then replaced as previously described. Figures 52–11 and 52–12 show steps in total stapedectomy.

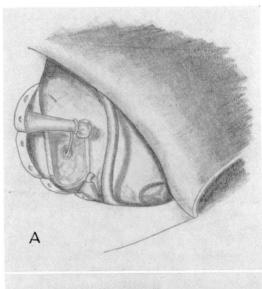

FIG. 52–11. Total stapedectomy. *A,* After the stapedius tendon is cut and the incudostapedial joint separated, the arch of the stapes is fractured by pushing inferiorly. *B,* The footplate is removed in segments after transection.

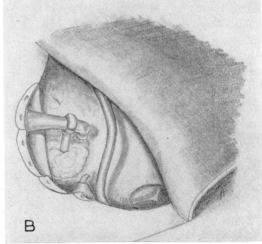

FIG. 52–12. Total stapedectomy. *A,* A preformed wire loop is used to replace the stapes after the oval window is sealed with Gelfoam or connective tissue. *B,* A Teflon piston replaces the stapes and is surrounded with Gelfoam to hold it and seal the oval window. Connective tissue may also be used as a seal.

Partial Stapedectomy with Piston (Shea)

This technique has proved useful in cases of obliterative otosclerosis. Bony regrowth is not uncommon with this form of the disease, and the piston was designed to prevent this regrowth from immobilizing the prosthesis. Teflon is used because of its inertness and the smooth, self-lubricating nature of its surface. Stainless steel has also been used and has some advantage because the steel produces a slight adsorption of bone immediately surrounding it and in this way resists fixation. The main disadvantage of the steel piston is that its length cannot be adjusted so that a variety of slightly differing sizes must always be kept available.

Some surgeons feel that any drilling on the otosclerotic focus will stimulate bone growth and rapid recurrence of the lesion (Fig. 52–13). These surgeons make a hole only large enough to admit the piston through the middle of the footplate with picks and chisel-knives. The experience of others has shown that removal of the mass of otosclerotic bone with burrs until the niche of the oval window is completely delineated is not associated with an increased incidence of bony regrowth. Because of this latter view, the following technique is recommended (Sooy).

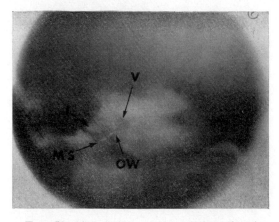

Fig. 52–13. Tomographic section showing regrowth of otosclerotic bone across the oval window (OW), resulting in recurrence of hearing loss. The metal strut (MS) is clearly shown to be attached to the incus (I). V, Vestibule. (Courtesy of Dr. Valvassori.)

The incudostapedial joint is separated and the crura fractured after sectioning of the stapedius tendon. Small cutting burrs used with constant irrigation are then employed to remove the mass of otosclerotic bone filling the oval window niche. The footplate itself is *not* opened but merely thinned to a degree equaling a slightly thick otosclerotic footplate. The bone debris is completely removed, and all bleeding is controlled. The footplate is then removed in a routine manner by transection and piecemeal removal with small angled picks. The oval window need not be opened to its normal extent, a 1- to 2-mm fenestra being sufficient. The distance to the incus is then measured and the piston placed so that the end lies just below the level of the oval window. The opening is then sealed with small pledgets of Gelfoam placed around the piston.

Complications of Stapedectomy. The major complication of stapedectomy is further loss due to cochlear damage. As mentioned before, this will occur in about 1% of cases. Some of the other factors reponsible for this secondary cochlear loss may be bone chips or bone dust in the vestibule, irrigation with an open oval window, rapid "uncorking" of the vestibule by removing the stapes in toto without a pressure-relief hole in the footplate, trauma with instruments to the vestibular contents, too rapid or violent aspiration of perilymph, and infection from bacteria entering or being implanted in the middle ear during surgical procedure.

Delayed cochlear losses seem to be associated with fistula developing in the membrane covering the oval window, sometimes associated with infection. In some instances this has led to meningitis. An occasional delayed hearing loss has seemed to be due to an immune response to foreign protein, although this is largely conjectural.

Tears of the tympanic membrane occasionally occur with creation of the tympano-meatal flap. These are repaired by approximation over Gelfoam or with a vein graft (see Myringoplasty, p. 840). Facial nerve paralysis sometimes occurs, but in most instances this is transient, being due to the local anesthesia. A persistent paresis may be due to scarring or pressure of the prosthesis on a bare facial nerve. This is corrected by removal of the prosthesis and replacement with a wire, which may be bent to fit around an overhanging facial nerve.

FENESTRATION

The anesthesia and skin preparation for fenestration are basically similar to that for stapedectomy. The operation microscope is used in this as in all temporal bone operations. The procedure is done through an endaural incision which is modified from that described in Chapter 50, Surgery in Chronic Ear Disease. The endaural incision is started inferiorly at the junction of the cartilaginous and bony canal, is carried up the posterior canal wall, and is then brought outward between the tragus and root of the helix for 1 to 2 cm. The lower half of the incision is carried to bone, while the upper portion extends to the level of the temporalis fascia to avoid incision of the temporalis muscle. To enlarge the external meatus, a semilunar piece of the cavum conchae is removed by a curved incision extending

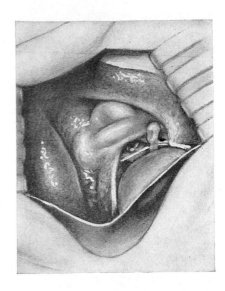

Fig. 52–15. The incus and the pyramidal eminence have been removed. The fenestra ovalis, with the stapes in situ, and the tympanic course of the facial canal are exposed to view. The head and neck of the malleus have been removed. The processus cochleariformis with the tendon of the tensor tympani muscle, the epitympanic course of the facial canal, and the roof of the vestibule are exposed to view. (Lempert, J.: Arch. Otolaryng., 66:35, 1957.)

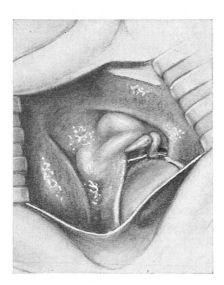

Fig. 52–14. The exposure and sharp definition of the external, superior, and posterior semicircular canals. The tympanomeatal cutaneous membrane has been created. The incudomalleolar joint, the anterior malleolar ligament, and the chorda tympani nerve are exposed to view. (Lempert, J.: Arch. Otolaryng., 66:35, 1957.)

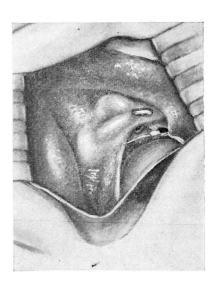

Fig. 52–16. The new oval window, with the utricle exposed to view, is seen in the dome of the vestibule. (Lempert, J.: Arch. Otolaryng., 66:35, 1957.)

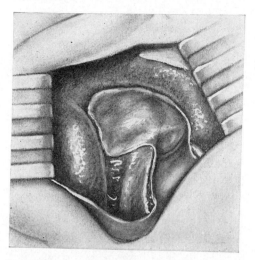

FIG. 52–17. The tympanomeatal membrane in position, with Shrapnell's membrane covering the entire fenestra nov-ovalis. (Lempert, J.: Arch. Otolaryng., 66:35, 1957.)

from the inferior end of the initial incision to the superior margin of the canal. This incision is carried through skin and cartilage to bone, and the segment of concha is discarded. A relaxing incision is then made in the anterior canal wall at the same level as the initial incision. This is started at the middle of the anterior canal wall and is carried posteriorly to meet the first incision. The periosteum is elevated, and after bleeding is controlled, a self-retaining retractor is placed. The operative steps are shown in Figures 52–14 to 52–17.

Preparation of the Tympanomeatal Skin Flap. The entire superior and posterior three fourths of the canal skin is used as a pedicle graft to cover the lateral semicircular canal fenestra and as much mastoid bone as possible. The flap is outlined with two incisions extending from the region of the tympanic annulus outward to the endaural incisions. One incision is made in the midportion of the anterior canal wall and meets the relaxing incision in the anterior canal wall; the other incision is carried up the posteroinferior canal to the start of the initial incision. The skin flap is elevated to the region of the annulus, care being taken not to tear it. The outer portion of the flap is thinned with scissors to aid in placement later. The flap is protected during the bone

dissection by packing it downward with paraffin gauze, which is in turn covered with a thin fiberboard flap protector.

Bone Dissection. Sufficient bone must be removed to expose the attic and mastoid antrum. The entire pneumatic system need not be exenterated, but the posterior canal should be lowered sufficiently to have complete exposure of the mastoid cavity. The antrum and attic are approached through the lateral attic wall, leaving the canal walls thin but intact. Motor-driven cutting burrs and continuous suction-irrigation with physiologic irrigating solution are used in this dissection. The tegmen is skeletonized and followed into the antrum and attic space, where the body and short process of the incus are usually the first landmarks to be seen. The head of the malleus, body of the incus and lateral semicircular canal are identified and exposed. The posterior canal wall is thinned by removing the air cells inferior to the antrum. The superior and posterior canal walls are removed with rongeurs to the point of attachment of the skin flap. The ridge of bone remaining across the attic space is called the "bridge." The skin flap is now elevated to the annulus, which is removed from the sulcus tympanicus to the region of the meatal incisions. The "bridge" is removed with rongeurs and curettes and the facial ridge lowered with diamond burrs. The incus is removed, as is the head of the malleus, after the neck is cut through with a malleus nippers. Any remaining ridges or protrusions of bone are smoothed with diamond burrs.

Creating the Fenestra. The prominence of the lateral semicircular canal is now well exposed. The fenestra is created in the ampullated end of the canal immediately above the stapes. The fenestra should be about the same size as the oval window, about 1.5 by 3 mm. The region of the fenestra is smoothed, still using suction-irrigation, with a diamond burr until the enchondral layer of bone is exposed. This enchondralization should extend from the facial canal over the entire prominence of the lateral canal for at least 5 mm in length. The actual margins of the fenestra are outlined with a small diamond burr by continuing the thinning process until a blue line outlines the fenestral site. This creates a bony cupula which will be fractured away intact in a dry field to open the fenestra. The margins of the fenestra are incised with the point of a fine knife and the cupula lifted with a pick or angled knife.

The skin flap is cleaned of any bone fragments and rotated down to lie over the fenestra. The remaining flap is smoothed over the bare bone of the attic and antrum. To secure good rotation, it may be necessary to make a small angle at the end of the anterior incision. The flap is invaginated mildly into the fenestra, and this is maintained by placing a cotton ball into the depression. This invagination seems to be a major factor in preventing bony closure of the fenestra. The cavity is then filled with Gelfoam and the endaural incision closed. A mastoid pressure dressing is applied to prevent hematoma.

Postoperative Management. Postoperatively, the fenestration patient will experience a period of disability due to the occurrence of serous labyrinthitis lasting from 7 to 14 days. This is marked initially by the onset of vertigo and nystagmus the day following surgery. This is most severe in the first 48 hours. As the vertigo lessens, the patient will notice a decrease in hearing as the cochlea becomes involved. At this point, the Weber test will begin to lateralize to the unoperated ear. These symptoms require hospitalization for an average of 7 days, during which time antiemetic and vestibular suppressant drugs are required to control these reactions.

The mastoid cavity is allowed to heal untouched for 3 weeks, after which bimonthly cleaning is instituted until epithelization is complete. Granulations are controlled with curettage and cautery with 50% silver nitrate solution. Gentian violet is used to dry areas of granulation, and antibiotic dusting powder is blown into the cavity to control infection. The cavity, when healed, will require inspection and cleaning at 6-month intervals from this point on. The patient is instructed to keep water out of his ear while bathing or shampooing. A cotton tampon covered with petrolatum is useful for this purpose. Swimming or other water sports are definitely contraindicated. Any water

entering the ear is best removed by rinsing with warm rubbing alcohol.

Complications of Fenestration. The major problem with fenestration, as with stapedectomy, is the loss of cochlear function due to labyrinthitis. This occurs in 4% of cases. Closure of the fenestra occurs in about 10%. This may be due to fibrous tissue proliferation within the bony labyrinth but is usually the result of bone regrowth. In these latter instances, reoperation is possible.

Injury to the facial nerve is a rare complication in these cases. This is usually transitory and secondary to the heat of the diamond burrs. In some instances a bone chip has impinged on the tympanic portion of the nerve. This is corrected by decompression of the nerve at the site of the injury. The nerve has occasionally been torn by a burr, in which case a graft should be placed immediately (see Facial Nerve Paralysis, Ch. 57).

A source of disability for some patients has been a persistent infection of the mastoid cavity. Every effort should be made to clear this because of the risk of extension of the infection to the labyrinth. In most of these cases revisional surgery of the mastoid accompanied by mastoid obliteration is indicated (see Surgery in Chronic Ear Disease, Ch. 50).

REVISION OF FENESTRATION

Today the best approach to the fenestration failure is with stapedectomy techniques. In these procedures, the stapes is removed, and the sound conduction mechanism is reconstructed with a prosthesis placed between the malleus handle and the oval window. Both preformed wire loops and Teflon pistons have been used for this purpose. With proper patient selection, at least 70% of this group may have their hearing restored to within 20 dB of measured bone conduction.

Patient Selection. The ideal patient for this procedure is one whose hearing improved temporarily after fenestration but regressed because of bony or fibrous closure of the fenestra. Those patients who had a good surgical result but because of poor bone conduction did not achieve serviceable hearing are also good candidates. Those patients who had no result from fenestration despite a patent fenestra as evidenced by a fistula sign are poor candidates. Less than 1 of 4 of this group will experience a hearing improvement with revision.

Operative Technique. Although this is a transcanal procedure as in stapedectomy, the incision must be modified because of the previous mastoid surgery. The incision originates below the fenestra and is brought back onto the facial ridge. The second limb of the incision is carried from the first onto the remaining posteroinferior canal wall as in stapedectomy (Fig. 52–18). The skin flap is elevated, and after the middle ear is entered by dissecting out the annulus, the posterior spine is removed to improve visualization of the oval window region.

The entire stapes is then removed and the ossicular mechanism reconstructed with a prosthesis extending from the malleus handle to the oval window. Sheehy has described the use of a preformed wire loop. A tunnel is formed by dissecting the drum from the malleus handle, through which the upper end of the wire prosthesis is placed so that it may be crimped around the handle. The lower end is placed in the middle of a compressed Gelfoam pad covering the oval window (Fig. 52–19).

A slightly easier method is to use a modified piston, the "house-top" piston, which

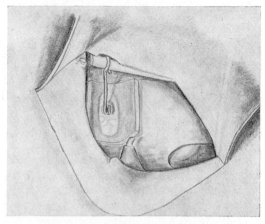

FIG. 52–19. Revision of fenestration. A preformed wire loop is placed between the malleus and the oval window after total stapedectomy (Sheehy).

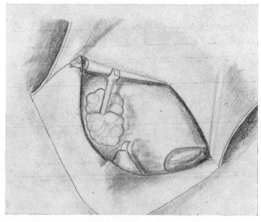

FIG. 52–20. Revision of fenestration. A Teflon piston is placed between the malleus and oval window after total stapedectomy (Shea).

attaches to the undersurface of the malleus by the clamping action of Teflon. The lower end of the piston is again placed in the middle of a compressed Gelfoam seal (Fig. 52–20).

In the unusual instance in which the malleus handle is missing, an incus homograft may be used. In this situation a tissue graft (vein or fascia) is used to cover the oval window and the incus placed as a columella, with the short process resting in the oval window and the articular surface under the drum membrane. This same technique may be used when the malleus is present, as de-

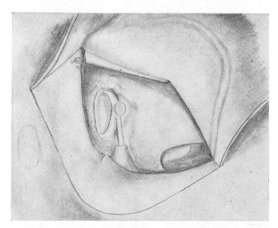

FIG. 52–18. Revision of fenestration. The middle ear is exposed by the indicated flap. Great care should be taken to avoid the fenestra.

scribed and illustrated in Chapter 50, Surgery in Chronic Ear Disease.

The skin flap is returned to its former position and dressed, as in stapedectomy. A common problem is a small gap in the region in which the posterior spine has been removed owing to flap shrinkage. A vein graft is used to fill this defect to prevent postoperative drum perforation.

A major contraindication to this procedure is the presence of infection of the mastoid cavity. This must be completely cleared before surgery, and in many instances a preliminary mastoid obliteration is advisable.

Cochlear loss will occur in about 1% of these procedures.

REFERENCES

Goodhill, V.: *Stapes Surgery for Otosclerosis.* New York, Hoeber Medical Division, Harper & Row, 1961.

Guild, S. R.: Histologic Otosclerosis. Ann. Otol., *53*:246, 1944.

Hough, J. V. D.: Partial Stapedectomy. Trans. Am. Acad. Ophthal. Otolaryng., *66*:412, 1962.

Hough, J. V. D.: Recent Advances in Otosclerosis. Arch. Otolaryng., *83*:379, 1966.

House, H. P.: Prefabricated Wire Loop-Gelfoam Stapedectomy. Arch. Otolaryng., *76*:298, 1962.

Lempert, J.: Fenestra Nov-ovalis Technique. Arch. Otolaryng., *66*:35, 1957.

Linthicum, F. H., Jr.: Correlation of Sensorineural Hearing Impairment and Otosclerosis. Ann. Otol., *75*:512, 1966.

Nager, G. T.: Sensorineural Deafness and Otosclerosis. Ann. Otol., *75*:481, 1966.

Panel on Technics and Results in Stapes Surgery. Arch. Otolaryng., *78*:546, 1963.

Reudi, L.: Pathogenesis of Otosclerosis. Arch. Otolaryng., *78*:469, 1963.

Reudi, L.: Histopathological Confirmation of Labyrinthine Otosclerosis. Laryngoscope, *75*:1582, 1965.

Reudi, L., and Spoendlin, H.: Pathogenesis of Sensorineural Deafness in Otosclerosis. Ann. Otol., *75*:525, 1966.

Schucknecht, H. F. (Ed): *Otosclerosis.* Boston, Little, Brown and Co., 1962.

Shambaugh, G. E., and Causse, J.: Ten Years' Experience with Fluoride in Otosclerotic (Otospongiotic) Patients. Ann. Otol., *83*:635, 1974.

Shea, J. J., Jr.: Fenestration of the Oval Window. Ann. Otol., *67*:932, 1958.

Shea, J. J., Jr.: Complications of the Stapedectomy Operation. Ann Otol., *72*:1109, 1963.

Shea, J. J., Jr., *et al.*: Teflon Piston Operation for Otosclerosis. Arch. Otolaryng., *76*:516, 1962.

Sheehy, J. L.: Stapes Surgery in Advanced Otosclerosis. Ann. Otol., *71*:601, 1962.

Sheehy, J. L.: Stapedectomy in the Fenestrated Ear. Arch. Otolaryng., *78*:574, 1963.

Sooy, F. A., *et al.*: Stapedectomy in Obliterative Otosclerosis. Ann. Otol. Rhinol. Laryngol., *73*:679, 1964.

Wolff, D., and Bellucci, R. J.: Otosclerosis. Arch. Otolaryng., *79*:571, 1964.

Chapter 53
Congenital Malformations of the Ear

The primordia of the external ear are the tissues of the first and second branchial arches. The middle ear is formed from the end of the first pharyngeal pouch and the surrounding mesenchyme, which also is part of the first and second branchial arches (see Anatomy and Embryology, Ch. 40). Since a failure in the development of one part influences the neighboring areas and all subsequent development, it is not surprising that congenital defects of the external and middle ear usually occur in combination and many times with congenital defects of other systems. Fortunately the labyrinth develops from an entirely different primordial tissue which is rarely influenced by maldevelopment of the middle ear (except the oval window region), so cochlear function is normal in most of these cases. This permits rehabilitation of hearing in most congenital defects of the ear.

The most commonly occurring defects are protrusion of the auricle (lop or outstanding ear) and macrotia (these are not associated with hearing loss and are discussed elsewhere); microtia; stenosis or atresia of the cartilaginous and/or bony external auditory canal; ossicular malformation; restricted or absent development of the middle ear or mastoid spaces; and preauricular fistula (which is discussed under cysts in Ch. 46, Tumors of the External and Middle Ear).

Although the etiologic factors influencing anomalous development of the ear are unknown, it has been established that drug intoxication occurring between the 28th and 42nd day after fertilization may result in anomalies. This was determined by a study of the large number of congenital defects produced by the drug thalidomide used in western Europe between 1958 and 1962. Genetic abnormality does not seem to be present in the majority of cases, with the major factor being intrauterine influences acting in the first trimester of pregnancy and particularly in the first six weeks of life. Unilateral involvement is reported more often than bilateral, and males are affected more often than females in a ratio of 2:1 to 5:1. It is possible that the more exposed male auricle causes this sex to seek medical attention more frequently. In bilateral cases, however, there is still a predominance of male incidence. The exact incidence of congenital defects of the ear is unknown, but obvious defects occur in at least 1 of 10,000 births and perhaps double this number.

CLASSIFICATION OF DEFECTS

The mechanism of origin of congenital anomalies of the ear does not permit a true classification, since there is a random association of defects of varying degrees and types. The most useful classification was given by Henner and is repeated here as a practical guide to therapy and prognosis. Figures 53–1 and 53–2 are included for comparative purposes.

Class I. In this category are those with the least abnormality. The external ear is shaped normally and is of near normal size.

cause of failure of hearing restoration in those operations utilizing the ossicular remnants for sound transmission.

A common anomaly, but one often unnoticed, is fixation of the malleus due to lack of differentiation of the anterior mallear ligament or persistence of a bony attachment of the anterior process of the malleus. This should be suspected in each case of ossicular chain fixation.

The tensor tympani tendon is usually present, serving, as does the cochleariform process, as a good surgical landmark. Malformation of the tensor tympani will accompany severe deformity of the malleus. The stapedius tendon may be absent as an isolated defect. In some instances, failure of differentiation will result in a bar of bone between the posterior tympanic wall and the stapes or long process of the incus.

RADIOGRAPHIC EXAMINATION

The standard projections of the temporal bone give only limited information in congenital defects of the ear. The abnormal middle ear with poor aeration and the absent external canal "window" does not give enough contrast with the dense labyrinthine block to furnish valid information about the ossicular anatomy. The most useful information gained from these views is the extent of pneumatization of the attic and mastoid and the position of the middle fossa dura in relation to the planned surgical approach to the attic.

The recently developed technique of body section radiography, particularly those employing the polytome, have made possible the exact prediction of tympanic anatomy. Using this technique, it is possible to demonstrate accurately the position of the oval window, the lateral semicircular canal, and the ossicular mass and the full extent of pneumatization. The value of this technique is inestimable for the evaluation, planning of management, and surgical correction of congenital ear disease.

MANAGEMENT

The patient with congenital ear disease presents a problem whose management de-

mands individual solution. Discovery of the condition usually takes place shortly after birth, which allows a generous period for evaluation and the education of the parents. Full advantage of this time should be made. These defects not only affect the communicative ability but also introduce a severe psychological handicap due to the disfigurement. With increasing demands on hearing as education advances, even a unilateral hearing loss may become a handicap. The seemingly minor problem of wearing eyeglasses can be difficult to solve for these patients.

The most urgent problem is that of hearing loss in bilateral involvement. Speech begins to develop during the first year of life, but hearing is necessary for this learning to occur. Delay of speech formation after the age of four presents a severe handicap from sensory deprivation during these critical years and may result in an educational problem even after hearing is regained. There is great reluctance to approach surgical correction before the age of 3 because of the increased risks of surgery and the problems of postoperative management. Accurate assessment of cochlear function is difficult before 3 or 4 years of age. In centers such as Oxford, England, however, where this work is done regularly, it is felt that the age of 2 is the ideal time to carry out surgical intervention.

Adequate screening methods are now available to obtain a close approximation of the hearing threshold in infants by free field measurement. If these tests indicate the possibility of a hearing deficit, a hearing aid (usually a bone conduction aid) should be fitted by the age of 6 months to provide the needed sensory environment for the development of sound appreciation and speech. Early hearing aid fitting will make possible the accurate assessment of cochlear function at a much earlier age.

A thorough pediatric examination is carried out to determine if other congenital abnormalities are present. No surgical procedure should be done until a complete evaluation has eliminated the possibility of circulatory anomalies because of the anesthetic risk when an unsuspected defect exists.

Radiographic examination of both ears is

carried out by age 2. This, combined with hearing function studies done by those experienced in the evaluation of children, will enable the physician to decide if operative correction of the hearing defect is possible and which ear offers the greater chance of success. Surgery, if elected, can then be done between the ages of 3 and 4.

If labyrinthine malformation accompanies that of the middle and external ear, a severe handicap exists which requires the services of all those engaged in auditory training, special education, and child psychology. In many of these cases, minor or major neurologic defects complicate the educational problem. A complete discussion of hearing rehabilitation is given elsewhere (see Audiology, Ch. 44), but in general, every available resource is often needed in the training of these patients.

Unilateral congenital malformation does not require early auditory training or early evaluation since the lack of hearing is not a factor in these cases. Unilateral hearing loss may be a definite handicap, especially as the upper levels of school are reached. If cochlear function is adequate, most otologists now agree that surgical correction of the hearing loss is of sufficient value to warrant the chance of failure and the surgical risks involved. This surgery should be done when anesthesia risks have become minimal and the child appreciates the need for surgical correction. These conditions have usually been met by the age of 8, and reconstruction may be undertaken any time thereafter. Class III patients and those with Treacher Collins syndrome have such a poor chance of hearing improvement that surgery should be done only in those patients with bilateral involvement.

The best resolution of the cosmetic problem has not yet been decided. There are many who feel that plastic reconstruction of the auricle is the solution which gives the most benefit to the patient. There are only a few plastic surgeons skilled in this difficult process of multiple operations, so that in the average situation, the patient, his parents, and the referring doctor do not feel the result has warranted the pain and effort involved. In this situation, the recommendation of a prosthesis is probably the best

solution. This problem is less critical in girls, who may adopt hair styles which hide the deformity. When a skilled plastic surgeon is available, reconstruction has much advantage to the patient. Although the plastic surgeons prefer to work in a "virgin" field, the external meatus cannot be varied in its position, creating the need for the initial surgery to be that for hearing restoration. Ideally the plastic surgeon and the otologic surgeon will work closely together in the planning and management of these cases.

TECHNIQUE OF SURGERY

Incision. In those patients without a significant external ear defect, the middle ear is approached as outlined for stapes surgery (see Otosclerosis, Chap. 52). Minor narrowing of the canal may be corrected by widening with burrs after elevation of the overlying skin. More severe stenosis or atresia in those cases with a near normal auricle will be approached through an endaural incision which incorporates some of the concha. In a case with microtia, the incision is placed over the area through which the canal will be formed.

Reconstruction of the Canal. Many surgeons will elect modified radical mastoidectomy in every case of congenital atresia of the external auditory canal, but the risk to an aberrant facial nerve is greatest with this approach. The method first suggested by Shambaugh and developed by Livingstone offers the greatest safety and least postoperative problem to the patient. The attic and mesotympanum are approached from directly lateralward, this direction of approach creating the ear canal, which is thus completely formed when the middle ear is exposed. Since the tympanic portion of the temporal bone has not formed in the majority of cases, the zygoma, the temporomandibular joint, and the temporal line are the landmarks for this dissection. Dissection of the canal is started at the junction of the middle fossa dura and the jaw joint. The bone over these structures is thinned but not removed. Keeping as far anterior as possible in the angle formed between these landmarks, the dissection is carried medially until the attic is reached. Enlargement of the

Chapter 54

Reconstruction of the Outstanding Ear (Otoplasty)

M. Eugene Tardy, Jr. and Oscar J. Becker

Anatomic and Pathologic Features

The normal ear is a thin, shell-like structure having definite depressions and projections (Fig. 54–1). Many variations are found which may still be considered within normal limits. It is only when the ear protrudes abnormally ("outstanding") or is absent that the defect is immediately noticeable. Large or small ears, which may be proportionately more deformed than an outstanding ear, may go unnoticed if they are placed in a normal relation to the head.

The normal *auricle,* or *pinna,* is described by Gray as ovoid with its larger end directed upward. The prominent rim of the auricle

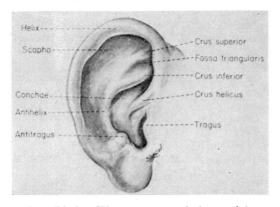

FIG. 54–1. The anatomy of the auricle.

is called the *helix*. Where the helix turns downward, a small projection, known as *Darwin's tubercle,* is frequently seen. This tubercle is evident about the sixth month of fetal life, when the whole auricle has a slight resemblance to that of a macaque monkey. This fact has caused much speculation and controversy among anthropologists, but as yet the significance of this tubercle is not clear. Another prominence parallel with and anterior to the helix is called the *anthelix;* this divides above into two *crura,* the *superior* and the *inferior,* between which is a shallow triangular depression, the *fossa triangularis*. Some authors refer to these two crura as the posterior and anterior crura. The narrow, curved depression between the helix and the anthelix is called the *scaphoid fossa,* or "boat-shaped ditch." The anthelix describes a curve around a deep cavity, the *concha,* which is divided into two parts by the crus or the beginning of the helix; the upper part is termed the *cymba conchae,* the lower part the *cavum conchae*. Anterior to the concha and projecting back over the external auditory meatus is a small pointed eminence, the *tragus,* so called because it is generally covered on its undersurface by a tuft of hair, resembling a goat's beard. Opposite the tragus and separated from it by the *intertragic notch* is a small tubercle, the

920

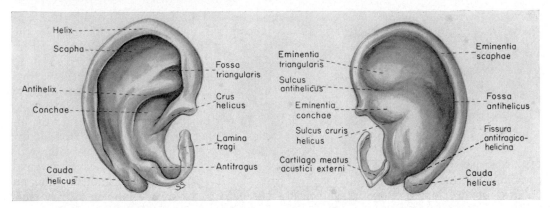

FIG. 54–2.   The cartilage of the auricle from the lateral (left) and medial (right) surfaces.

antitragus. Below this is the *lobule,* which is composed of areolar and adipose tissue with overlying epithelium. At the junction of the anthelix and the antitragus a small space exists, which may be deep in some ears and which is known as the *sulcus auriculae posterior.*

The auricle, with the exception of the lobules, is composed of a thin, flexible plate of yellow elastic fibrocartilage. The cartilage is 0.5 to 1 mm thick and is covered on each surface by integument intimately applied and having a minimum of subcutaneous tissue. The skin is closely adherent to the surface of the cartilage except on its posterior surface and along the helix.

The cartilage of the auricle (Fig. 54–2) is a single piece which gives form to the ear and outlines the landmarks previously mentioned. It is absent from the lobule and is deficient between the tragus and the beginning of the helix. At the anterior part of the auricle, where the helix bends upward, is a small projection of cartilage called the *spina helicis.* At the lower part of the helix the cartilage is prolonged downward as a tail-like process, the *cauda helicis,* which is separated from the anthelix by a fissure, the *fissura antitragohelicina.* The cranial aspect of the cartilage exhibits a transverse furrow, the *sulcus anthelicis transversus,* which corresponds to the inferior (anterior) crus of the anthelix and separates the *eminentia triangularis.* Another furrow exists at the central region of the concha, known as the *sulcus cruris helicis,* which corresponds to

the continuation of the helical rim and separates the concha into two portions, the *cavum conchae* and the *cymba conchae.*

The ligaments of the auricle consist of two sets: (1) extrinsic, which connect the auricle with the side of the head; and (2) intrinsic, which connect various parts of its cartilage to each other and to the external auditory meatus.

The muscles of the auricle likewise consist of two sets: (1) extrinsic, which connect it with the skull and scalp and move the auricle as a whole; and (2) intrinsic, which extend from one part of the auricle to another. Since these muscles are rudimentary, they have no particular surgical importance save for the abundant blood supply coursing within the musculature. In the infraprimate mammals, these muscles are particularly well developed and are important in turning the auricle toward the source of a sound.

The motor innervation is by the temporal branch and the posterior auricular branch of the facial nerve. The sensory nerves are the great auricular nerve from the cervical plexus, the auricular branch of the vagus nerve, the auriculotemporal branch of the mandibular nerve, and the lesser occipital nerve from the cervical plexus.

The arteries of the ear are composed of the posterior auricular, from the external carotid artery; the anterior auricular, from the superficial temporal artery; and a branch from the occipital artery. The veins accompany the corresponding arteries. The lymphatics drain into the periauricular nodes.

CORRECTION OF
PROTRUDING EARS

Etiologic Factors

Malformations of the auricle are not unusual and may range in severity from complete absence to macrotia. By far the most common deformity is the protruding ear (failure of development of the anthelical fold).

The embryonic origin of the external ear is still a controversial matter, but most observers agree that the six tubercles, or hillocks, of the first branchial groove, which appear about the fifth week of embryonic life, develop into the pinna. For convenience, these hillocks are numbered from one to six; three hillocks develop on the mandibular arch and three on the hyoid arch of the first branchial groove. The tragus is derived from mandibular hillock 2, the helix from mandibular hillocks 2 and 3, the anthelix from hyoid hillocks 4 and 5, and the antitragus from hyoid hillock 6. The lobule represents the lower end of the auricular fold.

At the end of the third month of embryonic life, the hillocks are well defined and the ear begins to assume definite form. According to Evans, it is at this time that the greatest number of malformations occur. The ear margin at this time is pointed, and because the crura of the anthelix are not formed, the ear protrudes from the head. Davis and Kitlowski stated that about the sixth fetal month the margin curls, forming the helix; the anthelix becomes more definitely folded, and its crura appear. It is the folding of the anthelix and the development of the crura that are responsible for bringing the ear closer to the head.

The protruding ear, therefore, is embryonically a congenital deformity, is inherited according to mendelian law, and may be a dominant or a recessive. Potter reported that a dominant gene may be transmitted through many generations. She revealed the transmission through five generations of a malformation in which the ears were extremely

cupped and protruding. A family tree embracing 92 members was obtained in the study. On the average, half of the members with this deformity had transmitted it to their children, while normal siblings married to normal persons had not transmitted the defect.

Therefore, the protruding ear in most instances is a congenital or hereditary deformity caused by maldevelopment of the anthelix. The angle between the concha and scapha is formed by the anthelix, and an absence or lack of development of the angle formed by the anthelix will result in a protrusion of the auricle away from the head. Since the angle of the anthelix determines the degree of protrusion of the ear, the pathologic condition would resolve itself into the type and development of the anthelix—that is, the more obtuse the angle, the more the ear projects (Fig. 54–3).

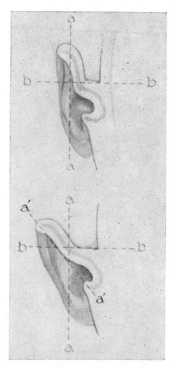

Fig. 54–3. The essential pathology of an outstanding ear. In the upper figure, the customary relation of the ear to the head is seen. The plane of the scapha, represented by *a–a* makes a right angle with the plane of the concha, indicated by *b–b*. In the lower figure, *a'–a'* is seen to make a much broader angle with *b–b*.

Other pathologic factors are encountered less frequently. A heavy concave concha will protrude the lower portion of the ear and is often accompanied by a thickened antitragus.

Congenital deformities of the helical rim are usually associated with a thin, flat ear which may or may not be protruding but is frequently lopped forward at the upper pole. If a deformed, everted superior crus accompanies this deformity, it produces a vertical projection of the upper pole to form the satyr type of ear.

The protruding (microtic) ear differs from the usual case of the protruding ear. The ear is folded on itself and is smaller than normal. This is almost invariably caused by a short (usually thickened) helix and a deformed anthelix. The conchal cartilage in some instances is heavier than normal or may appear so because of a superimposition of the anthelix over the concha.

Since little importance can be ascribed to the function of the auricle, it is only because of the deleterious psychological effect on the patient that protruding ears assume a clinical significance. Actually, according to comparative anatomists, the external ear in man is undergoing regression. In comparing the auricular muscles in man with those of animals with ears of similar type, a definite decrease in size, even to atrophy, is evident. In lower animals the auricle has real function in determining direction of sound and in protecting the internal auditory mechanism. Some animals on stimulation of the tragus will close the auditory canal by an infolding of the auricle to serve as a protection against water or insects. Henneberg and others observed that some mammals of the aquatic and semiaquatic group, such as the muskrat, seal, and beaver, can close the external ear when they are plunged into water. Rodents, moles, and other ground-burrowing animals are also capable of closing the external meatus.

The psychological effects of protruding ears vary with the sensitivity of the individual person. In almost all of the author's patients (and surprisingly enough, the effect was pronounced in children), a feeling of insecurity was evident, since this deformity, unlike most malformations, produces reactions of mirth in other people. To be constantly reminded of, and ridiculed about, a deformity will break all defense mechanisms of repression which the patient might have formed and subjects him to the development of an insecurity or inadequacy neurosis. Fortunately for these persons, this deformity can be corrected simply and satisfactorily, *preferably at an early preschool age, before any real psychological trauma can be inflicted*. Many who appear outwardly capable of rising above some defects may be sensitive about them and suffer inwardly. Other patients who are not at all sensitive about their appearance or defects may desire a correction of the ears purely for economic or social reasons.

In examining the normal ear from behind, it will be noted that the concha forms a 90-degree angle with the head. The scapha likewise forms an angle of approximately 90 degrees with the concha, but this may vary as much as 10 to 15 degrees and still be within normal limits, according to Young. The rim of the helix turns slightly outward. The angle between the scapha and the concha is formed by the anthelix, and in the absence or underdevelopment of the anthelix, the angle may become obtuse, thereby resulting in a protrusion of the auricle away from the head. Since the angle of the anthelix more or less determines the degree of protrusion of the ear, the pathologic condition would resolve itself into the type and development of the anthelix, i.e., the more obtuse the angle, the more the ear projects. The angle formed by the head and the helix is known as the auriculomastoid angle and is usually about 30 degrees.

Historical Survey

The earliest reference to the correction of protruding ears was by Dieffenbach in 1845, who advised removal of skin from the back of the ear followed by the suturing of the auricular cartilage to the periosteum of the mastoid bone.

Ely in 1881, Keen in 1890, and Monks in 1891 all described similar operations but added the removal of a cartilaginous section from the posterior surface of the auricle. Monks classified protruding ears into firm and soft cartilaginous types, the former requiring cartilage and skin excision, the latter only requiring skin excision. Haug in 1894, Joseph in 1896, and Morestin in 1903 described similar procedures; however, Morestin emphasized the complete sectioning of the cartilage from the superior to the inferior pole to prevent any recurrence of the protrusion.

A variety of complicated operations were later described. Gersuny in 1903 split the conchal cartilage into strips with removal of alternate sections. Payr in 1906 used a cross-shaped, pedunculated strip of cartilage and perichondrium which was passed under a loop of periosteum in the mastoid region. Ruttin in 1910 and Luthi in 1929 used fascia lata attached to the perichondrium at the inner edge of the helix and anchored it to periosteum over the mastoid. Alexander in 1928 recommended a longitudinal incision through the conchal cartilage. The cartilage was then overlapped and held in position with catgut sutures between the cartilage and postauricular fascia.

In 1937, Eitner recommended an operation similar to the Joseph and Morestin procedures. The skin and perichondrium were incised horizontally and then undermined before the longitudinal removal of the cartilage.

None of the procedures described can possibly result in a normal-appearing ear. The scapha projects abnormally, while the ear appears flattened against the head. On a lateral view, the concha often appears deformed, since sharp ridges and excess wrinkling of the skin are noted, along with absence of the anthelical fold.

The basic concept for the newer type of otoplasty was first described by Luckett, who in 1910 pointed out that the reason for protruding ears was the absence or underdevelopment of the anthelix. If a new anthelix were made, the prominence of the ear could be overcome; furthermore, on a lateral view a more normal-appearing ear would result without the distortions of the concha and absence of the normal anthelical fold. Luckett's operation consisted of removing a crescentic area of cartilage and skin from the posterior surface of the auricle

over the line of the proposed anthelix and everting the edges of cartilage by the use of a Lembert suture, thereby forming a new anthelix.

Davis in 1919 and again in 1937 emphasized Luckett's basic concepts, which also served as the basis for Barsky's operation in 1938. Davis and Kitlowski in 1937 published a method they had been using for correction of protruding ears which was based on the concepts of Luckett. They outlined the new anthelix along the inferior crus with brilliant green introduced by a needle through perforations in the skin from the anterior surface of the auricle. The skin on the posterior surface of the auricle which had been removed from both the conchal and the mastoid regions was discarded. The cartilage was split along the previously marked line and a section removed. The authors emphasized that the cartilage must be split through the entire length of the proposed anthelix to break its elasticity. Surgical gut sutures closed the perichondrium, and the edges were everted to form the new anthelix.

The objection to the Davis-Kitlowski procedure is that the normal postauricular sulcus is obliterated by the excessive removal of skin from the posterior surface of the auricle and from the mastoid region. Also, in the removal of cartilage only from the inferior crus, the superior crus may appear flat, and at times the ear will appear to lop forward at its upper pole.

The Davis-Kitlowski procedure led to a modification in 1940 by New and Erich, who used mattress sutures externally to help hold the form of the new anthelix. They also excised cartilage from the inferior crus but at times felt it necessary to remove a wedge of cartilage from the superior (posterior) crus to prevent the upper pole of the ear from falling forward. They cited Webster as stating that he had had satisfactory results without incising the cartilage but by merely shaving the cartilage in the region of the anthelix. New and Erich, however, stated that the ear can be folded back with greater ease if a narrow strip of cartilage is excised.

Young in 1944 described a method similar to, but an improvement of, the Davis-

Kitlowski procedures. He stated that if the section of cartilage forming the new anthelix were removed correctly, the scapha could be slipped over the concha, and thus no external mattress or internal gut sutures would be needed to hold the new fold of the anthelix. The excision of cartilage was made in the region of the superior crus rather than in the inferior crus, though Young expressed the belief that an incision is necessary in the inferior crus at times. No skin, other than the excess, is sacrificed from the postauricular sulcus.

Young's procedure is a decided improvement over the Davis-Kitlowski method for two reasons: (1) the main excision of cartilage is from the superior crus, giving the ear a better appearance; (2) no skin is sacrificed from the postauricular sulcus; thus, the ear is prevented from appearing too close to the head. The objection to Young's method is that a sharp ridge is produced in the region of the superior crus.

In 1947, McEvitt described a method similar to that used by Young. He advised the excision of cartilage at the anthelix and its crura and, in some cases, the placement of parallel incisions to break further the spring of the cartilage. He emphasized the necessity in some cases of excising part of the antitragus and of crosscutting the remaining portion, a detail which most reports fail to mention in correction of the extremely cupped type of ears. He stated that in correcting some of the similar types of protruding ears, he has lately tended to remove less and less cartilage, and at times none.

Pierce, Klabunde, and Bergeron in 1947 reported a procedure for correction of protruding ears which involved making eight to ten incisions almost through the cartilage. They stated the belief that the older operations leave a prominent ridge on the anterior surface of the auricle and that this new method gives an accurate representation of the normal fold. Five surgical gut sutures are used to hold back the anthelix fold and the ear. Excess skin is removed, and the remaining skin is sutured with Dermalon. This procedure represents an important advance, because it is an attempt to prevent sharp ridges on the anterior surface of the ear.

Recent Procedures

In 1949 and again in 1952, Becker described a method of correcting protruding ears based on the principle of incising the cartilage along natural lines, thereby allowing the ridges formed by those incisions to be hidden in the normal folds of the ear. The only excision of cartilage was made in the anthelix region. This excision was supplemented in cases of marked cupping and protrusion by the removal of a section of antitragus and in many cases by the removal of a section of cauda helicis. In other cases a section of the upper border of the superior crus under the helical rim was also removed.

The cartilage excision from the anthelix was continued by an incision extending through and along the inferior crus. This incision (after 1953) was extended up from the inferior crus to meet the incision along the helical rim which outlined the superior crus and superior border of the triangular fossa. If the cartilage was unusually firm, the superior crus cartilage was crosscut incompletely, that is, by incisions that did not completely transect the cartilage. The cartilage was then undermined for a few millimeters from the anterior surface of the auricle to prevent any wrinkling of the anterior skin and to help mobilize or round the borders of the incised and excised cartilage. The excess skin, which is always present in varying amounts, was removed and the incision closed. External mattress sutures were placed in the region of the anthelix and in some cases through the superior crus region. A drain was inserted and a fairly snug mastoid dressing applied.

The results of the foregoing procedure have been gratifying. However, occasionally the excision of cartilage from the anthelix left a slightly sharpened ridge. This was not objectionable to the patient but was disconcerting to the surgeon seeking perfection. Furthermore, to break the spring of the upper portion of the ear completely, the incision extending through the superior crus down through the fossa triangularis would sometimes leave a sharp ridge in the area near the juncture of inferior crus, triangular fossa, and new anthelix. To avoid this, the incision at the junction of anthelix, inferior crus, and triangular fossa was made incompletely through the cartilage. This was sometimes insufficient to break the spring of the firm, cartilaginous type of protruding ear, and to avoid cutting completely through in this area, Becker began depending on the incision along the inferior crus (sulcus anthelicis transversus). The incision was gradually extended to connect with the one along the upper pole of the superior crus. This maneuver allowed the incomplete transection of cartilage at the junction of the triangular fossa, inferior crus, and anthelix, thereby avoiding any sharpness in this area.

In 1956, Converse and coworkers presented a method of minimal removal of cartilage from the anthelix region by a new concept of thinning the cartilage so that it may be tubed in its lower portion. The incisions through the cartilage were the same as described, that is, along the natural folds, but instead of a section of cartilage being removed from the anthelix, the cartilage was thinned with a motor-driven brush and then rolled on itself with internal catgut fixation sutures. A section of cartilage was removed from the conchal side of the anthelix when necessary. This method of tubing the cartilage created a smoother anthelix than the method of excising cartilage. However, the incision through the fossa triangularis was retained by Converse.

A similar concept of using a burr to thin the cartilage of the superior crus was presented by Withers in 1955, but he retained the excision of cartilage from the anthelix.

Mattress Suture Otoplasty. During the mid-1960's a corrective otoplasty procedure, developed primarily by Mustardé, gained ready acceptance and wide popularity. Vertically positioned nonabsorbable mattress sutures were inserted to recreate the natural shelving curve of the antihelical fold, blending gently into the scaphoid fossa. The principal advantages of this cartilage-sparing technique were as follows:

1. No through-and-through cartilage incisions are necessary, thereby avoiding the potential sharp edges of other techniques.

2. Transperichondrial sutures may be positioned, test-tied, and then maintained (or replaced) as necessary to develop a natural

anthelix. This eliminates the commitment of cutting through cartilage, a noncorrectable action.

3. The procedure is rapid and relatively easy to learn and teach, requiring less dissection of the ear and avoiding surgical trauma.

4. The long-range results are quite satisfactory.

Since the introduction of the mattress suture otoplasty technique, the author (M.E.T.) has performed this procedure, with variations, in several hundred outstanding ears. Certain modifications have been introduced which lead to ease of operation and surgical safety. It must be emphasized that an operation is designed individually for each ear, dependent upon the existent deformity. Often a *combined* operation is accomplished, the basic mattress suture procedure being augmented by the dissection (O.J.B.) technique to achieve surgical correction and natural appearance. Ears are quite commonly asymmetric, and therefore asymmetric operations are necessary.

Detailed descriptions of the *dissection technique* of Becker and the *mattress suture technique* modified by Tardy and Tenta will follow. Mastery of the precise anatomy of the auricle (anterior and posterior), combined with a knowledge of the following two surgical procedures, will allow the surgeon wide latitude in achieving natural correction of the many varieties of outstanding ear. No single technique will suffice.

The Dissection Technique (Becker). The hair is shaved for a distance of 2.5 cm from the ear and is held away from the operative field with head drapes. The ears are washed with a detergent containing hexachlorophene followed by an antiseptic solution. With the patient lying on his back, the head is draped, and only one ear is exposed at a time. A comparison of the two ears is usually unnecessary during the operation, since one can judge with fair accuracy when the ears are evenly placed to the head.

Either local or general anesthesia may be used. A complete encirclement of the ear is made with injections of the local anesthetic agent, and additional solution is infiltrated on the posterior surface and the anterior surface of the anthelix, the injections in the latter two regions being primarily to facilitate the dissection and for hemostasis.

Before the anesthetic solution is injected, an outline of the proposed incisions is made on the anterior surface of the ear which will subsequently be transferred to the posterior surface during the surgery. The ear is pressed back toward the mastoid region, and an excess section of skin will appear on the posterior surface. An outline of this excess of skin can then be made with methylene blue. It is well to outline this excess of skin before an anesthetic solution is injected, since the ballooning of the tissues will interfere with the proper outline of the skin. The section of skin is then removed (Fig. 54–4, A).

The skin is dissected forward (toward the helical rim) just beyond the scaphoid eminence on the posterior surface of the auricle. Skin undermining should be kept to a minimum. Only that area which is necessary to expose the landmarks is undermined. The wide exposure shown on the illustrations is for diagrammatic purposes (Fig. 54–4, B).

After dissection of the skin, the following landmarks should be exposed by further dissection. The cauda helicis and the fissura antitragohelicina are exposed. The sulcus anthelicis transversus (inferior crus) is exposed by blunt dissection to remove the small intrinsic muscle which covers this area. The eminentia triangularis is exposed. The eminentia scapha is exposed down to the inferior crus.

A series of needles is now inserted from the anterior surface of the ear through the scaphoid fossa along its entire length. The lightly shaded dots represent the markings made under the helical rim at the depth of the scaphoid fossa and follow this fossa around the entire ear rim to the inferior crus.

The needle which was used to pierce the anterior surface of the auricle in the scaphoid fossa (under the helical rim) is noted to follow the scaphoid eminence from the bisection of the cauda helicis around to the inferior crus. It then follows the anterior border of the proposed anthelix, which is noted on the anterior surface of the ear when the ear is folded back into normal position (Fig. 54–4, C).

An incision through the cartilage is made along these markings. The cartilage should be cut completely through to the perichondrium on the anterior surface. It is then undermined with a fine flat scissors for about 4 or 5 mm, following completely around the incision. However, the lower pole is completely dissected free from the anterior skin so that it is detached for a distance of about 0.75 to 1 cm (Fig. 54–4, D). This allows the cartilage to curl on itself. The perichondrium over the center portion of the ear cartilage is completely removed by excision and scraping of the surface with a sharp scalpel (Fig. 54–4, E). The removal of the perichondrium helps turn the borders of the ear cartilage inward. The perichondrium along the edges of the incision is left attached to aid in the healing and adherence of the outer edges united by sutures. The lower free end of the cartilage is then sutured together with 0000 chromic catgut (Fig. 54–4, F).

An additional incision may be made through the eminentia triangularis if the upper pole of the ear seems to have any residual spring. The incision must not be completely through the cartilage at the lower end; otherwise, a sharp ridge will develop where the fossa triangularis meets the anthelix.

The skin incision is then sutured with interrupted black silk. An external mattress suture may be placed through the borders of the newly formed anthelix to help maintain its position on the anterior surface of the auricle. The mattress suture is tied without tension over a small roll of Adaptic dressing rolled on itself (Fig. 54–4, G, H). A narrow Penrose drain is usually inserted in the lower portion of the posterior incision and remains for 48 hours. Adaptic dressing is used to cover the ear and is followed by cotton packed into the convolutions. An external bandage is firmly applied.

In many cases a section of the antitragus is removed if the lower portion of the ear protrudes markedly. This area is just anterior to the lower pole which has been sutured. In other cases involving a large thick concha, it may be necessary to remove a section of conchal cartilage.

In cases in which the anthelix appears too

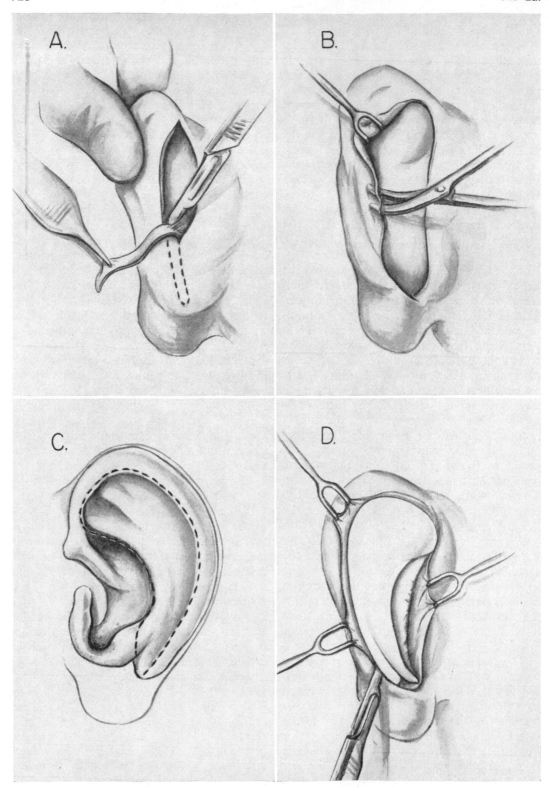

Fig. 54–4.

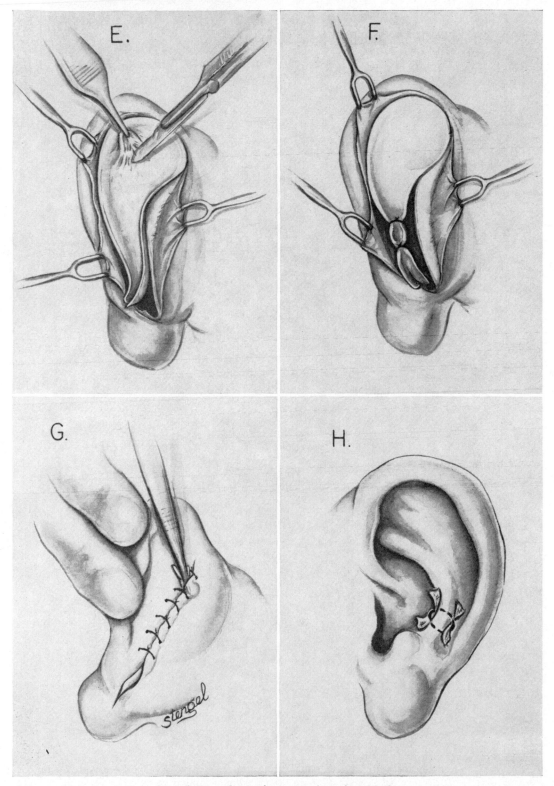

FIG. 54–4. Operative procedure (see text).

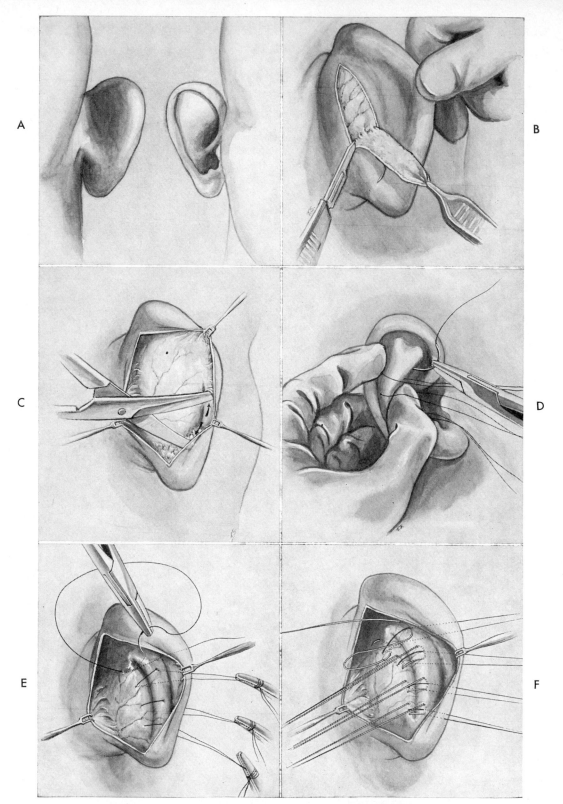

FIG. 54–5. *A*, Posterior and anterior outstanding ear deformity. *B*, Conservative excision of postauricular skin for surgical access. *C*, Conservative undermining of skin. *D*, Temporary silk sutures preplaced as guides to accurate placement of permanent buried transperichondrial mattress sutures. *E*, Preplaced temporary sutures indicate sites for mattress suture placement. *F*, Transperichondrial mattress sutures positioned and test-tightened to determine precise effect in creating new anthelical fold.

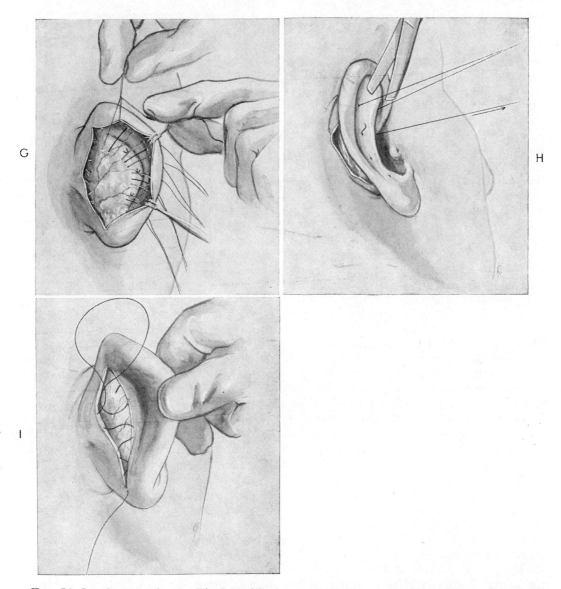

FIG. 54–5. *Continued*. *G*, Final positioning and ligation of transperichondrial mattress sutures. *H*, Preplaced temporary guide sutures removed. *I*, Postauricular incision closure with running intradermal monofilament suture.

prominent after this method has been used, or if the spring of the cartilage appears inadequately broken, the catgut sutures are removed and a narrow section of cartilage is removed from the center of the anthelix almost up to the inferior crus. The cartilage is then sutured together with catgut.

The dressings are changed on the second day. The drain is removed and a new bandage applied. On the fifth day the external mattress suture is removed, and the ears are again firmly rebandaged. On the eighth or ninth day, the postauricular sutures are removed, and a bandage is reapplied until the fourteenth day.

This method has been used in a large series of cases with excellent results. The method first described by the author (O.J.B.) in 1949 and again in 1952 resulted in a good correction. The two objections to the first procedure were that (1) the anthelix fold was sometimes too sharp, and (2) the spring at the juncture of the fossa triangularis and inferior crus, if it was completely cut through, would leave a sharpened ridge which was often objectionable. In many cases of protruding ears in which the cartilage was soft, this latter incision was made only partially through the cartilage, and a better result was obtained.

The present method of following up through the inferior crus and then curving along the scaphoid sulcus at its upper end eliminates the complete transection of the cartilage at the junction of the triangular fossa, anthelix, and inferior crus.

The undermining of the cartilage, the complete freeing of the lower border, and the removal of the perichondrium from the center portion of the cartilage (i.e., the section of cartilage remaining between the two lateral cut edges) help the cartilage to roll on itself to duplicate the natural curve of the anthelix. This is further reinforced by the catgut sutures and an external mattress suture.

If this method does not adequately correct the ear or if the anthelix is too prominent, then it is necessary to resect a section of cartilage from the new anthelix and/or from the conchal margin. In other cases it may be necessary to extend an incision

from the previous incision above the superior crus down through the eminentia triangularis.

A section of antitragus is removed when necessary.

An incision around the ear lobe, freeing its anterior attachment from the skin of the face, may also be necessary if the lobe itself projects abnormally after adequate excision of the antitragus.

The postauricular sulcus is not obliterated, as occurs following the procedure in which a large skin excision from the mastoid and conchal regions is necessary to hold the ear back in position.

Mattress Suture Otoplasty (Tardy). Following use of hexachlorophene shampoo and a facial prep the evening prior to surgery, application of Betadine solution completes the periauricular skin preparation. General endotracheal anesthesia is employed in children; adolescents and adults receive local infiltration anesthesia supplemented by continuously monitored intravenous analgesia. Apertured transparent plastic drapes allow frequent intraoperative auricular comparison to ensure symmetry of repair. Xylocaine, 1%, with 1:100,000 epinephrine (standard solution) infiltrates sparingly the postauricular subcutaneous tissues, aiding in dissection and promoting hemostasis (Fig. 54–5, *A*).

An incision adequate to expose the posterior surface of the neoanthelical fold is created in fusiform fashion (Fig. 54–5, *B*). It is unnecessary to remove a large portion of skin or to undermine extensively (Fig. 54–5, *C*). Minimal dissection thereby diminishes surgical trauma and promotes rapid healing, an advantage of mattress suture otoplasty. The posterior perichondrium is not stripped bare of subcutaneous tissue to facilitate postauricular scar formation in the posterior trough formed by the neoanthelical fold. This scar forms the eventual strength of the repair, relieving the buried mattress sutures of their original burden (revision operations will reveal the presence of this important sheet of scar, retaining the retropositional attitude of the ear even following removal of the mattress sutures). With the thumb and index finger the neoanthelical fold is sited and created, blending naturally into the posterior crus. Temporary marking sutures of 4–0 black silk are next passed from anterior to posterior (Fig. 54-5, *D, E*) to guide the precise ultimate position of placement of the permanent mattress sutures. Black silk siting sutures eliminate the disadvantages of marking with ink or sharp needles.

Using the silk sutures as a guide, transperichondrial horizontal mattress sutures of white 4–0 braided nylon are positioned sequentially (Fig. 54–5, *F*) from caudal to cephalic along the neoanthelical fold. It is essential that each suture encompass *both* the anterior and the posterior perichondrium in order to prevent ultimate tearing through of the suture. Seldom are less than four horizontal mattress sutures required, each sharing the retropositioning vector force until scar tissue cements the eventual position of the auricle. Each suture may be test-tightened to assess its effect (Fig. 54–5, *G*); unnatural fold appearance is avoided by the removal and repositioning of the suture until exact sculpture of the auricle is achieved, a considerable advantage of the technique.

The auricle with a deep cavum conchae may require excision of a semilunar segment of cartilage within the cavum conchae at this point to properly construct the neo-anthelix.

It is unnecessary to overcorrect the retropositioning of the auricle, as sufficient properly positioned sutures maintain the correction precisely (Fig. 54–5, *H*).

Following meticulous hemostasis, a continuous running intradermal monofilament nylon suture completes the postauricular skin closure (Fig. 54–5, *I*), thereby facilitating suture removal in 10 to 14 days. No drains are employed. Frequent comparison of the two ears during surgery ensures symmetry and exacting repair. Mineral oil–soaked cotton, gauze fluffs, and Kerlex wrap-around gauze comprise the support bandage, which is changed the morning following surgery and maintained thereafter for 36 to 72 hours. The use of nylon stocking caps during sleep is recommended to the patient to prevent inadvertent nocturnal trauma and displacement.

It is worthy of emphasis that the mattress suture procedure is frequently augmented by thinning, weakening, and even limited incision of cartilage to achieve natural and symmetrical results. Knowledge of one technique only is obviously inadequate.

REFERENCES

Aufricht, G.: Combined Nasal Plastic and Chin Plastic. Am. J. Surg., *25*:292, 1934.

Aufricht, G.: Total Ear Reconstruction, Preliminary Report. Plast. Reconstr. Surg., *2*:297, 1947.

Barsky, A. J.: *Principles and Practice of Plastic Surgery.* Baltimore, Williams & Wilkins Co., 1950.

Becker, O. J.: Surgical Correction of the Abnormally Protruding Ear. Arch. Otolaryng., *50*:541, 1949.

Becker, O. J.: Protruding Ears: Correction by Plastic Surgery. Illinois Med. J., *98*:196, 1950.

Becker, O. J.: Correction of the Protruding Deformed Ear. Br. J. Plast. Surg., *5*:187, 1952.

Brown, J. B., and Cannon, B.: Composite Free Grafts of Two Surfaces of Skin and Cartilage from the Ear. Ann. Surg., *124*:1101, 1946.

Brown, J. B., et al.: Surgical Substitutions for Losses of the External Ear; Simplified Local Flap Method of Reconstruction. Surg. Gynecol. Obstet., *84*:192, 1947.

Converse, J. M.: Reconstruction of the External Ear by Prefabricated Framework of Refrigerated Bone and Cartilage. Plast. Reconstr. Surg., *5*:148, 1950.

Converse, J. M., et al.: A Technique for Surgical Correction of Lop Ears. Trans. Am. Acad. Ophthal. Otolaryngol., *60*:551, 1956.

Davis, J. S., and Kitlowski, E. A.: A Method of Tubed Flap Formation. South. Med. J., *29*:1169, 1936.

Davis, J. S., and Kitlowski, E. A.: Abnormal Prominence of the Ears: A Method of Readjustment. Surgery, *2*:835, 1937.

Dieffenbach, J. F.: Die Operative Chirurgie. F. A. Bruckhaus, Liepzig, 1845.

Fraser, J. S.: Maldevelopments of the Auricle, External Acoustic Meatus and Middle Ear; Microtia and Congenital Meatal Atresia. Arch. Otolaryng., *13*:1, 1931.

Joseph, J.: Nasenplastik und sonstige Gesichtsplastik. Nebst einem anhang uber Mammaplastik und einige weitere Operationen aus dem Gebiete der Ausseren Korperplastik. Leipzig, Kabitzsch, 1931.

Luckett, W. H.: A New Operation for Prominent Ears Based on the Anatomy of the Deformity. Surg. Gynecol. Obstet., *10*:635, 1910.

Morestin, P. H. M.: De la Reposition et du Plissement Cosmétiques du de Pavillon de l'Oreille. Rev. Orthop., *4*:289, 1903.

New, G. B., and Erich, J. B.: Protruding Ears: A Method of Plastic Correction. Am. J. Surg., *48*:385, 1940.

Padgett, E. C.: Total Reconstruction of the Auricle. Surg. Gynecol. Obstet., *67*:761, 1938.

Peer, L. A.: Reconstruction of the Auricle with Diced Cartilage Grafts in a Vitallium Ear Mold. Plast. Reconstr. Surg., *3*:653, 1948.

Pierce, G. W.: Reconstruction of the External Ear. Surg. Gynecol. Obstet., *50*:601, 1930.

Potter, E. L.: A hereditary ear malformation transmitted through five generations. J. Heredity, *28*:255, 1937.

Wood-Jones, F., and I-Chuan, W.: The Development of the External Ear. J. Anat., *68*:525, 1934.

Young, F.: The Correction of Abnormally Prominent Ears. Surg. Gynecol. Obstet., *78*:541, 1944.

Chapter 55

Noninflammatory Diseases of the Labyrinth

Primary involvement of the cochlea, vestibular apparatus, or the eighth cranial nerve with spread to the contiguous structures is characteristic of this group of diseases. Unfortunately, the common involvement of the vestibular labyrinth and its widespread central nervous connections in systemic illness makes difficult the differentiation of symptoms due to this cause from those due to specific vestibular disease.

The principal subjective symptoms—vertigo, deafness, and tinnitus—are all common to this group of disorders, again creating problems of diagnosis. Rapid progress in methods of examination of cochlear and vestibular function has greatly aided in the differentiation of these diseases and thus removed a great deal of the confusion which was present in the past.

Vertigo and Dizziness. Vertigo is defined as a hallucination of movement. This may be a sensation of turning, spinning, falling, rocking, etc. Dizziness, although commonly used by the patient as a term to describe the above sensations, refers to less severe and distinct sensations of giddiness, faintness, confusion, blankness, or unsteadiness. This differentiation is important, since vertigo arises from disturbance of the vestibular end-organ, vestibular nerve, or vestibular nucleus. Dizziness may arise from mild disturbance of the vestibular apparatus but usually indicates disturbance in other regions.

An analogy given by Cawthorn helps to clarify the types of disturbance of the peripheral vestibular apparatus resulting in vertigo. This mechanism may be likened to a twin-engined airplane. When both engines are running normally and the controls are properly operating, the airplane flies on a straight course. If one engine suddenly fails, the plane is violently diverted off its course by the unopposed action of the normally running engine. By readjusting the controls, after a short period the pilot is able to fly on a straight course again, though turning or a sudden gust of wind will have a more disturbing effect than when the two engines are working normally. In another situation the faulty engine may start up again, and even if it does not return to its normal speed, all is well provided it runs steadily. However, should the faulty engine repeatedly fail and recover, the result will be more disturbing than having a dead engine. In another situation one engine may fail to work properly only when the airplane is in a certain position, such as in a steep bank to the left, but will return to normal as soon as the airplane straightens out. Finally, if one engine loses power slowly, the pilot almost imperceptibly is able to readjust the controls without deviating from his course.

The airplane engines may be directly compared to the set of vestibular end-organs in each labyrinth. Each of the types of failure may occur in man, resulting in each case with loss of equilibrium and a type of vertigo.

In evaluating vertigo, the history is of great importance. The following information should be elicited:

1. Whether the symptom experienced is true vertigo. If the complaint does consist of a sensation of motion or turning, the origin lies in the vestibular apparatus; otherwise, other regions must be subjected to examination and evaluation.

2. The pattern of the vertigo. It is important to note whether the attacks are spontaneous or precipitated by movement. The presence of paroxysmal attacks separated by periods of relative freedom from symptoms indicates a different pathologic condition than more or less continuous dizziness.

3. The degree of vertigo. Vertigo arising in the labyrinth is usually accompanied by nausea and often vomiting. Less specific forms may be milder and may arise from any part of the body.

4. The association of hearing loss or tinnitus with dizziness is a definite aid to localization. Complete audiometric evaluation is essential to the examination of the dizzy patient, since these diseases may affect the vestibular apparatus alone, the cochlear apparatus alone, or both together.

Tinnitus. This may be objective in rare instances (a sound which may be heard by the examiner) but is usually a subjective sensation of sound arising from within the head. Tinnitus may vary in intensity and may be continuous or intermittent. Subjectively loud and continuous tinnitus may produce a severe handicap to the individual.

Tinnitus is associated with hearing loss arising from disorders of the sound conduction system, the cochlea, or the neural pathways of the cochlear nerve. Patients describe the sound in various ways, but the examiner should attempt to obtain a description of the sound with which both the patient and the doctor is familiar. In general the sounds experienced will range from predominantly low frequencies (like a ventilating fan or sea shell sound) to wide-range white noise (a rushing sound commonly experienced in Meniere's disease) or high-pitched noise,

whistles, or insect sounds (which frequently may be matched on the audiometer).

Conductive hearing loss usually produces a low-pitched continuous sound which, if combined with inflammation, becomes pulsating. High-pitched continuous or intermittent tinnitus is associated with high tone hearing loss and is an important and early sign of drug intoxication (aspirin, digitalis, quinine, dihydrostreptomycin, etc.).

Pulsating low-pitched tinnitus without hearing loss is an important early symptom of glomus jugulare tumors of the middle ear. It is also associated with occlusive disease of the carotid artery, which will at times produce an audible bruit.

Other than relieving a conductive hearing loss, there is no effective treatment of tinnitus. Even section of the eighth nerve in most cases does not result in cessation of tinnitus. Patients suffering from this symptom deserve a full and honest explanation of the nature of the disorder so that natural anxiety does not cause exaggeration of the severity of the symptoms. Barbiturates and tranquilizers are rarely indicated for use in this condition, for in most instances patients are able to adapt to the presence of tinnitus and ignore it.

Examination and Differential Diagnosis. The main causes of vertiginous labyrinthine disturbance are:

1. Acute toxic labyrinthitis
2. Meniere's disease
3. Paroxysmal positional vertigo (postural vertigo)
4. Vestibular neuronitis
5. Vertebral-basilar artery insufficiency
6. Trauma
7. Tumor

The main types of disturbances to be differentiated from these diseases are the following:

1. Disease of the cerebellum, especially vascular disease and tumors
2. Disease of the proprioceptive system
3. Cerebral anoxemia, particularly mild arteriosclerosis, postural hypotension, and anemia
4. Endocrine disease, particularly hypothyroidism, and female hormonal disturbance
5. Epilepsy

Nonvertiginous labyrinthine disease affects primarily the cochlea and includes the following:

1. Congenital and neonatal hearing loss
2. Familial deafness
3. Presbycusis
4. Drug toxicity
5. Ototropic viral disease
6. Noise-induced hearing loss
7. Sudden idiopathic hearing loss
8. Otosclerosis

Examination of the patient with labyrinthine symptoms (vertigo, hearing loss, and tinnitus) should include caloric examination and hearing evaluation. The latter should consist of air and bone audiometry; speech audiometry; Békésy audiometry, when indicated; and determination of recruitment. If the examiner does not have the equipment to perform these tests, the patient should be referred to a Speech and Hearing center where they may be performed. In general, all patients with unilateral symptoms or findings or with widely differing findings in the two ears should have the complete battery of tests described above.

In recent times, electronystagmography has enabled accurate quantitative measurement of the ocular responses to caloric and rotatory tests of the vestibular apparatus and should be employed when available.

Radiographic examination of the inner ear includes the Stenvers view and the Town-Chamberlain view. These projections enable visualization of the petrous bone and internal auditory canal. In most instances polytomography is essential in the work-up of these problems.

In many cases complete neurologic examination and spinal fluid analysis are necessary to provide an exact diagnosis.

PRIMARILY VERTIGINOUS DISEASE OF THE LABYRINTH

Acute toxic labyrinthitis is the most common cause of vertigo seen by the otolaryngologist. The pathogenesis is indefinite, but it usually accompanies acute or subacute infections, especially of the nose and throat. The infection may be quite mild and still produce these symptoms. There is usually a gradual onset of vertigo which becomes maximal in 24 to 48 hours and then gradually subsides over a period of 7 to 10 days. In many patients, this pattern follows overindulgence with alcohol, drug intoxication, allergy, or debilitation. Often headache, fatigue, and a feeling of lightheadedness will accompany the vertigo.

The vertigo produced is not spontaneous but is brought on by head motion or position, particularly on looking up. Other than that produced by middle ear congestion in association with the upper respiratory infection, there is no hearing loss or tinnitus associated with this condition. Vestibular examination reveals in most instances a normal or hyperactive response to caloric stimulus.

The treatment of this condition is supportive while the underlying disease is treated. Since many times self-limited viral disease is present, only symptomatic treatment is indicated in these instances. This consists of the use of antivertiginous agents which are forms of antihistamines. The most potent suppressant of vestibular activity is promethazine, which has a common side effect of producing drowsiness.

Paroxysmal positional vertigo or postural vertigo is characterized by the sudden onset of vertigo and nystagmus when the head is placed in a certain position, usual hyperextended and to one side. Typically the symptoms ensue after a short latent period and soon disappear if the position is maintained. The disease is self-limited, with the symptoms disappearing in a few weeks, although they may recur. The diagnosis is made by placing the head in the offending position and observing the onset of nystagmus (see Tests of Vestibular Function, p. 937).

Although this condition has been attributed to utricular dysfunction and in many instances follows trauma, another form has been described occurring with posterior fossa lesions. This form (malignant positional vertigo) differs by the absence of a latent period before the onset of nystagmus which does not exhaust. Occlusive artery disease may also cause positional vertigo due to kinking of the vertebral artery when the head is placed in a position of hyperextension and rotation. Both of these possibilities must be kept in mind in cases of persistent positional vertigo.

30

Vestibular neuronitis, first described by Dix and Hallpike in 1952, is a form of epidemic neuritis, presumably of viral etiology, affecting the vestibular nerve. Characteristically, there is a sudden loss of vestibular function accompanied by severe vertigo, nausea, vomiting, and spontaneous nystagmus. Following the initially severe symptoms there is a gradual recovery, taking from 7 days to 3 weeks, leaving a residual loss of vestibular sensitivity. Audiometric examination shows no effect on the cochlea or its pathways.

Treatment consists of bedrest, sedation, and administration of antivertiginous agents. During convalescence the patient should be warned against sudden head motion which will induce vertigo. There is usually no permanent disability, although all individuals with unilaterally reduced vestibular function will have a latent tendency to vertigo and nystagmus. This is because of incomplete adaptation to the altered vestibular physiology.

Vertebral-basilar artery disease is an important cause of vertigo, usually without accompanying cochlear disturbance. Because the vestibular nuclei on the surface of the brain stem are more susceptible to arterial insufficiency than surrounding structures, these symptoms may persist for long periods before the nature of the disease becomes evident. With vertebral-carotid angiography it is possible to demonstrate these lesions and to provide an awareness of this condition.

The usual symptoms occur in individuals of an age prone to arteriosclerosis and consist of spontaneous short episodes of vertigo which are transient but recur frequently. These episodes may be precipitated by head position as described previously. With more severe hypoxia, increasing widespread effects occur, such as facial numbness or tingling, sensory disturbance of one or both sides of the body, or slurred speech. These episodes are extremely difficult to differentiate from threatened occlusion of the vestibular artery which causes more or less the same symptoms. In this instance, however, there should be a sudden loss of the high tones of hearing since the vestibular artery supplies the basal turn of the cochlea. Many of these patients are of an age in which this high tone loss will be already present.

Vestibular examination with hot and cold caloric testing will usually reveal a directional preponderance in the case of nuclear disease (see Tests of Vestibular Function, p. 938) and an end-organ loss to both hot and cold in disease of the vestibular artery.

Treatment is based on the nature of the arterial lesion causing the symptoms. This may range from anticoagulant therapy to prevent threatened occlusion in cases of insufficiency to endarterectomy in cases of occlusion of large arterial vessels. The diagnosis and treatment must be carried out with neurosurgical assistance.

Motion sickness may be defined as an abnormal response to the stimulus of motion, usually incurred in travel by car, boat, or airplane ("car sick," "sea sick," or "air sick"). The symptomatology varies in degree from sleepiness, sweating, and pallor to nausea and vomiting. Vertigo is not a symptom.

Investigation into the etiology of this condition has revealed no objective abnormality of the vestibular system. Many investigators feel that this condition represents an exaggerated response to stimulus on a psychogenic basis.

Treatment in severe cases is only through avoidance or cessation of the form of travel causing the symptoms. Sedation is only partially effective. In milder cases, drugs suppressing vestibular response, such as Dramamine or Phenergan, combined with sedatives or tranquilizers are effective.

LABYRINTHINE DISEASE AFFECTING BOTH VESTIBULAR AND COCHLEAR FUNCTION

Hemorrhage into the labyrinth, though rare, follows the usual patterns of stroke, with thrombosis usually occurring in early morning or shortly after rising and vascular rupture occurring with exertion or periods of hypertensive crisis. There is a sudden onset of severe, incapacitating vertigo, roaring tinnitus, and complete loss of hearing in the involved ear. These symptoms slowly recede over a period of 3 to 4 weeks, leaving a residual complete loss of response to caloric or sound stimuli.

The diagnosis of labyrinthine hemorrhage is presumptive when this picture is seen in a patient with the probability of antecedent vascular disease. It must be differentiated from an acute episode of Meniere's disease, which in most cases follows a much shorter course.

Treatment is supportive, but medical investigation of the vascular system is indicated to try to prevent episodes in other parts of the body.

Trauma to the labyrinth may range from concussion to fracture of the temporal bone.

CONCUSSION OF THE LABYRINTH AND BRAIN

Etiology. Concussion of the brain may follow such injuries as industrial, sport, or automobile accidents. Concussion of the brain may be associated with concussion of the internal ear or with fracture of the temporal bone. Concussion of the internal ear alone without associated concussion of the brain is improbable unless the injury is mild.

Pathology. Concussion of the brain is really compression of the brain substance. The cranial contents, brain, cerebrospinal fluid, and blood are all noncompressible, except that the blood may be forced out of the venous channels within the skull and to that extent relieve pressure. The skull itself is more elastic and, in the case of trauma by a severe enough fall or blow, is deformed from its usual shape. If the force applied is sufficiently sudden and severe, fracture takes place, but in any event there is compression. As an immediate result, the vessels enlarge, the circulation slows, and there is an exudate of serum and lymphocytes from the blood vessels. The lateral ventricles are compressed; the fluid is forced into the third ventricle and through the aqueduct of Sylvius into the fourth ventricle, producing a swirl and possibly affecting the vestibular nuclei. Degenerative changes may be variously localized. They are often in the vestibular or cochlear nuclei. About 40% of concussion cases have ear symptoms.

The histologic findings after head trauma are dilatation of the blood vessels and perivascular spaces, with slowing of the circulation; exudate into the perivascular spaces with eventual gliosis; and hemorrhages, petechial to massive, according to the severity of the trauma. Degenerative changes may occur in the vestibular centers.

Symptoms. The principal complaints of the postconcussion syndrome (without labyrinthine injury) are headache and dizziness; to these are added sleeplessness, irritability, inability to concentrate, and numerous others usually attributed to psychoneurosis and mostly subjective in type. Objectively, postural nystagmus, spontaneous nystagmus, and perverted induced nystagmus are evidence of injury or disease affecting the vestibular centers. A marked disparity in the amplitude of induced nystagmus or in its duration should also be considered objective evidence of imbalance in function and as supporting a claim of vertigo. A difference of one third or more in the duration or intensity of nystagmus may be taken as significant, especially if accompanied by irregularities in the turning tests, including past-pointing and falling, which of themselves would not be conclusive.

In order to differentiate peripheral from central lesions following head trauma, vestibular examination is essential. In a peripheral lesion in the absence of a suppurative process, spontaneous nystagmus and vertigo, which are more or less continuous, decrease and disappear in 2 or 3 weeks. The falling reaction is influenced by head position, being in the direction of the slow component of the spontaneous nystagmus, if present. Postrotational vertigo and nystagmus are about equal in duration. There is usually a concomitant loss of hearing as other evidence of peripheral pathologic condition. The patient feels worse when looking in the direction of the quick component of the nystagmus. The vertigo of a central lesion comes by "spells" over a long period of time. Head position and the direction of the spontaneous nystagmus, if present, have no influence on the direction of falling, which may be in the direction of the side of the lesion regardless of the head position.

If the blow or concussion causes fracture through the cochlea or semicircular canals, sudden and total deafness on the affected side, a staggering gait, and nystagmus will be the prominent symptoms. The nystagmus gradually subsides and altogether disappears in a few days or weeks (see Fracture of the Temporal Bone).

Prognosis. The prognosis in head injury should be guarded. In general the severity of the brain damage can be judged by the duration of the unconsciousness, disorientation, and amnesia. Young persons do better than those past middle age in whom the presence of arteriosclerotic changes is more frequent. If objective symptoms are present and disappear within 5 or 6 weeks, the outlook in general is good. If they persist for 6 months, there will probably be some permanent residua. The outcome of psychoneurosis depends on the severity of the injury, the relief of anxiety, the control of the environment, and many other factors.

Treatment. The early treatment of concussion cases consists of absolute rest and an ice bag to the head. To lower the intracranial tension, from 500 to 1000 ml of 10% dextrose solution or from 50 to 100 ml of 50% sucrose solution may be given intravenously. If there are cold extremities, weak pulse, and sweat, measures to combat surgical shock are necessary.

FRACTURE OF THE TEMPORAL BONE

Pathology. According to various reports, from 60 to 80% of all skull fractures are fractures of the base of the skull, especially of the middle fossa. The temporal bone is involved in over one third of the cases of basal skull fracture. The labyrinth is involved in 25%.

There are three different types of fracture of the temporal bone (Figs. 55–1 to 55–3), which may coexist: longitudinal, transverse, and rupture of the tip of the petrosa. Longitudinal fracture, the most frequent type, starts at the mastoid tegmen and crosses to the roof of the eustachian tube. It is usually linear; if branched, it may run to the external auditory canal or mastoid, rarely to the internal ear. In other words, it is usually a middle ear fracture. If the tympanic membrane is torn, there will be bleeding into the ear canal. The muscles, especially the tensor tympani, may be avulsed; often there will be dislocation of the incus. There are inner ear

hemorrhages only in the severe cases that are usually immediately fatal. About 30% of the patients with longitudinal fracture have conductive hearing loss. These fractures do not heal by bony union, owing to lack of regenerative power of the endochondral layer, and therefore may present a danger of meningitis from subsequent otitis media.

Transverse fractures start at the jugular fossa and cross the pyramid to its anterior surface, involving the vestibule and causing bleeding into the cochlea and semicircular canals. The middle ear will be intact unless the fracture extends through its medial wall.

A fissure or comminuted fracture of the posterior portion of the external auditory canal extending into the mastoid or antrum may result in emphysema over the mastoid. Injury to the lateral sinus occurs in 1% of these cases.

The seventh and eighth nerves may be injured by laceration or compression, usually after their entrance into the internal auditory canal. The facial nerve is reported to be involved in 7 to 45% of the cases of basal skull fracture. The sixth, third, and second cranial nerves may be injured.

Symptoms. Bleeding from one or both ears is reported as occurring in 25 to 75% of all cases of basal skull fracture. The bleeding ordinarily ceases after one or two days and may be profuse if from the tympanic artery or from a clot in the external auditory canal. Blood from external sources should be excluded.

Cerebrospinal fluid escaping from the ear is less common than bleeding from the ear. It always signifies fracture of the base of the skull with involvement of the temporal bone. The opening into the subarachnoid space usually occurs over the tegmen or in the sheaths of the seventh and eighth nerves in the internal auditory canal.

Brain substance in the external auditory canal is rare but, when present, is pathognomonic of a basal skull fracture involving the temporal bone.

Loss of taste on the anterior two thirds of the tongue occurs when the chorda tympani nerve is injured. Fracture of the bony portion of the external auditory canal is usually located in the posterosuperior wall. The

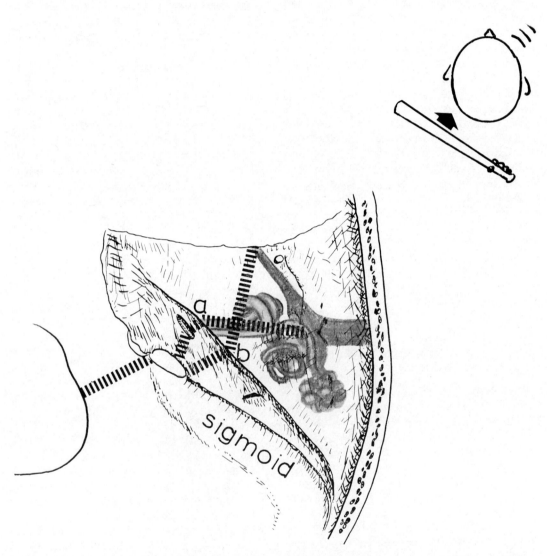

FIG. 55–1. Transverse fracture of the temporal bone (petrous fracture) (diagrammatic): *a*, the fracture line extends along the internal auditory canal, ending between the oval and round windows; *b*, the fracture crosses from the jugular foramen to the eustachian tube (see Fig. 55–4).

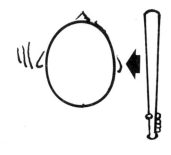

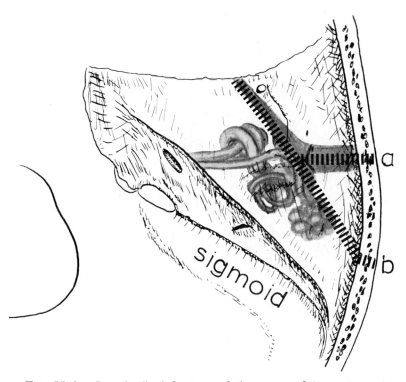

FIG. 55–2. Longitudinal fracture of the temporal bone (mastoidosquamosal fracture) (diagrammatic): *a*, the fracture extends along the external auditory canal, across the tegmen tympani, and along the eustachian tube; *b*, the fracture extends posteriorly along the tegmen mastoideum. (This may occur in combination with *a*.)

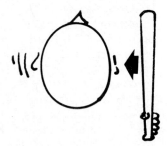

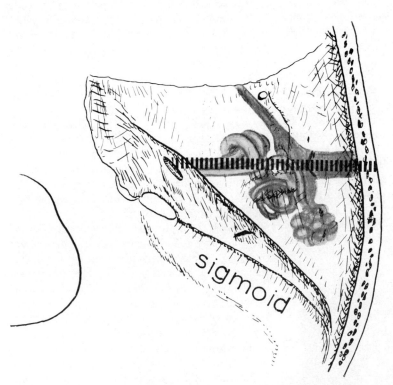

FIG. 55–3. Combined fracture of the temporal bone (axial fracture) (diagrammatic). The fracture involves the internal and external auditory canals.

tympanic membrane and contents of the middle ear, including the chorda tympani nerve, are involved frequently.

Facial paralysis will occur if the seventh nerve is injured. The paralysis is on the same side as the fracture. The sixth nerve is frequently involved in fractures through the middle fossa.

Hearing loss, partial or total, frequently accompanies fractures involving the temporal bone. The hearing loss may be due to injury of the eighth nerve or to hemorrhage or concussion within the cochlea. The hearing loss is in the same side as the lesion and is sensorineural unless the injury involves only the middle ear, resulting in a conductive hearing loss. Tinnitus is usually present.

Vestibular disturbances such as vertigo, nausea, vomiting, spontaneous nystagmus toward the normal side, and past-pointing are present if the vestibular apparatus is involved. Both the vestibular and auditory labyrinths are injured in the majority of cases. The vestibular disturbances gradually subside after several months. With complete destruction of the labyrinth, caloric tests of the affected ear show an absence of response after the subsidence of the acute phase.

Radiographic examination will disclose the fracture in most cases, although the fracture line may appear several weeks after the injury has occurred.

Diagnosis. In longitudinal fractures, blood and cerebrospinal fluid may be found in the

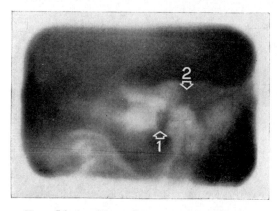

FIG. 55–4. Frontal tomograph of left ear with a fracture extending from the jugular fossa (arrow 1) through the labyrinth to the tegmen mastoideum (arrow 2). (This is diagrammed in Fig. 55–1, *b*.)

external canal. This is certain evidence of a fracture with a rupture of the dura. Redness of the superoposterior wall with other signs of fracture is significant. Hemotympanum or tear of the tympanic membrane is also significant if other signs of fracture are present. Functional tests reveal hearing loss, usually of the conductive type. Radiographic examination is reliable only if positive, since a negative film does not exclude fracture. Longitudinal fracture is by far the most common and in case of doubt is probably present.

In transverse fractures radiographic examination is more reliable (Fig. 55–4). The tympanic membrane is usually intact, but hearing is lost. The labyrinth does not respond to caloric or rotational stimulations.

Prognosis. The mortality rate varies between 5 and 10%. The first 24 to 48 hours are the most critical. Persistent coma indicates increasing danger.

In longitudinal fractures of the skull, about 8% of patients formerly died from meningitis extending from the nose, pharynx, or ear canal. In transverse fractures the death rate was about 15%, especially if there was a crack through the labyrinthine wall into the middle ear. Since the advent of the sulfonamides and antibiotics, the prognosis of skull fractures with a complicating meningitis has improved.

The great majority of skull fracture deaths are due to an acute increase in intracranial pressure. A dilation and fixation of the pupils gives a poor prognosis. The prognosis is better in children than in adults. There is permanent vestibular and auditory function loss in transverse fracture. In longitudinal fractures the prognosis is somewhat better.

Treatment. Complete bedrest is necessary with an ice cap to the head for the relief of headache. With fractures involving the external auditory canal or tympanic membrane, strict asepsis must be observed. The ear should be left entirely alone other than occasional observation. Packing of the ear should be avoided, but a cotton tampon may be placed in the concha to collect blood or spinal fluid. Spinal puncture may be done for the increased intracranial pressure. If in spite of spinal puncture there are still signs of increased pressure after 24 hours, such as unconsciousness, anisocoria, mydriasis on the injured side, and pathologic findings in the spinal fluid, decompression is indicated. Decompression is contraindicated if the patient is moribund, if there are many other fractures present, if there is another severe disease present, and in children generally.

MENIERE'S DISEASE
(IDIOPATHIC LABYRINTHINE HYDROPS)

In 1848 Prosper Meniere described the symptom complex bearing his name, illustrating the report by citing the case of a young girl who died from labyrinthine hemorrhage in order to prove definitely the anatomic origin of the symptoms. Knowledge of the pathologic process (although anticipated by G. Portmann, who likened the disease to glaucoma) was provided by Hallpike and Cairns in 1938, who reported the changes of dilatation of the endolymphatic system accompanied by degeneration of the sensory elements of the cochlea and vestibular apparatus. Since that time, microscopic examination of many involved temporal bones has clarified the exact pathologic picture, while the etiology remains obscure.

Pathology. Knowledge of the pathologic process in Meniere's disease has been gained by study of temporal bones of individuals suffering from this disease. The earliest findings are dilatation of the scala media of the cochlea and the saccule. This dilatation in the cochlea is evidenced by stretching of Reissner's membrane rather than of the basilar membrane. As the disease progresses, there is degeneration of the organ of Corti with loss of hair cell population. Tearing of Reissner's membrane with reattachment further out on the scala vestibuli has been demonstrated in a few temporal bones. Dilatation of the utricle and membranous semicircular canals is not often found, occurring late in the disease or in severe cases.

It has been demonstrated by electron microscopic study that the normal secretory endothelium of the endolymphatic sac has disappeared and been replaced with a simple flattened epithelium in patients with Meniere's disease. Some but not all human temporal bone specimens have demonstrated various degrees of narrowing and fibrosis of the vestibular aqueduct, reducing or obliterating the functional lumen of the endolymphatic duct. Valvassori has developed projections to visualize the vestibular aqueduct by polytomography and, together with others, has reported a high incidence of narrowing or nonvisualization of this structure in patients with Meniere's disease (Figs. 55–5 and 55–6).

The pathology is usually unilateral, but may become bilateral in as many as 25% of patients with longer durations of observation.

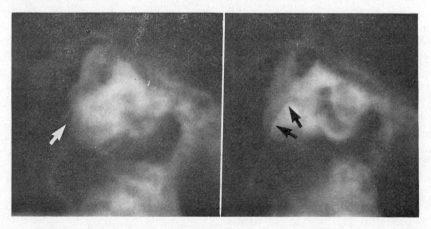

Fig. 55–5. Oblique tomographs of normal right ear. In the figure on the left, the arrow points to the notch where the endolymphatic sac enters the temporal bone. In a more medial section on the right, the arrows point to the course of the normal vestibular aqueduct.

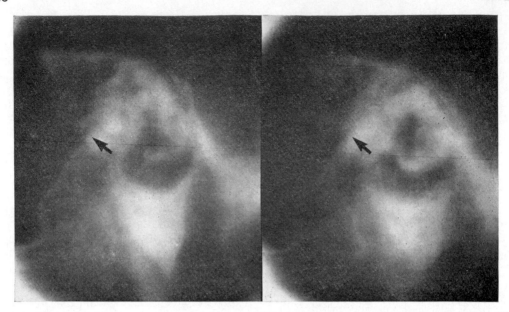

Fig. 55–6. Oblique tomographs of temporal bone of a patient with Meniere's disease. The planes of the sections correspond to those of the normal temporal bone above. In each of these views, the notch for the endolymphatic sac can be seen (arrows), but the vestibular aqueduct is narrowed to the point of obliteration.

Etiology. Although it is clear that this is a disease affecting the fluid physiology of the endolymphatic system, the origin of this disturbance has not been defined. It is not as yet known whether the primary disturbance is one of hypersecretion, hypoabsorption, or a disturbance of balance between both secretion and absorption. Also possible is a deficit of membrane permeability or alteration of osmotic pressure relationships. It is clear that all the energy required for the function of the cochlea is supplied by the stria vascularis and transported by the endolymph, showing that a rapid production of this fluid is needed. The exact site of absorption is not known, but most workers consider it to take place either in the endolymphatic sac or in the stria vascularis.

The most popular theories of etiology have been:

1. Local disturbance of salt and water balance, leading to "edema" of the endolymph.

2. Disturbance of the autonomic regulation of the endolymphatic system.

3. Local allergy of the inner ear, causing edema and disturbance in autonomic control.

4. Vascular disturbance of the inner ear especially of the stria vascularis.

5. Local labyrinthine manifestation of systemic metabolic disease involving either thyroid or glucose metabolism or both.

6. Alteration in the relationship between perilymphatic and endolymphatic pressure dynamics, which may be related to anatomic alterations in both the endolymphatic duct and the cochlear aqueduct.

7. Disturbance of the endolymphatic duct or sac, causing interference with absorption of endolymph. H. House has described a case with an otosclerotic focus blocking the endolymphatic duct which also showed distention of the membranous labyrinth.

This author's experience has led to yet another hypothesis concerning the pathogenesis of Meniere's disease. The concept is that of a primary (undefined) inflammatory or metabolic process acting on the endolymphatic sac and duct, which causes involution of the endothelium and functional narrowing or obliteration of the endolymphatic duct as seen by x-ray examination. These changes may be latent for varying periods of time but become manifest when stress acts upon the fluid systems of the inner ear. This stress will then result in hydrops because of the grossly impaired resorptive apparatus of the endolymphatic duct and sac. The more common stresses appear to be upper respiratory infection, particularly nasopharyngeal; metabolic alteration of thyroid or insulin function; allergic reaction, especially to food or tobacco; and acute emotional problems. Treatment based on this hypothesis has been successful in most patients in affording control of the symptomatology.

Symptoms. Meniere's disease has its onset usually in the third or fourth decade, affecting both sexes equally. It is characterized by active periods of variable length interspersed with longer periods of remission also of a variable length. The pattern of attacks and remissions is impossible to predict in the individual case, although the symptoms tend to become less severe over a period of years.

The symptoms experienced by the patient with Meniere's disease are typical and almost diagnostic. There is usually a period of intra-aural fullness or pressure which the patient may experience for weeks, days, or hours prior to the attack. This sensation is forgotten, however, because of the spontaneous, sudden onset of severe vertigo accompanied by nausea and vomiting. There is an almost unnoticed depression of hearing in the involved ear due to loud roaring tinnitus occurring with the onset of vertigo. The initial episode usually lasts for 2 to 4 hours, at which time the vertigo subsides, although there will be a persistent dizziness with head movement lasting for several hours. The hearing improves and the tinnitus lessens but does not disappear with the subsidence of the vertigo.

There is now a period of freedom from vertigo, during which the patient may notice increasing intra-aural pressure, fluctuation in hearing, and roaring tinnitus. These symptoms are then interrupted by another episode of spontaneous vertigo similar to the first but not as severe. The frequency of these episodes varies but usually they occur as often as once or twice a week or as little as once a month or less. In extreme cases they can occur daily.

Commonly following the above period, which lasts a few weeks, either spontaneous or treatment-induced remission occurs, during which time no symptoms are noted by the patient other than some loss of hearing in the involved ear. This remission does not prove to be permanent, however, with repetition of the above acute phase occurring in a few months. As this pattern of activity and remission goes on, the symptoms during the acute period are dulled by the gradual loss of responsiveness of the end-organ due to degeneration of the sensory elements.

Specific symptoms related to cochlear function occurring in Meniere's disease are:

1. *Fluctuating hearing loss.* The increased fluid pressure in the scala vestibuli and media interferes with acoustic transmission to the hair cell so the hearing efficiency varies with the degree of pressure increase.

2. *Diplacusis* (the perception of a different pitch in the involved ear than in the normal ear). This sensation is due to the tightening of the basilar membrane with increased pressure, changing its "tuning" and shifting the sound to a different set of nerve endings.

3. *Intolerance to loud sounds.* This is evidence of recruitment (see Physiology of Hearing, p. 675) and distortion occurring simultaneously in the involved ear.

Variants in symptomatology have been described and are occasionally encountered. *Lermoyez's syndrome* is one in which the hearing changes occur months or years before the first episode of vertigo. Another form has been described in which the vertigo may occur without affecting cochlear function. Since it has been shown that Meniere's disease affects the scala media primarily, this diagnosis is highly doubtful, and Meniere's disease should not be diagnosed without the typical findings relative to cochlear function described below.

Examination. Tests of cochlear function present a pattern which is typical of Meniere's disease. With the tests available today, diagnosis may be made even without the presence of vertigo, as in Lermoyez's syndrome, and treatment instituted early in its course. The tests to be employed are pure tone air and bone audiometry, speech audiometry, Békésy audiometry, and recruitment testing. Middle ear function, as demonstrated by tympanometry, is normal.

Pure tone audiometry reveals a perceptive hearing loss which in early cases involves the low tones primarily (a rising curve). With progressive destruction of hair cells, the curve becomes flat and then falling in late cases.

Speech audiometry reveals a loss of discrimination which is moderate in severity, usually averaging between 40 and 70%.

The *Békésy audiogram* shows a type II tracing (see Physiology of Hearing, p. 669), which indicates cochlear or hair cell damage.

Recruitment tests, such as Fowler's alternate binaural loudness balance test or the SISI (short increment sensitivity index), will show compete recruitment of the involved ear.

Caloric examination of the vestibular apparatus usually shows reduced function of the involved ear to both hot and cold stimuli.

Treatment. The forms of treatment available today may be divided into medical, conservative surgical, and destructive surgical. Since uninterrupted progression of the disease results in loss of cochlear function, every effort should be made to secure complete and lasting remission. To this end frequent and exhaustive examinations should be carried out and the patient instructed to report any recurrence of symptoms immediately. Medical treatment, as previously indicated, has centered around the various etiologic theories of Meniere's disease. The usual practice is to place a patient on several of these forms of treatment simultaneously, although many recommend proceeding from one form of treatment to another if remission does not occur. Because of the natural history of recurrent activity of the disease, it is extremely difficult to obtain an accurate estimate of the relative efficiency of the many forms of treatment.

1. *Electrolyte and Water Balance.* The earliest forms of systematized treatment attempted to control salt and water intake combined with diuresis, the Furstenberg regimen. This consisted of a high-protein, low-sodium diet combined with the use of ammonium chloride. Later modifications included the administration of potassium chloride to achieve lower serum sodium levels and carbonic anhydrase inhibitors.

In practice this method has proved difficult to control and is usually unacceptable to the patient outside of the hospital. Controlled study has thrown doubt on whether there is any effect on the ear in Meniere's disease, although some experienced clinicians find that it offers a definite measure of success. It has been estimated that at least 30% of the patients will respond.

2. *Vasodilator Treatment.* This has gained widespread acceptance, either in combination with the above regimen or alone. The two most commonly used drugs are nicotinic acid and histamine. Nicotinic acid should be used in flushing doses which must be individually determined and varies between 50 and 150 mg. The most consistent absorption will occur when it is given on an empty stomach, usually in the morning and before supper.

Histamine may be given subcutaneously or sublingually, the latter method being the most practical. In this method histamine diphosphate 0.275 mg/ml is dispensed in a dropper bottle and 2 to 4 drops placed sublingually twice a day before eating. Recent research indicates that histamine, other than achieving vasodilatation, may also affect the metabolism of the ground substance by influencing enzymatic control of the polymerization of mucopolysaccharides. The use of these agents in combination with the Furstenberg regimen has been reported to control as many as 70% of patients.

3. *Control of Autonomic Activity.* This has been less often advocated but is effective in some cases. Among those drugs employed are Banthine (methantheline bromide) and Bellergal (a combination of belladonna alkaloid and phenobarbital). These drugs are usually given four times a day and seem to be most helpful in the milder cases.

4. *Antihistamine Therapy.* Certain antihistamines have shown marked activity in suppressing labyrinthine activity. These drugs—Dramamine, Bonamine, Phenergan, and Antivert (Bonamine plus nicotinic acid) —probably have no effect on the disease directly but rather aid in reducing the vertiginous symptoms. Many have the somewhat beneficial side effect of inducing drowsiness.

5. *Other Drugs.* The emergence and disappearance of treatment recommendations has characterized the literature of Meniere's disease. Among the drugs advocated have been B complex vitamins, B_{12}, intravenous procaine, parenteral epinephrine, cortisone, stilbestrol, and many others. Another drug advocated is lemon bioflavonoid (lipoflavonoid) which has been studied statistically by Williams, who reports improvement in 90% of the patients receiving it. Follow-up study has not verified this degree of potency, however.

Conservative surgical treatment has received a recent reactivation owing to the development by William House of the endo-lymphatic-subarachnoid shunt operation which was conceived by Georges Portmann. This procedure attempts to control the endolymphatic hydrops by creating permanent drainage of the endolymphatic sac into the subarachnoid space. Although there is not as yet firm physiologic basis for this procedure, long-term results reported by Portmann and House indicate a consistent high percentage of success with this procedure. They indicate relief of vertigo in three fourths of the cases and improvement in hearing in one fourth. The greatest value of such a procedure is that, when effective, it prevents deterioration of cochlear function while allowing recovery of remaining function.

The operation consists of exposing the endolymphatic sac through a simple mastoidectomy in the area between the posterior semicircular canal and the lateral sinus (Fig. 55–7). The sac is then entered through an incision in its superior border (Fig. 55–8). An opening is made in the posterior wall to create a fistula or shunt between the endolymphatic sac and the subarachnoid space. A variety of techniques are employed to

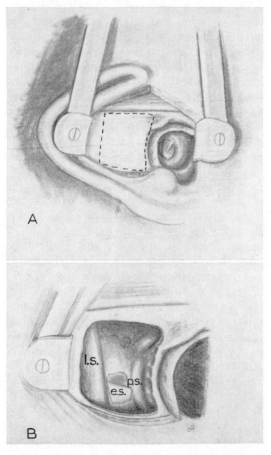

A

B

l.s.

ps.
e.s.

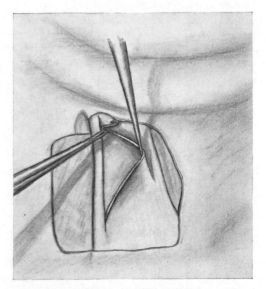

FIG. 55–7. *A,* Endolymphatic shunt operation. The dotted line encloses the area of mastoid cortex removed for exposure. *B,* The endolymphatic sac is located between the lateral sinus and the midpoint of the arch of the posterior semicircular canal.

FIG. 55–8. The endolymphatic sac is opened along its superior margin. A clip formed from a wire stapes replacement prosthesis is placed across the anterior (mastoid) wall of the sac. Drainage occurs by absorption into the mucosal lining of the mastoid.

maintain this opening. Portmann merely incises the posterior wall of the sac. Yamakawa-Naito excises the posterior wall, while Austin places a clip on the anterior wall, draining the sac into the mastoid. House employs a silicone rubber drain to maintain a fistula to the subarachnoid space.

An approach to the saccule through the stapes footplate has been advocated to achieve decompression of the endolymphatic system. This has the advantage of operative simplicity but does not seem to offer the same degree of success as the shunt operation, particularly in regard to hearing improvement.

Another conservative procedure employed for the relief of Meniere's disease is cervical sympathectomy. A procaine sympathetic block is used initially, followed by sympathectomy if the block showed improvement in symptoms. The initial results with this treatment were excellent, but with time a large percentage of patients showed return of symptoms. Sympathetic block is still used to treat sudden hearing loss by some, and there may be indication for this procedure in some bilateral cases.

Destructive treatment must be used in severe or unsuccessfully treated cases. The methods which are available today involve the use of either membranous labyrinthectomy or vestibular nerve section.

Membranous labyrinthectomy may be performed through the oval window, which is approached by a tympanotomy incision as described by Cawthorne. This has the advantage of simplicity and low morbidity. Unfortunately, symptoms may persist in as many as 5% of the cases owing to neuroepithelial remnants not destroyed because of the limitation of access provided by this approach. The operation consists of removing the stapes, fishing out the contents of the vestibule with picks and suction, and then replacing the stapes in the oval window.

The most popular means of membranous labyrinthectomy was also developed in part by Cawthorne and Day (Cawthorne-Day procedure); it exposes the vestibule by openings made in the superior and lateral semicircular canals at their common junction with the vestibule. The contents of the vestibule and both canals are then removed

with instruments and the openings closed with fascia. This procedure results in a low failure rate of less than 1%. Variations in these techniques have been described but do not seem to offer any advantages.

Intracranial section of the vestibular nerve offers complete control of symptoms without affecting cochlear function. Although it was originally performed as a neurosurgical procedure through the posterior cranial fossa, William House has described an approach through the middle cranial fossa which exposes the internal auditory canal from above. This allows inspection of the internal auditory meatus and provides sure identification of the vestibular divisions of the eighth nerve.

In those cases in which preservation of hearing is not a factor, the internal auditory meatus may be reached through the translabyrinthine approach also developed by William House (see Tumors of Cerebellopontine Angle).

Choice of Treatment in Meniere's Disease. Treatment in Meniere's disease must be directed not only at controlling the attacks of vertigo but also at preventing the associated progressive cochlear damage. To this end audiometry should be used at regular intervals, both in active and quiescent stages, in order to chart the effectiveness of treatment.

Initially, this author places all patients on therapy designed to relieve the individual stresses causing activation of the hydrops. Investigation preceding therapy includes estimation of thyroid function through T_3 and T_4 analysis; estimation of glucose metabolism by 5-hour glucose tolerance test; examination of the nose, paranasal sinuses, and nasopharynx to detect chronic infection; and estimation of the psychological status of the patient to detect any obvious anxiety or frustration. Sensitivity to allergens may be suspected by the pattern of attacks in relation to ingestion or exposure.

Most patients will exhibit some degree of hypothyroid state coupled with a flat glucose tolerance curve. Many will have active infection present, especially if seen during periods of activity of the disease. All patients are given a mixture of tri- and tetraiodothyronine in homeopathic dosage and placed on a high dosage of ascorbic acid. A high-protein, low-carbohydrate diet is advised. Local treatment of infection is instituted.

Patients are seen regularly at intervals of 1 to 3 months. They are asked to return immediately should symptoms appear. Since effective therapy requires not only control of vertigo but also maintenance of hearing, failure of the above regimen is signaled by either persistence of vertigo or worsening of hearing. Either of these findings indicates the necessity for surgical intervention.

Three surgical techniques may be employed. The endolymphatic shunt operation is used when there is polytomographic evidence of patency of the endolymphatic duct. If obliteration of the duct is present, vestibular nerve section by the middle fossa approach is indicated (see Surgery of Acoustic Neurinoma, p. 954–5). The third procedure which may be employed if hearing has been lost is labyrinthine destruction. The surest technique is the Cawthorne-Day procedure. Careful diagnosis is most important at this stage to rule out completely the possibility of acoustic neurinoma, since destruction will eliminate the vestibular signs which could signal the presence of such a lesion. If there is any doubt as to this possibility, a translabyrinthine exploration of the internal auditory canal should be carried out, since this will result in both elimination of symptoms and inspection of the area in question (see Surgery of Acoustic Neurinoma, p. 954–5).

Bilateral involvement with Meniere's disease is an especially difficult problem. Here, conservative surgical treatment of the most severe ear should be undertaken early before cochlear deterioration has proceeded to a severe level.

TUMORS OF CEREBELLO-PONTINE ANGLE

Space-occupying disease of the cerebellopontine angle may be caused by any of several tumors, all of which present with similar symptoms. They are considered here because they must be differentiated from other diseases causing unilateral hearing loss and dizziness, particularly Meniere's disease. New surgical approaches to the internal auditory canal have made it possible to remove these tumors with minimum morbidity, the hearing being saved in a few cases, creating the need for early and accurate diagnosis.

Pathology. The most commonly encountered tumor is acoustic neurinoma, accounting for 8.7% of intracranial tumors and 78% of tumors of the cerebellopontine angle; occurring less frequently are meningioma, cholesteatoma, and neruofibroma (von Recklinghausen's disease). The least frequently encountered tumors are benign or malignant gliomas of the brain stem or cerebellum. Rare instances of aneurysm of the basilar artery or its branches in the region have been reported.

Acoustic neurinoma is a slow-growing, benign tumor usually arising from the neurilemma sheath of the vestibular portion of the eighth cranial nerve within the internal auditory canal. Grossly the tumor is soft, often containing areas of necrosis, and is surrounded by a fibrous capsule. Microscopically the tumor is composed of streams of elongated spindle cells with fairly large nuclei and is accompanied by delicate fibers which parallel the long axis of the cells. There are usually areas in which the nuclei are arranged in rows, termed pallisading. Occasionally there are arrangements of nuclei resembling tactile corpuscles (Verocay bodies). The tumor grows slowly but may have periods of relatively rapid growth or may remain quiescent for many years. Although the tumor is not invasive, it causes destruction of the temporal bone and eventually involvement of the cerebellum and brain stem, accompanied by increase in intracranial pressure due to the progressive enlargement.

Symptoms. Although the onset of symptoms is usually insidious, rapid change in size due to hemorrhage or edema may cause sudden onset or worsening, making differentiation from Meniere's disease more difficult. The growth of the tumor within the internal auditory canal causes primary involvement of the eighth and seventh nerves. As the tumor enlarges beyond the internal auditory meatus, the fifth nerve becomes affected also.

The typical pattern is that of unilateral onset of tinnitus, followed by a slowly progressive hearing loss and symptoms of unsteadiness or dizziness. True vertigo may occur but is not as common. Some weeks or

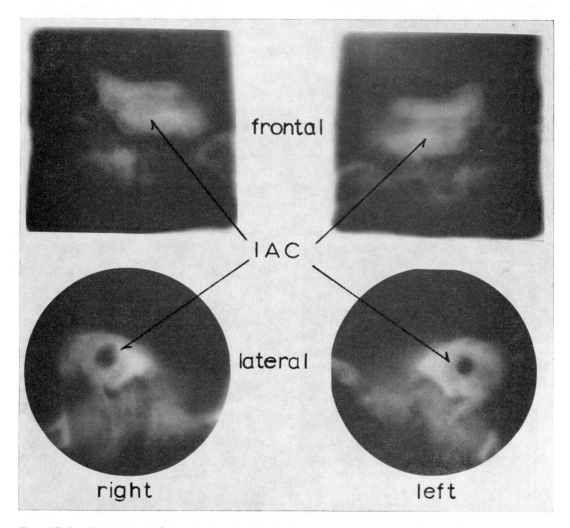

Fig. 55–9.   Frontal and lateral tomograms showing enlargement of the internal auditory canal on the right caused by a small acoustic neurinoma.

months later, numbness or paresthesias of the face may be noted. In late cases cerebellar signs, paralysis of the extremities, and head pain due to increased intracranial pressure may occur.

Diagnosis. In advanced cases the pattern of unilateral hearing loss, loss of vestibular function, and facial and trigeminal nerve involvement, coupled with radiographic evidence of enlargement of the internal auditory canal or erosion of the petrous bone, make the diagnosis of acoustic neurinoma or other space-occupying lesion relatively certain. Since surgical approaches have been developed which make possible the removal of small tumors without loss of cochlear function and the removal of larger tumors without loss of facial function, the early diagnosis of these lesions has become important. To this end an examination battery consisting of auditory, facial nerve, vestibular, and trigeminal function studies combined with delicate radiographic studies must be employed.

Audiometric examination consists of a battery of tests, including pure tone air and bone tests, speech discrimination, Békésy audiometry, SISI, and alternate binaural loudness balance tests. It has been shown that a high percentage of fibers of the auditory nerve may be lost before changes in pure tone thresholds occur, so that early cases may have little hearing loss. As hearing loss develops, it is a perceptive type and affects the high tones initially. Even with a small amount of pure tone loss, there is usually a great loss of discrimination, with the majority of cases being able to understand less than 30% of simple monosyllabic words. Békésy audiometry reveals a type III or IV tracing, indicating rapid fatigue or abnormal adaptation to steady tones. The SISI test and recruitment testing show normal responses in most cases. Middle ear function is normal.

Facial nerve testing in early cases is best done by testing lacrimal function and the threshold of taste to electric stimulation (see Facial Paralysis, p. 988). There will be diminished function of the involved side in the majority of cases. A sign described by House is numbness of the posterosuperior external auditory canal skin near the annulus due to involvement of the seventh nerve.

Vestibular testing reveals an end-organ type of paresis (diminished nystagmus to both hot and cold stimulus) in over 95% of the cases. In some cases, this is the only positive finding.

Trigeminal nerve testing should include light touch and pinprick as well as corneal reflex tests. Findings relative to the fifth nerve indicate extension beyond the internal auditory meatus and are an indication of the size of the tumor.

Radiographic examination should include Stenvers and Town-Chamberlain views, as well as a transorbital projection (Fig. 55–9). Laminography utilizing the polytome is of great value in early cases. Contrast media in the posterior fossa are used to outline the tumor to obtain an accurate estimate of its size and is of great diagnostic help in early cases which show no radiographic change (Fig. 55–10).

Spinal fluid protein determination should be carried out. Elevation of spinal fluid protein occurs in 70% of cases. Both false-

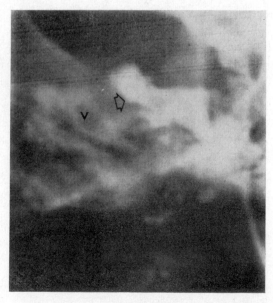

FIG. 55–10. Basal cisternogram with Pantopaque filling the right cerebellopontine angle. The tumor filling the internal auditory canal (arrow) prevents entry of the dye (*V*, vestibule).

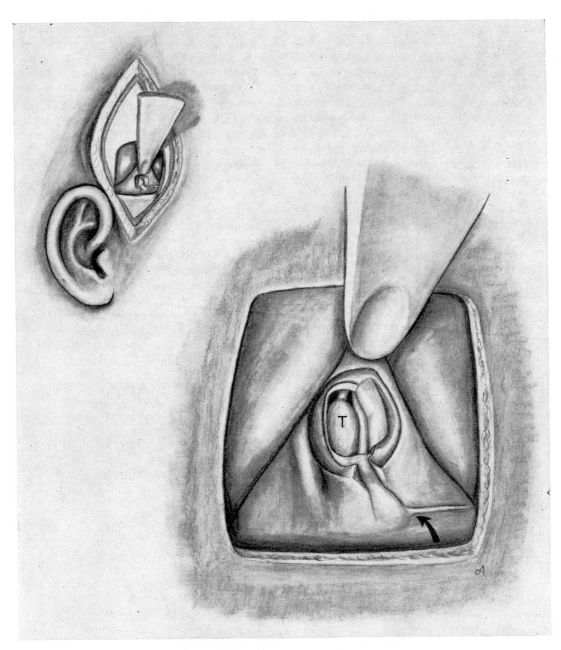

FIG. 55–11.   Middle fossa approach to internal auditory canal. The arrow indicates the junction of the greater superficial petrosal nerve with the geniculate ganglion. A small tumor of the vestibular nerve (*T*) has pushed the facial nerve anteriorly in the canal.

positive and false-negative findings occur in a significant number of cases.

The above findings constitute a distinct pattern making diagnosis absolute. Early cases, however, may show only a few of these signs, indicating the need for full testing in all cases of unilateral hearing loss. In some cases surgical exploration may be the only way to arrive at a diagnosis.

Treatment. The classic approach to tumors of the cerebellopontine angle has been neurosurgical through the posterior fossa, as developed by Cushing and Dandy. Recently William House has developed two microsurgical approaches to the internal auditory canal: one through the middle fossa which unroofs the canal, and a translabyrinthine approach which exposes both the posterior aspect of the canal and the cerebellopontine angle from anteriorly (Figs. 55–11 and 55–12).

The middle fossa approach to the internal auditory canal has the advantage of preserving labyrinthine function and allows the removal of small tumors or vestibular nerve section without sacrificing hearing. Larger tumors may not be removable from this approach, however, causing the development of the translabyrinthine approach. In this

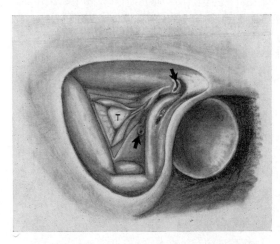

FIG. 55–12. Translabyrinthine approach to the internal auditory canal. The labyrinthine capsule has been removed, the opened portions of the superior and posterior semicircular canals being indicated by the arrows. The acoustic tumor (*T*) has invaded the cerebellopontine angle.

dissection, the entire vestibular system is removed, exposing the internal auditory canal from behind. At the same time the bony plate covering the posterior fossa dura is removed from the lateral sinus to the porus acusticus, giving excellent exposure of the cerebellopontine angle. This allows total removal of large tumors in most cases.

The advantages of these procedures are the markedly reduced morbidity and mortality compared to those in the classic neurosurgical approach because cerebellar damage and edema attendant to the latter are avoided. In addition, the facial nerve may be preserved in many of these cases, since it may be visualized in its normal intratympanic position and dissected free from the tumor. The use of the microscope and training in neurosurgical technique are necessary in the performance of these procedures, which are best carried out as a team effort between otologist and neurosurgeon.

LABYRINTHINE DISEASE AFFECTING HEARING PRIMARILY

Disorders of communicative abilities constitute a severe handicap and an increasingly severe social problem in this country. It has been estimated that between 5 and 10% of the population has a hearing impairment. Since this handicap becomes increasingly prevalent with age, the problem is even more acute than the overall statistics would indicate, as the incidence of hearing loss is greater than 130 per 1000 population in those 65 or over.

Congenital and Neonatal. These causes of hearing loss account for the majority of severe bilateral hearing impairment. These hearing losses are usually not detected until the age of 2 or after and then because of delayed speech development. Unilateral hearing loss may be present for many years until discovered during routine hearing testing or while trying to use the telephone on the involved side. In many instances congenital hearing loss may be associated with other anomalies, in some cases frequently enough to become syndromes. Often mental deficiency or cerebral palsy is associated with hearing loss, creating difficult problems of rehabilitation.

Etiology. Several distinct causes of congenital and neonatal hearing loss have been determined. It is most important to define these causes, because by this means a "high-risk" group of newborn children can be delineated and watched carefully so that much earlier diagnosis and institution of rehabilitative measures can be made. The most important of these causes are maternal rubella; drugs which are ototoxic, such as quinine, or associated with anomalous development, such as thalidomide taken during pregnancy; prematurity, especially when associated with hypoxia; traumatic delivery; and erythroblastosis fetalis. Congenital hereditary involvement may consist of hearing loss alone or may be combined to form distinct syndromes. Anatomically several types of malformation have been described. The Michel type is a complete lack of development of the inner ear. The Mondini-Alexander type shows only a primitive single curved tube representing the cochlea with similar maldevelopment of the vestibular system. In the Bing-Siebenmann type, the bony labyrinth is well formed, but the membranous labyrinth is not. The Schiebe type of malformation involves only the cochlea and saccule and is often accompanied by defects in pigmentation. A peculiar type is the Wardenburg syndrome, in which a white forelock, a prominent epicanthal fold, a widened intracanthal distance, and eyes of different colors (heterochromia iridis), as well as cochlear malformation, are found.

Diagnosis. Diagnosis of this form of hearing loss (Table 55-1) is usually made by inference from a history of nonprogressive bilateral hearing loss first discovered early in life. Delayed development of speech or motor function, as well as the presence of other congenital stigmata, is useful in arriving at this diagnosis. Extensive investigation into the family history should be made, and if possible, hearing tests should be given to the parents and siblings to determine if other members of the family exhibit a hearing loss. As mentioned earlier, those infants who fall into these etiologic categories form a high-risk group and should be observed carefully to determine the existence of a hearing loss so that auditory training may be instituted at the earliest possible age.

Treatment must be gauged by the severity of the hearing loss and the presence of associated deficiencies. (This will be discussed more fully under Management of Sensorineural Hearing Loss).

Familial deafness is a hereditary disease resulting in bilateral perceptive hearing loss as a dominant characteristic. These children are usually born with normal hearing, but during the school years, they suffer a fairly rapid deterioration of hearing in both ears.

Table 55-1.   Sensorineural Hearing Loss in Childhood

Infections	Function		Laterality
	Cochlear	Vestibular	
a. Meningitis	0	0	1 or 2
b. Mumps	0	0 or +	1 or 2
c. Measles	0	+	2
Congenital			
a. Genetic	0	+ — Recessive	1 or 2
	0	0 — Dominant autosomal	
b. Acquired	0	+	2
CNS	+	0	2
Ototoxic			
a. Neomycin	0	0	2

0 = Diminished or absent
+ = Normal
(Courtesy of Richard E. Marcus, M.D., Chicago, Illinois.)

The final hearing loss is variable but is usually quite severe. Special schooling and the fitting of binaural hearing aids is frequently required. Individuals with this type of hearing loss should be advised of the probability of their children suffering a similar affliction.

Presbycusis is by far the commonest affection of the hearing mechanism, so much so that loss of hearing with age has been accurately charted by statistical studies of a large population. The typical pattern is a gradual loss of the higher frequencies of hearing often associated with high-pitched tinnitus. In severe cases the speech frequencies of 2000 cps or lower may be affected.

The etiology of this condition has not been defined, but in the past it has been thought to be due to arteriosclerotic involvement of the stria vascularis. Rosen's studies of hearing acuity in Africa, however, tend to show that the major cause of this hearing loss is noise exposure, with only a small percentage of cases due to constitutional factors.

Symptoms are minimal in this group of patients because of the slow progress of the hearing loss. Advice is usually sought only at the urging of family or friends who are more aware of the problem than the patient.

Diagnosis is made in the typical picture of bilateral high-tone perceptive hearing loss in one of a proper age range. There is usually also a mild loss of discrimination, and if SISI and Békésy tests are done, they will show mild cochlear involvement. This problem does not cause unilateral involvement, and if this is present, another reason must be sought. Dizziness does not occur with this condition.

Treatment consists of evaluation of the hearing handicap of the patient and the fitting of a proper hearing aid if hearing loss exceeds a practical level. These patients should have hearing examinations at regular intervals both to follow any progression of the hearing loss and to note any change in the pattern of the hearing loss.

Ototrophic Viral Disease. Certain viruses may cause hearing loss due to toxic involvement of the cochlea. The most frequent of these is mumps, which is the usual cause of unilateral hearing loss in childhood, occurring in 0.4 per cent of all school children. Measles, pertussis, and influenza may affect either one or both ears. Occasionally viral pneumonia and viral upper respiratory infections are associated with perceptive hearing loss.

Examination of temporal bones in these cases shows extensive damage to hair cells and the stria vascularis.

Diagnosis is made through the history of perceptive hearing loss following one of the above illnesses.

Treatment is through aural rehabilitation in bilateral cases and counseling in unilateral cases. These latter patients will usually not benefit from hearing aids but should be trained in attentiveness. School children should have preferential seating to the front and side of the classroom to keep the good ear in the direction of the teacher's voice.

Drug Ototoxicity. Ototoxic side effects have been observed after exposure to chemicals of many classes. The frequency of this exposure has increased substantially in spite of concern with environmental protection and Federal Drug Agency concern with consumer protection. The most commonly encountered ototoxic drugs are:

Antibiotics: Streptomycin, dihydrostreptomycin, neomycin, kanamycin, gentamicin, vancomycin, polymyxin B, viomycin, and ristocetin

Diuretics: Ethacrynic acid and furosemide

Chemicals: Salicylates, quinine, antibrene, nitrogen mustard, carbon monoxide, mercury, arsenic, tobacco, gold, and alcohol

Chemically these agents may act in varied ways. Ototoxicity may appear rapidly with short-term exposure; it may occur more slowly during administration or exposure; or it may appear some time after cessation of exposure. Most of these drugs initially manifest as tinnitus, most often a high-pitched ringing. Although tinnitus may be the only manifestation, audiometric monitoring will usually show a progressive high-tone sensorineural hearing loss. Vestibular examination will often reveal loss of caloric response prior to or accompanying the hearing loss, especially with streptomycin and gentamicin. The insidious nature of these effects and their minimal symptomatology frequently result in severe functional loss before the patient or physician is alerted to the presence of ototoxicity. The ototoxic potential is increased many times if renal disease is present. These potent antibiotics are commonly used in the treatment of renal disease, thus greatly increasing the risk in this class of moribund patients. Neomycin has often been used in treating skin and bladder infections in infants and has produced its ototoxic effects by absorption across the inflamed surfaces.

Since hearing loss and vestibular paralysis are permanent in most cases, the thrust of care must be toward prevention. This is best achieved through avoidance of ototoxic agents when possible or through vestibular and hearing testing to detect the first appearance of toxicity in order to reduce or discontinue their use promptly.

The mode of action of ototoxic agents varies with the type of drug. The antibiotics generally cause hair cell damage which may be directed to the cells of the cristae and maculae or to the cells of the organ of Corti or both. Most observers feel that these drugs are concentrated in the endolymph and have a direct specific toxic effect. The diuretics listed have their effect upon the stria vascularis, creating effects similar to those seen in the renal tubules. Fluid accumulates between the intermediate cells of the stria, and there are changes in the microstructure of the secretory cells. Cessation of administration usually results in a rapid return to normal. It is felt that these agents affect primarily the sodium-potassium balance by interfering with the ATP transport mechanism. Other chemicals such as quinine, mercury, and lead have their primary effect on the neural pathways of hearing, including the spiral ganglion, eighth nerve, and cochlear nucleus. The site of action of aspirin has not yet been defined.

As new drugs appear, an increased occurrence of ototoxicity will undoubtedly follow. It will remain the responsibility of the otolaryngologist to detect these ototoxic drugs and to continue to alert the medical community to the dangers of ototoxicity.

Sudden Idiopathic Hearing Loss. This form of hearing loss has been described with increasing frequency in recent years. The typical patient presents with a history of an apoplectic onset of hearing loss often associated with transient vertigo and persistent tinnitus. Many of these patients will regain a portion of the lost hearing in the ensuing weeks or months, but in most a residual deficit remains. In the majority of cases, only one ear is affected.

The etiology of this condition is unknown, there being three likely possibilities: occlusion of the internal auditory artery by spasm or thrombosis, subclinical mumps (an increasing titer of mumps antibodies was demonstrated in a high percentage of one group of these patients), or a single episode of Meniere's disease, resulting in permanent loss of cochlear function.

Treatment is most effective if instituted within 48 hours of onset of the hearing loss. Bedrest is mandatory for the first week of treatment. During this period the use of anticoagulants (especially heparin), intravenous histamine in optimum dosage, and vasodilators, such as nicotinic acid or Arlidin, should be given. The most effective method of vasodilation is by stellate ganglion block administered daily for 7 days. After 7 to 10 days the patient may be ambulatory but should be kept on nicotinic acid and small doses of histamine until periodic (bimonthly) hearing testing reveals no further improvement.

Other Causes. Many types of systemic illness have been known to cause perceptive hearing loss through cochlear or neural involvement. The most frequently occurring are blood dyscrasias, multiple sclerosis, syphilis, carbon monoxide poisoning, lead poisoning, anemias, nephritis, diabetes, and metabolic diseases. These must all be kept in mind when a patient presents with hearing loss, especially when symptoms involving other systems are present.

MANAGEMENT OF SENSORINEURAL HEARING LOSS

Rehabilitation of the hearing handicapped is a complex problem, and experience in the past few years has taught the value of the multidisciplinary approach to its solution. Since World War II, an interdependence and reciprocal encouragement between workers in medicine (the generalist, obstetrician, pediatrician, neurologist, psychiatrist, and otologist) and those in nonmedical specialties (the audiologist, psychologist, hearing therapist, speech therapist, teacher for the hard of hearing and deaf, public health nurse, social case worker, social group worker, and vocational rehabilitation counselor) have developed. The common interest of these diversified occupations has brought about an integrative effort to bring help to the hearing handicapped.

The treatment of such a patient may be divided into four basic parts, which are individually different, depending upon the age of the individual. These categories are the assessment of the hearing loss and its effect on the patient, informing the patient of the nature of the handicap and the measures to be utilized in rehabilitation, institution of the planned program of care, and finally, follow-up of the patient's progress.

Audiologic Assessment. Evaluation of hearing loss must include not only determination of the patient's hearing acuity for pure tone sounds but also, more importantly, testing of discrimination. The latter test is most important because it indicates the direction that rehabilitation must take.

Hearing problems in children are especially difficult for the physician, not only in determining the degree of impairment but also in arriving at the decision as to whether hearing loss is present. Hearing loss occurring before or during the age of speech development has severe effects on auditory behavior, language development, and emotional maturation. These effects then may produce great difficulty in determining whether the lesion is peripheral, perceptive, or expressive. Not infrequently a child is observed with hearing loss, mental deficiency, emotional disturbance, and aphasia, illustrating the difficulty of this evaluation.

It is essential to detect hearing problems as soon as possible in order to provide the hard-of-hearing child with the proper guidance and counsel. To this end most speech and hearing centers have adapted the multidisciplinary approach with children, utilizing a staff which includes psychologists, social workers, neuropsychiatrists, and otologists, as well as audiologists.

The parents of these children will be puzzled over the need for this program. To them the child cannot hear and needs an operation or a hearing aid. Adding to their difficulty is a sense of guilt over the origin of the hearing loss. Many times the parents need more help than the child in adjusting to the situation in order to provide the home environment conducive to educational progress.

The emotional problems which occur with hearing loss in the adult constitute a major problem of therapy. Not only does hearing loss produce a threat to economic advancement in the male, but also it may become a symbol of sexual inadequacy for either sex. Since communication is the essence of all social behavior, this handicap also affects this aspect of life, often resulting in withdrawal from outside contacts. Resistance to rehabilitative efforts is also frequently present, presumably because of the blow to the ego produced by the obvious sign of handicap created by wearing a hearing aid. Complicating the above problems is the patient's frequent depressive conviction that hearing loss is always progressive, resulting finally in complete loss of hearing.

The foregoing incomplete list of doubts and fears of the patient facing a hearing handicap indicates the absolute necessity of a long and frank discussion. It is important for these patients to maintain hope, and to this end a discussion of the advances achieved through research in the field of communication is most helpful.

Hearing Aids. *Methods of Rehabilitation.* The evolution of the modern hearing aid has been a mainstay in the correction of hearing handicaps. Through the use of these devices, patients with hearing losses as severe as 70 dB may be helped. Hearing aids, however, have great limitations in their application to many patients, and these limitations must be understood by both physician and patient if hearing aids are to be correctly prescribed and successfully used.

The hearing aid is a tiny amplifying system with a limited and usually nonlinear frequency response. It has a limited output and, when driven beyond this, creates distortion. The microphone picks up unwanted noise as well as verbal communication and amplifies everything without discrimination. When worn at ear level, only a limited amount of gain may be used before feedback with its attendant sequela occurs, and when it is worn on the body to avoid this, a great deal of adventitial noise is created by friction with clothing.

As difficult as the above problems may seem, the chief limitation in the use of a hearing aid is in the patient with discrimination difficulty. The patient and his family must understand that amplification permits hearing softer sounds but will not make the understanding of speech any better, since the distortion of words occurs within the cochlea of the patient, and in fact if the aid is used with too much volume, it may even cause reduction in clarity. Unless this problem is fully understood by the patient, he will be disappointed in the partial benefits obtained and not infrequently discontinue use of the aid altogether. To help in overcoming this difficulty is the main indication for the use of binaural hearing aids which result in moderate improvement in discrimination as compared to unilateral amplification.

The greatest efficiency is obtained by the use of air conduction ear molds fitted in the canal. Occasionally the presence of a chronic ear infection contraindicates this use, and a bone conductor must be worn behind the ear. Irritation created by the ear mold and the accumulation of cerumen and debris necessitate frequent inspection and gentle cleaning of the canal. These follow-up examinations also allow evaluation of the patient's progress and should include close questioning of the patient to determine if other avenues of therapy need to be utilized.

Education of the Hearing Handicapped. The educational needs of those with a hearing loss are extremely complex and varied. The physician may be faced with the problem of a child with brain injury and total loss of hearing or an elderly patient with gradually increasing presbycusis now faced with the problem of learning to accept and use a hearing aid. The former patient will require the entire resources of a municipal or state-supported educational system to achieve effective rehabilitation and a useful adult life. The latter patient requires guidance and reassurance from his physician who understands the problems not only of hearing loss but also how this handicap is influenced by age.

The range of resources available include preferential seating in school, special classes in a normal school, special schools for handicapped children, and schools for the deaf. The American Hearing Society or similar groups usually offer classes for lip reading or general help to adults in adjusting to a compensated hearing loss, which are available in urban centers. Some speech and hearing centers will offer the same type of classes. The need for special education or classes cannot always be empirically determined, so that close follow-up of progress and performance is necessary in all age groups to evaluate the need for adjusting the educational program.

Unilateral Hearing Loss. Unilateral hearing loss is a common problem and one which is sometimes underestimated as to its impact on total hearing. Although the loss of function of one ear does not reduce the threshold for hearing, it does eliminate binaural appreciation of sound. This has two effects on hearing; the first is to markedly impair the sense of direction of the sound source. The second and more severe loss is that of the ability to separate conversation from background noise. This latter effect is particularly troublesome to students and to adults whose business requires this ability.

Both of these functions are carried out at a cortical level and depend on information arriving from both ears approximately equal in loudness sensitivity. The brain is then able to perceive and utilize small differences in phase and pitch to determine direction of sound and to cancel out unwanted background noise.

The usual method of compensating for this handicap is preferential seating in school and instructing adults to place themselves at work so that the better ear is toward the source of wanted sound and away from noise. It is also important to instruct these individuals as to the importance of concentrating on a speaker's lips in order to provide information which may be masked by the background noise.

Some individuals may be helped by the use of a hearing aid which may be worn in the most troublesome situations. This is possible when the loss is not too severe and poor discrimination in the affected ear will not adversely affect the total hearing by causing degradation of the wanted signal. The fitting of a hearing aid in unilateral hearing loss should certainly be considered and evaluated in those individuals with a particularly difficult hearing problem in their occupations. Among this group are school teachers, lawyers, sales people, and executives or others who participate in meetings at a conference table. These aids need not be worn constantly but only when the particular situation demands it.

REFERENCES

Altmann, F., and Kornfield, M.: Histological Studies of Meniere's Disease. Ann. Otol., 74:915, 1965.

Austin, D. F., and Hart, G. R.: Short Term Study of Endolymphatic Shunt Operation. Arch. Otolaryng., 81:359, 1965.

Austin, D. F.: Modern Diagnosis and Treatment of Acoustic Neuroma. Am. J. Med. Sci., 251:468, 1966.

Cawthorne, T. E.: The Treatment of Meniere's Disease. J. Laryngol., 58:363, 1943.

Cawthorne, T. E.: Labyrinthectomy. Ann. Otol., 69:1170, 1960.

Day, K. M.: Labyrinthine Surgery for Meniere's Disease. Laryngoscope, 55:617, 1943.

Derlacki, E. L.: Medical Management of Endolymphatic Hydrops. Laryngoscope, 75:1518, 1965.

DiGeorge, A. M., et al.: Waardenburg's Syndrome. Trans. Am. Acad. Ophthal. Otolaryng., 64:816, 1960.

Dix, M. R., and Hallpike, C. S.: The pathology, symptomatology and diagnosis of certain cancerous disorders of the vestibular system. Ann. Otol., Rhinol., Laryngol. 61:987, 1952.

Fick, I. A.: Sacculotomy for Hydrops. Laryngoscope, 75:1539, 1965.

Fields, W. S., and Alford, B. R.: *Neurological Aspects of Auditory and Vestibular Disorders.* Springfield, Ill., Charles C Thomas, Publisher, 1964.

Godlowski, Z. Z.: Endocrine Management of Allergy. Arch. Otolaryng., 71:513, 1960.

Goodhill, V.: The Nerve Deaf Child. Ann. Otol., 59:1123, 1950.

Hallpike, C. S., and Cairns, H.: Observations on the pathology of Meniere's syndrome. J. Laryng. & Otol., 53:625, 1938.

Harrison, M. S.: Endemic Vertigo-Vestibular Neuronitis. Brain, 85:613, 1962.

Heck, W., et al.: Comparison of Toxicity of Streptomycin and Dehydrostreptomycin. Ann. Otol., 62:101, 1953.

Hitselberger, W. E., and House, W. F.: Acoustic Neuroma Diagnosis. Arch. Otolaryng., 83:218, 1966.

House, H. P., et al.: Current Management of Hearing Loss in Children. Am. J. Dis. Child., 108:677, 1964.

House, H. P., and House, W. F.: Transtemporal Bone Removal of Acoustic Tumors. Arch. Otolaryng., 80:601, 1964.

House, W. F.: Subarachnoid Shunt for Drainage of Hydrops. Arch. Otolaryng., 79:338, 1964.

James, J. A.: Ultrasonic Therapy for Hydrops. Laryngoscope, 75:1552, 1965.

Karmody, C. C., and Schucknecht, H. F.: Deafness in Congenital Syphilis. Arch. Otolaryng., 83:18, 1966.

Lederer, F. L.: Hearing Loss from the Womb to the Tomb. Arch. Otolaryng., 74:391, 1961.

Lederer, F. L., and Austin, D. F.: Office Treatment of Hearing Loss. Mod. Treat., 2:1182, 1965.

Lindsay, J. R.: Positional Nystagmus in Otoneurological Diagnosis. Laryngoscope, 55:527, 1945.

McGee, T. M., and Olszewski, J.: Streptomycin and Dihydrostreptomycin Toxicity. Arch. Otolaryng., 75:295, 1962.

Meniere, M. P.: Maladies de l'oreille interne offrant les symptomes de la congestion cérébrale apoplectiforme. Gaz. Méd. Paris, 16:55, 88, 239, 279, 597, 1861.

Portmann, G.: Surgical Treatment of Vertigo. Laryngoscope, 75:1522, 1965.

Portmann, M.: Decompressive Opening of Endolymphatic Sac. Arch. Otolaryng., 79:328, 1964.

Proctor, C. A., and Proctor, B.: Understanding Hereditary Nerve Deafness. Arch. Otolaryng., 85:23, 1967.

Pulec, J. L., et al.: Technic of Posterior Fossa Myelography. Laryngoscope, 75:1572, 1965.

Quick, C. E.: Chapter 26 *In* Paparella, M. M., and Shumrick, D. A. (Eds.): *Otolaryngology.* Philadelphia, W. B. Saunders Co., 1973.

Rosen, S. T., et al.: Presbycusis Study. Ann. Otol., 71:727, 1962.

Schucknecht, H. F.: Meniere's Disease. Laryngoscope, *73*:651, 1963.
Shambaugh, G. E., Jr.: Surgery of the Endolymphatic Sac. Arch. Otolaryng., *83*:305,
1966.

Sheehy, J. L.: Vasodilator Therapy in Sensorineural Hearing Loss. Laryngoscope, *70*:885,
1960.
Wolff, D.: Malformations of the Ear. Arch.
Otolaryng., *79*:288, 1964.

Chapter 56

Industrial Noise Exposure and Hearing Loss

Meyer S. Fox

Historical Development. The problems created by industrial noise are of interest to the otolaryngologist because of the disturbing consequences resulting from noise exposure. In the worker, excessive noise produces a hearing loss; in industry, it produces an economic liability; and to society as a whole, it produces a social responsibility. This chapter discusses these various facets of occupational hearing loss. It is intended to indicate the essential knowledge of the problem and how hearing loss can be prevented or minimized in industry. Although the occupational hearing loss problem has been brought to the forefront in recent years, its existence has been known for over a century. It was long known that workers in certain noisy occupations, such as braziers, blacksmiths, railroad workers, and weavers, gradually developed hearing loss over the years of their employment. Likewise, the deafness occurring in branches of the military services were well known. Altogether too often, this hearing impairment accompanying years of employment was taken for granted and considered as a sign of a good worker.

In 1937, C. C. Bunch[1] published an extensive monograph on occupational deafness. He reviewed the previous studies and emphasized the medical, legal, and social problems which would arise. During World War II and thereafter, as modern industry developed and expanded, high-speed machines were introduced, mass production increased, and the resultant occupational noise became more intense and more frequent, thereby increasing the problems brought about by noise exposure. About this time several scientific groups of the military, medical, and acoustical professions decided to investigate the relations of hearing loss to noise exposure. In 1946 the Committee on Conservation of Hearing of the American Academy of Ophthalmology and Otolaryngology established a subcommittee, known as the Subcommittee on Noise in Industry, whose purpose and function was to study and report on the various aspects of the noise problem, its relation to hearing loss, and to make recommendations on how the hearing loss could be prevented or minimized. The Subcommittee on Noise in Industry and its Research Center over the years actively investigated the many aspects of the problem in its laboratories, in industrial environments, and by means of mass survey studies. The subcommittee published many reports and recommendations, including the Guide for Conservation of Hearing in Noise,[2] which is used for the establishment of industrial hearing conservation programs.

Two other interested groups, namely the American Standards Association, through its exploratory subcommittee Z-24-X-2, and the National Research Council and Armed Forces, through the Committee on Hearing and Bio-acoustics (CHABA), studied the relation of hearing loss to noise exposure with the purpose of setting damage risk criteria. The CHABA group concerned itself with the auditory and nonauditory effects of noise, not only upon persons in the military but also upon nonmilitary personnel working or living in areas close to airfields.

The economic stimulus to do something about the noise problem came as the result of a large number of hearing loss claims filed by workers in New York,[3] Wisconsin,[4] and elsewhere. The important challenge to do something about the noise problem resulted when the U.S. Department of Labor issued specific safety and health regulations under the Walsh Healey Act[5A] in 1969 and subsequently under the Occupational Safety and Health Act (OSHA)[5B] in April of 1971. These regulations specified noise criteria pertaining to permissible noise exposure limits for all employees working in noisy occupations. Violation of the federal noise criteria could result in severe penalties and closure of the plants. The primary objective of both the Walsh Healey and OSHA acts is hearing conservation. As the result of the workmen's compensation claims and the OSHA regulations, many diverse groups became actively interested and involved in the noise problems, including employers, unions, members of the legal and medical professions, legislative bodies, compensation boards, insurance carriers, and health and safety personnel.

Definitions. Occupational hearing loss can be defined as a hearing impairment of one or both ears, partial or complete, arising in, during the course of, and *as the result of one's employment.* It includes both acoustic trauma, as well as noise-induced hearing loss. The term *acoustic trauma* is often used to denote noise-induced hearing loss, as well as the sudden hearing loss resulting from intense blasts, explosions, gunfire, and direct trauma to the head or ears. These conditions, however, should be described by separate terms in order that one may logically distinguish between them. *Acoustic trauma,* denoting injury to the neural elements of the inner ear, should be reserved for the immediate hearing injury produced by one or a few exposures to sudden intense acoustic forms of energy, resulting from blasts, explosions, or direct trauma to the head or ear. It should be thought of as one single incident to which the worker relates the onset of the hearing loss. One or both ears may be affected, and it may involve the conductive as well as the sensorineural part of the ear. *Noise-induced hearing loss,* on the other hand, is used to describe the accumulative permanent loss of hearing, always of the sensorineural type, that develops over months or years of exposure to hazardous noise levels. Noise-induced hearing loss usually affects both ears equally in extent and degree. It should be kept in mind that the onset of the hearing loss, its progression and permanency, and the characteristics of the audiogram vary depending on whether the loss is noise-induced or due to acoustic trauma.

Noise is defined by the physicist as sound due to acoustic waves of random intensities and frequencies. As found in industry, noise represents unwanted sound and wasted energy. This wave motion is made up of pressure fluctuations that move outward from the source, usually vibrating at a speed of about 1100 feet per second. Two aspects of the pressure wave are important to the production of noise-induced hearing loss: (1) frequency, which is the number of fluctuations per second; and (2) sound pressure level, which indicates the magnitude of the fluctuations.

The frequency of the sound largely determines its pitch. Frequency is measured in vibrations per second or cycles per second, also designated as Hertz (Hz). The young adult with normal hearing can hear sounds ranging from as low as 20 Hz to as high as 16,000 to 20,000 Hz. Higher frequencies above 20,000 Hz are generally inaudible and are known as ultrasonics. Perhaps the most vital portion of the audible frequency range lies between 500 and 2000 Hz, the speech zone range. Hearing loss occurring in this frequency region is particularly important, because it handicaps the person in

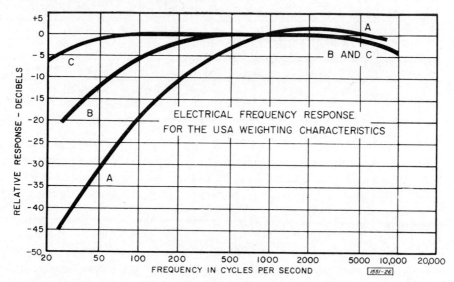

FIG. 56–1. Frequency-response characteristics in the USA Standard for Sound-Level Meters S1.4,, 1961. (From General Radio Company Handbook, West Concord, Mass., 1967.)

everyday activities and in communications with his family, friends, and coworkers.

Sound pressure level (SPL) is a measure of comparative amounts of sound. The sound pressure level of a noise is expressed in decibels. The decibel is a dimensionless unit based on the logarithm of the ratio of the sound pressure of the noise and a reference sound pressure. Noise analysis includes the measurement of sound pressure levels of various bands of frequencies in the noise. The analysis is made with a combination of a sound level meter and an octave band analyzer. The sound level meter is a device which reacts to the amplitude of sound pressure changes in the air so that objective quantitative measurements of sound levels can be made without analyzing the various frequency components. It is little more than an electronic ear which changes sound into electrical signals which can be measured. The sound level meter also has built-in weighting circuits—A, B, C—to indicate in a general way the frequency of the noise. A switch is provided for the selection of the circuit desired. The chief difference, as shown in Figure 56–1, is that the low frequencies below 500 Hz are filtered out by the A network, moderately so by the B network, and hardly at all by the C network. The A scale responds very much like the human ear, and

hence it has been adopted for noise measurements. A more complete and informative analysis of sound can be made using frequency wave analyzers. These devices, through the use of electronic filters, can measure the part of the energy in a complex sound wave which is present within a particular band of frequencies. By its use it is possible to determine not only the overall

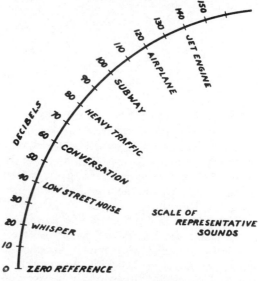

FIG. 56–2. Sound pressure levels re 0.0002 dynes/sq cm.

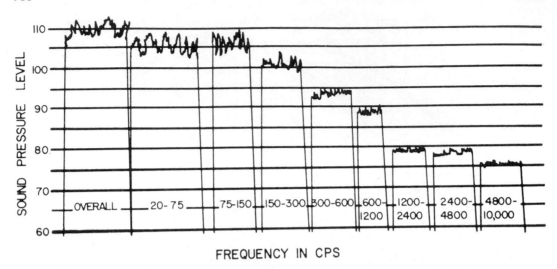

FIG. 56–3. Octave band analysis of a noise re 0.0002 dynes/sq cm.

intensity level of the sound but also the energy present in the various component sounds which go to make up the noise. The sound pressure levels of representative sounds and an octave band analysis of one kind of noise are shown in Figures 56–2 and 56–3.

For evaluating sudden impact sounds like those caused by artillery fire, drop hammers, punch presses, pneumatic tools, etc., which generate such swift powerful pulses that take place and die away before either the sound level meter or wave analyzer can measure them, the cathode ray oscilloscope, a peak meter, and high-speed photography have been used. The measurement of noise requires a high degree of skill. It should be undertaken only by personnel with training and experience in the use of appropriate equipment.

Effects of Noise. The known effects of noise exposure are of two types: *nonauditory effects,* which cause interference with communication by speech or which otherwise influence behavior; and *auditory effects,* which consist of temporary hearing loss and permanent hearing loss.

Nonauditory Effects of Noise Exposure. Perhaps the best understood nonauditory effect is interference with communication by speech. In industry the ability to communicate by speech is important. It is essential in employee training, in giving or under-

standing orders, in giving warning signals, and in other phases of plant operation. In addition, the inability to hear can be annoying to those concerned. It should be pointed out that many noises which are not intense enough to cause hearing loss may interfere seriously with communication by speech. The degree of interference depends primarily on two factors. The masking ability of the noise and the communication requirements of the situation, both of which can be measured.

The term speech interference level (SIL) is the measure of the interfering effect of noise on the ability of two people to converse. It is usually defined as the arithmetic average of the sound pressure level in the three octave bands 600 to 1200, 1200 to 2400, 2400 to 4800 Hz. These values may vary depending upon the distance at which the conversation is being carried out, the kind of voice, and environmental factors.

The annoyance caused by noise is an individual psychological reaction and depends a great deal upon the physical status, mental attitude, and personal motivation of the person or persons being annoyed. These factors are difficult to predict and defy objective measurements. In general, noises of high intensity, high frequency, and intermittency tend to be more annoying, but there are large individual differences in reaction. Annoyance itself is not a health hazard, and the fact that a noise is annoying does not establish it as a damage risk. Conclusions drawn from the most reliable tests of efficiency in performing mental and motor tasks under various conditions of noise exposure are that sudden and unfamiliar noise temporarily reduces efficiency, but that when an employee becomes accustomed to the noise, his efficiency returns to a previous non-noise performance level.

Studies have been reported describing the effects of noise upon health. The World Health Organization has defined health as a state of physical, mental, and social well-being. Schiff[6] reviewed the literature and reported on studies describing the effects of noise upon health. Cantrell[7] in a recent well-controlled investigation reported on biochemical changes resulting from prolonged exposure to intermittent noise. It is known that certain temporary changes occur in the human body as a result of noise exposure. Many of these changes are in the form of a stress reaction, but adaptation usually takes place without permanent effects. Long-term studies in these areas will be necessary to establish definite causal relationships to permanent health effects of workers.

Auditory Effects of Noise Exposure. When the normal ear is exposed to noise at damaging intensities for sufficiently long periods of time, a temporary depression of hearing results, disappearing after minutes or hours of rest. This temporary hearing loss is a physiologic phenomenon referred to as temporary threshold shift (TTS). It is believed to occur in the hair cells of the organ of Corti and may possibly be associated with metabolic changes in the hair cells, chemical changes in the inner ear fluids, or vascular changes in the inner ear. When the exposure is longer or the intensity greater or both, a stage is reached at which the hearing loss no longer returns to its original level. This is called noise-induced hearing loss or permanent threshold shift (PTS).

Studies by Glorig[8] and his staff have revealed the following important facts regarding temporary and permanent threshold shifts.

1. The temporary threshold shift (TTS) resulting from one day's exposure to noise levels of 100 dB or more may vary from no shift to 40 dB.

2. Typical industrial noise exposure produces the largest temporary shifts at 4000 and 6000 cycles per second.

3. Most of the temporary shift occurs during the first 2 hours of exposure.

4. The amount of temporary shift and its frequency location vary with the amount and frequency location of the permanent shift; i.e., the more the permanent change at any frequency, the less the temporary at that frequency.

5. Recovery from temporary threshold shift occurs mostly within the first hour or two after the noise exposure has ended.

6. There appears to be a distinct relationship between temporary and permanent threshold shifts: (*a*) a noise which does not produce a temporary hearing loss will not produce a permanent hearing loss; (*b*) the configuration of the audiogram seen in short temporary threshold shift will resemble that found when the permanent hearing loss is measured.

Experimental studies on temporary threshold shift have demonstrated that continuous exposure and interrupted exposure produce different effects in the ear. If a noise follows a pattern of 1 minute "on" and 1 minute "off," for example, the amount of temporary loss is just half that which is produced when the same noise is on continuously. If a similar effect occurs for permanent hearing loss and if employees are allowed relatively quiet periods at intervals throughout the day, then long-term changes in hearing will be less than changes produced by continuous exposure.

Noise Exposure and Other Factors Affecting Hearing. There are many factors that affect the degree and extent of hearing impairment found in cases of noise deafness. These are (1) intensity or loudness of the noise (sound pressure level), (2) type of noise (frequency spectrum), (3) period of exposure each day (duty cycle per day), (4) total work duration (years of employment), (5) individual susceptibility, (6) age of worker, (7) coexisting ear disease, (8) character of surroundings in which the noise is produced, (9) distance from source, and (10) position of each ear with respect to sound waves. The first four are the most important factors in noise exposure.

It has been observed that brief momentary exposures to high noise levels will usually not produce any significant hearing loss, while prolonged exposure to noise levels above 90 dBA may result in significant loss over the years. Thus, it is necessary to know not only "how much noise, but also what kind of noise and for how long." While a great deal has been learned about noise exposure and hearing loss as it applies to steady state noises, our knowledge about the hazard of impact noises, such as blasts, rifle fire, and drop hammers, to hearing is quite limited.

Characteristics of Permanent Hearing Loss. The early stage of noise-induced loss is characterized by a sharply localized dip in the threshold curve at the frequencies between 3000 and 6000 Hz, usually appearing first at 4000 Hz. In the early stages of noise-induced hearing loss, the worker may complain only of tinnitus, muffling of sound, discomfort in the ears, or a temporary depression of hearing, which is noted at work and upon leaving work but which clears after several hours away from the noise. Pain and vertigo are seldom encountered. As noise exposure continues, the loss spreads in both directions, but there is still little noticeable hearing effect on the subject. Impairment of hearing is usually not noticed until the hearing level of the speech frequencies—500, 1000, and 2000 Hz—average more than 25 dB (ANSI, 1969). Substantial losses may occur at frequencies from 3000 to 8000 Hz, producing no subjective awareness of a change in hearing. The onset and progress of noise-induced hearing loss are slow and insidious, and the worker is likely to be unaware of its existence or to disregard it. The hearing loss is of the sensorineural type quite similar in extent and degree in both ears. Otoscopically the eardrums appear normal.

Susceptibility Tests. Various attempts have been made to predict susceptibility to hearing loss as the result of noise exposure. It is obvious that such a test, if practical, would have great value. Most of these tests are based upon the use of temporary threshold shift procedures. Unfortunately, as of the present time, no practical susceptibility test has been developed which offers any degree of reliability or validity.

Sudden Loss. While noise-induced hearing loss is the result of repeated exposure over long periods of time, there are records[9] of cases in which the hearing loss was attributed to short-term exposures to sounds of high intensity. Attempts have been made to explain these unusual cases on the basis of special orientation or position of the ears to the sound source or stooping posture with the cervical spine held in an abnormal position, and by assuming these were cases of acoustic trauma rather than of noise exposure. However, the exact mode of production of the hearing loss in these cases remains unknown.

Presbycusis. Presbycusis is the loss of hearing which accompanies advancing age. This sensorineural hearing loss in older people has been attributed to atrophy of the end-organ, neural degeneration, vascular changes in the stria vascularis, or other changes in the inner ear.[10] Bunch[1] suggested that presbycusis is the accumulative effect of daily noise exposure over the years, which is responsible for the gradual deterioration. Glorig[8] has labeled this type of hearing loss as *sociacusis*. Studies performed at the Research Center, Subcommittee on Noise, and reported by Glorig and Davis[10] indicate that physical changes in the middle ear, occurring with age, lead to a conductive presbycusis. Rosen,[12] in a study of the hearing of a noise-free population in Africa, calls attention to the role of circulation, nutrition, heredity, tissue changes, climate, and the stress and strain of modern civilization, all of which may contribute to the time of onset and magnitude of presbycusis. Clinically it is usually difficult to distinguish between presbycusis and noise-induced hearing on the basis of the audiogram alone.

Coexisting Ear Disease. Ears with a pre-existing conduction lesion are less susceptible to noise damage than ears with normal hearing. This is explained by the concept that an existing conductive lesion will protect the ear, just as does an ear defender, and accordingly reduce the intensity of sound reaching the inner ear. These workers, therefore, should not be excluded from working in noisy areas. On the other hand, individuals with sensorineural hearing losses should be carefully evaluated and protected before exposure to intense noise levels. This is of particular importance with young apprentice individuals who may anticipate many years of noise exposure.

Character of Surroundings. The environment in which the worker is exposed to noise naturally assumes importance. Room acoustics play an important part. Sounding boards, reverberating chambers, and deflecting walls enhance prevailing noise. This is a problem of interest to acoustical and safety engineers who undertake to reduce the noise levels.

The position of each ear with respect to sound is of particular importance to military personnel exposed to explosions and gunfire and occasionally to an industrial worker whose job requires special orientation of the head in performing certain tasks. One ear may therefore receive a greater noise exposure, leading to a difference in hearing thresholds of the two ears. Likewise, the overall sound pressure level can be varied by altering the distance from the source of the sound.

Structural Changes in Noise-induced Hearing Loss. Reports concerning the histologic and postmortem studies of noise-induced hearing loss in humans have been few. The inner ear damage varies from minor changes in the hair cell endings to complete destruction of the organ of Corti. The exact process of production is not completely known, but it appears that overstimulation by noise for long periods of time produces metabolic changes and devascularization which eventually cause degenerative damage to the cell structure. In acoustic trauma the cochlear damage results from the intense vibration of the basilar membrane with its attached organ of Corti.

The hearing losses produced by noise and acoustic trauma have been studied experimentally in both humans and animals. Human experimentation has been primarily limited to studies of temporary threshold shift (TTS). Animal experimentation, as reported by Schuknecht,[13] has the advantage of lending itself to the study of temporary and permanent hearing losses and of the patho-

logic changes in the cochlea. Quantitative methods are used for evaluating the cochlear function and pathology in the animals, and the interrelationships of sound exposure, cochlear pathology, and hearing thresholds can be studied.

Experimental animal studies have indicated that high-intensity pure tones of high frequencies injure elements in the midbasal end of the cochlea and that low frequencies injure elements near the apex of the cochlea. Broad band noise of high intensity creates structural changes in the basal coil in the region serving the 4000 Hz area. Mild changes consist of disruption or degeneration of the outer hair cells and their supporting cells. More severe changes show degeneration of both outer and inner hair cells and flattening or complete loss of the organ of Corti.

Several explanations have been offered as to why the area which analyzes 4000 Hz is more vulnerable to noise exposure. Popular theories are that the anatomic structures at this region are more fragile and that it is the result of auditory acuity and the spectrum of sound stimulation. It is observed that the earliest frequency loss is usually about one half to one octave above the frequency range of the tonal stimulation. Since the threshold of hearing is more acute in the region between 1000 and 3000 Hz, it is reasonable to expect that industrial noises, because of their spectrum, would produce the earliest changes between 3000 and 4000 Hz.

MEDICOLEGAL ASPECTS OF THE INDUSTRIAL NOISE PROBLEM

Hearing loss resulting from noise exposure presents legal as well as medical problems. An understanding of the nature and extent of these problems must be preceded by some knowledge of the purpose, origin, development, and present-day status of workmen's compensation legislation.

Prior to the enactment of Workmen's Compensation Acts by the various states, an employee could obtain benefits for injuries due to industrial accidents mainly through a judgment at common law for damages. The faults of this last recourse were numerous. The employee was expected to assume a certain amount of on-the-job risk. In addition, there was the legal question as to whether the alleged injury was due to the negligence of the employer, the employee, or a fellow worker. Workmen's Compensation Acts were passed to eliminate much of this uncertainty by substituting wage loss or loss of earning capacity in place of negligence or fault as a basis for compensation.

Workmen's Compensation Acts originated in Germany and Great Britain in the latter part of the nineteenth century. In this country the first compensation legislation was enacted by the federal government for its employees in 1908. Wisconsin became the first state to have an effective Workmen's Compensation Act in 1911. The other states gradually followed, so that today all have some form of Workmen's Compensation statutes. While the original compensation laws covered only liability for wage loss resulting from disabling accidents at work, they were later amended to provide benefits for nondisabling accidents and occupational disease. Although the purpose and intent of the Compensation Acts of the various states might have some common features, they do vary considerably in their interpretation, coverage, schedule, and benefits.

Noise-induced hearing loss was not considered to be much of an industrial hazard or problem until 1947 when a large number of claims for alleged loss of hearing due to industrial noise exposure arose in the state of New York.[3] In 1950 hundreds of claims were filed in the state of Wisconsin.[4] Soon thereafter, cases appeared throughout the country. While loss of hearing resulting from sudden accidental acoustic trauma had previously been recognized and compensated, the new claims arising from noise exposure were met with surprise and resistance by industries and their insurance carriers. Alarmed and concerned, they felt that it was not the intent and purpose of existing legislation to compensate for a type of hearing impairment which resulted in neither wage nor time loss to the worker. These cases were therefore appealed to the higher courts of the various states. Between 1948 and 1953, decisions of the higher courts in the states of New York, New Jersey, Wisconsin, California, and Missouri and of the federal

courts of New York upheld the right of the worker to claim compensation for hearing loss arising from industrial noise exposure. Since that time, courts in other states have rendered similar opinions.

The causal relationship between noise and resulting hearing loss requires consideration of many complex acoustical, medical, audiological, and legal factors. Therefore, the otologist who examines and evaluates the industrial hearing loss cases must be properly informed, not only concerning the otologic aspects but also about the physical and legal aspects of the problem.

The otolaryngologist who appears as a medical expert in these cases must be an impartial and disinterested expert who will assist the courts and commissions in resolving the medical problem at hand. He must be objective and scientific and should not concern himself with the social and economic aspects of the problem. When, how much, or under what condition compensation is to be paid for loss of hearing are not matters for the medical man to decide. These are the functions of the commissions and courts.

The statements of the otolaryngologist should be based upon reasonable accepted otolaryngologic practices and not upon mere speculation. The words that throw the testimony into the category of speculation include "may," "possible," "could have been," "could be," "might," and "might have been." These are all terms of conjecture. As a rule, the opinions of the medical expert, when he is appearing before industrial commissions, need be based not upon medical certainty but rather upon reasonable medical probability. Probability applies to that which is so reasonable or well evidenced that it almost induces belief. In other words, the testimony should be based upon what the expert would ordinarily expect to find in the usual circumstances.

In order to establish a clinical diagnosis of noise-induced hearing loss and causal relationship to employment, the physician or otolaryngologist must consider the following factors:

1. The history of the hearing loss, its onset and progress.

2. The occupational history pertaining to

the type of work, years of employment, etc.

3. The noise studies to determine if the noise is of a type and of sufficient intensity and duration to cause hearing loss.

4. The results of the otologic examination.

5. The results of audiologic and hearing studies (pre-employment, periodic, and termination).

6. The ruling out of nonindustrial causes of hearing loss.

Numerous thorny medicolegal problems and questions accompanied the early claims of workers for alleged loss of hearing due to noise. Over the years many of these questions and problems have been settled by industrial and clinical studies, by laboratory investigations, and in some instances by compromise. There was an early demand on the part of industry, industrial commissions, courts, safety directors, and physicians for damage risk criteria. The original estimates of a dangerous level attempted to give a single number—the sound pressure level of the noise—which was supposed to represent the decibel level above which hearing loss would occur and below which the noise would not be hazardous to hearing. Clinical and industrial investigations soon revealed that noise-induced hearing loss depended upon other factors beside the overall noise level.

The Guide for Conservation of Hearing in Noise[2] had previously proposed standards for steady state noise exposure limits based on octave band analysis and exposure time. With the introduction of the OSHA regulations,[5] 90 dBA as a single overall number for an 8-hour day is used as a basis for hazardous noise exposure (see Table 56–1). Impulsive or impact noise is defined as sound with a rise time of not more than 35 milliseconds to peak intensity, measured at fast response, and a delay of not more than 500 milliseconds. It is recommended that exposure to impulsive noise should not exceed 140 decibels peak sound pressure.

It should be pointed out that, while it is desirable to protect the hearing of all workers at all frequencies, such a goal is not obtainable from a practical and operational standpoint. All hearing conservation programs have certain limits, and it is important to remember that the 90 dBA level was a compromise designed to protect the hearing of the majority of the workers for those frequencies necessary for speech (500, 1000, and 2000 Hz). It is estimated that by using the 90 dBA scale, about 90% of the workers will have these important frequencies protected during their work lifetimes. The National Institute for Occupational Safety and Health[14] has suggested that an 85 dBA exposure level would be more realistic and more effective in preventing hearing loss and that the 85 dBA level should be used as a guide for mandatory ear protection and hearing testing programs. Available studies show that about 40% of the industries have noise levels of 90 dBA or over. Many of the state

Table 56–1. Permissible Noise Exposures

Duration per Day (hours)	Sound Level dBA Slow Response	
8	90	When the daily noise exposure is composed of two or more periods of noise exposure of different levels, their combined effect should be considered rather than the individual effect of each, if the sum of the following fractions, C1/T1 + C2/T2 . . . Cn/Tn, exceeds unity, then the mixed exposure should be considered to exceed the limit value. Cn indicates the total time of exposure as a specified noise level, and Tn indicates the total time of exposure permitted at that level.
6	92	
4	95	
3	97	
2	100	
1½	102	
1	105	
½	110	
¼ or less	115	

Industrial, Noise and Hearing Conservation, National Safety Council, p. 308, 1975, Chicago Ill. 60611.

agencies through their hygiene or safety divisions are adopting safety codes which use the 90 dBA scale criteria.

The sensorineural hearing loss that results from noise exposure is similar to that found in many other instances without apparent cause. It is therefore difficult in any particular case without a base line pre-employment audiogram to state what part of the hearing loss can be attributed to the employment. The same problem presents itself where the employee has worked for numerous employers, each of whose employment might have contributed to the final hearing loss. Who is then to be held responsible for the hearing loss found at the time of the claim? Several states have arbitrarily settled this problem by enacting statutes or rules which hold the last employer who has contributed to the hearing loss responsible for the entire loss, unless by competent audiometric evidence the hearing level at the beginning of employment can be established. These rules and statutes have alerted industry to the need for pre-employment hearing tests of its workers.

Another important controversial medicolegal problem pertains to the various testing procedures used by physicians to determine the hearing ability of the claimant and the methods used to convert these readings into percentages of hearing impairment. After several years of studying the methods and procedures previously used, the Subcommittee on Noise of the Committee on Conservation of Hearing of the American Academy of Ophthalmology and Otolaryngology published its Guide for the Evaluation of Hearing Impairment[15] in 1959. The principles and recommendations therein were subsequently approved and incorporated into the Guide for Determination of Physical Impairments of the Ear, Nose, Throat and Related Structures published in the Journal of the American Medical Association in 1961.[16] These guides were the first officially approved formulas for determining percentage of hearing impairment. They provide a definitive method which is easily applied, can be understood by judge, examiner, or jury, and makes provision for the establishment of hearing impairment in one or both ears.

Because of its importance to the otolaryngologist the pertinent portion of the Guide is herewith reprinted below with permission of the editors of the Journal of the American Medical Association.

"Impairment," is here used in accordance with the definition of the American Medical Association, denoting a medical condition that affects one's personal efficiency in the activities of daily living. It is recognized that "disability," as used in various Workmen's Compensation Laws, involves nonmedical factors, since it may be related to actual or presumed reduction in ability to remain employed at full wages. Permanent impairment is, therefore, a contributing factor to, but not necessarily an indication of, the extent of a patient's permanent disability within the meaning of the Workmen's Compensation Laws.

The evaluation or rating of permanent impairment is a function of the physician alone and enters into the evaluation of permanent disability. The evaluation or rating of permanent disability is an administrative and not a medical responsibility and function.

Ideally, hearing impairment should be evaluated in terms of ability to hear everyday speech under everyday conditions; the term "impairment" will be used hereinafter in this sense only. The ability to hear sentences and repeat them correctly in a quiet environment is taken as sufficient evidence of satisfactory hearing for everyday speech. The hearing level* for speech should be estimated from measurements made with a pure tone audiometer. For this estimate, the Subcommittee recommends the simple average of the hearing levels at the three frequencies 500, 1000, and 2000 Hz.

In order to evaluate the hearing impairment, it must be recognized that the range of impairment is not nearly as wide as the audiometric range of human hearing. Audiometric zero, which is presumably the average normal hearing threshold level, is not the point at which impairment begins. If the

*The hearing level of the listener is the number of decibels that his threshold of hearing lies above the standard audiometric zero for that frequency. It is the reading on the so-called "hearing" dial of an audiometer that is calibrated according to ANSI(1969) or ISO(1964) levels.[17]

average hearing level at 500, 1000, and 2000 Hz is 25 dB or less, usually no impairment exists in the ability to hear everyday speech under everday conditions. At the other extreme, however, if the average hearing level at 500, 1000, and 2000 Hz is over 92 dB, the impairment for hearing everyday speech should be considered total (see Table 56–2). The Subcommittee on Noise recommended the following formula: for every decibel that the estimated hearing level for speech exceeds 25 dB, allow 1.5% up to the maximum of 100%. This maximum of 100% is reached at 92 dB (ANSI, 1969).

Recently, there has been some dissatisfaction with the AMA formula which is based only upon the average pure tone readings of the three frequencies 500, 1000, and 2000 Hz. It is felt that, in order to assess more accurately the hearing loss for speech under everyday conditions by means of pure tones, a modification of the AMA formula is warranted. It has been suggested that the 3000 Hz reading replace the 500 Hz reading in the computation.[14]

It should be pointed out that the formula used to determine the percentage of hearing impairment should *not* be modified or altered for the purpose of increasing or decreasing the amount of the compensation award. The final monetary award to the claimant will depend upon three factors: (1) the schedule of the number of weeks allowed for permanent total loss of hearing; (2) the monetary award for each week of the schedule; and (3) the formula used for evaluating the hearing impairment.

The formula used should be based upon scientific, medical, and audiological principles. The amount of compensation to be awarded is a matter for the commissions and legislative bodies to decide.

The Subcommittee on Noise recommended that any method for the evaluation of impairment include an appropriate formula for binaural hearing based on the hearing levels in each ear tested separately. Specifically, the Subcommittee on Noise recommended the following formula: the percentage of impairment in the better ear is multiplied by 5. The resulting figure is added to the percentage of impairment in the poorer ear, and the sum is divided by 6. The final percentage represents the binaural evaluation of hearing impairment. It is not the percentage of hearing loss. (See Table 56–2.)

The role of presbycusis in the evaluation of noise-induced hearing loss claims has received considerable attention. Several compensation boards have an arbitrary rule requiring a deduction for the threshold shift accompanying age. In those formulas or methods which do not use the 25 dB level as the beginning of impairment, often referred to as a low fence, or in which the 3000 and 4000 Hz frequencies are included in the evaluation, a deduction for the hearing loss accompanying age seems reasonable. However, in the Guides of the American Academy of Ophthalmology and Otolaryngology and the American Medical Association for the determination of hearing impairment, in which only the average of the three frequencies 500, 1000, and 2000 Hz and a low fence deduction of 25 dB is used, presbycusis does not become much of a factor. The reason for this is that the average threshold shift associated with age at the frequencies 500, 1000, and 2000 Hz that is to be expected in a group of normal men who have never been exposed to very loud noise is negligible at 40 years of age. It is not over 15 dB at 50 years and is 20 dB on the average at 65 years. Even the latter value is well below the level of 25 dB at which impairment of hearing of everyday speech is considered to begin. Therefore, the Committee on Conservation of Hearing of the American Academy of Ophthalmology and Otolaryngology has gone on record that no deduction should be made for presbycusis.[18]

In the discussion of noise exposure, it was pointed out that temporary threshold shift was related to the permanent hearing loss present. Attempts to establish the permanency of the hearing loss may be difficult if the claimant is working in noise at the time he presents himself for examination. The otolaryngologist must make sure that the claimant has been away from the noise for sufficient time to eliminate any contamination by temporary threshold shift. Some agencies, for economic and administrative reasons, require a 6-month removal or waiting period after termination of exposure to harmful noise before a claim can be filed.

Table 56–2. Example for Determining Percentage of Hearing Impairment (ANSI, 1969)

Hz	500	1000	2000	3000	4000	6000
Rt. (dB)	35	40	60	65	70	65
Lt. (dB)	40	50	60	70	75	70

Frequencies most important for
the understanding of speech.

Right Ear (dB)	Left Ear (dB)
35	40
40	50
60	60
———	———
135	150

$\dfrac{135}{3}$ dB $=$ 45 dB estimated hearing level for speech, right ear.

$\dfrac{150}{3}$ dB $=$ 50 dB estimated hearing level for speech, left ear.

To convert estimated hearing level for speech to % impairment of hearing:

Right Ear (dB)	Left Ear (dB)
45	50
−25	−25
———	———
20	25

20 dB $\times$ 1.5% $=$ 30% impairment   25 dB $\times$ 1.5% $=$ 37.5 % impairment

To convert the above monaural impairments to % binaural impairment, the formula is:

5 times % of hearing impairment in better ear: 5 $\times$ 30% $=$ 150%
Add % of hearing impairment in worse ear: 37.5%
                                                          ————————
                                                             187.5%

Divide the total by 6:

$\dfrac{187.5\%}{6} = 31.25\%$

The result is the % binaural impairment, or 31.5% in this case.

When a worker terminates his employment by retirement, his hearing status can be evaluated and the case closed. When no waiting period is required, there may be a tendency to file claims in an irresponsible fashion. Many of these repeated claims turn out to be nuisance claims in which the administrative, legal, and medical costs exceed the awards.

In 1966 the writer (M.S.F.), with the assistance of Mr. Ralph Gintz, Director of Workmen's Compensation of the State of Wisconsin, conducted a survey of all existing compensation statutes and rules in the United States and Canada.[19] The survey was updated in 1976. The purpose of these studies was to make a comparative analysis of the important provisions as they pertain to occupational hearing loss and particularly to learn how the hearing loss was determined and evaluated. Table 56–3 summarizes the most recent facts relative to the hearing loss statutes and rules as received from the various Industrial Accident Boards and Commissions* and from the 1974 edition of Workmen's Compensation Laws of the U.S. Chamber of Commerce.[20]

A comparative analysis of the existing Workmen's Compensation statutes and rules in the United States and Canada indicates great variances in the provisions pertaining to noise-induced hearing loss. All agencies recognize and compensate for hearing loss resulting from trauma. As of 1976 some 57 states and Canadian provinces have established legislation recognizing noise-induced hearing loss and providing for compensation for such loss.

The award for the hearing loss resulting from either trauma or noise exposure is usually determined by means of a schedule based upon total loss for one or both ears. Some agencies permit compensation based upon a wage loss, and in a few instances the award is computed as a percentage of the body as a whole.

The hearing threshold level is usually determined by means of pure tone air conduc-

tion audiometric testing procedures. Several agencies reported that they use the Guides of the American Academy of Ophthalmology and Otolaryngology and the American Medical Association; a few require the use of a specified formula or method, but most states rely on expert medical testimony. It is therefore important that the otologists become familiar with and use the Guides in the evaluation of hearing impairment in medicolegal cases. There are great variances in the schedules, in monetary awards, and in the relative value of one ear to both ears. It should be pointed out, however, that these are primarily the result of previous legislative judgment and decisions. Quite a few states will award compensation for tinnitus associated with the hearing loss, and most states provide the cost of a hearing aid, depending upon medical testimony. The question arises as to what, if any, consideration should be given to improvement with the use of a hearing aid. Several of the state agencies have indicated that a corrective factor is in order when there is improvement in the hearing ability with the use of a hearing aid. But the American Medical Association Guide emphasizes that impairment of hearing should be determined without benefit of the hearing aid. This recommendation is consistent with the general policy of determining impairment of body function without the use of any prosthetic device, and any benefit that results from the use of such a device should not be a mitigating factor in determining the hearing impairment.

A study of the survey of hearing loss statutes in the United States and Canada reveals numerous differences and areas of conflict and misunderstanding. These are problem areas in which the otolaryngologists are involved. The informed otolaryngologist is needed to help define and clarify areas of otologic involvement and to help develop uniform procedures based on recognized medical principles. The OSHA criteria and guidelines try to reduce hazardous noise exposure at its source, thereby preventing hearing loss. A national commission on Workmen's Compensation Laws was established under the provisions of the Occupational Safety and Health Act. This commission conducted a comprehensive study and

*It is inevitable that in a survey of this type changes will have occurred by the time of publication. It is therefore recommended that the reader check the latest information as to legislative or administrative changes in a particular jurisdiction.

Table 56-3. Comparative Provisions for Occupational Hearing Loss in Workmen's Compensation Cases
(After Fox.[19] Revised 1976)

Jurisdiction	Recognize Hearing Loss due to Noise	Specify Noise Level	Regulation for Ear Protection	Schedule in Weeks One Ear	Schedule in Weeks Both Ears	Maximum Compensation One Ear (traumatic)	Maximum Compensation Both Ears	Formula or Method Used	Waiting Period	Presbycusis Deduction	Compensation for Tinnitus	Compensation Nonorganic Hearing Loss	Provision for Hearing Aid	Credit for Improvement with Aid	COMMENTS
Alabama	Yes	No	No	53	163	$5,406	$16,526	°	No	°	°	°	°	No	Workmen's Compensation law administered by courts may use any criteria it deems appropriate to establish the degree of hearing loss.
Alaska	Yes	Yes	Yes	52	200	$7,280	$28,000	M.E.	No	°	Yes	Yes	Yes	No	Deduction for presbycusis can be made by the board upon sufficient evidence.
Arizona	P	–	–	20 months	60 months	$11,000	$33,000	A.M.A.	No	P	P	P	Yes	No	Noise-induced hearing loss compensated upon gradual injury theory.
Arkansas	Yes	No	No	40	150	$2,660	$9,975	M.E.	No	No	P	P	Yes	P	Credit for improvement with a hearing aid may be considered by the commission.
California	Yes	Yes	Yes	60	240	$3,157	$21,770	A.M.A. includes 3000 Hz	No		Yes	P	Yes	Yes	Uses a modification of the A.M.A. formula to include the 3000 Hz frequency.
Colorado	Yes	Yes	Yes	35	139	$2,940	$11,676	M.E.	No	Yes	Yes	P	Yes	No	Figures given are for so-called standard rating. The state has experienced large incidence of hearing loss claims.
Connecticut	Yes	No	No	52	156	$6,552	$19,656	M.E.	No	No	No	?	Yes	No	
Delaware	Yes	Yes	Yes	45	175	$5,625	$13,125	M.E.	No	No	?	?	Yes	?	?
Dist. of Columbia	Yes	–	–	52	200	$16,552	$63,660	A.M.A.	No	P	P	P	Yes	No	Figures given are taken from the U.S. Chamber of Commerce Report 1976.
Florida	Yes	Yes	Yes	40	150	$4,480	$16,800	M.E.	No	Yes	Yes	Yes	Yes	–	Question of award for presbycusis, tinnitus, and non-organic hearing loss is decided by judge of industrial claims.
Georgia	Yes	Yes	No	–	150	$5,700	$14,250	A.M.A.	6 months	No	No	No	Yes	No	The report applies only to noise-induced hearing loss claims. Traumatic hearing loss cases are handled differently.
Hawaii	Yes	Yes	No	52	200	$8,684	$33,400	A.M.A.	No	Yes	Yes	?	Yes	No	
Idaho	Yes	Yes	Yes	–	°	°	$14,437	A.M.A. & M.E.	P	?	Yes	Yes	Yes	No	Total loss of binaural hearing is equal to 35% of the whole man. Whole man is equal to 500 weeks of compensation.

State	1	2	3	4	5	6	7	8	9	10	11	12	Comments
Illinois	Yes	No	100	200	°	°	°	No	No	–	–	–	New statutes for occupational hearing loss became effective July 1, 1975. Partial permanent hearing loss compensable. The guidelines and formula have not been established. The amount of the award is based primarily upon the hearing loss and the percentage of weekly earnings.
Indiana	Not decided	No	75	200	$ 4,500	$12,000	M.E.	No	No	No	Yes	No	Noise-induced hearing loss is not specifically mentioned in the Indiana statutes.
Iowa	Yes	No	50	175	$ 7,350	$25,725	M.E.	No	P	Yes	Yes	No	
Kansas	Yes	No	30	110	$ 3,093	$11,341	M.E.	No	No	–	–	–	No definite requirement as to method for measuring loss of hearing. Formula used is a variation of the A.M.A. formula of 1942.
Kentucky	Yes	Yes	75	150	$ 7,200	$14,976	A.M.A.	No	No	P	P	Yes	Figures given are taken from the U.S. Chamber of Commerce report 1976. Provision for hearing aid and credit for improvement.
Louisiana	°	°					M.E.					°	Commission may award up to 100 weeks. Most questions not answered.
Maine	Yes	No	50	200	$7,070.50	$28,282	A.M.A.	6 months	*Yes	Yes	Yes	No	Deduction for presbycusis, ½ db for each yr. over 40.
Maryland	Yes	Yes	Based on bilateral loss	250 weeks	°	$14,655	A.M.A.	6 months	Yes	?	–	–	Schedule based upon binaural loss usually 250 weeks. On severe bilateral hearing loss can be increased to 333 wks, at rate of $117.24/wk. equivalent to $39,040.92.
Massachusetts	No	No	150	400	$ 4,500	$12,000	M.E.	No	P	P	Yes	No	Must be total loss in one or both ears to be compensable.
Michigan	Yes	No	°	°			M.E.	No	P	P	Yes	No	Legislation on Workmen's Compensation laws changes being considered. At the present time, must be total loss of hearing in one ear or both ears. Can be compensated on wage loss and inability to perform usual and customary work.
Minnesota	Yes	Yes	85	170	$11,475	$22,950	M.E.	No	No	P	Yes	No	
Mississippi	Yes	No	40	150	$ 2,520	$ 9,450	M.E.	No	No	Yes	Yes	No	Change in legislation being considered.
Missouri	Yes	No	40	148	$ 3,200	$11,840	A.M.A.	6 months	*Yes	No	Yes	Yes	Deduction for presbycusis ½ db after 40 yrs. of age. Credit given for improvement with the use of hearing aid.
Montana	Yes	Yes	40	200	$ 2,940	$14,700	A.M.A.	6 months	*Yes	No	Yes	No	Deduction for presbycusis ½ db for each year over 40 years of age.

* See "Comments" in far right-hand column
M.E.—Medical Evidence
P—Possible
A.M.A.—American Medical Association

977

Table 56-3 (*Continued*). Comparative Provisions for Occupational Hearing Loss in Workmen's Compensation Cases (After Fox.[19] Revised 1976)

Jurisdiction	Recognize Hearing Loss due to Noise	Specify Noise Level	Regulation for Ear Protection	Schedule in Weeks One Ear	Schedule in Weeks Both Ears	Maximum Compensation One Ear (traumatic)	Maximum Compensation Both Ears	Formula or Method Used	Waiting Period	Presbycusis Deduction	Compensation for Tinnitus	Compensation Nonorganic Hearing Loss	Provision for Hearing Aid	Credit for Improvement with Aid	COMMENTS
Nebraska	No	No	No	50	100	$ 5,000	$10,000	A.M.A.	No	No	Yes	Yes	Yes	No	
Nevada	Yes	Yes	Yes	°	°	°	$10,000	A.M.A.	No	No	Yes Medical basis	No	Yes	No	Uses A.M.A. guide. Total unilateral loss at 18% of body as a whole. Total bilateral loss at 35% of body basis.
New Hampshire	Yes	Yes	°No	52	214	$ 7,644	$31,458	A.M.A.	No	No	P	No	Yes	No	
New Jersey	Yes	No	No	75	200	$ 3,000	$ 8,000	Old A.M.A. formula most freq. used	No	No	Yes	Yes	Yes	No	Basis for tinnitus and nonorganic loss is the evaluation of the whole man and his subjective complaints. Processed about 1500 claims past 2 years. Frequently uses 1942 A.M.A. formula.
New Mexico	°No	No	No	40	150	$3,918.40	$14,694	M.E.		No	No		—	—	Only traumatic loss covered at this time. Legislative changes being considered.
New York	Yes	Yes	Yes	60	150	$ 5,700	$14,250	A.M.A.	6 months	No	Yes	Yes	Yes	No	Compensation for tinnitus if accompanied by hearing loss. Compensation for non-organic loss is on a case to case basis; if causally related cases are considered individually.
North Carolina	Yes	No	°Yes	70	150	$10,220	$21,900	A.M.A.	6 months	No	No	No	No	No	Compensation not payable if employee refused to wear ear protection devices.
North Dakota	Yes	Yes	Yes	50	200	$ 2,000	$ 8,000	M.E./ A.M.A.	Yes	No	No	No	Yes	Yes	Gives credit for improvement with hearing aid. Depends on medical evaluation.
Ohio	Yes	Yes	?	25	125	°°$ 2,325	°$11,625	°	No	Yes	Yes	P	Yes	No	No award made for less than permanent and total loss of hearing. Figures taken from the U.S. Chamber of Commerce Report 1976.
Oklahoma	Yes	No	No	100	200	$ 5,000	$10,000	M.E.	No	No	°Yes	°Yes	Yes	No	Considered as a series of traumatic incidents. Award for tinnitus and non-organic depends on medical evidence.

978

State														Comments
Oregon	Yes	Yes	60°	192°	$ 4,200	$13,440	Modified A.M.A.	Yes	No	Yes	P	Yes	–	Loss is measured in degrees—each degree is equal to $70.00 compensation. Uses formula that includes average of eight frequencies (from 250 through 3,000 Hz.) Award for tinnitus and non-organic loss depends upon medical testimony.
Pennsylvania	No	No	60	260	$11,220	$48,620	M.E.	No	No	No	No	No	–	For complete loss of hearing in both ears 66 2/3% of weekly wage with maximum $187/wk. for 260 weeks. Total loss of hearing one ear rated at 60 weeks.
Rhode Island	No	No	17	100	$ 765	$ 4,500	A.M.A.	Yes 6 months	Yes ½ db over age 40	No	No	Yes	No	
South Carolina	Yes	OSHA	80	165	$ 7,628	$15,733	M.E.	No	P	P	P	Yes	No	
South Dakota	Yes	No	50	150	$ 4,400	$13,200	M.E.	–	No	No	No	Yes	Yes	Credit for improvement with hearing aid.
Tennessee	Yes	OSHA	75	150	$ 6,375	$12,750	M.E.	No	–	–	–	–	–	
Texas	Yes	No	°None	150	–	$10,500	°	No	P.M.E.	P	No	Yes	No	Depend on medical evidence. Only bilateral loss compensated. Modification of A.M.A. method. No compensation for hearing loss in one ear.
Utah	Yes	Yes	50	100	Only Trauma	$10,323	M.E.	6 months	°Yes	Yes	No	Yes	No	Compensation for presbycusis ½ db over 40 years of age.
Vermont	No	OSHA	52	215	$ 4,732	$19,565	M.E.	No	No	No	No	P	No	
Virginia	Yes	No	50	100	$ 8,100	$16,200	Mod. A.M.A.	No	No	Yes	°Yes	Yes	No	
Washington	Yes	Yes			$ 2,400	$14,400	A.M.A.	No	No	Yes	Yes	Yes	No	
West Virginia	No	No			$10,380	$31,340	A.M.A.	No	P M.E.	?	No	Yes	No	Award for tinnitus, non-organic based on medical evidence. Each per cent is equivalent to 4 wks. × 2/3 of whole man. Unilateral total loss 15% = 60 wks. Bilateral total loss 45% = 180 wks.
Wisconsin	Yes	Yes	36	216	$ 2,052	$12,312	°	2 months	No	5% if related to hearing	P	Yes	No	Recent change in formula. Uses 1-2-3 Hz average with deductions of 35 db.

° See "Comments" in far right-hand column
M.E.—Medical Evidence
P—Possible
A.M.A.—American Medical Association

Table 56-3 (*Continued*). Comparative Provisions for Occupational Hearing Loss in Workmen's Compensation Cases (After Fox.[19] Revised 1976)

Jurisdiction	Recognize Hearing Loss due to Noise	Specify Noise Level	Regulation for Ear Protection	Schedule in Weeks One Ear	Schedule in Weeks Both Ears	Maximum Compensation One Ear (traumatic)	Maximum Compensation Both Ears	Formula or Method Used	Waiting Period	Presbycusis Deduction	Compensation for Tinnitus	Compensation Nonorganic Hearing Loss	Provision for Hearing Aid	Credit for Improvement with Aid	COMMENTS
Wyoming	Yes	No	No	40	80	$4,720.40	$9,440	M.E.	No	Yes	No	No	Yes	Not known	Deduction for presbycusis depends upon medical evidence.
U.S. Dept. of Labor	Yes	Yes	Yes		200 weeks	$28,360	$109,030		*						Federal employees compensation act provides for 200 weeks with a possible weekly maximum of $519.23. Additional compensation benefits possible if loss of earning results after 200 weeks. Use modified A.M.A. formula to include 3000 Hz frequency.
Puerto Rico	Yes	Yes	Yes	50	200	$2,250	$9,000	M.E.	No	No	P	P	Yes	No	Consideration for tinnitus and non-organic hearing loss on basis of medical testimony.
CANADIAN PROVINCES†															
Manitoba	Yes	Yes	Yes	Total Deafness 5%	*	*	*	*	No only before test	*	P	No	Yes	No	Deafness complete 1 ear 5%. Bilateral deafness 30%. Sudden, traumatic complete deafness 60%. Can be compensated on wage loss if there is no compensable hearing award. Uses the 4 freq. 500-1000-2000-3000 Hz. Deduction for presbycusis 0.5 db each year over 60. Possible compensation for tinnitus.

Province				Min %	Max %	°	Formula / frequencies	Noise-free period	Presbycusis	A.M.A.		M.E.		Comments
Nova Scotia	Yes	Yes	No	5%	30%	—	Average 500–1000—2000–3000 Hz	48 hrs before test	—	—	—	—	—	
Ontario	Yes	Yes	°No	°2.4%	°30%	—	500–1000—2000–3000 Hz	No	Yes ½ db each yr. over 60	P	No	Yes	No	See above.
Quebec	Yes	Dept. of Labour	No	°5%	°30%–60%	°	Average 500–1000—2000 Hz	½ db each yr. over 60	½ db each yr. over 60	P	No	Yes	No	5% one ear; 30% both ears. Post-traumatic total bilateral sudden loss 30%-60%. Uses 3 frequencies: 500-1000-2000. The amount of pension award depends upon several factors: The percentage of hearing loss, salary earned during past 12 months, the age of claimant. New Schedule being revised.
Saskatchewan	Yes	No / Dept. of Labour	No	°5%	°30%–60%	°	Average 500–1000—2000 cps	1 month	½ db each yr. over 60	P	No	Yes	No	Deafness complete 1 ear 5%. Bilateral deafness 30% sudden, traumatic complete deafness 60%.
Vancouver BC	Yes	Yes	Yes	3%	15%	°	500–1000—2000 Hz	No	No	No	No	Yes	No	Pensions payable depends upon hearing loss, age, wage earning and adaptability factor.

° See "Comments" in far right-hand column
M.E.—Medical Evidence
P—Possible
A.M.A.—American Medical Association

† The statutes and provisions in the Canadian Provinces show slight variations. In general, they compensate for noise-induced hearing loss and have specific guidelines for noise exposure and for the use of personal hearing protection devices. I am indebted to Dr. M. A. Hayley, Medical Specialist for Ear Claims with the Rehabilitation Services Division, Ontario, for furnishing the following information as to how Workmen's Compensation hearing loss claims are evaluated and compensated. In Ontario, the Minister of Labor and the Minister of Natural Resources have regulations relating to hazardous noise exposure. The minimum pension is awarded when there is a loss of 35 db ISO scale bilaterally. Total hearing loss is accepted as 80 db ISO bilaterally. To compute the bilateral hearing impairment, the poorer ear is rated according to the schedule and the better ear according to the scale multiplied by 5. The sum of the two gives the combined rating. The pension award is based upon the impairment and the workmen's earnings for the year prior to the evaluation. The Province has experienced a large number of claims; 1974: 986; 1975: 1,519.

evaluation of the existing Workmen's Compensation Laws to determine if such laws provided an adequate, prompt, and equitable system of compensation, as well as a safe place of employment for workers. The report of the commission published in 1972 called attention to various inadequacies and conflicts in many of the state statutes.[21]

INDUSTRIAL AUDIOMETRY AND HEARING CONSERVATION PROGRAMS*

Prior to World War II, hearing tests in industry were only occasionally performed using conversational and whispered voice or tuning fork tests, all of which gave a cursory estimate of an individual's hearing ability. The need for accurate quantitative measurements of hearing was not appreciated until large numbers of industrial compensation claims for loss of hearing occurred throughout the country. The combination of increased noise exposure and compensation claims produced the need for hearing conservation procedures in industry.

An industrial hearing conservation program has three primary objectives: (1) to conserve and minimize the hearing loss of the employees; (2) to comply with OSHA regulations; and (3) to prevent economic loss to the employer. The initiation of a hearing conservation program should be considered whenever persons have (1) difficulty in communicating by speech while they are in the noise; (2) head noises or ringing in their ears after working in noise for several hours; or (3) a loss of hearing that has the effect of muffling speech and certain other sounds after several hours of exposure to the noise. (This hearing loss is temporary and usually disappears in a few hours.)

Absence of pain should not be construed to mean absence of hearing loss. Pain and annoyance are not reliable indicators of a potential noise-induced hearing loss. Ulti-

*Portions of the material and recommendations in this chapter are reprinted with permission of the editors from the Guide for Conservation of Hearing in Noise, prepared by the Subcommittee on Noise of the Committee on Conservation of Hearing, American Academy of Ophthalmology and Otolaryngology, revised 1973.

mately, the analysis of noise exposure is the only completely satisfactory way of establishing the need for hearing conservation.

OUTLINE OF HEARING CONSERVATION PROGRAM

A hearing conservation program consists of three parts.
1. Analysis of noise exposure.
2. Control of noise exposure.
3. Measurement of hearing.

Assessment of Noise Exposure

In the analysis of noise exposure the following factors must be considered:
1. Overall noise level as measured on the A scale.
2. Composition of the noise.
3. Duration and distribution of exposure during a typical work day.
4. Total exposure time expected during a work life.

These are the four items previously discussed under noise exposure. Knowledge of each of these items is important in planning an effective program. Two noises may have the same overall noise level, for example, and yet the frequency composition may differ so that one may produce a hearing loss and the other may not. The daily duration and distribution of exposure may affect the extent and degree of the expected loss. Intermittent exposure is less hazardous than continuous exposure.

Noise level measurement should always be made at the approximate position of the employee's most exposed ear during normal operations. To take account of the noise level variations produced by changes in operational schedules or procedures, repeated measurements should be made during a single day, as well as on different days of the week.

Control of Noise Exposure

The control of noise exposure may be affected by either environmental control or personal protection of the exposed worker. Both of these approaches make possible the elimination or reduction of the noise entering the inner ear. The ideal hearing conservation program, as advocated by OSHA, is one which would be able to reduce or eliminate the hazardous noise at its source by proper designing of new machinery, by treatment of the existing machinery, or by acoustical isolation of noisy working areas. Unfortunately, in many instances the attainment of such ideals is not always practical from an engineering and an economic standpoint. Likewise, the revision or substitution of other industrial processes for noisy operations and the rotation of working personnel have met with objections from both the workers and the management.

Where the hazardous noise cannot be eliminated or reduced sufficiently by the above environmental controls, one can resort to the use of properly fitted ear protectors in an effort to reduce the noise levels reaching the inner ear. Two main varieties of ear protection have been developed and used: (1) the plug type that fits snugly into the external meatus of the ear, and (2) a cushion type (muff) held by a headband that lies around and over the ears. The ear plugs designed to occlude the ear canal are of many varieties and are made of soft rubber, neoprene, plastic, or cotton impregnated with wax. Dry cotton alone affords little or no protection despite common and frequent usage. Waxed cotton or silicone which can be shaped may be substituted for dry cotton. Material and shape otherwise have little to do with the effectiveness of ear plugs except

as they affect acceptance by the worker. Suitable ear defenders should be comfortable, effectively attenuate the noise, and have a low replacement cost. The ear plugs should not be made of rigid material which might injure the ear canal. The attenuation afforded by typical ear defenders is shown in Table 56–4.

Ear muffs are designed to cover the external ear. At frequencies above 1000 cps, muffs provide about the same protection as plugs. At frequencies below 1000 cps, certain correctly designed muffs provide more protection than plugs.

The choice of plugs, muffs, or both depends in part on the work situation. Will the employee's head be confined to a work space so small there is no room for muffs? Must he wear a hard hat in addition to ear protection? There are advantages and disadvantages to the use of either plugs or muffs, and before a choice is made between the two, all the circumstances of a particular job should be considered.

An employee's ears should be examined and his hearing tested at the time he is fitted with ear protectors. Plugs should be fitted individually for each ear; if the ear canals are not the same size or shape, they may require plugs of different size. To promote the acceptance of ear plugs, an employee should be allowed to choose from two or three different makes at the time he is fitted.

As with other kinds of personal protection (hard hats, safety glasses, safety shoes, or

Table 56–4.   Attenuation for the Eight Different Ear Protectors Tested
(in dB re zero of the audiometer)

Type	Frequency (cps)								
	125	250	500	1000	2000	3000	4000	6000	8000
Ear plugs									
A		21.9	25.0	25.9	33.4	38.0	41.2	33.0	37.5
B	15	15.9	16.2	21.3	28.8	33.7	33.7	32.9	39.1
C	8	16	16	19	23	29	27	34	40
Ear muffs									
A	8	23	30	32	33	40	39	39	38
B	19	30	38	38	42	44	45	40	35
C	7	13	23	31	34	34	12	10	35
Cotton	5	6	8	9	13	15	13	14	16

respirators), it may be difficult to convince employees that they should wear ear protectors. Successful personal protection programs are based on thorough indoctrination of personnel. An employee must be impressed with the importance of ear protection, that it makes good sense to protect one's ears and hearing, and convinced of the benefits to be gained from its consistent use.

Measurement of Hearing

The measurement of hearing ability is the most important part of a hearing conservation program. Both preplacement (often referred to as pre-employment) and periodic follow-up tests of hearing should be part of the program routine. The preplacement test should be made, if possible, at the time an employee is hired but in no case later than 90 days after hiring; the primary purpose of the preplacement test is to establish an auditory base line. Follow-up tests are made to provide a record of subsequent changes in hearing (due to accident, disease, age, noise exposure, etc.). A third aspect of the hearing program involves the disposition of cases whose audiograms show unusual changes as revealed by follow-up tests.

Preplacement Threshold Tests of Hearing Ability. Air conduction threshold tests are recommended for preplacement use in industry. The thresholds measured by these tests are the sound pressure levels at which certain pure tone test frequencies can just be heard. The recommended test frequencies are 500, 1000, 2000, 3000, 4000, and 6000 Hz. Any other additional frequencies may be added where local needs require same.

Preplacement threshold audiograms should be made for all employees, not only for those who are to work in noisy areas. From a practical and medicolegal standpoint, it is not good practice to streamline programs, limiting tests only to workers exposed to high noise levels. It is advisable to have a base line audiogram of all employees which can be followed throughout the years of employment. Such a record may show, for example, the presence of an early hearing loss of a type that is responsive to therapy. Detection and treatment of these non-noise-induced hearing losses will help pre-

vent their subsequent progress and the resulting loss of trained personnel.

If a preplacement audiogram shows an average hearing loss of more than 25 dB at 500, 1000, and 2000 Hz, the employee should be referred to a physician for otologic examination and placement evaluation. Such referral is also advised for employees whose audiograms show any unusual irregularity, particularly an abrupt loss beginning at 2000 cycles per second.

Whenever audiometric tests are given, the tester should ascertain that a period of at least 14 hours has elapsed since each subject's last noise exposure.

Follow-up Tests of Hearing Ability. Periodic follow-up hearing tests should be given yearly to persons stationed in areas where noise exposure exceeds the suggested hearing conservation level. The first threshold follow-up test should be given approximately 12 months after placement unless an earlier test is indicated. All follow-up tests should be made after as long a period of absence from noise as is practical (but at least 14 hours) to allow for as much recovery as possible from temporary threshold shifts produced during the previous work day.

A comparison should be made between the preplacement threshold audiogram and the follow-up audiogram. The OSHA guidelines recommend that if an employee's follow-up test shows a shift of 10 dB or more in the direction of increased hearing loss at frequencies 2000 Hz or lower, 15 dB at 3000 Hz, or 20 dB at 4000 and 6000 Hz, appropriate steps should be taken to conserve the employee's hearing. The hearing tests should be repeated within 1 month, and if the hearing loss persists, medical referral is advised. From a practical standpoint, if there is no greater change from the original preplacement reference audiogram, subsequent tests may be given at approximately yearly intervals, unless otherwise indicated. In ordinary noise exposure conditions, rechecks of hearing at yearly intervals have been found to be most practical and effective.

Records. The hearing conservation data card should provide space for the recording of the occupational and medical history, noise exposure information, history relating to employee's previous hearing status, and the audiograms. The usual audiogram charts supplied by audiometer manufacturers are designed for recording data in graphic form. These charts, however, are not flexible enough to be used effectively in the field of industrial audiometry. They do not provide the necessary space for the recording of important items already mentioned. Furthermore, since graphic records do not provide space for the recording of periodic hearing tests, a series of cards or charts will be required, making comparison between tests difficult, leading to the accumulation of bulky files with the possibility of records becoming lost or misplaced.

Audiometric Equipment and Procedures

Types of Audiometers. For industrial hearing testing programs, a simple but properly calibrated and maintained discrete air conduction audiometer is required. This may be a small portable or office model. Self-recording audiometers are also being used in industrial audiometric programs. The person being tested responds to the test tone by pressing a button. The button (switch) controls a mechanism in the audiometer which records the person's auditory threshold on a card. At periodic intervals the audiometer

larly, at least once a month. This check, known as a "biological calibration," consists of making audiograms for three or more young persons (less than 25 years of age) who have not had a history of previous ear disease or hearing loss. At each test frequency the average threshold of the young person should be within 5 dB of the audiometric zero; if not, the acoustical calibration of the audiometer is probably incorrect.

If the audiometer is not in correct acoustical calibration, it should be returned to the manufacturer for service and adjustment. In any case, an audiometer should be returned for service to the manufacturer or to an authorized service representative once a year. Inasmuch as ANSI and ISO standards for audiometers have replaced the old ASA 1951 zero reference level, it is extremely important that all audiograms be properly identified as to the reference level. The otolaryngologist must have this information available and also possess the knowledge to convert readings from one standard to another whenever it is necessary to do so.

Readings obtained on an audiometer calibrated to the ASA 1951 values may be converted to, and plotted as, readings of hearing threshold levels of the 1964 ISO values by adding the following numbers of decibels at the designated frequencies:

Frequency (Hz)	125	250	500	1000	1500	2000	3000	4000	6000	8000
db	9	15	14	10	10	8.5	8.5	6.0	9.5	11.5

automatically switches to another test frequency. When one ear has been tested, the recommended test tones are presented automatically in the same sequence to the other ear.

The self-recording audiometer has been found to provide excellent results in the industrial setting. Its major advantage is that it tends to reduce errors on the part of the test technician, less demands are made on the technician during the actual testing, and consequently less fatigue and errors are likely to result. Further, if several self-recording audiometers and test booths are available, up to four persons can be tested simultaneously by one technician.

Calibration of Audiometer. The accuracy of an audiometer should be checked regu-

Auditory Test Rooms and Booths. The importance of a satisfactory testing environment cannot be overemphasized. Hearing tests should be conducted in a room which meets the ANSI standards for background noise (S3.6–1960). An improper testing environment can and does produce inaccurate records of an individual hearing level because of the masking phenomenon. Hearing test rooms should be located in as quiet a place as possible, preferably within practical access but away from outside walls, elevators, heating and plumbing noises, waiting rooms, and busy hallways. Test rooms should be kept at a comfortable temperature. A fan or built-in ventilator should provide adequate ventilation and temperature control. Acoustical treatment of audiometry rooms may prove to be a difficult task and should be undertaken only with the help of an acoustical consultant. Prefabricated audiometry booths which are available have proved more satisfactory and are usually less expensive than either reconstructed rooms or sound-treated rooms.

Audiometric Technician. The person selected to be trained for the performance of industrial hearing tests should be an intelligent, interested, and well-motivated individual. This person, often referred to as an audiometric technician or audiometrist, can be selected from first-aid, safety, or personnel departments. Usually, nurses, or female employees are chosen for this assignment. However, because of rapid turnover of female employees, it is considered practical and desirable to train one or more male technicians to become acquainted with and to perform these duties. The technician's duties should be to perform only pure tone air conduction threshold tests and periodic rechecks, but these test results should aways be reviewed and evaluated by an otologist or audiologist. The audiometric technician should be able to show documentary evidence of satisfactory completion of a course of training as specified by the Intersociety Committee on Audiometric Technician Training.[22]

Medical Supervision and Responsibility for Program

Direct medical supervision of a hearing conservation program is highly desirable. The physician is responsible for the organization and administration of the testing program, as well as for checking and evaluating audiometric records. The physician himself does not perform all the operations necessary to conduct the program; he delegates responsibility for many of the technical activities to members of his staff and sets up standards or limits wherein they can operate semiautonomously. Whenever medical records show that control of noise exposures may be inadequate, the physician in charge so reports. The responsibility for making necessary noise measurements and for effecting further environmental noise exposure controls then devolves on the industrial hy-

gienist, members of the engineering or safety departments, or other persons assigned to the task. Although the actual operations of measurement and protection are performed by both medical and nonmedical personnel, the physician ultimately is responsible for the health of the employee.

Unsatisfactory hearing conservation programs may be the result of poor planning, noisy testing environments, the use of improperly trained technicians, questionable testing techniques, inadequate recordings, and particularly the lack of proper medical supervision. The practice on the part of some industries of merely making hearing tests on their employees without proper medical interpretation and supervision is to be condemned. This approach is not consistent with the practice of good medicine. Quite often the reliability and validity of these unsupervised records are often challenged in medicolegal proceedings.

The success of the hearing conservation program depends on the complete cooperation of employer and employee, medical directors, and those responsible for the health and safety of the workers. All groups stand to benefit equally from a hearing conservation program, and all groups should give the complete program their active support.

REFERENCES

1. Bunch, C. C.: The Neural Mechanism of Hearing; "Nerve Deafness" of Known Pathology or Etiology; Diagnosis of Occupational or Traumatic Deafness; Historical and Audiometric Study. Laryngoscope, *47*:615, 691, 1937.
2. Guide for Conservation of Hearing in Noise. Trans. Am. Acad. Ophthal. Otolaryng., *63*:236–8, 1959; revised, 1973.
3. A. Slawinski vs. Williams & Co., 298 N.Y. 546. B. Rosati vs. Dispatch Shop, 298 N.Y. 813.
4. A. Wojcik vs. Green Bay Drop Forge, 265 Wis. 38.
5. A. U.S. Department of Labor. "Safety and Health Standards," Federal Register, Superintendent of Documents, Washington, D.C. 20000. Vol. 34, No. 96, May 20, 1969, p. 7948.
   B. U.S. Department of Labor. Guidelines to the Department of Labors' Occupational Noise Standards for Federal Supply

Contracts (Bulletin 334), Superintendent of Documents, Washington, D.C. 20000. April, 1971.

6. Schiff, M.: Nonauditory Effects of Noise. Trans. Am. Acad. Ophthal. Otolaryng., 77:384, 1973.

7. Cantrell, R.: Prolonged Exposure to Intermittent Noise; Audiometric, Biochemical, Motor Psychological and Sleep Effects, Laryngscope Suppl. 1, Oct., 1974.

8. Glorig, A.: The Effects of Noise on Hearing. J. Laryngol. Otol., 25:447, 1961.

9. Lindsay, J. R.: Year Book of the Ear, Nose and Throat. Chicago, Year Book Medical Publishers, 1962-1963, p. 80.

10. Schuknecht, H. F.: Pathology of Slowly Progressive Sensorineural Deafness. Trans. Am. Acad. Ophthal. Otolaryng., 68:222, 1964.

11. Glorig, A., and Davis, H.: Age, Noise and Hearing Loss. Ann. Otol. Rhinol. Laryngol., 70:556, 1961.

12. Rosen, S.: High Frequency Audiometry in Presbycusis. Arch. Otolaryng., 79:18, 1964.

13. Schuknecht, H. F., and Davison, R. C.: Deafness and Vertigo from Head Injury. Arch. Otolaryng., 63:513, 1956.

14. Criteria for a Recommended Standard—Occupational Exposure to Noise. Washington, D.C., U.S. Department of Health, Education and Welfare. Cincinnati, Ohio, National Institute for Occupational Safety and Health, 1972.

15. Guide for the Evaluation of Hearing Impairment, A Report of the Committee on Conservation of Hearing. Trans. Am. Acad. Ophthal. Otolaryng., 63:2, 1959.

16. Guide to the Evaluation of Permanent Impairment of the Ear, Nose, Throat and Related Structures. J.A.M.A., 177:489, 1961; revised, 1971.

17. Specifications for Audiometers for General Diagnostic Purposes, S3.6—1969. ANSI, Inc., 1430 Broadway, New York, N.Y. 10018.

18. Reports of Committee on Conservation of Hearing. Trans. Am. Acad. Ophthal. Otolaryng., 68:116, 1964.

19. Fox, M. S.: Hearing Loss Statutes in the U.S. and Canada. National Safety News, Feb., 1976.

20. Analysis of Workmen's Compensation Laws. 1974 edition. Chamber of Commerce of the United States, 1615 H Street, N. W., Washington, D.C. 20006.

21. The Report of the National Commission on State Workmen's Compensation Laws, July 31, 1972. 1825 K Street, N.W., Washington, D.C. 20006.

22. American Industrial Hygiene Journal. 27: 303, 1966.

Chapter 57
Facial Nerve Paralysis

THE facial nerve is subject to disease at any point from its origin in the cerebral cortex to the motor end-plate in the face. The most common point of origin of facial nerve paralysis is within the temporal bone where the nerve lies within the long and tortuous fallopian canal. (See Facial Nerve, p. 636.)

FUNCTION OF THE FACIAL NERVE

The facial nerve leaves the medulla oblongata at its junction with the pons in two roots, the motor root and the intermediate nerve, which form a common trunk within the internal auditory canal. The motor root innervates the auricular muscles, the stylohyoid muscle, and the posterior belly of the digastric muscle by means of the posterior auricular nerve, which is given off immediately after leaving the stylomastoid foramen. The terminal branches then run forward to supply the muscles of facial expression.

The intermediate nerve contains special visceral afferent fibers (sensory) carrying taste sensation from the anterior two thirds of the tongue to the tractus solitarius; general somatic afferent fibers from some areas of the skin of the external auditory canal; proprioceptive fibers from the facial muscles; and efferent parasympathetic fibers arising from the superior salivatory nucleus and terminating at the lacrimal gland, the nasal mucosa, and the submandibular and sublingual glands.

The taste fibers leave the tongue with the lingual nerve but depart from the course of the lingual shortly before entering the middle ear as the chorda tympani nerve. The cell bodies of these fibers are grouped in the geniculate ganglion.

The greater superficial petrosal nerve is formed of parasympathetic fibers leaving the facial through the hiatus of the facial canal at the geniculate ganglion. This nerve runs in a groove across the floor of the middle fossa. It is joined by the sympathetic fibers of the deep petrosal nerve (from the carotid plexus) to form the nerve of the pterygoid canal (vidian nerve), which runs to the pterygopalatine ganglion where the parasympathetic fibers synapse. From the ganglion, fibers are distributed to the glands of the nasal and palatal mucosa, and to the lacrimal gland.

Other parasympathetic fibers join the chorda tympani to terminate in the submandibular ganglion. After synapse, the postganglionic fibers are distributed to the submandibular gland and to the sublingual gland.

PHYSIOLOGY OF NERVE INJURY

Nerve injuries are basically of two types, those resulting in wallerian degeneration and those without axonal degeneration. From the presence or absence of degeneration, three degrees of injury may be classified. *Neurotmesis* is an injury with anatomic disruption of the nerve trunk and complete degeneration distal to the point of injury. *Axonotmesis* is an injury of sufficient severity to result in nerve degeneration, but without disruption of the neurilemmal sheath or endoneural sheath. *Neurapraxia* is an injury resulting in loss of nerve transmission but without axonal degeneration or disruption of the nerve sheath.

Severe injury to a peripheral nerve results in a demyelinating process known as wallerian degeneration. This degeneration is limited proximally by the first uninvolved Schwann cell segment encountered, as seen by its cessation at the first proximal "node of Ranvier." The process proceeds distally for the entire extent of the nerve. In degeneration, the axon cylinders undergo fragmentation, while the myelin sheath dissolves into fat droplets. Macrophages remove the degenerated material, leaving an empty neurilemmal and endoneural sheath.

The neurilemmal and Schwann cells proliferate from both ends of the defect, attempting to bridge the defect. The neurofibrils begin to regenerate from the proximal segment at a slow rate (0.25 mm per day), attempting to cross the defect and enter the empty spaces in the nerve sheath. If successful, the growth rate increases to 3 or 4 mm per day. Failure of the regenerating neurofibrils to bridge the defect results in a tangled mass growing from the proximal stump, termed a neuroma. With successful regrowth of the neurofibrils, the myelin sheath is reformed by the Schwann cells, the entire process taking from 4 to 9 months, depending on the point of injury of the facial nerve.

Diagnosis

Interference with the function of the facial nerve will present different findings depending on whether the injury is central or peripheral.

Peripheral Lesions. The findings in peripheral disease of the facial nerve are on the same side as the lesion. They may include complete or partial loss of motion of the forehead; inability to close the eye (Bell's phenomenon is the turning of the eyeball upward and outward as the patient attempts to close the eye; partial loss may be indicated by widening of the palpebral fissure); inability to move the corner of the mouth, to pucker the lips, or to flare the nostril; a general sagging or flaccidity of the face with smoothing of the skin lines; loss of taste on the anterior two thirds of the tongue; and decrease in lacrimation.

Central Lesions. The findings in central disease involve the side opposite from that of the lesion. In supranuclear disease, there is a pattern of paralysis of the lower face with remaining function of the frontalis muscle due to bilateral cortical pathways for the nerve to the frontalis. There is loss of voluntary control, but not of emotional response as in laughing; Bell's phenomenon is not present in this group of cases.

Localization. Systems of locating the exact point of injury to the facial nerve by examination of the function of the various branches have often been described. The following tests of function are most helpful:

1. Lacrimation (greater superficial petrosal nerve). This branch is involved in lesions at or central to the geniculate ganglion. Lacrimation is best tested by folding strips of filter paper over the lower eyelids and comparing the rate of lacrimal secretion after a stimulus of sniffing ammonia (Schirmer test).

2. Stapedius muscle function. This test involves detecting changes in the impedance of the middle ear after a sound stimulus. Reflex contraction of the stapedius muscle is reflected back to the tympanic membrane, causing an increase in stiffness which is measured with an acoustic bridge. This test is not often used in office practice. (See discussion of Tympanometry, p. 765).

3. Taste (chorda tympani nerve). This function is best measured by comparing the threshold of taste sensation on the sides of the tongue 1 cm from the tip using galvanic stimulation. There is great variation in threshold sensitivity, but most individuals have a threshold of less than 50 microamperes of current.

4. Motor function to the face. This has been previously described.

Electrodiagnosis. The purpose of electrodiagnosis is to determine if nerve degeneration has taken place; if there is partial or complete loss of function; and to what degree the nerve remains excitable. Several methods of testing have been developed to answer these questions.

1. *Nerve Excitability.* In this test an electrode (cathode) is placed near the exit of the facial nerve at the stylomastoid foramen with an indifferent electrode at the base of the skull. Bipolar electrodes may also be used. Galvanic stimulation is given in the form of a 1 millisecond square wave. The amount of current required to stimulate the nerve is measured and compared to the opposite normal side.

A loss of excitability occurs with axon degeneration, which usually becomes complete within 4 or 5 days of onset. In some cases a needle electrode is used or the nerve trunk is exposed in order to determine absolutely that complete loss of excitability has occurred. Intensity-duration curves may be made by this technique to provide a modern controlled substitute for faradic-galvanic testing.

2. *Faradic-galvanic Stimulation.* This test was used widely in former times to determine whether nerve degeneration had occurred by finding the "reaction of degeneration." Faradic stimulation is by an interrupted high frequency current which stimulates normal nerve. With degeneration, this response is lost within 10 to 14 days. Galvanic current is a constant direct current. Normally there is greater response to the onset of cathodal current than anodal current. This is reversed with nerve degeneration, and the reaction becomes slow and sluggish.

In the *"reaction of degeneration,"* faradic current is of too short duration to stimulate the denervated muscle, so that loss of the normally more intense response to faradic stimulation is noted. Response to galvanic stimulation is present, but weak and sluggish with reversal of the normal polarity of response. This method of testing is only qualitative and has been shown to be subject to many errors of interpretation.

3. *Electromyography.* In this method, needle electrodes are placed in the muscles of the face, and the electrical activity is studied at rest and on attempted motion. At rest, normal muscle is lacking in electrical activity. After denervation, fibrillation (a constant irregular electrical activity) occurs within 12 days and continues until reinner-vation takes place. The presence of fibrillation at rest plus the lack of action potentials on voluntary movement will give quantitative information about the severity and extent of the nerve injury.

Etiology

The variety of causes of facial paralysis may be classified into the main groups of traumatic and atraumatic.

A. Traumatic
    1. Intracranial
        a. A transection in neurosurgical procedures within the cerebello-pontine angle
    2. Intratemporal
        a. Surgical division in operative procedures on the temporal bone
        b. Fracture of the temporal bone
    3. Extratemporal
        a. Surgical division in surgery of parotid gland or face
        b. Laceration of the face
B. Atraumatic
    1. Noninfectious
        a. Bell's palsy
        b. Melkersson's syndrome
        c. Tumors of cerebellopontine angle or facial nerve
    2. Infectious
        a. Otitis media
        b. Herpes zoster oticus

SPECIFIC DISEASES OF THE FACIAL NERVE

Bell's Palsy

Bell's palsy is a peripheral, unilateral, idiopathic paralysis of the facial nerve. It appears to be due to a primary vasospasm of the blood supply of the facial nerve. This leads to edema of the nerve, causing further secondary interference with capillary and lymphatic supply to the nerve and partial or complete loss of function.

The fibrous tissue surrounding the nerve as it leaves the stylomastoid foramen seems to be the point of constriction in Bell's palsy. Edema of the nerve and fibrous tissue interferes with venous and lymphatic drainage, causing further edema in a vicious circle.

Examination of the nerve at surgery may show hemorrhagic streaks in the nerve sheath, particularly near the stylomastoid foramen. When the sheath is opened, the nerve will usually bulge or herniate out of the opening proximal to the point of constriction but not distal. The bone surrounding the facial canal is often soft and hemorrhagic.

Only a few specimens of facial nerve tissue have been examined in cases of acute Bell's palsy, but several specimens of the chorda tympani have been examined. The microscopic picture usually shows edema of the nerve tissue and engorgement of capillaries, but without intraneural bleeding or infiltration with inflammatory cells. There may be fragmentation and demyelination of the axons, and in long-standing cases, fibrosis of the nerve will be seen.

Symptoms. The onset of the unilateral paralysis is usually sudden, frequently following exposure to cold, especially if a respiratory infection is present. At times, a severe shock or emotional disturbance seems to be the precipitating factor.

Various segments of the nerve may be involved, with symptoms depending on the location of involvement (see Diagnosis). The vertical segment is most often involved alone, with loss of taste the only accompanying disturbance with the facial paralysis. Pain, varying from slight to severe, is common during the initial days following paralysis. There is apparently a correlation between the severity of the pain and the severity of the paralysis.

Vertigo may be present in the early stages of the disease. This does not usually persist. Hyperacusis, loss of taste, and interference with lacrimation are of less frequent occurrence.

Treatment and Prognosis. Approximately 86% of the patients with Bell's palsy experience complete recovery. Studies utilizing tests of nerve excitability show that if complete degeneration occurs, complete recovery does not occur, and as many as 56% experience a residual deficit. If degeneration does not occur, over 85% recover full function. For this reason, nerve testing forms an important facet of management of Bell's palsy.

Treatment of Bell's palsy is not fully agreed upon today. Although three treatment modalities are commonly accepted— no treatment, use of corticosteroids, and surgical decompression of the facial nerve within its mastoid segment—the individual application of treatment and the timing of application serve as sources of controversy. The regime used at present by this author and its rationale are outlined below.

Incomplete Paralysis. Those patients presenting with an incomplete paralysis, usually of insidious onset, and without pain have a high probability of spontaneous complete recovery within 7 to 14 days. Nerve excitability testing is performed and repeated at biweekly intervals during the course of recovery. No specific therapy is prescribed. Ascorbic acid, 500 mg qid, is given to all patients with Bell's palsy for its antiviral activity.

Any patient who fails to improve over the first 7 days of observation or who shows worsening by electrical study or clinical evaluation is placed in the complete denervation treatment regime.

Complete Paralysis. These patients present with a history of rapid onset, often with pain over the mastoid region, and show complete loss of motion of the face on the involved side. If seen early, electrical study using excitability testing may not show alteration, but a lessening of nerve excitability over time is common. If untreated, these patients have a high probability of complete denervation with functionally incomplete recovery.

In past years, surgical decompression was felt to be indicated for these patients as soon as denervation was diagnosed through loss of nerve excitability. The work of Taverner in England and Adour in the United States has shown that the use of corticosteroids is as effective in producing an uneventful recovery as is surgical decompression. To employ steroids, glucose tolerance testing should be performed to eliminate those patients with diabetes or a prediabetic state from this form of therapy. Patients with history of ulcers also should not receive this form of treatment.

Oral prednisone is used, giving 60 mg per day for 5 days, 40 mg per day for 2 days,

20 mg per day for 2 days, and 10 mg for 1 day. Repeated nerve excitability testing is done three times weekly over the course of therapy. Improvement should be manifest within 4 days of the cessation of the oral prednisone. Those patients who show no change or worsening at 14 days are given a second course of prednisone as described above.

Patients who do not show response following the second course of prednisone and those for whom corticosteroids are contraindicated are advised to undergo surgical decompression of the facial nerve. Specific indications for surgical decompression are complete denervation as shown by electrical testing; paralysis persisting more than 4 to 6 weeks; incomplete return of function to normal within 60 days; recurrence of facial paralysis; and the persistence of severe retroauricular pain from onset of paralysis. The details of facial nerve decompression are given later in this chapter.

Melkersson's Syndrome

This is an unusual type of peripheral facial paralysis in which three findings occur: (1) facial paralysis, which may be familial, is often bilateral, and may show a tendency to relapse; (2) angioneurotic facial edema, especially of the lips; and (3) lingua plicata (furrowing of the tongue), which may not be present in all cases.

The etiology of this condition is probably similar to that of Bell's palsy, representing, however, a more widespread disturbance of the parasympathetic system over the distribution of the facial nerve.

The pathology encountered is similar to that in Bell's palsy, and the treatment is the same as outlined for that disorder.

Herpes Zoster Oticus (Hunt's Syndrome)

Herpes zoster is a viral disease most often affecting sensory nerves due to involvement of the ganglion. Involvement of the geniculate ganglion (first described by Ramsay Hunt in 1910) gives a characteristic group of symptoms.

After a prodromal period of malaise and slight fever, there is an onset of severe deep-seated ear pain. This is followed by a herpetic eruption over the drumhead, external meatus, and auricle. Facial paralysis is accompanied by impairment of lacrimation and salivation and loss of taste on the same side.

Often accompanying the above symptoms is involvement of the trigeminal and auditory nerves. Neurosensory hearing loss, vertigo, and tinnitus, as well as herpetic lesions of the face, result from this involvement.

The disease is usually short-lived with recovery in days to weeks. The pain may persist for several months, however.

Treatment is supportive and symptomatic. If the facial paralysis persists beyond 60 days without signs of recovery, decompression should be performed. In this case the horizontal segment and geniculate ganglion are decompressed.

Otitis Media

Facial paralysis may accompany both acute and chronic forms of otitis media, either from inflammatory edema of the nerve or by bony erosion and pressure from cholesteatoma.

Facial paralysis accompanying acute otitis media should be treated expectantly, as it usually recovers with subsidence of the infection.

Facial paralysis occurring in chronic otitis media is an indication for operative intervention. During this procedure the site of involvement of the facial nerve should be determined and the causative pathologic condition removed. Decompression of the nerve should be delayed, however, until postoperative observation reveals no return of function in 60 days.

Postsurgical Facial Paralysis

Facial paralysis following temporal bone surgery may have immediate or delayed onset. Since different therapy is indicated in the two cases, the need for observing facial nerve function immediately following any operation on the temporal bone is obvious.

Postsurgical paralysis of immediate onset must be presumed to be due to traumatic interruption of the facial nerve. Occasionally, local anesthetic agents will cause a temporary paralysis lasting for 2 to 3 hours after surgery. If this cause is proved not to be the case, immediate exploration of the facial nerve is indicated. After the site of injury is found, the nature of its extent is determined and appropriate measures taken to correct the injury. Usually one of two conditions are found: either compression of the nerve by a bone chip pushed into the fallopian canal, or an interruption of continuity due to a burr or curette. In the case of compression, removal of the bone chip usually results in return of function. If an interruption of the nerve is found, immediate grafting should be performed (see Facial Nerve Grafting, pp. 795–6).

Facial paralysis may occur after an interval of several days following temporal bone surgery. In this case there is no interruption of the nerve but rather an inflammatory interference with function. If tight packing was placed in the ear following surgery, this should be removed and medical treatment instituted. If there has been no return of function within 60 days, facial nerve exploration and decompression are then carried out.

SKULL FRACTURE

The facial nerve is frequently involved in fractures of the temporal bone. In a large percentage of these cases, cochlear function is lost, and the surgeon should make every effort to avoid the added handicap of facial deformity. Although expectant management has been advocated by some, recovery of function will be more rapid and complete if surgical debridement and repair are instituted early.

Consideration of the patient's general condition will determine when surgical exploration may be carried out. Radiographic examination and nerve branch testing are necessary to determine the site of the lesion. Transverse fractures frequently involve the internal auditory canal, which may be approached by techniques described under the treatment of acoustic neurinoma.

The use of corticosteroids and proteolytic enzymes to reduce swelling and promote the adsorption of blood and serum is indicated during the waiting period before surgery. If possible, exploration should be carried out within 60 days following the injury.

If cochlear function is preserved, any sound conduction lesion may be repaired at the same time as facial nerve surgery (see Tympanoplasty, Ch. 50).

Compressional fracture of the mastoid over the vertical portion of the facial nerve may occur in traumatic delivery. These cases should be decompressed as soon as possible, usually when the infant has reached a weight of 10 pounds.

HEMIFACIAL SPASM

This is an idiopathic condition of the facial nerve characterized by involuntary intermittent spasm of the face. It occurs in adult life and constitutes a severe handicap to the individual.

Many surgical treatments have been utilized for this condition, resulting in temporary relief only. Decompression, partial nerve section, complete nerve section, and nerve grafting have all given but partial or temporary relief in most cases. The most recent treatment to be described is "combing" of the nerve trunk following exposure of the vertical segment.

DECOMPRESSION OF
THE FACIAL NERVE

Decompression of the facial nerve is performed after preliminary simple mastoidectomy, which may be done through either an endaural or a postauricular incision. The mastoid dissection must extend from the aditus ad antrum to the mastoid tip, visualizing the short process of the incus and the digastric ridge in these respective regions. The procedure should be performed under magnification using the operation microscope.

The initial exposure of the facial nerve may be made either at the pyramidal portion below the short process of the incus or at the stylomastoid foramen (Fig. 57-1). In the former approach, the bone inferior to the horizontal semicircular canal and immediately posterior to the tip of the incus is carefully removed until the facial nerve

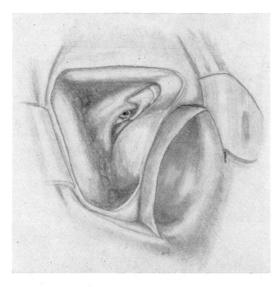

FIG. 57–1. Surgical exposure of mastoid and facial recess preparatory to facial nerve decompression.

is identified. The nerve is then followed in its descending course, leaving a thin shell of bone surrounding it. During this dissection at least 60% of the circumference of the nerve trunk should be skeletonized. The dissection is completed when the stylomastoid foramen is reached.

In the other method, the stylomastoid foramen is found by carefully following the digastric ridge forward toward its junction with the posterior canal wall. When the nerve has been identified, it is followed upward as described above until the second turn of the nerve has been reached inferior to the horizontal semicircular canal.

With diamond burrs and continuous irrigation, the skeletonized bone is further thinned vertically at both edges of the dissection. This allows the shell of bone covering the nerve to be lifted off like a flap to expose the nerve sheath with minimal chance of injury to the nerve.

When the entire vertical portion of the nerve has been exposed, the nerve sheath is slit open to allow the edematous nerve to expand freely (Fig. 57–2). This is done with a small sharp knife or tiny scissors.

In cases requiring dissection of the horizontal portion of the facial nerve and the

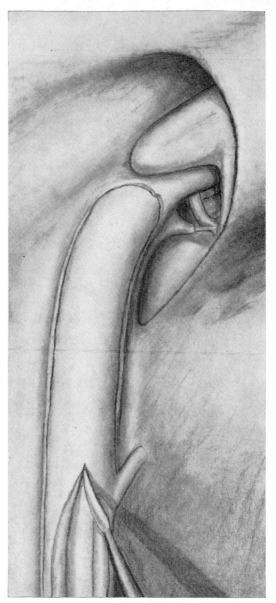

FIG. 57–2. Decompression of facial nerve. The nerve sheath is being slit with a tiny dissection blade.

geniculate ganglion, the mastoid dissection is carried forward into the attic area to expose the entire incus. Further bone is removed from the facial recess behind and below the short process of the incus until the middle ear course of the facial nerve can be visualized. The bone overlying the horizontal portion of the nerve and the geniculate ganglion may be removed and the sheath opened. It is important to do this dissection under sufficient magnification to avoid injury to the ossicular chain. It is sometimes necessary, however, to remove the incus to complete this dissection. If this last proves necessary, the incus may be replaced by transposing it to the stapes head (see Tympanoplasty, p. 843).

Following completion of this dissection, the wound may be closed primarily without drainage.

FACIAL NERVE GRAFTING

The principle of nerve grafting is to provide an intact neurilemmal sheath through which regenerating axons may travel without interference. To this end it is necessary to find the site of injury, to debride the injury, to provide a donor nerve of adequate size and length, and to place the graft in a fixed end to end position. Successful nerve grafts have been placed between the intracranial portion of the nerve and the main

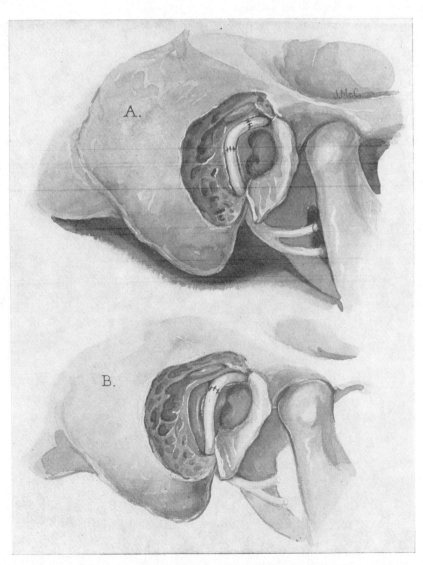

FIG. 57–3. *A,* A free nerve transplantation after the method of Ballance and Duel. *B,* A direct suture of the nerve ends with rerouting to shorten the course of the nerve.

trunk behind the parotid gland, which serves to illustrate the success which may be obtained by grafting techniques.

The site of the nerve injury is approached as described under decompression. After the nerve is identified, it is uncovered for several millimeters on either side of the injury. The nerve ends are then trimmed squarely with sharp techniques. If the injury has been present for some time, it will be necessary to remove the neuroma which forms on the proximal stump. The distance to be grafted is carefully measured.

A fresh graft is removed from either the greater auricular nerve in the neck or the lateral femoral cutaneous nerve in the thigh. Both of these nerves will supply a branchless graft of similar size to the facial nerve. The graft should be trimmed slightly longer than the defect to allow for shrinkage.

The graft is placed in the fallopian canal in exact end-to-end position (Fig. 57–3). Care should be taken to avoid twisting the graft. Usually fibrinous clotting of serum will secure the graft in position. Serum should not be allowed to accumulate between the nerve end and the graft. If the nerve does not rest in a bony bed, suturing of the nerve sheath may be used to secure the graft in position. One or two fine sutures are used for this purpose (7–0 black silk or nylon).

The nerve may be covered with gold leaf, vein, or fascia to protect it during healing. Tight packing should be avoided.

Usually intratemporal grafting results in return of function in 4 to 5 months. Upper facial (frontalis) function usually does not return, and some dysfunction (synkinesis) must be expected. During this period, heat, massage, and galvanic stimulation are of value to prevent atrophy and fibrosis of the facial muscles. Good results are to be expected in 90% of favorable cases.

REFERENCES

Adour, K. K.: Prednisone Treatment for Idiopathic Facial Paralysis. New Engl. J. Med., *287*:1268, 1972.

Alberti, P. W. R. M.: The Greater Auricular Nerve. Arch. Otolaryng., *76*:422, 1962.

Bull, T. R.: Taste and the Chorda Tympani. J. Laryngol., *79*:479, 1965.

Cawthorne, T.: Bell's Palsies. Ann. Otol. Rhinol. Laryng., *72*:774, 1963.

Danish Otolaryngologic Society Symposium: Management of Peripheral Facial Palsies. Arch. Otolaryng., *81*:441, 1965.

Kettel, K.: *Peripheral Facial Palsy*. Springfield, Ill., Charles C Thomas, Publisher, 1959.

Kettel, K.: Repair of Intratemporal Lesions of the Facial Nerve. Ann. Otol. Rhinol. Laryng., *72*:756, 1963.

Pulec, J. L., and House, W. F.: Facial Nerve Involvement and Testing in Acoustic Neuromas. Arch. Otolaryng., *80*:685, 1964.

Richardson, A. T.: Electrodiagnosis in Facial Palsies. Ann. Otol. Rhinol. Laryngol., *72*:569, 1963.

Taverner, D., et al.: Comparison of Corticotropin and Prednisone in Treatment of Idiopathic Facial Paralysis. Br. Med. J., *4*:20, 1971.

PART 5
BRONCHOESOPHAGOLOGY

James B. Snow, Jr.

Chapter 58
Introduction to Peroral Endoscopy

The advent of methods to visualize pathologic changes in the respiratory and alimentary tracts is undoubtedly the most important development in the care of patients with respiratory and alimentary diseases. Rational management of nearly all patients with pulmonary, upper respiratory, and digestive diseases requires endoscopic evaluation for diagnosis, and many commonly encountered disease processes are amenable to endoscopic management. Recent advances in lighting, flexibility, lens systems, photography, ventilation, anesthesia, and magnification have made the benefits of peroral endoscopy available to more patients than ever before. Peroral endoscopy continues to increase in diagnostic and therapeutic importance and has the widest acceptance by both the medical profession and the public that it has enjoyed throughout its history. Each advance stimulates new applications.

HISTORY

The history of peroral endoscopy extends into the last century. Manuel Garcia, a Spanish singing teacher living in London, was the first to report the visualization of the larynx with mirrors and reflected sunlight. His discovery, which was reported in 1855, was followed by the independent development in 1856 of direct laryngoscopy by Türck and Czermak in Vienna. In Freiburg in 1868, Adolph Kussmaul, an internist, looked into the esophagus with reflected light after studying the technique of a sword swallower (Huizinga). After this early inspiration, the relationship between esophagology and sword-swallowing has come to resemble the one between astronomy and astrology. Nevertheless, careful observation of the sword swallower reinforces the lessons on neck position relative to the trunk and head position relative to the neck. Gustave Killian, also in Freiburg, demonstrated the endoscopic feasibility of removal of foreign bodies from the tracheobronchial tree in 1897 and has been recognized as the "father of bronchoscopy" (Major).

Although Thomas Edison developed the electric lamp in 1878, the first distally lighted endoscope, the cystoscope, developed by Nitzi in 1879, utilized a platinum wire filament cooled by circulating water. At the turn of the century, Chevalier Jackson in Philadelphia introduced distally lighted laryngoscopes, bronchoscopes, and esophagoscopes, as well as telescopes with incandescent bulbs. His contributions to the whole understanding of bronchoesophagology were enormous, and he developed the art of the removal of foreign bodies from the air and food passages to an extent that there has not been any subsequent fundamental improvement (Jackson and Jackson).

RECENT ADVANCES

Distal incandescent bulbs in hollow or open endoscopes have been replaced by fiber illumination carriers which provide steady, dependable, bright lighting.

The early telescopes consisted of a series of small lenses separated by air spaces. These telescopes permitted viewing around angles, increasing the viewing angle, and subsequently magnification. Recently the telescopic rod lens system of the British optical physicist H. H. Hopkins of Reading University, in which the air-containing spaces between the conventional series of lenses are replaced with glass rods with polished ends separated by small "air lenses," has been applied to endoscopy. This new lens system is shown in comparison with the older lens system in Figure 58–1. This new system transmits much more light and allows a wider viewing angle and greater magnification. The depth and breadth of field is enhanced for detailed observation (Ward and coworkers).

The recent application of the principles that Lamm developed in 1930 in the trans-mission of an image through a coherent bundle of small flexible glass threads has permitted the development of a truly flexible endoscope. Hirschowitz and his associates applied the fiberoptic principle to the gastroscope in 1958, and Ikeda and his team, as well as others, applied it to bronchoscopy and esophagoscopy. Examinations with flexible endoscopes have become safer and more comfortable for the patient and better tolerated by his physicians. The fiberoptic bronchoscope has added greatly to the extent of the bronchial tree that can be visualized. Washings, brushings, curettage, and biopsy can be carried farther toward the periphery of the lung, especially in the upper lobes. Since the majority of early carcinomas of the bronchus arise in subsegmental bronchi of the third to sixth order of branching, this increased range is of critical importance. Visualization is often possible even if the bronchi are distorted, displaced, or stenotic. Longer, more detailed examinations can be carried out under local anesthesia. Fiberoptic bronchoscopy is reaching a level of perfection that brings it near to the safety and

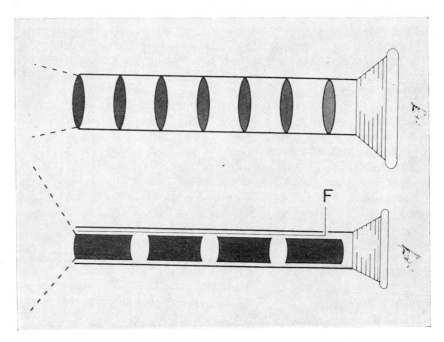

FIG. 58–1.   The Hopkins rod lens system compared to the conventional lens system; *F*—fiberoptic illumination. Note that glass rods are separated by air lenses in the Hopkins system (bottom). (Ward, P. H., *et al.*: Ann. Otol. Rhinol. Laryngol., *83*:754, 1974.)

effectiveness required for screening of selected populations.

Major contributions to documentation and teaching of bronchoesophagology have been made by Holinger with the Holinger-Brubaker camera. Marsh has contributed to the concepts of early detection of bronchogenic carcinoma and photography through fiberoptic bronchoscopes, although the image resolution is not entirely satisfactory with coherent bundle fiberoptics. Rayl's work with documentation through color television merits admiration. The best demonstration of endoscopic photography at this time has been achieved by Ward and others using the Hopkins rod lens telescope with surrounding fiber illumination and an antifog airflow system.

Microscopic evaluation and control of surgical procedures in the larynx has been developed under the leadership of Kleinsasser, Ono and Saito, Jako, and Strong. Kleinsasser has clearly pointed out the great possibilities of magnification in detecting early pathologic changes suggestive of malignancy. Laryngoscopy under microscopic control provides excellent exposure, brilliant illumination, binocular vision, bimanual instrumentation, and magnification for precise surgical manipulation (Strong).

Laser surgery of the larynx and bronchi has been introduced by Strong and appears to have important application in the precise removal of lesions of the vocal cord for restoration of the voice and control of squamous cell papillomas of the larynx, trachea, and bronchi (Strong and Jako; Strong and coworkers).

Through the application of developments in the physics of optics, endoscopy has entered into a period of rapid expansion of new information and new therapeutic techniques that make it as exciting as it must have been when Kussmaul, Killian, and Jackson first began to look into the previously dark interior. Today technical developments provide a new stimulus, just as they did at the turn of the century.

PREPARATION OF THE PATIENT

The patient should be carefully evaluated and prepared for peroral endoscopy. The present problem and all related and past medical problems should be assimilated. As in other surgery, specific inquiry regarding a personal or family history of a bleeding tendency should be made, and a survey of the blood clotting mechanism, including platelet count, prothrombin time, and partial thromboplastin time, should be obtained in addition to the complete blood count, serologic test for syphilis, blood urea nitrogen and glucose, and serum electrolytes. Of particular importance is the history of adverse reactions to drugs, especially to local anesthesia. A complete physical examination should be performed. Unless the endoscopy is a true emergency, as in the case of certain foreign bodies of the trachea and bronchi, the preoperative evaluation should include the appropriate radiographic studies. Posterior-anterior and lateral chest x-rays are a necessity, and depending on the clinical problem, roentgenograms of the lateral neck, laryngograms, laminograms of the larynx, xeroradiography, bronchography, upper gastrointestinal series with cinefluoroscopy of the swallowing function, and angiography may be indicated prior to the endoscopic procedure. Consultation with specialists in other fields should be obtained as indicated. If all of the information possible is available, the endoscopist will be in the best position to interpret the abnormal findings that he may encounter.

The psychological preparation should begin at the first contact with the endoscopist. The care in the history and physical examination, as well as the special diagnostic studies, instill confidence in the patient. The reasons for the endoscopic procedure should be presented in a thorough and rational way to gain the fullest understanding of the patient. The procedure should be described in positive terms. The possible benefits and risks should be discussed fully, and their ratio should be presented.

The patient should be admitted to the hospital at least one day prior to the endoscopic procedure. Food and fluids by mouth should be withheld for 8 hours prior to the procedure. The nature of the premedication depends on the type of anesthesia to be used.

As with other procedures on the respiratory and alimentary tracts, endoscopy may be accompanied by bacteremia. For this reason patients with structural defects of the heart as evidenced by a heart murmur should have prophylactic antibiotic therapy prior to and for a few days following endoscopy to prevent subacute bacterial endocarditis.

ANESTHESIA

The selection of local or general anesthesia for peroral endoscopy depends on a number of factors. At times no anesthesia is appropriate. In most adults either local or general anesthesia may be appropriate. Children are particularly sensitive to the toxicity of local anesthetics, so ordinarily they should receive either general anesthesia or no anesthesia. Wrapping of the child for restraint is still frequently employed, but the safety of general anesthesia in children has been satisfactorily demonstrated for direct laryngoscopy, bronchoscopy, and esophagoscopy. The greatest problem occurs in the child with an already compromised airway. Inhalation anesthesia is safer than intravenous agents in the presence of a compromised airway. If there is sufficient airway obstruction, it may not be possible to induce general anesthesia by inhalation. In such a situation either the procedure must be carried out without anesthesia, or a better airway must be established prior to the induction of anesthesia. An example of a situation in which anesthesia should not be employed is the child with complete obstruction of one bronchus by a foreign body, with atelectasis of that lung and compensatory emphysema of the other lung. Under these circumstances the bronchoscope must be inserted and the foreign body removed, for no other solution is available. On the other hand, the child with a bulky foreign body of the esophagus that compresses the membranous posterior wall of the trachea and produces upper airway obstruction can have endotracheal intubation carried out while awake, and then general anesthesia can be safely induced for the esophagoscopy and removal of the foreign body.

As a rule, general anesthesia is preferred for direct laryngoscopy, tracheoscopy, bronchoscopy, and esophagoscopy in infants and children. In direct laryngoscopy and tracheoscopy in infants and children, the procedure is usually indicated by abnormalities which are slight variations from normal. Gross variations from normal are not compatible with life. General anesthesia is preferred for these examinations so that the patient is relaxed. Accurate observations of these slight variations from normal can then be made (Snow). The specular examination of the respiratory tract can be followed advantageously by tracheography and bronchography under the same anaesthesia (Ferguson and Flake).

In adults local or general anesthesia may be used for any form of peroral endoscopy. Direct laryngoscopy for removal of lesions of the vocal cord to restore the voice and other procedures that require microscopic control are performed better under general anesthesia. Patients with large obstructive lesions, such as carcinoma of the larynx, are managed more satisfactorily as a general rule with local anesthesia. The patient with a compromised but barely adequate airway can protect the airway better under local anesthesia. A train of events is more likely to occur under general anesthesia leading to further compromise of the airway than would occur under local anesthesia. The patient's personality and ability to cooperate are factors in the selection of the type of anesthesia. Patients with a tendency toward gagging with indirect laryngoscopy often do not make good subjects for direct laryngoscopy under local anesthesia.

Bronchoscopy in the adult is usually satisfactorily performed under local anesthesia. Certainly local anesthesia is usually adequate for use with the flexible bronchoscope. Bronchoscopy for aspiration of obstructing secretions in patients with atelectasis is facilitated by the coughing that may occur under local anesthesia. Foreign bodies are generally removed more readily with general anesthesia. A careful search with a flexible bronchoscope for an occult lesion in a patient with cytology characteristic of a malignant neoplasm may require general anesthesia.

Esophagoscopy and gastroscopy in the adult with the flexible upper gastrointestinal panendoscope can ordinarily be performed with local anesthesia. Generally removal of foreign bodies of the esophagus and dilatation of esophageal strictures through open esophagoscopes are safer and more comfortable for the patient under general endotracheal anesthesia. Foreign body removal from the stomach with a flexible panendoscope is satisfactorily performed under local anesthesia.

Local Anesthesia

Local anesthetics are drugs that block nerve conduction anywhere in the nervous system. In order to be of practical value, their effect must be reversible but of sufficiently long duration to allow the procedure to be completed. The greatest hazard of local anesthetics is their toxicity. The ratio between the toxic dose and the effective dose is small. Most adverse reactions result from high blood levels due to overdosage rather than allergic reactions. Not only the total dose administered but also the route, concentration, and rate of application contribute to the resultant blood levels. Adriani and Campbell have shown that tetracaine and cocaine applied topically to the respiratory epithelium of the pharynx, trachea, and bronchi produce blood levels of the agent equal to 30% of the blood level obtained with intravenous administration. The absorption of topically applied local anesthetics is more rapid than from subcutaneous injection of these agents, and more toxic reactions occur when local anesthetics are applied topically than when they are infiltrated. The absorption is more rapid from pseudostratified ciliated columnar epithelium (respiratory epithelium), as in the trachea, than from stratified squamous epithelium, as in the esophagus. Unlike the situation with subcutaneously injected local anesthetics, the addition of epinephrine to the topically applied solution does not alter the rate of its absorption into the bloodstream.

Local anesthetic agents cause two types of toxic reactions. One is cardiovascular due to the direct depression of the myocardium and vasodilation. Depression of the myocardium and vasodilation lead to hypotension. The depression of the myocardium may result in asystole. The other is stimulation and subsequent depression of the central nervous system. The stimulation of the central nervous system produces restlessness, tremor, loquaciousness, and convulsions. The central nervous system stimulation is usually followed by profound depression and death due to respiratory failure. The two forms of toxicity appear to occur simultaneously and are additive. Support of respiration is the essential feature in the management of toxic reactions (Goodman and Gilman). Hypotension should be managed with intravenous sympathomimetic amines, and asystole should be managed by external cardiac massage. Convulsions should be controlled with neuromuscular blocking agents rather than central nervous system depressants, since the central nervous system stimulation is regularly and promptly followed by profound central nervous system depression.

Idiosyncratic and allergic reactions to local anesthetics are rare. Intolerance to local anesthetics is found in children, the aged, and debilitated and poor-risk individuals who cannot metabolize the agent at the usual rate. Contact dermatitis to tetracaine occurs not infrequently in medical personnel, and they should avoid skin contact with this agent.

Premedication for local anesthesia includes sedatives, narcotics, and cholinolytic agents. Barbiturates, when given prophylactically, protect animals from lethal doses of local anesthetics. Pentobarbital, a moderately long-acting barbiturate, is ideal for premedication for local anesthesia. In a dosage of 100 to 150 mg for a 70-kg adult, good psychic sedation is obtained without respiratory depression. Meperidine in a dose of 100 mg for a 70-kg adult adds a degree of relaxation to the effects of pentobarbital and produces a calm and cooperative patient without undue depression. These dosages must be reduced or even deleted, depending on the patient's age, debility, and pulmonary function. Atropine is the ideal cholinolytic agent for endoscopic procedures. Not only does it reduce the chance of adverse vagovagal reflexes during stimulation of the respiratory tract, but also it decreases secretion of the mucous membrane. Atropine may be given in a dosage of 0.6 mg in a 70-kg adult. The pentobarbital may be given orally 90 minutes before the procedure, and the meperidine and atropine may be given intramuscularly 45 minutes before the procedure.

The psychological preparation of the patient is as important as the premedication. Chevalier Jackson called it the "Sermon on Relaxation." The patient should be reassured that the procedure is designed for his benefit and that he will be able, with the aid of premedication and local anesthesia, to relax and cooperate in the procedure. One of the great advantages of local anesthesia is that it allows the surgeon and patient to cooperate in exploring the airway, since motion, source of secretion, and changes in contour during respiration are very important diagnostic clues.

Prior to the application of any local anesthetic agent, there must be in the operating room a laryngoscope, an endotracheal tube, and an anesthetic machine for the delivery of oxygen under positive pressure. The blood pressure should be monitored periodically, and an intravenous catheter should be securely in place. Only after these steps have been taken should the local anesthesia be applied. Once the topical application has been initiated, the patient must be monitored continuously and must not be left alone. The anesthetic should be applied in the operating room in which the operation is to be performed. All of the endoscopic instruments should be in readiness prior to the application of the anesthetic.

Cocaine, tetracaine, and lidocaine are the three topical local anesthetics in widest use for peroral endoscopy at this time. It is essential to be thoroughly familiar with the maximum safe dose of the agent to be used. Various estimates of the maximum safe dose for a 70-kg adult exist, but the following are suggested and adequate:

cocaine	100 mg
tetracaine	40 mg
lidocaine	100 mg

The smallest volume and the lowest concentration possible to accomplish the desired effect should be utilized. Subsequent applications should be made deliberately, so that the blood level will not rise above safe levels and so that each application will achieve maximum surface anesthesia.

The concentration of local anesthetics is customarily expressed in percentages. Tetracaine is effective in 0.5% and 1% solutions. Solutions of 1% are recommended for cocaine, and 1 or 2% solutions are recommended for lidocaine. It is absolutely essential to understand that a 1% solution means there is 1 g of the agent in 100 ml or *10 mg per ml*. In other words, 10 ml of a 1% solution of cocaine contains 100 mg. The safest way to handle a local anesthetic is to have only the maximum safe dose given to the operator. In other words, if the agent to be used is 1% cocaine and the maximum safe dose is considered to be 100 mg, the operator should ask for 10 ml of 1% cocaine and that exact amount should be poured into a graduated measuring glass. The operator should supervise the pouring of the agent. He should read the label of the stock solution and should verify that only the maximum safe dose has been delivered. It is then possible to calculate the dose applied at any time by subtracting the amount remaining in the graduated measuring glass from the maximum safe dose. Cocaine must not be injected. It should be tinted with methylene blue in the pharmacy as a further indication that it is not to be injected. Assuming 100 mg of cocaine is to be used as a topical agent in a 70-kg man for direct laryngoscopy or bronchoscopy, that amount should be enough for spraying the pharynx, for topical application into the piriform sinuses on cotton with Jackson cross-action forceps in the hope of establishing a conduction block of the superior laryngeal nerves, and for dropping the agent at first onto the vocal cords and then through them with a syringe and Abraham malleable cannula (Fig. 58–2). Not more than 1 ml or 10 mg should be applied at one time, and the applications should not occur more frequently than every 1 to 2 minutes. Less agent is needed if each application is given a chance to be effective before the next application. Once the larynx is anesthetized, the agent can be applied to the tracheobronchial tree more accurately. Positioning of the patient immediately after instillation of the agent into the tracheobronchial tree

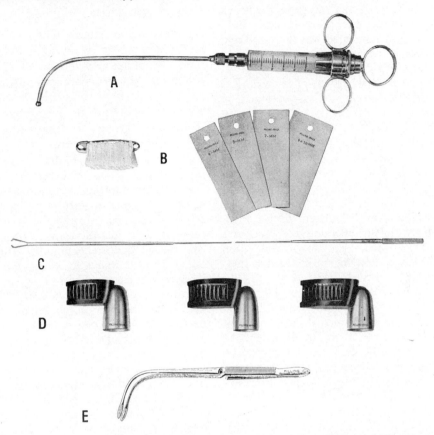

Fig. 58–2. *A*, Laryngeal syringe for introducing anesthetic solutions into the larynx by indirect laryngoscopy prior to peroral endoscopy. *B*, Bronchoscopic sponges—Metal patterns for making various size sponges from gauze bandage. *C*, Bronchoscopic sponge carrier. *D*, Lell bite blocks for infants, adults, and edentulous adults. *E*, Jackson cross-action forceps.

on to one elbow and then the other helps to distribute the agent to the bronchus on the same side. The maximum anesthetic effect of topically applied local anesthetics is not obtained until 5 to 10 minutes after the last application, and operative intervention should not begin until that latent period has elapsed.

Injection of a topical anesthetic agent into the lumen of the trachea through the crico-thyroid membrane has been advocated, but it is not without complication and should be employed when the anesthetic solution cannot be introduced through the lumen of the larynx.

Anesthesia for direct laryngoscopy and bronchoscopy can be enhanced by infiltration of 1 to 2 ml of 1% lidocaine in the area of the thyrohyoid membrane where the superior laryngeal nerves enter the larynx. Whenever agents for infiltration are to be used in conjunction with topical agents, the use of the topical agent should be completed, and any residuum and the vessel that contained it should be removed from the operating table before the injectable agent is brought into the operative field. In this way the chance of mistaking the topical agent for the injectable agent and injecting a topical agent such as cocaine is minimized. As with topical agents, the operator should specify the volume and concentration of the injectable agent he wishes to use, whether or not it should contain epinephrine, and if so, in what concentration. Epinephrine in a concentration of 1/100,000 is preferred. The operator must read the label on the stock solution, supervise the pouring, and verify that the amount requested was delivered and did not exceed the maximum safe dose.

Local anesthetic agents have been shown to interfere with the growth of bacteria and modify the bacteriologic data obtained at bronchoscopy. Tetracaine and lidocaine have an inhibitory effect on the culture of fungi and bacteria, including *Mycobacterium tuberculosis* (Conte and Laforet).

Bronchoscopy under local anesthesia with an open bronchoscope produces arterial pCO_2 levels below the preoperative level, and arterial pO_2 levels on room air are sometimes above those encountered preoperatively. These effects probably result from hyperventilation and increased cardiac output (Carden).

Bronchoscopy under local anesthesia with a flexible bronchoscope may be carried out through an open bronchoscope, tracheoscope, or nasal or oral endotracheal tube, or the flexible bronchoscope can be introduced alone. Hypoxia may occur under any of these circumstances if the flexible bronchoscope takes up too much of the airway. Oxygen may be delivered through a face mask over the oral or nasal endotracheal tube, and the flexible bronchoscope can be passed through a rubber diaphragm over the hole in the face mask. Likewise oxygen can be delivered through a side arm of the endotracheal tube, and the flexible bronchoscope may be passed through a rubber diaphragm over the lumen of the endotracheal tube. If the flexible bronchoscope is passed through an open bronchoscope or tracheoscope, oxygen can be delivered through the side arm of the open endoscope. If the flexible bronchoscope is introduced alone, supplementary oxygen may be supplied through a face mask.

Topical anesthesia for esophagoscopy may be obtained by spraying the pharynx and periodically giving the patient small measured sips of the topically active local anesthetic to swallow. Systemic absorption from the esophagus and the stomach is negligible if the mucous membrane is intact. If there is ulcerative disease of the esophagus or stomach, special care must be taken.

General Anesthesia

Inhalation anesthesia with halothane can be safely used for direct laryngoscopy in infants and children if the airway is not compromised. For bronchoscopy in infants and children, positive pressure ventilation or adequate spontaneous respiration can be maintained through the ventilating side arm of a Holinger bronchoscope. For esophagoscopy in infants and children, general endotracheal anesthesia is preferred.

General endotracheal anesthesia is preferred for direct laryngoscopy in which microscopic control, surgery for restoration of the voice, or dilatation are to be employed. The cuffed endotracheal tube of small but adequate size comes to rest in the interarytenoid fold and presents no great problem for most endolaryngeal surgery. Esophagoscopy with an open esophagoscope is usually performed under general endotracheal anesthesia, especially if foreign body removal or dilatation is required.

A number of general anesthetic techniques have been used in conjunction with the open bronchoscope. They include apnea with intermittent ventilation, apnea with delivery of oxygen through an endotracheal catheter, spontaneous respiration, cuirass ventilation or external chest compression, ventilation through an endotracheal tube alongside the bronchoscope, ventilation through the side arm of a bronchoscope, entrainment of gas through the bronchoscope with Sander's Venturi injector system, and injection of gas through the ventilating side arm of the bronchoscope as described by Carden.

Apnea under thiopental and succinylcholine after preoxygenation for 5 minutes allows 4 minutes of working time before reoxygenation is required. The arterial pCO_2 rises at a rate of 3 to 6 mm Hg per minute. Although blood gases may be maintained at acceptable levels in otherwise healthy individuals, the technique is not suitable for many patients with pulmonary pathology requiring bronchoscopy. This technique is no longer in common use.

Apnea with delivery of oxygen through an endotracheal catheter near the carina under thiopental and succinylcholine requires flow rates of 5 to 20 liters per minute. The oxygenation does not decrease with time because the diffusion through the alveoli is good. The pCO_2 increases at 0.9 to 4 mm Hg per minute, and the technique is limited by this factor.

General anesthesia with spontaneous ventilation through the bronchoscope has been widely used and is particularly suitable for bronchoscopy with halothane in children for therapeutic procedures, such as foreign body removal, as well as for diagnostic procedures. Nevertheless significant increase in the arterial pCO_2 may occur, and the pH may decrease. It is less suitable for adults than for children.

Ventilation by the use of a cuirass to produce negative or positive pressure about the chest and abdomen is not efficient and is not applicable to many patients. Hypoxia and hypercapnia result from the technique. It has generally been abandoned.

The use of a small endotracheal tube alongside the bronchoscope allows very satisfactory control of ventilation. The operator may work with a glass window occluding the bronchoscope or may have to occlude the bronchoscope with a thumb periodically. There is very little problem in the spatial accommodation of the bronchoscope and the endotracheal tube. Likewise, a bronchoscope with a ventilating side arm can be used with a glass window to occlude the bronchoscope, and the anesthetic gas and oxygen can be delivered through the ventilating side arm. More leakage of gas tends to occur with this method than with the endotracheal tube alongside the bronchoscope. With both of these methods, there is an increase in arterial pCO_2 when the window is removed to introduce instruments through the bronchoscope.

Sanders' Venturi injector system uses a small (16-gauge) high-pressure jet of oxygen in the long axis of the bronchoscope which causes entrainment of gas in the bronchoscope to ventilate the lungs (Sanders; Morales and coworkers; Smith). Figure 58–3 illustrates the equipment necessary. The oxygen jet is introduced intermittently at a predetermined pressure, usually 50 pounds per square inch or less. The oxygen jet en-

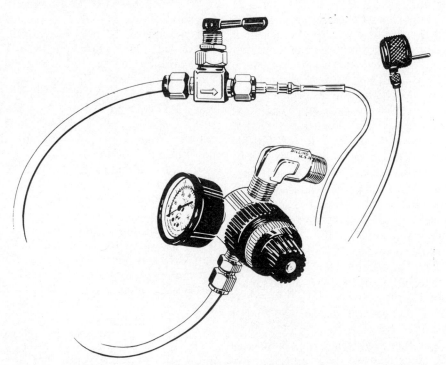

FIG. 58–3.   Sanders' Venturi injector system.

trains anesthetic gases being fed through the ventilating side arm, as well as air from the open proximal end of the bronchoscope. Hence 100% oxygen is not delivered to the lungs. The jet of oxygen is controlled by an on-off toggle valve, which is connected to a single-stage variable pressure regulator. The pressure regulator is supplied with oxygen under pressure. The system is more efficient with proximally expanded bronchoscopes. It does not work quite as well in patients in whom pulmonary compliance is below normal. Carden modified this system by eliminating the 16-gauge jet and utilizing a larger oxygen jet. This modification allowed the use of 100% oxygen and higher pressures at the proximal end of the bronchoscope. These systems may be used with intravenous agents, such as thiopental and succinylcholine, halothane entrainment, and 70% nitrous oxide and 30% oxygen (Carden).

General anesthesia is frequently needed for flexible bronchoscopy when the procedure is combined with other diagnostic procedures, such as biopsy of the nasopharynx; the search may be very long, as in occult primaries in cytologically positive patients, and the patient cannot tolerate a procedure under local anesthesia for psychological or other reasons. Fiberoptic bronchoscopes that measure 5 mm in diameter are in general use at this time. They contain channels for suctioning and passage of instruments. Application of positive pressure ventilation through the aspiration channel has proved dangerous because the tip of the flexible scope may make a tight seal with a segmental or subsegmental bronchus and produce a rupture of the parenchyma and pneumothorax (Britton and Nelson). If general anesthesia is to be employed, an endotracheal tube is inserted orally. The flexible bronchoscope is inserted through an adapter with a diaphragm across the lumen of the endotracheal tube. In this way an adequate seal is obtained for positive pressure ventilation during the general anesthetic. With a 5-mm flexible bronchoscope, endotracheal tubes larger than 32 French or 8.5 mm internal diameter must be used to prevent hypoxia, hypercapnea, and high end expiratory pressures. Smaller endotracheal tubes may be appropriate with the 2.7-mm flexible bronchoscopes.

EQUIPMENT

The armamentarium of peroral endoscopy is vast, and a comprehensive listing is not intended here. Special instruments have been developed for special purposes. A beginning student should study the instruments presented in Jackson and Jackson's *Bronchoesophagology*, as well as the recent catalogs of instrument manufacturers, to be aware of the special instruments available for particular endoscopic problems.

For direct laryngoscopy the standard Jackson laryngoscopes are useful in surveying the hypopharynx and larynx (Fig. 58-4, *A*). The distal tip of the spatular portion is blunt and is intended for insertion posterior to the epiglottis to the level of the false vocal cords. The proximal end of the tube has a dorsal sliding portion that is detachable, so that a bronchoscope can be introduced through the laryngoscope and the laryngoscope can be removed without disturbing the bronchoscope. The standard Jackson laryngoscope is available in the infant (internal diameter 10 mm and working length 7.5 cm), child (internal diameter 11.5 mm and working length 10.3 cm), adolescent (internal diameter 12 mm and working length 13.5 cm), and adult (internal diameter 14.5 mm and working length 13.5 cm) sizes. Holinger has designed an infant or newborn laryngoscope (internal diameter 8.0 mm and working length 6.2 cm) that is particularly useful in infants under 6 months of age. In the adult model of the standard Jackson laryngoscope, the handle is counterbalanced so that, when grasped properly, the spatular portion is maintained in the proper plane for inspection of the larynx. The standard Jackson laryngoscope does not permit adequate visualization of the anterior commissure in many patients. For visualization of the anterior commissure and laryngeal surface of the epiglottis, the Jackson anterior commissure laryngoscope is preferred (Fig. 58-4, *B*). It has a beveled distal end and is designed to be introduced below the false vocal cords, and this design permits excellent exposure of the ventricles, true cords, and

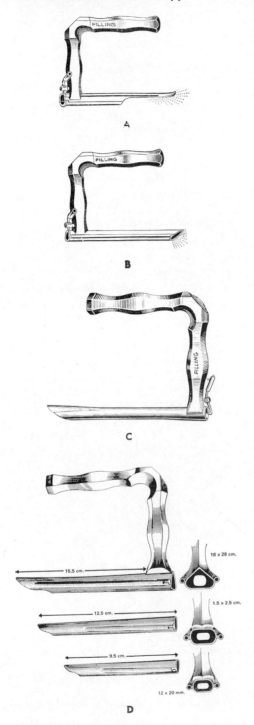

FIG. 58–4. Laryngoscopes. *A*, Standard Jackson laryngoscope. *B*, Jackson anterior commissure laryngoscope. *C*, Holinger anterior commissure laryngoscope. *D*, Jako laryngoscope.

anterior commissure. By rotating the handle 90 degrees so that the bevel will enter the glottis in the anterior-posterior plane, the subglottic area and trachea may be exposed. The Jackson anterior commissure laryngoscope is very suitable for operative work in the larynx. It is available in child (internal diameter 7 $\times$ 9 mm and working length 10.5 cm) and adult (internal diameter 10 $\times$ 11 mm and working length 14.8 cm) sizes. Holinger's hourglass modification of the anterior commissure laryngoscope incorporates the principle of the Yankauer postnasal speculum (Fig. 58–4, *C*). The distal end of the ventral surface of the tube rises obliquely and flares laterally. The proximal portion of the dorsal surface declines obliquely. It elevates the tuberculum of the epiglottis and provides additional working space for application of instruments.

Various laryngoscopes have been developed for laryngoscopy under microscopic control. The Jako laryngoscopes, in adolescent and adult sizes, provide excellent working conditions with the Zeiss operation microscope (Fig. 58–4, *D*). General anesthesia is used through a cuffed endotracheal tube. The laryngoscope is held by a Lewy laryngoscope holder which rests on a Mayo stand over the patient's chest. Binocular vision and bimanual manipulation are easily accommodated. Much endolaryngeal surgery which requires extensive manipulation, such as an arytenoidectomy, and which was formerly performed through the Lynch suspension laryngoscope is now performed under microscopic control.

The flexible laryngoscope is useful for viewing the larynx and for introducing endotracheal tubes in individuals in whom exposure of the larynx with a rigid laryngoscope is impossible or unadvisable, as may be the case in patients with trismus, temporomandibular arthritis, pharyngeal stenosis, and cervical spinal ankylosis and trauma.

The Jackson tracheoscope is an extralong anterior commissure scope for examination of the cervical trachea. It has a working length of 18 cm.

Modern open bronchoscopes, such as the C. L. Jackson and Holinger models, have expanded proximal ends and ventilating side arms (Fig. 58–5). The expanded proximal

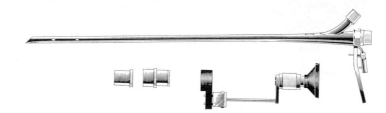

Fig. 58–5.   Holinger bronchoscope with ventilating side arm and lens system.

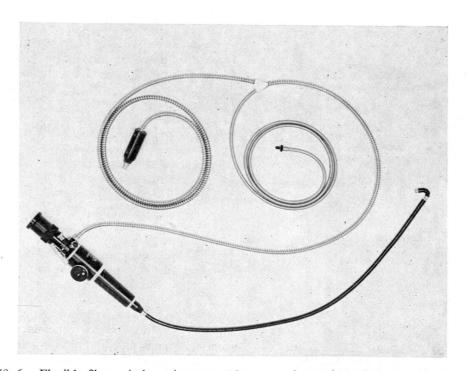

Fig. 58–6.   Flexible fiberoptic bronchoscope. (Courtesy of American Cystoscope Makers, Inc.)

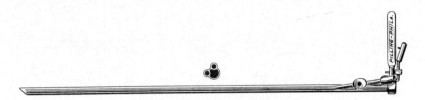

FIG. 58–7.   Standard Jackson esophagoscope.

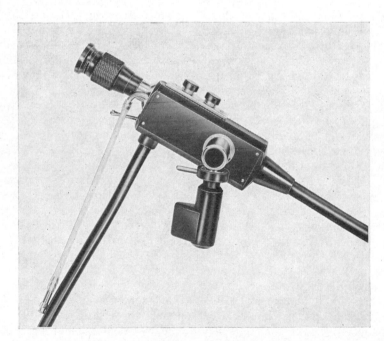

FIG. 58–8.   Upper gastrointestinal panendoscope (Courtesy of American
Cystoscope Makers, Inc.)

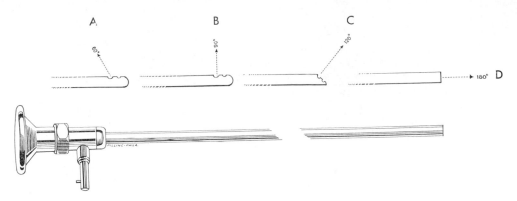

FIG. 58–9.   Bronchoscopic telescopes with conventional lens system. *A*, Retrospective, which is useful for viewing the upper lobe bronchi. *B*, Right angle, which is useful for viewing the upper lobe bronchi and the superior segmental bronchi of both lower lobes. *C*, Foroblique, which is useful for viewing the right middle lobe bronchus. *D*, Straight ahead.

ends improve visibility and allow visual centering by the operator with more ease. Instruments are introduced more easily into the funnel shape than into a cylindrical proximal end. A large ventilating side arm provides for the delivery of oxygen and anesthetic gases. Open bronchoscopes have fenestrations near the distal end to provide ventilation to the other lung when the distal end of the bronchoscope is in a bronchus. Open bronchoscopes are designated by the number of millimeters of internal diameter and the number of centimeters of length and range from 3–20 (3 mm × 20 cm) to 9–40 (9 mm × 40 cm).

Flexible bronchoscopes have an external diameter of 2.7, 4, and 5 mm and are 50 to 53 cm long (Fig. 58–6). The distal ends have a flexible angle of 200 to 270 degrees. The apical rotation to the right and left is 30 degrees in each direction. The field of vision varies from 62 to 80 degrees. There are channels for biopsy forceps and cytology brush and lavage and suction.

Open esophagoscopes are oval or round in cross section and range in size from 3.5–25 (3.5 mm internal diameter × 25 cm in length) to 9–53 (9 mm × 53 cm). A light carrier channel and an aspirating channel are built into the wall (Fig. 58–7). The oval open esophagoscopes, such as those designed by Mosher and Jesberg, are very suit-

able for foreign body removal, as well as for diagnostic procedures. The distal end of the Jesberg esophagoscope is thickened to form a protective edge and molded to a smooth Haslinger sled runner shape for safety and ease of introduction. The round open esophagoscopes are more appropriate for negotiating obstructions such as tumors and strictures and for their dilatation.

The flexible upper gastrointestinal panendoscopes have an external diameter of 10 to 12.5 mm and are 100 to 105 cm long (Fig. 58–8). The distal ends have a deflection capability of 270 degrees. The field of vision is 75 degrees. There are channels for biopsy and aspiration.

Modern laryngoscopes are made of tempered brass, stainless steel, and steel alloys, as are open bronchoscopes and esophagoscopes. The lighting is almost exclusively distal, and fiber illumination carriers are preferred.

Bronchoscopic telescopes of the conventional lens system with retrospective, right angle, foroblique, and straight ahead views extend the inspection that can be obtained with an open bronchoscope (Fig. 58–9). They are manufactured with a 5-mm external diameter and are 48 cm long. The viewing angle is 55 degrees. Telescopes with the Hopkins rod lens system are also used in open bronchoscopes and provide a brighter image and better resolution. They are available as forward, forward-oblique, and lateral telescopes with a 5.5-mm external diameter and a viewing angle of what appears to be 90 degrees. Both types utilize fiber illumination. The Hopkins telescopes are also available in a pediatric size with an outer diameter of 4 mm and the same angulations and viewing angle.

Tubes for application of suction are available in the size appropriate in length and diameter to the endoscope being used. Aspiration tubes are of the open-end and velvet eye type (Fig. 58–10). The open-end suction catheter applies stronger suction but is more traumatic. The velvet eye, because of its multiple openings, does not tend to pull mucous membrane into its lumen. Curved, flexible-tip aspiration tubes are very helpful in certain situations, such as aspiration of the upper lobe bronchi.

Forceps are required for manipulation, biopsy, and foreign body removal. Alligator forceps of various lengths and sturdiness are available for direct laryngoscopy, bronchoscopy, and esophagoscopy and are very useful in various manipulations (Fig. 58–11). Cupped, square, round, and oval basket and triangular forceps in various sizes and sturdiness are necessary for biopsy, depending on the clinical problem. Jackson papilloma forceps, which are blunt and duck-billed, allow removal of friable papillomas without trauma to the normal laryngeal structures. Foreign body removal has been greatly improved by the development of the center-action foreign body forceps. This design allows the blades to close without retraction into the tubular sheath of the forceps, as was the case with the Jackson and Jesberg forward grasping

forceps. Foreign body forceps have been developed to deal with nearly every type of object that has become a foreign body. The following partial list includes the type of forceps and the objects it is designed to remove: alligator grasping forceps for coins, buttons, meat, cloth, string, etc.; alligator rotation forceps for similar objects with a raised rim; Kahler grasping forceps for hard, irregular objects; ball forceps with cupped jaws for beads and toy jacks; Jackson sharp-pointed and dull rotation forceps for holding and pivoting foreign bodies with rings like safety pins; Jackson "sister-hook" forceps for delicate rotation and staples; C. L. Jackson head-holding forceps with canted crescentic jaws for grasping the head or shank of screws, nails, and tacks; side-lip forceps for inward rotation and ensheathing a point; Tucker tack and pin forceps which rotate the shaft of the foreign body into the axis of the endoscope; fenestrated, cupped grasping jaws for peanuts, nut meats, and beans; Jackson button forceps with long, sharp-pointed jaws for reaching into the holes of buttons; Jackson broad staple forceps for grasping both points of a staple; Tucker staple forceps with specially shaped angulated blades to permit withdrawal with both points of the staple into the beveled distal end of the endoscope; Clerf-Arrowsmith safety pin closer, in which a notched brace pushes the loop of the pin away from the jaws which grasp the limbs of the pin to approximate the point and the keeper; Jackson approximation forceps for bringing the sharp points of two pronged upholstery pins, paper fasteners, and tacks together; Gordon bead forceps for grasping spherical objects; Jackson globular object forceps for marbles,

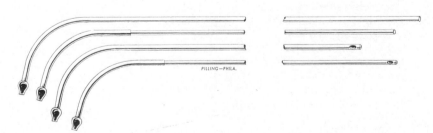

PILLING—PHILA.

Fig. 58–10.   Aspiration tubes. The upper two are open end aspiration tubes and the lower two, velvet eye (Pilling).

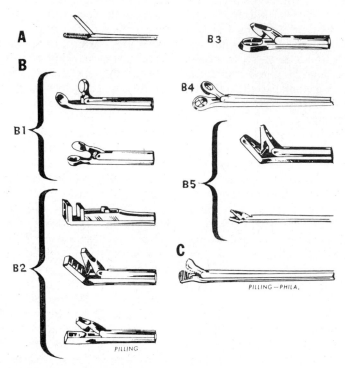

FIG. 58–11.   Endoscopic forceps. *A,* Alligator forceps. *B,* Biopsy forceps (Pilling): B1, straight and up-biting cupped; B2, right-angle, 45-degree, and straight square; B3, round; B4, oval; B5, straight and 45-degree triangular. *C,* Papilloma forceps (Pilling). *D,* Foreign body forceps: 1, center-action forceps of alligator rotation type; 1a, fenestrated forceps; 1b, Kahler forceps; 2, Jackson conventional foreign body forceps:

    A. ball forceps
    B. Jackson sharp-pointed rotation forceps
    C. Jackson dull rotation forceps
    D. sister-hook forceps
    E. C. L. Jackson head-holding forceps
    F. side-lip forceps
    G. Tucker tack and pin forceps
    H. fenestrated forceps
    I. Jackson button forceps
    J. Jackson broad staple forceps
    K. Tucker staple forceps
    L. Clerf-Arrowsmith safety pin closer
    M. Jackson approximation forceps
    N. Gordon bead forceps
    O. Jackson globular object forceps
    P. Jackson ring jaw globular object forceps
    Q. Jackson double-prong forceps
    R. Jackson flexible upper lobe bronchus forceps
    S. Jackson cylindrical object forceps
    T. Jackson cylindrical object forceps with teeth
    U. various expansile forceps
    V. C. L. Jackson pin-bending costophrenic forceps

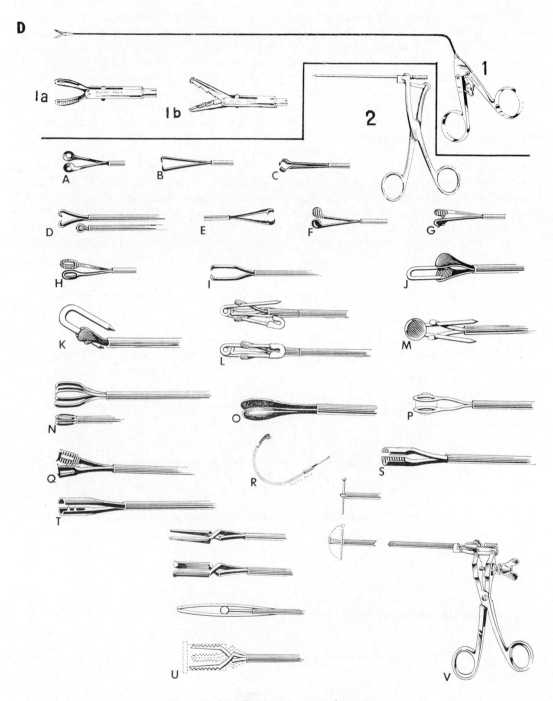

Fig. 58–11. Legend on opposite page.

ball bearings, and pebbles; Jackson ring jaw globular object forceps for beads; Jackson double-prong grasping forceps for teeth and similar objects; Jackson flexible upper lobe bronchus forceps for reaching 180 degrees around the corner; Jackson cylindrical object forceps; expansile forceps for introduction into a hollow object to grasp it from the inside with the dilating blades; C. L. Jackson pin-bending costophrenic forceps for removing straight pins from the periphery of the lung. A good magnet often solves an otherwise difficult foreign body removal problem (Fig. 58–12).

For dilatations various bougies are needed. For the larynx, Jackson triangular brass dilators are very useful. For the esophagus, Jackson steel-stem woven filiform bougies from size 8 to 40 French are necessary for

dilatation through the esophagoscope (Fig. 58–13). Plummer bougies from size 16 to 45 French may be passed over a thread but are now seldom employed. Tucker retrograde bougies from size 12 to 40 French are passed from the gastrostomy to the mouth in long strictures of the esophagus, as occur with lye burns. Dilatation blindly with Hurst mercury-filled bougies from size 16 to 60 French is infrequently used. Maloney's tapered modification of the Hurst bougies from size 20 to 60 French is more frequently employed.

For bronchoscopic diagnosis, special equipment for washing, such as the Lukens collecting tube, bronchial brushes, curettes, and aspirating needles, is needed.

Sponges and sponge carriers are required for topical anesthesia and for application of

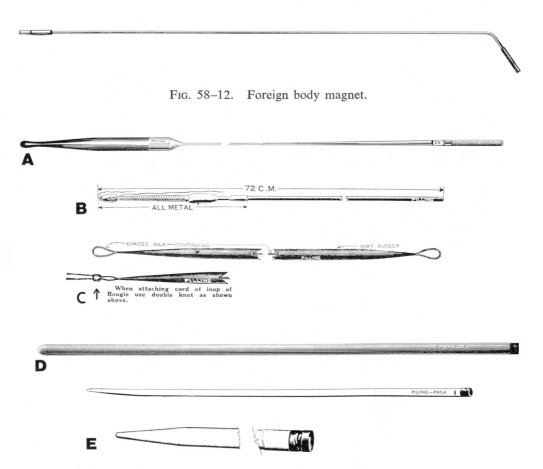

FIG. 58–12.   Foreign body magnet.

FIG. 58–13.   Esophageal bougies. *A*, Jackson steel-stem woven. *B*, Plummer. *C*, Tucker. *D*, Hurst. *E*, Maloney.

sympathomimetic amines to achieve vaso-constriction for visualization and control of bleeding (Fig. 58–2).

TECHNICAL FACTORS

Elective peroral endoscopy should be performed in the general operating rooms of a hospital. Endoscopic procedures should be carried out under the same circumstances as any other surgical procedure. All of the resuscitation facilities and personnel of a general operating suite should be available, just as with any other operative procedure.

Standard scrub facilities should be employed. Good overhead lighting must be available. Two dependable sources of suction must be available. Instruments should be autoclaved, gas-sterilized, or soaked for sterilization with the same care as in any other operative procedure. The operative team should include as a minimum the surgeon, the assistant, the instrument technician, and the circulating registered nurse. They must scrub, gown, and glove as in any other operative procedure. If local anesthesia is employed, it should be administered in the same room as the operative procedure.

In peroral endoscopy in which upper airway obstruction is actually present or could potentially develop, there should be an awareness that the degree of obstruction may be increased by the procedure. For this reason the operator must be prepared to relieve the obstruction promptly. A bronchoscope of the suitable size for the patient should be lighted. A sterile tracheotomy set as described by Maloney should always be at hand (McDowell and Maloney).

The patient's head and body should be draped. The head drape consists of a double layer of muslin 36 inches by 36 inches, one open prep towel, and one cuffed prep towel. The three elements of the drape are placed under the occiput, and the cuffed towel is wrapped about the head like a bandana and fastened with a towel clip. The body is draped with larger drapes in the usual manner.

It is convenient for a right-handed operator to sit with the stool slightly to the left of the long axis of the patient. The assistant should be at the operator's right. The fiber illumination source should be to the left of the patient's chest. The instrument table should be placed behind the operator so

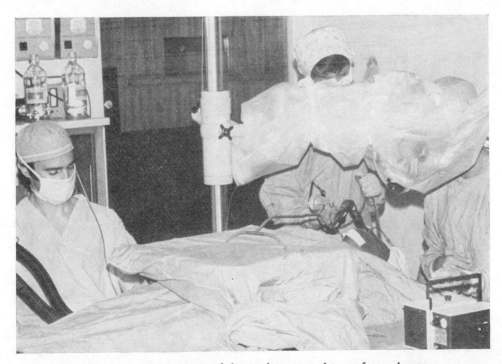

Fig. 58–14.   Arrangement of the equipment and team for endoscopy.

that the operator may have access to it and see the instruments and the specimens. The microscope should be positioned to the right-hand side. If general anesthesia is employed, the anesthesiologist can be at the patient's right-hand side, as illustrated in Figure 58–14.

The operator is seated on a backless stool. The height of the stool and the height of the table are adjusted so that the operator may lean forward to the endoscope from the hips with the back straight. The operator should not be required to take the right eye off of the operative field. Instruments including forceps, aspirating tube, spatula, scissors, dilators, applicators, knives, and syringes should be passed by the assistant, so that the tip of the instrument is placed into the endoscope and the handle is free for the operator to grasp. Most endoscopic instruments can be held like a pencil in the right hand of the assistant during the passing of the instrument to the operator, as illustrated in Figure 58–15. The tip can be accurately placed in the proximal end of the endoscope in this manner. As the instrument is brought out by the operator, the instrument is taken from him by the right hand of

the assistant, again as if the assistant were holding a pencil. Aspiration tubes, forceps, applicators, and so forth may all be passed in the same fashion. The instrument technician should keep the instrument table well organized.

The operating room should remain well lighted. The safety of the procedure is increased if the patient's color and general well-being can be monitored continuously. Not enough is gained in ability to see from working in a darkened room to make it worth the increased risk.

The patient should lie flat on the operating table. The top of the patient's shoulders should be at the point where the main portion of the table and the headrest break to allow maximum mobility of the head and neck. For direct laryngoscopy, the neck should be flexed upon the chest, and the head should be extended on the neck so that the chin points toward the ceiling. This position brings the larynx and cervical esophagus and trachea in a straight line with the thoracic esophagus and trachea. This Boyce position can be achieved with local or general anesthesia by positioning the head and the headrest of the operating table. It is the

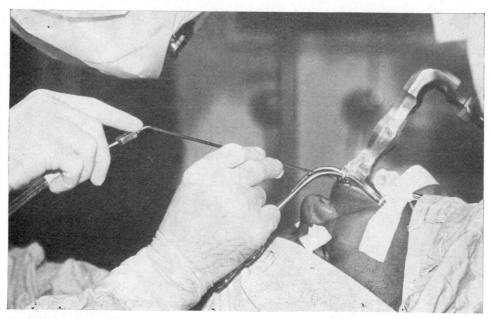

FIG. 58–15. Passage of endoscopic instruments to the operator. Note that assistant holds the instrument like a pencil and places the tip of the instrument in the endoscope so the operator may take the instrument by the handle.

correct position for atraumatic introduction of the laryngoscope, bronchoscope, and esophagoscope. In bronchoscopy with an open bronchoscope, the head must be lowered when the bronchoscope is in the trachea. Lowering the head is accomplished by adjusting the headrest of the table through the 36 × 36 inch muslin drape without contamination. As the right bronchus is entered, the head should be shifted toward the left. As the left bronchus is entered, the head should be shifted toward the right.

In esophagoscopy with an open esophagoscope, the head must be lowered as soon as the esophagoscope has reached the thoracic portion of the esophagus. As the esophagoscope is advanced toward the lower portion of the esophagus, the head should be shifted to the right to allow for the leftward course of the distal portion of the esophagus, and the head must be lowered below the level of the thorax to allow for the anterior course of the distal portion of the esophagus. Failure to adjust to the anatomic course of the esophagus makes advancement of the open esophagoscope difficult and increases the possibility of perforation.

REFERENCES

Adriani, J., and Campbell, D.: The Absorption of Topically Applied Tetracaine and Cocaine. Laryngoscope, 68:65, 1958.

Britton, R. M., and Nelson, K. G.: Improper Oxygenation during Bronchofiberscopy. Anaesthesiology, 40:87, 1974.

Carden, E.: Recent Improvements in Anesthetic Techniques for Use During Bronchoscopy. Ann. Otol. Rhinol. Laryngol., 83:777, 1974.

Conte, B. A., and Laforet, E. G.: Role of Topical Anesthetic Agent in Modifying Bacteriological Data Obtained by Bronchoscopy. New Engl. J. Med., 267:957, 1962.

Ferguson, C. F., and Flake, C. G.: Bronchography in the Diagnosis of Pediatric Problems. J.A.M.A., 164:518, 1957.

Goodman, L. S., and Gilman, A.: The Pharmacological Basis of Therapeutics. 3rd ed. New York, Macmillan Co., 1965.

Hirschowitz, B. I., et al.: Demonstration of a New Gastroscope, the Fibergastroscope. Gastroenterology, 35:50, 1958.

Holinger, P. H.: Photography of the Larynx, Trachea, Bronchi and Esophagus. Trans. Am. Acad. Ophthal. Otolaryng., 46:153, 1942.

Huizinga, E.: On Esophagoscopy and Sword-swallowing. Ann. Otol. Rhinol. Laryngol., 78:32, 1969.

Ikeda, S.: Flexible Bronchofiberscope. Ann. Otol. Rhinol. Larnygol., 79:916, 1970.

Jackson, C., and Jackson, C. L.: Bronchoesophagology. 2nd ed. Philadelphia, W. B. Saunders Co., 1959.

Jako, G. J.: Laryngoscope for Microscopic Observation, Surgery and Photography. Arch. Otolaryng., 91:196, 1970.

Kleinsasser, O.: Microlaryngoscopy and Endolaryngeal Microsurgery. Philadelphia, W. B. Saunders Co., 1968.

McDowell, D. E., and Maloney, W. H.: Acute Obstruction of the Upper Respiratory Tract. Arch. Otolaryng., 61:29, 1955.

Major, R. H.: A History of Medicine. Springfield, Ill., Charles C Thomas, Publisher, 1954.

Marsh, B. R., et al.: Flexible Fiberoptic Bronchoscopy: Its Place in the Search for Lung Cancer. Trans. Am. Broncho-Esophagol. Assoc., 1973, pp. 101–110.

Morales, G. A., et al.: Ventilation During General Anesthesia for Bronchoscopy; Evaluation of a New Technique. J. Thorac. Cardiovasc. Surg., 57:873, 1969.

Ono, J., and Saito, S.: Endoscopic Microsurgery of the Larynx. Ann. Otol. Rhinol. Laryngol., 80:479, 1971.

Rayl, J. E., and Rourke, D.: Application of Color Television in Bronchoesophagology. Trans. Am. Broncho-Esophagol. Assoc., 1974 (in press).

Sanders, R. D.: Two Ventilating Attachments for Bronchoscopes. Delaware Med. J., 39:170, 1967.

Smith, C. O'M. S., et al.: General Anesthesia for Bronchoscopy: The Use of the Sanders Bronchoscopic Attachment. Am. Thorac. Surg., 8:348, 1969.

Snow, J. B.: Clinical Evaluation of Noisy Respiration in Infancy. J. Lancet, 1966, pp. 504–509.

Strong, M. S.: Microscopic Laryngoscopy, A Review and Appraisal. Laryngoscope, 80:1540, 1970.

Strong, M. S., and Jako, H. J.: Laser Surgery in the Larynx. Ann. Otol. Rhinol. Laryngol., 81:791, 1972.

Strong, M. S., et al.: Bronchoscopic Carbon Dioxide Laser Surgery. Ann. Otol. Rhinol. Laryngol., 83:769, 1974.

Ward, P. H., et al.: Advances in Endoscopic Examination of the Respiratory System. Ann. Otol. Rhinol. Laryngol., 83:754, 1974.

Chapter 59
Direct Laryngoscopy

Direct laryngoscopy is the specular examination of the larynx. It employs direct visualization of the larynx, as opposed to the view obtained with a mirror at indirect laryngoscopy. The distinction becomes somewhat less precise with the ability to view the larynx with flexible laryngoscopes and bronchoscopes and laryngeal telescopes.

The image of the larynx is reflected from the laryngeal surfaces to the eye of the observer. The light source is usually located distally in laryngoscopes in current use, and the angle between the source of light impinging on the laryngeal surfaces and the beam of the reflected light is quite large. Under these circumstances, less light is reflected directly to the observer's eye, and the structures of the larynx take on a somewhat more natural color than they do in indirect laryngoscopy. In indirect laryngoscopy the light is reflected through the long axis of the hypopharynx, and the angle of incidence of light on the vocal cords is at right angles to the plane of their superior surfaces. Therefore, a greater amount of light is reflected from the true vocal cords toward the light source or the mirror in the pharynx, and a lesser amount is reflected to the mirror from other parts of the larynx where the light strikes the surface more tangentially. For these reasons the vocal cords look white on indirect laryngoscopy but have a more natural pink color at direct laryngoscopy. Certain photographic techniques in indirect laryngoscopy also project light down the long axis of the laryngoscope, and a maximum amount of light is reflected from the superior surfaces of the vocal cords, which are at right angles to the incidence of light. Therefore, some direct laryngoscopic photographs also portray the vocal cords as unnaturally white.

Indirect laryngoscopy can be applied to most children, just as it can to most adults. There are some individuals in whom the larynx can be seen with a mirror but not with an open tube, and there are others in whom direct laryngoscopy can be carried out but indirect laryngoscopy is not possible. In the presence of trismus, temporomandibular joint arthritis, pharyngeal stenosis, and cervical spinal ankylosis and trauma, the larynx may be visualized only with a flexible laryngoscope passed through the nose.

Indirect laryngoscopy and direct laryngoscopy provide quite a different view of the larynx. The view of the larynx with a mirror is somewhat more natural as far as endolaryngeal motion is concerned. Direct laryngoscopy is more meaningfully interpreted in the knowledge of the indirect laryngoscopic findings. Indirect laryngoscopy should be utilized to the fullest extent in every patient prior to the direct examination. Direct laryngoscopy is supplementary to indirect laryngoscopy and does not substitute for it.

Freehand sketches of the larynx are often helpful in communicating the findings at indirect and direct laryngoscopy. With indirect laryngoscopy a mirror image is seen, so that anterior parts appear to be posterior and vice versa, and right-sided parts appear on the left-hand side of the examiner and vice versa. At direct laryngoscopy the image is not reversed, and the true relationships to the rest of the patient's body are apparent. With indirect laryngoscopy, the image of the right vocal cord is on the examiner's left-hand side, while in direct laryngoscopy the right vocal cord is on the operator's right-hand side. Confusion is prevented by labeling the vocal cords right and left in drawings of images from both types of laryngoscopy. The telescope with the Hopkins rod lens system gives a direct rather than mirror image of the larynx.

RADIOLOGIC EVALUATION

Very important information can be obtained from the pre-endoscopic radiographic evaluation of the patient. The anterior-posterior and lateral radiographic view of the neck are particularly helpful. A great deal of important detail can be demonstrated on the lateral neck x-ray because of the contrast between the radiodensity of air and the soft tissue and skeleton of the larynx. The valleculae and lingual surface of the epiglottis are usually readily seen. The laryngeal surface of the epiglottis is crisply displayed and normally has a characteristic smooth, S-shaped contour (Fig. 59–1). The prominence of the soft tissue of the arytenoids can be defined, and the soft tissue densities of the false and true vocal cords stand out in relief from the radiolucency of the ventricles.

Laminagrams in the anterior-posterior plane provide a great deal of information about the endolaryngeal contour (Fig. 59–2). Submucosal masses that may be difficult to appreciate by indirect or direct laryngoscopy can be demonstrated. Changes in the bulk of the true and false vocal cords are particularly well displayed. The ventricles can be seen, and impingement on or obliteration of a ventricle is demonstrated in comparison to the opposite side. Laminagrams may be taken during quiet respiration and phonation on expiration, as well as phonation on inspiration, in which case the ventricles are seen particularly well. On phonation, the arytenoids glide medially and open the piriform sinuses. Likewise, the Valsalva maneuver dilates the ventricles and piriform sinuses and may demonstrate a

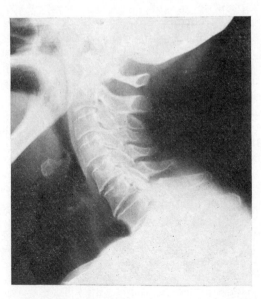

FIG. 59–1. Lateral neck x-ray that demonstrates an air-fluid level in a Zenker's diverticulum.

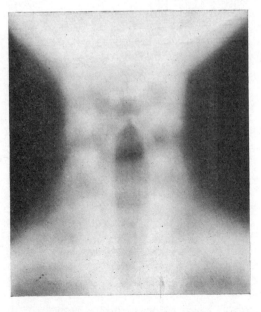

FIG. 59–2. Normal laminagram of the larynx during phonation. Note ventricles, true vocal cords, and subglottic configuration.

laryngocele. The ability to compare the two sides of the larynx at the same anterior-posterior level on the same film is especially useful. Laminagrams are very helpful in demonstrating subglottic extension of tumors that may be difficult to demonstrate by indirect or direct laryngoscopy. The normal, symmetrical, concave subglottic contour during phonation becomes asymmetrical with subglottic extension of tumor. The upper trachea is also available for evaluation on a laminagram. Laminagrams should be performed prior to direct laryngoscopy. After direct laryngoscopy it is difficult to differentiate between edema produced by the trauma of the instrumentation and biopsy from that which might have existed prior to the surgery. In addition to changes in the soft tissue contour that can be seen on laminagrams, destruction of the laryngeal cartilages, particularly the thyroid cartilages, may be seen in advanced malignant tumors of the larynx. Neurologic lesions of the larynx can also be demonstrated by virtue of the lack of symmetry and the reduced

range of motion of the true vocal cords that they produce.

Laryngograms using positive contrast material after topical anesthesia of the larynx also provide a great deal of information on the endolaryngeal contours and mobility (Fig. 59–3). Abnormalities of motion and pliability of the tissues are more readily recognized with the application of surface contrast material, such as an iodized oil, and fluoroscopic monitoring. Neurologic lesions resulting in pooling of secretion in the piriform sinuses and abnormalities of vocal cord motion on phonation and deep inspiration are readily demonstrated. Surface lesions resulting in erosion and ulceration retain small quantities of dye and are demonstrated in that way. Pathologic irregularity of the surface epithelium from any cause may be detected. On the lateral view, the smooth contour of the valleculae and lingual surface of the epiglottis are well shown. Likewise, irregularity of the laryngeal surface of the epiglottis may be sharply defined. On the anterior-posterior view, the true and false vocal cords and the arytenoid prominences are nicely delineated. The vocal cords are seen to have a flat superior surface and a concave inferior surface. The false vocal cords are seen to have a flat inferior surface and a convex superior surface. The definition of the true vocal cords can be enhanced by phonation. The ventricles fill with the contrast material and are readily seen on phonation on expiration and particularly well on phonation on inspiration and the Valsalva maneuver. The piriform sinuses are best seen during phonation when the arytenoids have glided medially to open them fully. The subglottic contour is well outlined in the anterior-posterior view. As with laminagrams, laryngograms should be obtained prior to the endoscopic procedure.

Xeroradiography has had very useful application to the larynx because of its ability to differentiate between small differences in the radiodensity of structures and to enhance the sharpness of edges. Xeroradiography is a process that utilizes electrically charged selenium-coated aluminum plates which develop positive and negative charges in a pattern that varies according to the radiodensity of the tissue through which

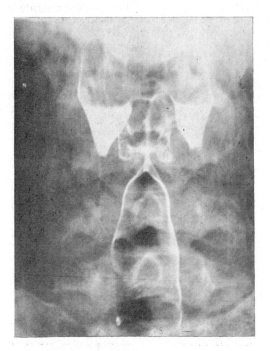

Fig. 59–3. Normal laryngogram of the larynx during phonation. Note piriform sinuses, ventricles, true vocal cords, and subglottic configuration.

the x-rays pass. The plates are dusted with a cloud of negatively charged, fine blue plastic powder, and the image is formed (Holinger and coworkers). The image produces a vertical electrical field with enhanced borders which can be transferred to paper electrostatically. The delicate pattern brings out details that are more difficult to delineate with standard radiographic techniques. In laryngeal xeroradiography, voltages of between 120 and 125 kv are utilized. The lateral view of the larynx is particularly informative. Structures of the right and the left side can often be separated from each other in the contour map of the larynx that is produced.

Contrast studies of the pharynx and esophagus with barium, iodized oil, or water-miscible contrast material frequently provide information critical to the most informed approach to direct laryngoscopy. Lesions of the larynx may secondarily invade the esophagus, and lesions of the esophagus may invade the larynx. In certain circumstances the upper gastrointestinal study with contrast material and cinefluoroscopy of the swallowing function provide valuable positive or negative information. Certainly they are an essential part of the evaluation of patients with paralyses of the vocal cords, masses in the neck, and large laryngeal or hypopharyngeal tumors with or without complaints of odynophagia and dysphagia.

ENDOSCOPIC ANATOMY OF THE LARYNX

As the base of the tongue is elevated by the laryngoscope, the free superior edge of the epiglottis comes into view. With more elevation of the base of the tongue, the glossoepiglottic fold can be seen between the base of the tongue and the lingual surface of the epiglottis. The glossoepiglottic fold separates the two valleculae. The valleculae are lined with mucous membrane which has loose areolar tissue in the lamina propria and can be lifted from surrounding tissue with some ease. The base of the tongue is mainly composed of lymphoid tissue, and there are fairly prominent crypts in the lingual tonsils. The base of the tongue and

valleculae are richly supplied with seromucinous glands. Superficial veins are often prominent in the base of the tongue and valleculae. The surface epithelium varies from nonkeratinizing stratified squamous epithelium to pseudostratified ciliated columnar epithelium. The lingual surface of the epiglottis, the superior part of the laryngeal surface of the epiglottis, the true vocal cords, and the piriform sinuses are lined by stratified squamous epithelium, while the rest of the endolarynx is lined with respiratory epithelium. It is not possible to distinguish nonkeratinizing stratified squamous epithelium from respiratory epithelium with the naked eye or with magnification from light reflected from the epithelial surface.

The free edge of the epiglottis is convex, and its epithelium is closely applied to the cartilage and is part of a true mucoperichondrium. The yellow color of the fibroelastic cartilage of the epiglottis shows through at its free margin. The mucous membrane is loosely applied to the cartilage on the lingual surface of the epiglottis. The lingual surface is soft, and the epithelium moves independent of the cartilage. The mucous membrane is closely applied to the laryngeal surface. The cartilage contains many small dehiscences, and the mucoperichondrium on the laryngeal surface tends to dip into these defects in the cartilage. The surface therefore has a somewhat stippled appearance. The tuberculum is a prominent structure in the midline of the epiglottis on the laryngeal surface. It is produced by the configuration of the cartilage just superior to the petiole and begins 1 cm superior to the true vocal cords. When it is very large, the tuberculum may obscure the anterior commissure on indirect laryngoscopy.

The aryepiglottic folds extend from the lateral margins of the epiglottis to the arytenoids. A thin ribbon of muscle, the aryepiglottic muscle, is contained in each fold, and together they tilt the epiglottis posteriorly on contraction. These muscles are not ordinarily visible at direct laryngoscopy. One may at times see the cuneiform cartilages of Wrisberg in the posterior aspect of the aryepiglottic folds just deep to the mucous membrane. They may be made visible with slight pressure on the mucous membrane.

The aryepiglottic folds indicate the line of demarcation of the vestibule of the larynx or the endolarynx from the piriform sinuses. As the name indicates, the piriform sinuses are pear-shaped. The apex of the pear is directed inferiorly. The piriform sinuses lead toward the opening of the esophagus like a funnel. Each piriform sinus lies between the lamina of the thyroid cartilage and the arytenoid cartilage. On deep inspiration the piriform sinuses tend to be obliterated. On phonation the arytenoids are rotated medially and glide medially and open the piriform sinuses. The internal branch of the superior laryngeal nerve which mediates sensation to the interior of the larynx lies deep to the mucous membrane of the anterior wall of the piriform sinus and can be anesthetized with a conduction block through the intact mucous membrane by topical application of a local anesthetic.

The false vocal cords have a convex superior surface and a flat inferior surface. The false vocal cords contain numerous seromucous glands in the lamina propria and have a somewhat knobby or cobblestone appearance as compared to the true vocal cords. The false vocal cord may be easily compressed with the tip of the laryngoscope to enable visualization of the entire superior surface of the true vocal cord, which extends almost to the lamina of the thyroid cartilage. The lateral retraction of the false vocal cord gives an excellent view of the length and width of the ventricle.

The superior surface of the true vocal cord is flat, and the undersurface is concave. The anterior two thirds of the true vocal cord is membranous, and the posterior one third is composed largely of the vocal process of the arytenoid. The mucous membrane is closely applied to the vocal process medially, and the yellow color of the cartilage may be seen with pressure on its medial surface. The vocal cords are attached to the thyroid cartilage at the anterior commissure. The lamina propria of the free edge and the superior and inferior surfaces of the true vocal cord have a unique histologic arrangement. There is a potential space between the internal elastic lamina which is applied to the vocalis muscle (thyroarytenoid muscle) and the external elastic lamina. This space, known as *Reinke's space*, is limited on the superior surface of the true vocal cord by the superior linea arcuata and on the inferior surface of the vocal cord by the inferior linea arcuata. Reinke's space extends from the vocal process of the arytenoid to the anterior limit of the true vocal cord. In the presence of a lesion of the free edge of the true vocal cord, this space fills with fluid and tends to protect the underlying vocalis muscle from injury when superficial lesions of the mucous membrane are excised.

On phonation the vocal cords approximate firmly. On deep inspiration the arytenoids glide laterally and rotate laterally so that the vocal processes of the arytenoids are directed laterally and create a somewhat diamond-shaped glottis.

The internal diameter of the upper airway is smallest at the cricoid cartilage. The size of endotracheal tubes and bronchoscopes that can be inserted atraumatically is limited by the internal diameter of the cricoid cartilage. The internal diameter of the subglottic area increases as the lumen encompassed by the cricoid cartilage is passed.

INDICATIONS FOR DIRECT LARYNGOSCOPY

Direct laryngoscopy is indicated to elucidate clinical problems associated with the voice and the larynx. Patients who present with hoarseness that has persisted for 2 to 3 weeks in whom the larynx cannot be seen by indirect laryngoscopy or in whom an adequate explanation for the hoarseness cannot be identified by indirect laryngoscopy should have direct laryngoscopy to rule out a lesion that might be apparent on direct laryngoscopy but not on indirect laryngoscopy, such as a subglottic neoplasm. As a general rule, all new growths and discrete lesions of the larynx should be biopsied to exclude carcinoma. Direct laryngoscopy is generally considered the only safe and appropriate method for biopsy of the larynx. If a malignant tumor is suspected, the objective of direct laryngoscopy is not only to obtain tissue for diagnosis but also to determine the gross extent of the tumor so that the patient's therapy can be planned.

Restoration of the voice by the removal of polyps of the vocal cords and vocal nodules and the biopsy of contact ulcers are carried out at direct laryngoscopy, usually under general anesthesia and microscopic control. Likewise, papillomas and other benign tumors of the larynx are removed at direct laryngoscopy.

Direct laryngoscopy is indicated in cases of suspected or proven foreign bodies of the larynx to find and remove the foreign body. Many foreign bodies of the larynx can only be removed after a tracheotomy has been performed. A tracheotomy may be necessary to establish and maintain an adequate airway and to induce general anesthesia for the laryngoscopic removal of the foreign body.

Patients with trauma to the neck may require direct laryngoscopy as well as tracheoscopy and esophagoscopy to determine the extent and severity of the trauma. If blunt trauma to the neck is associated with hemoptysis or subcutaneous emphysema, laryngoscopy and tracheoscopy are indicated, even if the appearance of the larynx at indirect laryngoscopy is not significantly abnormal, to exclude the possibility of a trachea fracture or separation. In patients in whom the endolarynx has been distorted by trauma, a tracheotomy is usually performed. Following tracheotomy, direct laryngoscopy can be performed under general anesthesia to assess the damage and to plan the reconstruction of the larynx. Such reconstructions may require performance of a laryngofissure for repair of the mucous membrane of the endolarynx, reduction of cartilaginous fractures, and insertion of an internal mold of the larynx. In less severe trauma in which there may be fractures of the cartilages with little mucous membrane laceration and displacement, an internal mold may be inserted at direct laryngoscopy.

Patients with vocal cord paralysis of undetermined etiology should be evaluated with direct laryngoscopy in addition to radiography of the skull, chest, esophagus, and larynx and a thyroid scan. The laryngoscopy should be combined with bronchoscopy, esophagoscopy, and examination of the nasopharynx. It is important to differentiate between vocal cord paralysis and cricoarytenoid arthritis by testing the passive mobility of the arytenoid. In acute vocal cord paralysis, there is no limitation of passive manipulation of the arytenoid with a laryngeal spatula. In cricoarytenoid arthritis, the limitation of motion is severe. It must be borne in mind that some degree of limitation of cricoarytenoid joint fixation occurs with long-standing vocal cord paralysis.

Direct laryngoscopy is indicated in patients who present with a mass of undetermined etiology in the neck. After a careful history is taken and physical examination made, with scrutiny of the salivary glands, nasopharynx, pharynx, hypopharynx, and larynx, radiography of the paranasal sinuses, neck, chest, and esophagus, and thyroid scan, direct laryngoscopy should be carried out in conjunction with bronchoscopy, esophagoscopy, and nasopharyngoscopy, with random biopsies of the nasopharynx. Occult lesions of the laryngeal surface of the epiglottis, the piriform sinuses, and the postcricoid and subglottic areas might be overlooked if the evaluation of the larynx depended only on indirect laryngoscopy.

The evaluation of noisy breathing in infants requires endoscopic evaluation, including laryngoscopy. Airway obstruction at any point between the anterior nares and the smallest bronchioles may produce respiratory noise or stridor. Prior to the endoscopic evaluation, it is important to try to determine the anatomic site of the lesion. The phase of respiration in which the noise occurs depends primarily on the location of the obstruction (Snow). In the lower respiratory tract where dilatation of the airway occurs during inspiration and contraction of the airway occurs during expiration, partial obstruction will tend to produce noise more prominently during expiration. The upper portions of the respiratory tract do not vary in size with the phases for respiration. The diameter of the upper airway is fixed by virtue of its cartilaginous skeleton. With partial obstruction in the upper airway, inspiration with its negative intraluminal pressure tends to pull soft tissue toward the center of the lumen and increase the degree of obstruction. The noise is more prominent on inspiration. Expiration with its positive intraluminal pressure tends to push aside obstructing soft tissue. Tracheal obstruction produces noise on inspiration and expiration and results in a to-and-fro stridor.

Likewise, the relative lengths of the phases of respiration depend primarily on the location of the obstruction for the same reasons. The relative length of inspiration tends to be greater in upper respiratory obstruction, and the relative length of expiration tends to be greater in lower respiratory obstruction.

Among the well-recognized causes of upper respiratory obstruction encountered in the immediate neonatal period are bilateral choanal atresia; the Pierre Robin syndrome of cleft palate, hypoplasia of the mandible, and a relatively large tongue; bilateral vocal cord paralysis and subluxation of the arytenoids secondary to traumatic delivery; laryngomalacia or the exaggerated infantile larynx; stenosis and atresia of the larynx or web of the larynx; cyst of the larynx; subglottic hemangioma; intrinsic tracheal lesions, such as tracheomalacia, absence of tracheal rings, and tracheal stenosis; and extrinsic tracheal compression, including tumors of the thyroid, thymus, esophagus, and mediastinum and vascular rings. Tetany of the newborn with laryngospasm is usually recognized by other characteristics of this condition. Newborns with tracheoesophageal fistulas certainly have noisy respiration due to aspiration but usually no true airway obstruction.

In addition to the phase of respiration in which the noise occurs and the relative length of inspiration and expiration, differential points in determining the site of the lesion include the presence or absence of hyperextension of the neck, the quality of the voice or cry, the presence or absence of difficulty in feeding, the amount of intercurrent pulmonary infection, and auscultation of the point of maximum intensity. Hyperextension of the neck is more likely to be present in supraglottic obstruction and extrinsic tracheal obstruction. This sign is usually present in retropharyngeal abscesses

and in vascular rings and tumors compressing the trachea. Hyperextension of the neck is unlikely in intrinsic laryngeal obstruction. The quality of the voice tends to be normal unless the true vocal cords are deformed. For example, bilateral vocal cord paralysis is associated with a normal cry, while laryngeal webs usually produce profound hoarseness.

Difficulty in feeding occurs with extrinsic lesions of the esophagus and trachea, such as mediastinal tumors, and with vascular rings, such as the double aortic arch and the right aortic arch with the left ligamentum arteriosum. Other vascular malformations, such as the anomalous innominate artery and the anomalous left common carotid artery, produce tracheal obstruction without esophageal compression (Fearon and Shortreed). An aberrant right subclavian artery may produce esophageal compression without tracheal compression. Stridor due to neurologic abnormalities resulting from infantile myasthenia gravis, brain stem gliomas, and encephalitis is likely to be associated with difficulty in feeding. A tracheoesophageal fistula will also result in extreme feeding difficulties. On the other hand, laryngeal obstruction and extrinsic tracheobronchial obstruction are rarely associated with feeding problems. However, any infant who is severely dyspneic is likely to aspirate fluids. The presence of intercurrent pneumonitis tends to occur more frequently with tracheal and bronchial obstruction and is rare, for example, with laryngomalacia.

Auscultation of the chest and neck for the point of maximum intensity of the stridor is likely to give valuable information as to the site of the obstruction. In addition, there may be signs of obstructive emphysema or atelectasis distal to the point of obstruction.

Helpful radiographic studies in the elucidation of stridor in infancy and childhood include the lateral neck and posterior-anterior and lateral chest x-rays. A lateral neck x-ray may demonstrate an unsuspected retropharyngeal mass or a hypopharyngeal or esophageal foreign body. The lateral chest film gives a good view of the tracheal air column, which may be compressed anteriorly with the vascular rings. Mediastinal masses may be apparent on these films. Evidence of obstructive emphysema or atelectasis may be present on the posterior-anterior film. A water-miscible radiopaque esophagogram may demonstrate a tracheoesophageal fistula, an esophageal foreign body, or compression of the esophagus by mediastinal cysts and tumors and vascular rings. Tracheography and bronchography at the time of laryngoscopy, tracheoscopy, and bronchoscopy yield valuable information in extrinsic as well as intrinsic obstruction of the tracheobronchial tree (Ferguson and Flake).

The circumstances under which the stridor is first encountered, together with information on the location of the lesion, prepares the endoscopist for dealing effectively with the problem. In the delivery room, choanal atresia and the Pierre Robin syndrome will produce immediate respiratory difficulty. If either of these problems exists in a newborn who is making respiratory effort but inadequately ventilating the lungs, an oral airway relieves the obstruction. Exposure of the vocal cords with a laryngoscope will relieve the obstruction of laryngomalacia with its prolapse of the flexible epiglottis and arytenoids into the glottis on inspiration. Although subglottic hemangiomas may produce upper airway obstruction at birth, they are likely to be asymptomatic until the infant has had his first upper respiratory infection. Subglottic hemangiomas may be recognized endoscopically as purplish masses below the true vocal cords. They should not be biopsied because of the likelihood of uncontrolled bleeding in the trachea. Corticosteroid therapy results in reduction in the size of the lesion and is the treatment of choice (Cohen and Wang).

Laryngomalacia is the most common cause of stridor in the newborn and improves with time. If a newborn infant has stridor but has adequate ventilatory exchange to maintain life, endosocopic evaluation should be postponed. If there is gradual improvement, the investigation may be limited to radiographic studies. Should the degree of airway obstruction become worse or fail to improve within 2 to 3 months, the endoscopic evaluation should be carried out. Tracheomalacia is recognized endoscopi-

cally by the improvement in exchange that occurs once the weak area is passed with the bronchoscope. Tracheomalacia also improves with time. Tracheal stenosis is recognized by the inability to pass the bronchoscope beyond it. Absence of tracheal rings appears as stenosis, but the bronchoscope passes it easily. Tracheoscopy may demonstrate a pulsatile compression of the anterior and lateral walls of the trachea due to the vascular malformations. Tracheography also demonstrates the tracheal compression. Angiography definitely delineates the type of vascular malformation present (Seda and Snow).

Finally, direct laryngoscopy should be carried out in each bronchoscopy to avoid overlooking an upper airway problem that may be related to or exist in addition to the lower respiratory symptoms or signs. Likewise, direct laryngoscopy is utilized whenever possible to establish an airway by endotracheal intubation or insertion of a bronchoscope prior to a tracheotomy for upper airway obstruction, so that the tracheotomy can be converted from an emergency procedure to one which can be carried out in a calm and orderly fashion.

TECHNIQUES

Two techniques of direct laryngoscopy are in general use. In one, a laryngoscope of the standard Jackson or anterior commissure type is held in the left hand of the right-handed operator. This technique is appropriate for diagnostic procedures in which relatively more movement of the laryngoscope is needed. It is also employed for various therapeutic purposes. In the other technique, the laryngoscope is held by a self-retaining device, and microscopic control and general anesthesia are utilized. This technique is more appropriate for therapeutic purposes but is also important diagnostically. In the latter method, precision of observation or manipulation is relatively more important than mobility of the scope and field of vision. In the latter method, bimanual manipulation can be carried out, and the method is more appropriate to long and extensive manipulation (Fig. 59–4).

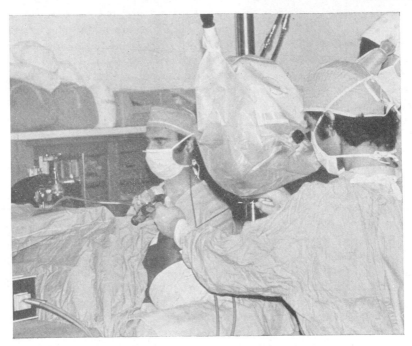

FIG. 59–4.   Direct laryngoscopy under microscopic control.

Often the two methods are combined so that the initial survey of the hypopharynx and larynx is carried out with a hand-held laryngoscope, and then a self-retaining device and microscopic control are used for the evaluation of the mucous membrane or the endolaryngeal surgery.

The patient should be placed in the Boyce position. The standard Jackson laryngoscope is held in the left hand by grasping the vertical portion of the handle with four fingers and resting the thumb at the angle between the vertical and horizontal portions of the handle. The fiber illumination cord is laid over the left wrist to have it out of the way. The laryngoscope is held in the left hand of a right-handed operator in order to leave the right hand free for delicate manipulations through the laryngoscope. The operative field is viewed with the right eye of the right-handed operator, so that the operator's head is as far to the left as possible to avoid interference with the passage and manipulation of the instruments (Fig. 59–6) during continuous viewing through the laryngoscope. The upper lip is retracted by the index finger of the right

hand. The tip of the laryngoscope is passed along the left side of the base of the tongue, and the base of the tongue, valleculae, and free edge and lingual surface of the epiglottis are inspected. The distal end of the laryngoscope is passed posterior to the epiglottis, and the laryngeal surface of the epiglottis and the endolarynx are inspected. The standard Jackson laryngoscope is advanced to the false vocal cords. In order to expose the endolarynx as fully as possible, it is necessary to lift the laryngoscope. The proximal portion of the laryngoscope may come in contact with the upper teeth, but the teeth must not be used as a fulcrum. The posterior hypopharyngeal wall and each piriform sinus are inspected. Under local anesthesia the motion of the vocal cords may be observed by having the patient phonate and take deep breaths.

The anterior commissure laryngoscope is inserted, using the same technique, to the level of the glottis to view the true vocal cords, anterior commissure, and ventricles. The motion of the true vocal cords is again evaluated. The false vocal cords are retracted laterally with the beveled tip of the

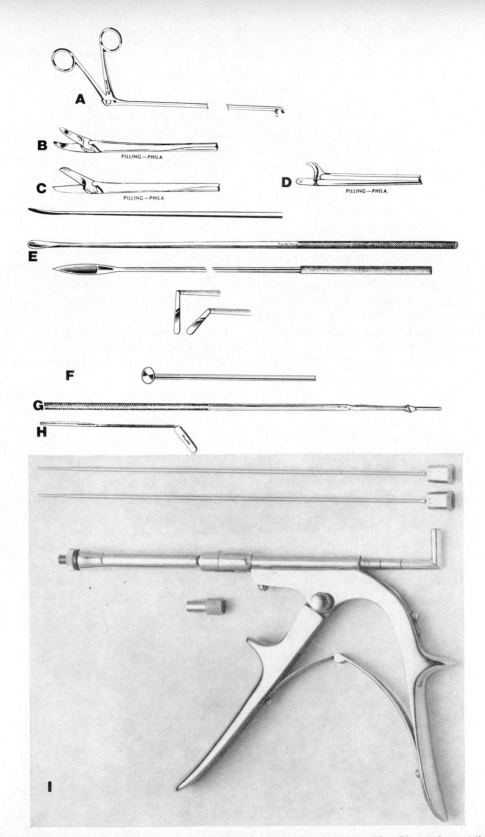

FIG. 59–5. Laryngeal instruments: *A*, cupped biopsy forceps (see Fig. 58–11 for additional forceps configuration); *B*, curved scissors; *C*, straight scissors; *D*, shears; *E*, spatula; *F*, knife, dissectors, and saw; *G*, knife handle for disposable blades; *H*, dilators; *I*, Arnold-Bruening syringe. (*A* to *H* courtesy of Pilling Co., Philadelphia. *I* courtesy of Storz Surgical Instruments, St. Louis.)

laryngoscope to inspect the ventricles. The handle of the laryngoscope is rotated 90 degrees to the right and insinuated through the true vocal cords in order to inspect the subglottic area. The piriform sinuses can often be more satisfactorily inspected with the anterior commissure laryngoscope than with the standard Jackson laryngoscope.

It is important to develop the routine of a thorough inspection of every square centimeter of the hypopharynx and larynx to avoid overlooking a lesion.

If observation under magnification, prolonged and extensive manipulation, or surgery for restoration of the voice are required, the Jako laryngoscope is inserted to the level of the glottis, and the Zeiss microscope with the straight head and 400-mm objective lens is brought into position.

Bacterial conjunctivitis and tuberculous keratitis can result from contamination of the endoscopist's eyes during laryngoscopy and bronchoscopy. The operator and all who look through laryngoscopes and bronchoscopes must protect their eyes, by wearing eyeglasses, from sputum that could be coughed into them (Fig. 59–6). Plane lenses may be worn by those not requiring refraction. The eyeglasses should be worn with the face mask for a sufficient period of time prior to the endoscopic procedure so that the lenses will be warmed by the operator's breath and will not become fogged by the condensation of water vapor from the operator's or the patient's breath. Care must be taken not to look over the lenses as some tend to do. The optical properties of eyeglasses are far superior to plastic shields, and eyeglasses do not interfere with the positioning of the operator's head or manipulation of the instruments.

DIRECT LARYNGOSCOPY IN MANAGEMENT OF DISEASES OF THE LARYNX

Laryngitis

There are few instances in which direct laryngoscopy is appropriate for the treatment of acute laryngitis except to establish an airway by introduction of an endotracheal tube or bronchoscope prior to a tracheotomy in severe upper respiratory obstruction due to epiglottiditis or laryngotracheobronchitis. The successful use of endotracheal tubes in epiglottiditis may make the need for tracheotomies for this condition less frequent in the future. Occasionally laryngeal diphtheria is still seen. Smears and cultures of the larynx may be taken at direct laryngoscopy, but direct laryngoscopy for this

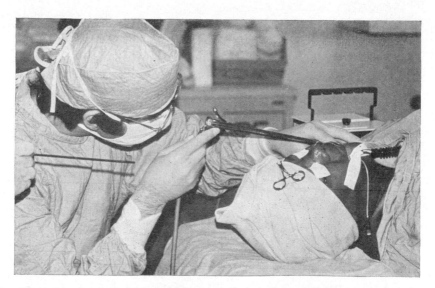

FIG. 59–6.   Note that the operator is wearing eyeglasses to protect his eyes from contamination with sputum if the patient should cough.

purpose is usually not indicated in the acute infectious forms of laryngitis.

Patients with chronic inflammatory diseases of the larynx do require direct laryngoscopy for biopsy and culture. Hyperplastic and ulcerative lesions of the larynx must be biopsied to exclude carcinoma and to determine the etiology of the granulomatous process. Laryngeal tuberculosis, syphilis, histoplasmosis, blastomycosis, and sarcoidosis may be diagnosed with biopsy. The diagnosis of Wegener's granulomatosis may be suggested by a biopsy that shows vasculitis. The fungal infections and tuberculosis may be identified by culture of the tissue removed or from swabs of the ulcerated areas. Characteristically, tuberculosis involves the posterior half of the larynx, while carcinoma tends to occur in the anterior half of the glottis. Laryngeal tuberculosis ordinarily does not occur except in the presence of open cavitary pulmonary tuberculosis. Even when the diagnosis of tuberculosis has been established from smear or culture of the sputum, the hyperplastic or ulcerative lesion in the larynx must be biopsied, because carcinoma can only be excluded by biopsy. Occasionally pulmonary tuberculosis and carcinoma of the larynx coexist.

Structural Changes in the Larynx Secondary to Abuse and Misuse of the Voice

Polyps. Polyps of the true vocal cords are most frequently due to using the voice too loudly and too long or in a way that traumatizes the mucous membrane. Polyps may also occur as an allergic manifestation or as a result of the inhalation of irritants, such as cigarette smoke. The surface epithelium is characteristically normal in a vocal cord polyp, and the pathologic change is in the lamina propria, where there is marked edema. If the condition is chronic and produces hoarseness, the polyp may be removed at direct laryngoscopy. If the polyp is thought to be caused by misuse or abuse of the voice or a faulty habit of phonation, voice therapy should precede and follow surgical removal of the polyp to prevent recurrence. Direct laryngoscopy under microscopic control is the method of choice, and the lesion is re-

moved by multiple precise applications of sharp, cupped forceps (Fig. 59–7) so as to produce a smooth free edge and superior and inferior surfaces of the involved vocal cord. Care should be taken not to tear the mucous membrane adjacent to the point of forceps application. When cupped forceps are being applied to edematous mucous membrane, the bite should not be larger than one half of the circumference of the forceps cutting edge. In other words, the tissue should not extend into the cup beyond the equator of the cup, or the cutting efficiency will be reduced and the adjacent mucous membrane will be torn. The unwanted tissue is precisely trimmed away with multiple discrete bites and not torn or stripped away. The removal should not include any fibers of the vocalis muscle. If both vocal cords have polypoid degeneration that reaches to the anterior commissure, the polypoid tissue can be removed from only one vocal cord at a time. The polypoid tissue must be removed from the other vocal cord 6 weeks later to avoid the development of a web at the anterior commissure, as can occur if both vocal cords are denuded of epithelium at the anterior commissure at the same time.

Vocal Nodules. Vocal nodules are caused by misuse and abuse of the voice, in particular by using the voice too loudly and too long and using a fundamental frequency that is unnaturally low. Vocal nodules occur in children as well as adults. In children, they are likely to occur in robust athletic boys, 8 to 12 years of age, who yell a great deal. The voice may be pitched unnaturally low in men for the affectation of authority. It is done by women for the affectation of sexiness, and it is probably done by young boys to identify with older males in the family or community. Vocal nodules are condensations of hyaline connective tissue in the lamina propria at the junction of the anterior one third and the posterior two thirds of the free edge of the true vocal cord. These nodules produce hoarseness and a breathy quality to the voice. In adults, these lesions may be removed at direct laryngoscopy under general anesthesia and microscopic control to restore the voice.

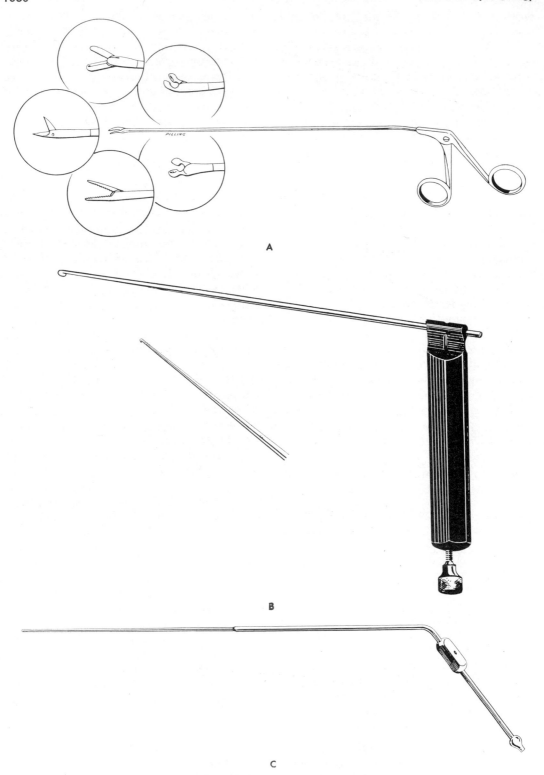

FIG. 59–7. Laryngeal instruments for microsurgery: *A*, forceps and scissors;
B, knife and hook; *C*, aspiration tube.

Both nodules can be removed at the same time. Each nodule is removed precisely with cupped forceps, and trauma to the surrounding normal tissue is avoided. The technique is the same as described for polyps of the vocal cord. The removal should not include any fibers of the vocalis muscle. It is necessary to begin voice therapy prior to the surgery. If the underlying misuse of the voice is not corrected, the nodules will recur. In children, surgical removal is not usually necessary because the vocal nodules will regress on voice therapy, which consists of voice rest, reduction in intensity and duration of voice production, and elevation of the fundamental frequency.

Contact Ulcers. Contact ulcers of the larynx are thought to result from misuse and abuse of the voice, particularly in the form of a sharp glottal attack or unusually rapid attainment of maximum intensity at the onset of phonation. They occur unilaterally or bilaterally over the vocal process of the arytenoid. The presence of these lesions causes mild pain on phonation and swallowing and varying degrees of hoarseness. The ulcers have a shaggy, granular base. They should be carefully biopsied at direct laryngoscopy to exclude the possibility of carcinoma. Voice therapy is important to correct the underlying misuse of the voice. However, prolonged voice rest is required for contact ulcers to heal. A minimum of 6 weeks of absolute voice rest is usually necessary. Individuals who develop contact ulcers must recognize the limitation in the durability of their voice and with experience can judge their vocal activities to remain free of recurrent ulcers. Prolonged ulceration leads to the formation of a nonspecific granuloma. These lesions produce varying degrees of hoarseness. They are responsive to prolonged voice therapy. They tend to recur after surgical removal.

Benign Tumors

Benign tumors of the larynx may be removed at direct laryngoscopy. Large bulky tumors deep to the lamina propria of the mucous membrane may require a thyrotomy for removal. Squamous cell papillomas of the larynx may be removed at direct laryngoscopy under general anesthesia with Jackson papilloma forceps. These blunt, duckbilled forceps are used to avoid damage to the surrounding normal tissue. The friable papillomas come away from the surrounding tissue with little or no force.

A 50-W carbon dioxide laser has also been used by Strong to vaporize juvenile papillomas in the larynx and tracheobronchial tree through a Jako laryngoscope and a ventilating bronchoscope (Strong and Jako; Strong and coworkers, 1974). General anesthesia with a nonflammable anesthetic is delivered through an endotracheal tube or the ventilating side arm of the bronchoscope. The tidal flow of gases keeps the trachea and bronchi free of steam and smoke. It results in very precise removal of the lesion with minimum trauma to surrounding tissue. It is bloodless, and no serious complications have been reported. It has been used to remove vocal cord keratosis, carcinoma in situ, vocal nodules, and polyps of the vocal cords, as well as papillomas. Its greatest advantage over conventional techniques is the bloodless removal of papillomas from the tracheobronchial tree. It does not prevent the recurrence of papillomas.

Malignant Tumors

Any discrete lesion of the larynx must be biopsied to exclude carcinoma. The biopsy may be carried out under local or general anesthesia. If the lesion is large, the biopsy can be accomplished satisfactorily under local anesthesia with the standard Jackson or anterior commissure laryngoscope. If the lesion is small or if there is generalized leukoplakia, general anesthesia and magnification may be required to select the areas to be biopsied. Painting the epithelium under inspection with 2% toluidine blue produces supravital staining of areas of erosion and ulceration and indicates the areas most likely to yield the diagnosis of carcinoma (Strong and coworkers, 1970). Toluidine blue has an affinity for nucleic acids. Atypical and dysplastic mucous membrane and keratosis do not fix the dye, while carcinoma in situ and superficial carcinoma stain deeply.

In biopsying suspected carcinoma of the larynx, firm pieces of tissue should be obtained. If the tissue that has been removed is firm when gently held between the index finger and thumb, it is quite likely that the tissue will yield the diagnosis of carcinoma. On the other hand, normal mucous membrane is soft and semigelatinous.

The information necessary for definitive treatment of the patient with suspected carcinoma of the larynx should be gathered at direct laryngoscopy. The extent of the tumor must be carefully determined by inspection, palpation, and application of toluidine blue. In the presence of a glottic lesion, it should be determined whether the lesion is limited to a freely movable vocal cord; in such a case, the patient can be treated with irradiation therapy. Likewise, in the more advanced lesion it should be determined whether a partial or a total laryngectomy is indicated. Particular attention should be given to the degree of subglottic extension and involvement of the other side of the larynx. In supraglottic lesions, information on possible invasion of the pre-epiglottic space and the margin between the tumor and the true vocal cords should be evaluated to decide if a supraglottic partial laryngectomy is feasible. Likewise, with piriform sinus lesions, the possibility of an extended supraglottic partial laryngectomy should be considered. The decision for or against conservative surgery for carcinoma of the larynx in a particular patient must, of course, take into consideration the general health, age, and pulmonary function of the patient, as well as the radiographic evaluation of the larynx.

Stenosis of the Larynx

The location and extent of the laryngeal and subglottic stenosis may be determined at direct laryngoscopy in conjunction with the indirect laryngoscopic and radiologic findings. The causes of laryngeal stenosis include congenital malformations, trauma, infection, and complications of respiratory therapy. Supraglottic stenosis is frequently of traumatic origin and may respond well to supraglottic partial laryngectomy. Subglottic stenosis is frequently iatrogenic and may be relieved by resection and anastomosis of the trachea to the larynx or trachea to trachea. Glottic stenosis may be severe enough to interfere with both voice production and respiration. In a milder form, it may consist of a web at the anterior commissure and produce hoarseness but no respiratory problem. Arytenoidectomy performed endoscopically or through a thyrotomy is often appropriate management in the more severe forms of glottic stenosis. Dilatation, particularly when combined with local depot corticosteroid injections, has been helpful in some patients, as have long indwelling stents and molds. Excision of webs of the anterior commissure with the insertion of keels is a well-established and effective technique which can be carried out endoscopically.

Foreign Bodies of the Larynx

Foreign bodies that are likely to be retained in the larynx may be either sharp and pointed, sticking into the mucous membrane, or large, irregular, and soft, being caught between the vocal cords in laryngospasm. Foreign bodies of the larynx produce coughing and shortness of breath. There may be pain on swallowing, phonation, or even deep inspiration. There may be hoarseness or aphonia. Usually a laryngeal foreign body may be seen at indirect laryngoscopy, but if it lodges subglottically, as grass and sandburs are likely to do, or if it enters a ventricle, it may be hidden. A lateral neck x-ray may help locate radiopaque foreign bodies. A thin, flat foreign body will come to rest in the antero-posterior or sagittal plane between the vocal cords. In the esophagus, such a foreign body will be in the coronal plane. Foreign bodies of the hypopharynx are likely to come to rest in the valleculae or piriform sinuses.

A frequently fatal foreign body of the larynx is a bolus of meat aspirated by the intoxicated adult. After it is aspirated, the bolus of meat is caught firmly between the vocal cords in laryngospasm. There may be complete or nearly complete occlusion of the airway. Death takes place rapidly unless a prompt tracheotomy is performed. This "cafe coronary" may be distinguished from a myocardial infarction by the respiratory effort without exchange and the marked suprasternal, intercostal, and subxiphoid retraction.

Foreign bodies of the larynx produce sufficient laryngospasm to make their removal difficult. Often, general anesthesia is required. Even with a nonobstructive foreign body, a tracheotomy may be required as the first step in removing the foreign body. After the tracheotomy has been performed, general anesthesia can be induced with the endotracheal tube introduced through the tracheostomy. This method is particularly appropriate in managing subglottic foreign bodies. The standard Jackson laryngoscope is very suitable for foreign body removal. The anterior commissure laryngoscope is more suitable for foreign bodies in the ventricles, subglottic area, and piriform sinuses. Alligator forceps are appropriate for the removal of nearly all laryngeal foreign bodies. The foreign body is exposed, grasped, disengaged, and removed through the laryngoscope or as a trailing foreign body.

REFERENCES

Cohen, S. R., and Wang, C. I.: Steroid Treatment of Hemangioma of the Head and Neck in Children. Ann. Otol. Rhinol. Laryngol., 81:584, 1972.

Fearon, B., and Shortreed, R.: Tracheobronchial Compression by Congenital Cardiovascular Anomalies in Children. Ann. Otol. Rhinol. Laryngol., 72:949, 1963.

Ferguson, D. F., and Flake, C. G.: Tracheographic and Bronchoscopic Studies as Aids in Diagnosis of Congenital Malformations of the Tracheobranchial Tree and Aortic Arch in Infants and Children. Ann. Otol. Rhinol. Laryngol., 63:1056, 1954.

Holinger, P. H., et al.: Xeroradiography of the Larynx. Ann. Otol. Rhinol. Laryngol., 81: 806, 1972.

Seda, H. J., and Snow, J. B.: Diagnostic Considerations in Anomalous Innominate Arteries. Ann. Otol. Rhinol. Laryngol., 78:511, 1969.

Snow, J. B.: Clinical Evaluation of Noisy Respiration in Infancy. J. Lancet, 85:504, 1965.

Strong, M. S., et al.: Bronchoscopic Carbon Dioxide Laser Surgery. Ann. Otol. Rhinol. Laryngol., 83:769, 1974.

Strong, M. S., et al.: Toluidine Blue in Diagnosis of Cancer of the Larynx. Arch. Otolaryng., 91:515, 1970.

Strong, M. S., and Jako, G. J.: Laser Surgery in the Larynx. Ann. Otol. Rhinol. Laryngol., 81:791, 1972.

Chapter 60
Bronchology

New information in bronchology has developed rapidly in recent years because of major advances made in the instrumentation of bronchoscopy. Bronchoscopy is now performed for the evaluation of patients with diseases of the respiratory system more frequently than ever before. The importance of direct visualization of the pathologic changes in the tracheobronchial tree and of the ability to take specimens from the lumen of the respiratory tract for culture and histopathologic study cannot be overemphasized. They are the basis for rational management of patients with diseases of the respiratory system.

The reader is referred to Chapter 58, Introduction to Peroral Endoscopy, for a discussion of recent advances in equipment, preparation of the patient, and anesthesia which apply to bronchoscopy.

ANATOMY OF THE TRACHEOBRONCHIAL TREE

The trachea is a cartilaginous and muscular tube lined with pseudostratified ciliated columnar epithelium that extends from the cricoid cartilage to its bifurcation into the right and left bronchi. Its length averages 12 cm in men and 10 cm in women. The average anterior-posterior diameter is 13 mm, and the average transverse diameter is 18 mm. The respiratory epithelium lining the trachea has numerous goblet cells and a prominent basement membrane. There is no muscularis mucosae but rather a promi-

nent layer of elastic fibers in the lamina propria called the internal elastic membrane. Seromucous glands are generally found posteriorly and in the submucosa, with fat and loose connective tissue between cartilages. The lumen is supported by approximately 18 incomplete rings of hyaline cartilage, which in cross section are rounded internally and flat externally. The open ends of these C-shaped cartilages are directed posteriorly. Some of the rings branch and join adjacent rings. The posterior part of the tracheal wall is composed of the trachealis muscle, which connects the free ends of the C-shaped cartilages. Although some of these smooth muscle fibers run longitudinally, most fibers are directed transversely. A fibroelastic membrane which blends into the perichondrium of the cartilages extends across the open segments and connects adjacent cartilages to each other and the first tracheal cartilage to the perichondrium of the cricoid cartilage. The cartilages are wider than the space between them.

One half of the trachea is in the neck, and one half is in the mediastinum. The trachea is in the midline in the neck but deviates slightly to the right in the mediastinum just above its bifurcation. The trachea is quite elastic, and its length and position vary with the position of the head and neck.

The lowest tracheal ring extends inferiorly and posteriorly between the right and left bronchi and produces a sharp ridge internally, the carina. The right bronchus has six to eight cartilages over its 2.5-cm length,

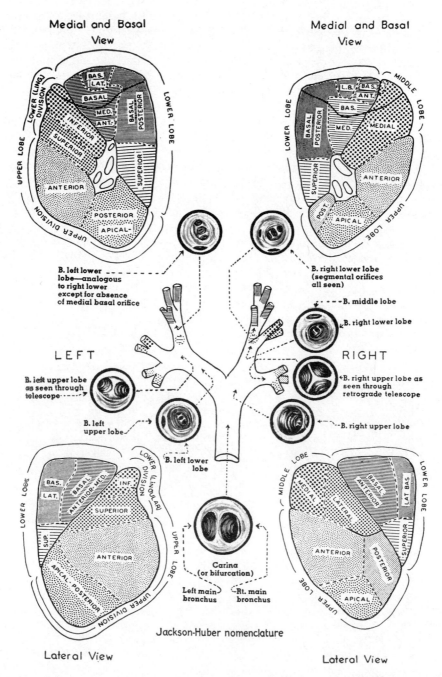

FIG. 60–1.   Schema showing the tracheobronchial tree, the bronchopulmonary segments, and the endoscopic landmarks.

while the left bronchus has 9 to 12 carti- lages and is nearly 5 cm long in the adult. The lumen of the right bronchus is one fourth larger in cross section than the left bronchus, and its long axis deviates 25 de- grees laterally, while the long axis of the left bronchus deviates 45 degrees to the left from the midline. The right and left bronchi are designated primary bronchi. The right and left bronchi are cylindrical and have the same histologic or structural elements as the trachea. As the bronchi divide and become smaller, the walls become thinner, the cartilages become irregular in shape and disappear in bronchi that are 1 mm in diameter, and the muscular components of the bronchi become relatively more promi- nent.

The right lung is divided into three lobes and the left lung into two lobes. The right lung is divided into the upper, middle, and lower lobes and the left into the upper and lower lobes. Each lobe has a secondary or lobar bronchus. Each lobe is covered by visceral pleura which projects into deep fis-

International Congress of Anatomists (Scott- Brown and Ballantyne).

The lung is fundamentally the aggregate of all of the branchings of the bronchus. The right upper lobe has three segments, the apical (B1), posterior (B2), and anterior (B3) segments. The right middle lobe has a lateral (B4) segment and a medial (B5) segment. The right lower lobe has an apical (superior) (B6) segment and four basal segments. The basal segments are the medial basal (B7), anterior basal (B8), lateral basal (B9), and posterior basal (B10). The left upper lobe has two divisions correspond- ing to the right upper and the right middle lobes. The superior division has an apical- posterior (B1-2) segment and an anterior (B3) segment. The inferior division or lingula has a superior (B4) segment and an inferior (B5) segment. The left lower lobe has an apical (superior) (B6) seg- ment and four basal segments. The basal segments are the medial basal (B7), ante- rior basal (B8), lateral basal (B9), and posterior basal (B10).

Right Lung

Lobes	Segments	
Upper	Apical	B1
	Posterior	B2
	Anterior	B3
Middle	Lateral	B4
	Medial	B5
Lower	Apical (superior)	B6
	Medial basal	B7
	Anterior basal	B8
	Lateral basal	B9
	Posterior basal	B10

Left Lung

Lobes	Segments	
Upper — Superior division	Apical-posterior	B1-2
	Anterior	B3
Upper — Inferior division (lingula)	Superior	B4
	Inferior	B5
Lower	Apical (superior)	B6
	Medial basal	B7
	Anterior basal	B8
	Lateral basal	B9
	Posterior basal	B10

sures between lobes to the hilus. Each lobe is subdivided into bronchopulmonary seg- ments. These segments have a tertiary bronchus and a discrete blood supply. The tertiary bronchi and their bronchopulmonary segments have been named by Jackson and Huber and numbered by Boyden as illus- trated in Figure 60–1. There is variation in the nomenclature and numbering, and the one presented here is based on the Nomina Anatomica adopted in 1960 by the Seventh

Variations in the arrangement of the sec- ondary and tertiary (segmental) bronchi do occur. Although the branching from the up- per lobe bronchi to form the segmental bron- chi is more constant than the branching from the lower lobe bronchi, a not too in- frequent anomaly is the origin of the apical segment from the trachea rather than the right upper lobe bronchus (Harris). Often two segmental bronchi of the right upper lobe may arise from a short common stem.

The size of a bronchopulmonary segment may be larger or smaller than expected. In the lower lobe bronchi, the apical (superior) and medial basal segments are almost as constant as the upper lobe segments, while more variation occurs with the anterior basal, lateral basal, and posterior basal segments. In nearly 50% of the specimens, a branch arises from the posterior aspect of the lower lobe bronchus between the apical (superior) segmental and basal segmental bronchi or inferior to the anterior basal segmental bronchus. Agenesis of a lung or lobe or segment occurs, as do congenital tracheo-esophageal fistulas with or without esophageal atresia. A rare anomaly is the incomplete separation of trachea and esophagus or the esophagotrachea as described by Atkins.

The divisions of the tracheobronchial tree are fundamentally dichotomous. The trachea divides into 23 bronchial dichotomies. Dichotomies 1 through 16 are conductive bronchioles, and 17 through 22 are transi-

would be designated B1a1 and B1a2. The next order receives the lower case letter designation, and the one after that receives the arabic numeral designation with alternation to the periphery. Somewhat arbitrarily, the more superior divisions are given the a and 1 designations, and the inferior divisions are given the b and 2 designations. If the divisions do not seem to be related in a superior-inferior manner, a counterclockwise order is used in the right lung, and a clockwise order is used in the left lung as viewed from the anterior. The minor carina or crest between bronchial divisions is designated by hyphenation, so that the crest between bronchus B1a1 and bronchus B1a2 in the left lung would be designated LB1a1–2. This system is needed to describe the location of peripheral lesions, since fourth and sixth order bronchi can be visualized with flexible bronchoscopy (Ikeda).

The cadaveric dimensions of the tracheobronchial tree, as tabulated by Chevalier Jackson, are:

	Adult Male	Adult Female	Child	Infant
Diameter of trachea (mm)	14 × 20	12 × 16	8 × 10	6 × 7
Length of trachea (cm)	12	10	6	4
Length of right bronchus (cm)	2.5	2.5	2	1.5
Length of left bronchus (cm)	5	5	3	2.5
Length from upper teeth to trachea (cm)	15	13	10	9
Length from upper teeth to secondary bronchus (cm)	32	28	19	15

tional bronchioles with increasing alveolation. Number 23 is the alveolar sac (Weibel).

A letter and number system has been developed by Boyden to designate the segmental (tertiary) bronchi and their dichotomous branchings. The right lung is designated R, and the left lung is designated L. The segmental bronchi on each side are designated B1 through B10, as indicated above and in the chart on page 1036. The system alternates the use of lower case letters, a and b, and arabic numerals, 1 and 2, beginning with the quaternary bronchi. For example, the apical segment of the right lung is designated B1. Its subsegmental branches are designated B1a and B1b. The next order of branching of bronchus B1a

ENDOSCOPIC ANATOMY

As the endoscopic view of the anatomy unfolds, the tracheal rings can be seen through the respiratory epithelium. The trachea is narrowed somewhat where the thyroid gland partially surrounds it. The innominate artery's pulsation may be seen crossing the anterior wall obliquely from inferiorly on the left to superiorly on the right. The arch of the aorta makes an impression on the left lateral wall just above the carina. The trachea deviates slightly to the right just above the carina. The carina appears as a sharp vertical crest that is to the left of the midline of the trachea. It moves on respiration and cardiac pulsation.

The right bronchus is larger than the left and appears to be more of a continuation of the trachea than the left bronchus. The bronchi expand in length and diameter with inspiration and contract with expiration.

As the right bronchus is entered, the sharp vertical crest of the right upper lobe bronchus is encountered in the lateral wall of the right bronchus. The orifice of the right upper lobe bronchus is superior to the crest. Unless there is atelectasis of the middle or lower lobe or these lobes have been removed surgically, the contents of the right upper lobe bronchus cannot be visualized without a flexible bronchoscope or a right-angle or retrospective telescope. With these telescopes, the apical (B1), posterior (B2), and anterior (B3) segmental bronchi and their subsegmental (fourth order) bronchi can be seen. The orifice of the apical (B1) segmental bronchus is located superiorly in the right upper lobe bronchus. The orifice of the posterior (B2) segmental bronchus is located posteriorly, and the orifice of the anterior (B3) segmental bronchus is located anteriorly. The three segmental bronchi are of approximately equal size, and the distal end of the upper lobe bronchus appears to trifurcate (see inset in Figure 60–1).

The transverse crest of the middle lobe bronchus arises from the anterior wall of the right bronchus slightly counterclockwise to 12 o'clock. The middle lobe bronchus is anterior to the crest and can be inspected with an open bronchoscope or more effectively with a flexible bronchoscope or a foroblique telescope. The minor carina separating the lateral (B4) segmental bronchus from the medial (B5) segmental bronchus is oblique from the left anteriorly to the right posteriorly.

The right lower lobe bronchus is a continuation of the right bronchus. Its five segmental bronchi can be seen with an open bronchoscope, but the contents of the apical (superior) (B6) segmental bronchus cannot be seen without a flexible bronchoscope or right-angle telescope. The medial basal (B7) segmental bronchus arises independently from the anterior medial wall of the right lower lobe bronchus. As a general rule, the anterior basal (B8), lateral basal (B9), and posterior basal (B10) segmental bronchi

arise in an oblique row that extends from anterior laterally to posterior medially, with the anterior basal (B8) segmental bronchus being most anterior and the posterior basal (B10) being most posterior. The apical (superior) (B6) segmental bronchus arises from the posterior wall of the right lower lobe bronchus more proximally than the other right lobe segmental bronchi and just distal to the take-off of the right middle lobe bronchus.

The left bronchus is nearly twice as long as the right bronchus, although the diameter is less. The crest of the left upper lobe bronchus is found running obliquely from inferior laterally to superior medially on the lateral wall of the left bronchus. The orifice of the left upper lobe bronchus is proximal to the crest, and its contents may be inspected with the flexible bronchoscope and foroblique and right-angle telescopes. The minor carina between the superior division and the inferior division is transverse. The superior division subdivides into the superiorly placed apical-posterior (B1–2) segmental bronchus and the inferiorly placed anterior (B3) segmental bronchus. The inferior division (lingula) subdivides into the superiorly placed superior (B4) segmental bronchus and the inferiorly placed inferior (B5) segmental bronchus.

The left lower lobe bronchus is a continuation of the left bronchus. Its four or five segmental bronchi can be seen with an open bronchoscope, but the contents of the apical (superior) (B6) segmental bronchus cannot be seen without a flexible bronchoscope or a right-angle telescope. The medial basal (B7), anterior basal (B8), lateral basal (B9), and posterior basal (B10) segmental bronchi arise in an oblique row that extends from anterior laterally to posterior medially with the medial basal (B7) segmental bronchus most anterior and the posterior basal (B10) segmental bronchus most posterior. The Jackson and Huber terminology uses the term anterior-medial basal segmental bronchus, and Boyden designates it B7–8. The subdivision of the anterior-medial basal (B7–8) bronchus into the medial basal (B7) and the anterior basal (B8) bronchi can usually be seen with an open bronchoscope. The apical (superior)

(B6) segmental bronchus arises from the posterior wall of the left lower lobe bronchus more proximally than the other left lower segmental bronchi and just distal to the take-off of the left upper lobe bronchus.

INDICATIONS FOR BRONCHOSCOPY

Bronchoscopy is a primary method of investigating the problem in patients with diseases of the respiratory system. Along with the history, physical examination, and radiography, it is indicated in nearly all patients with respiratory diseases that are not self-limited and of short duration. It is appropriate in all patients with respiratory diseases in which the etiology and pathologic process are not clearly understood. It is specifically indicated in the diagnosis of patients with unexplained chronic cough, sputum production, stridor, wheezing, hemoptysis, shortness of breath on a noncardiac basis, suspected foreign body, paralysis of a vocal cord, a mass in the neck thought to be metastatic carcinoma, auscultatory evidence of tracheal, mediastinal, endobronchial, and pulmonary parenchymal disease, sputum cytology suggestive or diagnostic of a malignant tumor, and esophageal and thyroid diseases secondarily involving the tracheobronchial tree.

More particularly, the radiologic findings of segmental, lobar, or pulmonary atelectasis; compensatory or obstructive emphysema; localized parenchymal densities, such as pneumonitis, masses, and coin lesions; cavitary lesions; pleural effusion; mediastinal masses except an aortic aneurysm; and radiopaque foreign bodies are specific indications for investigation of the problem with bronchoscopy.

The differential diagnosis of diseases of the respiratory system is often dependent on bacteriologic, cytologic, and histopathologic specimens gathered at bronchoscopy.

Bronchoscopy for therapeutic purposes is indicated for aspiration in atelectasis and for tracheobronchial secretions that cannot be handled by the patient; removal of benign endobronchial tumors, such as papillomas, osteochondromas, lipomas, and neurofibromas; removal of foreign bodies and broncholiths; drainage of lung abscess; dilatation of bronchial stenosis; and aspiration in bronchiectasis.

Contraindications to bronchoscopy exist but must be evaluated in each patient individually. Contraindications to bronchoscopy are aortic aneurysms, bleeding tendencies, and recent massive hemoptysis of any cause. Relative contraindications are acute respiratory infections and cardiac decompensation. Aortic aneurysms can be ruptured at bronchoscopy with open bronchoscopes; however, bronchoscopy with a flexible bronchoscope should be safe. Likewise, patients with cervical spinal ankylosis or trauma or trismus may have bronchoscopy safely accomplished with a flexible bronchoscope. Patients with bleeding tendencies should not have bronchoscopy because of the possibility of its initiating intraluminal hematomas or bleeding that could not be controlled. Such patients have developed a cast of clotted blood throughout the tracheobronchial tree. Unless the indication for bronchoscopy is very pressing for therapeutic reasons, bronchoscopy should be postponed until the cause of the bleeding tendency has been identified and corrected. Bronchoscopy is contraindicated after recent massive hemoptysis because of the possibility of initiating another massive bleed. Usually after a few days, bronchoscopy can be carried out safely. At times the clinical picture of massive atelectasis with dyspnea, temperature elevation, and cyanosis may follow hemoptysis and may require emergency bronchoscopy to remove an obstructive clot.

Bronchoscopy should be avoided in acute respiratory infections, particularly in children, because of the possibility of producing edema of the respiratory tract that might interfere with adequate ventilation. The young child with a history of possible foreign body aspiration and an active respiratory infection presents a difficult problem in differential diagnosis, and it is hard to decide whether to perform bronchoscopy or not.

Patients with severe cardiovascular diseases and cardiac decompensation or arrhythmias are at special risk with peroral endoscopy, and the possible benefits and risks should be carefully considered. The additional exertion at bronchoscopy could lead to a greater degree of decompensation.

RADIOLOGIC DIAGNOSIS

Radiographs of the chest in the posterior-anterior and lateral projections may demonstrate pulmonary or mediastinal masses; segmental, lobar, and pulmonary atelectasis; lobar and pulmonary emphysema of both the acute or chronic and the compensatory or obstructive types; cavitary lesions; coin lesions; parenchymal densities, such as pneumonitis; the honeycomb appearance of bronchiectasis; pleural effusion; and radiopaque foreign bodies. Atelectasis and obstructive or compensatory emphysema suggest bronchial obstruction and are of special concern to the endoscopist. Atelectasis may occur distal to any cause of bron-

chial obstruction. If the atelectasis is massive, as with the collapse of a lobe or lung, compensatory emphysema occurs in the other lobes or lung. Obstructive emphysema may occur with any form of partial bronchial obstruction.

Oblique roentgenograms of the chest are helpful in demonstrating lesions that lie posterior to the heart. Lateral decubitus roentgenograms demonstrate pleural fluid, and apical lordotic roentgenograms demonstrate lesions at the apices of the lungs.

Tomograms of the lung are very helpful in demonstrating parenchymal pulmonary masses and cavities in what appear to be mass lesions on plane films. Tomograms of the trachea are particularly important in demonstrating tumors of the trachea (Karlan and coworkers).

Bronchography is the technique of coat-

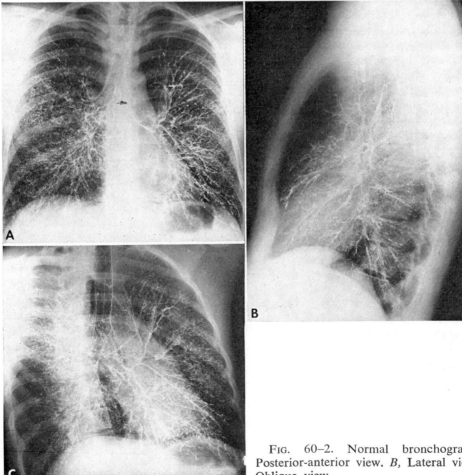

FIG. 60–2. Normal bronchogram. *A*, Posterior-anterior view. *B*, Lateral view. *C*, Oblique view.

ing the lining of the tracheobronchial tree with a radiopaque substance to demonstrate its morphology. Iodized oil, barium, water-miscible iodine compounds, and tantalum powder [for tracheography; still experimental (Stitik and Proctor)] have been used for this purpose (Fig. 60–2). The technique is useful in demonstrating bronchiectasis, lung abscess, bronchial stenosis, compression of the trachea and bronchi, as with vascular malformations (congenital rings), congenital malformations of the tracheobronchial tree, including tracheoesophageal fistulas, and bronchopleural fistulas. Although it is generally not a good way to prove the presence or absence of a foreign body, it has been used to demonstrate the point of obstruction in a segmental bronchus due to a foreign body. It is also helpful in demonstrating which segmental bronchus is involved in a parenchymal lesion.

The information gained from bronchography complements the information gained from bronchoscopy. Ordinarily bronchoscopy is performed first. In children, the bronchography can be carried out under the same general anesthesia as that used for the bronchoscopy. Performing bronchoscopy first allows the removal of secretions, so that filling of segmental and subsegmental bronchi is improved.

Bronchography provides important guidance to the correct bronchopulmonary segment in the bronchoscopic and postural drainage of lung abscess. It also provides critical information in the diagnosis of bronchiectasis. It is difficult to establish the diagnosis of bronchiectasis without bronchography. It is necessary to determine which segments and lobes are affected, so that surgical resection or conservative treatment with bronchoscopic and postural drainage can be effectively carried out.

Lung scans are helpful in differentiating pulmonary emboli from other parenchymal lesions.

TECHNIQUE

The technique of direct laryngoscopy, which is utilized for the introduction of the open bronchoscope, as well as the flexible bronchoscope at times, is discussed in Chapter 59.

The open bronchoscope is passed to a right-handed operator with the handle of the bronchoscope turned to the right, the leading edge of the bevel of the bronchoscope held vertically for introduction through the vocal cords. The assistant holds the bronchoscope at its midpoint like a pencil and places the distal tip of the bronchoscope in the laryngoscope. The operator takes hold of the handle and advances the bronchoscope after shifting his right eye from the field of view through the laryngoscope to the field of view through the bronchoscope. Once the bronchoscope is in the trachea, the handle of the laryngoscope is rotated to the left, and the slide of the laryngoscope is removed so that the laryngoscope can be removed. The assistant reassembles the laryngoscope by putting the slide back in place so that it will be in readiness should it be needed later in the procedure. The head is lowered from the Boyce position to the level position or a slightly dependent position. The upper lip is protected by the fingers of the left hand as the bronchoscope is steadied by the thumb and index and third fingers of the left hand at the level of the teeth, while the fourth and fifth fingers of the left hand rest on the teeth or hard palate. The handle of the bronchoscope or its proximal end is manipulated by the right hand as it is advanced. If manipulation through the bronchoscope is to be carried out, the operator performs this with his right hand and fixes the bronchoscope to the teeth or hard palate with his left hand. There is a tendency for the bronchoscope to be withdrawn by the respiratory motions, so it is important to fix the bronchoscope to the teeth or hard palate at the desired level before biopsy or foreign body forceps application is attempted.

The trachea is inspected by carrying the bronchoscope through a rotary course as it is advanced so that the entire circumference of the trachea can be seen. The trachea is studied for intrinsic lesions and for external compression. The carina is evaluated for its position, sharpness, and mobility on respiration and cardiac contraction. Enlarged lymph nodes and masses displace the carina, make its leading edge dull, and broaden its base. The respiratory and cardiac movements may be damped under such circumstances.

The decision whether to examine the right bronchus or the left bronchus first depends on a number of factors. As a general rule, the right bronchus and its subdivisions are inspected first. If the known clinical problem is in the distribution of the left bronchial tree, the left bronchus and its subdivisions may be inspected first so that the most essential portion of the examination is carried out first. It should be emphasized that the objective is to do a thorough and comprehensive examination of the tracheobronchial tree in each patient, but depending on a number of factors, including the patient's tolerance, it is at times prudent to proceed expeditiously with the gathering of the critical information. Contrary to this concept, there are situations in which the most critical maneuver, such as a biopsy, should be postponed until the inspection of the rest of the tracheobronchial tree has been completed because the subsequent bleeding may interfere with visualization.

As the right bronchus is entered, the head and neck are moved to the left a small distance to provide a more direct passage of the bronchoscope distally in the long axis of the right bronchus. The handle of the bronchoscope is rotated to the right so that the tip of the bevel will enter the right bronchus. After the bronchoscope has entered the right bronchus, the handle is rotated to the left so that the orifice of the right upper lobe bronchus may be inspected. Since the right bronchus is short, the proximal margin of the right upper lobe orifice is at approximately the same level as the carina. After the crest of the right upper lobe bronchus is identified, the proximal edge of the bevel of the bronchoscope is withdrawn to the superior margin of the orifice of the right upper lobe bronchus. The right-angle or retrospective telescope is passed by the assistant to the operator in the same manner as the bronchoscope and instruments are passed, and the contents of the right upper lobe bronchus are inspected. Biopsy of lesions in the bronchi

of the upper lobes is carried out through a flexible bronchoscope or with the Jackson flexible, curved, upper lobe forceps.

The handle of the bronchoscope is rotated posteriorly so that the anterior wall may be inspected, and the bronchoscope is advanced to identify the crest of the middle lobe bronchus. The orifice lies anterior to the crest. The middle lobe bronchus may be inspected with the open bronchoscope. It can be entered with a 6-mm open bronchoscope in the adult, the foroblique telescope, or the flexible bronchoscope. Lowering the head more may facilitate the examination of the contents of the right middle lobe bronchus.

As the bronchoscope is advanced to inspect the right lower lobe bronchus and its segmental bronchi, the head may have to be elevated slightly. The right-angle telescope is introduced to view the contents of the apical (superior) (B6) segmental bronchus of the right lower lobe.

As the bronchoscope is withdrawn, the head and neck are shifted back to the midline and then to the right as the left bronchus is entered to provide a more direct passage of the bronchoscope distally in the long axis of the left bronchus. At first the handle of the bronchoscope is rotated to the left so that the tip of the bevel will enter the left bronchus. After the bronchoscope has entered the left bronchus, the handle is rotated to the right to inspect the orifice of the left upper lobe bronchus. After the crest of the left upper lobe bronchus is identified, the proximal edge of the bevel of the bronchoscope is withdrawn to the superior margin of the orifice of the left upper lobe bronchus. The foroblique, right-angle, or retrospective telescope is inserted, and the contents of the left upper lobe bronchus are inspected.

The bronchoscope is advanced to inspect the left lower lobe bronchus and its segmental bronchi. The right-angle telescope is introduced to view the contents of the apical (superior) (B6) segmental bronchus of the left lower lobe.

The bronchoscope is withdrawn to just below the carina. Bronchial washings are usually taken from each bronchial tree separately. Normal saline, 5 to 10 ml, is injected through the bronchoscope and aspirated. The specimen is submitted for bacterial culture and sensitivities, acid-fast smear and culture, fungus culture, and cytologic examination. More limited areas of the bronchial tree may be washed, brushed, curetted, or randomly biopsied through the flexible bronchoscope. Specific segmental bronchi corresponding to radiographic abnormalities may be cannulated for the gathering of specimens.

Lesions projecting into the bronchus may be biopsied with little risk. Biopsy of endobronchial lesions is more adequately carried out through an open bronchoscope if the lesion can be visualized with an open bronchoscope. A large sample of tissue can be given to the pathologist, and bleeding and other complications are more easily controlled. Such biopsies can also be carried out through the instrument channel of the flexible bronchoscope. More peripheral lesions can be identified and biopsied with the flexible bronchoscope (Marsh and coworkers).

Abnormal bronchial mucous membrane may be biopsied but with more caution. The best site can be determined with telescopic magnification. Biopsies over the carina or interbronchial crests must be performed very carefully and only a very superficial specimen obtained to prevent perforation of the bronchus.

Lung biopsy may be performed through the bronchoscope with acceptable complication rates (Andersen). The most common indication is diffuse, bilateral, parenchymal pulmonary disease which defies diagnosis by other means. It is performed by inserting flexible blunt biopsy forceps as far as possible so that it can be felt to engage a small peripheral bronchus. If pain occurs, the assumption is that the pleura has been touched, and no biopsy is taken. If there is no pain, the forceps are opened on inspiration and closed on expiration. The procedure may be complicated by bleeding, pneumothorax, and mediastinal emphysema. Specimens are taken only from one lung because of the possibility of pneumothorax. It is not done in suppurative disease because of the possibility of establishing a bronchopleural fistula and emphysema.

Bronchial brushing, usually performed through the instrument channel of the flexible bronchoscope, is a method for obtaining bacteriologic, cytologic, and histopathologic specimens from the periphery of a suspicious segment of the lung with tiny brushes with nylon or steel bristles (Fennessy). It is applicable to lesions beyond the view of the flexible bronchoscope. It can be complicated by pneumothorax or bleeding. Curettage may be used in a similar manner through the instrument channel of the flexible bronchoscope to obtain histopathologic specimens. The procedure may be complicated by pneumothorax and bleeding. Both of these techniques find their greatest application in the diagnosis of bronchogenic carcinoma.

The various methods of introducing the flexible bronchoscope, as well as the anesthesia for it, have been discussed in Chapter 58. The advancement of the flexible bronchoscope is carried out with ease. The control of the direction of the tip varies somewhat with various manufacturers; however, all have a control in the handle for angulation in one plane. Apical rotation may be achieved by rotating the entire instrument on itself or may be built in as a second control. Each anatomic area in the tracheobronchial tree is inspected with the knowledge of the anatomy in mind (Ikeda; Marsh and coworkers).

The endoscopic procedure should be described in positive terms for the medical record. There is no such thing as a "negative" bronchoscopy. Even if no abnormality is found, the fact that the tracheobronchial tree has a normal appearance is important clinical information. A statement should be made about each bronchopulmonary segment to indicate whether it was normal, abnormal, or not seen. The size and type of instruments used should be recorded.

ENDOSCOPIC MANAGEMENT OF DISEASES OF THE RESPIRATORY TRACT

Ventilation and drainage of the tracheobronchial tree are necessary for normal function. The tracheobronchial tree is cleared of secretions by the movement of the trachea and bronchi during the respiratory cycle and by the movement of the mucous blanket by ciliary action. The ciliary action may fail to maintain clearance because the mechanism is overwhelmed by too much bronchial secretion and pulmonary exudate or because of injury to the ciliary mechanism, as occurs in chronic inhalation of irritants and acute viral infections. Another cause of failure is some form of mechanical obstruction, such as stenosis, foreign body, and viscous secretions. If these clearance mechanisms fail, cough occurs, and the tussive squeeze and bechic blast are employed (Huizinga). If the cough is not effective in clearance because of the magnitude of the bronchial

or pulmonary pathologic process(es), neurologic defects, or general debility, atelectasis may occur.

Atelectasis

Collapse of bronchopulmonary segments, lobes, and the whole lung is amenable to bronchoscopic removal of obstructing tissue, secretions, and foreign bodies, as well as dilatation of structures (Fig. 60–3). The longer atelectasis persists, the greater the chance of irreversible damage to the lung parenchyma. Local anesthesia is particularly

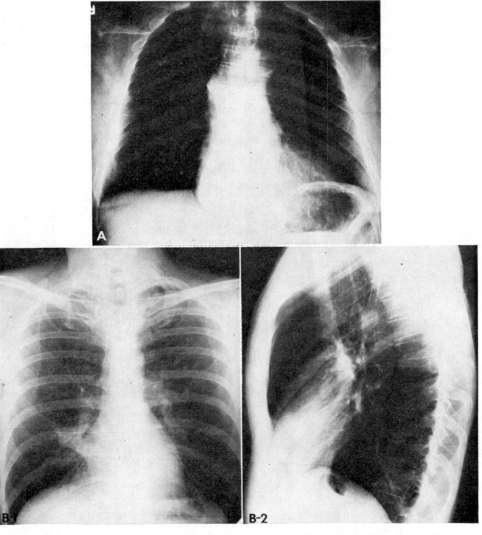

FIG. 60–3. Chest roentgenograms in atelectasis. *A,* Discoid in both lower lobes. *B,* Right middle lobe: posterior-anterior view and lateral view.

appropriate for bronchoscopy for the treatment of atelectasis due to retained viscous secretions, because the coughing produced is helpful in bringing secretions within view of the open bronchoscope. Although direct application of suction with a large lumen aspirating tube can be better accomplished with an open bronchoscope, flexible bronchoscopy is also effective and appropriate in high-risk critically ill patients and in those patients with cervical vertebrae ankylosis or trauma, trismus, and other factors interfering with open bronchoscopy (Lindholm).

Cystic Fibrosis

Cystic fibrosis (fibrocystic disease of the pancreas or mucoviscidosis) is a generalized hereditary disease with respiratory aspects characterized by tenacious sputum, progressive pulmonary fibrosis, and emphysema (Fig. 60-4). The difficulty in handling the tenacious bronchial secretion often results in atelectasis. The peripheral bronchi are most likely to be obstructed, and the atelectasis is often subsegmental. The clearance of the tenacious sputum is dependent on a vigorous cough. Treatment such as

tracheotomy which interferes with the effectiveness of the cough in clearing small bronchi aggravates the problem and is contraindicated. Bronchoscopy for aspiration of tracheobronchial secretions is often of definite benefit, but usually the obstructive process is too far in the periphery to be approached with an open bronchoscope in a child. When indicated, the bronchoscopy should be carried out without anesthesia and as gently and quickly as possible.

Bronchiectasis

Bronchiectasis is a disease that develops in the young. There was a sharp decline in the incidence of bronchiectasis from 1950 to 1960, and this decline has been attributed to the introduction of broad-spectrum antibiotics. Bronchiectasis more frequently involves the left lung than the right. The diagnosis is established with bronchography. Bronchoscopy plays a somewhat lesser role in the treatment of bronchiectasis now than in the past. Many patients with bronchiectasis are well controlled with intermittent broad-spectrum antibiotic therapy and postural drainage (Field). Conservative pulmo-

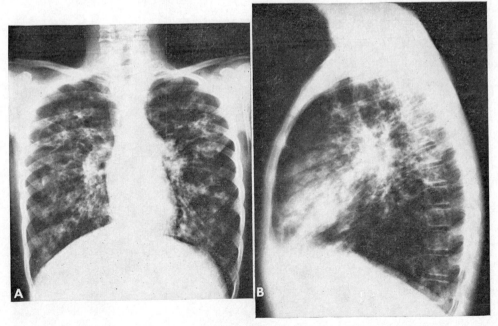

FIG. 60-4. Posterior-anterior (A) and lateral (B) chest roentgenograms of a patient with advanced cystic fibrosis.

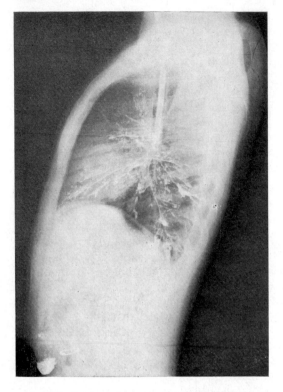

FIG. 60–5. Bronchogram demonstrating bronchiectasis in the right middle and lower lobes of a 10-year-old child with a 5-week sojourn of a deciduous tooth in the right bronchus.

nary resections are helpful to a few patients with bronchiectasis. Bronchoscopic aspiration of purulent secretions is indicated in those few patients who cannot be controlled on antibiotic therapy and postural drainage and who have too multisegmental bronchiectasis to have pulmonary resection. Since some bronchiectasis is secondary to foreign bodies, all patients with bronchiectasis should have diagnostic bronchoscopy initially (Fig. 60–5).

Lung Abscess

The treatment of lung abscess is prolonged antibiotic therapy with the agent to which the responsible microorganism is sensitive, chest percussion, and postural drainage and bronchoscopic drainage (Fig. 60–6). Emphasis in diagnosis is placed on differentiating primary lung abscesses, whether they be bacterial or fungal, from those occurring in association with systemic or local diseases (Huizinga). Bronchoscopy is indicated for diagnostic purposes to rule out a bronchogenic carcinoma or a foreign body, to obtain a culture, and for therapeutic purposes to provide drainage of the abscess by aspiration of the appropriate segmental bronchus

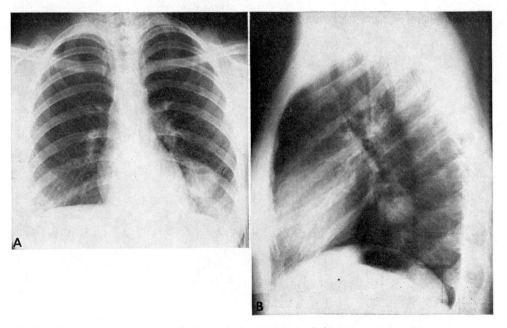

FIG. 60–6.   Lung abscess in the left lower lobe. Note air fluid level. *A*, Posterior-anterior view. *B*, Lateral view.

as determined by plane films of the chest and bronchography.

Benign Endobronchial Tumors

Benign tumors of the bronchus may be removed through an open bronchoscope. Papillomas, fibromas, lipomas, and chondromas are amenable to endobronchial resection. Adenomas usually require segmental resection. Tumors with narrow pedicles are more suitable for endobronchial resection than broad-based, vascular lesions. Amyloidosis produces endobronchial masses that can be satisfactorily resected at bronchoscopy.

Malignant Tumors of the Tracheobronchial Tree

The most common malignant tumor of the trachea and bronchus is squamous cell carcinoma. Bronchogenic carcinoma has assumed epidemic proportions, with 65,000 deaths per year in the United States. It is far more prevalent in men than in women and is etiologically related to the smoking of tobacco. Undifferentiated carcinomas, adenocarcinomas, and alveolar or bronchiolar carcinoma also occur in the lung. Bronchial adenomas are also malignant tumors of the lung. The pathogenesis of squamous cell carcinoma (40 to 50% of the total) passes through stages of squamous metaplasia, dysplasia, carcinoma in situ, and invasive carcinoma (Watson). It usually arises in the larger bronchi but can arise in the periphery. Undifferentiated or oat cell carcinoma (30 to 50% of the total) also usually arises in the larger bronchi but can occur more distally. Adenocarcinoma (10 to 20% of the total) is more frequently found in the periphery of the lung. Alveolar or bronchiolar carcinoma (5 to 10% of the total) tends to arise in the periphery and be multicentric. Metastasis from all types occurs through lymphatics and to a lesser extent through the bloodstream, and the lymph nodes of the mediastinum, neck, and abdomen become involved.

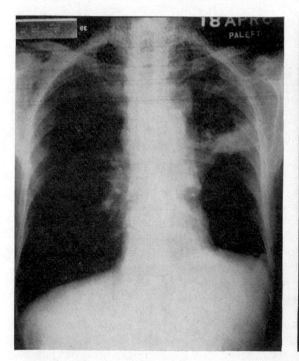 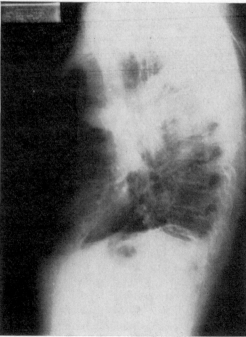

FIG. 60–7. Posterior-anterior and lateral roentgenograms of a 60-year-old man with left vocal cord paralysis. Bronchoscopy, cytology, and scalene node biopsy were not diagnostic, but poorly differentiated carcinoma was proved at mediastinoscopy.

Clinical manifestations include the symptoms of cough, pain, hemoptysis, and weight loss and the signs of bronchial obstruction, such as pneumonitis and atelectasis (Fig. 60-7). Diagnosis is based on history, physical findings, radiographic evidence, sputum cytology, bronchoscopy, and mediastinoscopy (Carlens; Marsh and coworkers).

In recent years the trend in therapy has been to define through bronchoscopy, mediastinoscopy, and other means the resectability of the tumor, so that only approximately 50% of patients with bronchogenic carcinoma are considered candidates for surgical therapy, and only approximately 25% of patients with bronchogenic carcinoma undergo resection. Lobectomies are more commonly employed than pneumonectomies. The overall 5-year survival rate is approximately 8%. Radiation therapy and chemotherapy play a major role in current therapy.

Suspected carcinoma of the bronchus is the most frequent indication for bronchoscopy today. At bronchoscopy for bronchogenic carcinoma, an attempt must be made to locate the tumor, prove the diagnosis histopathologically or cytologically, and determine the extent of the neoplasm and thereby its resectability. The position of the lesion and the distances from endobronchial landmarks must be specifically documented.

Mediastinal Tumors

Mediastinal tumors may compress, distort, or invade the tracheobronchial tree. Mediastinitis may result from mediastinal, esophageal, or tracheobronchial tumors, penetrating wounds of the chest, and esophagoscopy and may produce a mass lesion that similarly affects the tracheobronchial tree. Chronic mediastinitis may be due to fungal infections and tuberculosis. Histoplasmosis commonly involves the mediastinal lymph nodes. Mediastinal emphysema may result from a tracheobronchial lesion but usually does not compress or distort the tracheobronchial tree. Hemorrhage into the mediastinum and superior vena caval obstruction produce mediastinal compression syndromes which have generally little effect on the tracheobronchial tree. Primary tumors of the mediastinum include neurogenic tumors, teratodermoids, thymomas, and lymphomas. Cysts of the mediastinum are classified as pericardial, bronchogenic, enterogenous, and others (Oldham and Sabiston). Malignant tumors from other parts of the body frequently metastasize to the mediastinum.

Neurogenic tumors include neurofibromas, neurilemomas, ganglioneuromas, neurogenic sarcomas, neuroblastomas, sarcomas, paragangliomas, and pheochromocytomas and are the most common primary tumors in the mediastinum. In adults they are usually benign, but in children there is a greater chance that they will be malignant. The typical location is in the posterior mediastinum.

Teratodermoids are composed of several tissue types and tend to be benign in the mediastinum. They are characteristically located in the anterior mediastinum. They become manifest in adult life and may contain teeth and hair.

Thymomas are more common in adults than in children and are associated with myasthenia gravis. They may be benign or malignant. Thymomas arise in the superior or anterior mediastinum.

Lymphomas may occur primarily in the mediastinum or as a part of disseminated lymphoma. Hodgkin's disease and lymphosarcoma may present as primary mediastinal tumors. Lymphomas usually occur in the anterior mediastinum.

Thyroid tumors frequently invade the anterior mediastinum. The diagnosis is established with radioactive iodine scanning. Parathyroid tumors occur in the anterior and superior mediastinum.

Bronchogenic cysts originate from elements of the ventral foregut and are usually located near the trachea or bronchi. Usually there is no connection with the respiratory lumen. Bronchogenic cysts are rare in infancy but may produce severe respiratory distress by compressing the trachea or bronchi (Gerami and coworkers). Enteric or enterogenous cysts (reduplication cysts) originate from the dorsal foregut and are located in the posterior mediastinum in close relationship to the esophagus.

Foreign Bodies of the Tracheobronchial Tree

Foreign bodies of the tracheobronchial tree occur mainly in children, particularly in those under 2 years of age. Small objects capable of being aspirated should be kept out of the reach of small children. Children under 6 years of age should not be given peanuts or other nuts. Watermelon seeds, tacks, nails, pins, and bones are other common foreign bodies found in young children. Carelessness in one form or another accounts for most foreign body accidents (Jackson and Jackson). Carelessness can take the form of permitting children to play while eating, haphazard preparation of food, putting inedible substances like watermelon seeds, nails, tacks, and pins in the mouth, failure to close safety pins, and using the teeth to remove small objects from other objects, like a grass burr from gloves. Children being cared for by older children, which occurs more commonly in the lower socioeconomic groups, seems to be a factor.

Physicans should advise against allowing children under 6 years of age to eat nuts. Keeping small objects out of the reach of small children should be emphasized. Children should not run, scuffle, or laugh while eating.

While sharp foreign bodies are likely to lodge in the palatine tonsil, lingual tonsil, valleculae, or larynx, smooth objects like peanuts and other nuts, kernels of corn, watermelon seeds, beans, peas, and plastic toys pass through the larynx into the tracheobronchial tree.

The entrance of a foreign body into the tracheobronchial tree produces severe spasmodic cough which is often accompanied by cyanosis. The coughing lasts for approximately 30 minutes and subsides. During this period, the foreign body travels from one part of the tracheobronchial tree to another and more frequently than not finally lodges

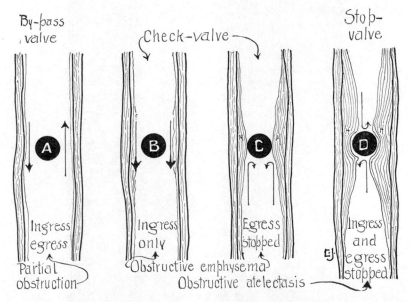

Fig. 60–8.   Valve mechanisms in bronchial obstruction. *A*, Bypass valve permits the passage of air on inspiration and expiration. No distal collapse or emphysema develops. *B, C*, Expiratory check or one-way valve permits the ingress of air during inspiration (*B*) but prevents the egress of air during expiration (*C*) owing to contraction of the bronchus. This form of obstruction traps air in the lung distal to the foreign body, and the repetition of this process with each respiratory cycle produces obstructive emphysema. *D*, Inspiratory check or stop valve prevents the movement of air on inspiration or expiration. Absorption of the air distal to the obstruction results in atelectasis (Jackson, C.: *Bronchoscopy and Esophagoscopy*. Philadelphia, W. B. Saunders Co., 1950.)

in the right bronchus. The right bronchus is the site of predilection for foreign bodies, because the carina is slightly to the left of the midline, the right bronchus is larger in diameter than the left, and the right bronchus is a more direct extension of the trachea than is the left bronchus. As the foreign body comes to rest, the coughing abates, and a latent period begins in which the patient is relatively free of symptoms. The family often assumes that the foreign body has been coughed out and may not report to the physician. The physician may also make the same assumption; however, careful auscultation of the chest at this time may demonstrate an expiratory wheeze and other signs of bronchial obstruction.

A foreign body in the bronchus may produce a bypass valve, an expiratory check or one-way valve, or an inspiratory check or stop valve (Fig. 60–8). The most common mechanism is the one-way valve, through which air may enter the bronchus distal to the foreign body during inspiration but may not escape from the lung on expiration. This type of valve obstruction produces emphysema distal to the foreign body. The obstructive emphysema can be demonstrated by increased resonance and decreased breath sounds on physical examination.

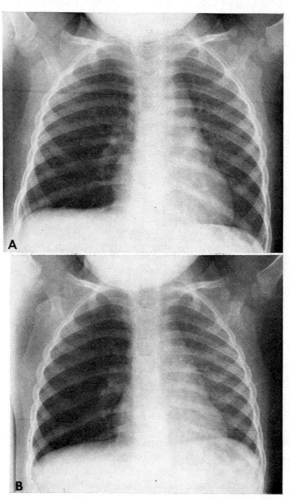

FIG. 60–9. Inspiratory (*A*) and expiratory (*B*) posterior-anterior chest roentgenograms demonstrating obstructive emphysema of the right lung due to a peanut in the right bronchus. The difference between the two lung fields becomes more marked on expiration.

Radiographically, obstructive emphysema may not be apparent on films taken on inspiration, but it becomes apparent on films taken in expiration as the unobstructed lung empties. For this reason inspiratory and expiratory posterior-anterior chest films are taken in a patient with a suspected foreign body (Fig. 60–9). In expiratory films, the lung distal to the foreign body becomes radiolucent as compared to the rest of the lung or the other lung. On expiration the mediastinum shifts away from the side that has the obstruction. The thoracic cage remains in greater expansion, as evidenced by the separation of the ribs from each other, and the diaphragm's excursion during expiration is limited. These changes are easily demonstrated on fluoroscopy of the chest, and a permanent cine record can be made. This clinical picture is the characteristic one seen with aspiration of a peanut.

The stop valve that completely occludes the bronchus on inspiration and expiration causes the rapid development of a more serious pathophysiologic state. Atelectasis of the lung distal to the foreign body occurs due to absorption of the air remaining in the lung. The whole lung is likely to be obstructed with the aspiration of a bean or

pea. Beans and peas are hygroscopic and swell as water is absorbed. They tend to obstruct the bronchus completely. With atelectasis of the lung containing the foreign body, the mediastinum shifts toward the atelectatic lung, and the unobstructed lung develops compensatory emphysema. The atelectatic lung is useless for ventilatory exchange, and the respiratory efficiency of the emphysematous lung is greatly reduced. Such patients are in severe respiratory distress within 30 minutes following the aspiration of a bean or pea. Cyanosis is often present, and rapid cardiorespiratory failure occurs unless the foreign body is removed. Limited expansion of the chest on the side of the obstruction is evident on inspection. Percussion of the chest is dull, and breath sounds are absent on the affected side. Radiographically atelectasis with a shift of the mediastinum and compensatory emphysema of the other lung can be demonstrated (Fig. 60–10).

Large foreign bodies of the trachea may result in very rapid suffocation. A young child, otherwise well, who collapses at play is very likely to have a tracheal foreign body. Smaller tracheal foreign bodies, such as watermelon seeds, may move in the trachea on each inspiration and may produce an audible slap and a palpatory thud as the foreign body strikes the subglottic area on expiration. Radiography is not usually helpful with tracheal foreign bodies. By listening at the open mouth and by palpating the trachea, one can confirm the diagnosis of a tracheal foreign body by these telltale physical signs.

Some characteristic clinical presentations of patients with foreign bodies have been presented, but the clinical features in a given patient depend on the size, shape, and character of the foreign body, the size and age of the patient, how long the foreign body has been present, and the location of the foreign body in the tracheobronchial tree. Vegetable foreign bodies produce severe inflammatory reactions in the respiratory tract. These reactions occur rapidly and are particularly severe with peanuts and nuts. Peanuts produce a very severe tracheobronchitis, the so-called arachidic bronchitis. After the latent period of approximately 24

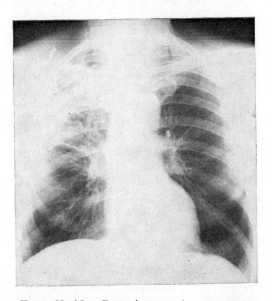

FIG. 60–10. Posterior-anterior roentgenogram of the chest in a patient with right upper lobe pneumonitis secondary to a peanut in the right upper lobe bronchus.

hours, the patient develops a cough productive of purulent sputum and fever. On the other hand, metallic and plastic foreign bodies that cause partial obstruction of a bronchus may be tolerated for long periods. Grass heads (inflorescences) present a special problem because of their tendency to migrate toward the periphery of the lung owing to the ratchet action of their barbs during the respiratory cycle (Clery and coworkers). Inflorescences usually descend into the right bronchus. The inflorescences of Timothy grass are usually classed as nonextrusive, while those of barley are extrusive and penetrate lung, pleura, and chest wall to form a sinus. Symptoms of severe pneumonitis often occur within 24 hours of the aspiration. The foreign bodies often require thoracotomy for removal. A long indwelling foreign body of the bronchus may produce bronchiectasis, recurrent pneumonitis, lung abscess, and emphysema.

In a patient in whom the history of an episode of choking, cough, or difficulty breathing is thought to be due to aspiration of a foreign body, the situation usually demands investigation of that possibility with bronchoscopy. Even when no foreign body is found on bronchoscopy, it is wise to keep an open mind about the possible presence of a foreign body. The possible presence of a foreign body of the tracheobronchial tree can be investigated by bronchoscopy, but it cannot be categorically excluded by bronchoscopy. In the patient suspected of having a tracheobronchial foreign body in whom no foreign body is found at bronchoscopy, repeat bronchoscopy is indicated if the symptoms, physical signs, and radiography do not return to normal.

In patients in whom the history, physical examination, or radiologic evidence point toward a foreign body, it is very helpful to obtain a duplicate object to study its mechanical properties and the problems involved in the removal of that foreign body. A well thought-out plan for removal may make the difference between successful management and a more complicated problem.

Most bronchial foreign bodies do not present a need for urgent intervention, and one may take time to prepare the patient optimally and to gather those items of equipment that might be particularly useful in the problem at hand. In a patient with a foreign body indwelling more than 24 hours, attention to adequate hydration and control of the febrile reaction resulting from secondary infection with antibiotic therapy and of other coincident medical problems makes the removal safer and more likely to be successful.

General anesthesia is used in most pediatric and adult patients for foreign body removal, but local anesthesia in adults and no anesthesia in children have advocates and are appropriate in some cases. For example, in the child with atelectasis of one lung due to a bean in the bronchus and compensatory emphysema of the other lung, anesthesia cannot be induced by inhalation, and bronchoscopy without anesthesia provides the only solution to this problem.

The size of the ventilating bronchoscope should be appropriate to the size of the patient. It should be small enough in diameter to reach the level of the foreign body and yet provide as large a working lumen as possible. Forceps specifically designed for each type of foreign body should be utilized. Many foreign body forceps are listed and illustrated in Chapter 58.

Once the foreign body has been visualized, it is important to avoid any maneuver that might displace the foreign body distally and thereby make its subsequent removal more difficult. Surrounding secretions should be gently suctioned away, and the foreign body should be studied to achieve the best exposure and to determine the best position of the bronchoscope for forceps application. Sharp or pointed foreign bodies may require disengagement from the mucous membrane prior to withdrawal. In general, the distal tip of the bronchoscope should be as close as possible to the foreign body without touching it or without interfering with the space needed for application of the particular forceps appropriate to that foreign body. This whole matter has been greatly simplified by the development of center-action foreign body forceps in many styles. Nevertheless, careful consideration should be given to the plane in which the forceps is opened and the manner in which it is advanced to encompass the foreign body.

As a general rule, foreign bodies of the bronchus are removed by placing the distal ends of the forceps beyond the equator of the foreign body so that it cannot be propelled distally as the forceps is closed. Ideally, the application of forceps should be carried out under constant visual monitoring. Care must be taken to avoid crushing fragile foreign bodies such as peanuts. The fragmentation of foreign bodies greatly complicates the problem because it creates several smaller foreign bodies. As a general rule, bronchial foreign bodies are withdrawn through the bronchoscope, but in some instances the foreign body is too large to be brought out through the bronchoscope and must be removed as a trailing foreign body. This method of foreign body removal is carried out by gently withdrawing the foreign body to the bevel of the bronchoscope and then fixing the relationship of the forceps and bronchoscope with the thumb and index finger of the left hand, which is also holding the bronchoscope. The forceps, bronchoscope, and foreign body are then removed as one unit. Chances of success in withdrawing the unit is best during the inspiratory phase of the respiratory cycle. The longer axis of the cross section of the foreign body should be rotated into the anterior-posterior plane at the level of the glottis so that the foreign body will not be sheared from the forceps by the vocal cords.

Some foreign bodies which are small enough to enter through the cricoid cartilage either produce subglottic swelling or expand, owing to their hygroscopic nature, sufficiently to make their exit through the cricoid cartilage impossible. Under these circumstances, a tracheotomy should be performed so that the foreign body may be removed as a trailing foreign body with a bronchoscope that has been introduced through the tracheostomy. In such a situation, the tracheotomy should be maintained until the subglottic edema subsides.

With the advances brought about by relatively safe general anesthesia, good illumination with ventilating bronchoscopes, and center-action forceps, most bronchial foreign bodies may be removed safely on the first effort. As a general rule, the endoscopic time utilized in an attempt at foreign body removal should be limited to 30 minutes. Thereafter, the chance of endobronchial and subglottic edema requiring a tracheotomy greatly increases. The risk of leaving the foreign body for a while longer must be weighed against the risk of the effects of undue endoscopy trauma. At times endoscopic manipulation can be carried out for 50 or 60 minutes under general anesthesia for foreign body removal without untoward sequelae. Someone in the operating room should be appointed to keep the endoscopic time and inform the operator gently of the time elapsed. After a certain period of unsuccessful manipulation, it may be better to wait for a day or two and try again once the reaction to the initial manipulation has subsided.

In the past there was considerable interest in and enthusiasm for fluoroscopic guidance for the removal of opaque foreign bodies located so far in the periphery of the lung that they cannot be removed under direct vision through the bronchoscope (Fig. 60–11). A double-tube, double-plane fluoroscope is required so that the guidance can alternately be furnished in two planes. It requires very close cooperation between an endoscopist and a radiologist trained in these techniques to minimize the mortality and morbidity of fluoroscopic bronchoscopy. Single-plane fluoroscopy is rarely helpful in foreign body removal. There is considerable question as to whether patients with peripheral foreign bodies are not equally well managed with a thoracotomy if the foreign body cannot be removed under direct vision through the bronchoscope.

Tracheal foreign bodies may produce little or no respiratory distress and then suddenly become impacted in the subglottic area. With the introduction of the bronchoscope, they can be bypassed or displaced into the distal portion of the trachea. With bulky tracheal foreign bodies, it may be necessary to bypass the foreign body with the bronchoscope and insert it into a bronchus to ventilate the patient. Tracheal foreign bodies may be missed by inadvertently bypassing them.

After a foreign body of the tracheobronchial tree has been removed, it is necessary to reintroduce the bronchoscope and inspect

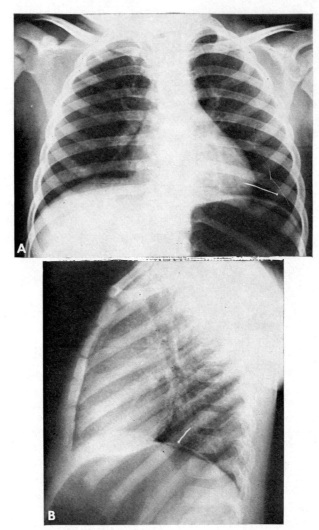

FIG. 60–11. Posterior-anterior (*A*) and lateral (*B*) chest roentgenograms of a patient with a straight pin in the left lower lobe bronchus.

the whole tracheobronchial tree for a second foreign body.

In looking for a foreign body, it is important to know what part of the foreign body is likely to be seen and what to look for. Pointed foreign bodies, such as nails, tacks, and pins, are almost always situated with the point directed superiorly, and it is the point one must look for, not the whole foreign body. The point must be ensheathed in the bronchoscope or enclosed in the blades of the forceps before traction is made to prevent perforation of the bronchus. If the point is already embedded in the mucous membrane, the foreign body must be pushed distally with the forceps to disengage the point. It is often more helpful to grasp the shaft near the point rather than the point with Tucker tack and pin forceps, which tend to align the long axis of the foreign body with the long axis of the bronchoscope.

Wood screws usually lodge with the head proximally situated and are difficult foreign bodies to remove because there are no forceps spaces around the head for application of the forceps blades. The tips of head-holding forceps may be passed over the head of the screw to obtain a secure grasp.

Hollow foreign bodies may also have no external forceps spaces but may be very satisfactorily handled by placing one blade of an alligator forceps inside and one outside. Expanding hollow object forceps are usually too large to use through a bronchoscope.

Complications are relatively rare after the prompt removal of foreign bodies, and recovery is generally rapid. The resolution of the obstructive emphysema, if present initially, should occur in 24 to 48 hours. All other physical or radiographic signs of the foreign body should progressively disappear. If that is not the case, repeat bronchoscopy should be carried out.

The recovery after removal of a long indwelling foreign body is more variable but is often surprisingly complete and prompt. Recovery depends on the amount of permanent bronchiectasis, bronchial stenosis, and lung necrosis produced.

REFERENCES

Andersen, H. A.: Lung Biopsy via the Bronchoscope. Ann. Otol. Rhinol. Laryngol., *79*: 931, 1970.

Atkins, J. P.: Laryngeal Problems of Infancy and Childhood. Pediatr. Clin. North Am., *9*:1125, 1962.

Boyden, E. A.: *Segmental Anatomy of the Lungs.* New York, McGraw-Hill Book Co., 1955.

Carlens, E.: Mediastinoscopy. Ann. Otol. Rhinol. Laryngol., *74*:1102, 1965.

Clery, A. P., *et al.*: Problems Associated with Aspiration of Grass Heads (Inflorescences). J.A.M.A., *71*:1478, 1959.

Fennessy, J. J.: Bronchial Brushing. Ann. Otol. Rhinol. Laryngol., *79*:924, 1970.

Field, C. E.: Bronchiectasis. Third Report on a Follow-up Study of Medical and Surgical Cases from Childhood. Arch. Dis. Child., *44*:551, 1969.

Gerami, S., *et al.*: Obstructive Emphysema due to Mediastinal Bronchogenic Cysts in Infancy. J. Thorac. Cardiovasc. Surg., *58*:432, 1969.

Harris, J. H.: Clinical Significance of the Tracheal Bronchus. Am. J. Roentgen., *79*: 228, 1958.

Huizinga, E.: The Tussive Squeeze and the Bechic Blast of the Jacksons. Ann. Otol. Rhinol. Laryngol., *76*:923, 1967.

Ikeda, S.: Flexible Bronchofiberscope. Ann. Otol. Rhinol. Laryngol., *79*:916, 1970.

Jackson, C., and Huber, J. F.: Correlated Applied Anatomy of the Bronchial Tree and Lungs with a System of Nomenclature. Dis. Chest, *9*:319, 1943.

Jackson, C., and Jackson, C. L.: *Bronchoesophagology.* Philadelphia, W. B. Saunders Co., 1950.

Karlan, M. S., *et al.*: Diagnosis of Tracheal Tumors. Trans. Am. Broncho-esophagol. Assoc., 1973, pp. 79–88.

Lindholm, C. E.: Flexible Fiberoptic Bronchoscopy in the Critically Ill Patient. Ann. Otol. Rhinol. Laryngol., *83*:786, 1974.

Marsh, B. R., *et. al.:* Flexible Fiberoptic Bronchoscopy: Its Place in the Search for Lung Cancer. Trans. Am. Broncho-esophagol. Assoc., 1973, pp. 101–110.

Marsh, B. R., *et al.*: Flexible Fiberoptic Bronchoscopy: Its Place in the Search for Lung Cancer. Ann. Otol. Rhinol. Laryngol., *82*: 757, 1973.

Oldham, H. M., and Sabiston, D. C.: Primary Tumors and Cysts of the Mediastinum. Monogr. Surg. Sci., *4*:243, 1967.

Perlman, L. V., *et al.*: Clinical Classification and Analysis of 97 Cases of Lung Abscess. Am. Rev. Resp. Dis., *99*:390, 1969.

Scott-Brown, W. G., and Ballantyne, J.: *Diseases of the Ear, Nose and Throat.* Vol. I. London, Butterworths, 1965.

Stitik, F. P., and Proctor, D. F.: Tracheography with the Experimental Contrast Agent Tantalum. Trans. Am. Broncho-esophagol. Assoc., 1973, pp. 138–144.

Watson, W. L.: *Lung Cancer.* St. Louis, Mo., C. V. Mosby Co., 1968.

Weibel, E.: *Morphometry of the Lung.* New York, Academic Press, 1963.

Chapter 61
Esophagology

The development of the flexible fiberoptic upper gastrointestinal panendoscopes has allowed the application of esophagoscopy and gastroscopy to more patients with upper gastrointestinal diseases than ever before. Just as the flexible bronchoscope extends the depth of the search, the flexible panendoscope extends the examination of the upper gastrointestinal tract to the duodenum. The flexible endoscope's safety and its tolerance by patients have greatly increased the applicability of the specular examination of the upper gastrointestinal tract.

ANATOMY OF THE ESOPHAGUS

The esophagus is a vertical muscular tube that extends from the hypopharynx to the stomach. It measures 23 to 25 cm in length in the adult. It begins at the lower border of the cricoid cartilage or approximately the level of the sixth cervical vertebra. It passes through the neck, superior mediastinum, and posterior mediastinum anterior to the cervical and thoracic vertebrae. It terminates at the cardiac orifice of the stomach at the level of the eleventh thoracic vertebra. It passes through the esophageal hiatus of the diaphragm at the level of the tenth thoracic vertebra. The esophageal hiatus of the diaphragm is elliptical and is located anterior, superior, and to the left of the aortic hiatus of the diaphragm. It transmits the vagus nerves and some small esophageal vessels, as well as the esophagus.

In the neck the esophagus is in the midline but veers slightly to the left. In the mediastinum it returns to the midline at the level of the fifth thoracic vertebra. In the inferior portion of the mediastinum, it deviates to the left as it passes anteriorly into the esophageal hiatus of the diaphragm. Of very considerable importance are the flexures in the anterior-posterior plane that correspond to the convexity of the bodies of the cervical vertebrae and the concavity of the bodies of the thoracic vertebrae. The abdominal portion of the esophagus, which is only 1.25 cm long, is in the esophageal groove on the posterior surface of the left lobe of the liver. The left and anterior surfaces of the abdominal esophagus are covered with peritoneum.

In the neck, the esophagus is posterior to the trachea. It is in contact with the common carotid arteries. The recurrent laryngeal nerves lie in the angle between the esophagus and the trachea. The thoracic duct lies on its left side. Both lobes of the thyroid gland come in contact with the esophagus, but the area of contact is greater on the left side because the esophagus veers slightly to the left in the neck. In the superior mediastinum, the esophagus passes posterior to and to the right of the arch of the aorta and then descends on the right side of the descending aorta until the inferior portion of the mediastinum is reached, and then it passes anterior to and very slightly to the left of the aorta. The left bronchus crosses and indents the esophagus anteriorly inferior to the arch of the aorta. The thoracic duct is posterior to the lower portion of the esophagus. It passes to the right of the esophagus and is posterior to it at the level of the fourth thoracic vertebra as it passes to the left side of the esophagus to enter the neck. The azygos vein is to the right side of the esophagus in the thorax. The right vagus nerve descends posterior to the esophagus, and the left vagus nerve descends anterior to the esophagus.

The esophagus is lined by thick nonkeratinizing stratified squamous epithelium. The lamina propria is thin and has fine interlacing fibers, fibroblasts, and histiocytes with occasional solitary lymphoid nodules. The muscularis mucosae appears to be a continuation of and takes the place of the elastic layer of the pharynx. Its smooth muscle fibers are arranged longitudinally. The muscularis mucosae becomes thicker in the lower one third of the esophagus. The submucosa consists primarily of thick collagenous and coarse elastic fibers and contains mucous glands and Meissner's plexus. The muscle is composed of an inner circular layer and an outer longitudinal layer. The circular layer is continuous with the inferior constrictor of the pharynx. The longitudinal fibers are arranged proximally into three fascicles. One fascicle is attached anteriorly to the cricoid cartilage, and one fascicle on each side is continuous with the musculature of the pharynx. Distally the three fascicles blend together to form a uniform layer. Auerbach's myenteric plexus lies between the two layers. The muscle is striated in the upper third, partly striated and partly smooth in the middle third, and nearly all smooth in the lower third. The outer coat or fibrosa consists of loose fibroelastic tissue. It is not a true serosa like that found in the gastrointestinal tract distal to the esophagus.

The glands of the esophagus are of particular interest. They are divided into submucosal and mucosal glands. The submucosal glands extend into the submucosa as tubuloalveolar end-pieces. The secretory portions are composed only of mucous cells in man. The mucosal or cardiac glands have branched terminal portions similar to the glands in the cardiac portion of the stomach. They are confined to the lamina propria and are only of the mucus-secreting type.

ENDOSCOPIC ANATOMY

Normally the lumen of the esophagus is collapsed and has a flattened or stellate configuration. The wall of the esophagus is thin. The diameter of the esophagus is reduced at four points: the cricopharyngeus muscle, the crossing of the aorta, the crossing of the left bronchus, and the diaphragm. Its lumen is slightly larger just before it enters the diaphragm. The average distances to these points from the upper incisor teeth, according to age, are shown in Figure 61–1.

The cricopharyngeus muscle periodically relaxes and contracts. This dilation and closure can be viewed through an esophagoscope placed posterior to the cricoid cartilage. The impressions of the arch of the aorta and the left bronchus are not easily seen endoscopically. The hiatus is usually apparent as an anteriorly placed oblique narrowing. As the hiatus is passed, the stellate pattern of the esophagus disappears, and the deeper red gastric mucosa with its prominent rugae is seen.

INDICATIONS FOR ESOPHAGOSCOPY

Esophagoscopy is a primary method of investigating the problem in patients with diseases of the esophagus. Together with the history, physical examination, and radiography, it is indicated in nearly all patients with unexplained symptoms and signs of esophageal and mediastinal diseases. Esophagoscopy is required to prove the diagnosis of many diseases of the esophagus. It is appropriate in all patients with alimentary diseases in which the etiology and pathologic process are not clearly understood. Esophagoscopy is specifically indicated in the diagnosis of patients with dysphagia, odynophagia, aphagia, a sensation of a lump or sticking sensation in the throat, neck masses thought to be metastatic carcinoma, vocal cord paralysis, retrosternal pain, heartburn, hematemesis and other evidence of gastrointestinal bleeding, regurgi-

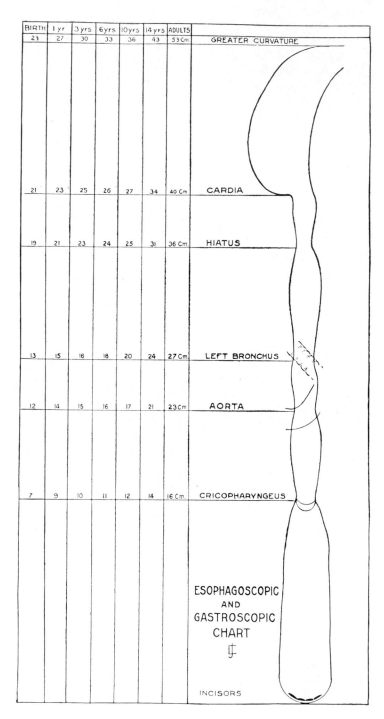

BIRTH	1 yr	3 yrs	6 yrs	10 yrs	14 yrs	ADULTS	
23	27	30	33	36	43	53 Cm.	GREATER CURVATURE
21	23	25	26	27	34	40 Cm.	CARDIA
19	21	23	24	25	31	36 Cm.	HIATUS
13	15	16	18	20	24	27 Cm.	LEFT BRONCHUS
12	14	15	16	17	21	23 Cm.	AORTA
7	9	10	11	12	14	16 Cm.	CRICOPHARYNGEUS

ESOPHAGOSCOPIC
AND
GASTROSCOPIC
CHART

INCISORS

FIG. 61–1.   Distances from the upper incisor teeth to esophageal landmarks. (Jackson, C., and Jackson, C. L.: *Bronchoesophagology*. Philadelphia, W. B. Saunders Co., 1950.)

tation, vomiting, suspected foreign body, caustic ingestion, aspiration following nocturnal regurgitation, and radiographic evidence of intrinsic or extrinsic esophageal obstruction, esophageal stenosis, vascular anomalies, tracheoesophageal fistulas, esophageal diverticula, peptic esophagitis, peptic ulcer of the esophagus, achalasia, varices, and foreign bodies.

The differential diagnosis of diseases of the esophagus is usually dependent on radiographic findings, motility studies and observations, and histopathologic specimens gathered at esophagoscopy.

Esophagoscopy for therapeutic purposes is indicated in patients with foreign bodies, achalasia, pulsion diverticula, and stenosis of various causes. Esophagoscopy provides the opportunity for dilatation of strictures due to congenital webs, infectious processes, caustic ingestions, peptic esophagitis, trauma, foreign bodies, esophageal surgery, and scleroderma, as well as the insertion of indwelling tubes of various types in carcinoma of the esophagus.

Contraindications to esophagoscopy exist but must be evaluated individually in each patient. Perforation of the esophagus from previous esophagoscopy is a relative contraindication, particularly if the perforation resulted from what seemed to be an atraumatic esophagoscopy. Massive bleeding from esophageal varices within the last 24 to 48 hours in a patient in whom the bleeding appears to have ceased usually contraindicates esophagoscopy for several days. Likewise, recent perforation of the esophagus from trauma or spontaneously, as in the Mallory-Weiss syndrome, would dictate against esophagoscopy until the healing process is mature. Cervical ankylosis or trauma may contraindicate open esophagoscopy but is not a contraindication to flexible esophagoscopy. Trismus may contraindicate both open and flexible esophagoscopy unless the esophagoscope can be passed through a nasal cavity. The presence of a bleeding tendency is a relative but not an absolute contraindication to esophagoscopy. If the bleeding tendency can be corrected, it is appropriate to do so before diagnostic or therapeutic esophagoscopy is undertaken.

RADIOLOGIC DIAGNOSIS

Radiographic evaluation of patients with diseases of the esophagus is especially rewarding. As a general rule, the radiographic evaluation should precede the endoscopic evaluation. Usually the radiographic evaluation begins with plane roentgenograms of the chest in the posterior-anterior and lateral projections. Such roentgenograms may demonstrate mediastinal masses or widening, pulmonary masses, aspiration pneumonitis, atelectasis, obstructive or compensatory pulmonary emphysema, mediastinal emphysema, pleural effusion, and radiopaque foreign bodies.

Radiography of the neck in the anterior-posterior view and particularly in the lateral view is of great help in evaluating patients with lesions of the cervical esophagus. A good lateral neck roentgenogram, in which the neck is slightly extended on the thorax, the head is extended on the neck, and the shoulders are displaced inferiorly by asking the patient to reach toward the knees, provides a great deal of information about the cervical esophagus. The distance between the cervical vertebrae and the larynx and trachea may be evaluated for swelling in this area. Radiopaque foreign bodies of the cervical esophagus can be visualized, and changes in the cervical esophagus, such as intraluminal air around a nonradiopaque foreign body, may give a clue to the presence of a foreign body. Paraesophageal swelling and air can be seen on this view in the presence of a perforation of the esophagus. Displacement of the larynx and trachea due to neoplasms of the esophagus is readily appreciated in the lateral neck roentgenogram. Cervical spine changes, such as osteophytes that may produce dysphagia, can also be detected.

The esophagus is an ideal organ, with its relatively large lumen and thin wall, for radiographic evaluation with contrast material. Barium sulfate suspensions of various consistencies have been used for this purpose, but water-miscible iodized solutions or iodized oil can also be used. The water-miscible solutions are particularly appropriate if there is some question as to the presence of a perforation. Water-miscible or oily preparations are preferred over barium sulfate suspensions by some radiologists in patients in whom aspiration into the tracheobronchial tree is likely. Various consistencies of barium sulfate are particularly useful because of their ability to bring out mucosal details.

The esophagus should ordinarily be evaluated fluoroscopically as part of an evaluation of the upper gastrointestinal tract that includes the pharynx, hypopharynx, esophagus, stomach, and duodenum. In patients in whom disease of the esophagus is suspected, a cinefluoroscopic study should be obtained. Many details of esophageal mobility, contour, and mucosal pattern are better evaluated with cinefluoroscopy than with live or still radiography. It also provides a permanent record with which to monitor the progress of the disease process or the effectiveness of therapeutic measures. Contrast studies of the esophagus are useful in demonstrating atresia, stenosis, tracheoesophageal or bronchoesophageal fistulas, external compression due to vascular anomalies and cervical and mediastinal masses, diverticula, congenital shortening of the esophagus, achalasia, intrinsic masses, foreign bodies, varices, peptic esophagitis, esophageal ulcers, hiatal hernias, gastric reflux, Schatzki rings, presbyesophagus, scleroderma, and perforation.

The endoscopist is in a much better position to interpret the esophageal findings in the light of the radiographic findings. Furthermore, the endoscopic procedure can be conducted with greater safety with knowledge of the structural and functional state of the esophagus and associated structures. Therefore, as a general rule, the radiographic evaluation is carried out prior to the endoscopic evaluation. Motility studies are ordinarily carried out after the endoscopic examination because of the necessity of introducing the recording equipment.

TECHNIQUE OF ESOPHAGOSCOPY

Esophagoscopy may be performed with an open esophagoscope or with a flexible esophagoscope or panendoscope. The examination should be performed in the operat-

ing room, and the patient should not have taken anything to eat or drink for 8 to 12 hours prior to the examination. Premedication, as described in Chapter 58, should be administered, and this premedication will ordinarily include a sedative (pentobarbital), a narcotic (meperidine), and a cholinolytic agent (atropine). Local anesthesia is very satisfactory for esophagoscopy performed with a flexible esophagoscope and is often satisfactory for esophagoscopy with an open esophagoscope. However, general anesthesia with an endotracheal tube is preferred for the majority of patients requiring open esophagoscopy. Local anesthesia can be achieved by spraying the pharynx with measured quantities of a topical anesthetic and letting the patient sip measured quantities of a topical anesthetic. The application of 40 mg of tetracaine as 4 ml of a 1% solution is very satisfactory. In the use of general anesthesia with an endotracheal tube, the introduction of the esophagoscope is facilitated by the use of a neuromuscular blocking agent, such as succinylcholine, and temporary deflation of the cuff of the endotracheal tube. Introduction of the open esophagoscope in a paralyzed patient under general anesthesia is safer than any other technique in preventing perforation of the cervical esophagus. Certainly general anesthesia is preferred for the removal of foreign bodies of the esophagus.

The patient who is under local anesthesia is encouraged to swallow the lubricated flexible esophagoscope, and it is gently advanced. The position of the patient is not critical with the flexible esophagoscope.

The position of the patient for open esophagoscopy is the same as for open bronchoscopy. The patient is placed in dorsal recumbency with the neck flexed on the chest and the head extended on the neck. The superior surface of the patient's shoulders should be at the edge of the main portion of the operating table so that the head and neck may be manipulated freely on the headrest. It is important to keep in mind that the cervical esophagus is virtually vertical in the Boyce position; therefore, the open esophagoscope should be held nearly vertically. The tip and shaft of the esophagoscope are lubricated with sterile mineral oil prior to introduction. The upper lip is retracted with the third and fourth fingers of the left hand of a right-handed operator, and the esophagoscope is steadied with thumb and index finger of the left hand. The proximal end of the esophagoscope is held like a pencil with the fingers of the right hand. The right eye is used by a right-handed operator to look into the esophagoscope so that the instruments can be manipulated through the esophagoscope under continuous visualization without the operator's head being in the way.

As the esophagoscope is introduced to the level of the junction of the hypopharynx and esophagus, gentle pressure may be applied through the tip of the esophagoscope with the thumb of the left hand to the posterior aspect of the signet ring portion of the cricoid cartilage. As one observes the entrance of the esophagus in this position, the cricopharyngeus muscle will periodically open and close in the patient under local anesthesia. As the cricopharyngeus muscle relaxes, one can see several centimeters into the lumen of the esophagus. The esophagoscope is gently advanced only during a period of relaxation of the cricopharyngeus muscle. It should not be forced while the cricopharyngeus muscle is in contraction. An esophagoscope is never advanced unless there is a distinct lumen ahead. Often considerable patience is required at this site. It is essential to be patient here, because this site is the one most frequently perforated. The position of the patient must be correct as described above for safe passage of the esophagoscope.

Under general anesthesia in which the patient has been paralyzed with a neuromuscular blocking agent, such as succinylcholine, the esophagus will be patent any time the cricoid cartilage is displaced anteriorly, and the esophagoscope may be advanced gently.

As one advances through the cervical esophagus and into the superior portion of the thoracic esophagus, the esophagoscope is maintained in a nearly vertical position. As one continues to advance the esophagoscope, it begins to impinge upon the posterior wall of the esophagus. The head is lowered gradually, and it is possible to advance the esophagoscope through the midportion of the thoracic esophagus. At this stage of the examination the head, neck, and chest are resting on parts of the table which are all in the same plane. In the lower one-third of the esophagus, the esophagoscope begins to impinge on the posterior wall of the esophagus again, and the head must be lowered to allow the esophagoscope to be advanced. Lowering of the head is required because of the slightly anterior course of the esophagus in its lower one third. At this point in the examination, the head is depressed relative to the thorax. It is also necessary at this time to move the head to the right because the esophagus is deviating to the left in its lower one third. The course of the esophagus through the diaphragm and the esophagogastric junction must be negotiated gently and only if a lumen lies ahead of the esophagoscope. The esophagoscope should be aimed for the patient's left anterior superior iliac spine as one looks for the hiatal esophagus. The esophageal lumen appears as a slit or a rosette where the esophagus goes through the diaphragm. In some patients, particularly if there is dilatation of the thoracic esophagus, it may be difficult to find the hiatus. It will usually appear as an oblique slit from 10 to 4 o'clock. Once the hiatus is found, the abdominal esophagus and cardia are easily passed if they are normal. Many congenital and acquired abnormalities occur in this area which predispose to perforation of the esophagus unless gentleness, care, patience, and judgment are exercised. As the stomach is entered, the gastric juice usually flows down the esophagoscope, and the color and texture change of the mucosa can be noted. The stomach can be safely entered with the esophagoscope in the vast majority of patients, but occasionally it is not possible to visualize the gastric mucosa safely with an open esophagoscope. There is no disgrace in using the good judgment to recognize this situation.

Perforation of the esophagus is a catastrophic complication and should be avoided by the use of the most conservative judgment, particularly in the manipulation of an open esophagoscope.

In withdrawing the esophagoscope, the opportunity to look at everything again should be taken. The esophagoscope can be rotated gently about the fixed point of the operator's left hand to give a more panoramic view of the interior of the esophagus as the esophagoscope is withdrawn.

ENDOSCOPIC DIAGNOSIS AND MANAGEMENT

Diverticula of the Esophagus

Diverticula of the esophagus are categorized by location and the mode of development, as well as whether they are true or false diverticula. Pulsion diverticula are generally false diverticula in the sense that they are composed of mucosa and submucosa but do not contain a muscle layer. Pulsion diverticula are more common and are located at the junction of the hypopharynx and the esophagus and just above the diaphragm. Traction diverticula are true diverticula in that they are composed of all layers of the esophageal wall and may be located anywhere along the course of the esophagus but characteristically develop in the midthoracic portion. Pulsion diverticula are thought to be related to disordered motility of the esophagus and to congenital or acquired weakness in the muscular walls of the hypopharnyx or esophagus. (Cross and coworkers). Traction diverticula are thought to result from inflammatory processes adjacent to the esophagus, with secondary involvement of the esophageal wall in the scar contracture that subsequently occurs. Tuberculosis of the mediastinal lymph nodes is often given as an etiologic factor. Traction diverticula tend to be less symptomatic than pulsion diverticula of the hypopharynx and are often found incidentally on radiographic studies of the upper gastrointestinal tract.

Pulsion diverticula of the hypopharynx are frequently referred to as Zenker's diverticula; although they develop in areas of the hypopharynx where there are muscular defects between the oblique fibers of the inferior constrictor muscle of the pharynx and the transverse fibers of the cricopharyngeus muscle, they produce symptoms by compressing the cervical and superior portion of the thoracic esophagus and are customarily called esophageal diverticula. "Pharyngoesophageal diverticula" is a more appropriate term and is gaining in popularity. Pharyngoesophageal diverticula tend to occur in older patients and are nearly always on the left side. These diverticula produce varying degrees of dysphagia, noisy swallowing, and regurgitation of undigested food into the pharynx. The diverticulum tends to remain full following eating and empties into the hypopharynx when the patient lies down and goes to sleep. Aspiration pneumonitis is a frequent complication and often the presenting complaint. The diverticulum tends to enlarge with time and generally will become large enough to completely obstruct the cervical and superior portion of the thoracic esophagus by external compression. The diagnosis is easily made radiographically with a swallow of barium sulfate suspension (Figure 61-2). Gastroesophageal

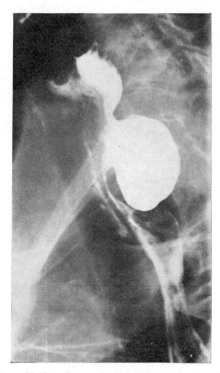

FIG. 61–2.   Lateral view of contrast radiography of a Zenker's diverticulum. Note aspiration of contrast material.

reflux and hiatus hernia are often associated with pharyngoesophageal diverticula and are thought by some to play an etiologic role in their development.

Although patients with pharyngoesophageal diverticula are often dehydrated and debilitated from nutritional deprivation and recurrent aspiration pneumonia, appropriate preparation for surgery can be carried out and the surgery performed with acceptable risk. Small diverticula should be resected before they become large and produce debilitation.

Esophagoscopy should be carried out prior to the resection to aspirate the contents of the diverticulum, to exclude the possibility of neoplasm which occasionally occurs, and to inspect the cervical esophagus for any related problem (Garlock and Richter). With large diverticula it is easier to enter the diverticulum with the esophagoscope than it is to enter the esophagus, and care must be taken to avoid perforation. The esophagoscope may be left in the esophagus during the resection of the diverticulum to avoid resecting too much of the esophageal wall (Figure 61-3). A transverse incision is made between the cricoid cartilage and the clavicle on the left side with the neck extended and the head rotated to the right. The sternocleidomastoid muscle is retracted laterally, and the left lobe of the thyroid gland is retracted medially. The diverticulum is approached by retracting the contents of the carotid sheath laterally. The diverticulum is dissected superiorly to its neck and transected. The pharyngoesophageal mucous membrane is closed with interrupted sutures of slowly absorbed material with the knots in the lumen. The musculature is approximated as a separate layer, and a soft rubber drain is inserted. A cricopharyngeal myotomy may be performed at the same time. Some have advocated cricopharyngeal myotomy for the smaller diverticula on the assumption that the etiology is incoordination in the swallowing mechanism with contraction of the constrictors after closure of the cricopharyngeus muscle (Ellis and coworkers).

An endoscopic approach for the resection of the party wall between the esophagus and the diverticulum was originally described by Dohlman and subsequently used by Holinger with an acceptable complication rate (Holinger and Schild). This technique, which can be used under local anesthesia, appears to be more appropriate for the severely debilitated patient who cannot be improved with conservative management in preparation for the external approach. The endoscopic approach has not

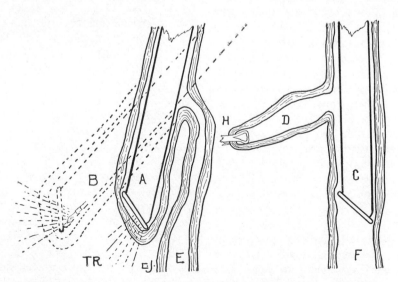

FIG. 61–3.   *A,* Esophagoscopic inspection of a pharyngoesophageal diverticulum. *B,* Esophagoscope placed in the esophagus for resection of the diverticulum. (Jackson, C., and Jackson, C. L.: *Bronchoesophagology.* Philadelphia, W. B. Saunders Co., 1950.)

gained popularity, and the external approach is generally preferred.

Pulsion diverticula of the lower esophagus tend to be less symptomatic but may at times require resection with a long extramucosal esophagomyotomy.

Spasm of the Cricopharyngeus Muscle

A number of central nervous system diseases may result in spasm of the cricopharyngeus muscle. The problem was first recognized in patients with bulbar poliomyelitis in whom deglutition was not possible and in whom cricopharyngeal myotomy resulted in marked improvement in their swallowing ability (Kaplan). Subsequently this entity has been recognized in patients with bulbar paralysis of many causes, including cerebrovascular accidents, intracranial trauma and neoplasms, and multiple sclerosis, as well as radical resections of the pharynx and larynx. Similar clinical pictures occur in muscular dystrophy, myasthenia gravis, dermatomyositis, and the myopathy of thyrotoxicosis. Cricopharyngeal muscle spasm may be accurately diagnosed by esophageal motility studies (Blakely and coworkers). Normally the pharyngoesophageal sphincter is open during contraction of the constrictor muscles of the pharynx. If this opening fails to occur, the diagnosis is suspected. Similar information can be obtained more easily with a barium swallow in which no barium enters the esophagus. In such patients, if esophagoscopy is normal, the empirical use of cricopharyngeal myotomy is worthwhile. Cricopharyngeal myotomy is frequently utilized at the time of radical resection of the pharynx and partial resection of the larynx to prevent this type of dysphagia.

Achalasia

Achalasia is characterized by lack of peristalsis in the thoracic esophagus and failure of the inferior sphincter to relax. Its etiology is undetermined. Although it is thought to result from neuromuscular abnormalities, it remains unclear whether the primary neural lesion is in the wall of the esophagus, vagus nerve, or brain stem (Cassella and coworkers). Certainly disintegration and absence of ganglion cells of Auerbach's plexus can be found throughout the thoracic esophagus and appear to be responsible for the lack of peristalsis. There is no structural change associated with the lack of relaxation of the inferior sphincter. A similar disease due to destruction of the myenteric plexus by neurotropic toxins produced by the leishmanial forms of *Trypanosoma cruzi* occurs in South America. Megaesophagus associated with South American trypanosomiasis or Chagas' disease occurs mainly in central Brazil (Köberle).

Progressive dilatation of the esophagus above the inferior sphincter is the hallmark of achalasia. The esophagus retains food and fluid and tends to allow emptying only when the intraluminal pressure is greatly elevated. Aspiration of retained food and fluids occurs in the recumbent position, particularly at night during the patient's sleep. Pulmonary complications secondary to aspiration may occur and lead to progressive pulmonary disability. Carcinoma of the esophagus probably secondary to chronic inflammation occurs not infrequently, particularly in those with long-standing untreated achalasia (Wychulis and coworkers).

Achalasia is fairly common and occurs with an equal incidence in men and women. Although it may occur in children or at any age, the majority of patients with achalasia first develop symptoms between 30 and 50 years of life.

The predominant symptom is dysphagia, and the presence of regurgitation and substernal pain vary from patient to patient. Initially solid food is handled more readily than liquids. Later liquids are handled with greater ease. Cold fluids tend to cause more difficulty than warm ones. Some patients seem to be relieved by drinking enough fluid to raise the intraluminal pressure sufficiently to open the lower sphincter. Regurgitation occurs mainly at night in the recumbent position and while asleep. Substernal pain is usually mild and is less bothersome than the full feeling. Weight loss, pulmonary complications, and polyarthritis occur periodically.

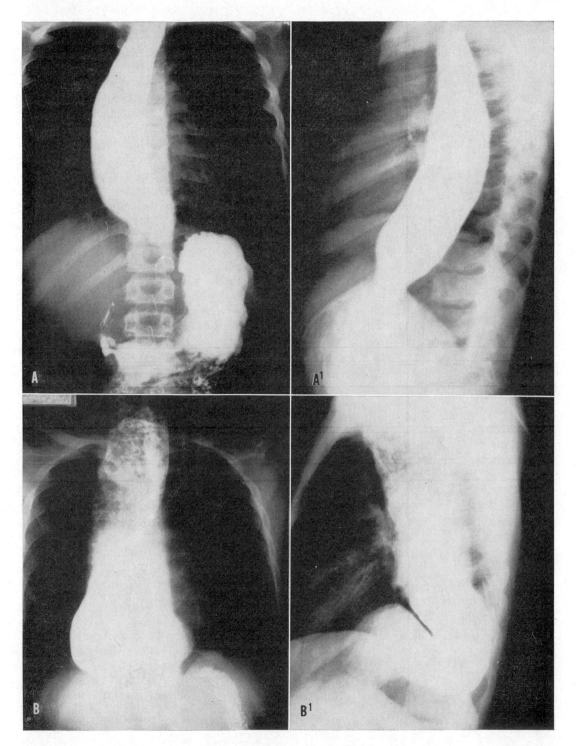

FIG. 61–4.   Contrast radiography in achalasia. *A,A'*, Type I. *B,B'*, Type II with a sigmoid fold of the esophagus.

The diagnosis is based on radiographic findings, esophageal motility studies, esophagoscopy, and the methacholine test. Roentgenograms of the chest may show widening of the mediastinum due to distention of the esophagus. An air fluid level may be seen in the esophagus. Absence of the gastric air bubble is characteristic of achalasia. With a swallow of barium sulfate suspension, the dilatation of the esophagus can be demonstrated (Fig. 61-4). The distal end tapers to form a funnel-shaped pattern with a conelike portion that narrows over a short distance with a beaklike projection into the nonrelaxed portion (type I). As the disease progresses, the esophagus may develop a sigmoid shape and fold on itself posteriorly (type II). In the early stages the radiographic differentiation from carcinoma is difficult. Esophageal motility studies are of interest in that they show slight elevation of pressures in the esophagus due to distention and small increases in pressure throughout the esophagus with swallowing. In contrast to normal function, swallowing does not induce relaxation of the inferior esophageal sphincter. In a few patients, a mass spasm occurs in swallowing, and this peculiarity has been designated vigorous achalasia (Sanderson and coworkers, 1967). Definitive diagnosis requires esophagoscopy to differentiate it from carcinoma and to rule out the fairly frequent development of carcinoma in achalasia.

Cholinomimetic drugs, such as methacholine, in small doses produce exaggerated responses in the esophagus in achalasia, apparently because of the lack of cholinergic innervation (Cannon's law of denervation) (Hightower and coworkers). Small doses produce a strong contraction, which may be painful but not effective in emptying the esophagus.

Medical treatment of achalasia has not been effective. Sedation before meals and tranquil eating conditions may be helpful. Local anesthetics in the esophagus have not produced desired results. Anticholinergic and cholinolytic drugs would be expected to aggravate the basic problem but are of no practical value anyway. Amyl nitrite does relax the smooth muscle of the esophagogastric sphincter but is of no real help clinically.

Two forms of treatment are in current use: dilatation and esophagomyotomy. Dilatation has been carried out in a number of different ways. Dilatation may be performed with woven bougies of the Jackson type at the initial diagnostic esophagoscopy if no significant mucosal lesion is found. Subsequently the use of mercury-filled bougies of the Hurst or Maloney type may prove effective. Often only with forceful dilatation with the Tucker pneumatic mercury bougies under fluoroscopic guidance is significant relief obtained. After forceful dilatation, relief may last for short or long periods of time, but most patients require monthly dilatations. The risk is considerable with mechanical, hydrostatic, or pneumatic dilatation (Sanderson and coworkers, 1970). Iatrogenic perforation eventually occurs in 2 to 4% of patients, and death occurs in one half of these. Since dilatation must be repeated frequently and involves risk, esophagomyotomy, introduced by Heller in 1913, for the treatment of achalasia, has steadily gained in popularity. It is now carried out through a thoracic approach, and a longitudinal incision is made through the muscular layers from the stomach to well above the site of narrowing. Although the procedure is occasionally complicated by reflux esophagitis which may go on to stricture formation, most patients are greatly benefitted by the procedure. A trial with dilatation is appropriate except in children and in the adult with a tortuous, greatly dilated esophagus or vigorous achalasia.

Diffuse Spasm of the Esophagus

Diffuse spasm of the esophagus is characterized by pain rather than dysphagia. The pain is substernal and may be severe. It tends to radiate to the back, neck, shoulders, and arms and to mimic cardiac pain. It may occur under tension, while eating, or during sleep. Patients with diffuse spasm of the esophagus tend to be tense and depressed. Patients with this condition are usually past middle life, and it is more common in men than women. The diagnosis may be elusive because the spasm may not be present during radiographic or esophageal motility studies. The radiographic picture with contrast material has been described as the corkscrew esophagus, curling of the esophagus, pseudomuscular hypertrophy, and pseudodiverticulosis. The spasm is more prominent in the lower one third of the esophagus. The degree of spasm may vary from point to point and produce the picture of an irregular string of beads. The contractions may be repetitive and prolonged. Occasionally barium may be propelled proximally, and this phenomenon has been termed the elevator esophagus.

The esophagogastric sphincter does not produce obstruction in diffuse spasm of the esophagus, and it behaves normally in response to distention and deglutition (Code and coworkers).

Treatment should emphasize explanation and reassurance. Sedation, nitrites, and amphetamines are helpful.

Esophageal Varices

Esophageal varices result from hypertension in the portal venous system. Intrahepatic obstructive diseases account for more than 90% of patients with portal hypertension. Portal cirrhosis secondary to chronic alcoholism is the most common cause of intrahepatic obstructive disease, and cirrhosis has become the eighth most common cause of death in the United States. Other causes of intrahepatic obstruction include posthepatitis cirrhosis, biliary cirrhosis, Wilson's disease, neoplasms, and schistosomiasis. Extrahepatic causes of portal hypertension include portal vein thrombosis, congenital atresia and stenosis, and extrinsic pressure.

Increased pressure in the valveless portal vein produces enlargement of collateral circulation. Esophageal varices develop through shunting of blood through the right and left gastric (coronary) veins to the esophageal veins (Fig. 61-5). The esophageal veins become huge in the submucosa of the distal end of the esophagus. Rupture of these veins produces massive, difficult to control bleeding. Bleeding from esophageal varices is the most common cause of death from upper gastrointestinal bleeding.

Esophageal varices produce one symptom, bleeding, which may be manifest by hematemesis or melena. In patients with cirrhosis and portal hypertension, the presence of varices suggests that the bleeding is from the varices. The upper gastrointestinal series with a barium sulfate suspension is a safe and reliable means of demonstrating esophageal varices. Esophageal varices produce smooth but irregular indentations of the esophageal lumen extending as high as the middle one third of the esophagus (Fig.

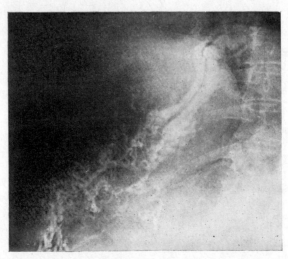

FIG. 61–5.   Splenoportogram which demonstrates the collateral circulation to the esophageal varices.

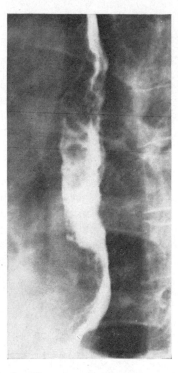

Fɪɢ. 61–6.   Contrast radiography which demonstrates extensive esophageal varices.

61-6). Barium contrast studies of the stomach and duodenum also help differentiate varices from other causes of upper gastrointestinal bleeding. Information gained by esophagogastroscopy ensures the most accurate diagnosis (Conn and coworkers, 1967). It is often difficult to differentiate mucosal folds from varices, and there is considerable observer variation in the endoscopic diagnosis of esophageal varices (Conn and coworkers, 1965). Varices appear as compressible, mucosa-covered, smooth masses, often with little color variation from surrounding mucosa. Esophagoscopy with the flexible panendoscope is the best means of determining whether the varices are actually bleeding. Esophagogastroscopy is the only reliable method of establishing the diagnosis of hemorrhagic gastritis or the uncommon Mallory-Weiss syndrome.

Steps to correct shock by blood and fluid replacement must be taken before radiographic studies and esophagogastroscopy are undertaken.

The bleeding may be controlled by the use of esophageal balloon tamponade, and this control is considered presumptive evidence that the esophageal varices are the sites of bleeding. This approach has always been open to question and is not relied upon as much as esophagoscopy. The Sengstaken-Blakemore triple-lumen, double-balloon tube is fairly effective. The distal spherical balloon is inflated and pulled against the diaphragm with mild continuous traction. The long cylindrical balloon is inflated to compress the varices in the distal esophagus. The central lumen is used to irrigate the stomach for the removal of blood and monitoring the degree of control of the hemorrhage. Other nonoperative approaches include intravenous posterior pituitary extract and esophagogastric hypothermia. Posterior pituitary extract reduces portal hypertension and blood flow by constricting the splanchnic arterioles. The rationale for esophagogastric hypothermia is that it reduces the digestive activity of the gastric juice and reduces gastric blood flow. These nonoperative techniques do not appear to influence the mortality rate of bleeding from esophageal varices and have been used mainly as temporizing measures to allow preparation of the patient for a portacaval shunt. Since two thirds to three fourths of patients managed in this fashion die before coming to a portacaval shunt, there has been considerable recent enthusiasm for emergency surgery. Two forms of emergency surgery have been advocated: transesophageal varix ligation and emergency portacaval shunt. Both operations are effective in stopping bleeding, but both frequently result in hepatic decompensation. Transesophageal varix ligation must be followed later by an elective portacaval shunt to prevent subsequent hemorrhages. Transesophageal varix ligation and emergency portacaval shunt each result in a survival rate from the initial hemorrhage of approximately 50%. Since the 5-year survival is approximately 40% with emergency portacaval shunts and approximately 20% with transesophageal varix ligation, emergency portacaval shunts have been favored (Orloff).

Scleroderma

Scleroderma is a progressive chronic disease of unknown etiology which results in diffuse sclerosis of the connective tissue of the skin and other organs. Its peak incidence is in the third and fourth decades. It is twice as common in women as men. Initially there may be an inflammatory phase. Collagen throughout the body becomes hypertrophic and dense. The epidermis and its appendages atrophy. It is associated with Raynaud's phenomenon and polyarthritis. There may be diffuse calcinosis, and pulmonary cysts and fibrosis occur. Renal and cardiac involvement are associated with a poor prognosis.

The esophagus, small intestine, and colon become involved in approximately 20% of patients with scleroderma. Dense fibrous tissue replaces the smooth muscle, and motor disturbances, dilation, and stricture formation develop. The esophagus becomes stiff, peristalsis diminishes, and there may be reflux of gastric contents leading to esophagitis and distal narrowing.

The symptoms of esophageal involvement are dysphagia, regurgitation, and substernal pain. The diagnosis is based on the general manifestations of the disease. The esophageal involvement can be demonstrated and monitored with upper gastrointestinal contrast radiography and esophageal motility studies (Brindley) (Fig. 61-7).

Corticosteroid therapy is of value in controlling the initial inflammatory stage but is not of value in the chronic state. Esophageal dilatation is of value in patients with strictures but is hazardous. The rigidity of the esophagus requires that great care be taken in performing esophagoscopy and dilatation.

Dermatomyositis

Dermatomyositis is a rare disease with similarities to scleroderma. It produces polymyositis and cutaneous changes. Scleroderma and systemic lupus erythematosus with chronic skin changes may simulate dermatomyositis. Of all the so-called collagen diseases, the incidence of dysphagia is highest in dermatomyositis. Sixty to 80% of patients with dermatomyositis complain of it. The sensation of dysphagia is referred to the pharynx. Radiography of the upper gastrointestinal tract with contrast material demonstrates diminished or absent peristalsis and frequent aspiration. Esophageal motility studies also demonstrate a lack of peristaltic activity, but the inferior sphincter protects effectively against reflux of gastric contents. The similarity of the radiographic and esophageal motility findings makes the differential diagnosis from scleroderma difficult (Donaghue and coworkers). Stiffening of the esophagus is a less prominent feature of dermatomyositis, and ulcerative esophagitis and stricture formation are less common than in scleroderma. The dysphagia in dermatomyositis is apparently due to the degree of myositis and is improved with corticosteroid therapy.

Esophageal Neoplasms

Benign neoplasms of the esophagus are very rare compared to malignant ones. Less than 1% of esophageal neoplasms are benign. They include leiomyoma, lipoma, hemangioma, and papilloma. Of these, the leiomyoma is the most common and has a 3 to 1 male to female incidence. The majority of these tumors arise in the inferior one

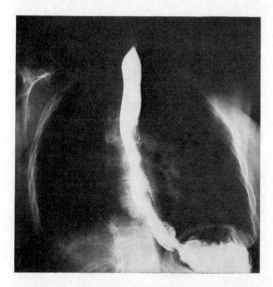

FIG. 61-7. Contrast radiography of the esophagus in scleroderma showing dilatation.

third of the esophagus and occur before the fifth decade. Dysphagia, regurgitation, and aspiration may occur. A smooth filling defect or later the appearance of extrinsic compression can be found on contrast radiography of the esophagus. They may contain calcification. At esophagoscopy the mass is mobile and covered with normal mucosa. With large lesions extrinsic compression may occur. Biopsy under these circumstances is inadvisable (Sweet and coworkers). These tumors may be excised at thoracotomy without incising the mucosa.

Lipomas appear as polypoid intraluminal lesions and produce dysphagia, regurgitation, and aspiration. An intraluminal filling defect on contrast radiography of the esophagus is characteristic, and endoscopic resection is very satisfactory.

Hemangiomas of the esophagus are very rare. They may bleed. Localized resection has been the treatment of choice in the past for bleeding hemangiomas, but corticosteroid therapy would be expected to produce satisfactory regression of these lesions. Papillomas may be removed endoscopically. Granular cell myoblastomas also occur in the esophagus and can be resected conservatively at thoracotomy (Farrell and coworkers).

Squamous cell carcinoma is the predominant primary malignant neoplasm of the esophagus. Although adenocarcinomas occur in the lower one third of the esophagus, they are most often the result of superior invasion from a primary neoplasm of the stomach. Leiomyosarcomas and the still more rare rhabdomyosarcomas occur in the young.

Squamous cell carcinoma of the esophagus is more common in South Africa, China, Japan, Puerto Rico, Russia, and the Dutch West Indies than in the United States. In the United States it is more frequent in blacks than in Caucasians, particularly in the lower socioeconomic groups. Possible etiologic factors include hot liquids, hot, spicy, and coarse foods; strong alcoholic beverages; cigarette, cigar, and pipe smoking; and excessive ethanol intake. Predisposing conditions include achalasia, hiatus hernia, caustic and other strictures, and the Plummer-Vinson syndrome. Carcinoma of the esophagus is rare before 40 years of age, with the highest incidence in the seventh decade. It is far more common in men than women, except that carcinoma of the cervical esophagus is more common in women than men in those areas where the Plummer-Vinson syndrome is common. Esophageal carcinoma accounts for 1% of cancer deaths in women and 4% of cancer deaths in men in the United States.

Carcinoma occurs more frequently in the middle one third and the lower one third of the esophagus than in the upper one third. This neoplasm may present as a hard intraluminal mass or as an infiltrating process that produces widespread rigidity of the esophagus and surrounding structures. Metastasis occurs to regional lymph nodes, supraclavicular and celiac lymph nodes, the liver, lungs, and bones. Esophageal carcinoma produces dysphagia for solid foods at first and then for liquids. The dysphagia is usually accompanied by weight loss. Cough may result from regurgitation and aspiration or direct invasion of the tracheobronchial tree by the tumor. Recurrent laryngeal nerve paralysis is a frequent finding.

The diagnosis is suspected when the radiographic contrast study of the esophagus demonstrates a filling defect, ulceration, interference with peristalsis, abrupt narrowing of the lumen, and dilatation superior to the narrowing (Fig. 61-8). Esophagoscopy is required to establish the histologic diagnosis and to exclude other possibilities and may be helpful in palliation with the introduction of an indwelling tube (Celestin). Biopsy of the lesion may be difficult when there is considerable narrowing of the lumen by infiltration of the tumor. Inflammatory tissues may overlie the tumor. Biopsy is, of course, not without risk of perforation. Bronchoscopy should be performed in lesions of the upper and middle thirds of the esophagus to rule out tracheobronchial extension of the tumor (Leon and coworkers).

Surgical treatment of patients with carcinoma of the esophagus is discouraging, in part because of the advanced state of the lesion when the diagnosis is established (Leon and coworkers). Radiation therapy is used for palliation, preoperative treatment, and cure. The cure rate is disappointing, but many patients receive effective palliation from radiation therapy. Chemotherapy has not been particularly helpful. Useful palliative measures should be tried in the following order: nasogastric or cervical esophagostomy tube feedings, indwelling esophageal tubes, and gastrostomy. Radiation therapy is complicated by esophagitis, perforation, hemorrhage, stenosis, radiation pneumonitis, and tracheoesophageal or bronchoesophageal fistulas. Relative contraindications to radiation therapy include mediastinitis, tracheal and bronchial involvement or tracheoesophageal or bronchoesophageal fistulas, and extensive distant metastasis.

Carcinoma metastatic from other organs, particularly the breast, involves the esophagus and produces stenosis and dysphagia (Polk and coworkers). Other primary sites are the pharynx, pancreas, testes, prostate, and liver.

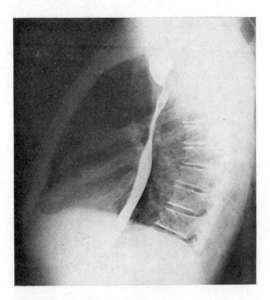

Fig. 61–8. Contrast radiography which demonstrates an annular constriction with sharp, irregular edges due to carcinoma of the upper one third of the esophagus.

Foreign Bodies

The constrictor muscles of the pharynx are very strong and can force large and irregular objects into the esophagus. Since the muscular activity of the upper portion of the esophagus is very weak, foreign bodies are likely to lodge just below the cricopharyngeus muscle. Ninety-five percent of esophageal foreign bodies come to rest in this location. The next most common site is just superior to the esophagogastric junction. Other likely locations are the indentations of the esophagus caused by the arch of the aorta and the left bronchus.

Foreign bodies of the esophagus are common in young children and are likely to occur whenever a child places an inedible object in the mouth. Foreign bodies are also common in the older age group, particularly in edentulous individuals who appear to be less proprioceptive to the presence of bones and other inedible objects in their food. Preexisting esophageal disease, particularly strictures, predisposes to the retention of foreign bodies, and at times food that is not very carefully chewed becomes a foreign body. Coins, campaign buttons, bones, safety pins, toy jacks, plastic toys, and boluses of meat are common foreign bodies.

Foreign bodies of the esophagus can be prevented by careful food preparation, careful chewing, scrutiny of food in the mouth, particularly while eating chicken, fish or pork, not placing inedible objects in the mouth, keeping safety pins closed while not in use, and keeping small inedible objects out of the reach of small children.

Foreign bodies coming to rest just inferior to the cricopharyngeus muscle produce dysphagia and pain in the suprasternal area on swallowing. Rough and sharp foreign bodies may produce an abrasion or laceration of the pharynx or esophagus and pass on through the gastrointestinal tract, in which case the pain on swallowing subsides within 24 hours. Persistent pain on swallowing which the patient localizes to the suprasternal area is very suggestive of a foreign body. Sharp foreign bodies are likely to result in perforation of the esophagus, and perforation may occur initially or toward the end of the 24 hours of the foreign body's sojourn in the esophagus. The longer a foreign body is retained in the esophagus, the more likely perforation of the esophagus will occur. Occasionally the symptoms relative to the esophagus are minimal, and a long indwelling foreign body is discovered in the evaluation of a child with failure to thrive. The presence of a bulky foreign body may produce extrinsic compression of the trachea through its posterior membranous wall, and the patient may present with the symptoms and signs of upper respiratory tract obstruction.

The history is of paramount importance. The patient who presents with a history of the ingestion of an inedible substance places the physician in a position of having to prove whether or not a foreign body is retained. Radiopaque foreign bodies can be identified in many instances with a lateral neck roentgenogram (Fig. 61-9). On this same roentgenogram, radiopaque foreign bodies of the palatine tonsils, lingual tonsils, valleculae, and piriform sinuses can be visualized. Evidence of nonopaque foreign bodies of the esophagus may also be found, such as an increase in the distance between the cervical vertebrae and the larynx and trachea or air in the cervical esophagus. If the foreign body cannot be located on the lateral neck roentgenogram, posterior-

anterior and lateral chest roentgenograms may demonstrate a radiopaque foreign body. If the foreign body cannot be located in this manner, a contrast study of the esophagus with a barium sulfate suspension or a water-miscible radiopaque solution may demonstrate the foreign body. A small pledget of cotton saturated with a radiopaque fluid may hang on a sharp foreign body. If a foreign body can be located without the use of barium sulfate, the subsequent removal is made easier because the presence of flecks of white barium make many small foreign bodies more difficult to see at esophagoscopy.

Often the patient's perception of the sensation of a foreign body persists in spite of a lack of radiographic evidence of a foreign body. The safest course is to exclude the possibility of a foreign body with open esophagoscopy. As mentioned, patients with abrasions or lacerations of the pharynx or esophagus usually become asymptomatic within 24 hours.

There are actually two problems in the patient with a history of ingestion of a foreign body: (1) Has the foreign body been retained in the pharynx or esophagus, or has it passed into the stomach? (2) If it has been retained in the pharynx or esophagus, where is it?

Regarding the first problem, it is general-

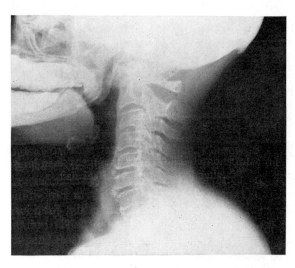

FIG. 61–9.   Lateral neck roentgenogram which demonstrates the vertebra of a fish in the cervical esophagus.

ly true that foreign bodies that reach the stomach will pass through the gastrointestinal tract without difficulty, even in the case of sharp objects such as straight pins and open safety pins. In the child with the history of ingestion of a radiopaque foreign body, a single anterior-posterior roentgenogram which encompasses everything from the base of the skull to the pubis is particularly useful. If the object is radiopaque and can be demonstrated in the stomach radiographically, the patient's stools can be examined by the parent by crushing them for 5 days until the foreign body is recovered. If it has not been recovered in 5 days, another roentgenogram should be obtained to locate the foreign body. If the foreign body is sharp like a straight pin, the progress of the foreign body through the gastrointestinal tract should be followed with daily abdominal roentgenograms. If a sharp foreign body passes beyond the stomach but does not make progress for a day or two, a laparotomy for its removal should be performed. Foreign bodies of the stomach which do not progress, and this situation is likely to occur with foreign bodies that are too long to negotiate the first curve of the duodenum, should be removed with a flexible upper gastrointestinal panendoscope.

Regarding the second problem, the endoscopic removal of a foreign body is much more likely to be safe and successful if the exact location of the foreign body is known prior to esophagoscopy.

A foreign body of the esophagus is removed more safely with an open esophagoscope and under general endotracheal anesthesia. An esophagoscope appropriate for the size of the patient should be used. The oval lumen Jesberg esophagoscopes are particularly useful for foreign body removal. Care must be taken not to override or pass distal to a foreign body. Sharp foreign bodies can be driven through the esophageal wall under these circumstances.

Once the foreign body has been visualized, it is important to avoid any maneuver that might inadvertently displace it distally. Surrounding secretions should be gently suctioned away, and the foreign body should be studied to achieve the best exposure and to determine the best forceps application and the best strategy for removal. Forceps specifically designed for each type of foreign body should be utilized. In general, the distal tip of the esophagoscope should be as close as possible to the foreign body without touching it or without interfering with the space between the distal tip of the esophagoscope and the foreign body needed to apply the forceps appropriate to that foreign body. More room exists for forceps application during inspiration if the patient is initiating his own respiration.

Sharp foreign bodies must be disengaged from the esophageal mucosa prior to withdrawal. In the removal of a sharp foreign body, such as an open safety pin, with its point directed proximally, the foreign body must be displaced distally to disengage it. As a general rule, the point of a sharp foreign body should be ensheathed in the lumen of the esophagoscope for removal. It is often helpful to grasp the shaft near the point, rather than grasping the point, with forceps such as the Tucker tack and pin forceps with side jaws which tend to align the long axis of the foreign body with the long axis of the forceps and esophagoscope. Other ways of removing open safety pins include closing the pin before removal and carrying the pin with rotation forceps distally into the stomach and rotating the pin so that it can be removed with the point trailing.

The forceps should be applied to esophageal foreign bodies under constant visual monitoring. Care must be taken to avoid grasping mucosa between the forceps and the foreign body in order to avoid perforation of the esophagus. As a general rule, esophageal foreign bodies must be withdrawn as a trailing foreign body rather than brought out through the esophagoscope. The removal of a trailing foreign body is carried out by gently withdrawing the foreign body to the level of the esophagoscope and then fixing the relationship of the forceps and the esophagoscope with the thumb and index finger of the left hand, which is also holding the esophagoscope, as the forceps, esophagoscope, and foreign body are removed as one unit. Under these circumstances, the esophagoscope serves as a leading edge to prevent the proximal mucosa from shearing the foreign body from the forceps. Some irregular objects like toy jacks are removed by grasping the knobbed end lightly with ball forceps with cupped jaws and tumbling the jack from one esophageal wall to the next.

After the foreign body has been removed, the esophagus is re-entered to make sure there is no second foreign body and to inspect the esophagus for trauma and predisposing factors such as stenosis. Occasionally whole grapes and other foods are retained as foreign bodies. After the foreign body has been removed, such patients should have upper gastrointestinal contrast studies with cinefluoroscopy to exclude an underlying abnormality of the esophagus.

Forcing the foreign body into the stomach by eating bread and blind removal of cervical esophageal foreign bodies with Foley catheters and other forms of the probang are condemned for the following reasons: foreign bodies are often multiple; a smooth, opaque foreign body may be accompanied by a nonopaque sharp foreign body; esophageal foreign bodies are often associated with previously unrecognized esophageal abnormalities; and safe methods for removal of foreign bodies through open esophagoscopes exist (Ritter). The use of proteolytic enzymes to digest meat foreign bodies has been abandoned because of the mortalities associated with their use (Ritter).

Caustic Ingestion

Ingestion of caustic material usually occurs accidentally in children, but it also occurs in adults who attempt suicide or who are victims of homicide. Basic caustics include sodium hydroxide found in household lye, as in drain cleaners like Drano and Liquid Plumr, sodium carbonate (washing soda), sodium metasilicate (automatic dishwashing powder), and ammonia. Acid caustics include nitric acid, hydrochloric acid, bichloride of mercury, sulfuric acid, silver nitrate, and phenol. Sodium hypochlorite, as found in household chlorine bleach like Clorox at a concentration of 5.2%, has the potential to cause a burn severe enough to result in stricture formation but probably is not a clinically important agent (Hook and Lowry).

Lye and other caustics penetrate tissue deeply and produce liquefaction necrosis that may extend through all layers of the esophagus, depending on the amount and concentration ingested. Acid caustics produce a coagulation necrosis which tends to limit the deep penetration of the acid. Nevertheless, strong acids produce severe burns that result in severe strictures. Initially the burn may demonstrate hyperemia, erosion, ulceration, or perforation. The luminal surface changes in the esophagus are very prominent by 24 hours. In burns in which ulceration occurs, repair by the formation of granulation tissue occurs, and the phase during which granulation tissue lines the lumen of the esophagus may last for 2 to 3 weeks or longer. Circumferential scarring and subsequent scar contracture become apparent from 3 to 6 weeks following the cautic ingestion and continue for several weeks or months thereafter.

Lye is ingested as granules and in liquid form. Granular lye left in the reach of a small child or spilled on the floor is dangerous because an infant or child old enough to pick up the granules may sustain a very severe burn from ingestion of just one granule. Liquid caustics placed in familiar containers like soft drink bottles are particularly tempting to youngsters. Prevention depends on proper storing and handling of these ubiquitous and powerful substances. New parents must be made aware of the need to baby-proof their homes by either doing without these caustics or storing and controlling them with great care. Parents must also be aware of the danger of allowing a toddler to run unsupervised in a home in which young children do not live and in which proper precautions have not been taken. Disposal of these agents by workmen and others in residential areas is another source of grief. These agents should be packaged in containers with child-proof caps.

Characteristically youngsters with ingestion of corrosive agents present with burns of the lips and oral cavity and are drooling and refuse to accept food or fluids. There may be burns of the hands, and they should be washed thoroughly to avoid burns of the eyes. Antidotes are not effective and may induce vomiting; therefore, they should be avoided. Fever and substernal or abdominal pain are ominous signs of possible perforation. Laryngeal burns may result in sufficient upper respiratory obstruction to require a tracheotomy.

The correlation between the degree of burn of the lips, oral cavity, and pharynx and the esophageal burn is poor. There may be no burns of the lips, mouth, and pharynx and yet a massive burn of the esophagus. Likewise, severe oral cavity and pharyngeal burns may occur without esophageal burns.

In the first 24 hours after caustic ingestion, the patient should be supported with parenteral fluids and observed for mediastinitis, tracheoesophageal fistula, gastric perforation, peritonitis, pneumonia, and laryngeal edema. At approximately 24 hours after the burn, esophagoscopy under general endotracheal anesthesia should be performed to determine if there is a burn of the esophagus (Cardona and Daly). If a burn is encountered, the esophagoscopy is terminated, and no attempt is made to pass the burned area with the esophagoscope for fear of perforating the esophagus. If no burn is found at esophagoscopy, the patient may be discharged from the hospital, usually in 2 or 3 days, as soon as the oral and pharyngeal burns heal sufficiently to allow an adequate oral intake of fluid. If a burn is encountered at esophagoscopy, a small polyethylene nasogastric tube should be inserted for feeding and maintenance of the esophageal lumen. Corticosteroid therapy should be initiated and continued for 6 weeks, and a broad-spectrum antibiotic such as ampicillin should be given until the radiographic contrast studies of the esophagus demonstrate that the mucosa has healed. An esophagogram should be performed at 3 weeks. Once the patient is able to swallow liquids, usually 3 to 4 days after the burn, the antibiotic is given orally for its topical effect in the area of granulation tissue. Liquids by mouth are allowed, but food containing particulate matter which might be retained in the granulation tissue is withheld until there is con-

trast radiographic evidence of mucosal healing. The next esophagogram is performed for any clinical indication and routinely at 6 weeks. If evidence of stricture formation is present after the corticosteroid therapy has been terminated, bouginage is started. In severe burns, the feeding tube is not removed until the risk of stricture formation is passed. A feeding tube or string must be kept in the patient with a developing stricture to prevent the complete loss of the lumen.

In 1920, Salzer introduced early bouginage in the treatment of caustic burns of the esophagus. In the first few days after the burn, bouginage is initiated and continued for weeks or months (Salzer). It is not thought to be safe to combine this method with corticosteroid therapy. In animal experiments, the combination of corticosteroids and dilatation after a burn results in a high mortality rate (Haller and Backman). The Salzer method gained considerable popularity in the past because of the high percentage of successful results. The efficacy of this method of treatment was based on the low rate of stricture formation in patients who had not had esophagoscopic confirmation of a burn.

Patients with corrosive strictures of the esophagus may be managed with dilatation or reconstruction of the esophagus. Dilatation may be accomplished with prograde mechanical methods, the retrograde mechanical method of Tucker, and the hydrostatic method with mercury-filled bougies. With short single strictures, the first dilatation is appropriately carried out in a prograde fashion with woven bougies of the Jackson type passed through the esophagoscope. If this method works well, subsequent dilatations may be performed with Maloney's mercury-filled bougies on a regular weekly or biweekly basis, the ultimate plan being to increase the diameter and the interval between dilatations. In more difficult strictures, injection of triamcinolone diacetate into the stricture followed by immediate dilatation has proved helpful (Mendelsohn and Maloney).

In patients with more severe and extensive corrosive strictures of the esophagus, retrograde dilatation with Tucker bougies is safer and more effective (Tucker). The Tucker bougie is made of soft rubber that is tapered at each end and surrounds a cord which runs the length of the bougie and is looped at each end. This method requires a gastrostomy and consists essentially of drawing the bougies from the stomach through the esophagus and out of the mouth. In order to establish a loop through the esophagus, strong silk suture (No. 2) is passed through the left nasal cavity and into the pharynx. It is swallowed over a 24-hour period, and the distal end is recovered from the stomach through the gastrostomy. The two ends are tied together under the clothing, and the loop of silk is maintained between dilatations. At the time of dilatation, a bougie and a new silk suture are attached to the old silk at the gastrostomy. The silk in the pharynx is brought out of the mouth. The traction of the silk suture is made within the mouth in the long axis of the esophagus to avoid trauma to the epiglottis and base of the tongue. The bougies are drawn up through the stricture in tandem. The force used in pulling the bougie decreases the diameter of the bougie. Each one is left in the area of the stricture for a brief period so that it is allowed to return to its original diameter and exert its maximum dilating effect. The new silk suture is drawn through the nose and tied under the clothing to the end coming out of the gastrostomy so that the loop of silk will be ready for the next dilatation. The dilatation may be repeated as frequently as necessary, and the interval varies from a week to a month or more, depending on the stricture's behavior.

Patients with extensive persistent strictures that do not respond to Tucker retrograde bouginage are candidates for a colonic bypass procedure. The right side of the colon with an attached segment of terminal ilium may be brought through a retrosternal tunnel, and the ilium is anastomosed to the cervical esophagus.

Carcinoma of the esophagus occurs far more frequently in individuals with lye strictures than in the general population. The diagnosis is often very difficult due to the associated scarring and inaccessibility of the lesion for biopsy.

Esophagogastric Junction

The normal pressure relationships of the lower esophagus and stomach favor gastroesophageal reflux. The pressure in the stomach is above atmospheric pressure, and the pressure within the esophagus is below atmospheric pressure. The anatomic basis for the lower esophageal sphincter has been elusive, but the physiologic existence of the sphincter is well established. A high intraluminal pressure zone extends over approximately 3.5 cm at the level of the diaphragm. A pressure inversion point (PIP) is located at the level of the diaphragm. Above that point, intraluminal pressure decreases with inspiration, and below that point intraluminal pressure increases with inspiration. The pressure in the PIP is higher than that in the stomach or esophagus, and this high pressure zone is the lower esophageal sphincter. After deglutition as the peristaltic wave passes downward, the pressure in the high pressure zone falls precipitously.

Diaphragmatic Hernia

Diaphragmatic hernias are divided into sliding or hiatal and paraesophageal or parahiatal hernias. Sliding hernias result in movement of the esophagogastric junction above the diaphragm and are often associated with reflux of gastric contents into the esophagus. In paraesophageal hernias, the esophagogastric junction remains at the level of the diaphragm, and there is no incompetence of the sphincter. Sliding hernias are much more common than paraesophageal hernias. Paraesophageal hernias develop more frequently in the elderly than in the young.

The defect in paraesophageal hernias is in the esophageal hiatus to the left of the esophagus. The hernia sac and fundus of the stomach pass into the thorax. On eating, the thoracic stomach becomes distended and produces pain. Patients reduce their food intake to avoid the pain and lose weight. Incarceration can occur with ne-

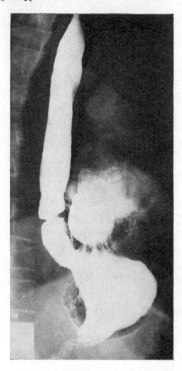

FIG. 61–10. Contrast radiography of a paraesophageal hernia.

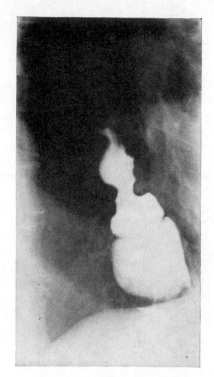

FIG. 61–11. Contrast radiography of a hiatal hernia.

crosis and perforation. The diagnosis is made with upper gastrointestinal contrast radiography (Fig. 61-10). The thoracic stomach fills readily. Even on a chest roentgenogram, the diagnosis may be suggested by gas in the thoracic stomach above the diaphragm. The hernia ring may be repaired after reduction of the hernia through an abdominal approach. The results of this surgery are excellent.

Sliding hiatal hernias result from weakness of the phrenoesophageal ligament, and the esophagogastric junction, cardiac portion of the stomach, and peritoneum move superiorly through the esophageal hiatus of the diaphragm (Fig. 61-11). With inflammation and scarring, the sliding nature of the hernia may be lost, and the cardiac portion of the stomach may become fixed above the diaphragm. This situation is associated with a shortened esophagus. Hiatal hernias as such probably do not cause symptoms but are related to peptic esophagitis if there is reflux of gastric contents.

Peptic Esophagitis

Reflux of gastric contents into the esophagus contributes to the development of an inflammatory reaction in the esophageal mucous membrane which may proceed to ulceration and stricture formation. The relationship of sliding hiatal hernias to the reflux of gastric contents remains unclear. The frequency of occurrence of hiatal hernias in probably one quarter of the population far exceeds the frequency of reflux of gastric contents. Even in patients with hiatal hernia, the incidence of reflux of gastric contents is less than 30%. The uncertainty regarding the roles of hiatal hernia, gastric reflux, and peptic esophagitis is compounded by the fact that reflux of gastric contents does not necessarily produce symptoms or esophagitis in normals or those with esophagogastric incompetence. The presence of a short esophagus had been stressed in the past as an etiologic factor in peptic esophagitis, but a short esophagus is usually the result of chronic esophagitis. Very rarely a true congenital short esophagus occurs in infancy and is associated with a nonsliding hiatal hernia, regurgitation, hemorrhage, and stricture formation. There is a strong relationship between duodenal ulcer and peptic esophagitis. Peptic esophagitis occurs in roughly 30% of patients with peptic ulcers, and peptic ulcers occur in 16% of patients with peptic esophagitis (McHardy). Both conditions can be thought of as a part of the peptic diathesis. Peptic esophagitis does not appear to be related to ulcerative colitis or Crohn's disease.

The early changes in peptic esophagitis are limited to the epithelium and lamina propria. Leukocyte and plasma cell infiltration, edema, and hyperemia increase the thickness of the lamina propria. Epithelial erosion, pseudomembranous formation, and ulceration penetrating into the muscularis occur in the more advanced stage. Finally, fibrosis and acanthosis of the surface epithelium become prominent as the stricture forms. Deep ulceration is frequently referred to as Barrett's ulcer and tends to occur in areas of the distal esophagus lined with columnar epithelium. It is not clear whether the presence of columnar epithelium

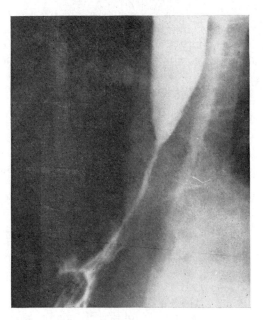

FIG. 61–12. Contrast radiography which shows a stricture of the lower one third of the esophagus due to peptic esophagitis.

in the esophagus is a congenital anomaly or an acquired condition.

The symptoms of peptic esophagitis are dysphagia, substernal pain or heartburn, and regurgitation or water brash. The heartburn is aggravated by stress, spicy foods, alcoholic beverages, vomiting, leaning forward, and nasogastric intubation.

The diagnosis of peptic esophagitis is confirmed by changes in the contrast radiography of the lower esophagus, such as erosion or ulceration, spasm, and narrowing, as well as the often associated hiatal hernia and reflux of gastric contents (Fig. 61-12). Esophagoscopy is required to establish the diagnosis and exclude other causes. Characteristically the mucosa is red and friable and bleeds easily, and there may be patches of gray-white fibrinous exudate.

Treatment should consist of a bland diet with frequent small feedings, antacids at frequent intervals, and postural instruction, which should include sitting erect during meals, avoiding postprandial recumbency for 2 hours, no food at bedtime, and elevation of the head of the bed with shock blocks. Stricture formation is satisfactorily managed with bouginage at esophagoscopy initially followed by hydrostatic bouginage with the Maloney mercury-filled bougies. Since the stricture tends to be limited to the lamina propria, the results of bouginage are more satisfactory than in the corrosive strictures where the muscular layers of the esophagus are involved.

Surgical repair of sliding hiatal hernias requires transabdominal repair of the diaphragmatic crura and closure of the angle of His by suturing the fundus of the stomach to the left lateral border of the esophagus. In patients with coexistent peptic ulcer and gastric hypersecretion, vagotomy and pyloroplasty may be performed at the same time. A transthoracic approach is required in those patients with a shortened esophagus. Another surgical approach to peptic esophagitis is the fundoplication of Nissen, in which the fundus of the stomach is wrapped completely around the distal esophagus and sutured on the right side of the esophagus (Nissen and Rossetti). The high intraluminal gastric pressure compresses the esphagus and prevents reflux of gastric contents. Disadvantages of this procedure, which is very effective in eliminating peptic esophagitis, are interference with emptying of the esophagus in the first few months requiring dilatation in some, feeling of fullness after meals, distention, increased borborygmi, increased passage of flatus, and inability to eructate or vomit.

Several Miscellaneous Conditions

In 1929 Mallory and Weiss described massive upper gastrointestinal bleeding due to a longitudinal tear through or below the esophagogastric junction following alcoholic binges. Retching characteristically precedes the hematemesis. The differential diagnosis includes esophageal varices, hemorrhagic gastritis, and peptic ulcer. Another form of emetogenic injury is the Boerhaave syndrome of spontaneous rupture of the esophagus.

Cushing ulcers or stress ulcers following intracranial trauma or extensive burns may also occur in the esophagus and can bleed or perforate and result in mediastinitis.

The Plummer-Vinson syndrome (Paterson-Kelly syndrome or sideropenic dysphagia) is a confusing association of dysphagia, iron deficiency anemia, upper esophageal webs, glossitis, cheilitis, spoon-shaped, brittle fingernails, splenomegaly, and a 10% incidence of postcricoid and oral cavity carcinoma. It tends to occur in older edentulous women of Scandinavian or Irish heritage. Not all patients have all of the findings, and the syndrome probably describes a broad range of related conditions. Treatment consists of administration of iron and vitamins and esophageal dilatation.

Congenital webs of the esophagus occur more commonly in the middle third of the esophagus but may also occur in the upper and lower thirds (Fig. 61-13). In the vast majority of such patients, dilatation is a satisfactory form of treatment.

The lower esophageal ring of Schatzki is believed to cause dysphagia in older people, although the majority of patients with nar-

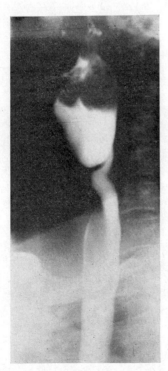

FIG. 61-13. Contrast radiography of a congenital web of the upper one third of the esophagus.

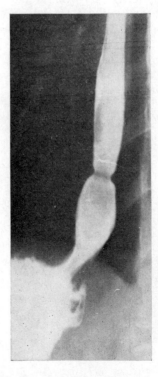

FIG. 61-14. Contrast radiography of a Schatzki ring.

rowing of the esophagus a few centimeters above the esophagogastric junction are asymptomatic (Fig. 61-14). This radiographic finding occurs in 6% of patients examined with contrast studies of the upper gastrointestinal tract. There is no anatomic, pathologic, or endoscopic correlate to this radiographic finding. Dysphagia on the basis of this ring is relieved by peroral bouginage (Postlethwait and Sealy).

Strictures of the esophagus have occurred in patients with epidermolysis bullosa dystrophica and benign mucous membrane pemphigoid (Schild and coworkers; Minkin and coworkers).

COMPLICATIONS OF ESOPHAGOSCOPY

The two major complications of esophagoscopy are bleeding and perforation. Bleeding is likely to follow biopsy or dilatation. It can be of sufficient magnitude to require replacement of blood. Preoperative evaluation of the blood coagulability should include platelet count, prothrombin time, and partial thromboplastin time to avoid esophagoscopy in the presence of an uncontrolled bleeding tendency.

Vulnerable areas for perforation during esophagoscopy are the hypopharynx just above the cricopharyngeus muscle, the cervical esophagus, and proximal to the esophagogastric junction. The hypopharynx and cervical esophagus are likely to be perforated during introduction of the open esophagoscope by impinging the distal tip of the esophagoscope onto the cervical vertebrae. The esophagus just above the esophagogastric junction is likely to be injured because of difficulty in determining the course of the esophagus, particularly when there is a hiatal hernia, short esophagus, stricture, or achalasia. Occasionally when the esophagoscope touches the diaphragm, violent movement of the diaphragm may cause perforation of the esophagus. Most perforations of the esophagus are associated with foreign body removal and disease of the esophagus which makes it more vulnerable to perforation. Perforation may occur with biopsy of the esophagus because of its thin wall and with dilatation. All types of dilatation carry the risk of perforation. Although bouginage through an esophagoscope under direct vision with mechanical dilators is rarely associated with perforation, it is always a possibility, particularly if the stricture is near the esophagogastric junction. Pneumatic dilatation is relatively risky. Hydrostatic dilatation with the mercury-filled rubber bougies of the Hurst and Maloney

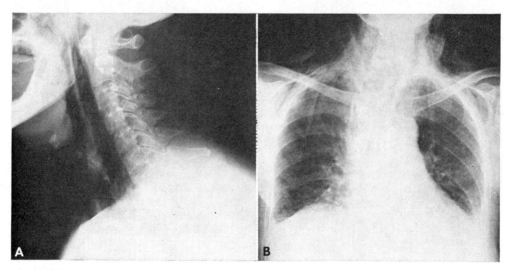

Fig. 61–15. Roentgenograms of a patient with perforation of the esophagus which demonstrate mediastinal and subcutaneous emphysema. *A,* Lateral view of neck. *B,* Posterior-anterior view of chest.

types is usually safe in the patient who has recently had mechanical dilatation through the esophagoscope without difficulty. They cannot be used safely in a patient whose problem has not been studied endoscopically. Although retrograde bouginage is safer than other methods in multiple and extensive strictures, this method can result in perforation by splitting of the esophagus longitudinally if used too aggressively.

Perforation of the esophagus usually makes itself manifest within 24 hours after esophagoscopy. It is prudent to prevent the patient from taking anything by mouth and to maintain him on intravenous fluids until one is fairly sure perforation has not occurred.

Perforation of the cervical esophagus and hypopharynx is characterized by steady pain and tenderness in the neck. Swelling and subcutaneous crepitus can be palpated. The subcutaneous emphysema can also be demonstrated radiographically. Subsequently the infection extends into the mediastinum. Treatment includes high intravenous doses of broad-spectrum antibiotics, such as ampicillin, and exploration and drainage of the paraesophageal area through a low transverse cervical incision. Repair of the perforation is usually not feasible.

Perforations of the thoracic esophagus are more serious and are characterized by high fever, tachycardia, hypotension, pain in the chest radiating to the back, tenderness on sternal pressure, and subcutaneous emphysema in the neck. Chest roentgenograms will demonstrate mediastinal widening and emphysema and unilateral or bilateral pleural effusion (Fig. 61-15). Water-miscible contrast media may be given to define the exact point of perforation. Thoracotomy and drainage of the mediastinum are essential. In early injuries, the esophagus may be repaired. The patient should be maintained on hyperalimentation and given nothing my mouth. The mortality associated with nonoperative management of perforation of the esophagus has repeatedly been shown to be greater than that in patients in whom early drainage of the mediastinum has been carried out (Palmer and Wirts).

REFERENCES

Blakely, W. R., et al.: Section of the Cricopharyngeus Muscle for Dysphagia. Arch. Surg., 96:745, 1968.

Brindley, G. V.: Neuromuscular Disorders of the Esophagus. Surg. Clin. North Am., 52: 319, 1972.

Cardona, J. C., and Daly, J. F.: Current Management of Corrosive Esophagitis. Ann. Otol., 80:521, 1971.

Cassella, R. R., et al.: Achalasia of the Esophagus: Pathologic and Etiologic Considerations. Ann. Surg., 160:474, 1964.

Celestin, L. R.: Permanent Intubation in Inoperable Cancer of the Oesophagus and Cardia: A New Tube. Ann. R. Coll. Surg. Engl., 25:165, 1959.

Code, C.F., et al.: An Atlas of Esophageal Motility in Health and Disease. Springfield, Ill., Charles C Thomas, Publisher, 1958.

Conn, H. O., et al.: Observer Variation in Endoscopic Diagnosis of Esophageal Varices. New Engl. J. Med., 272:830, 1965.

Conn, H. O., et al.: Fiberoptic and Conventional Esophagoscopy in the Diagnosis of Esophageal Varices. Gastroenterology, 52: 810, 1967.

Cross, F. S., et al.: Esophageal Diverticula. Associated Neuromuscular Changes in the Esophagus. Arch. Surg., 83:525, 1961.

Dohlman, G., and Mattsson, O.: The Endoscopic Operation for Hypopharyngeal Diverticula. Arch. Otolaryngol., 71:744, 1960.

Donaghue, F. E., et al.: Esophageal Defects in Dermatomyositis. Ann. Otol., 69:1139, 1960.

Ellis, F. H., et al.: Cricopharyngeal Myotomy for Pharyngoesophageal Diverticulum. Ann. Surg., 170:340, 1969.

Farrell, K. H., et al.: Granular Cell Myoblastoma of the Esophagus: Incidence and Surgical Treatment. Ann. Otol., 82:784, 1973.

Garlock, J. H., and Richter, R.: Carcinoma in a Pharyngo-esophageal Diverticulum: A Case Report. Ann. Surg., 154:259, 1961.

Haller, J. A., and Backman, K.: The Comparative Effect of Current Therapy on Experimental Caustic Burns of the Esophagus. Pediatrics, 34:236, 1964.

Heller, E.: Extramuköse Cardioplastik beim chronischen Cardiospasmus mit Dilatation des Oesophagus. Mitt. Grenzgeb. Med. Chir. 27:141, 1913.

Hightower, N. C., et al.: A Comparison of Effects of Acetyl-beta-methyl-choline Chloride (Mecholyl) on Esophageal Intraluminal

Pressure in Normal Persons and Patients with Cardiospasm. Gastroenterology, 26:592, 1954.

Holinger, P. H., and Schild, J. A.: Zenker's (Hypopharyngeal) Diverticulum. Ann. Otol. Rhinol. Laryngol., 78:679, 1969.

Hook, C. T., and Lowry, L. D.: Effect of Chlorine Bleach on the Esophagus: A Review and Study. Ann. Otol., 83:709, 1974.

Kaplan, S.: Paralysis of Deglutition; Postpoliomyelitis Complication Treated by Section of Cricopharyngeus Muscle. Ann. Surg., 133:572, 1951.

Köberle, F.: Megaesophagus. Gastroenterology, 34:460, 1958.

Leon, W., et al.: Carcinoma of the Esophagus. Ann. Thorac. Surg., 11:583, 1971.

McHardy, G.: Reflux Esophagitis. Ann. Otol., 81:761, 1972.

Mendelsohn, H. J., and Maloney, W. H.: The Treatment of Benign Strictures of the Esophagus with Cortisone Injection. Ann. Otol., 79:900, 1970.

Minkin, W., et al.: Esophageal Stenosis in Benign Mucous Membrane Pemphigoid. Ann. Otol., 82:384, 1973.

Nissen, R., and Rossetti, M.: Surgery of the Cardia Ventricule. CIBA Symposium, 11: 195, 1963.

Orloff, M. J.: Emergency Portacaval Shunt: A Comparative Study of Shunt, Varix Ligation and Non-surgical Treatment of Bleeding Esophageal Varices in Unselected Patients with Cirrhosis. Ann. Surg., 166:456, 1967.

Palmer, E. D., and Wirts, C. W.: Survey of Gastroscopic and Esophagoscopic Accidents. J.A.M.A., 164:2010, 1957.

Polk, H. C., et al.: Dysphagia and Esophageal

Stenosis: Manifestations of Metastatic Mammary Cancer. Cancer, 20:2009, 1967.

Postlethwait, R. W., and Sealy, W. C.: Experiences with the Treatment of 59 Patients with Lower Esophageal Web. Ann. Surg., 165:786, 1967.

Ritter, F. N.: Questionable Methods of Foreign Body Treatment. Ann. Otol., 83:729, 1974.

Salzer, H.: Frühbehandlung der Speiseröhrenverätzung. Wien. Klin. Wochenschr., 33: 307, 1920.

Sanderson, D. R., et al.: Syndrome of Vigorous Achalasia: Clinical and Physiologic Observation. Dis. Chest, 52:508, 1967.

Sanderson, D. R., et al.: Achalasia of the Esophagus: Results of Therapy by Dilation, 1950–1967. Chest, 58:116, 1970.

Schild, J. A., et al.: Esophageal Stricture Associated with Epidermolysis Bullosa Dystrophica. Laryngoscope, 72:510, 1972.

Sengstaken, R. W., and Blakemore, A. H.: Balloon Tamponade for the Control of Hemorrhage from Esophageal Varices. Ann. Surg., 131:781, 1950.

Sweet, R. H., et al.: Muscle Wall Tumors of the Esophagus. J. Thorac. Surg., 27:13, 1954.

Tucker, G. F.: Cicatricial Stenosis of the Esophagus with Particular Reference to Treatment for Continuous String Retrograde Bouginage with the Author's Bougie. Ann. Otol., 33:1180, 1924.

Weiss, S. and Mallory, G. K.: Lesions of Cardiac Orifice of the Stomach Produced by Vomiting. J.A.M.A., 98:1353, 1932.

Wychulis, A. R., et al.: Achalasia and Carcinoma of the Esophagus. J.A.M.A., 215:1638, 1971.

Chapter 62
Gastroscopy and Duodenoscopy

The development of the flexible upper gastrointestinal panendoscope has made it possible to visualize all portions of the stomach and duodenum and to take biopsies and other specimens without significant risk or discomfort to the patient. Peroral endoscopy has been extended to include visualization and canalization of the papilla of Vater for pancreatography and cholangiography (Oi).

A semiflexible gastroscope was introduced in 1932 by Rudolph Schindler. The distal tip was flexible, and the proximal portion was rigid. It provided a side view through a system of multiple lenses. Some portions of the stomach could not be seen. In 1958 Hirschowitz and his colleagues introduced a fully flexible gastroscope which employed fiberoptic image transmission and later fiber illumination (see Fig. 58–8). Side-viewing and forward-viewing endoscopes have been developed. The field of view has been widened to 75 degrees, and the tip can be deflected 270 degrees. The upper gastrointestinal panendoscopes have been lengthened to 100 cm so that the ligament of Treitz can be reached. A channel for suction, irrigation, inflation, biopsy, cytology brushing, injection, snares, and cautery has been incorporated.

Side-viewing instruments are required for visualization and cannulation of the papilla of Vater. Both wide-angle forward-viewing and side-viewing panendoscopes are needed in approximately 10% of patients to see into deep pockets in deformed duodenal bulbs (Belber).

INDICATIONS

Gastroscopy and duodenoscopy are frequently indicated in patients with symptoms of diseases of the esophagus. They are often indicated in the peptic diathesis, even when the problem appears to be limited to peptic esophagitis. They are specifically indicated in upper gastrointestinal bleeding, neoplasms of the stomach, peptic ulcer, unexplained iron deficiency anemia or occult blood in the stools, unexplained chest or abdominal pain, gastric outlet obstruction, and radiographic abnormalities of the stomach and duodenum. Gastroscopy is a useful technique for removing foreign bodies of the stomach that will not pass into the duodenum. Duodenoscopy is useful in transduodenal pancreatography and cholangiography (Oi). It provides a safe means of obtaining biopsies of the mucous membrane of the small bowel in the investigation of inborn errors of digestion. Tumors of the pancreas and biliary system that involve the papilla can be diagnosed by biopsy. Gastroscopy and duodenoscopy are contraindicated in the presence or probable presence of a perforated viscus and in a patient in shock. Stenosis of the esophagus is a contraindication to gastroscopy and duodenoscopy.

TECHNIQUE

The premedication and local anesthesia appropriate to gastroscopy and duodenoscopy have been discussed in Chapter 58.

The examination is performed with the patient in the left lateral position. The panendoscope is introduced into the mouth and advanced as the patient swallows the distal tip of the instrument. The lubricated endoscope is gradually advanced through the esophagus and into the stomach. The entire interior of the stomach can be inspected.

The duodenal bulb can be entered in nearly all patients in whom the lumen is large enough or can be dilated sufficiently to admit the panendoscope. The mucosa of the duodenum is paler than the gastric mucosa. The duodenal bulb (cap, first portion, or superior portion) is 3 to 7 cm long and tapers gently. It terminates at the superior flexure of the duodenum, and the descending or second portion of the duodenum begins. The inner angle of the curve between the bulb and the descending portion is the superior duodenal angle. The papilla of Vater is located on the inner or left wall of the descending portion and may be seen with side-viewing panendoscopes. The papilla has a covering fold, and occasionally bile may be seen coming from it spontaneously. The inferior flexure of the duodenum and the inferior angle are less prominent than the superior ones. The circular folds (valves of Kerckring) begin 2.5 to 5 cm beyond the pylorus and become more prominent beyond the papilla of Vater. Duodenal motility is more rapid than gastric motility and may be peristaltic or antiperistaltic.

The papilla of Vater can be cannulated for injection of radiocontrast material to fill the pancreatic duct, common bile duct, cystic duct, gall bladder, and intrahepatic ducts (Oi). The pancreatic duct can be filled more easily than the biliary system. Pancreatography is technically successful in approximately 70% of the patients in whom it is attempted, and cholangiography is possible in approximately 40%. The tip of the cannula must be turned superiorly to inject the dye into the biliary system. The main pancreatic duct can be visualized from head to tail, and secondary branches are frequently seen. The diameter of the pancreatic duct measures 1 to 6 mm in the head and 1 to 3 mm in the tail. The injection should be monitored continuously with fluoroscopy

to limit the amount of dye used to the amount needed. The contrast material clears in a few minutes. The accessory pancreatic duct has not been successfully cannulated. Significant complications have not been found in the literature, but mild transient elevation of the serum amylase occurred in Oi's patients after pancreatography. Significant findings such as stones and tumors have been demonstrated in patients with negative oral or intravenous cholangiograms, and transduodenal cholangiograms have been obtained in patients with serum bilirubins greater than 20 mgm%.

DIAGNOSIS OF DISEASES OF THE STOMACH AND DUODENUM

The history plays a very important part in the diagnostic process in upper gastrointestinal disorders. It is the fundamental process in diagnosis, and through concentration on the history, the individuality of the patient is emphasized. Nowhere is this more important than in gastroenterology. The interrelation of organic and psychosomatic disorders in the gastrointestinal tract demands this concentration. The social and occupational history are of as paramount importance as the pain, aching, cramping, vomiting, diarrhea, constipation, and evidence of bleeding. The location and radiation of pain and its relationship to eating, exercise, stress, body position, and bowel movements must be explored. The patient's experience with the relief of his symptoms must be known. Historical factors suggesting anxiety, neurosis, and interpersonal conflicts must be considered.

The esophagus does not lend itself to physical examination, but inspection, palpation, percussion, and auscultation of the abdomen and the anal and rectal examination provide very valuable information.

Radiography of the abdomen, stomach, and duodenum consistently provides reliable information in patients with upper gastrointestinal disorders. Flat plates of the abdomen provide a wealth of information, and contrast radiography of the esophagus, stomach, and duodenum focuses attention on the areas for subsequent endoscopic evaluation and confirmation of the diagnosis.

The endoscopic findings in the stomach have been well documented. Acute gastritis without bleeding is rarely appreciated endoscopically and is difficult to recognize unless there are erosions. The hemorrhagic variety of acute gastritis is often seen endoscopically in the differential diagnosis of upper gastrointestinal bleeding and is characterized by multiple bleeding points associated with erosion of the mucosa. Chronic gastritis of the hypertrophic type produces a cobblestone appearance to the mucosa that is not unlike that seen in lymphoma of the stomach. Atrophic gastritis including that associated with pernicious anemia is characterized by pale, green-gray mucosa with prominent blood vessels. In giant hypertrophy of gastric mucosa (Menetrier's disease), the rugae are very large and stiff, and the secretion of mucus is profuse. The appearance of peptic ulcers differs from erosions on the basis of the depth of the lesion. Erosions do not extend beyond the glandular portion of the mucosa, while ulcers penetrate the muscularis mucosae and submucosa. Most benign gastric ulcers occur on the lesser curvature in the prepyloric area.

Adenomatous polyps are compact rounded masses of glandular tissue and are generally not considered true neoplasms (Monaco and coworkers). Benign submucosal tumors include leiomyomas, fibromas, and lipomas. They are not easily biopsied.

Carcinoma produces ulcers with greater surrounding induration. The distinguishing features are the raised edge of the ulcer and its greater diameter.

Bleeding from esophageal varices, peptic ulcers, gastritis, and carcinoma can often be distinguished at endoscopy. It can be carried out during a lull in the bleeding or during active bleeding.

Duodenal ulcers, duodenitis, and duodenal deformity are the major abnormalities in the duodenum. They often coexist. Most duodenal ulcers occur within 3 cm of the pylorus. Only 10% are beyond the superior flexure. More ulcers occur on the superior wall of the bulb than on its inferior wall. Most duodenal ulcers are small; 85% are 1 cm in diameter or less. The most common deformity of the bulb is a midbulb constriction that can go on to a contraction ring and produce pseudodiverticula on either side.

Neoplasms of the duodenum are very rare. Benign adenomas composed of cells of Brunner's glands are the most common type (River and coworkers). Lipomas and leiomyomas are usually submucosal. Malignant neoplasms are very rare and include adenocarcinomas, lymphoblastomas, sarcomas, and carcinoid tumors. Malignant tumors of the pancreas, kidney, and gall bladder secondarily invade the duodenum. Blood coming from the papilla of Vater is suggestive of biliary cancer.

With pancreatography, tumors may obstruct the duct at any point from the head to the tail of the gland. Dilatation of the duct occurs distal to carcinoma in the head of the pancreas. Stenosis due to chronic inflammation has been demonstrated, but the pancreatogram is usually normal in chronic pancreatitis. Gall stones can be demonstrated in the common duct and in the gall bladder with cholangiography. Tumors may completely obstruct the common duct, and hepatomas may compress the common duct and gall bladder and distort the intrahepatic ducts. Cholangitis cannot be satisfactorily demonstrated with this technique.

GASTROSCOPY FOR FOREIGN BODIES

Most foreign bodies that reach the stomach will pass through the gastrointestinal tract without difficulty. Even sharp foreign bodies like straight pins will ordinarily progress through the gastrointestinal tract in 24 to 48 hours without incident. The stools may be crushed for 5 days to recover the foreign body. Cathartics should not be given, and the diet should not be altered, because the normal intestinal contents are the best vehicle for the foreign body. If it has not been recovered in 5 days, its progress should be monitored radiographically. In the case of sharp foreign bodies, their progress should be monitored daily. If progress of a sharp foreign body stops for 24 hours, a laparotomy should be performed to remove the foreign body.

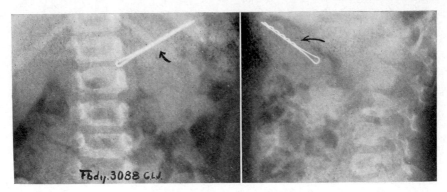

Fody.3088 CU.

FIG. 62–1.   Foreign body of the stomach. This "bobby pin" in a child's stomach
is too long to make the turn into the duodenum.

Some foreign bodies of the stomach cannot advance because they are too long to make the turn into the duodenal bulb (Fig. 62–1). These foreign bodies may be removed with the flexible upper gastrointestinal panendoscope. Forceps for grasping the foreign body may be passed through the instrument channel, and it may be removed as a trailing foreign body.

The need for magnets in the removal of gastric foreign bodies has been reduced because of the ease with which they are removed by the flexible upper gastrointestinal panendoscope; however, their use should be kept in mind for special problems.

It is important to make sure, by careful radiography in the anterior-posterior and lateral views, that the foreign body is in the stomach and not already in the duodenum or colon. General anesthesia should be used for children, but foreign body removal from the stomach may be satisfactorily performed in adults with local anesthesia.

REFERENCES

Belber, J. P.: Endoscopic Examination of the Duodenal Bulb. A Comparison with X-ray. Gastroenterology, 61:55, 1971.

Hirschowitz, B. I., et al.: Demonstration of a New Gastroscope, the "Fiberscope." Gastroenterology, 35:50, 1958.

Monaco, A. P., et al.: Adenomatous Polyps of the Stomach. A Clinical and Pathologic Study of 153 Cases. Cancer, 15:456, 1962.

Oi, I.: Fiberduodenoscopy and Endoscopic Pancreatocholangiography. Gastrointest. Endoscop., 17:59, 1970.

River, L., et al.: Benign Neoplasms of the Small Intestine. A Critical Comprehensive Review with Reports of 20 New Cases. Internatl. Abstr. Surg., 102:1, 1956.

Chapter 63
Mediastinoscopy

Mediastinoscopy is a technique for examination and biopsy of lesions arising in the mediastinum and metastatic to the mediastinum. It has been found to be of great value in establishing a histologic diagnosis in granulomatous lesions of the mediastinal lymph nodes, sarcoidosis, and lymphosarcoma and in determining the resectability of carcinoma of the lung.

Contributions to the solution of the problem of resectability of carcinoma of the lung in an individual patient are made with physical examination, as in finding a paralysis of a vocal cord or evidence of distant spread of the tumor; radiographically, as in finding pleural fluid; cytologically, in the examination of pleural fluid; endoscopically, as in finding broadening or fixation of the carina and invasion of the esophagus; and surgically, as in scalene node biopsy (Daniels). All of these methods except scalene node biopsy continue to provide help in solving this problem in an individual patient; however, mediastinoscopy is the most definitive method of determining resectability in the large number of patients in whom the other methods are not helpful or applicable. Many patients whose carcinoma of the lung is too advanced for resection are spared a thoracotomy by this relatively safe and effective technique.

In 1954 Harkens and coworkers described a unilateral exploration of the superior mediastinum with a standard Jackson laryngoscope and increased the rate of demonstration of bronchogenic carcinoma in lymph nodes to 40%. Carlens in 1959 presented the technique of midline mediastinoscopy, which opened the right and left paratracheal areas, as well as the superior and middle mediastinum, to inspection and biopsy. The method has reduced the percentage of unresectable cases at thoracotomy from 40% to 10% and has become one of the primary methods for investigating primary and metastatic diseases of the mediastinum.

ANATOMY OF THE MEDIASTINUM

The mediastinum contains all of the thoracic viscera except the lungs and pleurae. It serves as a partition between the two pleurae. The mediastinum is bounded anteriorly by the sternum, posteriorly by the thoracic vertebrae, superiorly by the thoracic inlet, and inferiorly by the diaphragm. It is divided into superior and inferior divisions at the superior aspect of the pericardium. The superior division is known as the superior mediastinum (Fig. 63–1). The inferior division is subdivided into the anterior mediastinum, middle mediastinum, and posterior mediastinum. The anterior mediastinum is anterior to the pericardium. The middle mediastinum contains the pericardium and heart, and the posterior mediastinum is posterior to the pericardium.

The superior mediastinum contains the aortic arch, the innominate artery, the left common carotid artery, the left subclavian artery, the right and left innominate veins, the upper half of the superior vena cava, the bronchi. The bronchopulmonary lymph nodes are at the hilum of each lung, and the pulmonary lymph nodes are in the substance of the lung.

The afferents to the tracheobronchial lymph nodes drain the lungs and bronchi, trachea, and heart, as well as the anterior and posterior mediastinal lymph nodes. Their efferents form the right and left bronchomediastinal trunks, which empty, respectively, into the right lymphatic duct and the thoracic duct.

The lymphatics of the lung are composed of a deep and a superficial system. The deep lymph vessels accompany the pulmonary vessels. In the larger bronchi are a subepithelial network in the lamina propria and a peribronchial network. In the smaller bronchioles, there is only one network. The superficial lymph vessels course on the visceral surfaces of the lungs and enter lymph nodes at the hilum. The deep system of lymph vessels enters the tracheobronchial lymph nodes. According to Nohl, the collecting sites in the deep system are first at the pulmonary (intersegmental) lymph nodes, second at the bronchopulmonary (hilar) lymph nodes, then at the bronchial (bifurcation) lymph nodes, and finally at the tracheal (paratracheal) lymph nodes. The three lobes on the right follow this pattern and stay on the right side. The right upper lobe drains to the right tracheal (paratracheal) or azygos lymph node. The middle and lower lobes drain to the azygos lymph node via the bronchial (bifurcation) lymph nodes (Fig. 63–3). The lower left lobe drains to pulmonary (intersegmental) and bronchopulmonary (hilar) lymph nodes, and then the efferents go to the paraesophageal lymph nodes, bronchial (bifurcation) lymph nodes, or ductus lymph nodes and at this level tend to cross to the right side. The left lower lobe tends to drain to the right upper tracheal (paratracheal) lymph nodes,

THE SPREAD OF CARCINOMA OF THE BRONCHUS

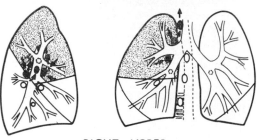

RIGHT UPPER

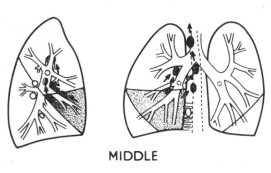

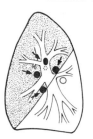

MIDDLE

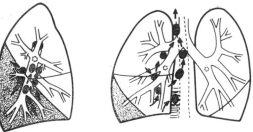

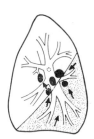

LOWER

FIG. 63–3. Lymphatic drainage from the right lung. (Nohl, H. C.: Thorax, *11*:172, 1965.)

THE SPREAD OF CARCINOMA OF THE BRONCHUS

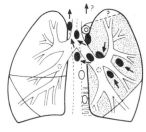

LEFT UPPER

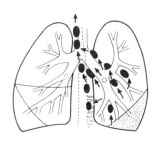

LEFT LOWER

FIG. 63–4. Lymphatic drainage from the left lung. (Nohl, J. C.: Thorax, *11*:172, 1965.)

and drainage from the left upper lobe may go to the right or left (Fig. 63–4). Approximately 20% of Carlens' patients have been demonstrated with mediastinoscopy to have contralateral metastases which would not have been detectable during thoracotomy. Of course, normal lymphatic flow patterns may be altered with disease, and there may be rerouting and reversal of flow with lymphatic blockage.

INDICATIONS

Mediastinoscopy is an important diagnostic procedure in hilar adenopathy and mediastinal masses. Its yield in the diagnosis of bronchogenic carcinoma is better than bronchoscopy, cytology, and scalene node biopsy (Preciado and coworkers). Mediastinoscopy is indicated in nearly all patients with apparently resectable carcinoma of the lung. If no positive nodes are obtained at mediastinoscopy, the chance of resectability is very high (90%) (Reynders). Positive biopsies are more likely to be obtained at mediastinoscopy with large, centrally located parenchymal lesions. The chance of biopsies being positive for carcinoma is low with peripherally located coin lesions. Most causes of nonresectability in carcinoma of the lung can be found in the superior mediastinum. Actually 85 to 95% of inoperable patients have infiltration or metastasis to the mediastinum.

Some authorities advocate mediastinoscopy to determine the resectability of carcinoma of the esophagus in the same manner as is done for carcinoma of the bronchus (Efskind).

Mediastinoscopy has proved particularly helpful in establishing the diagnosis of sarcoidosis. The success rate attained in diagnosing sarcoidosis has been 96%. It is equally useful in granulomatous lymphadenitis due to *Mycobacterium tuberculosis,* fungi, and the pneumoconioses. Hodgkin's disease is often limited to the superior mediastinum and can be diagnosed with mediastinoscopy. Metastases to the mediastinum from neoplasms in distant organs are frequently found at mediastinoscopy, and these primary sites include the larynx, breast, and prostate.

Therapeutic indications for mediastinoscopy have included dividing constricting paratracheal conglomerations in sarcoidosis, right vagotomy for pain from hypertrophic osteoarthropathy in association with inoperable lung cancer, insertion of a cardiac pacemaker for atrial triggered stimulation, resection of parathyroid adenoma, and removal of a bullet (Ward and coworkers; Carlens, 1965).

Mediastinoscopy does not provide access to the thymus gland because of its location anterior to the left innominate vein. Likewise, there is an inferior limit to mediastinoscopy. Although dissection may be carried 4 to 5 cm along the anterior and lateral walls of the bronchi, extension of the dissection to the subaortic and subcarinal lymph nodes involves too much risk.

Contraindications include aortic aneurysm, innominate artery aneurysm, pharyngoesophageal diverticulum, previous mediastinoscopy, and severe tracheal deviation. Superior vena cava obstruction is a relative contraindication.

TECHNIQUE

Carlens has consistently advocated general endotracheal anesthesia for mediastinoscopy, and it is very satisfactory. Local infiltrative anesthesia has also proved satisfactory. A general anesthetic allows controlled ventilation. The mediastinal space is wider. There is no distention of the veins and less bleeding. The risk of mediastinal emphysema and pneumothorax if the pleura is perforated is lessened.

Mediastinoscopes have been designed by Carlens, Tucker, and others. The Tucker mediastinoscope is an oval, tapered, 13-cm long tube with diameters of 2.25 cm and 1.5 mm proximally and 2 and 1.2 cm distally (Tucker). The distal tip is beveled. The sides are slotted at the proximal end for easy introduction of instruments. It has twin, distal, fiber illumination which gives bright light and reduces shadows. The handle extension allows application of self-retaining laryngoscope holders (Fig. 63–5).

The patient's neck is extended on the thorax, and the head is extended on the neck, so that the patient is in the same position as

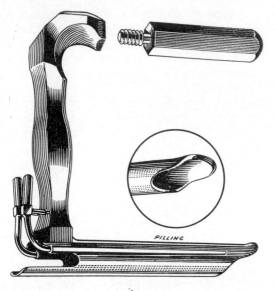

FIG. 63–5.   Tucker mediastinoscope.

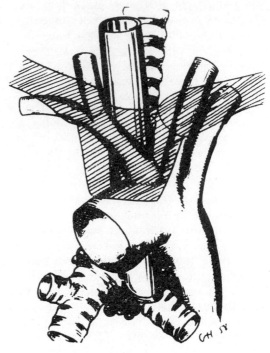

FIG. 63–6.   Position of the mediastinoscope.
(Carlens, E.: Dis. Chest., *36*:343, 1959.)

for a tracheotomy. This position brings more of the trachea out of the thorax and makes it relatively more superficial. The depth of intrathoracic dissection is reduced in this way. A 4- to 5-cm transverse incision is made between the cricoid cartilage and the suprasternal notch inferior to the thyroid isthmus. The pretracheal fascia is incised, and the dissection is continued bluntly on the anterior wall of the trachea (Fig. 63–6). With blunt dissection with the finger, the innominate artery, arch of the aorta, left carotid artery, and pulmonary artery can usually be easily identified. The rest of the dissection is done under direct vision, and care is taken not to go deeper than one can see. The risk of exploring the area anterior to the left innominate vein, including the thymus gland, is too great because it is not accessible to direct vision.

The right bronchial artery crosses the anterior tracheal wall 8.7% of the time, and the left bronchial artery crosses anterior to the trachea 2% of the time (Cauldwell and coworkers). The great arteries close to the trachea are safer to work around than the veins that lie anterior to them, because the arteries are easier to palpate and less fragile. One must stay posterior to the innominate artery at all times. The innominate artery is easy to palpate; it runs obliquely from the right superiorly to the left inferiorly. It forms a "V" with the left common carotid artery as it arises from the arch of the aorta. The dissection is carried posterior to the arch of the aorta. The pulmonary arteries are the anterior, lateral, and inferior limits of the dissection. No attempt should be made to dissect them from the bronchi.

The main lymphatic drainage of the lungs and esophagus leads to nodes close to the trachea, so that the critical nodes for diagnosis are available in the area immediately adjacent to the trachea.

The right paratracheal space contains the right recurrent laryngeal nerve, right vagus nerve, azygos vein, and right pulmonary artery, while the left paratracheal space contains the left recurrent laryngeal nerve, left common carotid artery, aortic arch, right bronchial artery, left bronchial artery, and left pulmonary artery.

Standard laryngeal forceps may be used for biopsy, and a Matthew forceps may be used for dissection. Open and velvet eye aspirating tubes are needed. The most critical instrument is the needle and syringe for aspiration. A 15-cm shaft with a 23-gauge needle on a 3-ml Luer-Lok syringe serves very well. Each tissue to be biopsied must be tested with aspiration to exclude the possibility of biopsying a vessel wall. Veins and lymph nodes have a similar appearance. Tissue selected for biopsy must be cut through cleanly with the biopsy forceps without torsion, which might tear thin-walled vessels adherent to the lymph node.

Tucker advocates monitoring of the right radial pulse by the anesthesiologist to avoid cerebrovascular accidents from compression of the innominate artery.

Complications of mediastinoscopy include hemorrhage, subcutaneous emphysema, pneumothorax, perforation of the trachea, bronchus, or esophagus, cardiac arrhythmia, fever, mediastinitis, tracheitis, cerebrovascular accidents, upper respiratory obstruction, chylomediastinum, wound infection, air embolism, tumor seeding and spread, and recurrent laryngeal and vagus nerve injury. There are more deaths from mediastinoscopy than have been reported (Tucker).

REFERENCES

Carlens, E.: Mediastinoscopy. A Method for Inspection and Tissue Biopsy in the Superior Mediastinum. Dis. Chest., *36*:343, 1959.

Carlens, E.: Mediastinoscopy. Ann. Otol., *74*:1102, 1965.

Cauldwell, E. W., et al.: The Bronchial Arteries: An Anatomic Study of 150 Cadavers. Surg. Gynecol. Obstet., *86*:395, 410, 1948.

Daniels, A. C.: Method of Biopsy Useful in Diagnosing Certain Intrathoracic Diseases. Dis. Chest., *16*:360, 1949.

Efskind, L.: Carcinoma of the Lower Portion of the Esophagus. Acta Chir. Scand. (Suppl.), *245*:157, 1959.

Harkens, D. E., et al.: A Simple Cervicomediastinal Exploration for Tissue Diagnosis of Intrathoracic Disease with Comments on Recognition of Inoperable Carcinoma of the Lung. New Engl. J. Med., *251*:1041, 1954.

Nohl, J. C.: *The Spread of Carcinoma of the Bronchus*. London Lloyd-Luke Medical Books, 1962.

Preciado, M. C., et al.: Mediastinoscopy: A Review of 450 Cases. Laryngoscopy, *83*: 1300, 1973.

Reynders, H.: Mediastinoscopy in Bronchogenic Cancer. Dis. Chest., *45*:606, 1964.

Tucker, J. A.: Mediastinoscopy: 300 Cases Reported and Literature Reviewed. Laryngoscopy, *82*:2226, 1972.

Ward, P. H., et al.: Interesting and Unusual Lesions Encountered during Mediastinoscopy. Ann. Otol., *80*:487, 1971.

Index

Antibody(ies), blocking, 105
  reaginic, 105
  relation to immunity, 537
Antigen(s),
  human tumor, 531–533
  tumor-specific, 529
Antihelix, 609
Antimetabolites, 545
Antineoplastic agents, cell life cycle and, 544
  head and neck and, 547
  mode of action of, 545
  site of action of, 544
  toxicity of, 545
Anti-streptolysin O titer, 143
Antitragus, 609
Antrochoanal polyp, 232
Antrum, mastoid, 605, 657
  maxillary, 650, 651
Anvil. See *Incus*.
AOR, 768
Aperature, piriform, 1
Apex, petrous, 661
Apex nasi, 47
Aphasia, 581
  classification of, 583–584
  congenital, 581–582
  in adults, 583–584
  in children, 583
Aphonia, 437, 588. See also *Larynx, functional disorders of*.
APR, 768
Apsithyria, 437
Aqueduct, cochlear, 606
  of Sylvius, 939
  vestibular, 662, 668
Arabinosylcytosine, 545
Arches, branchial, first, 648, 649, 905
  second, 648, 649
Arcuate eminence, 653
ARD, 133
Area, Killian-Jamieson, 447
Areflexia, 750
Arteritis, cranial, 118
  temporal, 118
Artery(ies), auditory, internal, 606, 634
  auricular, 634
    anterior, 921
    posterior, 921
  auriculotemporal, 634
  caroticotympanic, 634
  carotid, 493
    external, 634
  cochlear, 634
  cricothyroid, 335
  infrahyoid, 335
  innominate, 1087, 1088
  laryngeal, superior, 331
  maxillary, external, 634
    internal, tympanic branch of, 605
  meningeal, middle, 606
  petrosal, 634
  pharyngeal, ascending, 634
  stapedial, 649, 910
  stylomastoid, 634
  temporal, superficial, 921

thyroid, inferior, 335, 447
  superior, 335, 446–447, 493
tympanic, 634
vestibulocochlear, 634
Arthritis, cricoarytenoid, 435, 1023
  rheumatoid, 435
Articulary defects, 573
Articulation, defects of, 575–578
ASO, 143
Asthma, bronchial, 112
  etiologic agents in, 112
  obstructive, symptoms of, 112–113
  treatment of, 113
Atelectasis, bronchoscopy and, 1044–1045
Atelectatic otitis, 827
Atresia plate, 907, 910, 911
Attenuator, 759
Attic, 612, 657
Attic space, 612
Audiogram, 759
  pre-employment, 972
Audiology, brain stem response and, 769
  electrodermal responses and, 769
Audiometer, 759–760
  biological calibration of, 985
Audiometric zero, 972
Audiometrist, 760, 987
Audiometry, admittance, 808
  air conduction, 760–762
  Bekesy, 767
  bone conduction, 762–764
  children and, 767–771
  diagnostic, 765–767
  impedance, 808
  play, 769
  pure tone, 760–764
  speech, 764–765, 770
Auditory area, 759
Auditory canal, atresia, 905
  external, 662, 907
    adenoma of, 795–796
    anatomy of, 609
    benign tumors of, 795–796
    carcinoma of, 801–802
    cerumen and, 780–782
    exostosis of, 795
    foreign bodies, 783
    inflammation of, 783–788
      treatment of, 785–788
    keratosis obliterans and, 788–789
    osteoma of, 795
  internal, 606, 647, 657, 661, 662, 668, 710
    radiology of, 658
  self-cleaning property of, 609
  stenosis of, 905–907
Auditory cortex, pure tone thresholds and, 703
Auditory-evoked electrophysiologic responses, 698–700
Auditory-evoked responses, central, 700–702
Auditory neuronal population, 696
Auditory oculogyric reflex, 768
Auditory pit, 637
Auditory placodes, 637
Auditory system, central pathways, 696–704
  anatomy of, 696